...k of
...Medicine

ON

FICP, FICA
Med)

...Medicine
...Education and

Director
LRS Institute of Tuberculosis and Respiratory Diseases
Sri Aurobindo Marg
New Delhi, India

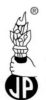

JAYPEE BROTHERS MEDICAL PUBLISHERS (P) LTD

**New Delhi • St Louis (USA) • Panama City (Panama) • Ahmedabad • Bengaluru
Chennai • Hyderabad • Kochi • Kolkata • Lucknow • Mumbai • Nagpur**

Published by

Jitendar P Vij

Jaypee Brothers Medical Publishers (P) Ltd

Corporate Office

4838/24 Ansari Road, Daryaganj, New Delhi - 110002, India, Phone: +91-11-43574357, Fax: +91-11-43574314

Registered Office

B-3 EMCA House, 23/23B Ansari Road, Daryaganj, New Delhi - 110 002, India
Phones: +91-11-23272143, +91-11-23272703, +91-11-23282021
+91-11-23245672, Rel: +91-11-32558559, Fax: +91-11-23276490, +91-11-23245683
e-mail: jaypee@jaypeebrothers.com, Website: www.jaypeebrothers.com

Offices in India

- **Ahmedabad**, Phone: Rel: +91-79-32988717, e-mail: ahmedabad@jaypeebrothers.com
- **Bengaluru**, Phone: Rel: +91-80-32714073, e-mail: bangalore@jaypeebrothers.com
- **Chennai**, Phone: Rel: +91-44-32972089, e-mail: chennai@jaypeebrothers.com
- **Hyderabad**, Phone: Rel:+91-40-32940929, e-mail: hyderabad@jaypeebrothers.com
- **Kochi**, Phone: +91-484-2395740, e-mail: kochi@jaypeebrothers.com
- **Kolkata**, Phone: +91-33-22276415, e-mail: kolkata@jaypeebrothers.com
- **Lucknow**, Phone: +91-522-3040554, e-mail: lucknow@jaypeebrothers.com
- **Mumbai**, Phone: Rel: +91-22-32926896, e-mail: mumbai@jaypeebrothers.com
- **Nagpur**, Phone: Rel: +91-712-3245220, e-mail: nagpur@jaypeebrothers.com

Overseas Offices

- **North America Office, USA,** Ph: 001-636-6279734, e-mail: jaypee@jaypeebrothers.com, anjulav@jaypeebrothers.com
- **Central America Office, Panama City, Panama,** Ph: 001-507-317-0160, e-mail: cservice@jphmedical.com
  Website: www.jphmedical.com

Textbook of Pulmonary Medicine

© 2010, D Behera

This book has been published in good faith that the material provided by author is original. Every effort is made to ensure accuracy of material, but the publisher, printer and editors will not be held responsible for any inadvertent error(s). In case of any dispute, all legal matters are to be settled under Delhi jurisdiction only.

First Edition: 1995

Second Edition: 2010

ISBN 978-81-8448-749-7

Typeset at JPBMP typesetting unit

Printed at Replika Press Pvt. Ltd.

Contents

VOLUME 2

Chapter 16

Chronic Obstructive Pulmonary Diseases

DEFINITION

There used to be (and still is) a great deal of confusion in the use of the terms chronic bronchitis, emphysema, and chronic obstructive disease. The clinical term "emphysema" in USA was equivalent to chronic bronchitis in Great Britain. To add further to the confusion, it was suggested in 1961 that bronchial asthma, chronic bronchitis, and emphysema should be considered as different expression of one disease and the term "chronic nonspecific lung disease (CNLD)" should be used for this. Both endogenous (host) and exogenous (environment) factors were thought to play a role (Dutch hypothesis). A hereditary predisposition to develop allergy and bronchial hyperreactivity were considered to be important denominators of disease susceptibility. Although there are still proponents of this hypothesis, over the years with better understanding of the pathophysiologic processes of these diseases, it is clear that these entities are distinct even if they have common features like airflow obstruction, and similar manifestations like cough, wheezing and dyspnea, etc. However, sometimes, in a few minorities of patients, it may not be possible to distinguish one from the other and they may coexist.[1-6] Recently, American Thoracic Society has tried to rationalize some of these confusions.[7]

CHRONIC BRONCHITIS

Chronic bronchitis is defined as chronic or recurrent (coughing of sputum on most days during at least three consecutive months in two successive years) bronchial mucus hypersecretion resulting in chronic expectoration when other causes such as bronchiectasis or tuberculosis have been excluded.[1,8] Chronic bronchitis is further subdivided into (i) simple chronic bronchitis with chronic or recurrent mucoid hypersecretions; (ii) chronic or recurrent mucopurulent bronchitis when the sputum is persistently or intermittently mucopurulent; and (iii) chronic obstructive bronchitis, when there is air flow limitation as measured by physiological measurements.

EMPHYSEMA

Emphysema is defined pathologically as "a condition of the lung characterized by abnormal, permanent enlargement of air spaces distal to the terminal bronchioles, accompanied by the destruction of their walls, and without obvious fibrosis". Destruction in emphysema is defined as nonuniformity in the pattern of respiratory airspace enlargement so that the orderly appearance of the acinus and its components is disturbed and may be lost.[4]

CHRONIC OBSTRUCTIVE PULMONARY DISEASES

Chronic obstructive pulmonary disease (COPD) is defined as a disorder characterized by abnormal tests of expiratory flow that do not change markedly over periods of several months of observation. This qualification is intended to distinguish COPD from bronchial asthma. The other synonyms for the term include chronic obstructive lung disease (COLD), chronic obstructive airway disease (COAD), and chronic airflow obstruction (CAO). The airflow obstruction may be structural or functional. Specific causes of airflow obstruction such as localized diseases of the upper airways, bronchiectasis, and cystic fibrosis are excluded. Bronchial hyperreactivity may be present in patients with COPD. Some degree of reversibility is also possible, although the extent is not as much as that is possible with bronchial asthma.

Three disorders are incorporated in COPD: emphysema, peripheral airway disease, and chronic bronchitis.[5] Any individual patient may have one or all of these conditions, but the dominant clinical feature in COPD is always impairment, or limitation of expiratory airflow. Earlier, bronchial asthma was considered under COPD. However, with better understanding of the complex pathophysiology of bronchial asthma and because of the fact that most patients of bronchial asthma has a reversible element, the condition is separated from COPD. In 1995, the American Thoracic Society has included only chronic bronchitis and emphysema under COPD.[7] It is to be emphasized that in many patients with chronic obstructive pulmonary disease, a significant reversible component may be present, and on the other hand, some patients with bronchial asthma may go on to develop irreversible airflow obstruction indistinguishable from COPD.

Several different definitions exists for COPD:

The American Thoracic Society (ATS) defines COPD as *"A disease state characterized by the presence of airflow limitation due to chronic bronchitis are emphysema; the airflow obstruction is generally progressive, may be accompanied by airway hyperreactivity that may be partially reversible".*[7]

The European Respiratory Society (ERS) defines COPD as *"reduced maximum expiratory flow and slow forced emptying of the lungs, which is slowly progressive and mostly irreversible to present medical treatment".*[8]

The Global initiative for Chronic Obstructive Lung Disease (GOLD) classified COPD as *"a disease state characterized by airflow limitation that is not fully reversible. The airflow limitation is usually both progressive and associated with an abnormal inflammatory response of the lungs to noxious particles or gases".*[9]

For these three different definitions, however, the precise classification of airflow limitation, reversibility, and severity of disease varies. In addition, the definitions and diagnoses of chronic bronchitis, emphysema, and asthma also can vary.

The airflow limitation and reversibility are defined as follows:

Disease Severity

Severity of COPD has typically been described using the degree of lung impairment. However, ideally this should include factors such as arterial blood gas levels, time and distance walked, sensation of dyspnea, and body mass index. COPD is classified into the following:

a) ATS criteria

　Stage 1—$FEV_1 \geq 50$ percent of predicted

　Stage 2— FEV_1 35 to 49 percent of predicted

　Stage 3—$FEV_1 < 35$ percent of predicted

b) ERS criteria

　Mild—$FEV_1 \geq 70$ percent of predicted

　Moderate—FEV_1 50 to < 80 percent of predicted

　Severe—$FEV_1 < 50$ percent of predicted

c) GOLD criteria (See later for clinical severity)

　Stage 1—$FEV_1 \geq 80$ percent of predicted

　Stage 2—FEV_1 30 to < 80 percent of predicted

　Stage 3—$FEV_1 ,< 30$ percent of predicted

PERIPHERAL AIRWAY DISEASE

A number of morphologic abnormalities are reported in patients with COPD. These are inflammation of the terminal and respiratory bronchioles, fibrosis of the airway walls with narrowing, and goblet cell metaplasia of the epithelium. There may be considerable variation in the distribution and severity of these changes among individuals. Structure function correlation suggest that these changes contribute to air flow obstruction in severe COPD, but their importance is secondary to emphysema. In cigarette smokers prone to develop emphysema, pathological changes in the peripheral airways precede the development of emphysema. It has been suggested that inflammatory and other changes in these airways may represent early or preclinical COPD and may be responsible for subtle pulmonary function abnormalities

Origin of criterion	Criterion for airflow limitation	Criterion for reversibility
ATS 1991[10]	FEV_1/FVC ratio of less than the fifth percentile	FEV_1 increase of 200 ml and 12% above baseline
ERS, 1995[8]	Males:FEV_1/VC ratio below 88% predicted Females: FEV_1/VC ratio below 89% predicted	> 10% improvement in predicted FEV_1
GOLD 2001[9]	FEV_1/FVC ratio of less than 70%	FEV_1 increase of 200 ml, and 12% improvement from baseline FEV_1 for treatment with either corticosteroids or bronchodilators

although there is no physical impairment. However, these relationships are not confirmed by long-term studies and their clinical relevance remains uncertain.

ASTHMATIC BRONCHITIS

The term was described in 1987, by Burrows[11] who identified a subgroup in their COPD patients who were predominantly women with higher survival rates and with a slower decline of lung function than the emphysematous subgroup. Many of them had positive skin tests and wheezing was a prominent symptom. It was suggested that the disorder appears to depend on an "asthmatic predisposition." These subjects are either atopic or had not smoked as much as the emphysematous group does. The 10 year mortality in them is about 10 percent as against 60 percent in the emphysematous group. The term has not been used by many other investigators and should better be avoided. Some people use the term for those chronic bronchitis who present with wheezing as prominent symptoms. In United States, the term is used for individuals with chronic asthma who, when exposed to chronic irritation such as cigarette smoke, may develop chronic productive cough, which is a feature of chronic bronchitis. This is otherwise known as the *asthmatic form of COPD*. The spectrum of COPD is shown schematically in Figure 16.1.[7] The figure is a classic Venn diagram used to describe the overlapping disease entities included in the definition of COPD and the potential clinical subcategories. A Venn diagram is commonly used to describe the overlap between emphysema, chronic bronchitis and asthma in COPD. The key feature that unites these three diseases is the physiologic phenomenon of obstruction to forced expiratory airflow represented in this diagram as the area within the rectangle. Patients may have mild or early lung disease without airflow obstruction (areas 1, 2 and 11), indicating persons at risk for acquiring permanent lung damage. Other airway diseases such as cystic fibrosis and some interstitial diseases such as hypersensitivity pneumonitis can also have expiratory airflow obstruction (area 10), but they are not included in the definition of COPD.

PREVALENCE AND MORTALITY

Even if there are great variations in the prevalence and mortality for COPD, which may partly be due to differences in diagnostic patterns and labels of diagnosis,[12-15] it is currently the sixth leading cause of death and 12th leading cause of morbidity worldwide.[16] The entity is the one that is rising the most rapidly. As per prediction of the World Health Organization, by the year 2020 COPD is expected to be the third leading cause of death and the fifth leading cause of disability.[17] Reasons for the dramatic increase in COPD include reduced mortality from other causes, like cardiovascular diseases in the industrialized countries and infectious diseases in developing countries, along with a marked increase in smoking, and environmental pollution in developing countries.

In almost all countries from which figures are available, the male mortality rate is much higher than the females and is shown in Figure 16.2.[18] This can be explained by the overall prevalence of smoking in males. There is also a steady increase in mortality with increasing urbanization. The highest mortality is reported during winter Similarly there is a steady increase in the mortality with descending socioeconomic class, which may reflect the differences in tobacco consumption. The available mortality data as shown in the figure may be slightly higher because deaths from asthma and extrinsic, allergic alveolitis are included.

Although precise data on prevalence are scanty, COPD is more frequent in industrialized countries than in developing ones. Like all chronic diseases, COPD is strongly associated with age, and thus, the prevalence and incidence have risen constantly over the last decade. It is estimated that approximately 14 million people in the United States have COPD. In the third US National Health and Nutrition Examination Survey (NHANES III), airflow obstruction was found in approximately 14 percent of white male smokers and in 3 percent of white male nonsmokers.[19] In females, the figures are slightly lower in white female smokers and for black male smokers. COPD is now the fourth leading cause of death in that country. As prevalence of cigarette smoking halved among British males during the period 1950-1990, there was a slight reduction in the prevalence of persistent cough and phlegm in middle-aged men from about 25 percent in the 1950s and 1960s to about 15 percent in 1990, with no change among middle aged females.[20,21] National Health Survey during 1994 to 1995 in Canada showed a prevalence rates of chronic bronchitis por emphysema as follows; 4,6 percent in the age group 55 to 64 years; 5 percent in the 65 to 74 group and 6.8 percent in subjects over 75 years.[22] A rising trend in hospital admissions of COPD is also noted in Italy and Finland.[23] Calculations of the distribution of disability-adjusted life years (DALYS), i.e. the sum of life years lost due to premature death and of the years lived with disability; showed that in 1990, COPD accounted for 2.1 percent of DALYS, ranking 12th among the most

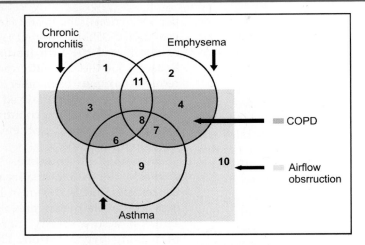

FIGURE 16.1: Venn diagram showing COPD

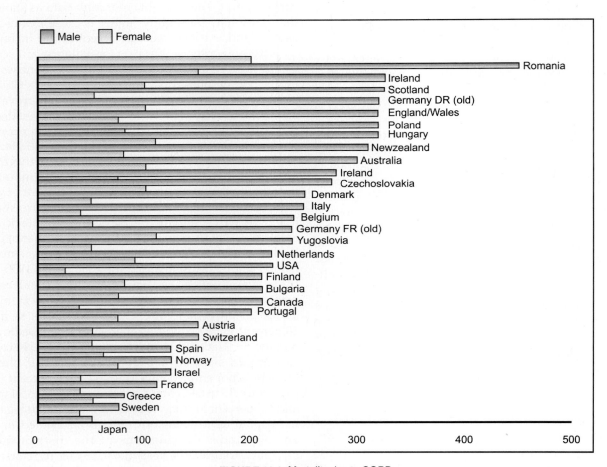

FIGURE 16.2: Mortality due to COPD

TABLE 16.1: Prevalence of chronic bronchitis (%) in different countries[12]

Country	Males			Females		
	Total	S	NS	Total	S	NS
Africa	0.3-35	9.7	-	0.2-40.4	-	-
Australia	6.3-21.4	17.2	-	-		
China	-	11.7	9.2	3.4	-	-
France	-	25.4	16.0	-	26.5	8.1
Finland	-	32.7	12.0	-	-	-
India	-	32.0	0.66-6	-	33-53	0.44-5.8
Italy	13.1	-	-	2.8	6.0	1.0
Japan	5.8	-	-	3.1-5.5	12.5	4.4
Morocco	10.7-20.2	-	-	-	-	-
Netherlands	-	-	-	5.5	12.5	4.4
New Mexico	8.8-15.7	-	-	8.9-15.9	-	-
Nepal	17.6	18.6	3.0	18.9	20.8	13.8
Poland	15.2-24.2	21.0	5.4	5.3-10.4	10.8	5.3
Sudan	23.5-26	-	-	-	-	-
Sweden	2.2	-	-	1.5	-	-
Switzerland	4.5	-	-	8.0	-	-
Tunisia	10.4	-	-	7.6	-	-
USA	6.5-21.2	8.4-40.3	2.4-13.8	4.1-9.4	7.9-19.8	3.5-9.4
UK	13.9-17.0	-	-	8.0-8.8	-	-
USSR (Former)	11.3-20.3	-	-	6.1-12.3	-	-

S-smokers; NS-nonsmokers

common causes. These figures are expected to increase up to 4.1 percent and to move to 5th rank by 2020.[24]

The prevalence study from many countries utilizes the British Medical Research Council questionnaire and is summarized in Table 16.1.[12] The data suggests that the prevalence of chronic bronchitis remains a common problem in many countries. There is some evidence that a reduced prevalence has been achieved in some European countries, including Poland, and in other countries of the world the prevalence is declining. The prevalence/incidence of chronic bronchitis in India as reported by different workers has been shown in Table 16.2.[25-31]

ETIOLOGY

SMOKING

Various retrospective and prospective studies have proved unequivocally that chronic bronchitis and emphysema are closely related to smoking and smoking is the most important factor in the etiology of COPD.[32-36] One of the major risk factors for developing COPD is cigarette smoking.[37] The benefits of smoking cessation seen in the improvement in pulmonary function test results have been well documented[37,38] although little is known about the effects of smoking cessation on the changes in the inflammatory response in the lung. The major importance of COPD as a component of chronic

morbidity has been recognized in the UK as early as the early twentieth century. Its relationship with atmospheric pollution and dust was also realized since that time. Numerous surveys have shown that much higher rates of cough and sputum in smokers than in nonsmokers with the incidence being increased with the degree of smoking. Recent studies have shown that smoking lower tar cigarettes does not necessarily reduce the prevalence of cough and sputum. However, smoking cessation usually leads to decreased symptoms and the number of exacerbations and dyspnea, at least in the early stages of the disease. The most important evidence of association of smoking with that of chronic bronchitis was first evident from the classic study by Doll and Peto[39] and Doll et al.[40] The incidence of smoking related chronic bronchitis has been reported subsequently from all over the world as will be seen from Tables 16.1 and 16.2. The incidence has been as high as 52 percent in some series (Table 16.1). The risk of mortality and morbidity increases with the amount smoked. Heavy smokers have 2 to 25 time greater mortality than that in nonsmokers. Those who inhale deeply have a higher mortality. The incidence decreases after stopping smoking early in the course of the disease. Although earlier studies were in men, subsequent studies showed that susceptibility is the same in either sex, if they smoke. A high incidence of chronic bronchitis has been reported from India in women smokers, which varied between 33 to 52 percent. Both

TABLE 16:2. Prevalence of chronic bronchitis in India[25-31]

Population	Age (Yr)	Total No	M(%)	F(%)	Total(%)
			Prevalence of chronic bronchitis		
Delhi University	14-55	656	7.0	5.0	6.0
AIIMS campus	All	2366	1.23	0.56	1.0
Kanpur	-	900	-	-	11.0
Ludhiana	17-64	473	12.5	-	12.5
Delhi	-	993	8.0	4.3	6.3
Patna	-	14910	2.12	1.33	1.77
Madras	-	817	1.4	2.7	1.59
Rural Kurali	-	1401	3.36	2.54	3.0
Rural Delhi	-	1001	4.7	3.5	4.2
Rural UP	30	1140	6.67	4.48	5.7
Rural Punjab	-	7132	0.84	0.61	0.74
Rural Bhiwani	-	278	21.8 (S)	-	
PGI attendants (Chandigarh)	-	3046	20 (S) 5.2 (NS)	4.1(NS)	
Chandigarh (Teachers)	-	743	8.2(S) 0.6(NS)	1.2(NS)	
Chandigarh city	-	2825	10(S) 1.0(NS)	1.6(NS)	
South India (Telgu)	Adult	374	33.3(Chutta)	32.7(Chutta)	33
Shimla	18-80	446	32(S) 5.8(NS) 6.0(NS)	52(S)	
Chandigarh (Rural)	-	1569	10.4(S) 4.1(NS) 5.0(NS)	23(S)	
Chandigarh	Adult	2372	0.9(NS)	1.6(NS)	
Mullanpur	Adult	1171	4.10(NS)	4.96(NS)	
Bombay	-	4129	-	-	2.3-5
Gujrat (Railway workshop)	>20	108	-	-	16.7
Udaipur (Talc industry)	-	202	-	-	13.36
Orissa	24-62	105	-	-	2.9
Bikaner (Wool workers)	>21	200	-	-	7
Kashmir	>15	560	7.56	7.81	7.68

bidi and cigarette as well as reverse smoking of home made "chuttas" are associated with the development of chronic bronchitis.[41-43] Mortality in pipe and cigar smokers is lower than that in cigarette smokers. For cigar smokers the ratio of excess mortality compared with nonsmokers has varied from 1 to 4 in different series; for pipe smokers from 1 to 9; in most studies the ratio has been about 2.[44,45] Filter-tipped cigarettes are less deleterious.[46]

Although a number of the above studies have shown a strong relationship between smoking and COPD, in many a high proportion of nonsmokers also develop COPD. In these subjects, the role of childhood infection, pollution, hyperreactivity and effect of climates have been proposed (see below).

The effects of smoking on the airways are the best and most documented in medical literature. There is an inverse relationship between cigarette consumption and expiratory flow rates. However, a significant number of patients, in spite of being active smokers show no lung function abnormalities. In the patients who smoke and are susceptible to the effects of smoke, cessation of smoking slows down the speed of pulmonary function deteriorations to that of nonsmokers, but do not normalize the lung function. A prospective study of early stages of the development of COPD in London working men showed that FEV_1 falls gradually over a life time, but in many smokers clinically significant airflow obstruction never develops.[47] In susceptible people, however, smoking causes irreversible obstructive changes. If a susceptible smoker stops smoking, he will not recover his lung function, but the average further rates of loss of FEV_1 will revert to normal. Therefore, severe, and fatal obstructive lung disease can be prevented by screening smokers lung function in early middle age if those with reduced function can stop smoking. Inflammatory process and chronic mucus hypersecretion do not cause chronic airflow obstruction to progress more rapidly. These are thus two largely unrelated disease processes chronic airflow obstruction and mucus hypersecretion including inflammatory process. Other lung function abnormalities including a faster decline in PEFR, FEV_1 and diffusing capacity have been reported in smokers than in nonsmokers.[48-54] Airway resistance also increases following smoking of even only one cigarette.[55-57] A steeper decline with age in smokers compared to ex-smokers or nonsmokers have also been reported. The twenty-first Report of the Surgeon General of the US Public Health Service on the Health consequences published in 1990 reemphasizes the reduction of respiratory symptoms and illness that follows cessation. For persons without clinically evident chronic obstructive pulmonary disease, lung function can be expected to improve by approximately 5 percent shortly after cessation, and the accelerated age-related decline of function returns to that of never smokers. For persons with overt COPD, immediate benefits of cessation for mortality have not been demonstrated. In fact, mortality rates from COPD tend to be higher for former smokers than for continuing smokers, presumably reflecting cessation by persons with symptomatic disease. The inflammatory process present in the airway mucosa of current smokers may persist after smoking cessation in subjects who continue to have symptoms of chronic bronchitis.[58] A highly significant quantitative relationship has been reported between pack-years of smoking and functional impairment.[59]

Tobacco smoking accounts for 80 to 90 percent of the risk of developing COPD.[34] The smoking attributable fraction of COPD mortality in USA during the 1980's was 0.850 for men and 0.694 for women.[36]

PASSIVE SMOKING

It is increasingly being believed that passive smoking, also known as environmental tobacco smoke (ETS), or second hand smoke, is related to various respiratory disorders. The 1984 report of the Surgeon General of USA had shown a significant correlation between parental smoking and bronchitis or pneumonia in young children.[34] In older children, the data is conflicting. A number of other studies have shown a small but significant decrease of lung function in children of smoking mothers. Smoking in the household has been found to be strongly associated with continuing asthma symptoms in young children. Continuing symptoms more than 3 years after an attack of acute bronchiolitis in children is significantly associated with maternal

smoking. Some, but not all studies have demonstrated minor changes in adults. The effect of cigarette smoke may begin at an early age. There is an increase in respiratory illness and diminished lung function in children passively exposed to parental smoking.[60-64] Even infants of smoking parents have more respiratory illness than infants of nonsmokers[65] and and pneumonia at that age may predispose to chronic bronchitis in later life.[66,67] The significance of these findings for the later development of COPD are uncertain at this moment. In the absence of smoking in adult life the effects of passive smoking may not be very important.

α_1-Antitrypsin Deficiency

One of the most significant breakthroughs in the field of COPD in the past 30 years was the discovery of a close association between an inherited deficiency of a protein in the blood called the α_1-antitrypsin (AAT). It is the only known genetic disorder that leads to COPD. AAT deficiency accounts for less than 1 percent of COPD in USA.[7] This deficiency is an autosomal hereditary disorder in which there are low levels of α_1-antitrypsin in serum and lungs, with a high risk of development of panlobular emphysema in the third to fifth decade. There is an increased risk of development of liver disease in the childhood associated with this condition. The enzyme is synthesized and secreted by the hepatocytes and to a lesser extent by the mononuclear phagocytes, and then is released into the blood from which it then diffuses into the lungs.[68] AAT is a glycoprotein coded for by a single gene on chromosome 14. It is a serine protease inhibitor with primary function of inhibiting neutrophil elastase. Emphysema results from an imbalance between the neutrophil elastase in the lung and the anti-elastases. While the former has the capability of destroying elastin and other tissue components, the later is responsible for protecting the lung from elastase. This concept is known as the "elastase-antielastase balance hypothesis of emphysema." The concept has been proved both in humans and animal experiments. According to the theory, either an excess of protease or a deficiency in the amount of functional activity of anti-proteases (or both) can lead to the development of emphysema.

At least 75 alleles of the α_1-antitrypsin gene have been identified[69] and categorized into the protease inhibitor (Pi) system. These alleles can be categorized into four groups according to the α_1-antitrypsin levels in the serum.[70] They are:

(1) **Normal**. This is associated with normal serum levels of α_1-antitrypsin with normal function.

(2) **Deficient**. This is associated with serum α_1-antitrypsin levels < 35 percent of average normal levels.

(3) **Null**. In this type there is no detectable α_1-antitrypsin protein in serum.

(4) **Dysfunctional**. In this type α_1-antitrypsin is present but does not function normally.

The normal and deficient α_1-antitrypsin alleles are designated from A to Z on the basis of their electrophoretic mobility. The family of normal α_1-antitrypsin alleles is referred to as M (M1, M2, and M3) and are found in approximately 90 percent of the population. The most deficiency allele associated with emphysema is the Z allele. The α_1-antitrypsin phenotype, therefore, is made up of the two parental alleles and is referred to as the Pi phenotype. α_1-antitrypsin variants are inherited as codominant alleles. The most common phenotype is PiMM (PiM2M3) and the most common deficient phenotype associated with a high risk for the disease is PiZZ. The specific mutations responsible for many forms of α_1-antitrypsin deficiency have been identified. The abnormal Z allele is associated with replacement glutamic acid by lysin at position 342 as a result of a single base mutation from GAG to AAG. This substitution results in alteration of the three dimensional configuration of the molecule. Thus, it aggregates in the rough endoplasmic reticulum of the hepatocyte and consequently a decreased secretion of AAT occurs from the liver to about 15 percent of the normal.[71,72]

By convention, the serum α_1-antitrypsin levels have been expressed in units of mg/dl (commercial standards) or µM (true laboratory standards). The normal values of serum AAT are 150 to 350 mg/dl or 20 to 48 µM. Levels of 80 mg/dl (11 µM) have been considered to be the threshold serum level above which the quantity is sufficient to protect the lung and below which the individual has an increased chance of emphysema compared with the general population. PiZZ homozygotes have levels of 2.5 to 7 µM (mean, 16% of normal), and PiSS homozygotes have levels of 13 to 33 µM (mean, 52% of normal). In contrast, individuals who are heterozygous have reduced concentrations with the extent of reduction depending on the phenotype. Thus PiSZ will have values of 8 to 19 µM (mean, 37% of normal) and PiMZ will have values of 12 to 35 µM (mean, 57% of normal). They do not appear to be at increased risk for COPD, in family studies and in surveys in some populations of COPD patients, however there is an increased frequency of heterozygotes.[73] There is some evidence that MS heterozygotes may have an increased frequency of nonspecific airways hyperreactivity.[74] Subjects with Pi null phenotype, by definition, have

serum values of 0. The deficient null alleles are very rare, together representing less than 1 percent of all α_1-antitrypsin alleles. They are at a very high risk of developing emphysema since there is no α_1-antitrypsin to protect their lungs.

Epidemiological studies indicate that a threshold value of 11 αM or about 35 percent of the average normal level, is sufficient to protect the lungs. It follows therefore, that individuals who are at greater risk are PiZZ homozygotes, the null homozygotes, and, occasionally PiSZ heterozygotes. PiSS homozygotes and other heterozygotes like PiMZ, and PiMS, do not appear to be at increased risk. Severe AAT deficiency leads to premature emphysema of the panacinar type with more severe affection at the bases, and is often associated with chronic bronchitis and occasionally with bronchiectasis.[75] Individuals with a PiZZ phenotype who smoke cigarettes are at increased risk, become symptomatic earlier with dyspnea occurring at a median age of about 40 years. The same will be about 53 years in cases of nonsmokers. Smokers with AAT deficiency and COPD will have a life expectancy that is approximately 10 years less than the nonsmokers with this condition. The rate of decline of FEV_1 is also more in them with a decline in excess of 100 ml/year. Severity of lung disease varies considerably. Patients who are detected on population surveys only live longer to the age of 80 or 90 years. Airflow obstruction occurs more in men. Other risk factors are asthma, recurrent respiratory infections, and familial factors.[76] Liver disease associated with α_1-antitrypsin deficiency is less common than emphysema and occurs in less than 10 percent of the PiZZ phenotypes. The most common manifestation is neonatal hepatitis. Other presentations include unexplained chronic liver disease in older children, and cirrhosis and hepatoma in adults.[77,78]

Many Indian studies have tried to examine the role of alpha-1-antitrypsin deficiency in the causation of COPD and is summarized by Malik et al.[79] The heterozygote state (intermediate) was found to be 10.3 to 23.3 percent and homozygous (severe) state in 2.8 to 20 percent of cases of COPD.

AIR POLLUTION

The interrelationship of COPD and pollution associated with the London "smogs" that became notorious in the later parts of 19th century through the early 1960s is well reported in literature. Incomplete combustion of coal with emission of black smoke and sulfur dioxide and production of tar with sulfuric acid resulted in a smoke/fog/SO_2 mixture that was associated with a marked increases in sudden deaths, hospital admissions, illness in bronchitis patients with reduction in lung function and urban excess of morbidity and mortality from chronic airway disease.[80-83] Subsequently many cross sectional studies suggest that air pollution of whatever origin is responsible for respiratory symptoms and reduced lung function.[81] Surveys conducted in Lancaster, Burbank, Long Beach, Mumbai, Netherlands and many other places, compared the importance and nature of air pollution with lung function. The town of Lancaster was considered a clean area as opposed to Burbank, known for its pollution due to oxidants, and to the town of Long Beach, characterized by the presence of petrochemical plants causing pollution due to particles, hydrocarbons, and sulfur dioxide. The percentage of patients with diminished airflows was significantly higher in the polluted areas of Burbank and Long Beach than the Lancaster area. Another longitudinal survey in Netherlands compared the expiratory flows of subjects in rural areas free of air pollution and another area, Vlaardingen, polluted by refineries releasing sulfur monoxide and smoke. It was demonstrated that the mean reduction in vital capacity and the mean expiratory flow in ml/year was higher in the polluted than in the non-polluted area. A study from Mumbai has reported a high prevalence of cough, dyspnea, or both in nonsmokers (13%) and was attributed to the industrial pollution.[84]

Indoor air pollution due to domestic cooking and heating has been associated with chronic respiratory symptoms as reported from many developed and developing countries.[85-93] In a large study from India Behera and Jindal[89] has reported the incidence of chronic bronchitis to be about 3 percent in nonsmoking rural Indian women exposed to domestic cooking fuels. The effect is more marked in women using biomass fuel. These women also had reduced ventilatory functions, particularly FVC.[91] These fuels produce respiratory irritants such as oxides of nitrogen, sulphur dioxide, and unburnt hydrocarbons (soot particles). Soot particles that are generated more with firewood cooking *chulla* are probably more hazardous in causing changes of chronic bronchitis as well as airways obstruction. Such pollution itself does not produce chronic bronchitis to a large extent independent of smoking, except one study from Nepal, which reported a high incidence due to domestic smoke pollution.[92,93] Nonetheless, indoor air pollution is an important cause of chronic bronchitis, particularly in nonsmoking women.[90]

There is of course, an interrelationship of pollution with smoking; the effects are at least additive and may in some circumstances be synergistic.

OCCUPATION

The universality of the smoking habit in working men and women and its strong casual role in the genesis of COPD has tended to overshadow the potential contribution of occupational exposures. However, recent evidence from cross sectional and longitudinal studies, both community based, and workplace related, points to a casual role in association with or independently of cigarette smoking.[94,95] Occupational exposures to dusts alone or to dusts and in association with fumes and vapors are independent risk factors for the development of COPD.[94] There are also occupational exposures in which smoking has the effect of amplifying the exposure risk. In a longitudinal study over 12 years period in 575 men, aged 30 to 54 years, working in the Paris area, the yearly reduction of FEV_1 was reported to be significantly higher, by 10 to 20 ml per year; in the subjects exposed to occupational air pollutants, whatever their smoking level was. Details are discussed in the chapter on Occupational lung diseases.

CHILDHOOD LUNG DISEASES

Data from retrospective and longitudinal studies suggest that childhood illnesses may be responsible for respiratory diseases in adulthood. The prevalence of lung involvement was shown to be higher in subjects with parents who had sustained respiratory tract infections in their childhood. The mother's smoking also seems to increase the prevalence of respiratory symptoms. Retrospective studies suggest that paediatric lung diseases account for an important risk factor of obstructive disease developing in adult life, whether the parents were smokers or not.[96-101]

There is increasing evidence also from longitudinal studies for an association between acute respiratory tract infection of the lower respiratory tract in childhood and the occurrence of COPD in adulthood. This association has been consistent in many studies. However, it is not very clear whether the association is causal or noncausal and whether the effect is epidemiologically important.[96-100] While studies by Burrows et al[96] have shown a direct relationship between respiratory infections during childhood and development of COPD in adults during later life, English studies.[97,98] have largely excluded the contribution of childhood respiratory infection in the causation of adult chronic respiratory diseases. Social and environmental factors have a major influence on the incidence and severity of acute respiratory tract infection in children. Among these factors are low birth weight, nutritional status, and the effect of passive smoking, indoor pollution, crowding, and ambient temperature. These factors may be responsible indirectly for the development of COPD later in life.

In contrast to findings in children, there is inconsistent evidence as to whether acute respiratory tract infection in adults is associated with COPD.[101-103] There is no such reliable evidence to suggest that the lower respiratory tract infection initiates the onset of COPD, although intercurrent infections are important causes of increased morbidity in patients with established COPD. These episodes do not seem to cause permanent loss of lung function. Influenza epidemics have been associated with increased mortality in patients with COPD and other infectious agents causing acute respiratory tract infection might similarly affect mortality rates.

It was suggested that alcohol, may be a causative factor for COPD. However, it is difficulty to differentiate an alcohol effect from that linking to smoking. Studies have reported opposite conclusions. If there is an effect, it is probably minor.

The predictors of probability of developing COPD was reported in a population of men and women aged 16 to 74 years in Tecumseh over a period of 18 years. The findings are summarized in Table 16.3.[104]

TABLE 16.3: Age adjusted risk factors for COPD

Documented	Not documented
Airflow limitation	Drinking habits
Smoking habits	Social class
Chronic bronchitis	Physical measurements
Respiratory symptoms	Genetic markers
History of infections	
Familial respiratory diseases	

The most important factors were age, daily cigarette consumption, possible alterations of smoking habits and the observed value of FEV_1.

BRONCHIAL HYPERRESPONSIVENESS

With normal aging process there is a fall in FEV_1 of about 25 ml/year in healthy nonsmokers over the age of 30 years. In smokers the fall is about 50 ml/year. However, certain smokers show a markedly decline in FEV_1 of more than 50 ml/year and these are the subgroups who later on develop COPD. Although factors which result in such an accelerated rate of decline in lung functions are not known, Dutch investigators have proposed a "Dutch hypothesis"[105] which suggested that an allergic constitution might predispose chronic smokers to severe chronic airflow obstruction. These investigators proposed that an "asthmatic constitution" underlay the development of chronic airflow limitation. This asthmatic

"constitution" consists of a predisposition to atopic disease, eosinophilia, and airway hyperresponsiveness. According to the hypothesis, smoking is only an extrinsic factor that is superimposed on this constitutional susceptibility leading on to chronic airflow limitation. This view has subsequently been found favor with many investigators who believe that hyperreactivity is a contributing factor in the causation of COPD.[106-113] It has been shown that smokers have a higher level of IgE levels,[114] and there is a correlation of eosinophilia in the peripheral blood with that of smoking.[115] Smokers have a high prevalence of certain markers of atopy compared to controls.

Nonspecific hyperreactivity of the airways is reported in smokers in many studies although its possible role in the development is unclear.[7] This reactivity might stem from the airway inflammation that typically seen in smoking related COPD. In the Lung Health Study, nonspecific airway hyperreactivity was noted in 85.1 percent of women than men (58.9%). While 46.6 percent of women responded to 5 mg/ml or less of methacholine, only 23.9 percent of men responded to the same dose, a number almost half of that of women. In both sexes, degree of airflow obstruction was highly correlated with severity of airflow obstruction but not with age.[113]

DEMOGRAPHIC AND OTHER VARIABLES

There is higher prevalence of respiratory symptoms in men. Mortality rates for COPD are higher in whites than in nonwhites. Morbidity and mortality rates are inversely related to socioeconomic status and are higher in blue collar than white-collar workers.[7] COPD may also aggregate in families suggesting a genetic link.[116] It is suggested that dietary fish intake perhaps reduces the susceptibility to COPD as is evident that asthma is extremely low in Eskimoes. Britton reported that a high dietary intake of ω-3 fatty acids may protect cigarette smokers against COPD.[117]

NATURAL HISTORY OF COPD

As mentioned in the previous section, the FEV_1 in asymptomatic healthy nonsmokers declines by 25 to 30 ml per year at about the age of 35 years. The rate of decline is steeper for smokers and the rate of fall is directly proportional to the severity of smoking.[118] The decline in function occurs in a slowly accelerating curvilinear path. In most subjects, the loss is uniform, and in some it develops in stages. There is a direct relationship between the initial FEV_1 level and the slope of FEV_1 decline.[119] The relationship is also direct with the initial FEV_1/FVC particularly in men.[120] The fall in PEFR in both the symptomatic and asymptomatic males showed a decline of about 5L/min/year. The fall was negligible in women over a period of 10 years, both symptomatic and asymptomatic.[121] Other risk factors are age, lifetime smoking history, and the number of cigarettes currently smoked.[122,123] Acute chest illness, which is common in COPD, decreases lung function for about 3 months.[119] The role of mucus hypersecretion on the mortality is unclear.[124-126] It was earlier believed that small airways (those less than 2 mm in diameter) obstruction as calculated from closing volumes, closing capacity, and the slope of the alveolar plateau derived from a single breath nitrogen test may be good predictors of development of COPD subsequently. However, it is proved now that this is not so.[127] Ventilatory function tests indicating emphysema (DLCO, FRC, TLC) predict survival in a minor way.[128]

After smoking cessation, a small amount of lung function is regained. About 35 percent of subjects in the Lung Health Study who stopped smoking, for one year showed an increase in postbronchodilator FEV_1 of about 57 ml in opposed to 38 ml who did continued smoking.[129] Thereafter, the rate of lung function decline slows to approximately that seen in never smokers of the same age.[51,130] Other reports suggest that subjects who have a more rapid decline in lung function can be defined by greater loss of FEV_1 or FEV_1/FVC ratio.[120,131] Smoking cessation improves prognosis regardless of age.[132]

PATHOGENESIS

There has been a lot of research on how smoking damages the lung.[55-57,133-151] The damage affects many elements in the respiratory tract, including mucus secreting cells, cilia, bronchial muscles, small airways, and alveoli. Mucosal glands undergo hypertrophic changes in response to smoking with resultant excess mucus secretion. Ciliotoxic action of smoke affects the mucociliary-blanket and predisposes to accumulation of mucus in the bronchial tree. This in turn will predispose to superinfection with resultant mucosal edema, and infiltration with inflammatory cells, which will further exacerbate airway obstruction. The effect on the bronchial smooth muscle tone may be mediated by irritant receptors and this may be a reflex-induced phenomenon. It has been demonstrated that even smoking of one cigarette increases the airway resistance, which can be blocked effectively by atropine. The effects on small airways and alveoli are mediated by inadequately antagonized enzymatic action by proteases (particularly elastase). Smoking recruits inflammatory cells to the lungs including neutrophils, monocytes, and macrophages.

Macrophages also produce neutrophil chemoattractants stimulated by smoking and direct release of elastase can also occur directly from neutrophils due to smoke.[152-156] Some other cells like platelets, smooth muscle cells, and mast cells also release elastase. Antiproteases are inactivated by highly active oxidants in tobacco smoke, which may also directly damage connective tissue and by active oxygen radicals released from stimulated phagocytes. Repair mechanisms may also be inhibited. Smoking may also decrease the maximal surface tension of surfactant, leading to overdistention of alveoli, and interfere with gas absorption through the surfactant layer.

Thus smoking results in an overproduction of proteases (i.e. elastase). Further, it inactivates the anti-elastases. Thus there is an imbalance between the protease-antiprotease with resultant excess action of protease, which leads on to the destruction.[157-159]

There has been a renewed interest in the "Dutch hypothesis", (see above) which suggested that there is an atopic element in susceptibility to tobacco smoke.[149-151] There is evidence both for and against this proposition. Increased bronchial hyperresponsiveness, elevated serum IgE levels, and intermittent sputum eosinophilia in COPD patients is not uncommon. There is also a significant inverse relationship in the individual patient between PEFR and variations in sputum levels of IgE, histamine, and SRS-A. Although, all these findings suggest the contribution of atopic elements, it is relatively small compared with the overwhelming and potentially lethal long-term effect of tobacco smoke in inducing COPD.

Earlier it was thought that the underlying mechanism of airways obstruction was mucus hypersecretion. It was believed that smoke inhalation was responsible for mucus hypersecretion because of bronchial irritation and mucus gland hypertrophy—"the British Hypothesis", which in turn induces recurring bronchial infections leading to chronic bronchitis and obstructive lung disease. This concept was challenged in 1977 by Fletcher and Peto,[51] who suggested that smoking gives rise to two different lung diseases. One is due to hypertrophy of mucus glands responsible for mucus hypersecretion and recurring bronchial infections. The other is an airway disease with emphysema, leading to airflow limitation and respiratory failure. Both conditions differ in regard to susceptibility to cigarette smoke, which accounts for 50 percent for hypertrophy of mucus glands, and to 10 to 15 percent for airway obstruction. Smoking cessation stops mucus hypersecretion and prevents further excessive exacerbations, but it does not restore the airflow limitation. Similar conclusions have been reported by other workers subsequently. Moreover, numerous structure-function correlative studies have failed to identify a close relationship between airflow obstruction and mucous gland hyperplasia.

The obstruction to airflow in emphysema is primarily due to the collapse of the airways as a result of loss of radial support of their walls normally provided by the elastic recoil of the lung tissue. Other contributory factors include decreased elastic recoil of the lungs resulting in a decreased driving force. Emphysema is invariably associated with chronic bronchitis (except the hereditary type) and peripheral airways disease, which further contribute to airflow obstruction in emphysema.

Conceptually, airflow, like the pressure determines flow in any hydraulic system applied or the resistance encountered, which can be expressed as:

Flow = Pressure/Resistance

This concept can be extended for chronic airflow limitation as under

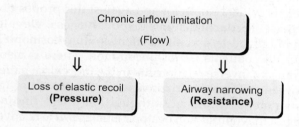

In the lungs, pressure is generated by elastic recoil, which is diminished or lost resulting in generation of less pressure; and resistance is determined by airways caliber, which is narrowed. Thus the flow is diminished as a net effect.

MECHANISMS OF AIRWAY OBSTRUCTION IN COPD

In normal lungs the resistance of the peripheral bronchi and bronchioles is much less than that in the larger airways.[160] However, in COPD, the peripheral airways are the major site of increased resistance.[161] At least three mechanisms account for the increase in peripheral airways resistance in patients with COPD. (i) The loss of elastic recoil of the lungs in emphysema allows the airways to narrow;[162-162C] (ii) the airways narrow because the supporting alveolar attachments are destroyed by the emphysematous process;[163] and (iii) the inflammatory process in the airways thickens the wall and narrows the lumen of the distal airways. However, the explanation based on the first two mechanisms has been challenged,[161,163] although these changes do occur in COPD. Perhaps these two changes in

lung parenchyma are less important than the inflammatory process that occurs in the wall and lumen of the distal airways.[164,165] The parenchymal destruction play less important role in airways obstruction because (a) it is present in a moderate to severe form in patients with normal airways function; (b) It tends to increase in prevalence rather than in severity as lung function is reduced; and (c) it is not affected by maneuvers that should lower the resistance of poorly supported airways. When tissues are damaged, exudation of plasma and cells occur from the vascular space into the tissue where the damage has occurred. Plasma derived proteins in the exudate are activated and potent mediators are generated from the complement, kinin, coagulation, and fibrinolytic systems. These mediators along with others generated in the tissue from mast cells, nerve endings, and damaged cell membranes control the exudation associated with inflammatory response. The structural changes that occur include tissue swelling, because of vascular congestion and fluid accumulation from the vascular compartment into the interstitial space. These changes are associated with leucocyte and mononuclear cell migration into the damaged area and the exudative material is organized. Shedding of epithelial cells occur into the bronchial lumen accompanied by excess mucus secretion. There will be an increase in the smooth muscle and other connective tissue in the subepithelial structure leading to contraction of the tissue and fixed narrowing of the airway lumen.[166] The extent and severity of the inflammatory response in the peripheral airways correlates with deterioration in airway function. Thus, the inflammatory process in the peripheral airways provides the structural basis for the excessive deterioration in airways function seen in heavy smokers.[164-170]

Over the last years, many studies have aimed at better redefining the airway inflammatory changes that are associated with COPD, the diagnostic umbrella comprising emphysema, small airways disease, and chronic bronchitis (CB). The reappraisal of inflammation of the airways as a fundamental part of the disease was possible by capitalizing, on one side, on the different tools that are available for evaluating airway inflammation from more to less invasive or noninvasive (e.g. BAL or sputum) and, on the other side, on the recent progresses in immunology and leukocyte biology.[171] In the majority of studies on the cellular bases of COPD, findings from bronchial biopsy specimens, BAL fluid (BALF) samples, and induced sputum (IS) samples were analyzed. The IS sample examination is a well-tolerated, effective method for the analysis of bronchial cellular response. Several studies performed in patients with COPD revealed the role of neutrophils, macrophages, and

CD8-positive lymphocytes in the pathogenesis of this disorder. Long-term smoke exposure causes similar changes in the IS cell profile with features of neutrophil and macrophage activation. It is difficult to establish the macrophage phenotype, since these cells represent a heterogeneous population with different stages of activation. The most stable surface markers seem to be the following: (i) the transferrin receptor CD71; (ii) the adhesion associated molecules CD11a, CD11b, and CD11c; (iii) the intercellular adhesion molecule-1 (CD54); and (iv) the receptor to lipopolysaccharide-CD14. As shown in the investigation of the BALF from smokers, cigarette smoke alters the expression of the above markers. However, the analysis of IS samples in patients with COPD revealed no significant differences in cell count and macrophage phenotypes between active smokers and ex-smokers.[172]

Neutrophils have been known for a long time as the major component of sputum in CB and COPD patients[173] and consistently their role in intraluminal inflammation has been confirmed, but new and important information has been added on the mechanisms of polymorphonuclear leukocyte recruitment and on their activities in the derangement of the airways and lung parenchyma. Moreover, what was really new and exciting was the observation of a role for mononuclear cell-mediated inflammation also in COPD patients. Lymphocytes and monocytes/macrophages are found in increased numbers and in the activated state in the bronchial submucosa of CB and COPD patients.[174,175] It is a picture that somehow resembles that found in the bronchi of asthmatic patients, but differs with the situation in asthma patients, in COPD patients the causative agents and the characteristics (e.g. T helper-1 vs T helper-2 cytokine profile) of this reaction are still unclear.[176] Moreover, the interaction between the mononuclear and the polymorphonuclear part of airway inflammation is just starting to be addressed, with evidence of the role of chemokines and chemokine receptors.[177,178] Beginning with these observations, the research focused on the possible molecular mechanisms causing airway inflammation, trying to identify the possible targets for new treatment approaches. Many researchers think that neutrophil chemotaxis is the key. As a follow-up to this concept, the hypothesis that by inhibiting, or reducing, the neutrophil influx into the airways one should be able to reduce the burden of airway inflammation and, thus, to change the natural history of the disease, has arisen. Chemotaxis is a biological phenomenon whereby a cell type migrates through barriers (e.g. vessel walls or epithelial layers) and tissues toward a site of inflammation or infection. Thus, it represents a useful biological phenomenon since it allows for the allocation of resources (i.e. cells and cell products) in a short time to the place where they are needed. The cells migrating to the site of chemotaxis will initiate and maintain the inflammatory processes, which may switch up self-maintaining circuits and become chronic and irreversible, causing tissue derangement and organ failure. In the case of COPD, although cigarette smoke is the cause of the disease in most patients and smoke is able to induce neutrophil chemotaxis,[179,180] one of the characteristics is the continuing maintenance of the airway inflammatory picture after smoking cessation. Chemotaxis is also a complex and multistep process in which, under a variety of stimuli, different cell types produce either the chemotactic factors or the factors that induce their production, other cells migrate through margination, deformation, and rolling adhesion mediated by adhesion molecules, and the mediators of chemotaxis and their receptors have interplay. As an example, a long list of molecules, each of them produced by different cell types, are able to exert a chemotactic activity for neutrophils: classic chemoattractants such as C5a, leukotriene (LT) B4, platelet-activating factor, and formyl-methionyl-leucyl-phenylalanine; chemokines such as interleukin (IL)-8, growth-related oncogene (GRO)-α, GRO-β, and GRO-γ; and other recently recognized factors.[181-183] IL-8 and LTB4 are identified as neutrophil chemotactic factors in the sputa of COPD patients and is demonstrate that a mouse antibody antagonist of IL-8 and an antagonist of LTB4 receptor may inhibit *in vitro* neutrophil chemotaxis. Similarly, an LT synthesis inhibitor has been shown to be ready for further clinical studies, and other compounds are being tested.[184-186] This evidence means that if chemotaxis is the key factor in the airway inflammation of patients with COPD, there are compounds that can block it, thus opening new avenues for the treatment of this deadly disease. Together with antichemotactic drugs, many new compounds or classes of compounds are presently in development for the treatment of COPD, such as antioxidants, protease inhibitors, adhesion molecule inhibitors, and new anti-inflammatory drugs.[185,186] All of these new approaches have their rationale in cellular and molecular mechanisms of the inflammatory components in COPD that are taken as targets for the proposed treatment, but there are still a number of problems to be solved. For the anti-chemotactic drugs, the first problem is to identify the important mediators of chemotaxis that drive neutrophils into the airways of COPD patients. Neutrophilic chemotactic factors such as, IL-8, LTB4, and GRO-α have been identified in COPD patients at different levels, in BAL,[187-190] sputum,[191-193] serum[194] and lung tissue.[195] There is a need to clearly identify the chemotactic factors that, among many others, may be more important in COPD patients, and/or are more easily inhibited in their functional activity. As an example, Beeh and colleagues observed that the pretreatment of neutrophils with the combination of both of the antichemotactic drugs (i.e. anti-IL-8 and anti-LTB4 receptor) reduced the sputum-induced chemotaxis by roughly 45 percent, which was less than the combined effect of either drug alone, thus suggesting the presence in the sputa of other, yet unidentified, neutrophil chemoattractants. Chemotaxis may be quantitatively assayed *in vitro* using the chemotaxis chamber[196] or chemotactic factors may be identified by immunoenzymatic methods. In both cases, methodologic problems that are caused by the presence of the natural inhibitors of some chemotactic factors[197] or by the possible confounding effects of dithiothreitol on sputum sol assays[198,199] may occur. In addition, it is possible that at different sites (e.g. larger vs smaller airways) the "cocktail" of chemotactic factors varies. The different proportions of the various chemotactic factors that are detected would then be due to the methodology used to obtain solutes from the airways (e.g. sputum, sampling more proximal airways, or BAL, sampling also the lower respiratory tract). Exacerbations of COPD, or subtypes of them (e.g. bacterial), may be associated with a set of chemotactic signals that is different from that driving neutrophilic inflammation during the stable state, a difference that can be hypothesized also for the other COPD patient groups such as current smokers vs former or never-smokers.[189,200,201] Severe and mild-to-moderate stages of the disease are associated with different cellular inflammatory bronchial infiltrates[202] and also may be characterized by distinct sets of chemotactic factors. The genetic background of patients is probably important, as the same agent (i.e. cigarette smoke) could cause different molecular responses in patient subpopulations sharing particular alleles for one or more chemotactic factors. After identifying and antagonizing the relevant neutrophil chemotactic factors, and certainly IL-8 and LTB4 are good candidates, one should ask to what extent the airway inflammation in COPD patients would be reduced. Together with variable bronchospasm and hyper-reactivity, the features of COPD causing airflow limitation comprise a substantial reduction in the caliber and number of small airways, the loss of alveolar attachments causing air trapping, exaggerated mucus production,

and the presence of airway inflammatory infiltrates.[176] Neutrophils and their products contribute to all these features, but other cell types (e.g. macrophages, lymphocytes, or eosinophils) are surely also involved in the genesis of airway inflammation. At least other cell types, such as macrophages, could surrogate some activities of neutrophils in COPD.[203] Thus, the suppression only of the neutrophil-dependent part of inflammation, even if possible, may be not be sufficient to cure COPD while it could have also serious side effects on bacterial infection susceptibility. Since one of the targets of the anti-chemotactic strategies seems to be IL-8 or its receptor, it should be remembered that the chemokine system is redundant, with many molecules sharing overlapping effects and acting through the same surface receptors,[204] and it may be difficult to inhibit *in vivo* chemotaxis significantly by blocking just one chemokine or receptor. Lastly, it has been demonstrated that old drugs that are used worldwide, such as theophylline exert similar activities claimed for the new antichemotactic drugs, directly or indirectly.[205] Thus, the antichemotaxis approach is probably not ready for prime time in the treatment of COPD. Despite all of the above-mentioned limitations, it represents a very good working hypothesis, introducing for the first time the concept of an etiologic treatment that would counteract the noxious effects of the neutrophilic inflammatory burden in the airways of COPD patients.

COPD is a debilitating inflammatory disease of the lungs characterized by an increased presence of neutrophils and macrophages in the airways of affected patients. Neutrophils produce proteinases such as neutrophil elastase, matrix metalloproteinases, and cathepsins that may lead to emphysema and mucous hypersecretion. Recruitment of neutrophils to the airways requires their adhesion to pulmonary and bronchial epithelial cells and subsequent migration into the airways and alveoli. Previous studies have indicated that airway secretions from patients with cystic fibrosis, bronchiectasis, or COPD contain chemoattractants for neutrophils. However, the contribution of different neutrophil chemoattractants may vary between different diseases, or even in different stages of the same disease.

Understanding the mechanisms leading to airway neutrophilia in COPD is important, since several chemoattractants may serve as targets for future anti-inflammatory drugs. These anti-inflammatory agents may potentially reduce the rate of decline of lung function in these patients by ameliorating neutrophil-mediated tissue destruction. Several neutrophil chemotactic factors have been implicated, including interleukin

(IL)-8, tumor necrosis factor and leukotriene B$_4$ (LTB$_4$), with a predominant role for IL-8 in cystic fibrosis, LTB$_4$ in bacterial exacerbations of COPD, and a combination of both IL-8 and LTB$_4$ in bronchiectasis. Moreover, unlike IL-8, LTB$_4$ has also been shown to prolong neutrophil survival by inhibiting apoptosis.

There is still ongoing debate about the benefit of inhaled or oral corticosteroids in patients with stable COPD. While corticosteroids have no effect on neutrophilic inflammation they may influence cytokine levels, or neutrophil survival and activation. Hence, only steroid-naive patients are chosen to exclude a possible influence of concomitant anti-inflammatory treatment on sputum chemotaxis. Neutrophilic inflammation is a major feature of COPD. Several factors in bronchial secretions have been identified as chemoattractants for neutrophils. IL-8 and LTB$_4$ are important cytokines as chemoattractants for neutrophils in bronchial secretions from patients with COPD, and suggest that specific inhibitors may have therapeutic potential in COPD.[206]

PATHOLOGY

Several of the abnormalities in chronic bronchitis and emphysema occur in large bronchi (airways with cartilages in their walls and more than 2 mm in diameter), bronchioles (no cartilages in their walls and less than 2 mm internal diameter), and parenchyma. Since emphysema and chronic bronchitis are invariably associated in the same patient, it is common to find changes in all the above three components, although one or the other change may predominate.

The important change in the large bronchi is the hypertrophy of the mucus secreting glands in the subepithelial layer that are enlarged and are thought to secrete most of the mucus found in the airways.[207] The hypertrophy can be measured as the thickness of the gland layer in histological sections and comparing it to that of the bronchial wall and is expressed as Reid index.[208] The mucus gland size can also be assessed by measurement of absolute gland area or by volume proportion of the glands, both of which have a better correlation with antemortem quantification of sputum production than the Reid index.[209] The mucous gland hypertrophy is mainly seen in the larger bronchi and is uniformly distributed throughout the lungs. The mucus secreting goblet cells are also increased in number in the large as well as in the bronchioli.[210] Bronchial muscle hyperplasia is present in patients with COPD. The exact proportion varied from zero to universal, but most studies show an increased average amount of muscle in patients with chronic bronchitis and COPD. The increasing

amount of muscle may be responsible for the airway hyperreactivity seen in these patients. It may also thicken the bronchial wall and impinge upon the lumen. Inflammatory changes with infiltration of chronic inflammatory cells are also common. Focal squamous metaplasia occurs in about 2/3rd of the smokers and the intensity of tobacco use (packs per day) rather than the number of pack years is more important factor in promoting squamous metaplasia.[211,212]

The changes in the bronchioles are referred to as "small airway disease or bronchiolitis. The lesions are variable and are thought to be the most important cause of mild chronic airflow limitation.[213-217] Inflammation is the most important change in the smaller airways. The inflammation is mild and chronic inflammatory cells dominate. It is suggested that obstruction to airflow is due to exudation of edema fluid that displaces the surfactant of bronchioles rendering them unstable as they narrow and close easily. They would open with more difficulty. Release of inflammatory mediators may also directly or reflexly constrict bronchiolar muscles. Goblet cell metaplasia is another characteristic finding in the bronchioles. Normally, about 1 percent or less of the lining cells of bronchioles is mucus-secreting cells. An increase in their number probably reflects a response to inflammation. Bronchiolar fibrosis and bronchiolar muscle hyperplasia have both been associated with airflow obstruction. They are probably due to inflammation and exert their effect by narrowing the airways. Bronchiolar deformity with tortuosity and irregularity is common and has a good correlation with airflow obstruction. Destruction of cartilage in some subsegmental bronchi has been described. Macroscopically there may be some exaggeration of the normal longitudinal folds of mucous membrane in the larger airways and a development of transverse folds in the more peripheral bronchi, which can be seen on bronchograms. Diminished alveolar attachment is common.

Thus, changes in the bronchial tree in chronic bronchitis can be summarized as:
1. Central airway lesions
   (a) Mucus gland enlargement
   (b) Muscle hyperplasia
   (c) Bronchial wall thickening and encroachment on the bronchial lumen
   (d) Inflammation
2. Bronchiolar lesions (bronchiolitis, small airway or peripheral airway disease)
   (a) Inflammation
   (b) Fibrosis
   (c) Increased muscle

(d) Goblet cell metaplasia

(e) Mucus plugging

(f) Loss of alveolar attachment and bronchiolar deformity

(g) Bronchiolar narrowing

(h) Bronchiolar obliteration

3. Acinar changes (see below).

Parenchymal destruction results in emphysema.[5,157, 218-224] Depending on its severity, emphysema can be diagnosed in a variety of ways including naked eye examination, by dissecting microscope examination of the lung slice fixed in inflation, by light microscopic examination of thick or thin stained mounted sections and by scanning electron microscopic observation. Emphysema is recognized as a subcategory of respiratory airspace enlargement, which is described below.

Respiratory Airspace Enlargement

1. Simple airspace enlargement
   (a) Congenital
   (b) Acquired
2. Airspace enlargement with fibrosis
3. Emphysema
   (a) Centriacinar
   (b) Panacinar
   (c) Distal acinar.

In simple airspace enlargement the pattern of the acinus is maintained without any destruction. Congenital airspace enlargement occurs in Down's syndrome or congenital lobar inflation, whereas acquired forms include compensatory hyperinflation, and the uniform airspace enlargement associated with aging. The later may be a combination of age and effect of environment. Since the change is almost universal it is suggested that they should be regarded as normal. This is otherwise known as senile emphysema.

Other air space enlargements associated with fibrosis include honeycombed interstitial pulmonary fibrosis, those associated with tuberculosis, sarcoidosis, or eosinophilic granuloma.

The three subtypes of emphysema that are recognized are:[223]

(a) *Centriacinar Emphysema*. This is otherwise known as proximal acinar emphysema because the proximal part of the acinus (respiratory bronchiole) is involved predominantly. This is probably secondary to bronchiolitis resulting in destruction and distension of alveolar walls due to air trapping. It is commoner at the lung apices. There are two subdivisions of this type. The first one is classically associated with smoking and airflow obstruction, and also referred as *centrilobular emphysema*. The other type is associated with inhalation of coal dust and other mineral dusts and result in dilatation of respiratory bronchioles with accumulation of dust-laden macrophages in and around the respiratory bronchioles. This has been referred to as *focal emphysema*. However, in these patients the term pneumoconiosis is preferable.

(b) *Panacinar or Panlobular Emphysema*. In this subtype all components of the acinus are involved about equally. This form is commonly associated with α_1 antiprotease deficiency. It may also occur in bases of the lung in patients with centrilobular emphysema, and as an incidental finding in older individuals.

(c) *Distal Acinar Emphysema*. The distal parts of the acinus, namely the alveolar ducts and sacs, are predominantly involved in this type. This is associated with secondary interlobular septa, and therefore, is also known as *paraseptal emphysema*. The distal acinus abuts on pleura, vessels, and airways, and the emphysema is worse in these regions.

Additional subtypes of emphysema have been suggested, but there is no reason for this, since there is considerable overlap between these types. When emphysema becomes severe, it is difficult to classify it into any one of the above-described types. The severity of emphysema is best correlated with airflow obstruction such as FEV_1. Patients who have significant physical impairment due to COPD usually exhibit at least moderately severe emphysema on autopsy. Occasionally, such patients have only mild emphysema, and, rarely, it is absent.

The capillary bed is thin or atrophied in chronic bronchitis. The pulmonary artery of smokers differ from that of nonsmokers in that in the former there are increased numbers of transacted muscular arteries of < 200 μm in diameter, medial hypertrophy, and more intimal thickening. These changes are probably hypoxia induced and have a good correlation with degree of emphysema and small airway changes. Major pulmonary embolism or thrombosis is a frequent finding in patients dying with cor pulmonale. However, these are not universal.

Although right ventricular hypertrophy and pulmonary hypertension are commonly associated with COPD, varying degrees of left ventricular hypertrophy can be seen in 25 to 60 percent of patients dying with chronic bronchitis. This is seen in association with right ventricular hypertrophy.

The diaphragmatic muscle mass and weight is decreased with increasing emphysema.

CLINICAL FEATURES OF COPD

Symptoms

Patients with COPD are usually smokers with a smoking history of at least 20 cigarettes per day for 20 years or more before they are symptomatic. The usual presentation is at the fifth decade of life.[225] The characteristic symptoms of chronic bronchitis are cough with expectoration, wheeze, and breathlessness.[226-228] The cough and expectoration are usually exacerbated from time to time particularly more during the winter. The presence of cough and expectoration is more common in men than women and in early stages, the patient may not be aware of its presence unless questioned in more detail. The sputum is usually mucoid, purulent, or mucopurulent depending upon the superimposed infection. The sputum can be purulent even in the absence of infection, because of increased amounts of neutrophils. The intensity of cough gradually increases till it becomes troublesome. At the early stages, cough is increased in fog, cold, and damp weather.

Wheeze and dyspnea may at first be noticed during cold, damp weather and gradually increase in severity, which will persist throughout the year with periodic exacerbations. The wheezing may not be responsive to oral/inhaled steroids or beta-adrenergic agonists and inhaled anticholinergic agents. The response is never complete with the degree of reversibility being less than 20 percent.

Pure emphysema is mainly manifested as breathlessness and wheezing, cough and expectoration are less important symptoms. The patient gives a history of progressive dyspnea, sometimes starting apparently after a mild infection and following exertion or exercise.[229-231] Airflow obstruction causes dyspnea and by the time this present, the FEV_1 is about 1 liter or less than 50 percent of the predicted value. The course progresses over the next 5 years or more with further loss of FEV_1. The patient will try to breathe with pursed lips to utilize the respiratory muscles maximum.[232] He/She becomes a respiratory invalid and dies of respiratory failure.

Since emphysema and chronic bronchitis almost always coexist, except in the rare instance of hereditary emphysema, all or most of the above-described symptoms are seen together. It may be possible that either chronic bronchitis or emphysema is the predominant disease in a particular patient. However, there are certain differences in the clinical course of the two entities. While cor pulmonale is more common in chronic bronchitis,

this is less common in emphysema except terminally. Respiratory failure is the common mode of death of emphysema patients. The emphysema patient maintains a near normal PaO_2 and normal $PaCO_2$ by hyperventilation until a late stage of the disease. On the other hand, chronic bronchitis have frequent cor pulmonale with heart failure and hypoxia. For these reasons, chronic bronchitis are often called "blue bloaters" and emphysema patients are called "pink puffers". The progressive alveolar wall destruction in emphysema leads to formation of bullae. Weight loss is a common feature in overt emphysema. Exercise limitation is an important symptom in these subjects. This may be due to dyspnea or leg fatigue or a combination of the two. In the advanced stage of the disease, chronic hypoxemia is responsible for peripheral muscle atrophy, related to deconditioning and poor nutrition of the patient.[229, 233-236] High wasted ventilation and oxygen cost of ventilation may further be responsible for the weight loss.

Physical Signs

The general physical examination may be normal in early stage of the disease. However in later stages, there will be emaciation, cyanosis, polycythemia, edema, and raised jugular venous pressure, if there is associated cor pulmonale and heart failure.[237]

The chest is often barrel shaped with kyphosis, increased anteroposterior diameter, ribs being set more horizontally, prominent sternal angle and wide subcostal angle. These changes are permanent. Due to the elevation of sternum, the distance between the suprasternal notch and the cricoid cartilage is reduced from the normal 3 to 4 finger breadths. One may feel a inspiratory tracheal tug due to the contraction of low, flat diaphragm.[237] The movement of the chest wall is reduced with limited expansion. The patient may use his accessory muscles of respiration. In drawing of the suprasternal and supraclavicular fossae and of the intercostal muscles result from swings in intrathoracic pressure. Jugular venous pressure may be seen during expiration. In the more severe cases, the costal margins, will be drawn inwards on inspiration, paradoxically, due to the pull of the low, flattened diaphragms.[238] Chest percussion will reveal findings of hyperinflation with obliteration of cardiac and liver dullness. Elsewhere, the note will be hyperresonant. Breath sounds will have a prolonged expiratory phase with a uniformly diminished intensity. Fine inspiratory crepitations and rhonchi are commonly heard. Forced expiratory time will be prolonged and is usually more than 6 seconds against a normal value of 4 seconds or less.[239]

Because of hyperinflation, apex beat will be difficult to feel. The characteristic heave of right ventricular hypertrophy may be felt. The second heart sound may be exaggerated; best heard in the second or third spaces, when there is associated pulmonary hypertension. The heart sounds in general may be difficult to auscultate because of overlying hyperinflation. There may be a third heart sound and right-sided gallop rhythm. Functional tricuspid incompetence murmur with a diastolic gallop rhythm is not uncommon in the presence of cor pulmonale with cardiac failure. Other features of hypercapnia may be obvious.

Liver may be palpable because of the push by the low diaphragm. Tender hepatomegaly is common in the presence of cardiac failure.

Complications like pneumonias, cor pulmonale, and respiratory failure are common in these patients. These are discussed subsequently. Pneumothorax may occur as a result of rupture of bullae in emphysema.

INVESTIGATIONS

1. *Roentgenographic examination.*[240-245] A plain skiagram in both posteroanterior and lateral view is necessary for the evaluation of patients with suspected COPD. The lung is over inflated with flattened diaphragms and tubular heart. The maximum curvature of the right diaphragmatic dome is less than 1.5 cm and placed low above which the posterior portions of the 11th or even 12th ribs may be visible. The hilar vessels are enlarged. Peripheral vascular shadows are thin, straight, or even lost as they are deranged or destroyed by advancing emphysema. Presence of regional hyperluscency (bullae) and vascular attenuation are confirmatory of emphysema. In advanced cases, obvious bullae are fairly common. The bullae are identified by fine hairlike margins and lack of vascular shadows. The bullae may be quite stable or may enlarge progressively causing compression of the lung with crowding of vessels. Sometimes the enlargement is so much that the entire lung is hyperluscent without any recognizable normal lung, and is known as the "vanishing lung syndrome". Most often this condition is confused with a large pneumothorax. The later may be differentiated by the absence of the compressed medial margin of the lung. However, the bullae may rupture themselves giving rise to secondary pneumothorax.

On a lateral film, there will be a large retrosternal air space; 3 cm below the manubrium the horizontal distance from the posterior surface of the aorta to the sternum exceeds 4.5 cm. This will be clearer in whole lung tomograms.

Sometimes the chest skiagram may show persistent, irregular lung shadows, which are thought to be due to scarring and destruction secondary to infections. Patients with complicated cor pulmonale and cardiac failure will have cardiomegaly, enlarged and dilated pulmonary arteries.

Five radiologic criteria have been described to diagnose emphysema.[244] They are:

(i) a retrosternal space (greatest distance from the sternum to the anterior heart silhouette) more than 2.54 cm (lateral radiograph); (ii) regular or irregular hyperluscency of lung fields reflecting attenuated pulmonary vessels; (iii) low (mid diaphragm below tenth posterior intercostal space) and flat diaphragm (for two thirds of their length) on lateral films; (iv) low (mid diaphragm below tenth posterior intercostal space) and flat (for two thirds of their length) on PA radiograph; and (v) bullae—one or more clear walled lesions not considered to be a cavity. Radiologic emphysema is considered to be present when two criteria are present.[244] (Figs 16.3 to 16.14).

Fluoroscopic examination of the chest will reveals a low and flat diaphragm with limited excursions. There may be a paradoxical movement upwards during inspiration due to the upward drag of the costal margins during this phase of the respiration. This paradoxical movement differs from that due to phrenic nerve palsy in the way that while in the later inspiratory sniffing gives rise to a sharp upward movement of the convex diaphragm, in the former the movement is slight in a flattened diaphragm. Screening will also be able to detect the enlarged pulmonary trunk.

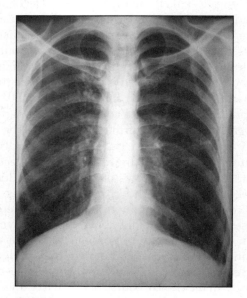

FIGURE 16.3: COPD. Note classical changes

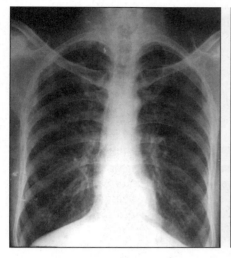

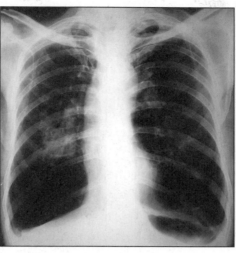

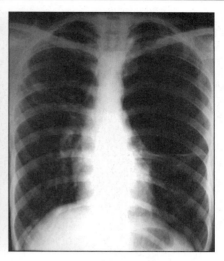

FIGURE 16.4: Changes of emphysema along with increased bronchovascular marking due to associated chronic bronchitis

FIGURE 16.5: CXR PA view showing evidence of COPD. Note the hyperinflated lungs, bullae on either side, tubular heart, low and flat diaphragm

FIGURE 16.6: COPD with bulla

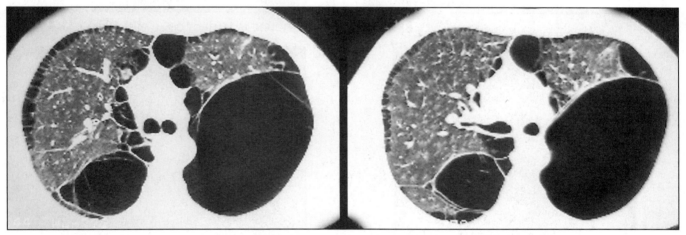

FIGURE 16.7: CT Chest - Para-septal and Bullous emphysematous lesions

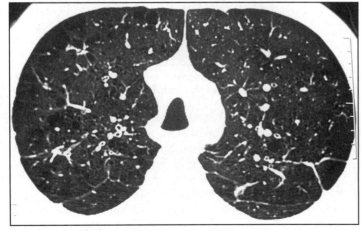

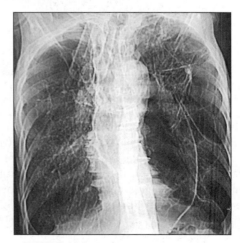

FIGURE 16.8: CT scan of chest in a case of emphysema showing peripheral proning

FIGURE 16.9: CXR - Bullous lung disease

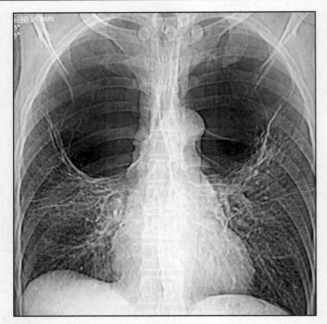

FIGURE 16.10: CXR - Bullous lung disease. Note it is not a case of COPD

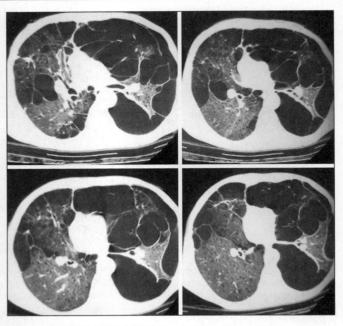

FIGURE 16.11: HRCT Chest - Bullous lung disease

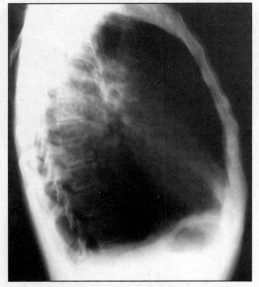

FIGURE 16.12: Lateral skigram of chest in a case of COPD (Emphysema). Note there is increased ratrostemal transluscency

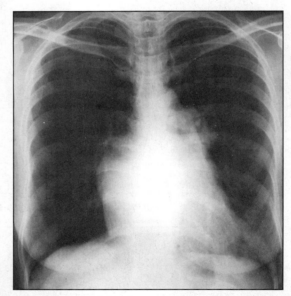

FIGURE 16.13: Mcleods syndrome mimicking COPD. Note there is hyperiuscency, but the right pulmonary artery is hypoplastic

Although bronchography is not necessary or routinely indicated in the diagnosis of COPD, bronchograms will show irregular, narrowed, and distorted bronchi. There is often irregularity in the peripheral filling with the contrast material being pooled in dilated bronchioles. There will be a diminution in the number of side branches of bronchi. Apparent diverticula may be visible in large bronchi because of the accumulation of contrast material in the mouths of hypertrophied mucous glands.[245]

The radiological studies have limited sensitivity for the detection of emphysema, and the correlation of roentgenography abnormalities with the severity of airflow obstruction or of anatomic emphysema is imperfect.

Computerized tomography is usually not necessary routinely in patients with uncomplicated emphysema.[246] Emphysema is characterized on CT by the presence of localized areas of abnormally low attenuation without

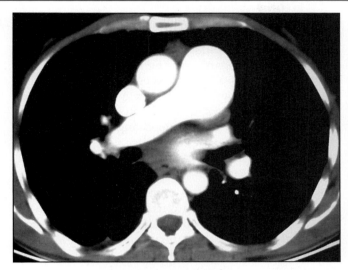

FIGURE 16.14: CT scan of chest showing emphysema

surrounding walls or with very thin (1 mm or less in diameter) walls. It is possibly the best method currently for assessing gross lung morphology short of having the pathologic specimen. CT may show evidence of emphysema in patients with normal chest radiograph.[247-253] However, CT assessment of emphysema is influenced by a number of factors including the type of scanner, the thickness of the sections, the window level, width at which the images are photographed and there is a significant intra- and inter-observer variability of the interpretation. Another disadvantage of CT is that localized areas of destruction measuring less than 0.5 cm in diameter are often missed. Therefore mild emphysema can be missed.[253] Nonetheless, while CT is not most perfect, it is currently the most accurate method for diagnosing emphysema *in vivo*.[246]

(2) *Pulmonary function testing*. Pulmonary function evaluation not only establishes the diagnosis of COPD but also assesses the severity of the disease and is helpful in following its progress.[254,255] The abnormalities consist of a reduction in the FEV_1, and in the ratio of the FEV_1 to the FVC. Although many other parameters of expiratory flow can be calculated from the spirogram, they usually provide no extra useful diagnostic information beyond that is obtained from the above two. It is desirable to perform spirometry in all individuals with unexplained dyspnea and/or in whom COPD is suspected. It has been advocated that all individuals at risk of developing COPD (habitual smokers) be screened regularly by spirometry to detect mild abnormalities with the idea that smoking cessation and early treatment may prevent severe disease. Repeat spirometry should be

performed following medications to determine to what extent the disease is reversible and to provide guidelines for rational therapy. The failure of FEV_1 to improve acutely after bronchodilator inhalation does not preclude a long-term beneficial effect of either bronchodilators or steroids. Up to 30 percent of patients will show some reversibility of about 15 percent or more of FEV_1 following inhalation of a beta-agonist aerosol. However, absence of a bronchodilator response during a single test does not justify withholding bronchodilator therapy.

Other abnormalities of pulmonary function tests include an increase in the total lung capacity and residual volume, and a reduction in the diffusing capacity for carbon monoxide (DL_{CO}). The later is reduced because of the loss of alveolar capillary bed. It is decreased in proportion to the severity of emphysema.[256-260] The measurement of lung volumes and of the DL_{CO} may be helpful in the initial evaluation of patients suspected of having COPD. In subsequent follow-ups, forced expiratory spirometry alone is usually sufficient to demonstrate the response to therapy, or to explain symptomatic deterioration. The increased TLC and residual volume in COPD is due to hyperinflation of the lungs, which is due to several factors.[261-263] These include a loss of elastic recoil resulting in overstretching of the lung tissue. The other contributors include a reflex reaction by which the patient breaths at higher functional residual capacity in an attempt to maintain the airways patency and air trapping due to a failure to maintain a patent airway.

COPD is also associated with abnormalities in lung mechanics (compliance and airflow resistance), and abnormalities of various tests of ventilation distribution. The ventilatory response to hypoxia appears to be depressed in some chronically hypoxemic patients.[264-268] Similarly, the ventilatory drive to carbon dioxide is also depressed in these patients particularly in whom who have CO_2 retention.[264, 269,270] However, these tests are not necessary on a routine basis.

A reduction in exercise tolerance is common in these patients, although routine evaluation of exercise capacity is unnecessary.[271-277] Such a test may be indicated when there is consideration for the need for supplemental oxygen therapy or when one is considering for additional causes of disability in patients whose exercise tolerance seems out of proportion to the limitation of airflow.

Any impairment of oxygen uptake and carbon dioxide elimination by the lung is detected by arterial blood gas analysis. COPD is characteristically associated with hypoxemia of varying degree and in advanced stages, with hypercarbia. These blood gas abnormalities are due to a combination of factors.[278-281] These include a combination of factors like $\dot{V}/\dot{Q}$ mismatch, alveolar hypoventilation, and shunts. Hypercarbia is observed with increased frequency as the FEV_1 falls below 1L. Blood gas abnormalities worsen during acute exacerbations, sleep, and exercise.[282-284] The usual abnormalities are chronic respiratory acidosis with hypoxemia; acute respiratory acidosis; acute on chronic respiratory acidosis. Concomitant use of steroids or diuretics may alter the picture.

(3) *Other laboratory tests.* The detection of secondary polycythemia by periodic measurements of hemoglobin or hematocrit levels suggests chronic hypoxemia and indicates to assess the need for oxygen therapy. The degree of polycythemia may be related to the level of carboxyhemoglobin due to smoking and the values lessen on stopping smoking.[285-287] However, if the patient is having poor nutrition, the polycythemia may be absent which is not an uncommon with Indian patients.

The common finding in electrocardiogram is the clockwise rotation of the heart about the anteroposterior and vertical axes. This will be reflected as right axis deviation in the standard leads, an RS pattern in the chest leads extending to the left as far as V5 or V6. The RS pattern may also be seen in aVL, and a QR pattern may be seen in aVF. If the heart is very long and thin, aVR and aVF may be indistinguishable. Changes of cor pulmonale may be present if the patient develops pulmonary hypertension, and the ECG changes are discussed in the concerned chapter. The presence of right ventricular hypertrophy in the electrocardiogram suggests the need for arterial blood gas analyses and supplemental oxygen.[288-291]

Recurrent purulent sputum is very frequent in COPD. Although they are suspected of infectious in origin, the precise etiology of these episodes remains speculative. In the absence of clinical or radiographic signs of pneumonia, bacterial or viral cultures of sputum usually provide little useful information. However, when infective exacerbations are there, the usual organisms grown are *Streptococcus pneumoniae* and *Haemophilus influenzae*.[292-295] Other oropharyngeal flora like Moraxella catarrhalis and viral infections[296] may cause exacerbations. In the outpatient setting, routine cultures or Gram staining are not necessary.

In a very small percentage of cases COPD is associated with α_1-antitrypsin deficiency. This disorder should be suspected in patients who develop severe COPD at a relatively young age, especially if they have affected siblings or parents, and have smoked occasionally or not at all. The diagnosis can be made by measurement of the serum α_1-antitrypsin level specifically, or from plasma electrophoresis when the tiny

sharp peak in the α_1-globulin region is absent. This is discussed in detail above.

Measurement of pulmonary pressure is not required routinely. The pressure may be normal in less severe disease at rest, but rises excessively on exercise. Pathological studies have shown a good correlation between the degree of emphysema and small airway disease and the hypertensive changes in pulmonary vasculature.

Differential Diagnosis

Most often the diagnosis of chronic bronchitis and emphysema is quite straightforward. However, on occasions it becomes very difficult to differentiate it from bronchial asthma particularly when the patient is relatively young and nonsmoker. The important differentiating points are shown in Table 16.4.

TABLE 16.4: Differentiation between asthma and COPD

Bronchial asthma	COPD
1. The patient is relatively young	Usually the subject is in his middle age or older
2. Nonsmoker	Invariably smokers
3. History of atopy or other family members having similar problem	Atopy is not essential
4. In between symptom free	Symptoms are invariably persistent and more in winter
5. Wheezing is the main symptoms	Cough, sputum and dyspnea are predominant symptom
6. Response to bronchodilators and steroid therapy is excellent	The response may not be that dramatic[297]
7. Eosinophilia, sputum eosinophils and positive skin tests to common allergens usual	Unusual
7. Cor pulmonale unusual	Common as a complication
8. Chronic CO_2 retention and hypoxia not seen except in acute severe asthma	Possible
9. Reversibility to bronchodilators is characteristic	There may be some reversibility but usually not more than 20 percent
10. Diffusing capacity normal	Low
11. Prognosis usually good	Downhill course

The points mentioned in each category are not absolute and may be present or absent in either condition.

However, confusion may occur in elderly patients where asthma and COPD may be difficult to differentiate.[298] For many years, asthma has been considered a disease of childhood or young adulthood, although it is not uncommon in the elderly.[299] Elderly asthmatic patients mainly include subjects who acquired the disease during childhood or adolescence and whose disease progressed over time or relapsed after periods of remission; however, the first manifestations of asthma may also occur in the late adulthood or after 65 years of age. The reasons why asthma is rarely diagnosed in the elderly are unclear. The presumed low prevalence of asthma in the elderly can be attributed to greater difficulties encountered when providing a correct diagnosis of asthma in the elderly as opposed to the younger population.[299,300] It is likely that factor pertaining to aging play a significant role. This may be, at least in part, attributed to a blunted perception of symptoms at this age.[301] In addition, physician may overlook respiratory symptoms or, when noted, may not be properly evaluated with functional assessment;[302] however, underestimation of the prevalence of asthma may be due to confusion with COPD. In fact, asthma and COPD share clinical and functional similarities, although their pathologic presentations differ considerably and the two syndromes are, indeed, different diseases.[303] Finally, one cannot exclude the simultaneous occurrence of the two pathologic conditions, given the high prevalence of asthma and COPD and the fact that a smoking habit may be present in both entities. Taken together, these observations imply clinical and therapeutic consequences, in that correct treatment may be omitted or delayed in the elderly population.[304] It is important, therefore, to promptly recognize and, when possible, distinguish the two diseases in order to provide appropriate treatment. Asthma in the elderly is frequently confused with COPD. Misdiagnosis can be related to older age and to greater degree of disability. Asthma in patients with mild functional impairment may be underdiagnosed in spite of overt respiratory symptoms suggestive of asthma. Of asthmatic patients, COPD had been improperly diagnosed in 19.5 percent, whereas 27.3 percent of asthmatic patients do not report any previous diagnosis of asthma. The main correlates of misdiagnosis are older age and disability. Conversely, underdiagnosis is associated with better functional conditions, expressed by spirometry, even when wheezing or a significant response to the bronchodilator test occurred.[298]

PROGNOSIS

A number of factors have been identified to influence the ultimate prognosis of COPD.[128,305-320] Long-term prospective studies in patients with severe COPD with FEV_1 of less than 1 liter, have shown that 5 and 10 year survival rates are 69 and 40 percent respectively. The presence of radiological evidence of emphysema or of bullae in one study resulted in five-year mortalities of 53 percent and 70 percent respectively. Right ventricular failure carries a poor prognosis with a five year mortality

of 65 to 80 percent reported in different studies. Right ventricular systolic pressure of > 35 mm Hg, FEV_1 of < 30 percent of predicted and age > 70 years are other poor prognostic factors.[315]

Three risk factors have been useful in predicting the outcome of a patient with COPD: age, smoking status, and FEV_1. The studies of prognosis in the National Institutes of Health Intermittent Positive Pressure Trial[311] confirmed the findings of earlier studies that age and initial FEV_1 are powerful predictors of outcome. The diffusing capacity and the total lung capacity are weak predictors of survival. The only consistent predictor of decline in FEV_1, besides the initial FEV_1, is the bronchodilator response of the patient. The larger the response, the slower the decline in FEV_1, and this relation is not dependent on the initial FEV_1. In persons with FEV_1 of less than 0.75 L, the approximate mortality rate at 1 year is 30 percent and at 10 year 95 percent.[310] However, some patients with severe airflow obstruction may survive longer, and even up to 15 years. Some other data suggest that next to cessation of smoking, a higher degree of reversibility of airflow obstruction and a lower degree of airway reactivity are the two most important predictors of a slower decline in FEV_1. The asthmatic bronchitis group of patients survives for much longer than patients with typical COPD, a 10-year mortality of 10 percent versus 60 percent, respectively.[11] Recent studies have identified other predictors like alveolar-arterial oxygen gradient greater than 41 mm Hg, ventricular arrhythmias, and atrial fibrillation.[314] Most often death in COPD generally occurs as a result of a medical complication, such as acute respiratory failure, severe pneumonia, pneumothorax, cardiac arrhythmia, or pulmonary embolism.

Although it is well established that oxygen therapy is beneficial for overall survival of patients with COPD (see below), the response differs depending on the initial oxygen values, age, and pulmonary pressure at the time of initiation of such a therapy.[317-320]

STAGING OF COPD

The mortality and morbidity of COPD has a strong correlation with FEV_1. Therefore COPD severity has been staged on the basis of the severity of airflow obstruction, which utilizes the American Thoracic Society statement on interpretation of lung function.[321] Accordingly severity of COPD can be staged into:

- Stage I FEV_1 of 50 percent or more of predicted
- Stage II FEV_1 of 35 to 49 percent of predicted
- Stage III FEV_1 of < 35 percent of predicted.

Patients with stage I COPD usually do not have severe hypoxemia, and arterial blood gas analysis is not required. For stages II and III arterial blood gas measurements should be done. Most patients of COPD will be of stage I type. Patients of this stage if complain of dyspnea, should be investigated further. Stage II patients are only a minority. These patients have a significant impact on quality of life and medical care. They need evaluation by a respiratory physician. Stage III patients also include a minority of COPD cases and need specialized care.[7]

MANAGEMENT

PREVENTION MEASURES

(1) *Smoking and Pollution*. COPD is a disease caused by smoking in susceptible individuals. Also certain work environments and air pollution play an additional modifying role, but nothing is as important as smoking as an external preventable factor. Smoking is the greatest international killer and tobacco use is the preventable cause of death in developed countries and is quickly gaining that distinction in developing countries.[322,323] An ambitious campaign should be undertaken to curtail the addiction of smoking. Smoking must be stopped completely in all symptomatic patients and certainly in those with objective abnormalities on pulmonary function testing. *Stopping smoking is of fundamental importance to the successful management of all stages of COPD.* If stopped early in the natural course of the disease, the airway injury may reverse,[324] and the rate of decline in ventilatory function will slow to a rate equivalent to age related changes.[325-327]

To achieve success in smoking cessation, patient education and physician participation are perhaps the most important.[328] Unfortunately many patients with COPD are either unaware of the fact that smoking is hazardous for them. In a study conducted by Behera[329] it was found that most patients with chronic bronchitis still continue to smoke despite they are seen by physicians who fail to impress upon them to quit smoking. Other studies have shown that continuous abstinence even in patients with symptoms after counselling may not be very high and may be as low as only 27 percent. In follow-up periods ranging from 6 months to 7 years.[330] Factors associated with continued smoking varies among patients and may include nicotine addiction, conditioned response to smoking associated stimuli (work and social situations), psychosocial problems (depression, poor education, low income, and vigorous campaign for sell by tobacco companies. Therefore, successful cessation programs involve multiple interventions.[331-337] The caring physician must show strong but sustained interest in smoking cessation. Physician counseling perhaps is important for any successful cessation program. As a first step, the physician and the patient must identify the patients stage of readiness for stopping smoking.

Five stages have been identified from smoking to nonsmoking status.[338] These stages are (a) preconteplation, (b) conteplation, (c) preparation, (d) action, and (e) maintenance. The clinician's role is to help the patient to follow these stages and should ensure that interventions are tailored to the stage of the patient. Besides the physician, a strong social support system is required to sustain long-term abstinence. Support may come from professionals, as well as from family and friends. Group smoke cessation clinics are also helpful adjuncts. Other components of smoking cessation include behavior therapy, additional counseling, adjunctive pharmacologic treatment, and relapse prevention.

Pharmacologic intervention is an attractive adjunct in smoking cessation programs. Most often the smoker says "can I get some replacement for smoking"? Nicotine is the ingredient in smoking which is primarily responsible for addictive potential.[334] It is estimated that with each cigarette smoked; about 1 to 2 mg of nicotine is delivered to the lungs. Because of rapid absorption and a short half-life of 2 hours, regular smoking causes nicotine accumulation. Smoking withdrawal causes unpleasant side effects in most quitters.[333] The symptoms are anxiety, irritability, difficulty in concentration, anger, fatigue, drowsiness, depression, and sleep disruption. Many patients also complain of constipation, fullness in abdomen and many other vague complaints. These reactions are most often observed during the first week of cessation. Nicotine replacement after smoking cessation will reduce with these withdrawal symptoms in those with addictive potentials and enhances abstinence in a dose-dependent manner. Highly dependent smokers are those who usually smoke more than one pack of cigarettes per day and they usually require their first smoking material within 30 minutes of getting up from bed. They also cannot resist smoking in places where it is forbidden. Physical dependence can also be assessed by Fagerstrom tolerance questionnaire.[339]

Various nicotine preparations include nicotine chewing gums,[335] and transdermal nicotine patches.[340] Short-term success has been varying between 18 to 77 percent and they are about twice as effective as those with placebo. Long-term success rates (more than 6 months) varied between 22 to 42 percent. When nicotine replacement therapy is combined with adjuvant programs like group or individual counselling produces better results. Patients who fail to obstante during the first two weeks of smoking cessation programs are unlikely to succeed and additional programs are necessary for them. Clonidine (an alpha$_2$-adrenergic agonist) may enhance abstinence, but long-term effects are not well studied. The anxiolytic drug, buspirone, may reduce withdrawal symptoms. Hypnosis is another helpful adjunct for smoking cessation programs.

Hazards in the work environment should also be eliminated. Dusts inhaled by grain and cotton workers, miners and other dusty-atmosphere workers, fumes from solvents and paint industries and other possible pollutants in the environment should be identified and eliminated if possible.

(2) VACCINES. The patient with COPD is especially more susceptible to influenza infection. Thus, influenza virus vaccine is recommended each fall, particularly if epidemics are expected.[341] Progressively pure and potent multivalent vaccines are now widely used each fall in many countries with a change in vaccine strains necessary because of the antigenic shifts which are characteristic of influenza A viruses. The use of oral amantadine during the influenza season is an effective alternative and, in fact, more effective in preventing or modifying early stages of disease than the vaccine itself. Both can be used. Amantadine can also modify the early stages of developing influenza.

Even though controversial, polyvalent pneumococcal vaccine is useful in affording at least some degree of protection against a common pneumonia organism, i.e. *Streptococcus pneumoniae*, in susceptible individuals. Pneumococcal vaccine is recommended only once. It at least reduces the risk of bacteremia. Both the pneumococcal and influenza vaccines can be administered at the same time for convenience and efficiency.

The vaccines are discussed in more detail in the chapter on pneumonias.

PHARMACOLOGIC THERAPY

The classes of drugs, which are most useful in the management of COPD, are bronchodilators, anti-inflammatory drugs (corticosteroids), mucolytics, antimicrobials and other ancillary drugs.

(1) Bronchodilators

Bronchodilators play a role in many patients with COPD because of a degree of bronchial hyperreactivity, which is present in many patients.[342-344] Many patients with COPD have a reversible component to their airflow obstruction, as evidenced by an increase in FEV1 following use of an inhaled bronchodilator even if not

to the extent that is seen in bronchial asthma.[342] The bronchodilator may be useful in promoting airflow by its capability of dilating obstructed airways by combating increased muscular tone (bronchospasm) and may also help in preventing reflex bronchoconstriction which occurs as a response to a variety of nonspecific stimuli. In addition to improvement in symptoms, regular use may improve prognosis.[343] The rate of decline of FEV1 also decreases with the use of bronchodilators.[344]

Three main classes of bronchodilators are in use in COPD: theophyllines, Beta-agonists, and ipratropium bromide.

(a) *Theophylline*. Theophylline preparations are a major class of oral and parenteral bronchodilators used in the management of acute exacerbations and maintenance therapy of COPD.[345-370] Both short-acting and long-acting preparations are widely used. Theophylline is not only a bronchodilator, but has a beneficial effect on respiratory muscle fatigue particularly the diaphragm.[353,356] Theophylline is also partially effective in blocking bronchial hyperreactivity to methacholine, histamine, and antigen stimulation.[355,356] Long-term use of theophylline improves various parameters of lung function including vital capacity, FEV$_1$, minute ventilation and gas exchange.[357] The drug improves dyspnea and improves exercise performance in patients with advanced COPD.[358,359] Finally, theophylline is a mild respiratory stimulant, which might be helpful in patients with a decreased respiratory drive.[360] A small, but statistically significant improvement in cardiac function, pulmonary artery pressure, and renal function is also noted in some patients.[361-364] Other nonrespiratory effects, which may be beneficial, include improved ciliary function.[365] The pharmacology, and toxicity of the drug has been discussed in the previous chapter.[367] Theophylline also possesses some anti-inflammatory properties.[368] Recent information suggests that adding theophylline to the combination of salbutamol and ipratroipum can result in maximum benefit in stable cases of COPD.[369,370] The dosage of oral theophylline for the average nonsmoking, reasonably healthy adult is 10 to 12 mg/kg/day in divided doses. Smoker may require up to 50 percent larger dosages, whereas hypoxemic patients or those with hepatic insufficiency may require a 25 to 50 percent reduction in dosage. Its interaction with other drugs has been discussed previously. In acute exacerbations, the drug can be used in same dosages as used for management of acute bronchial asthma.[366] The drug is commonly used as an adjunct with oral/inhaled sympathomimetic bronchodilators for the maintenance therapy of COPD.

(b) *Sympathomimetic bronchodilators.* The beta-adrenergic agonists are the keystones of therapy in patients with obstructive airways disease.[371-377] Because they can improve mucociliary clearance and serve prophylactically to protect against bronchospasm produced by various stimuli, they may be of value even if they do not cause improvements of spirometric values.[378] Aerosol formulations provide the optimal therapy for chronic outpatient use. In most patients, the metered-dose inhaler (MDI) is preferred, whereas for inpatient therapy powered nebulizers are often used. The MDI can be kept in the pocket or purse and used for emergencies to overcome shortness of breath. A more useful role of this drug is the regular dosing 3 or 4 times a day for maintenance management. Oral drugs can be used for this purpose also. The problem with MDI is its proper use by the patients.[378] Although many patients are unable to use it optimally, repeated instructions result in a satisfactory outcome in the majority of cases. In those, who can not use it properly, a spacer will be useful. Optimal use of MDI results in not more than 10 percent of the dose being deposited in the lung, while as much As 85 percent is deposited in the oropharynx. The use of a large volume reservoir may increase the amount deposited in the lungs to 15 percent, while reducing the oropharyngeal deposition to 5 percent. A powered nebulizer unit will result in about 10 percent of the initial dose being deposited in the lung, whereas only about 10 percent will be deposited in the mouth and pharynx, and about 80 percent of the dose will remain in the apparatus or is lost into the atmosphere. The desired strategy of giving a bronchodilating aerosol is to deliver a small amount of active agent into the airways for effective bronchodilatation. Patients should be taught to inhale from mid-lung volume so that the airways are open in order to allow deep penetration and deposition. Inhalation should be at a slow flow rate with a pause at the end of inspiration followed by exhalation against pursed lips, again to promote deposition of small particles. Separating two inhalations by 10 to 20 minutes also offers better bronchodilatation than by rapidly sequencing the two inhalations. Attention to the details of proper use of the MDI and carefully instructing the patient about overuse allows one to draw maximum benefits of these potent agents and to minimize side effects or abuse.

Patients with COPD have an increased risk of cardiovascular disease. Despite the clinical benefits of long-acting β-agonist agents in the treatment of COPD, patients may be at an increased risk of cardiovascular toxicity, including tachyrhythmia due to β-adrenergic stimulation. Treatment with salmeterol, 50 μg bid, does not increase the risk of cardiovascular AEs in this population of COPD patients compared with placebo.[379]

(c) *Anticholinergics.* Ipratropium bromide is a proven bronchodilator with efficacy in certain patients suffering from chronic bronchitis and emphysema.[380-385] The drug is delivered either as a metered dose inhaler or as a nebulized aerosol. It directly acts in the airways to block acetylcholine uptake at cholinergic receptors. This results in bronchodilatation primarily in the large airways, which differs from the mechanism of action of other currently available bronchodilators. The recommended dose of the MDI aerosol is 2 puffs (40 μg) 4 times daily. Systemic side effects such as those seen with atropine are greatly reduced because of the low lipid solubility and poor absorption, particularly across blood-brain barrier. Recently, oxytropium bromide has also been used.[385,386]

Oxytropium bromide has also been found effective in COPD.[386,387] Recently tiotropium bromide has become available that has many advantages. Apart from an improvement in trough FEV_1—the primary outcome—clinically relevant outcomes such as quality of life and dyspnea were significantly better in the treatment group, which increases one's confidence that tiotropium was clinically beneficial.

Studies have shown impressive effects of tiotropium. It is probably the most potent bronchodilator yet for COPD. In part, its potency may be attributed to its unique selectivity for M1 and M3 muscarinic receptors, a feature that ipratropium and all other available antimuscarinic agents lack. With a nominal duration of action of 24 hrs, and probably much longer,[388] tiotropium is by far the longest-acting bronchodilator of any class. Apart from the convenience of once daily dosing for patients, the long duration of action ensures that significant bronchodilation is maintained around the clock. If patients use tiotropium consistently, their FEV_1 would never fall to baseline. Out of interest, one can calculate the potential magnitude of this effect in relation to the natural decline in lung function from available data. The trough FEV_1 increased by a mean of 115 mL in the group that received tiotropium for 1 year, while that of subjects who received placebo declined by 38 mL, giving an overall treatment effect of 153 mL. If the mean annual decline in FEV_1 of this population is 38 mL, an amount which accords with other reports,[389,390] then an increase in trough FEV_1 of 153 mL due to tiotropium use would correspond to the amount the FEV_1 would otherwise be expected to decline in 153/38 years, approximately 4 years. It would be as if their FEV_1 had been restored to its level 4 years previously. This calculation is quite speculative, of course, and it cannot be said that patients will survive

4 years longer if they use tiotropium; there are no data on the effects of tiotropium on survival at this time. Nor are there definitive data that use of tiotropium decreases the rate of decline of lung function or the frequency of important events such as acute exacerbations; such studies are ongoing. But the data do suggest that tiotropium will become an important addition to our therapy for this common and highly symptomatic disease.

Inhaled bronchodilators such as β_2-agonists and anticholinergic agents have different modes of action, and they have been used as the main pharmacotherapy for stable patients with COPD. A balance of activity between the sympathetic (adrenergic) and parasympathetic (cholinergic) autonomic nervous systems maintains the airway smooth muscle tone. Bronchodilation may be obtained either by stimulating the adrenergic receptors with β_2-agonists, or by inhibiting the action of acetylcholine at muscarinic receptors with anticholinergic agents. In terms of the acute bronchodilating effects of β_2-agonists and anticholinergic agents, both drugs have been reported to be similarly effective. However, exercise capacity and dyspnea have recently become the major treatment end points in patients with COPD, since they are considered as directly related to the patient's quality of life.

Although the effects of selective β_2-agonists on exercise capacity are controversial in COPD patients, negative reports appear to be more prevalent. Furthermore, the dose-dependent effects of β_2-agonists have not been observed for exercise capacity, unlike those for FEV_1. On the other hand, with regard to anticholinergic agents, it has been previously demonstrated that their effects on exercise capacity in COPD patients depended on the dose administered and the type of exercise performance tests that had been carried out. In particular, it has been reported that a cycle endurance test is much more sensitive in detecting the effects of oxitropium bromide on exercise capacity than are the 6-min walking test and progressive cycle ergometry in patients with COPD. Therefore, when comparing the effects of β_2-agonists and anticholinergic agents on exercise capacity, it is considered that the lower doses may not have a meaningful impact on the variables measured, and that a submaximal endurance test would be suitable for detecting the changes. Therapy with both salbutamol and ipratropium bromide improved exercise capacity, as evaluated by the endurance time, and reduced dyspnea similarly in patients with COPD. In addition, the effects of the different bronchodilators on exercise capacity varied within individuals, and a complex mechanism

may be responsible for the different effects of these two bronchodilators on exercise capacity vs airflow limitation. These results support the conclusion that both types of inhaled bronchodilators can be used as first-line drugs for the treatment of stable patients with COPD.[391]

(d) *Anti-inflammatory drugs.* Considerable controversy exists regarding the use of corticosteroids in COPD. However, some evidence indicates that these drugs offer both subjective and objective benefit to a substantial number of patients.[392-397] A dose equivalent of 40 mg prednisolone given daily for two weeks resulted in a significant benefit in a controlled clinical trial in patients with advanced emphysema by Mandella et al. A therapeutic trial of steroids should be given to such patients guided by symptoms and objective measurements of FEV_1 and FVC. If objective benefits are gained, corticosteroids should be continued until maximum benefit occurs. After maximum benefit is reached, the drug should be tapered to the lowest dose, which will maintain this predominant benefit. This might be alternate day steroid or a small morning dose. Inhaled steroids are not as effective as oral steroids in COPD. If there is no benefit, the drug should be discontinued. One must be very careful to monitor the side effects of corticosteroids since the patients are usually elderly. These are discussed earlier in the previous chapter.

Nedocromil sodium has also been tried by some investigators.

(e) *Antibiotics.* Antibiotics have been used extensively for years to treat acute exacerbations of chronic bronchitis, as well as for prophylaxis in stable chronic bronchitis. However, their value for either purpose has not yet been established. A number of studies have attempted to define the role of bacterial infections on the course and prognosis of COPD.[101-103,398-400] Although it is well known that bacterial invasion of the lower airways commonly occurs in these patients, the importance of this infection, apart from causing exacerbations of symptoms like increased cough and expectoration, remains unknown. Patients who already have lung disease are at special risk for pneumonia because natural defense mechanisms of the airways are reduced. Pneumonia in patients with COPD may be either community-acquired, or hospital acquired. Two organisms, *Haemophilus influenzae*, and *Streptococcus pneumoniae*, have been cultured from sputum and transtracheal aspirates more frequently and in greater numbers from patients with acute exacerbations of chronic bronchitis. *Haemophilus influenzae* strains are almost always nonencapsulated and nontypable. The other organisms that are isolated include anaerobes, staphylococci, and other Gram-negative organisms. However, apart from the first two microorganisms the significance of colonization by other organisms is unknown. Short-term antimicrobial therapy directed specifically against these two organisms has most often been used. The value of such short-term treatment is difficult to assess, although few carefully controlled and properly designed studies reported so far failed to show any clear cut benefit. On the other hand, a few patients have repeated exacerbations due to bacterial infection and do benefit clearly from anti-microbial therapy. Prophylactic therapy has not been shown to arrest deterioration of pulmonary function over time or to decrease symptoms.

Since the value of antimicrobial therapy is doubtful in most patients, any drug chosen for this purpose must be economical and nontoxic. The most suitable agents are ampicillin, amoxycillin, tetracycline, erythromycin, trimethoprim-sulfamethoxazole, and cefaclor, etc. Culture and sensitivity are not indicated, neither they are accurate and may be misleading. Most physicians would prescribe an antimicrobial at the first sign of sputum purulence, i.e. yellow or green sputum, with accompanying increased cough and fever. Antibiotics are of proven value in the presence of infection like the presence of fever, leukocytosis, or a change in the chest radiograph.[401-403] It is probably best to have the patient initiate therapy at the first sign of infection, and to report to the physician about the response. Such use will shorten the symptomatic period, reduce days lost from work, and probably prevent or shorten hospitalizations. In many instances, no infectious agent can be found to explain an exacerbation of purulent bronchitis. In these cases a viral infection is the most likely cause.

(f) *Other drugs*. (i) It is difficult to treat the abnormal mucus production.[404] Sympathomimetic bronchodilators and theophylline stimulate mucociliary clearance, and these drugs are useful for any obstructive disease syndrome accompanied by impaired mucokinesis. There is also evidence that corticosteroid therapy can improve mucokinesis.

Oral expectorants are commonly used for the treatment of cough and expectoration. These include guaifenesin, terpine hydrate, ammonium and other salts, organic iodide and ipecac.[405,406] N-acetylcysteine is available both as an oral agent and aerosol.[407] However, the value of such agents has not been demonstrated in objective studies. A recent controlled clinical trial has shown that iodinated glycerol can be useful in reducing cough frequency; cough severity, and chest discomfort, and increases ease in bringing up sputum. A feeling of well being was observed in some patients with advanced

COPD.[405] Genetically engineered DNAse has been useful in cystic fibrosis. However the usefulness in COPD is not yet clear.

(ii) Diuretics are useful for edema formation, which may occur with or without heart failure. Thiazides are preferable to loop diuretics because they do not promote calcium wasting. Digitalis is not useful in isolated right heart failure, but can be used to combat supraventricular tachyarrhythmias. Calcium channel blockers are probably more effective than cardiac glycosides in controlling arrhythmias and do not cause bronchospasm. Beta-blockers are contraindicated in patients with any bronchospastic disorder. Angiotensin-converting-enzyme (ACE) inhibitors are also useful. Digoxin is not of use in cor pulmonale and congestive heart failure unless there is associated left ventricular disease. All these drugs must be used with caution since they are likely to precipitate electrolyte imbalance, dehydration, hypotension, myocardial ischemia, and arrhythmias. It is to be remembered that most such patients are usually elderly individuals with impaired drug clearance, and most often associated with hypoxemia, potentials of side effects increases further. If they occur, the drug regimen must be modified.

(iii) Many other drugs have been used to relieve dyspnea, particularly dihydrocodeine, in the "pink puffer" type of COPD, i.e. those patients with the highest respiratory drives and most intense dyspnea. An effective dose is 5 to 15 mg three or four times daily.[408] Other drugs are already discussed in earlier chapter on dyspnea.

(iv) Psychoactive agents may be necessary in some of these patients because of depression, anxiety, insomnia, or pain. These drugs are potentially respiratory depressants.[409] Benzodiazepines are well tolerated in mild to moderate COPD, but can be suppressive in severe disease, especially during sleep. The safer hypnotics are sedating antihistamines, and chloral hydrate. Antidepressants may also have the advantage of improving sleep. Diazepam may particularly be harmful in these patients. Respiratory stimulants have no proven value in COPD.

(v) Recent developments in basic genetics have made genetic therapy possible in subjects with alpha-1-antitrypsin deficiency emphysema.[410] Alpha-1-antitrypsin augmentation therapy is beneficial in nonsmoking, younger patients with severe alpha-1-antitrypsin deficiency and associated emphysema. Such therapy is not indicated in common forms of COPD. Alpha-1-antitrypsin gene delivery is still an experimental system and is yet to be applied to human disease.[411]

(vi) Nutrition. There is some concern that a high carbohydrate may increase the carbondioxide production, which may not be acceptable in these patients.[412] On the other hand, poor nutritional status may be an important factor in muscle wasting in some of these subjects. Therefore, a balance must be struck between these two so as to supplement a correct diet to these patients. It has been suggested that patients with COPD might benefit from a high - lipid, low-carbohydrate diet due to the reduced respiratory quotient.

(g) *Oxygen therapy*. Supplemental oxygen is one of the most common drugs used in treating patients with COPD and Tarpy and Celli have reviewed the topic recently.[413] Both long-term and short-term studies have proved beyond doubt that supplemental oxygen therapy is useful in the treatment of COPD in certain situations.[414-426] The goal of such therapy is to prevent hypoxic tissue damage, which results from arterial hypoxemia. When other diseases complicate COPD, like reduction in cardiac output or hematocrit, tissue hypoxia results from inadequate oxygen delivery of oxygen to tissues. Such deficiencies will require therapy aimed at the underlying basic condition. Arterial hypoxemia is one of the most serious manifestations of COPD and is at present is the only acceptable indication for oxygen therapy. The immediate goal, of such therapy is to increase arterial oxygenation to acceptable levels.

In general, oxygen therapy in COPD is used in 2 situations: (i) in acutely ill hospitalized patients; and (ii) in chronically ill patients who are not in the hospital.

(i) OXYGEN THERAPY FOR ACUTELY ILL PATIENTS
The indication of oxygen therapy in such situation is when the PaO_2 is less than 60 mm Hg. The goal of oxygen therapy in this situation is to increase PaO_2 to at least 60 mm Hg, equivalent to an arterial oxygen saturation of nearly 90 percent. If the PaO_2 is increased beyond 65 mm Hg, there is a very minor increase in the arterial oxygen content. Therefore, little purpose is served by increasing PaO_2 to values greater than 80 mm Hg, and oxygen doses that will do so should generally be avoided. The dose of oxygen that will increase PaO_2 to 65 to 80 mm Hg in a given patient with COPD can vary greatly, depending on the severity of the initial hypoxemia, and the precise nature of the physiological disturbance. Attaining the correct dose is best done by trial and error, starting at a given dose, measuring the PaO_2 and adjusting the flow accordingly. In severe COPD, it generally takes 20 to 30 minutes for a steady state to be achieved after a change in the inspired gas mixture, so that arterial blood gas should not usually be sampled at shorter intervals after changes in oxygen dose.

Oxygen therapy and associated increase in PaO_2 may produce CO_2 retention, with an increase in $PaCO_2$. This is a potentially serious problem in that CO_2 retention may produce coma. There is no way to predict whether or not a given patient will develop such complication of rising $PaCO_2$ with oxygen therapy. However, it generally occurs in very sick patients with PaO_2 of less than 40 mm Hg and with an elevated $PaCO_2$ while breathing room air. The accurate way to assess the effect of oxygen therapy on $PaCO_2$ is to measure both PaO_2 and $PaCO_2$ repetitively. If there is a rise in $PaCO_2$, oxygen therapy should be used cautiously. CO_2 produces central nervous system disturbances by changes in brain pH, which in turn depends on the brain bicarbonate levels. CO_2 narcosis, therefore, cannot be predicted on the basis of the $PaCO_2$, since there is no correlation between such changes and a particular $PaCO_2$. To diagnose CO_2 narcosis serial clinical observation is essential. In hypoxemic patients who develop CO_2 retention with oxygen therapy, an attempt should be made to increase PaO_2 without causing an increase of $PaCO_2$ sufficient to cause drowsiness or stupor. Often it will be possible to produce clinically significant increases in PaO_2 that do not reach the ideal goal of 65 mm Hg, but are not associated with disturbances of consciousness. Severe hypoxemia may cause, death whereas disturbances associated with severe CO_2 retention are not usually lethal. In severe hypoxemia the first priority should be to increase PaO_2 and if excess oxygen is given and the patient develops CO_2 narcosis, the inspired oxygen concentration should be reduced, but not never to room air since abrupt cessation of all oxygen therapy can produce fatal hypoxemia. If adequate oxygenation cannot be achieved without progressive hypercapnia, mechanical ventilation may be required.

In emergency situations, the application of the above principle may not be possible. Patients are frequently encountered with respiratory distress of causes that are not entirely clear at the time they are first seen. Oxygen therapy may have to be undertaken without the prior knowledge of blood gas values. If such patients do not have COPD, short-term oxygen therapy is without risk, and doses up to 100 percent oxygen can be used safely. If, however, COPD is a diagnostic possibility, such high dose therapy carries the risk of carbon dioxide narcosis and should be avoided. The lower the oxygen dose, the less is the risk of CO_2 retention. Inspired concentrations of less than 40 percent of oxygen are uncommonly associated with rapidly rising $PaCO_2$, and it is rare with inspired concentrations of less than 30 percent. Therefore, when blood gas results are not available, patients suspected of having COPD should be given oxygen concentrations of 24 to 40 percent. It is best to start with the lowest dose and to increase only when there is clinical or laboratory evidence that this should be done. These inspired concentrations are usually achieved by nasal flows of 1 to 5 L liters/min. Measurements of arterial blood gas is essential during therapy.

In general there are 2 methods of delivering oxygen at a concentration of equal or less than 40 percent. Nasal prongs are convenient because they do not interfere with eating and conversation. Varying oxygen flow can vary the oxygen dose, but the precise inspired concentration achieved depends on the patient's ventilation and breathing pattern. The inspired oxygen concentration in percent (FiO_2) can be roughly calculated as:

$$FiO_2 = 20 + 4 \times O_2 \text{ flow (L/min)}$$

At flows of 4 L/min or more, oxygen should be humidified, and at lower flows it is not required. The other methods of administration of oxygen are Venturi masks. Though they interfere with eating and conversation, and the patient may feel "suffocated", fixed, known inspired oxygen concentrations ranging from 24 to 50 percent can be delivered. Oxygen at concentrations greater than 40 percent can only be administered by masks (i.e. polymasks), which can deliver up to 90 percent. These systems are potentially dangerous in patients with COPD.

(ii) Oxygen therapy in chronic lung disease.

In hypoxemic COPD patients, long-term oxygen supplementation has clearly been demonstrated to prolong survival and improve quality of life in the large randomized controlled trials of the Nocturnal Oxygen Therapy Trial (NOTT) Group in the USA, and of the MRC Working Party on Long-term Domiciliary Oxygen therapy in the UK.[414,415] These studies have confirmed the previous findings in smaller uncontrolled trials that oxygen could improve some physiologic variables of pulmonary hemodynamics and showed that a correlation exists between the prognostic effect of oxygen therapy and the duration of oxygen used daily. Both these studies have demonstrated decreases in hematocrit and pulmonary vascular resistance. All patients showed a significant improvement in neuropsychological function tests and in the subjective perception of their quality of life including exercise tolerance. The effects of this treatment on survival and the improvement in quality of life are impressive. The benefit is greatest if the treatment is applied at least 18 hours/day. It is said, "no oxygen is

TABLE 16.5: Indications for long-term oxygen therapy

I. *Continuous oxygen*
- Resting PaO_2 of 55 mm Hg or less or oxygen saturation of 88% or less
- Resting PaO_2 of 56-59 mm hg or oxygen saturation of 89% in the presence of any of the following:
  - Dependent edema suggesting congestive heart failure
  - P pulmonale on the electrocardiogram (p wave > 3 mm in standard leads II, III, or aVF)
  - Polycythemia (hematocrit (> 56%)
II. *Noncontinuous oxygen* (oxygen flow rate and number of hours per day must be specified)
- During exercise: Resting PaO_2 of 55 mm Hg or less or oxygen saturation of 88% or less with a low level of exertion
- During sleep: Resting PaO_2 of 55 mm Hg or less or oxygen saturation of 88% or less with associated complications such as pulmonary hypertension, daytime somnolence, and cardiac arrhythmias.

bad, oxygen for some of the time is better, but oxygen for most of the time is the best". However, there is no evidence of benefit for long-term oxygen therapy used less than 12 hours/day.

The indications of long-term oxygen therapy are summarized in Table 16.5.

Patients who fulfil these criteria should receive continuous oxygen therapy as close to 24 hours/day as possible. There is no proof that oxygen therapy of less than 15 hours a day is beneficial in COPD. The dose should be sufficient to raise resting PaO_2 to 65 to 80 mm Hg (saturation, 91 to 95%). The dose should be increased by 1 L/min while the patient is sleeping or exercising to eliminate hypoxemic episodes. The adequacy of daytime resting oxygen dose should be assessed periodically.

Before deciding long-term oxygen therapy, the patient must be evaluated at least in a stable condition for about 4 weeks and repeat blood gas analysis is made. He must also quit smoking. The American Thoracic Society recommends that measurement of resting PaO_2 after 30 minutes of air breathing, not pulse oxymetry (oxygen saturation), be the clinical standard for initiating long-term oxygen therapy. Settings should be adjusted for rest, exertion, and sleep to meet the individual patient's needs. Availability, and affordability are other considerations of long-term oxygen therapy.

Some COPD patients develop PaO_2 of less than 60 mm Hg during sleep or exercise, although the value is adequate during rest. Although, it is not clear whether supplemental oxygen may be helpful in these situations.

The only practical way of delivering home oxygen to patients is by nasal prongs. Recently, prongs that supply oxygen only during inspiration have been developed to conserve oxygen. Oxygen can also be delivered directly to the sublaryngeal trachea through a chronic trans-tracheal cannula. Sources of home oxygen include compressed gas cylinders, concentrators, and the liquid oxygen system. Each has its own advantages and disadvantages. Domiciliary oxygen has been proved safe and devoid of any side effects. Details of oxygen therapy, the mode of administration, and toxicity are dealt with in more detail in subsequent chapters.

Supplemental oxygen is routinely used in the treatment of cardiorespiratory disorders associated with hypoxemia because it reduces pulmonary artery pressure and prolongs life.[414,427] During air breathing, most hypoxemic patients with chronic airways obstruction (CAO) complain of breathlessness both at rest and during exercise. Although there is ample evidence that supplemental oxygen may improve exercise tolerance and dyspnea during exercise in patients with CAO,[428-430] its effect on dyspnea at rest has received little attention. Liss and Grant[431] administered air and oxygen-enriched gas mixtures via nasal cannulas to eight CAO patients at rest to test the hypothesis that any reduction of dyspnea in these patients was due to the effect of gas flow on nasal receptors rather than to increased PaO_2 or decreased ventilation. They found no significant effect of inspired oxygen concentration, gas flow, or PaO_2 on breathlessness, which was assessed by a visual analog score (VAS). The oxygen-enriched air, however, was administered through the nasal cannula for only 5 min, and ventilation was not measured. In contrast, Swinburn and colleagues,[432] who administered 28 percent oxygen though a facemask for 10 min to 12 hypoxemic CAO patients, found a significant decrease in both severity of dyspnea (VAS) and minute ventilation (VE). They attributed the improvement in dyspnea to a reduction in the hypoxic drive to breathing, as reflected by the decreased VE. The latter, however, would also be expected to reduce the degree of dynamic pulmonary hyperinflation with a concurrent reduction in inspiratory load due to a decrease in intrinsic positive end-expiratory pressure (PEEPi)[433] and improvement of the mechanical advantage of the inspiratory muscles,[434] contributing to the reduction in dyspnea sensation with hyperoxic breathing. In fact, dynamic hyperinflation (DH) is probably the main cause of dyspnea in patients with CAO.[433,435] During 30 percent oxygen breathing, patients with chronic airway disease receiving long-term oxygen may benefit from hyperoxic breathing at rest, since it decreases the ventilation and the degree of DH, with concurrent improvement of dyspnea sensation.[436]

(h) *Respiratory care and rehabilitation.* These modalities are valuable adjunctive therapy in the care of patients with COPD. Patient, family and other caregivers should be trained in these modalities. These include measures for lung expansion (incentive spirometry), bland aerosol and humidity therapy, medicated aerosol therapy, chest physical therapy and breathing exercises.[437-449]

Besides lessening the airflow limitation and managing hypoxia and infection, the important goal of managing COPD is to decrease respiratory symptoms and improve quality of life. Many patients with COPD are unable to enjoy life to the full extent because of shortness of breath and exercise intolerance. Pulmonary rehabilitation program involves an integrated approach with an objective of improving the quality of life, well being, health status, reduction of respiratory symptoms, increased exercised tolerance, and functional activities such as walking, increased independence, enhanced ability to perform daily activities, improved psychological function, with less anxiety and depression, and increased feelings of hope, control, and self esteem.

Incentive spirometry is a technique to encourage the patient to take a sustained, deep breath, using a measuring device for direct visual feedback. It is indicated as an aid to facilitate lung expansion in hospitalized patients to treat and prevent lung collapse, particularly postoperatively. The deep breathing maneuvers stimulates cough and removal of secretions. Use of IPPB in hospital settings may be useful as in the management of atelectasis; to provide frequent periodic deep breathing for patients with acute respiratory failure in an attempt to avoid intubation or re-intubation as a temporary measure; and for delivery of aerosol medications. Chest physical therapy or chest physiotherapy consists of the use of postural drainage, chest percussion, and vibration as well as cough and deep breathing with the belief that these measures will facilitate mobilization and clearance of secretions from the airways, leading to improvement in pulmonary function. Breathing exercises encourage the patient to inspire slowly and to expire through pursed lips with simultaneous relaxation of the neck and upper thoracic muscles. Such exercises may be effective by increasing the patient's tidal volume, decreasing the respiratory rate, and lowering the FRC, thereby improving the efficiency of gas exchange and reducing the work of breathing.

The most common and distressing symptoms in COPD are dyspnea resulting in limitation of activity. The objectives of pulmonary rehabilitation are to control and alleviate symptoms and pathophysiologic complications and to achieve optimal ability to carry out activities of daily living. Several physical rehabilitation techniques are utilized to increase the dyspnea-limited level of activity or to decrease the degree of dyspnea associated with the same level of activity. These include exercise reconditioning, inspiratory muscle retraining, breathing retraining, energy conservation, nutritional management, smoking cessation programs, and psychosocial management.

Since breathlessness is an important and most often disabling symptom in patients with COPD, breathing retraining is an essential component of pulmonary rehabilitation programs. The goal is to help the patient to relieve and control breathlessness and to counteract physiologic abnormalities like hyperinflation of the chest. Retraining techniques include diaphragmatic and pursed-lips breathing to improve the ventilatory pattern by slow respiratory rate and increased tidal volume, to prevent dynamic airway compression, to improve respiratory synchrony of abdominal and thoracic musculature, and to improve gas exchange. Although there is an improvement in the physiological measurements, clinical improvement in symptoms is consistent findings. The most consistent physiological findings have been an increase in the tidal volume and a decrease in the respiratory rate. Blood gases also do improve.

Many patients adopt the pursed-lips breathing to be more beneficial of their own and pursue this method of breathing. Specific instruction can be given to improve dyspnea. They are to be instructed to breath in slowly and deeply through the nose; to purse the lips lightly as if to whistle; then to breath out slowly through the pursed lips, taking twice as long to exhale as to inhale. Indian patients can be trained to pronounce slowly "OM" which may be more acceptable and practicable in the socioreligious melliue.[450] Leaning forward, with arms resting on the patient's thighs or on a Table or other hard surface, may also help some patients in relieving dyspnea. Diaphragmatic breathing is often combined with pursed-lips breathing in which the patient learns to coordinate expansion of the abdominal wall with inspiration. Some studies has reported a detrimental effect of diaphragmatic breathing.[451]

Patients can be trained in an outpatient pulmonary rehabilitation program involving regular exercise on a bicycle. Incremental symptom-limited exercise testing (1-min increments of 10 W) may be performed on an electronically braked cycle ergometer. Increases in neuromuscular coupling, aerobic capacity, and tolerance to dyspnogenic stimuli and possibly breathing retraining are likely to contribute to the relief of both exertional dyspnea and leg effort after exercise training.[452]

(i) *Ventilatory support.* Ventilatory assistance may be required on an elective basis or in a nonselective manner.[453-456] Standard medical therapy often is not enough to reduce hypercapnia, alleviate dyspnea, to improve stamina poor quality of life in patients with severe COPD. They are most often need hospitalization with respiratory failure and respiratory acidosis with increased mortality. Thus, they are potential candidates of mechanical ventilatory support. Although there have been numerous studies evaluating the efficacy of elective mechanical ventilation in COPD, the results have been variable and the conclusions controversial.[457] Routine elective use of ventilatory support in ambulatory patients with COPD with hypercapnia is not recommended at present. However, patients who require emergency institution of mechanical ventilation for acute exacerbation may require more than short-term (nonelective) mechanical ventilation. The difficulty in these patients is weaning them off the ventilator because of the severity of the underlying condition and associated altered respiratory mechanics. In such cases a tracheostomy may be required. There is no simple, reliable way to predict inability to wean from the ventilator, nor there is a precise definition of chronic ventilator dependency. These involve a number of health care issues including the economics and ethical problems.

(j) *Lung volume reduction surgery.* A number of surgical procedures have been adopted to reduce dyspnea and improving the exercise tolerance in patients with emphysema.[458] These include tracheostomy, autonomic denervation, pneumoperitoneum, costchondrectomy, thoracoplasty, and bullectomy. Lung reduction surgery, otherwise known as reduction pneumoplasty is the latest surgical procedure to receive a great deal of attention after the recent refinement of the procedure with reduced amounts of complications by Cooper and his co-workers.[459,460] Following the procedure marked improvement occur in the physiological parameters including blood gas changes. Although the exact mechanism of such improvements occur is not known, it is possibly due to an improvement in the mechanical function of the chest wall, increased effective elastic recoil of the lung, and/or changes in the cardiopulmonary interdependence, reduced hyperinflation, reduced functional residual capacity from the more than normal values seen in emphysematous patients. A majority of the LVRS patients survived for = 3 years. Among survivors, dyspnea and lung function benefits were seen. Baseline BMI and postoperative LOS were significantly associated with survival.[461,462]

COPD and other allied conditions are the fourth-leading cause of death in the United States.[463] Emphysema affects approximately 2 million Americans.[464] When advanced, emphysema causes severe dyspnea that markedly diminishes quality of life.[465] Despite medical therapy, the course of advanced disease is slowly but relentlessly progressive. In the 1950s, Brantigan and Mueller[466] proposed that excision of the most hyperinflated and destroyed portions of the emphysematous lung might improve lung elastic recoil, reduce airflow limitation, and improve chest wall mechanics. However, the unilateral partial lung reduction, combined with radical hilar stripping, resulted in high mortality, limited clinical success, and general lack of acceptance. Based on the work of Brantigan and Mueller,[466] Cooper et al developed and initiated a procedure for bilateral lung volume reduction surgery (LVRS) at Barnes-Jewish Hospital in 1993. Published results of LVRS during the 1990s have been encouraging. The short-term efficacy of LVRS in selected patients has been demonstrated, and mechanisms of improvement have been described.[467-484] However, the value of LVRS has remained controversial due to varied patient selection, inconsistent utilization of preoperative rehabilitation, differences in surgical methods, incomplete follow-up data, varying degrees of benefit, and a lack of long-term results in published reports.[485,486] Patients with severe emphysema seek relief of dyspnea, improved functioning, and better quality of life from LVRS. Studies of LVRS limited to short-term follow-up have demonstrated improvements in physiologic measurements following surgery. A smaller number of short-term studies evaluating dyspnea and patient-perceived PF have also demonstrated improvements in these parameters after LVRS, but most studies have emphasized the assessment of physiologic parameters. Only a minority of patients referred for surgery is considered candidates for surgery.

A paucity of data describing long-term outcomes following LVRS exists. A recent study provided insight into the durability of LVRS: Flaherty and colleagues.[484] at the University of Michigan described a cohort of 89 consecutive patients who underwent bilateral LVRS during the interval of 1994 through 1998. The 30-day postoperative mortality rate was 5.6 percent, and a total of 16 patients died during the 3 year follow-up period. All survivors who completed testing initially showed improvement in dyspnea following LVRS, compared to their preoperative post-rehabilitation baseline, although the average improvement waned over time. The majority of patients demonstrated improvement in FEV_1, and the mean FEV_1 was significantly improved throughout follow-up, although the FEV_1 did trend downward over time. Of the 46 patients eligible for follow-up at 3 years after LVRS, 34 patients (74%) completed testing. Ten of the 34 patients had an FEV_1 at least 200 mL greater than

the preoperative baseline, and half of these had an FEV_1 > 400 mL above baseline. The average 6 min walk distance improved throughout the follow-up period. These significant improvements in dyspnea, lung function, and exercise capacity suggest that select patients have meaningful outcomes through at least 3 years after surgery.

Another recent study by Gelb and colleagues[487] described follow-up of a cohort of patients through 4 years after bilateral LVRS in 1995, with the most detailed long-term data described at 3 years after surgery. The subset of 26 nonconsecutive patients included in the study were able to complete rigorous preoperative physiologic testing, while the study excluded 56 other patients who underwent LVRS but did not have detailed testing. The included and excluded patients had similar preoperative pulmonary function results. Actuarial survival was 96 percent at 1 year after surgery and 69 percent at 3 years after surgery. The study found that 46 percent of surviving patients had an improved modified MRC dyspnea score at 3 years after surgery. However, the study did not specify that the baseline dyspnea measurements were made after completion of a preoperative comprehensive pulmonary rehabilitation program. Since medical therapy can improve dyspnea scores, some of the improvements may have been due to medical therapy. Nineteen of the 26 patients were considered to be short-term (1 year after LVRS) physiologic responders (FEV_1 improved > 200 mL or FVC improved > 400 mL compared to baseline), and 9 of these patients met the responder criteria through at least 3 years after surgery. Improvements in maximal expiratory airflow were accompanied by improvements in lung elastic recoil and airway conductance. This study provided a physiologic rationale for long-term improvements in airflow obstruction.

Yusen et al[488] designed a large prospective cohort study in a tertiary care urban university-based referral center to assess the first 200 patients undergoing bilateral LVRS (from 1993-1998), with follow-up through the year 2000. They used preoperative pulmonary rehabilitation and bilateral stapling LVRS. Each patient served as his own control, initially receiving optimal medical management including exercise rehabilitation before undergoing surgery. Preoperative postrehabilitation data were used as the baseline for comparisons with postoperative data. The primary end points were the effects of LVRS on dyspnea (modified Medical Research Council dyspnea sale), general health-related quality of life (Medical Outcomes Study 36-Item Short-Form Health Survey [SF-36]), patient satisfaction, and survival. The secondary end points were the effects of LVRS on pulmonary function, exercise capacity, and supplemental oxygen requirements.

The 200 patients accrued 735 person-years (mean ± SD, 3.7 ± 1.6 years; median, 4.0 years) of follow-up. Over the three follow-up periods, an average of > 90 percent of valuable patients completed testing. Six months, 3 years, and 5 years after surgery, dyspnea scores were improved in 81 percent, 52 percent, and 40 percent of patients, respectively. Dyspnea scores were the same or improved in 96 percent (6 months), 82 percent (3 years), and 74 percent (5 years) of patients. Improvements in SF-36 physical functioning were demonstrated in 93 percent (6 months), 78 percent (3 years), and 69 percent (5 years) of patients. Ninety six percent of the patients reported good-to-excellent satisfaction (6 months), 89 percent for 3 years, and 77 percent of patients for 5 years. The FEV_1 was improved in 92 percent (6 months), 72 percent (3 years), and 58 percent (5 years) of patients. Changes in dyspnea and general health-related quality-of-life scores, and patient satisfaction scores were all significantly correlated with changes in FEV_1. Following surgery, the median length of hospital stay in survivors was 9 days. The 90-day postoperative mortality was 4.5 percent. Annual Kaplan-Meier survival through 5 years after surgery was 93 percent, 88 percent, 83 percent, 74 percent, and 63 percent, respectively. During follow-up, 15 patients underwent subsequent lung transplantation. In this stringently selected patients group, the authors concluded that LVRS resulted in substantial beneficial effects over and above those achieved with optimized medical therapy. The duration of improvement was at least 5 years in the majority of survivors. However. Other published reports did not show these good results.[489-492]

The physiologic benefits associated with LVRS provide a rationale for the improved dyspnea and general health-related quality of life and high satisfaction reported by patients. Patients almost certainly had complex physiologic changes beyond an increase in FEV_1. Thus, the measured improvements in quality of life and dyspnea following surgery are probably partially explained by other physiologic changes that were not measured as part of this study.[493]

Defining what constitutes a successful outcome after LVRS is complex. The complexity arises in part from limited understanding of dyspnea and quality of life, and the enigmatic interactions between major medical interventions and patient perceptions. The sustained improvement in patient-perceived PF and dyspnea and high patient satisfaction after surgery partially define the success of LVRS in this group of patients. Use of measured lung function as the sole outcome to assess LVRS is inadequate.[477,484,494,495] Although physiologic parameters such as FEV_1 are relatively easy to follow, they are only surrogate markers of the improvement in dyspnea, functional status, and quality of life sought by patients disabled by severe emphysema. Too often, the success or the failure of an intervention is focused on surrogate outcomes (e.g. FEV_1). Incorporation of comprehensive pulmonary rehabilitation, a mainstay of therapy for most patients with far-advanced emphysema,[496] is an important preoperative intervention. Preoperative rehabilitation improves functioning and allows patients to confirm their desire for surgery based on their new baseline state. Preoperative rehabilitation with graded exercise effects no significant change in lung function.[474,475,482,483] However, the 6 min walk distance, dyspnea, and perceived PF improved with rehabilitation, also consistent with other studies.

The impact of LVRS on the mortality of patients with severe emphysema cannot be accurately determined without using an external control group. The four published randomized controlled trials of LVRS vs medical therapy demonstrated, as expected, a higher short-term mortality in the surgical arms compared to the mortality in the medical arms, mainly due to post-operative complications.[474,475,484,497] However, these studies demonstrated significantly better postoperative pulmonary function, exercise capacity, and subjective health status in the surgical treatment arms compared to the medical treatment arms. The four published studies did not assess long-term outcomes.

(j) *Transplantation.* Lung transplantation in patients with end-stage lung disease has now become a valid therapeutic option.[498,499] The last decade has seen lung and heart-lung transplantation move from experimental procedures to clinical treatments. Heart-lung transplants, single and double lung transplants have been possible in patients with emphysema and α-1-antitrypsin deficiency. The details of lung transplantation have been discussed subsequently.

SPECIAL PROBLEMS IN COPD

SLEEP AND COPD

Patients with COPD have higher prevalence of insomnia, excessive daytime sleepiness, and nightmares compared to the general population and the effect is independent of the use of theophyllines or beta-agonists.[500] Oxygen desaturation during sleep, particularly at REM sleep, is common in COPD. This is clinically associated with daytime hypoxemia, blunted chemosensitivity while awake, severe pulmonary function abnormalities, and chronic carbon dioxide retention. However, none of these parameters is a good predictor of sleep desaturation. The possible explanation of this desaturation is suggested to be either due to reduced ventilation during sleep, or ventilation-perfusion imbalance, or both. This REM associated drops in oxygen saturation is associated with increase in pulmonary artery pressure.[501,502] Patients with COPD also have increased premature ventricular contractions during sleep.[503] The overall survival of patients with COPD is reduced in whom there is a sleep-associated desaturation.[504,505] Although COPD and obstructive sleep apnoea can coexist, the incidence of later is not increased in COPD.[502] However, if both disorders coexist, there is more likelihood of development of pulmonary hypertension and right heart failure.

Nocturnal oxygen should be used in patients who have significant desaturation (88% or less) during sleep. This can be predicted from daytime hypoxia (paO_2 < 55 mm Hg). Measurement of nocturnal oxygen saturation in patients with COPD having daytime paO_2 > 60 mm Hg is not required, except in the presence of polycythemia or cor pulmonale. Full plethysmography is indicated in patients with symptoms suggestive of coexisting obstructive sleep apnea.

COPD AND AIR TRAVEL

Air travel in commercial airplanes exposes the passengers to hypobaric hypoxia, since aircrafts cabins are not usually pressurized to sea levels. It may be all right for normal passengers or with compensated, mild COPD patients, but those who have severe uncompensated COPD may face problem with including severe hypoxemia.[506,507] Dyspnea, wheezing, chest pain, cyanosis, and right heart failure will manifest this. Physical exertion during flights can also increase the risk of exacerbation of symptoms.

The cabin pressure limits for a passenger aircraft is 10,000 feet (3048 mtrs), but usually the aircrafts are pressurized to between 5000 to 7000 feet (1524-2134 mtrs). For the preflight evaluation of most patients, the evaluation should be made at 8000 feet (2438 mtrs) of altitude above sea level. This level is a realistic "worst case scenario" evaluation. This assessment includes estimation of the expected degree of hypoxia at altitude, identification of co-morbid disease(s), and provision of oxygen prescription if necessary. This includes hypoxia inhalation testing, and the use of regression formulae. In the hypoxia inhalation test, the subject is exposed to hypoxic gas mixtures equivalent to 8000 feet altitude (15.1% oxygen fraction) for a minimum of 15 minutes. During the test, the patient is assessed for clinical evaluation, electrocardiographic changes, and arterial blood gas changes.[508] Accordingly a decision regarding supplemental oxygen will be taken. Those patients already on oxygen should increase their oxygen by 1 or 2L/min while in flight.

SURGERY IN COPD

Evaluation of any surgery in COPD patients should identify the goal of surgery and should determine the risk-benefit ratio. This will depend on several factors like the indication of surgery, site and type of surgery, experience of the surgeon, type of anesthesia, and the severity of respiratory impairment, and associated co-morbid diseases.[509-516] The risk factors are identified by history, clinical examination, chest skiagram, and a number of pulmonary and cardiovascular tests.

The incidence of postoperative complications varies. The subject is dealt in more detail in the chapter on physiology. In brief, ophthalmologic procedures carry a low mortality rate of below 1 percent. However, use of narcotics, sedatives and general anesthesia increase the risk. Cough should be of concern in these patients since that will increase the intraocular pressure, which the ophthalmologist will not like. Head and neck procedures involve the risk of manipulation of the airways. The complications will include sleep-associated disorders in COPD, aspiration, direct inflammation, compression, compromise of the airways, and accumulation of secretions. These may increase the risk in COPD patients. Orthopedics procedures have a special risk of venous thromboembolism. Urologic, gynecologic, colorectal procedures, retroperitoneal and renal surgery in patients with stage II or III COPD that are likely to be short and/or unlikely to involve intraoperative complications should be performed under local or epidural anesthesia whenever possible. Lengthy abdominal or pelvic surgery using general anesthesia may be associated with increased risk in COPD. Patients with a FEV_1 of less than 1L are at increased risk for complications and may require perioperative ventilatory support. However there is no absolute contraindication for lower abdominal surgery. Upper abdominal surgery poses a higher risk of complication for all patients. The risk is more in subjects who are obese, smokers, heart disease, and old age. In these patients the morbidity may be as high as 80 percent and the mortality rate is around 3 to 5 percent. The problems are related to the shift of the respiratory pump from the diaphragm to the accessory muscles, due to a non-pain-related reflex, mucus hypersecretion, airway closure, and lung or chest wall restriction. Laparoscopic surgery decreases the operative risk.

COPD is the most common cause of preoperative pulmonary dysfunction in patients undergoing cardiac surgery. Cessation of smoking should precede surgery by a minimum of 8 weeks. Inhaled beta-2-agonists and anticholinergics bronchodilators can be used for management. Monitoring of theophylline should be carried out in these patients. Most patients will require mechanical ventilation and there may be special problems in ventilatory management in such patients. Major abdominal vascular surgery is associated with high postoperative complications because of usual association of moderate to severe degree of COPD. Prolonged mechanical ventilation (> 24 hours) may be required because of high incidence of heavy smoking, preoperative arterial hypoxemia, and major intraoperative blood loss.

Bronchoscopy in COPD is usually safe unless COPD is severe, although some degree of hypoxemia is imperative. Supplemental oxygen should be used in such situations. Thoracoscopy is better tolerated than open thoracotomy. Thoracotomy will have transient adverse effect on lung function for several months. Pneumonectomy may permanently reduce all lung functions by 40 to 50 percent, which may be devastating to patients with COPD. Therefore, other minimizing surgical procedures can be tried like wedge resection (0-10% functional decrease); segmentectomy (5-10% loss of lung function); and lobectomy (10-20% loss of lung function) whenever possible. If the resected region has no function there is no decrease except the temporary loss of thoracotomy, rather it is beneficial. Relative risk and acceptable lung function parameters are discussed in earlier chapters.

COPD patients undergoing surgery should be managed in a proper planned manner. Smoking cessation should be there at least 8 weeks prior to surgery. Aggressive treatment of lung dysfunction includes bronchodilators including theophylline, corticosteroids, and antibiotic as indicated. Patients with stage II or III COPD should be admitted to the hospital before surgery for detailed evaluation, patient education, and aggressive therapy. During the intraoperative period, although there are a number of physiological changes, there is not much of a problem since they are usually put on ventilators and monitoring is carried out with pulse oximetry and end-tidal carbon dioxide monitoring. In the postoperative period, the immediate problems are respiratory muscle dysfunction, acidosis, hypoxemia, and hypoventilation. It is therefore necessary to closely monitor these patients. Subsequently deep breathing maneuvers including intermittent positive pressure breathing, and incentive spirometry, chest physiotherapy are necessary.

GENERAL APPROACH TO MANAGEMENT OF COPD

A general approach to the management of COPD in outpatient setting is summarized below.
  I. Establish the diagnosis and symptomatic assessment.
 II. Smoking cessation should be achieved as completely as possible.
III. Encourage exercise, healthy life-style and immunization.
 IV. Treatment of obstruction by pharmacologic therapy (see below).
  V. Assessment of hypoxemia and if needed oxygen to be prescribed.
 VI. Assessment of response to therapy.
VII. Depending upon VI above, patient may be referred for multidisciplinary rehabilitation programs/life long monitoring and care.
VIII. Patient education.

The American Thoracic Society has recommended a step-by- step pharmacologic therapy for COPD which is shown in Table 16.6.

The American Thoracic Society also has put for the guidelines for indications for hospitalization, admission into the ICU and discharge criteria. These are summarized in Table 16.7.

PRINCIPLES OF MANAGEMENT IN THE INPATIENT

Stepwise therapy is to be instituted. The basic principle has already been outline above. To start with the cause of exacerbation is to be identified like infection, sedative use, and the therapy is directed accordingly. Regulated oxygen therapy is the basic requirement in most of these patients. A beta-2-agonist aerosol or nebulization is started as the first line of therapy. Injectable drugs (adrenaline, salbutamol, or terbutaline) may be tried subcutaneously. Inhaled/nebulized ipratropium bromide may be added if necessary. If there is no response then injectable theophylline is added. In places injectable theophylline is tried as the first line therapy because of its ease of administration and low cost. However, the drug is potentially toxic and this fact is to be taken into account. Steroid may be tried when the above regimen fails. However, if no response is forthcoming, the drug is to be withdrawn as soon as possible. Antibiotic and mucokinetics are usually necessary. Methods to mobilize secretions are to be employed which include direct coughing, or through physical methods including IPPB and nasotracheal suctioning in appropriate situations.

Assisted ventilation is usually required in two situations: (a) when there is respiratory muscle fatigue

TABLE 16.6: Step-by-step pharmacologic therapy[7]

I. *Mild, variable symptoms*
  - Selective beta$_2$-agonist metered dose inhaler (MDI) aerosol, 1-2 puffs every 2-6 hours as needed. Maximum dose 8-12 puffs over 24 hours

II. *Mild to moderate continuing symptoms*
  - Ipratropium MDI aerosol, 2-6 puffs every 6-8 hrs; not to be used more frequently
  - Plus selective beta-2-agonist MDI aerosol, 1-4 puffs every 6 hrly, for rapid relief, when needed or as regular replacement

III. *If no response to step II, or there is mild to moderate increase in symptom*
  - Add sustained release theophylline, 200-400 mg twice daily or 400-800 mg at bed times for nocturnal bronchospasm And/or
    Consider sustained release salbutamol 4-8 mg twice daily or at bed time only
  - Consider mucokinetic agent

IV. *If control of symptoms suboptimal*
  - Consider a course of oral corticosteroid (e.g. prednisolone) up to 40 mg/day for 10-14 days.
    - If improvement occurs, taper to low daily or alternate-day dose, e.g. 7.5 mg
    - If no improvement occurs stop abruptly
    - If appears to be helpful, consider inhaler steroid, particularly if there is evidence of hyperreactivity

V. *Severe exacerbation*
  - Increase beta$_2$-agonist dosage (MDI with spacer 6-8 puffs every 1/2-2 hrs or inhalant solution, every 1/2 to 2 hrs or subcutaneous administration of epinephrine or salbutamol or terbutaline, 0.1-0.5 ml
  And/or
  - Increase ipratropium dosage (MDI with spacer) 6-8 puffs every 3-4 hrs or inhalant solution every 4-8 hrs
  And
  - Intravenous theophylline to make serum level to 10-12 mg/ml
  And
  - Methyl prednisolone intravenous 50-100 mg starts followed by the same dose every 6-8 hrly; taper as soon as possible (hydrocortisone can be used instead)
  And add
  - Antibiotic, if indicated
  - Mucokinetic agent if sputum is very viscous

TABLE 16.7: Hospitalization indications of COPD[7]

Hospitalization
1. Acute exacerbations (increased dyspnea, cough or sputum production) with one or more of the following:
   - Inadequate response to outpatient management
   - Inability to walk between rooms
   - Inability to eat or sleep due to dyspnea
   - Conclusion by physician and family that the patient cannot manage at home with supplementary home care not immediately available
   - High-risk co-morbid pulmonary, or nonpulmonary conditions
   - Prolonged progressive symptoms before emergency visit
   - Altered mentation
   - Worsening hypoxemia
   - New or worsening hypercarbia
2. New or worsening cor pulmonale unresponsive to outpatient management
3. Planned invasive surgical or diagnostic procedure requiring analgesics sedatives that may worsen pulmonary function
4. Co-morbid conditions like severe steroid myopathy, acute vertebral compression fracture that have caused lung function worsening

ICU Admission
1. Severe dyspnea that responds inadequately to initial emergency therapy
2. Confusion, lethargy, or respiratory muscle fatigue (paradoxical diaphragmatic motion)
3. Persistent or worsening hypoxemia despite supplemental oxygen or severe/worsening respiratory acidosis (pH, 7.30)
4. Assisted mechanical ventilation is required, either by endotracheal intubation ornon-invasive techniques.

and progressive worsening of respiratory acidosis and/or altered mental status despite aggressive pharmacologic therapy and other nonventilatory support; (b) clinically significant hypoxemia which develops despite providing supplemental oxygen by usual techniques. The selection of ventilatory device is wide and the clinician can choose his own including endotracheal intubation, oral or nasal mask ventilation, and negative pressure ventilation. Most clinicians advocate positive pressure inflation, although some investigators report success with negative pressure ventilation. Major risks associated with positive pressure ventilation include ventilator-associated pneumonia, pulmonary barotrauma, laryngotracheal complications associated with intubation, and/or tracheostomy. Other specific problems of such ventilations peculiar to COPD include overventilation resulting in acute respiratory alkalosis, systemic hypotension and the creation of intrinsic positive end-expiratory pressure (PEEP) or auto-PEEP, especially if the expiratory time is inadequate or if dynamic airflow obstruction exists. The three ventilatory modes most widely used in COPD are: assist-control ventilation (ACV); intermittent mandatory ventilation (IMV); and pressure support ventilation (PSV). Noninvasive assisted ventilation has been tried with success in COPD also. Most patients of COPD who required mechanical ventilation for acute bronchospasm, fluid overload, oversedation or inadvertent hyper-oxygenation can be successfully extubated without going through weaning. However, some patients with COPD intubated for respiratory failure may require weaning. The most important factors for successful weaning include neuromuscular reserve capacity relative to respiratory load, cardiovascular performance, oxygenation, and psychological factors. Sometimes, weaning may be very difficult.

OUTCOME MEASUREMENTS IN COPD

The proportion of patients with COPD who show a significant bronchodilator response increases cumulatively with the number of times the test is performed.[517-519] Approximately 80 percent of patients with COPD will exhibit a significant bronchodilator response over the course of three separate challenges, so a single bronchodilator challenge is not a reliable assay of responsiveness. Besides this, there may be benefits that are not measured by the FEV_1 response itself, shown in many studies.[520,521] Patients who are "poor responders" in terms of their first FEV_1 response to an agent may nevertheless experience significant symptomatic relief and improved quality of life from regular use of the same. Some authors believe that "the test does not accurately predict whether benefits may be achieved with maintenance ... therapy and therefore should not be used to guide decisions to prescribe a bronchodilator therapy."

The second point concerns how one should evaluate the benefits of a treatment for COPD. The main problem with using the FEV_1 is that it correlates only poorly with clinically relevant outcomes. Jones et al[522] have shown that it bears little relationship to quality of life. In acute studies, it has been quite difficult to show that an improvement in FEV_1 correlates with an acute improvement in symptoms such as dyspnea or exercise tolerance[523] that one certainly would expect. Why else would patients use (and sometimes overuse) bronchodilators when they are dyspenic? The explanation for this paradox may be that the FEV_1 is a maneuver that does not correspond to any common breathing activity except perhaps sneezing or blowing out candles. It is a rather poor if convenient surrogate. Perhaps the reduction of hyperinflation, e.g. inspiratory capacity[520] will be a better surrogator, which we simply do not know at this time.

There is not a reliable, convenient surrogate marker for the clinical benefit of any agent in COPD. There are now several appropriate, specific, and well-validated clinical outcomes. Instruments such as measures of quality of life, dyspnea, and effort tolerance have the advantage that they are clinically relevant to COPD and can detect changes over quite short periods of time. Their drawback is that they are time consuming and subject to the skill of the experimenter and the cooperation of the subject. Their noise-to-signal ratio is fairly high, so their sensitivity to subtle changes is low.

Other important clinical outcomes include the use of health-care resources such as unscheduled visits to doctors or emergency departments, acute exacerbations of COPD, and mortality. These events are highly relevant to both health and health-care costs. They have the advantage that each can be captured with confidence although they remain susceptible to some subjectivity. How certain can one be that the event was related to COPD rather than to one of the comorbidities that are common in the COPD population? Other disadvantages are that these events, particularly mortality, are relatively uncommon, so a large and expensive trial over a fairly prolonged period of time may be required to detect a significant treatment effect with statistical confidence. One is mindful, too, that a treatment can, in theory, have benefit by improving quality of life, for example, without increasing survival, and *vice versa*.

For all of these reasons, a wide range of outcomes, including both physiologic and clinical end points, is needed before one can understand whether and how a novel therapeutic agent may be of clinical benefit to patients. Despite the above-mentioned difficulties, it is good that many current trials include clinical end points.[524]

Recently, the Global Initiative for COPD and WHO-India had developed guidelines for the management of COPD and they are shown as Appendix-I and II respectively.

REFERENCES

1. Ciba Guest symposium Report. Terminology, definitions and classification of chronic pulmonary emphysema and related conditions. Thorax 1959;14:286-99.
2. Aspen conference report of committee on definition of emphysema. Am Rev Respir Dis 959;79:114.
3. Medical Research Council. Definitions and classification of chronic bronchitis for clinical and epidemiological purposes. Lancet 1965;1:775-79.
4. Snider GL, Kleinerman J, Thurlbeck WM, Bengali ZH. The definition of emphysema. Report of a National Heart, Lung and Blood Institute, Division of Lung diseases workshop Am Rev Respir Dis 1985;132:182-85.
5. American Thoracic Society. Standards for the diagnosis and care of patients with chronic obstructive pulmonary disease (COPD) and asthma. Am Rev Respir Dis 1987;137:225-44.
6. Snider GL. What's in a name. Respiration 1995;62: 297-301.
7. American Thoracic Society. Medical section of the American Lung association. Standards for the diagnosis and care of patients with chronic obstructive pulmonary disease. Am J Respir Crit Care Med 1995;152:S77-S120.
8. Siafakas NM, Vermeire P, Pride NB, et al. Optimal assessment and management of chronic obstructive pulmonary disease (COPD): The European Respiratory Society Task Force. Eur Respir J 1995;8:1398-1420.

9. World Health Organization. The GOLD global strategy for the management and prevention of COPD. Available at www.goldcopd.com. Accessed March 16, 2001.

10. American Thoracic Society. Lung function testing: Selection of reference values and interpretive strategies. Am Rev Respir Dis 1991;144:1202-18.

11. Burrows B. Differential diagnosis of chronic obstructive pulmonary disease. Chest 1990;97:16S-18S.

12. American Thoracic Society. Chronic bronchitis, asthma, and pulmonary emphysema: A statement by the Committee on Diagnostic Standards for Nontuberculous Respiratory Diseases. Am Rev Res Dis 1962;85: 762-68.

13. The rise in chronic obstructive pulmonary disease mortality. Am Rev Respir Dis 1989;140(Suppl) S3-S107.

14. Thom TJ. International comparisons in COPD mortality. Am Rev Respir Dis 1989;140(Suppl):S27-S34.

15. Woolcock AJ. Epidemiology of chronic airways disease. Chest 1989;96(Suppl) 302S-06S.

16. Murray CJ, Lopez AD. Global morality, disability and the contribution of risk factors: Global burden of disease study. Lancet 1997;349:1436-42.

17. Murray CJ, Lopez AD. Alternative projection of mortality by cause 1990-2020: Global burden of disease study. Lancet 1997;349:1498-1504.

18. Thom TJ. International comparisons in COPD mortality. Am rev Respir Dis 1989;140:S27-S34.

19. Centers for Disease Control and Prevention. Current estimates from the National Health Interview Survey, 1995. Vital and health statistics. Washington DC. Government Printing Office, (DHHS publication no. (PHS) 1996;96-1527.

20. Strachan DP. Epidemiology: A British perspective. In Calverley P, Pride N (Eds): Chronic Obstructive Pulmonary Disease. London, Chapman & Hall, 1995;47-68.

21. Cook DG, Kussick SJ, Shaper AG. The respiratory benefits of stopping smoking. J Smoking Related Dis 1990;1:45-58.

22. Lacasse Y, Brooks D, Goldstein RS. Trends in the epidemiology of COPD in Canada, 1980 to 1995. COPD and Rehabilitation Committee of the Canadian Thoracic Society. Chest 1999;116:306-13.

23. Viegi G, Scognamiglio A, Baldacci S, Pistelli F, Carrozzi L. Epidemiology of Chronic Obstructive Pulmonary Disease (COPD). Respiration 2001;68:4-19.

24. Murray CJ, Lopez AD. Mortality by cause for eight regions of the world: Global Burden of Disease Study. Lancet 1997;349:1269-76.

25. Malik SK. Profile of chronic bronchitis in North India- The PGI experience (1972-1985). Lung India 1986;4:89-100.

26. Kamat SR, Godkhindi KD, Shah VN, et al. Prospective 3 year study of health morbidity in relation to air pollution in Bombay, India. Methodology and early results upto 2 years. Lung India 1984;2:1-20.

27. Bachani D. Chronic airflow limitation in talc industry: Role of age, smoking habits, and dust exposure. Ind J Chest Dis All Sc 1984;26:220-24.

28. Behera D, Malik SK. Chronic respiratory disease and peak expiratory flow rates in rural Oriya females—A preliminary communication. Lung India 1988;6:127-28.

29. Gupta SK, Singh SK. A study on the prevalence of chronic bronchitis in workers exposed to smoke and irritant fumes in a railway workshop. Ind J Chest Dis All Sc 1992;34:25-28.

30. Kumar S, Kochar SK, Sabir M, Saksena HC. Pulmonary disorders in wool workers in Bikaner, Rajsthan. Lung India 1992;10:65-68.

31. Qureshi KA. Domestic smoke pollution and prevalence of chronic bronchitis/asthma in a rural area of Kashmir. Ind J Chest Dis All Sc 1994;36:61-72.

32. Crofton J. Chronic airways disease: The smoking component. Chest 1989;96(Suppl):349S-54S.

33. Higgins MW, Thom T. Incidence, prevalence, and mortality: Intra- and intercountry differences. In MJ Ensley, Saunders NA (Eds): Clinical epidemiology of chronic obstructive pulmonary diseases. Marcel Dekker: New York, 1990;23-43.

34. Surgeon General of the United States. The health consequences of smoking: Chronic obstructive lung disease. Washington DC: US department Health and Human Services, DHHS Publication No. 1984;84-50205.

35. Sherril DL, Lebowitz MD, Burrows B. Epidemiology of chronic obstructive disease. Clin Chest Med 1990;11: 375-88.

36. Davis RM, Novotny TE. The epidemiology of cigarette smoking and its impact on chronic obstructive lung disease. Am Rev Respir Dis 1989;140:S82-S84.

37. National Institutes of Health. Global initiative for chronic obstructive lung disease. Bethesda, MD: National Institutes of Health, National Heart, Lung, and Blood Institute, April 2001; Publication No. 2701.

38. Murray RP, Anthonisen NR, Connett JE, et al. Effects of multiple attempts to quit smoking and relapses to smoking on pulmonary function: Lung Health Study Research Group. J Clin Epidemiol 1998;51,1317-26.

39. Doll R, Peto R. Mortality in relation to smoking: 10 years observation on British doctors. Br Med J 1976;2: 1525-36.

40. Doll R, Gray R, Hafner B, Peto R. Mortality in relation to smoking; 22 years observation on female British doctors. Br Med J 280:967.

41. Malik SK. Chronic bronchitis—North India. Chest 1977;72:800.

42. Behera D, Malik SK. Chronic bronchitis and respiratory function impairment in chutta smokers (reverse smoking). Ind J Chest Dis All Sc 1984;26:26-29.

43. Malik SK. Chronic bronchitis and ventilatory impairment in bidi smokers. Ind J Chest Dis All Sc 1977;19:21-26.

44. Olsen HC, Gilson JC. Respiratory symptoms, bronchitis and ventilatory capacity in men: An Anglo-Danish comparison, with special reference to differences in smoking habits. Br Med J 1960;1:450-56.

45. Higgins ITT. Tobacco smoking, respiratory symptoms and ventilatory capacity: Studies in random samples of the population. Br Med J 1959;1:325-29.

46. Rimington J. Phlegm and filters. Br Med J 1972;2: 262-64.

47. Fletcher CM, Peto R, Tinker C, Speizer FE. The natural history of chronic bronchitis and emphysema. Oxford University Press. 1976; Chapter 1.

48. Behera D, Malik SK. Chronic respiratory disease in Chandigarh teachers. A follow up study. Ind J Chest Dis 1987;29:25-28.

49. United States Public Health Service. The Health consequences of smoking. US Department of Health, Education, and Welfare Washington, 1967.

50. Bates DV. The fate of the chronic bronchitis: A report of the 10 years follow up in the Canadian Department of Veterans Affairs coordinated study of chronic bronchitis. Am Rev Respir Dis 1973;108:1043-65.

51. Fletcher C, Peto R. The natural history of chronic airflow obstruction. Br Med J 1977;1:1645-48.

52. Higgins ITT, Gilson JC, Ferris BG, et al. Chronic respiratory disease in an Industrial town: A nine years follow up study. Preliminary report. Am J Publ Health 1968;58:1667-76.

53. Camilli AE, Burrows B, Knudson RJ, et al. Longitudinal changes in forced expiratory volume in one second in adults. Effects of smoking and smoking cessation. Am Rev Respir Dis 1987;135:794-99.

54. Van Ganse WF, Ferris BG, Cotes JE. Cigarette smoking and pulmonary diffusing capacity (transfer factor). Am Rev Respir Dis 1972;105:30-41.

55. Nadel JA, Comroe JH. Acute effects of inhalation of cigarette smoke on airway conductance. J Appl Physiol 1961;16:713-16.

56. Guyatt AR, Berry G, Alpers JH, et al. Relationship of airway conductance and its immediate change on smoking to smoking habits and symptoms of chronic bronchitis. Am Rev Respir Dis 1970;101:44-54.

57. Miller JM, Sproule BJ. Acute effects of inhalation of cigarette smoke on mechanical properties of the lungs. Am Rev Respir Dis 1966;94:721-26.

58. Turato G, Di Stefano A, Maestrelli P, et al. Effect of smoking cessation on airway inflammation in chronic bronchitis. Am J Respir Crit Care Med 1995;152:1262-67.

59. Burrows B, Knudson RJ, Cline MG, Lebowitz MD. Quantitative relationships between cigarette smoking and ventilatory function. Am Rev Respir Dis 1977; 115:195-205.

60. Tager IB, Weiss St, Munoz A, et al. Longitudinal study of the effect of maternal smoking on pulmonary function in children. New Engl J Med 1983;309:699-703.

61. Ware JH, Dockery DW, Spiro A, et al. Passive smoking, gas cooking, and respiratory health of children living in six cities. Am Rev Respir Dis 1984;129:366-74.

62. Charlton A. Children's coughs related to parental smoking. Br Med J 1984;288:1647-49.

63. Weiss St, Tager Ib, Speizer FE. The health effects of involuntary smoking. Am Rev Respir Dis 1983;128: 933-42.

64. O' Conner GT, Weiss ST, Tager IB, Speizer FE, et al. The effect of passive smoking on pulmonary function and nonspecific bronchial responsiveness in a population based sample of children and young adults. Am Rev Respir Dis 1987;135:800.

65. Collery JRT, Holland WW, Corkhill RT. Influence of parental smoking and parental phlegm on pneumonia and bronchitis in early childhood. Lancet 1974;2:1031-34.

66. Colley JRT, Douglas JWB, Reid DD. Respiratory disease in young adults. Influence of early childhood respiratory tract illness, social class, air pollution, and smoking. Br Med J 1973;3:195-98.

67. Kiernan KE, Colley JRT, Douglas JWB, Reid DD. Chronic cough in young adults in relation to smoking habits, childhood environment and chest illness. Respiration 1976;33:236-44.

68. Crystal RG. Alpha-1-antitrypsin deficiency, emphysema, and liver disease: genetic basis and strategies for therapy. J Clin Invest 1990;85:1343-52.

69. Guidelines for the approach to the patient with severe hereditary alpha-1-deficiency. Am Rev Respir Dis 1989;140:1494-97.

70. Brantly MT, Nukiwa T, Crystal RG. Molecular basis of alpha-1-deficiency. Am J Med 1988;84:13-31.

71. Weinberger SE. Recent advances in pulmonary medicine. First of two parts. New Engl J Med 1993;328:1389-97.

72. Crystal RG, Brantly ML, Hubbard RC, et al. The alpha-1 antitrypsin gene and its mutations: Clinical consequences and strategy for therapy. Chest 1989;95:196-208.

73. Feld RD. Heterozygosity of alpha-1 antitrypsin: A health risk ? Crit Rev Clin Lab Sc 1989;27:461-81.

74. Townley RG, Southard JG, Radford P, et al. Association of MS Pi phenotype with airway hyperresponsiveness. Chest 1990;98:594-99.

75. Snider GL. Pulmonary disease in alpha-1 antitrypsin deficiency. Ann Intern Med 1989;111:957-59.

76. Silverman EK, Pierce JA, Province MA, Rao DC, Campbell EJ. Variability of pulmonary function in alpha-1-antitrypsin deficiency: Clinical correlates. Ann Intern Med 1989;111:982-91.

77. Erikson S, Carlson J, Velez R. Risk of cirrhosis and primary liver cancer in alpha-1-antitrypsin deficiency. New Engl J Med 1986;314:736-39.

78. Perlmuter DH. The cellular basis of liver injury in alpha-1-antitrypsin deficiency. Hepatology 1991;13:172-85.

79. Malik SK, Khatri GK, Sehgal S. Alpha-1-antitrypsin deficiency in chronic lung disease patients. Ind J Chest Dis All Sc 1977;19:188-91.

80. Reid DD. Air pollution as a cause of chronic bronchitis. Proc Royal Soc Med 1964;57:965.

81. Crofton J, Douglas A. Respiratory diseases (3rd edn). Oxford. Blackwell Scientific publications, 1981;350.

82. Chretien J. Pollution (atmospheric, domestic, and occupational) as a risk factor for chronic airways disease. Chest 1989;96(Suppl):316S-17S.

83. Crapo J, Miller FJ, Mossmann B, Pryor WA, Kiley JP. NHLB Workshop summary. Environmental lung diseases. Relationship between acute inflammatory responses to air pollutants and chronic lung disease. Am Rev Respir Dis 1992;145:1506-12.

84. Kamat SR, Patil JD, Gregart J, Dalal N, Deshpande JM, Hardikar P. Air pollution related respiratory morbidity in central and north-eastern Bombay. J Assoc Physicians India 1992;40:588-93.

85. Higgins BG, Francis HC, Yates CJ, et al. Effects of air pollution on symptoms and peak expiratory flow measurements in subjects with obstructive airways disease. Thorax 1995;50:149-55.

86. Samet JM, Marbury MC, Spengler JD. Health effects and source of indoor air pollution. Part I. Am Rev Respir Dis 1987;136:1486-08.

87. Anderson HR, Limb ES, Bland TM, et al. Health effects an air pollution episode in London, December 1991. Thorax 1995;50:1188-93.

88. Samet JM, Marbury MC, Spengler JD. Health effects and source of indoor air pollution. Part I. Am Rev Respir Dis 1988;137:221-42.

89. Behera D, Jindal SK. Respiratory symptoms in Indian women using domestic cooking fuels. Chest 1991;100:385-88.

90. Behera D. Health effects of indoor air pollution due to domestic cooking fuels. Ind J Chest Dis All Sc 1995;37:227-38.

91. Behera D, Jindal SK, Malhotra H. Ventilatory function in nonsmoking rural Indian women using different cooking fuels. Respiration 1994;61:89-92.

92. Pandey MR. Prevalence of chronic bronchitis in a rural community of the Hill region of Nepal. Thorax 1984;39:331-36.

93. Pandey MR. Domestic smoke pollution and chronic bronchitis in a rural community of the Hill region of Nepal. Thorax 1984;39:337-39.

94. Becklake MR. Occupational pollution. Chest 1989;96(Suppl):372S-77S.

95. Sharp JT, Paul O, McKean H, Best WR. A longitudinal study of bronchitic symptoms and spirometry in a middle aged, male industrial population. Am Rev Respir Dis 1973;108:1066-87.

96. Burrows B, Knudson RJ, Lebowitz MD. The relationship of childhood respiratory illness to adult obstructive airway disease. Am Rev Respir Dis 1977;115:751-60.

97. Pride NB. Role of infection, in chronic bronchitis in nonsmokers. Eur J Respir Dis 1982;63:43-50.

98. Phelan PD. Does adult chronic obstructive lung disease begin in childhood? Br J Dis Chest 1984;78:1-9.

99. Shaheen SO, Barker DJP. Early lung growth and chronic airflow obstruction. Thorax 1994;49:533-36.

100. Samet JM, Tager IB, Speizer FE. The relationship between respiratory illness in childhood and chronic airflow obstruction in adulthood. Am Rev Respir Dis 1983;127:508-23.

101. Colley JRT, Miller DL. Acute respiratory infections. Chest 1989;96(Suppl):355S-60S.

102. Edelman NH, Kaplan RM, Buist AS, et al. Chronic obstructive pulmonary disease. Chest 1992;102:Suppl:243S-56S.

103. Murphy TF, Sethi S. Bacterial infection in chronic obstructive pulmonary disease. Am Rev Respir Dis 1992;146:1067-83.

104. Murray JF. Chronic obstructive airway disease. Chest 1989;96(Suppl):301S-78S.

105. Orie NG, Sluiter K, De Varies K, Tammeling GH, Witkop J. The host factor in chronic bronchitis. In NG Orie, HJ Sluiter (Eds): Bronchitis. Royal Vangorcum, Assen, Netherlands, 1961;43-59.

106. O'Connor GT, Sparrow D, Weiss ST. The role of allergy and nonspecific airway hyperresponsiveness in the pathogenesis of chronic obstructive pulmonary disease. Am Rev Respir Dis 1989;140:225-52.

107. Pande JN. Bronchial hyperreactivity, annual rate of decline in FEV_1 and chronic airflow obstruction: Relationship with smoking. Ind J Chest Dis All Sc 1984;26:203-04.

108. Koyama H, Nishimura H, Mio T, et al. Bronchial responsiveness and acute bronchodilator response in chronic obstructive pulmonary disease. and diffuse panbronchiolitis. Thorax 1994;49:540-44.

109. Pande JN, Guleria R. (Editorial) Bronchial hyperreactivity in chronic obstructive airways disease. Ind J Chest Dis All Sc 1992;34:163-65.

110. Suri JC, Dar A, Goel A. A sty of bronchial reactivity in relation to baseline pulmonary functions in patients with chronic bronchitis. Ind J Chest Dis All Sc 1992;34:167-73.

111. Srinivasan S, Jindal SK, Malik SK. Influence of baseline airway obstruction and degree of smoking on bronchial reactivity in smokers. Ind J Chest Dis All Sc 1988;30:78-83.

112. Verma VK, Cockroft DW, Dosman JA. Airway responsiveness to inhaled histamine in chronic obstructive airway disease. Chronic bronchitis vs emphysema. Chest 1988;94:457-61.

113. Taskin DP, Altose MD, Bleeker ER, et al. Lung Health Study Research Group. The Lung Health Study: Airway responsiveness to inhaled methacholine in smokers with mild to moderate airflow limitation. Am Rev Respir Dis 1992;145:301-10.

114. Annesi I, Oryszozyn MP, Fretti C, et al. Total circulating IgE and FEV_1 in adult men: An epidemiological longitudinal study. Chest 1992;101:642-48.

115. Burrows B, Hasan FM, Barbee RA, Halonen M, Lebowitz M. Epidemiologic observations on eosinophilia and its relation to respiratory disorders. Am Rev Respir Dis 1980;122:708-19.

116. Kauffmann F, Kleisbauer JP, Cambon-De-Mouzon A, et al. Genetic markers in chronic airflow limitation: A

genetic epidemiologic study. Am Rev Respir Dis 1983;127:263-69.

117. Britton J. Dietary fish oil and airways obstruction. Thorax 1995;50(Suppl 1):S11-S15.

118. Snider GL, Faling LJ, Rennard SI. Chronic bronchitis and emphysema. In Murray JF, Nadel JA (Eds): Text book of respiratory medicine. WB Saunders: Philadelphia 1994;1342.

119. Burrows B, Knudson RJ, Camilli AE, Lyle SK, Lebowitz MD. The horse racing effect and predicting decline in forced expiratory volume in one second from screening spirometry. Am Rev Respir Dis 1987;135:788-93.

120. Burrows B. Airway obstructive diseases: Pathogenetic mechanisms and natural histories of the disorders. Med Clin North Am 1990;74:547-60.

121. Burrows B, Bloom JW, Traver GA, Cline MG. The course and prognosis of different forms of chronic airway obstruction in a sample from general population. New Engl J Med 1987;317:1309-14.

122. Peto R, Speizer FE, Cochrane AL, et al. The relevance in adults of airflow obstruction but not of mucus hypersecretion, to mortality from chronic lung disease: Results from 20 years of prospective observation. Am Rev Respir Dis 1983;128:491-500.

123. Ebi-Kryston KL. Predicting 15 years chronic bronchitis mortality in the Whitehall study. J Epidemiol Commun Health 1989;168-72.

124. Lange P, Nyboe J, Appleyard M, Jensen G, Schnohr P. Relation of ventilatory impairment and of chronic mucus hypersecretion to mortality from obstructive lung disease and from all causes. Thorax 1990;45:579-85.

125. Buist AS, Vollmer WM, Johnson LR. Does the single breath N_2 test identify the susceptible individual? Chest 1984;85:10S.

126. Anthonisen NR. Prognosis in chronic obstructive lung disease; Results from multicenter clinical trials. Am Rev Respir Dis 1989;133:S95-S99.

127. Anthonisen NR, Connett JE, Kiley JP, et al. Lung Health Study Group. The effects of smoking intervention and the use of an inhaled anticholinergic bronchodilator on the rate of decline of FEV_1: The Lung Health Study. JAMA 1994;272:1497-1505.

128. Camilli AE, Burrows B, Knudson RJ, Lyle SK, Lebowitz MD. Longitudinal changes in forced expiratory volume in one second in adults: Effects of smoking and smoking cessation. Am Rev Respir Dis 1987;135:794-97.

129. Higgins MW, Keller JB, Baker M, et al. An index of risk for obstructive airways disease. Am Rev Respir Dis 1982;125:144-51.

130. Postma DS, Sluiter HJ. Prognosis of chronic obstructive pulmonary disease: The Dutch experience. Am Rev Respir Dis 1989;140:S100-S05.

131. Flenley DC. Pathogenesis of pulmonary emphysema. QJ Med 1986;61:901-09.

132. Janoff A, Pryor WA, Bengali ZH. Effect of tobacco smoke components on cellular and biochemical pro-

cesses in the lung. Am Rev Respir Dis 1987;136: 1058-64.

133. Weitz JI, et al. Increased neutrophil elastase activity in cigarette smokers. Ann Int Med 1987;107:680-82.

134. Giamonna ST. Effect of cigarette smoke and plant smoke on pulmonary surfactant. Am Rev Respir Dis 1967;96:539-41.

135. Balbi B, Aufiero A, Pesci A, et al. Lower respiratory tract inflammation in chronic bronchitis: Evaluation by bronchoalveolar lavage and changes associated with treatment with immucytal, a biological response modifier. Chest 1994;106:819-26.

136. Snider GL. The pathogenesis of emphysema- Twenty years of progress. Am Rev Respir Dis 1981;124:321-25.

137. Janoff A. Elastases and emphysema. Current assessment of the protease-antiprotease hypothesis. Am Rev Respir Dis 1985;132:417-33.

138. Costabel U, Maire K, Teschler H, Wang YM. Local immune components in chronic obstructive lung disease. Respiration 1992;59:(Suppl 1):17-19.

139. Sanguinetti CM. Oxidant/antioxidant imbalance: Role in the pathogenesis of COPD. Respiration 1992;59(Suppl 1):20-23.

140. Thurlbeck WM. Pathology of chronic airflow obstruction. Chest 1990;97(Suppl)6S-10S.

141. Matsuba K, Thurlbeck WM. Diseases of the smaller airways in chronic bronchitis. Am Rev Respir Dis 1973; 107:552-58.

142. Thurlbeck WM. Aspects of chronic airflow obstruction. Chest 1977;72:341-49.

143. Fletcher C, Pride N. Definition of emphysema, chronic bronchitis, asthma and airflow obstruction. 25 years on from the Ciba Symposium. Thorax 1984;39:81-85.

144. Petty TL (Guest Editor). Diagnosis and treatment of chronic obstructive pulmonary disease. Chest 1990; 97(Suppl):1S.

145. Nadel JA. Role of enzymes from inflammatory cells on airway submucosal gland secretion. Respiration 1991; 58(Suppl 1):3-5.

146. Huchon G. Risk factors for chronic bronchitis and chronic obstructive lung disease. Respiration 1991;58 (Suppl 1):10-12.

147. Bianco S, Sestini P. Hyperreactivity and bronchial obstruction. Respiration 1991;58(Suppl 1):30-33.

148. Sluiter HJ, Koeter GH, de Monchy JGR, et al. The dutch hypothesis (chronic nonspecific lung disease) revisited. Eur Respir J 1991;4:479-89.

149. Neurohumoral mechanisms in obstructive lung disease: Role of inhaled anticholinergic agents. Chest 1987;91 (Suppl):35S.

150. Linden M, Bo Rasmussen J, Piitulainen E, et al. Airway inflammation in smokers with non-obstructive and obstructive chronic bronchitis. Am Rev Respir Dis 1993;148:1226-32.

151. Lusuardi M, Capelli A, Cerutti CG, Spada EL, Donner CF. Airways inflammation in subjects with chronic

bronchitis who have never smoked. Thorax 1994; 49:1211-16.

152. Turato G, Di Stefano A, Maestrelli P, et al. Effect of smoking cessation on airway inflammation in chronic bronchitis. Am J Respir Crit Care Med 1995;152: 1262-67.

153. Postma DS, Renkema TEJ, Noordhoek JA, et al. Association between nonspecific bronchial hyper-reactivity and superoxide anion production by polymorphonuclear leukocytes in chronic airflow obstruction. Am Rev Respir Dis 1988;137:57-61.

154. Venge P, Rak S, Steinholtz L, Hakansson L, Lindblad G. Neutrophil function in chronic bronchitis. Eur Respir J 1991;4:536-43.

155. Snider GL. Emphysema: The first two centuries and beyond a historical overview, with suggestions for future research: Part 1 and 2. Am Rev Respir Dis 1992;146:1334-44 and 1615-22.

156. Dash S, Sen S, Behera D. High neutrophil myeloperoxidase activity in smokers. Blood 1991;77:1619.

157. Behera D, Dash S, Sen S. Neutrophil count and myeloperoxidase activity in Indian Bidi smokers. Respiration 1994;61:269-73.

158. Macklem PT, Mead J. Resistance of central and peripheral airways measured by a retrograde catheter. J Appl Physiol 1967;22:395.

159. Hogg JC, Macklem PT, Thurlbeck WM. Structure and nature of airway obstruction in chronic obstructive lung disease. N Engl J Med 1968;278:1355-60.

160. Butler J, Caro CG, Alcola R, Dubois AB. Physiological factors affecting airways resistance in normal subjects and in patients with obstructive airways disease. J Clin Invest 1960;39:584-91.

161. Dayman H. Mechanics of airflow in health and in emphysema. Clin Invest 1951;30:1175-90.

162. McLean KH. The histology of localized emphysema. Australas Ann Med 1957;6:282-94.

162A. McLean KH. The histology of generalized pulmonary emphysema. II. Diffuse emphysema. Australas Ann Med. 1957;6:203-17.

162B. McLean KH. The histology of generalized pulmonary emphysema. I. The genesis of the early centrolobular lesion: Focal emphysema. Australas Ann Med 1957; 6:124-40.

162C. McLean KH. The pathology of acute bronchiolitis A study of its evolution. II. The repair phase. Australas Ann Med 1957;6:29-43.

163. McLean KH. The pathogenesis of pulmonary emphysema. Am J Med 1958;25:62-74.

164. Cosio M, Ghezzo H, Hogg JC, et al. The relation between structural changes in small airways and pulmonary function changes. N Engl J Med 1978; 298:1277-81.

165. Wright JL, Lawson LM, Pare PD, Kennedy S, Wiggs B, Hogg JL. The detection of small airways disease. Am Rev Respir Dis 1984;129:989-94.

166. Hogg JC. Mechanisms of airways obstruction in COPD. Pulm Perspectives 1990;7(2):1-3.

167. Wright Casio M, Wiggs B, Hogg JL, et al. Morphologic grading scheme for membranous and respiratory bronchioles. Arch Pathol Lab Med 1985;109:163-65.

168. Berend N, Wright JL, Therlbeck WM, Marlin GE, Woolcock AJ. Small airway disease: Reproducibility of measurements and correlation with lung function. Chest 1981;79:263-66.

169. Petty TL, Silvers GW, Stanford RE, Baired MD, Mitchell RS. Small airway pathology is related to increased closing capacity and abnormal slope of phase III in excised human lung. Am Rev Respir Dis 1980;121: 449-56.

170. Baile EM, Wright JL, Parre PD, Hogg JL. The effect of acute small airway inflammation on pulmonary function in dogs. Am Rev Respir Dis 1982;126:298-301.

171. Balbi B. COPD: Is chemotaxis the key? Chest 2003; 123:983-86.

172. Domagaa-Kulawik J, Maskey-Warzchowska M, Kraszewska I, Chazan R. The cellular composition and macrophage phenotype in induced sputum in smokers and ex-smokers with COPD. Chest 2003;123:1054-59.

173. Chodosh S. Examination of sputum cells. N Engl J Med 1970;282,854-57.

174. Saetta M, Di Stefano A, Maestrelli P, et al. Activated T-lymphocytes, and macrophages in bronchial mucosa of subjects with chronic bronchitis. Am Rev Respir Dis 1993;147,301-06.

175. Di Stefano A, Turato G, Maestrelli P, et al. Up-regulation of adhesion molecules in the bronchial mucosa of subjects with chronic obstructive bronchitis. Am J Respir Crit Care Med 1994;149,803-10.

176. Jeffery PK. Structural and inflammatory changes in COPD: A comparison with asthma. Thorax 1998;53, 129-36.

177. Di Stefano A, Capelli A, Lusuardi M, et al. Decreased T lymphocyte infiltration in bronchial biopsies of subjects with severe chronic obstructive pulmonary disease. Clin Exp Allergy 2001;31,893-902.

178. Saetta M, Mariani M, Panina-Bordignon P, et al. Increased expression of the chemokine receptor CXCR3 and its ligand CXCL10 in peripheral airways of smokers with chronic obstructive pulmonary disease. Am J Respir Crit Care Med 2002;165,1404-09.

179. ML Janoff A. Possible mechanisms of emphysema in cigarette smokers: Release of elastase from human polymorphonuclear leukocytes by cigarette smoke condensate *in vitro*. Am Rev Respir Dis 1978;117, 317-25.

180. Sato E, Koyama S, Takamizawa A, et al. Smoke extract stimulates lung fibroblasts to release neutrophil and monocyte chemotactic activities. Am J Physiol 1999; 277,L1149-L1157.

181. Holland SM, Gallin JL. Neutrophils crystal. In RG West, JB Weibel ER (Eds): The lung scientific foundations (2nd edn). Lippincott-Raven: Philadelphia, PA, 1997;877-90.

182. Pan ZZ, Parkyn L, Ray A, et al. Inducible lung-specific expression of RANTES: Preferential recruitment of neutrophils. Am J Physiol 2000;279,L658-L666.

183. Parmar JS, Mahadeva R, Reed BJ, et al. Polymers of alpha(1)-antitrypsin are chemotactic for human neutrophils: A new paradigm for the pathogenesis of emphysema. Am J Respir Cell Mol Biol 2002;26,723-30.

184. Gompertz S, Stockley RA. A randomized, placebo-controlled trial of a leukotriene synthesis inhibitor in patients with COPD. Chest 2002;122,289-94.

185. Barnes PJ. Chronic obstructive pulmonary disease. N Engl J Med 2000;343,269-80.

186. Pauwels RA, Buist S, Calverley PMA, et al. Global strategy for the diagnosis, management and prevention of chronic obstructive pulmonary disease: NHLBI/WHO Global Initiative for Chronic Obstructive Lung Disease (GOLD) workshop summary. Am J Respir Crit Care Med 2001;163,1256-76.

187. Riise GC, Ahlstedt S, Larsson S, et al. Bronchial inflammation in chronic bronchitis assessed by measurements of cell products in bronchial lavage fluid. Thorax 1995;50,360-65.

188. Pesci A, Balbi B, Majori M, et al. Inflammatory cells and mediators in bronchial lavage of patients with chronic obstructive pulmonary disease. Eur Respir J 1998;12, 380-86.

189. Balbi B, Majori M, Bertacco S, et al. Inhaled cortico-steroids in stable COPD patients: Do they have effects on cells and molecular mediators of airway inflammation? Chest 2000;117,1633-37.

190. Tanino M, Betsuyaku T, Takeyabu K, et al. Increased levels of interleukin-8 in BAL fluid from smokers susceptible to pulmonary emphysema. Thorax 2002;57, 405-11.

191. Keatings VM, Collins PD, Scott DM, et al. Differences in interleukin-8 and tumor necrosis factor-alpha in induced sputum from patients with chronic obstructive pulmonary disease or asthma. Am J Respir Crit Care Med 1996;153,530-34.

192. Mikami M, Llewellyn-Jones CG, Bayley D, et al. The chemotactic activity of sputum from patients with bronchiectasis. Am J Respir Crit Care Med 1998;157, 723-28.

193. Traves SL, Culpitt SV, Russell REK, et al. Increased levels of the chemokines GRO and MCP-1 in sputum samples from patients with COPD. Thorax 2002;57,590-95.

194. Seggev JS, Thornton WH Jr, Edes TE. Serum leukotriene B4 levels in patients with obstructive pulmonary disease. Chest 1991;99,289-91.

195. De Boer WI, Sont JK, van Schadewijk A, et al. Monocyte chemoattractant protein 1, interleukin-8, and chronic airways inflammation in COPD. J Pathol 2000;190, 619-26.

196. Boyden SE Jr. The chemotactic effects of mixtures of antibody and antigen on polymorphonuclear leuko-cytes. J Exp Med 1962;115,453-66.

197. Marshall LJ, Perks B, Ferkol T, et al. IL-8 released constitutively by primary bronchial epithelial cells in culture forms an inactive complex with secretory component. J Immunol 2001;167,2816-23.

198. Pignatti P, Delmastro M, Perfetti L, et al. Is dithiothreitol affecting cells and soluble mediators during sputum processing? A modified methodology to process sputum. J Allergy Clin Immunol 2002;110,667-68.

199. Kelly MM, Leigh R, Horsewood P, et al. Induced sputum: Validity of fluid-phase IL-5 measurement. J Allergy Clin Immunol 2000;105,1162-68.

200. Rutgers SR, Postma DS, Ten Hacken NH, et al. Ongoing airway inflammation in patients with COPD who do not currently smoke. Thorax 2000;55,12-18.

201. Lusuardi M, Capelli A, Cerutti CG, et al. Airways inflammation in subjects with chronic bronchitis who have never smoked. Thorax 1994;489,1211-16.

202. Di Stefano A, Capelli A, Lusuardi M, et al. Severity of airflow limitation is associated with severity of airway inflammation in smokers. Am J Respir Crit Care Med 1998;158,1277-85.

203. Hautamaki RD, Kobayashi DK, Senior RM, et al. Requirement for macrophage elastase for cigarette smoke-induced emphysema in mice. Science 1997;277, 2002-04.

204. Mantovani A. The chemokine system: Redundancy for robust outputs. Immunol Today 1999;20,254-57.

205. Culpitt SV, de Matos C, Russell RE, et al. Effect of theo-phylline on induced sputum inflammatory indices and neutrophil chemotaxis in chronic obstructive pulmonary disease. Am J Respir Crit Care Med 2002;165,1371-76.

206. Beeh KM, Kornmann O, Buhl R, Culpitt SV, Giembycz MA, Barnes PJ. Neutrophil chemotactic activity of sputum from patients with COPD role of interleukin 8 and leukotriene B_4. Chest 2003;123:1240-47.

207. Thurlbeck WM. Pathology of chronic obstructive pulmonary disease. Clin Chest Med 1990;11:389-404.

208. Reid L. The pathology of emphysema. Lloyd-Luke, 1967, London.

209. Jamal K, Cooney TP, Fleetham JA, Thurlbeck WM. Chronic bronchitis. Correlation of morphological findings to sputum production and flow rates. Am Rev Respir Dis 1984;129:719-22.

210. Lumsden AB, McLean A, Lamb D. Goblet and Clara cells of human distal airways. Evidence for smoking induced changes in their numbers. Thorax 1984;39: 844-49.

211. Peters EJ, Morice R, Benner SE, et al. Squamous metaplasia of the bronchial mucosa and its relationship to smoking. Chest 1993;103:1429-32.

212. Dye JA, Adler KB. Effects of cigarette smoke on epithelial cells of the respiratory tract. Thorax 1994;49: 825-34.

213. Jeffery PK. Histological features of the airways in asthma and COPD. Respiration 1992;59(Suppl 1):13-16.

214. Wohl MEB, Chrenick V. Bronchiolitis. Am Rev Respir Dis 1978;118:759-81.
215. Wright JL, Cagle P, Churge A, Colby TV, Myers J. Diseases of the small airways. Am Rev Respir Dis 1992;146:240-62.
216. Kuwano K, Bosken CH, Pare PD, et al. Small airways dimensions in asthma and in chronic obstructive pulmonary disease. Am Rev Respir Dis 1993;148:1220-25.
217. Beinert T, Brand P, Behr J, Vogelmeier C, Heider J. Peripheral airspace dimensions in patients with COPD. Chest 995;108:998-1003.
218. Fiaux GW, Gilloly M, Stewart JA, Hulmes DJS, Lamb D. Collagen content of alveolar wall tissue in emphysematous and nonemphysematous lungs. Thorax 1994;49:319-26.
219. Nagai A, Yamawaki I, Takizawa T, Thurlbeck WM. Alveolar attachments in emphysema of human lungs. Am Rev Respir Dis 1991;144:888-91.
220. Nagai A, Thurlbeck W. Scanning electron microscopic observations of emphysema in humans. A descriptive study. Am Rev Respir Dis 1991;144:901-08.
221. Thurlbeck WM. Overview of the pathology of emphysema in human. Clin Chest Med 1983;4;337-50.
222. Hogg JC, Wright JL, Wiggs BR, et al. Lung structure and function in cigarette smokers. Thorax 1994;49:473-78.
223. Verbeken EK, Cauberghs M, Mertens I, et al. The senile lung: Comparison with normal and emphysematous lungs: 1. Structural aspects. Chest 1992;101:793-99.
224. Verbeken EK, Cauberghs M, Mertens I, et al. The senile lung: Comparison with normal and emphysematous lungs: 2. Functional aspects. Chest 1992;101:800-09.
225. Buist AS, Connett JF, Miller RD, et al. Chronic obstructive pulmonary disease early intervention trial (Lung Health Study). Baseline characteristics of randomized participants. Chest 993;103:1863-72.
226. Medical Research Council. Standardized questionnaires on respiratory symptoms. 1960;2:1665.
227. Wijkstra PJ, Ten Vergert EM, Van Altena, et al. Reliability and validity of the chronic respiratory questionnaire (CRQ). Thorax 1994;49:465-67.
228. Badgett RG, Tanaka DJ, Hunt DK, et al. The clinical evaluation for diagnosing obstructive lung disease in high risk patients. Chest 1994;106:1427-31.
229. Palange P, Forte S, Felli A, et al. Nutritional state and exercise tolerance in patients with COPD. Chest 1995;107:1206-12.
230. O'Donnel DE. Breathlessness in patients with chronic airflow limitation: Mechanisms and management. Chest 1994:106:904-12.
231. Mahler DA, Faryniarz K, Tomlinson D, et al. Impact of dyspnoea and physiologic function on general health status in patients with chronic obstructive pulmonary disease. Chest 1992;102:395-401.
232. Hanafin E. The pattern of respiratory muscle recruitment during pursed lip breathing. Chest 1992;101:75-78.
233. Van der Schans CP, de Jong W, de Vries G, et al. Oxygen consumption of respiratory muscles of patients with COPD. Chest 1994;105:782-89.
234. Shindoh C, Hida W, Kikuchi Y, et al. Oxygen consumption of respiratory muscles of patients with COPD. Chest 1994;105:790-97.
235. Frankfort JD, Fischer CE, Stansbury DW, McArthur DL, Brown CE, Light RW. Effects of high- and low-carbohydrate meals on maximum exercise performance in chronic airflow obstruction. Chest 1991;100:792-95.
236. Ryan CF, Road JD, Buckley PA, Ross C, Whittaker JS. Energy balance in stable malnourished patients with chronic obstructive pulmonary disease.. Chest 1993;103:1038-44.
237. Campbell EJM. Physical signs of diffuse airways obstruction and lung distension. Thorax 1969;24:1.
238. Stubbing DG, Mathur PN, Roberts RS, Campbell EJM. Some physical signs in patients with chronic air flow obstruction. Am Rev Respir Dis 1982;125:549-52.
239. Kern DJ, Patel SR. Auscultated forced expiratory time as a clinical and epidemiologic test of airway obstruction. Chest 1991;100:636-39.
240. Kilburn KH, Warshaw RH, Thornton JC. Do radiographic criteria for emphysema predict physiologic impairment? Chest 1995;107:1225-31.
241. Simon G, Medei VC. Chronic bronchitis: Radiological aspects of a 5 year follow-up. Thorax 1962;17:5-8.
242. Sanders C. The radiographic diagnosis of emphysema. Radiol Clin North Am 1991;29:1019-30.
243. Thurlbeck WM, Simon G. Radiological appearance of the chest in emphysema. Am J Radiol 1978;130:429-40.
244. Sultinen S, Christoforidis AJ, Klugh GA, et al. Roentgenologic criteria for the recognition of non-symptomatic pulmonary emphysema. Am Rev Respir Dis 1965;91:69-76.
245. Musk AW, Gandevia B, Palmer FJ. Peripheral pooling of bronchographic contrast material: Evidence of its relationship to smoking and emphysema. Thorax 1978;33:193-200.
246. Muller ML (Ed). CT diagnosis of emphysema. It may be accurate, but is it relevant? Chest 1993;103:329-30.
247. Hruban RH, Meziane MA, Zerhouni EA, et al. High resolution computed tomography of inflation-fixed lungs: Pathologic radiologic correlation of centrilobular emphysema. Am Rev Respir Dis 1987;136:935-40.
248. Miller RR, Muller NL, Vedal S, Morrison NJ, Staples CA. Limitations of computed tomography in the assessment of emphysema. Am Rev Respir Dis 1989;139-980-83.
249. Kuwano K, Matsuba K, Ikeda T, et al. The diagnosis of mild emphysema: Correlation of computed tomography and pathology scores. Am Rev Respir Dis 1990;141:169-78.

250. Begin RO, Filion R, Ostiguy G. Emphysema in silica- and asbestos-exposed workers seeking compensation: A CT scan study. Chest 1995;108:647-56.

251. Watanuki Y, Suzuki S, Nishikawa M, Miyashita A, Okubo T. Correlation of quantitative CT with selective alveolobronchogram and pulmonary function tests in emphysema. Chest 1994;106:806-12.

252. Klein JS, Gamsu G, Webb WR, Golden JA, Muller NL. High resolution CT diagnosis of emphysema in symptomatic patients with normal chest radiographs and low diffusing capacity. Radiology 1992;182:817-21.

253. Bense L, Lewander R, Eklund G, Odont D, et al. Nonsmoking, Non-alpha-1-antitrypsin deficiency-induced emphysema in nonsmokers with healed spontaneous pneumothorax, identified by computed tomography of the lungs. Chest 1993;103:433-38.

254. Bates DV. Respiratory function in disease (3rd edn). WB Saunders: New York 1989;172-87.

255. Buist AS, Van Fleet DL, Ross BB. A comparison of conventional spirometric tests and the test of closing volume in an emphysema screening center. Am Rev Respir Dis 1973;107:735-43.

256. Shepard RH, Cohn JE, Cohen G, et al. The maximal diffusing capacity of the lung in chronic obstructive disease of the air ways. Am Rev Tuberc 1955;71:249-59.

257. Morrison NJ, Abboud RT, Muller NL, et al. Comparison of single breath carbon monoxide diffusing capacity and pressure volume curves in detecting emphysema. Am rev Respir Dis 1989;141:1179-87.

258. Bedell GN, Ostiguy GL. Transfer factor for carbon monoxide in patients with airways obstruction. Clin Sc 1967;32:239-48.

259. West WW, Nagai A, Hodgkin JE, Thurlbeck WM. The National Institute of Health intermittent positive pressure breathing trial- pathology studies. Am Rev Respir Dis 1987;135:123-29.

260. Thurlbeck WM, Hendersen JA, Fraser RC, Bates DV. Chronic obstructive lung disease. Medicine 1970;49:81.

261. Hugh-Jones P, Whimster W. The aetiology and management of disabling emphysema. Am Rev Respir Dis 1978;117:343-78.

262. Emmanuel G, Briscoe WA, Cournand A. A method for the determination of the volume of air in the lungs; measurement in chronic pulmonary emphysema. J Clin Invest 1961;40:329-37.

263. Prasad J, Kataria S, Behera D, Bansal SK. Total lung capacity estimation: Comparison of radiologic and Helium dilution methods. Lung India 1990;8:191-94.

264. Flenly DC, Millar JS. Ventilatory response to oxygen and carbon dioxide in chronic respiratory failure. Clin Sc 1967;33:319-34.

265. Bradly CA, Fleetham JA, Anthonisen NR. Ventilatory control in patients with hypoxemia due to obstructive lung disease. Am Rev Respir Dis. 1979;120:21-30.

266. Kawakami Y, Irie T, Shida A, Yoshikawa T. Familial factors affecting arterial blood gas values and respiratory chemosensitivity in chronic obstructive pulmonary disease. Am Rev Respir Dis 1982;125:420-25.

267. Fleetham JA, Arnup ME, Anthonisen NR. Familial aspects of ventilatory control in patients with chronic obstructive pulmonary disease. Am Rev Respir Dis 1984;129:3-7.

268. Berry RB, Mahutte CK, Kirsch JL, Stansbury W, Light RW. Does the hypoxic ventilatory response predict the oxygen induced falls in ventilation in COPD? Chest 1993;103:820-24.

269. Altose MD, McCauley WC, Kelsen SG, Cherniack NS. Effects of hypercapnia and inspiratory flow resistive loading on respiratory activity in chronic airways obstruction. J Clin Invest 1977;59:500.

270. Stone PJ, Morris TA III, Franzblau C, Snider GL. Hypercapnic ventilatory response in patients with lung disease: improved accuracy by correcting for ventilatory ability. Respiration 1995;62:70-75.

271. Belman MJ. Exercise in chronic obstructive pulmonary disease. Clin Chest Med 1986;7:585-97.

272. Carter R, Nicotra B, Blevins W, Holiday D. Altered exercise gas exchange and cardiac function in patients with mild chronic obstructive pulmonary disease. Chest 1993;103:745-50.

273. Vaz Fragoso CA, Clark T, Kotch A. The tidal volume response to incremental exercise in COPD. Chest 1993;103:1438-41.

274. Postma DS, Van Altena R, Kraan J, Koeter GH. Relation of lung function, maximal inspiratory pressure, dyspnoea and quality of life with exercise capacity in patients with chronic obstructive pulmonary disease. Thorax 1994;49:468-72.

275. Marin JM, Hussain NA, Gibbons WJ, et al. Relationship of resting lung mechanics and exercise pattern of breathing in patients with chronic obstructive lung disease. Chest 1993;104:705-11.

276. Pollock M, Roa J, Benditt JO, Celli BR. Estimation of ventilatory reserve by stair climbing: A study in patients with chronic obstructive lung disease. Chest 1993;104: 1378-83.

277. LoRusso TJ, Belman MJ, Elashoff JD, Koerner SK. Prediction of maximal exercise capacity in obstructive and restrictive pulmonary disease. Chest 1993:104:1748-54.

278. Whipp BJ. Carotid bodies in humans. Thorax 1994; 49:1081-84.

279. Ayers SM, Gianneli S. Causes of hypoxemia in patients with obstructive pulmonary emphysema. Am J Med 1965;39:422-28.

280. West JB. Causes of carbon dioxide retention in chronic lung disease. New Engl J Med 1971;284:1232-36.

281. Bentiveglio LG, Beerel F, Stewart PB, et al. Studies of regional ventilation and perfusion in pulmonary emphysema using xenon-133. Am Rev Respir Dis 1963;88:315-29.

282. Vos PJE, Folgering HTM, Van Herwaarden CLA. Sufficient indication of nocturnal oxygen desaturation and breathing pattern in COPD patients from a single night study. Resp Med 1995;89:615-16.

283. Baldwin DR, Bates AJ, Evans AH, Bradbury SP, Pantin CFA. Nocturnal oxygen desaturation and exercise induced desaturation in subjects with chronic obstructive pulmonary disease. Resp Med 1995;89:599-601.

284. Enarson DA, Newman SC, Fan RL, Macarthur C. Chronic airways obstruction leading to chronic hypoxemic respiratory failure: An estimate of the size and trend of the problem in Canada. Bull Int Union Tuberc Lung Dis 1991;66:113-23.

285. Hume R. Blood volume changes in chronic bronchitis and emphysema. Br J Haematol 1968;15:131-39.

286. Smith JR, Landaw SA. Smokers polycythaemia. New Engl J Med 1978;298:6-10.

287. Balter MS, Daniak N, Chapman KR, Sorba SA, Rebuck AS. Erythropoietin response to acute hypoxemia in patients with chronic pulmonary disease. Chest 1992;102:482-85.

288. Roger TK, Sheedy W, Waterhouse J, Howard P, Morice AH. Haemodynamic effects of atrial natriuretic peptide in hypoxic chronic obstructive pulmonary disease. Thorax 1994;49:233-39.

289. Render ML, Weinstein AS, Blausein AS. Left ventricular dysfunction in deteriorating patients with chronic obstructive pulmonary disease. Chest 1995;107:162-68.

290. Volterrani M, Scalvini S, Mazzuero G, et al. Decreased heart rate variability in patients with chronic obstructive lung disease. Chest 1994;106:1432-37.

291. Schulman LL, Lennon PF, Wood JA, Enson Y. Pulmonary vascular resistance in emphysema. Chest 1994;798-805.

292. Murphy TF, Sethi S. Bacterial infection chronic obstructive pulmonary disease. Am Rev Respir Dis 1992;146: 1067-83.

293. Monso E, Ruiz J, Rossel A, et al. Bacterial infection in chronic obstructive lung disease. A study of stable and exacerbated outpatients using the protected specimen brush. Am J Respir Crit Care Med 1995;152:1316-20.

294. Sachs APE, Koeter GH, Groenier KH, et al. Changes in symptoms, peak expiratory flow, and sputum flora during treatment with antibiotics of exacerbations in patients with chronic obstructive lung disease in general practice. Thorax 1995;50:758-63.

295. Paz HL, Wood CA. Pneumonia and chronic obstructive lung disease. What special considerations does this combination require? Postgrad Med 1991;90:77-86.

296. Fox R, French N, Daris L, et al. Influenza immunization status and viral respiratory tract infection in patients with chronic airflow limitation. Respir Med 1995;89: 559-61.

297. Kesten S, Rebuch AS. Is the short-term response to inhaled beta adrenergic agonist sensitive or specific for distinguishing between asthma and COPD? Chest 1994;1042-45.

298. Bellia V, Battaglia S, Catalano F, Scichilone N, Incalzi RA, Imperiale C, Rengo F. Aging and disability affect misdiagnosis of COPD in elderly asthmatics The SARA study. Chest 2003;123:1066-72.

299. Burrows B, Barbee RA, Cline, MG, et al. Characteristics of asthma among elderly adults in a sample of the general population. Chest 1991;100,935-42.

300. Lee HY, Stretton TB. Asthma in the elderly. Br Mmed J 1972;4,93-95.

301. Connolly MJ, Crowley JJ, Charan NB, et al. Reduced subjective awareness of bronchoconstriction provoked by methacholine in elderly asthmatic and normal subjects as measured on a simple awareness scale. Thorax 1992;47,410-13.

302. Patterson CJ, Dow L, Teale C. Prevalence of under-diagnosed airflow limitation in acute elderly admission. Age Ageing 1996;25(suppl 1):27.

303. Magnussen, H, Richter, K, Taube C. Are chronic obstructive pulmonary disease (COPD) and asthma different diseases? Clin Exp Allergy 1998;28(Suppl 5):187-94.

304. Enright PL, McClelland RL, Newman AB, et al. Underdiagnosis and undertreatment of asthma in the elderly: Cardiovascular Health Study Research Group. Chest 1999;116:603-13.

305. Antonisen NR, Wright EC, Hodgkin JE. Prognosis in chronic obstructive lung disease. Am Rev Respir Dis 1986;133:14-20.

306. Peto R, Speizer FE, Cochrane AL, et al. The relevance in adults of airflow obstruction, but not of mucus hypersecretion, to mortality from chronic lung disease: Results from 20 years of prospective observation. Am Rev Respir Dis 1983;128:491-500.

307. Speizer FE. Overview and summary. The rise in chronic obstructive pulmonary disease mortality. Am Rev Respir Dis 1989:140(Suppl):S106-S107.

308. Hentel W, Longfield AN, Vincent T, Filley GF, Mitchell RS. Fatal chronic bronchitis. Am Rev Respir Dis 1963;87:216-27.

309. Anthonisen NR. Prognosis in chronic obstructive pulmonary disease. Results from multicenter clinical trials. Am Rev Respir Dis 1989;140(Suppl):S95-S99.

310. Hodgkin JE. Prognosis in chronic obstructive pulmonary disease.. Clin Chest Med 1990;11:555-69.

311. West WW, Nagai A, Hodgkin JE, Thurlbeck WM. The National Institute of Health Intermittent Positive Pressure Breathing trial—Pathology Studies. III. The diagnosis of emphysema. Am Rev Respir Dis 1987;135: 123-29.

312. Rieves RD, Bass D, Carter R, Griffith JE, Norman JR. Severe COPD and acute respiratory failure. Correlates for survival at the time of tracheal intubation. Chest 1993;104:854-60.

313. Cote TR, Stroup DF, Dwyer DM, Horan JM, Peterson DE. Chronic obstructive pulmonary disease. A role for altitude. Chest 1993;103:1194-97.

314. Fuso L, Incalzi RA, Pistelli R, et al. Predicting mortality of patients hospitalized for acutely exacerbated chronic obstructive pulmonary disease. Am J Med 1995;98: 272-77.

315. Dallari R, Barozzi G, Pinelli G, et al. Predictors of survival in subjects with chronic obstructive pulmonary disease treated with long term oxygen therapy. Respiration 1994;61:8-13.

316. Cooper CB. Life expectancy in severe COPD. (Editorial). Chest 1994;105:335-57.

317. Pierre EP, Jamart J, Machiels J, Smeets F, Lulling J. Prognosis of severe hypoxemic patients under long term oxygen therapy. Chest 1994;105:469-74.

318. Dubois PEP, Jamart J, Machiels J, Smeets F, Lulling J. Prognosis of severe hypoxemic patients under long term oxygen therapy. Chest 1994;105:469-74.

319. Dallari R, Barozzi G, Pinneli G, et al. Predictors of survival in subjects with chronic obstructive pulmonary disease treated with long term oxygen therapy. Respiration 1994;61:8-13.

320. Skwarski K, MacNee W, Wraith PK, Silwinski P, Zielinski J. Predictors of survival in patients with chronic obstructive pulmonary disease treated with long term oxygen therapy. Chest 1991;100:1522-27.

321. American Thoracic Society. Lung function testing: Selection of reference values and interpretative strategies (Statement). Am Rev Respir Dis 1991;144:1201-18.

322. Soffer A. The greatest international killer. Chest 1992;101:1-2.

323. Samet JM. The 1990 report of the Surgeon General: The health benefits of smoking cessation. Am Rev Respir Dis 1990;142:993-94.

324. Swan GE, Hodgkin JE, Roby T, et al. Reversibility of airways injury over a 12-month period following smoking cessation. Chest 1992;101:607-12.

325. Banner AS. The war against cigarette smoking: The final battles. Chest 1994;106:662-63.

326. Jarvis MJ. Smoking cessation: Time for action. Thorax 1995;50(Suppl 1):S22-S24.

327. Anthonisen NR, Connett JE, Kiley JP, et al. Effects of smoking intervention and the use of inhaled anticholinergic bronchodilator on the rate of decline of FEV1: The lung Health Study. JAMA 1994;272:1497-1505.

328. Moxham J, Munro A. The BTS and Doctors for Tobacco law: Working towards ending tobacco advertising. Thorax 1995;50:6-8.

329. Behera D. Attitude of chronic bronchitic patients towards smoking. Lung India 1992;10:138-39.

330. Pederson I, Williams J, Lefooe N. Smoking cessation among pulmonary patients as related to type of respiratory disease and demographic variables. Can J Publ Health 1980;71:191-94.

331. Edmunds M, Conner H, Jones C, Gorayeb R, Waranch H. Evaluation of multicomponent group smoking cessation programme. Prev Med 1991;20:404-13.

332. Koltke TE, Battista RN, DeFriese GH. Attributes of successful smoking cessation interventions in medical practice: A meta-analysis of 39 controlled trials. JAMA 1988;259:2882-89.

333. Rennard SI. Smoking and health: A physician responsibility. A statement of the Joint Committee on Smoking and Health. Chest 1995;108:1118-21.

334. Lee EW, D'Alonzo GE. Cigarette smoking, nicotine addiction, and its pharmacologic treatment. Arch Intern Med 1993;153:34-48.

335. Tang JL, Law M, Wald N. How effective is nicotine replacement therapy in helping people to stop smoking? Br Med J 1994;308:21-26.

336. Smoking cessation. Role of nicotine dependence. Chest 1988;93(Suppl):33S-78S.

337. Nett LM. A team approach to nicotine dependency treatment. Chest 1991;100:1484-85.

338. Prochaska JO, Goldstein MG. Process of smoking cessation. Clin Chest Med 1991;12:727-35.

339. Fagerstrom KO, Schneider NG. Measuring nicotine dependance: A review of the Fagerstrom Tolerance Questionnaire. J Behav Med 1989;12:159-82.

340. Fiore MC, Jorenby DE, Baker TB, Kenford SL. Tobacco dependence and the nicotine patch: Clinical guidelines for effective use. JAMA 1992;268:2687-94.

341. Wilson R. Influenza vaccination (Editorial). Thorax 1994;49:1079-80.

342. COMBIVENT Inhalation Aerosol Study Group. In chronic obstructive pulmonary disease, a combination of ipratropium and albuterol is more effective than either agent alone. Chest 1994;105:1411-19.

343. Anthonisen NR, Wright EC, IPPB Trial Group. Response to inhaled bronchodilators in COPD. Chest 1987;91:36S-39S.

344. Chang JT, Moran MB, Cugell DW, Webster JR. COPD in the elderly: A reversible cause of functional impairment. Chest 1995;108:736-40.

345. McNicholas WT, Mulloy E. Role of theophylline in severe chronic obstructive pulmonary disease. Postgrad Med J 1991;67(Suppl 4):S30-S33.

346. Addis GJ. What use is steady-state theophylline in severe chronic obstructive pulmonary disease: A preliminary report. Postgrad Med J 1991;67(Suppl 4): S34-S35.

347. Jenne JW. What role for theophylline? Thorax 1994; 49:97-100.

348. Fink G, Kaye C, Sulkes J, Gabbay U, Spitzer SA. Effect of theophylline on exercise performance in patients with severe chronic obstructive pulmonary disease. Thorax 1994;49:332-34.

349. Ramsdell J. Use of theophylline in the treatment of COPD. Chest 1995;107:206S-09S.

350. Eaton ML, Green BA, Church TR, et al. Efficacy of theophylline in "irreversible" airflow obstruction. Ann Intern Med 1980;92:758-61.

351. Jenne JW (Guest Ed). Rationale for the use of theophylline in COPD: Bronchodilatation and beyond. Chest 1987;92(Suppl):1S.

352. Mitenko PA, Ogilive RI. Rational intravenous doses of theophylline. N Engl J Med 1973;289:600-03.

353. Murciano D, Aubier M, Lecocguic Y, et al. Effects of theophylline on diaphragmatic strength and fatigue in patients with chronic obstructive pulmonary disease. N Engl J Med 1984;311:349-53.

354. Aubier M, Troyer AD, Simpson M, et al. Aminophylline improves diaphragm contractility. N Engl J Med 1981;305:249-52.

355. Gustaffson B, Perrson CGA. Effect of different bronchodilators on smooth muscle responsiveness to contractile agents. Thorax 1991;46:360-65.

356. Pauwels R, Van Renterghem D, Van der Straeten M, et al. The effect of theophylline and enorphylline on allergen induced bronchoconstriction. J allergy Clin Immunol 1985;76:583-90.

357. Murciano D, Aucair M, Parienti R, et al. A randomized controlled trial of theophylline in patients with severe chronic obstructive pulmonary disease. New Engl J Med 1989;320:1521-25.

358. Guyatt GH, Townsend M, Pugsley SO, et al. Bronchodilators in chronic airflow obstruction: effect on airway function, exercise capacity, and quality of life. Am Rev Respir Dis 1987;135:1069-74.

359. Mahler DA, Matthay RA, Snyder PE, et al. Sustained release theophylline reduces dyspnoea in nonreversible obstructive airway disease. Am Rev Respir Dis 1985;131:22-25.

360. Gorini M, Duranti R, Misuri G, et al. Aminophylline and respiratory muscle interaction in normal humans. Am Rev Respir Dis. 1994;149:1227-34.

361. Matthay RA, Mahler DA. Theophylline improves global cardiac function, and reduces dyspnoea in chronic obstructive pulmonary disease. J allergy Clin Immunol 1986;78:793-99.

362. Mathay RA, Berger NJ, Davies R, et al. Improvement in cardiac performance by oral long-acting theophylline in chronic obstructive pulmonary disease. Am Heart J 1982;104:1022-66.

363. Parker JO, Kelkar K, West RO. Hemodynamic effects of aminophylline on cor pulmonale. Circulation 1966;33:17-25.

364. Maren TH. The additive renal effects of oral aminophylline and trichlormethiazide in man. Clin Res 1961;9:57.

365. Iravani J, Melville GN. Theophylline and mucocilliary function. Chest 1987;92:38S-43S.

366. Kino R, day RO, Pierce GA, Fulde GWO. Aminophylline in the emergency department: Maximizing safety and efficacy. Chest 1991;100:1572-77.

367. Derby LE, Jick SS, Langlois JC, et al. Hospital admissions for xanthine toxicity. Pharmacotherapy 1990;10:112-14.

368. Sullivan P, Bekir S, Jaffar Z, et al. Antiinflammatory effects of low dose oral theophylline in atopic asthma. Lancet 1994;343:1006-08.

369. Karpel JP, Kotch A, Zinny M, Pesin J, Alleyne W. A comparison of inhaled ipratropium, oral theophylline plus inhaled beta-agonist, and the combination of all three in patients with COPD. Chest 1994;105:1089-94.

370. Nishimura K, Koyama H, Sogiura N, et al. The additive effects of theophylline on a high dose combination of inhaled salbutamol and ipratropium bromide in stable COPD. Chest 1995;107:652-56.

371. Popa VT. Clinical pharmacology of adrenergic drugs. J Asthma 1984;21:183-207.

372. Postma DS. Inhaled therapy in COPD: What are the benefits? Respir Med 1991;85:447-49.

373. Lofdahl CG, Svedmyr N. Beta-agonists- Friends or foes? Eur Respir J 1991;4:1161-65.

374. Ziment I. The beta agonist controversy. Impact in COPD. Chest 1995;107:196S-205S.

375. Kumar A, dev G, Steele D. Nonbronchodilator effect of pirbuterol and ipratropium in chronic obstructive pulmonary disease. Chest 1995;107:173-78.

376. Nava S, Crotti P, Currieri G, Fracchia C, Rampulla C. Effect of a beta-2 agonist (broxaterol) on respiratory muscle strength and endurance in patients with COPD with irreversible airway obstruction. Chest 1992;101:133-40.

377. Thomas P, Pugsley JA, Stewart JH. Theophylline and salbutamol improve pulmonary function in patients with irreversible chronic obstructive lung disease. Chest 1992;101:160-65.

378. Behera, D. Aerodynamics of aerosol deposition in lungs: Both in therapeutics and disease. Cardiothorac J 1995;1:12-19.

379. Ferguson GT, Funck-Brentano C, Fischer T, Darken P, Reisner C. Cardiovascular safety of salmeterol in COPD Chest 2003;123:1817-24.

380. Siefkin AD. Inhaled ipratropium bromide in the management of chronic obstructive pulmonary disease. Intern Med 1989;10:3.

381. Gross NJ, Skorodin MS. Role of the parasympathetic nervous system in airway obstruction due to emphysema. N Engl J Med 1984;311:421-25.

382. Ikeda A, Nishimura K, Koyama H, Izumi T. Bronchodilating effect of combined therapy with clinical dosage of ipratropium bromide and salbutamol in stable COPD: Comparison with ipratropium bromide alone. Chest 1995;107:401-05.

383. Guleria R, Behera D, Jindal SK. Comparison of bronchodilatation produced by an anticolinergic (Ipratropium bromide), a beta-adrenergic agent (fenoterol) and their combination in patients with chronic obstructive airway disease—An open trial. J Assoc Physicians Ind 1991;39:680-82.

384. Sandralee A, Hershey B, Maxwell SL, et al. Is an anticholinergic agent superior to a beta$_2$ agonist in improving dyspnoea and exercise limitation in COPD? Chest 1995;108:730-35.

385. Wesseling G, Mostert R, Wouters FM. A comparison of the effects of anticholinergic and beta₂ agonist and combination therapy on respiratory impedance in COPD. Chest 1992;101:166-73.

386. Tamaoki J, Chiyotani A, Tagaya E, Sakai N, Konno K. Effect of long term treatment with oxitropium bromide on airway secretion in chronic bronchitis and diffuse panbronchiolitis. Thorax 1994;49:545-48.

387. Koyama H, Nishimura K, Ikeda A, Izumi T. A comparison of bronchodilating effect of oxytropium bromide and fenoterol in patients with chronic obstructive lung disease. Chest 1993;104:1743-46.

388. Disse B, Speck GA, Rominger KL, et al. Tiotropium (Spiriva): Mechanical considerations and clinical profile in obstructive lung disease. Life Sci 1999;64,457-64.

389. Anthonisen NR, Connett JE, Kiley JP, et al. The effects of smoking intervention and the use of an inhaled anticholinergic bronchodilator on the rate of decline of FEV₁: The Lung Health Study. JAMA 1994;272,1497-1505.

390. Pauwels RA, Lofdahl CG, Laitinen LA, et al. Long-term treatment with inhaled budesonide in persons with mild chronic obstructive pulmonary disease who continue smoking. N Engl J Med 1999;340,1948-53.

391. Oga T, Nishimura K, Tsukino M, Sato S, Hajiro T, M Mishima M. A comparison of the effects of salbutamol and ipratropium bromide on exercise endurance in patients with COPD. Chest 2003;123:1810-16.

392. Mandella LA, Manfreda J, Warren CPW, et al. Steroid response in stable chronic obstructive pulmonary disease. Ann Intern Med 1982;96:17-21.

393. Clarke SW. Chronic bronchitis in the 1990s: Up-to-date treatment. Respiration 1991;58(Suppl 1):43-46.

394. Weir DC, Gove RI, Robertson AS, Berge PS. Response to corticosteroids in chronic airflow obstruction: Relationship to emphysema and airway collapse. Eur Rerspir J 1991;4:1220.

395. Dompeling E, van Schayck CP, van Grunsven PM, et al. Slowing the deterioration of asthma and chronic obstructive pulmonary disease observed during bronchodilator therapy by adding inhaled corticosteroids: A 4-years prospective study. Ann Intern Med 1993;118:770-78.

396. Ziment I. Pharmacologic therapy of obstructive airways disease. Clin Chest Med 1990;11:461-86.

397. de Jong JW, Postma DS, van der Mark TW, Koeter GH. Effect of nedocromil sodium in the treatment of nonallergic subjects with chronic obstructive pulmonary disease. Thorax 1994;49:1022-23.

398. Leeder SR. Role of infection in the cause and course of chronic bronchitis. J Infect Dis 1975;131:731-42.

399. McHardy VU, Inglis JM, Calder MA, Crofton JW. A study of infective and other factors in exacerbation of chronic bronchitis. Br J Dis Chest 1980;74:228-38.

400. Tager I, Speizer FE. Role of infection in chronic bronchitis. N Engl J Med 1975;292:563-71.

401. Anthonisen NR, Manfreda J, Warren CPW, et al. Antibiotic therapy in exacerbations of chronic obstructive pulmonary disease. Ann Intern Med 1987;106:194-204.

402. Rodnick JE, Gude JK. The use of antibiotics in acute bronchitis and acute exacerbations of chronic bronchitis. West J Med 1988;149:347-51.

403. Schlick W. Selective indications of use of antibiotics: When and what. Eur Respir Rev 1992;2:187-92.

404. Airway mucin. Am Rev Respir Dis 1991;144(Suppl):S1.

405. Petty TL. The national mucolytic study: Results of a randomized double blind placebo controlled study of iodinated glycerol in chronic obstructive bronchitis. Chest 1990;97:75-83.

406. Tabusso G. Task Group on Mucoactive drugs. Recommendations for guidelines on clinical trials of mucoactive drugs in chronic bronchitis and chronic obstructive lung disease. Chest 1994106:1532-37.

407. Vecchiarelli A, Dottorini M, Pietrella D, et al. Macrophage activation by N-acetyl-cystine in COPD patients. Chest 1994;105:806-11.

408. Johnson MA, Woolcock AA, Geddes DM. Dihydrocodeine for breathless in "pink puffer". Brit Med J 1983;286:675-77.

409. Robinson RW, Zwillich C. The effects of drugs on breathing during sleep. In Kryger MH, Roth T, Dement WC (Eds): Principles and practice of sleep medicine. WB Saunders: Philadelphia, 1989;501-12.

410. Knowlton AA. Current concepts in transcription, translation, and the regulation of gene expression: A primer for the clinician. Chest 1995;107:241-48.

411. Knoell DL, Wewers MD. Clinical implications of gene therapy for alpha-1 antitrypsin deficiency. Chest 1995;107:535-45.

412. Talpers S, Romberger DJ, Bunce SB, Pingleton SK. Nutritionally associated increased carbon dioxide production: Excess total calories vs high proportion of carbohydrate calories. Chest 1992;102:551-55.

413. Tarpy SP, Celli BR. Long term oxygen therapy. New Engl J Med 1995;333:710-14.

414. Nocturnal Oxygen Therapy Trial Group: Continuous or Nocturnal Oxygen Therapy in Hypoxemic Chronic Obstructive Lung Disease. Ann Intern Med 1980;93:391-98.

415. The Medical Research Council Working Party: Long-term domiciliary oxygen therapy in chronic hypoxic cor pulmonale complicating chronic bronchitis and emphysema. Lancet 1981;i:681-86.

416. Weitzenblum E, Apprill M, Oswald M. Benefits from long term oxygen therapy in chronic obstructive pulmonary disease patients. Respiration 1992;59(Suppl 2):14-17.

417. Findley LJ, Whelan DM, Moser KM. Long-term oxygen in COPD. Chest 1983;671-74.

418. Cooper CB, Howard P. An analysis of sequential physiologic changes in hypoxic cor pulmonale during long term oxygen therapy. Chest 1991;100:76-80.

419. Samsel RW, Schumacker PT. Oxygen delivery to the tissues. Eur Respir J 1991;4:1258-67.

420. Howard P, de Haller R. Domicilliary oxygen- by liquid or concentrator? Eur Respir J 1991;4:1284-87.

421. Soler M, Michel F, Perruchoud AP. Long-term oxygen therapy for cor pulmonale in patients with chronic obstructive pulmonary disease. Respiration 1991;58 (Suppl 1):52-56.

422. Fletcher EC, Donner CF, Midgren B, et al. Survival in patients with day time PaO_2 > 60 mm Hg with and without nocturnal oxyhaemoglobin desaturation. Chest 1992;101:649-55.

423. Cottrelli JJ, Openbrier D, Lave JR, Paul C, Garland JL. Home oxygen therapy: A comparison of 2- vs 6-month patient reevaluation. Chest 1995;107:358-61.

424. Campbell EJM. Oxygen therapy in diseases of chest. Br J Dis Chest 1964;58:149-57.

425. Berg BW, Dillard TA, Rajagopal KR, Mehm WJ. Oxygen supplement during air travel in patients with chronic obstructive pulmonary disease. Chest 1992;101:638-41.

426. Hagarty EM, Skorodin MS, Stiers WM, Jessen JA, Bellingon EC. Performance of a resorvoir nasal cannula (Oxymizer) during sleep in hypoxemic patients with COPD. Chest 1993;103:1129-34.

427. Ashutosh K, Mead G, Dunsky M. Early effects of oxygen administration and prognosis in chronic obstructive pulmonary disease and cor pulmonale. Am Rev Respir Dis 1983;127,399-404.

428. Woodcock AA, Gross ER, Geddes DM. Oxygen relieves breathlessness in "pink puffers." Lancet 1981;1:907-9.

429. Swinburn CR, Wakefield JM, Jones PW. Relationship between ventilation and breathlessness during exercise in chronic obstructive airways disease is not altered by prevention of hypoxaemia. Clin Sci 1984;67,515-19.

430. Davidson AC, Leach R, George RJD, et al. Supplemental oxygen and exercise ability in chronic obstructive airways disease. Thorax 1988;43,965-71.

431. Liss HP, Grant BJB. The effect of nasal flow on breathlessness in patients with chronic obstructive pulmonary disease. Am Rev Respir Dis 1988;137,1285-88.

432. Swinburn CR, Moulo H, Stone TN, et al. Symptomatic benefit of supplemental oxygen in hypoxemic patients with chronic lung disease. Am Rev Respir Dis 1991;143, 913-15.

433. Milic-Emili J. Intrinsic PEEP. In Vincent JL (Eds): Yearbook of intensive care and emergency medicine Springer-Verlag. Berlin: Germany 1994,477-81.

434. Bellemare F, Grassino A. Force reserve of the diaphragm in patients with chronic obstructive pulmonary disease. J Appl Physiol 1983;55,8-15.

435. Eltayara L, Becklake MR, Volta CA, et al. Relationship between chronic dyspnea and expiratory flow limitation in COPD patients. Am J Respir Crit Care Med 1996;154,1726-34.

436. Alvisi V, Mirkovic T, Nesme P, Guérin C, Milic-Emili J. Acute effects of hyperoxia on dyspnea in hypoxemia patients with chronic airway obstruction at rest. Chest 2003;123:1038-46.

437. Donner CF, Braghiroli A, Patessio A. Can long-term oxygen therapy improve exercise capacity and prognosis? Respiration 1992;59(Suppl 2):30-32.

438. Stewart AG, Howard P. Indications for long-term oxygen therapy. Respiration 1992;59(Suppl 2):8-13.

439. Brain JD. Aerosols and humidity therapy. Am Rev Respir Dis 1980;122:(Suppl):17.

440. Sutton PP, Pavia D, Bateman JRM, Clarke SW. Chest physiotherapy: A review. Eur J Respir Dis 1982;63:188.

441. Rochester DF, Goldberg SK. Techniques of respiratory therapy. Am Rev Respir Dis 1980;122(Suppl):133-56.

442. American Thoracic society. Pulmonary rehabilitation. Am Rev Respir Dis 1981;124:663-66.

443. Curtis JR, Deyo RA, Hudson LD. Pulmonary rehabilitation in chronic respiratory insufficiency: Health-related quality of life among patients with chronic obstructive pulmonary disease. Thorax 1994;49:162-70.

444. Keilty SEJ, Ponte J, Fleming TA, Moxnham J. Effects of inspiratory pressure support on exercise tolerance and breathlessness in patients with severe stable chronic obstructive pulmonary disease. Thorax 1994;49:990-94.

445. Reardon JZ, Awad ER, Normandin E, et al. The effect of comprehensive outpatients pulmonary rehabilitation on dyspnoea. Chest 1994;105:1046-52.

446. Renston P, Dimarco AF, Supinski GS. Respiratory muscle rest during nasal BIPAP ventilation in patients with stable severe COPD. Chest 1994;105:1053-60.

447. Haggerty MC, Wooley RS, Nair S. Respi-care: An innovative home care programme for the patient with chronic obstructive pulmonary disease. Chest 1991; 100:607-12.

448. Emery CF, Leatherman NE, Burker EJ, Macintyre NR. Psychological outcomes of a pulmonary rehabilitation programme. Chest 1991;100:613-17.

449. Punzal PA, Ries AL, Kaplan RM, Prewitt LM. Maximum intensity exercise training in patients with chronic obstructive pulmonary disease. Chest 1991:100:618-23.

450. Malik SK, Singh P. Recitation of 'Om': a useful breathing exercise for patients with chronic obstructive pulmonary diseases. Bull PGI 1982;16:119-121.

451. Willeput R, Vashaudez JP, Landers D, et al. Thoracoabdominal motion during chest physiotherapy in patients affected by chronic obstructive lung disease. Respiration 1983;44:204-14.

452. Gigliotti F, Coli C, Bianchi R, Romagnoli I, Lanini B, Binazzi B, Scano G. Exercise training improves exertional dyspnea in patients with COPD Evidence of the role of mechanical factors. Chest 2003;123:1794-1802.

453. Gigliotti F, Spinelli A, Duranti R, et al. Four weeks negative pressure ventilation improves respiratory function in severe hypercapnic patients. Chest 1994; 105:87-94.

454. Corrado A, de Paola E, Messori A, Bruscoli G, Nutini S. The effect of intermittent negative pressure

ventilation and long term oxygen therapy for patients with COPD: 4 years study. Chest 1994;105:95-99.

455. Leger P, Bedicam JM, Comette A, et al. Nasal intermittent positive pressure ventilation: Long term follow up in patients with severe chronic respiratory insufficiency. Chest 1994;105:100-05.

456. Campbell EJM. Management of respiratory failure. Br Med J 1964;2:1328.

457. Fernadez E, Tanchoco-Tan M, Make BJ. Methods to improve respiratory muscle function: Seminars in respiratory medicine. Pulmonary Rehabilitation 1993;14:446-65.

458. Benditt JO, Albert RK. Lung reduction surgery: Great expectations and a cautionary note. Chest 1995;107: 297-98.

459. Cooper JD. Technique to reduce air leak after resection of the emphysematous lung. Ann Thorac Surg 1994;57:1038-39.

460. Trulock F, Cooper JD. Reduction pneumoplasty for COPD. Chest 1994;106:52S.

461. Appleton S, Adams R, Porter S, Peacock M, Ruffin R. Sustained improvements in dyspnea and pulmonary function 3 to 5 years after lung volume reduction surgery. Chest 2003;123:1838-46.

462. Takayama T, Shindoh C, Kurokawa Y, Hida W, Kurosawa H, Ogawa H, Satomi S. Effects of lung volume reduction surgery for emphysema on oxygen cost of breathing. Chest 2003;123:1847-52.

463. National Center for Health Statistics. National vital statistics report. Centers for Disease Control and Prevention. Hyattsville, MD, 2002;(50):16.

464. American Thoracic Society. Standards for the diagnosis and care of patients with chronic obstructive pulmonary disease. Am J Respir Crit Care Med 1995; 152,S77-S121.

465. McSweeny A, Grant I, Heaton R, et al. Life quality of patients with chronic obstructive pulmonary disease. Arch Intern Med 1982;142,473-78.

466. Brantigan O, Mueller E. Surgical treatment of pulmonary emphysema. Am Surg 1957;23,789-804.

467. Cooper J, Trulock E, Triantafillou A, et al. Bilateral pneumectomy (volume reduction) for chronic obstructive pulmonary disease. Thorac Cardiovasc Surg 1995;109,106-19.

468. Keenan R, Landreneau R, Sciurba F, et al. Unilateral thoracoscopic surgical approach for diffuse emphysema. Thorac Cardiovasc Surg 1996;111,308-16.

469. Martinez F, Montes de Oca M, Whyte R, et al. Lung-volume reduction improves dyspnea, dynamic hyperinflation, and respiratory muscle function. Am J Respir Crit Care Med 1997;155,1984-90.

470. McKenna R Jr, Brenner M, Fischel R, et al. Should lung volume reduction surgery for emphysema be unilateral or bilateral? Thorac Cardiovasc Surg 1996;112,1331-39.

471. McKenna RJ, Brenner M, Gelb AF, et al. A randomized, prospective trial of stapled lung reduction vs laser bullectomy for diffuse emphysema. Thorac Cardiovasc Surg 1996;111,317-21.

472. Sciurba FC, Rogers RM, Keenan RJ, et al. Improvement in pulmonary function and elastic recoil after lung-reduction surgery for diffuse emphysema. N Engl J Med 1996;334,1095-99.

473. Criner G, Cordova FC, Leyenson V, et al. Effect of lung volume reduction surgery on diaphragm strength. Am J Respir Crit Care Med 1998;157,1578-85.

474. Criner G, Cordova F, Furukowa S, et al. Prospective randomized trial comparing bilateral lung volume reduction surgery to pulmonary rehabilitation in severe chronic obstructive pulmonary disease. Chest 1999; 160,2018-27.

475. Geddes D, Davies M, Koyama H, et al. Effect of lung-volume-reduction surgery in patients with severe emphysema. N Engl J Med 2000;343,239-45.

476. Gelb A, Zamel N, McKenna R, et al. Mechanism of short term improvement in lung function after emphysema resection. Am J Respir Crit Care Med 1996; 154,945-51.

477. Brenner M, McKenna R, Gelb A, et al. Dyspnea response following bilateral thoracoscopic staple lung volume reduction surgery. Chest 1997;112,916-23.

478. O'Donnell D, Webb K, Bertley J, et al. Mechanisms of relief of exertional breathlessness following unilateral bullectomy and lung volume reduction surgery in emphysema. Chest 1996;110,18-27.

479. Kotloff R, Tino G, Palevsky H, et al. Comparison of short-term functional outcomes following unilateral and bilateral lung volume reduction surgery. Chest 1998;113,890-95.

480. Stammberger U, Thurnheer R, Bloch K, et al. Thoracoscopic bilateral lung volume reduction for diffuse pulmonary emphysema. Eur J Cardiothorac Surg 1997;11,1005-10.

481. Young J, Fry-Smith A, Hyde C. Lung volume reduction surgery (LVRS) for chronic obstructive pulmonary disease (COPD) with underlying severe emphysema. Thorax 1999;54,779-89.

482. Cooper JD, Patterson GA, Sundaresan RS, et al. Results of 150 consecutive bilateral lung volume reduction procedures in patients with severe emphysema. Thorac Cardiovasc Surg 1996;112,1319-29.

483. Pompeo E, Marino M, Nofroni I, et al. Reduction pneumoplasty vs respiratory rehabilitation in severe emphysema: A randomized study. Ann Thorac Surg 2000;70,948-54.

484. Flaherty KR, Kazerooni EA, Curtis JL, et al. Short-term and long-term outcomes after bilateral lung volume reduction surgery: Prediction by quantitative CT. Chest 2001;119,1337-46.

485. Holohan T, Handelsman H. Lung-volume reduction surgery for end-stage chronic obstructive pulmonary disease. Agency for Health Care Policy and Research. Rockville, MD: publication No. 96-0062, 1996.

486. The National Emphysema Treatment Trial Research Group. Rationale and Design of The National Emphysema Treatment Trial: A prospective randomized trial of lung volume reduction surgery. Chest 1999; 116,1750-61.

487. Gelb AF, McKenna RJ, Brenner M, et al. Lung function 4 years after lung volume reduction surgery for emphysema. Chest 1999;116,1608-15.

488. Yusen RD, Lefrak SS, Gierada DS, Davis GE, Meyers BF, Patterson GA, Cooper JD. A prospective evaluation of lung volume reduction surgery in 200 consecutive patients. Chest 2003;123:1026-37.

489. Gelb AF, McKenna RJ Jr, Brenner M, et al. Lung function 5 years after lung volume reduction surgery for emphysema. Am J Respir Crit Care Med 2001;163, 1562-66.

490. Flaherty K, Kazerooni EA, Curtis JL, et al. Short-term and long-term outcome after bilateral lung volume reduction surgery: Prediction by quantitative computed-tomography. Chest 2001;119,1337-46.

491. Bloch KE, Georgescu C, Russi EW, et al. Gain and subsequent loss of lung function after lung volume reduction surgery in cases of severe emphysema with different morphologic patterns. J Thorac Cardiovasc Surg 2002;123,845-54.

492. Hamacher J, Bloch KE, Stammberger U, et al. Two years' outcome of lung volume reduction surgery in different morphologic emphysema types. Ann Thorac Surg 1999;68,1792-98.

493. Leyenson V, Furukawa S, Kuzma AM, et al. Correlation of changes in quality of life after lung volume reduction surgery with changes in lung function, exercise, and gas exchange. Chest 2000;118,728-35.

494. Yusen R. What outcomes should be measured in patients with COPD? Chest 2001;119,327-28.

495. Moy ML, Ingenito EP, Mentzer SJ, et al. Health-related quality of life improves following pulmonary rehabilitation and lung volume reduction surgery. Chest 1999;115,383-89.

496. Ries A, Kaplan R, Limberg T, et al. Effects of pulmonary rehabilitation on physiologic and psychosocial outcomes in patients with chronic obstructive pulmonary disease. Ann Intern Med 1995;122,823-32.

497. National Emphysema Treatment Trial Research Group. Patients at high risk of death after lung-volume-reduction surgery. N Engl J Med 2001;345,1075-83.

498. Cremona G, Higenbottam T, Wallwork J. Transplantation for end stage lung disease. Respiration 1991;58 (Suppl 1):22.

499. Wanke TH, Merkle M, Formanek D, et al. Effect of lung transplantation on diaphragmatic function in patients with Dillard TA, Moores LK, Bilello KL, Phillips YY. Thorax 1994;49:459-64.

500. Klink M, Quan S. Prevalence of reported sleep disturbances in a general population and their relationship to obstructive airway disease. Chest 1987;91:540-46.

501. Levi-Valensi P, Weitzenblum E, Rida Z, et al. Sleep related desaturation and daytime pulmonary haemodynamics in COPD patients. Eur Respir J 1992;5:301-07.

502. Fletcher E Luketi R, Miller T, Fletcher J. Exercise haemodynamics and gas exchange in patients with chronic pulmonary obstructive disease, sleep desaturation, and a day time paO_2 above 60 mm Hg. Am Rev Respir Dis 1989;140:1237-45.

503. Douglas N, Flenly D. Breathing during sleep in patients with chronic obstructive lung disease. Am Rev Respir Dis 1990;141:1055-70.

504. Connaughton J, Catteralli K, Elton R, Stradling J, Douglas N. Do sleep studies contribute to the management of patients with severe obstructive pulmonary disease? Am Rev Respir Dis 1988;138:341-44.

505. Fletcher E, Donner C, Midgren B, et al. Survival in COPD patients with daytime PaO_2 > 60 mm Hg with and without nocturnal oxyhaemoglobin desaturation. Chest 1992;101:649-55.

506. Dillard TA, Berg BW, Rajagopal KR, Dooley JW, Mehm WJ. Hypoxemia during air travel in patients with chronic obstructive pulmonary disease. Ann Intern Med 1989;111:362-67.

507. Dillard TA, Moores LK, Bilello KL, Phillips YY. The preflight evaluation: A comparison of the hypoxic inhalation test with hypobaric exposure. Chest 1995;107:352-57.

508. AMA Commission on Emergency Medical Services. Medical aspects of transportation aboard commercial aircraft. JAMA 1982;247:1007-11.

509. Kroenke K, Lawrence VA, Theroux JF, Tuley MR, Hilsenbeck S. Postoperative complications after thoracic and major abdominal surgery in patients with and without obstructive lung disease. Chest 1993;104:1445-51.

510. Merli GJ, Weitz HH. Approaching the surgical patient: Role of the medical consultant. Clin Chest Med 1993;14:205-10.

511. Zibrak JD, O'Donnell CR. Indications for preoperative pulmonary function testing. Clin Chest Med 1993; 14:227-36.

512. Ford GT, Rosenal TW, Clergue F, Whitelaw WA. Respiratory physiology in upper abdominal surgery. Clin Chest Med 1993;14:237-52.

513. Celli BR. Perioperative respiratory care of the patient undergoing upper abdominal surgery. Clin Chest Med 1993;14:253-61.

514. Sykes LA, Bowe EA. Cardiorespiratory effects of anaesthesia. Clin Chest Med 1993;14:211-26.

515. Gracey DR, Divertie MB, Didier EP. Preoperative pulmonary preparation of patients with chronic obstructive pulmonary disease. Chest 1979;76:123-29.

516. Celli BR, Rodriguez KS, Snider GL. A controlled trial of intermittent positive pressure breathing, incentive spirometry, and deep breathing exercise in preventing pulmonary complications after abdominal surgery. Am Rev Respir Dis 1984;130:12-15.

517. Anthonisen NR, Wright EC. Bronchodilator response in chronic obstructive pulmonary disease. Am Rev Respir Dis 1986;133,814-19.

518. Gross NJE, Skorodin MS. Cholinergic bronchomotor tone, estimates of its amount in comparison to normal. Chest 1989;96,984-87.

519. Nisar M, Earis JE, Pearson MG, et al. Acute bronchodilator trials in chronic obstructive pulmonary disease. Am Rev Respir Dis 1992;146,555-59.

520. Tantucci C, Duguet A, Similowski T, et al. Effect of salbutamol on dynamic hyperinflation in chronic obstructive pulmonary disease patients. Eur Respir J 1998;12,799-804.

521. Mahler DA, Donohue JF, Barbee RA, et al. Efficacy of salmeterol xinafoate in the treatment of COPD. Chest 1999;115,957-65.

522. Jones PW, Quirk FH, Baveystock CM, et al. A self-complete measure of health status for chronic airflow limitation: The St George's Respiratory Questionnaire. Am Rev Respir Dis 1992;145,1321-27.

523. Mahler DA, Harver A. Clinical measurement of dyspnea. Dyspnea, Futura Publishing. Mt Kisco: NY, 1990,75-126.

524. Gross JN. Outcome Measurements in COPD. Are We Schizophrenic? Chest 2003;123:1325-27.

APPENDIX 1

Global Strategy for the Diagnosis, Management, and Prevention of Chronic Obstructive Pulmonary Disease. GOLD Executive Summary. Updated 2007.

www.goldcopd.org; American Journal of Respiratory and Critical Care Medicine 2007;176:532-55.

Chronic obstructive pulmonary disease (COPD) remains a major public health problem. It is the fourth leading cause of chronic morbidity and mortality in the United States, and is projected to rank fifth in 2020 in burden of disease worldwide, according to a study published by the World Bank/World Health Organization. Yet, COPD remains relatively unknown or ignored by the public as well as public health and government officials. In 1998, in an effort to bring more attention to COPD, its management, and its prevention, a committed group of scientists encouraged the US National Heart, Lung, and Blood Institute and the World Health Organization to form the Global Initiative for Chronic Obstructive Lung Disease (GOLD). Among the important objectives of GOLD are to increase awareness of COPD and to help the millions of people who suffer from this disease and die prematurely of it or its complications. The first step in the GOLD program was to prepare a consensus report, *Global Strategy for the Diagnosis, Management, and Prevention of COPD*, published in 2001. The present, newly revised document in 2007 follows the same format as the original consensus report, but has been updated to reflect the many publications on COPD that have appeared. GOLD national leaders, a network of international experts, have initiated investigations of the causes and prevalence of COPD in their countries, and developed innovative approaches for the dissemination and implementation of COPD management guidelines.

The present information is on the basis of the 2007 update.

The guideline has emphized the following facts:

1. COPD is characterized by chronic airflow limitation and a range of pathologic changes in the lung, some significant extrapulmonary effects, and important comorbidities that may contribute to the severity of the disease in individual patients.

2. In the definition of COPD, the phrase "preventable and treatable" has been incorporated following the American Thoracic Society/European Respiratory Society recommendations to recognize the need to present a positive outlook for patients, to encourage the health care community to take a more active role in developing programs for COPD prevention, and to stimulate effective management programs to treat those with the disease.

3. The spirometric classification of severity of COPD now includes four stages: stage I, mild; stage II, moderate; stage III, severe; stage IV, very severe. A fifth category, "stage 0, at risk," that appeared in the 2001 report is no longer included as a stage of COPD, as there is incomplete evidence that the individuals who meet the definition of "at risk" (chronic cough and sputum production, normal spirometry) necessarily progress on to stage I. Nevertheless, the importance of the public health message that chronic cough and sputum are not normal is unchanged.

4. The spirometric classification of severity continues to recommend use of the fixed ratio post-bronchodilator FEV_1/FVC < 0.7 to define airflow limitation. Using the fixed ratio (FEV_1/FVC) is particularly problematic in patients with milder disease who are elderly because the normal process of aging affects lung volumes. Post-bronchodilator reference values in this population are urgently needed to avoid potential overdiagnosis.

5. Section 2, BURDEN OF COPD, provides references to published data from prevalence surveys to estimate that about 15 to 25 percent of adults aged 40 years and older may have airflow limitation classified as stage I mild COPD or higher and that the prevalence of COPD (stage I, mild COPD and higher) is appreciably higher in smokers and ex-smokers than in nonsmokers, in those over 40 years compared with those younger than 40, and higher in men than in women. The section also provides new data on COPD morbidity and mortality.

6. Cigarette smoke is the most commonly encountered risk factor for COPD and elimination of this risk factor is an important step toward prevention and control of COPD. However, other risk factors for COPD should be taken into account where possible, including occupational dusts and chemicals, and indoor air pollution from biomass cooking and heating in poorly ventilated dwellings—the latter especially among women in developing countries.

7. The section on pathology, pathogenesis, and pathophysiology, continues with the theme that inhaled cigarette smoke and other noxious particles cause lung inflammation, a normal response which appears to be amplified in patients who develop COPD. The section has been considerably updated and revised.

8. Management of COPD continues to be presented in four components: (*1*) assess and monitor disease, (*2*) reduce risk factors, (*3*) manage stable COPD, and (*4*) manage exacerbations. All components have been updated on the basis of recently published literature. Throughout it is emphasized that the overall approach to managing stable COPD should be individualized to address symptoms and improve quality of life.

9. In Component 4, Manage Exacerbations, a COPD exacerbation is defined as "an event in the natural course of the disease characterized by a change in the patient's baseline dyspnea, cough, and/or sputum that is beyond normal day-to-day variations, is acute in onset, and may warrant a change in regular medication in a patient with underlying COPD."

10. It is widely recognized that a wide spectrum of health care providers is required to ensure that COPD is diagnosed accurately, and that individuals who have COPD are treated effectively. The identification of effective health care teams will depend on the local health care system, and much work remains to identify how best to build these health care teams. A section on COPD implementation programs and issues for clinical practice has been included but it remains a field that requires considerable attention.

DEFINITION

Chronic obstructive pulmonary disease (COPD) is a preventable and treatable disease with some significant extrapulmonary effects that may contribute to the severity in individual patients. Its pulmonary component is characterized by airflow limitation that is not fully reversible. The airflow limitation is usually progressive and associated with an abnormal inflammatory response of the lung to noxious particles or gases.

The chronic airflow limitation characteristic of COPD is caused by a mixture of small airway disease (obstructive bronchiolitis) and parenchymal destruction (emphysema), the relative contributions of which vary from person to person. Airflow limitation is best measured by spirometry, because this is the most widely available, reproducible test of lung function.

Because COPD often develops in longtime smokers in middle age, patients often have a variety of other diseases related to either smoking or aging.[1] COPD itself also has significant extrapulmonary (systemic) effects that lead to comorbid conditions.[2] Thus, COPD should be managed with careful attention also paid to comorbidities and their effect on the patient's quality of life. A careful differential diagnosis and comprehensive assessment of severity of comorbid conditions should be performed in every patient with chronic airflow limitation.

Spirometric Classification of Severity and Stages of COPD

For educational reasons, a simple spirometric classification of disease severity into four stages is recommended (Table A1.1). Spirometry is essential for diagnosis and provides a useful description of the severity of pathologic changes in COPD. Specific spirometric cut points (e.g. post-bronchodilator FEV_1/FVC ratio < 0.70 or FEV_1 < 80, 50, or 30% predicted) are used for purposes of simplicity; these cut points have not been clinically validated. A study in a random population sample found that the post-bronchodilator FEV_1/FVC exceeded 0.70 in all age groups, supporting the use of this fixed ratio.[3] However, because the process of aging does affect lung volumes, the use of this fixed ratio may result in overdiagnosis of COPD in the elderly, especially in those with mild disease.

TABLE A1.1. Spirometric classification of chronic obstructive pulmonary disease severity based on post-bronchodilator FEV_1

Stage I: mild	FEV_1/FVC < 0.70
	$FEV_1 \geq 80\%$ predicted
Stage II: moderate	FEV_1/FVC < 0.70
	$50\% \leq FEV_1 < 80\%$ predicted
Stage III: severe	FEV_1/FVC < 0.70
	$30\% \leq FEV_1 < 50\%$ predicted
Stage IV: very severe	FEV_1/FVC < 0.70
	$FEV_1 < 30\%$ predicted *or* $FEV_1 < 50\%$ predicted plus chronic respiratory failure[*]

[*] Respiratory failure: Arterial partial pressure of oxygen (Pa_{O2}) < 8.0 kPa (60 mm Hg) with or without arterial partial pressure of CO_2 (Pa_{CO2}) > 6.7 kPa (50 mm Hg) while breathing air at sea level.

The characteristic symptoms of COPD are chronic and progressive dyspnea, cough, and sputum production. Chronic cough and sputum production may precede the development of airflow limitation by many years. This pattern offers a unique opportunity to identify smokers and others at risk for COPD, and to intervene when the disease is not yet a major health problem. Conversely, significant airflow limitation may develop without chronic cough and sputum production.

Stage I: mild COPD: Characterized by mild airflow limitation (FEV_1/FVC < 0.70, $FEV_1 \geq 80\%$ predicted). Symptoms of chronic cough and sputum production may be present, but not always. At this stage, the individual is usually unaware that his or her lung function is abnormal.

Stage II: moderate COPD: Characterized by worsening airflow limitation (FEV_1/FVC < 0.70, $50\% \leq FEV_1 < 80\%$ predicted), with shortness of breath typically developing on exertion and cough and sputum production sometimes also present. This is the stage at which patients typically seek medical attention because of chronic respiratory symptoms or an exacerbation of their disease.

Stage III: severe COPD: Characterized by further worsening of airflow limitation ($FEV_1/FVC < 0.70$, $30\% \le FEV_1 < 50\%$ predicted), greater shortness of breath, reduced exercise capacity, fatigue, and repeated exacerbations that almost always have an impact on patients' quality of life.

Stage IV: very severe COPD: Characterized by severe airflow limitation ($FEV_1/FVC < 0.70$, $FEV_1 < 30\%$ predicted *or* FEV_1 < 50% predicted plus the presence of chronic respiratory failure). Respiratory failure is defined as an arterial partial pressure of O_2 (Pa_{O2}) less than 8.0 kPa (60 mm Hg), with or without an arterial partial pressure of CO_2 (Pa_{CO2}) greater than 6.7 kPa (50 mm Hg) while breathing air at sea level. Respiratory failure may also lead to effects on the heart such as cor pulmonale (right heart failure). Clinical signs of cor pulmonale include elevation of the jugular venous pressure and pitting ankle edema. Patients may have stage IV COPD even if their FEV_1 is greater than 30 percent predicted, whenever these complications are present. At this stage, quality of life is very appreciably impaired and exacerbations may be life threatening.

Although asthma can usually be distinguished from COPD, in some individuals with chronic respiratory symptoms and fixed airflow limitation it remains difficult to differentiate the two diseases. In many developing countries, both pulmonary tuberculosis and COPD are common.[4] In countries where tuberculosis is very common, respiratory abnormalities may be too readily attributed to this disease.[5] Conversely, where the rate of tuberculosis is greatly diminished, the possible diagnosis of this disease is sometimes overlooked. Therefore, in all subjects with symptoms of COPD, a possible diagnosis of tuberculosis should be considered, especially in areas where this disease is known to be prevalent.[6]

MANAGEMENT OF COPD

Introduction

An effective COPD management plan includes four components: (*i*) assess and monitor disease, (*ii*) reduce risk factors, (*iii*) manage stable COPD, and (*iv*) manage exacerbations. Although disease prevention is the ultimate goal, once COPD has been diagnosed, effective management should be aimed at the following goals:

- Relieve symptoms
- Prevent disease progression
- Improve exercise tolerance
- Improve health status
- Prevent and treat complications
- Prevent and treat exacerbations
- Reduce mortality.

These goals should be reached with minimal side effects from treatment, a particular challenge in patients with COPD because they commonly have comorbidities. The extent to which these goals can be realized varies with each individual, and some treatments will produce benefits in more than one area. In selecting a treatment plan, the benefits and risks to the individual, and the costs, direct and indirect, to the individual, his or her family, and the community must be considered.

Patients should be identified as early in the course of the disease as possible, and certainly before the end stage of the illness when disability is substantial. Access to spirometry is key to the diagnosis of COPD and should be available to health care workers who care for patients with COPD. However, the benefits of community-based spirometric screening, of either the general population or smokers, are still unclear.

Educating patients, physicians, and the public to recognize that cough, sputum production, and especially breathlessness are not trivial symptoms is an essential aspect of the public health care of this disease.

Reduction of therapy once symptom control has been achieved is not normally possible in COPD. Further deterioration of lung function usually requires the progressive introduction of more treatments, both pharmacologic and nonpharmacologic, to attempt to limit the impact of these changes. Exacerbations of signs and symptoms, a hallmark of COPD, impair patients' quality of life and decrease their health status. Appropriate treatment and measures to prevent further exacerbations should be implemented as quickly as possible.

Component 1: Assess and Monitor Disease

KEY POINTS

- A clinical diagnosis of COPD should be considered in any patient who has dyspnea, chronic cough or sputum production, and/or a history of exposure to risk factors for the disease. The diagnosis should be confirmed by spirometry.
- For the diagnosis and assessment of COPD, spirometry is the gold standard because it is the most reproducible, standardized, and objective way of measuring airflow limitation. A post-bronchodilator $FEV_1/FVC < 0.70$ confirms the presence of airflow limitation that is not fully reversible.
- Health care workers involved in the diagnosis and management of patients with COPD should have access to spirometry.
- Assessment of COPD severity is based on the patient's level of symptoms, the severity of the spirometric abnormality, and the presence of complications.

- Measurement of arterial blood gas tensions should be considered in all patients with FEV_1 < 50% predicted or clinical signs suggestive of respiratory failure or right heart failure.
- COPD is usually a progressive disease and lung function can be expected to worsen over time, even with the best available care. Symptoms and objective measures of airflow limitation should be monitored to determine when to modify therapy and to identify any complications that may develop.
- Comorbidities are common in COPD and should be actively identified. Comorbidities often complicate the management of COPD, and vice versa.

Initial Diagnosis

A clinical diagnosis of COPD should be considered in any patient who has dyspnea, chronic cough or sputum production, and/or a history of exposure to risk factors for the disease (Table A1.2). The diagnosis should be confirmed by spirometry.

TABLE A1.2. Key indicators for considering a diagnosis of chronic obstructive pulmonary disease

Consider COPD, and perform spirometry, if any of these indicators are present in an individual. These indicators are not diagnostic themselves, but the presence of multiple key indicators increases the probability of a diagnosis of COPD. Spirometry is needed to establish a diagnosis of COPD.

Dyspnea that is	Progressive (worsens over time)
	Usually worse with exercise
	Persistent (present every day)
	Described by the patient as an "increased effort to breathe," "heaviness," "air hunger," or "gasping"
Chronic cough	May be intermittent and may be unproductive
Chronic sputum production	Any pattern of chronic sputum production may indicate COPD
History of exposure to risk factors, especially,	Tobacco smoke
	Occupational dusts and chemicals
	Smoke from home cooking and heating fuels

Definition of abbreviation: COPD = chronic obstructive pulmonary disease.

ASSESSMENT OF SYMPTOMS

Dyspnea, the hallmark symptom of COPD, is the reason most patients seek medical attention and is a major cause of disability and anxiety associated with the disease. As lung function deteriorates, breathlessness becomes more intrusive. Chronic cough, often the first symptom of COPD to develop[7] and often predating the onset of dyspnea, may be intermittent, but later is present every day, often throughout the day. In some cases, significant airflow limitation may develop without the presence of a cough. Patients with COPD commonly raise small quantities of tenacious sputum after coughing bouts. Wheezing and chest tightness are nonspecific symptoms that may vary between days, and over the course of a single day. An absence of wheezing or chest tightness does not exclude a diagnosis of COPD. Weight loss, anorexia, and psychiatric morbidity, especially symptoms of depression and/or anxiety, are common problems in advanced COPD.[8,9]

Medical History

A detailed medical history of a new patient known or believed to have COPD should assess the following:
- Exposure to risk factors
- Past medical history, including asthma, allergy, sinusitis, or nasal polyps; respiratory infections in childhood; other respiratory diseases
- Family history of COPD or other chronic respiratory disease
- Pattern of symptom development
- History of exacerbations or previous hospitalizations for respiratory disorder
- Presence of comorbidities, such as heart disease, malignancies, osteoporosis, and muscloskeletal disorders, which may also contribute to restriction of activity[10]
- Appropriateness of current medical treatments
- Impact of disease on patient's life, including limitation of activity, missed work and economic impact, effect on family routines, feelings of depression or anxiety
- Social and family support available to the patient
- Possibilities for reducing risk factors, especially smoking cessation.

Physical Examination

Although an important part of patient care, a physical examination is rarely diagnostic in COPD. Physical signs of airflow limitation are usually not present until significant impairment of lung function has occurred,[11,12] and their detection has a relatively low sensitivity and specificity.

Measurement of Airflow Limitation (Spirometry)

Spirometry should be undertaken in all patients who may have COPD. Spirometry should measure the volume of air forcibly exhaled from the point of maximal inspiration (FVC) and the volume of air exhaled during the first second of this maneuver (FEV_1), and the ratio of these two measurements (FEV_1/FVC) should be calculated. Spirometry measurements are evaluated by comparison with reference values[13] based on age, height, sex, and race (use appropriate reference values; e.g., *see* Reference 13). Patients with COPD typically show a decrease in both FEV_1 and FVC. The presence of airflow limitation is defined by a post-bronchodilator FEV_1/FVC < 0.70. This approach is pragmatic in view of the fact that universally applicable reference values for FEV_1 and FVC are not available. Where possible, values should be compared with age-related normal values to avoid overdiagnosis of COPD in the elderly.[14] Using the fixed ratio (FEV_1/FVC) is particularly problematic in patients with milder COPD who are elderly because the normal process of aging affects lung volumes.

Assessment of COPD Severity

Assessment of COPD severity is based on the patient's level of symptoms, the severity of the spirometric abnormality (Table A1.1), and the presence of complications such as respiratory failure, right heart failure, weight loss, and arterial hypoxemia.

Additional Investigations

For patients diagnosed with stage II, moderate, COPD and beyond, the following additional investigations may be considered.

Bronchodilator Reversibility Testing

Despite earlier hopes, neither bronchodilator nor oral glucocorticosteroid reversibility testing predicts disease progression, whether judged by decline in FEV_1, deterioration of health status, or frequency of exacerbations[15,16] in patients with a clinical diagnosis of COPD and abnormal spirometry.[16] In some cases (e.g. a patient with an atypical history such as asthma in childhood and regular night waking with cough or wheeze), a clinician may wish to perform a bronchodilator and/or glucocorticosteroid reversibility test.

Chest X-ray

An abnormal chest X-ray is seldom diagnostic in COPD unless obvious bullous disease is present, but it is valuable in excluding alternative diagnoses and establishing the presence of significant comorbidities, such as cardiac failure. Computed tomography (CT) of the chest is not routinely recommended. However, when there is doubt about the diagnosis of COPD, high-resolution CT scanning might help in the differential diagnosis. In addition, if a surgical procedure such as lung volume reduction is contemplated, a chest CT scan is necessary because the distribution of emphysema is one of the most important determinants of surgical suitability.[17]

Arterial Blood Gas Measurement

In advanced COPD, measurement of arterial blood gases while the patient is breathing air is important. This test should be performed in stable patients with FEV_1 < 50 percent predicted or with clinical signs suggestive of respiratory failure or right heart failure.

α_1-Antitrypsin Deficiency Screening

In patients of Caucasian descent who develop COPD at a young age (< 45 yr) or who have a strong family history of the disease, it may be valuable to identify coexisting α_1-antitrypsin deficiency. This could lead to family screening or appropriate counseling.

Differential Diagnosis

In some patients with chronic asthma, a clear distinction from COPD is not possible using current imaging and physiologic testing techniques, and it is assumed that asthma and COPD coexist in these patients. In these cases, current management is similar to that of asthma. Other potential diagnoses are usually easier to distinguish from COPD (Table A1.3).

TABLE A1.3. Differential diagnosis of chronic obstructive pulmonary disease

Diagnosis	Suggestive Features
COPD	Onset in midlife Symptoms slowly progressive Long history of tobacco smoking Dyspnea during exercise Largely irreversible airflow limitation
Asthma	Onset early in life (often childhood) Symptoms vary from day to day Symptoms at night/early morning Allergy, rhinitis, and/or eczema also present Family history of asthma Largely reversible airflow limitation
Congestive heart failure	Nonspecific basilar crackles on auscultation Chest X-ray shows dilated heart, pulmonary edema Pulmonary function tests indicate volume restriction, not airflow limitation
Bronchiectasis	Large volumes of purulent sputum Commonly associated with bacterial infection Coarse crackles/clubbing on auscultation Chest X-ray/CT shows bronchial dilation, bronchial wall thickening
Tuberculosis	Onset all ages Chest X-ray shows lung infiltrate Microbiological confirmation High local prevalence of tuberculosis
Obliterative bronchiolitis	Onset in younger age, nonsmokers May have history of rheumatoid arthritis or fume exposure CT on expiration shows hypodense areas
Diffuse panbronchiolitis	Most patients are male and nonsmokers Almost all have chronic sinusitis Chest X-ray and HRCT show diffuse small centrilobular nodular opacities and hyperinflation

Definition of abbreviations: COPD = chronic obstructive pulmonary disease; CT = computed tomography; HRCT = high-resolution computed tomography.

These features tend to be characteristic of the respective diseases, but do not occur in every case. For example, a person who has never smoked may develop COPD (especially in the developing world where other risk factors may be more important than cigarette smoking); asthma may develop in adult and even elderly patients.

Ongoing Monitoring and Assessment

Monitor disease progression and development of complications: COPD is usually a progressive disease. Lung function can be expected to worsen over time, even with the best available care. Symptoms and objective measures of airflow limitation should be monitored to determine when to modify therapy and to identify any complications that may develop.

Follow-up visits should include a physical examination and discussion of symptoms, particularly any new or worsening symptoms. Spirometry should be performed if there is a substantial increase in symptoms or a complication. The development of respiratory failure is indicated by a $Pa_{O_2} < 8.0$ kPa (60 mm Hg) with or without $Pa_{CO_2} > 6.7$ kPa (50 mm Hg) in arterial blood gas measurements made while breathing air at sea level. Measurement of pulmonary arterial pressure is not recommended in clinical practice as it does not add practical information beyond that obtained from a knowledge of Pa_{O_2}.

Monitor pharmacotherapy and other medical treatment: To adjust therapy appropriately as the disease progresses, each follow-up visit should include a discussion of the current therapeutic regimen. Dosages of various medications, adherence to the regimen, inhaler technique, effectiveness of the current regime at controlling symptoms, and side effects of treatment should be monitored.

Monitor exacerbation history: Frequency, severity, and likely causes of exacerbations should be evaluated. Increased sputum volume, acutely worsening dyspnea, and the presence of purulent sputum should be noted. Severity can be estimated by the increased need for bronchodilator medication or glucocorticosteroids and by the need for antibiotic treatment. Hospitalizations should be documented, including the facility, duration of stay, and any use of critical care or intubation.

Monitor comorbidities: Comorbidities are common in COPD and may become harder to manage when COPD is present, either because COPD adds to the total level of disability or because COPD therapy adversely affects the comorbid disorder. Until more integrated guidance about disease management for specific comorbid problems becomes available, the focus should be on identification and management of these individual problems.

Component 2: Reduce Risk Factors

KEY POINTS

- Reduction of total personal exposure to tobacco smoke, occupational dusts and chemicals, and indoor and outdoor air pollutants are important goals to prevent the onset and progression of COPD.
- Smoking cessation is the single most effective—and cost-effective—intervention in most people to reduce the risk of developing COPD and stop its progression (**Evidence A**).
- Comprehensive tobacco control policies and programs with clear, consistent, and repeated nonsmoking messages should be delivered through every feasible channel.
- Efforts to reduce smoking through public health initiatives should also focus on passive smoking to minimize risks for nonsmokers.
- Many occupationally induced respiratory disorders can be reduced or controlled through a variety of strategies aimed at reducing the burden of inhaled particles and gases.
- Reducing the risk from indoor and outdoor air pollution is feasible and requires a combination of public policy and protective steps taken by individual patients.

Smoking Prevention and Cessation

Comprehensive tobacco control policies and programs with clear, consistent, and repeated nonsmoking messages should be delivered through every feasible channel, including health care providers, community activities, and schools, and radio, television, and print media. Legislation to establish smoke-free schools, public facilities, and work environments should be developed and implemented by government officials and public health workers, and encouraged by the public.

Smoking Cessation Intervention Process

Smoking cessation is the single most effective—and cost-effective—way to reduce exposure to COPD risk factors. All smokers—including those who may be at risk for COPD as well as those who already have the disease—should be offered the most intensive smoking cessation intervention feasible. Even a brief (3 min) period of counseling to urge a smoker to quit results in smoking cessation rates of 5 to 10 percent.[18] At the very least, this should be done for every smoker at every health care provider visit.[18,19]

There are guidelines for smoking cessation. A Clinical Practice Guideline published by the US Public Health Service[20] recommends a five-step program for intervention (Table A1.4), which provides a strategic framework helpful to health care providers interested in helping their patients stop smoking (20-23).

TABLE A1.4. Brief strategies to help the patient who is willing to quit

1. Ask: Systematically identify all tobacco users at every visit.
   Implement an office wide system that ensures that, for *every* patient at *every* clinic visit, tobacco use status is queried and documented.
2. Advise: Strongly urge all tobacco users to quit.
   In a clear, strong, and personalized manner, urge every tobacco user to quit.
3. Assess: Determine willingness to make a quit attempt.
   Ask every tobacco user if he or she is willing to make a quit attempt at this time (e.g. within the next 30 d).
4. Assist: Aid the patient in quitting.
   Help the patient with a quit plan; provide practical counseling; provide intratreatment social support; help the patient obtain extratreatment social support; recommend use of approved pharmacotherapy except in special circumstances; provide supplementary materials.
5. Arrnage: Schedule follow-up contact.

   Schedule follow-up contact, either in person or via telephone.

PHARMACOTHERAPY

Numerous effective pharmacotherapies for smoking cessation now exist[20,21,24] (Evidence A), and pharmacotherapy is recommended when counseling is not sufficient to help patients quit smoking. Numerous studies indicate that nicotine replacement therapy in any form (nicotine gum, inhaler, nasal spray, transdermal patch, sublingual tablet, or lozenge) reliably increases long-term smoking abstinence rates.[20,25]

The antidepressants bupropion[26] and nortriptyline have also been shown to increase long-term quit rates [24,25,27], but should always be used as one element in a supportive intervention program rather than on their own. The effectiveness of the antihypertensive drug clonidine is limited by side effects.[25] Varenicline, a nicotinic acetylcholine receptor partial agonist that aids smoking cessation by relieving nicotine withdrawal symptoms and reducing the rewarding properties of nicotine, has been demonstrated to be safe and efficacious.[28-30] Special consideration should be given before using pharmacotherapy in the following selected populations: people with medical contraindications, light smokers (<10 cigarettes/d), and pregnant and adolescent smokers.

Occupational Exposures

Although it is not known how many individuals are at risk of developing respiratory disease from occupational exposures in either developing or developed countries, many occupationally induced respiratory disorders can be reduced or controlled through a variety of strategies aimed at reducing the burden of inhaled particles and gases [31-33].

The main emphasis should be on primary prevention, which is best achieved by the elimination or reduction of exposures to various substances in the workplace. Secondary prevention, achieved through surveillance and early case detection, is also of great importance.

Indoor and Outdoor Air Pollution

Individuals experience diverse indoor and outdoor environments throughout the day, each of which has its own unique set of air contaminants and particulates that cause adverse effects on lung function.[34] Although outdoor and indoor air pollution are generally considered separately, the concept of total personal exposure may be more relevant for COPD. Reducing the risk from indoor and outdoor air pollution is feasible and requires a combination of public policy and protective steps taken by individual patients. At the national level, achieving a set level of air quality standards should be a high priority; this goal will normally require legislative action. Reduction of exposure to smoke from biomass fuel, particularly among women and children, is a crucial goal to reduce the prevalence of COPD worldwide. Although efficient nonpolluting cooking stoves have been developed, their adoption has been slow due to social customs and cost.

The health care provider should consider COPD risk factors, including smoking history, family history, exposure to indoor/outdoor pollution, and socioeconomic status, for each individual patient. Those who are at high risk should avoid vigorous exercise outdoors during pollution episodes. Persons with advanced COPD should monitor public announcements of air quality and be aware that staying indoors when air quality is poor may help reduce their symptoms. If various solid fuels are used for cooking and heating, adequate ventilation should be encouraged. Under most circumstances, vigorous attempts should be made to reduce exposure through reducing workplace emissions and improving ventilation measures, rather than simply using respiratory protection to reduce the risks of ambient air pollution. Air cleaners have not been shown to have health benefits, whether directed at pollutants generated by indoor sources or at those brought in with outdoor air.

Component 3: Manage Stable COPD

KEY POINTS

- The overall approach to managing stable COPD should be individualized to address symptoms and improve quality of life.
- For patients with COPD, health education plays an important role in smoking cessation (Evidence A) and can also play a role in improving skills, ability to cope with illness, and health status.
- None of the existing medications for COPD have been shown to modify the long-term decline in lung function that is the hallmark of this disease (Evidence A). Therefore, pharmacotherapy for COPD is used to decrease symptoms and/or complications.
- Bronchodilator medications are central to the symptomatic management of COPD (Evidence A). They are given on an as-needed basis or on a regular basis to prevent or reduce symptoms and exacerbations.
- The principal bronchodilator treatments are β_2-agonists, anticholinergics, and methylxanthines used singly or in combination (Evidence A).
- Regular treatment with long-acting bronchodilators is more effective and convenient than treatment with short-acting bronchodilators (Evidence A).
- The addition of regular treatment with inhaled glucocorticosteroids to bronchodilator treatment is appropriate for symptomatic patients with COPD with an FEV_1 < 50 percent predicted (stage III, severe COPD, and stage IV, very severe COPD) and repeated exacerbations (Evidence A).
- Chronic treatment with systemic glucocorticosteroids should be avoided because of an unfavorable benefit-to-risk ratio (Evidence A).
- In patients with COPD, influenza vaccines can reduce serious illness (Evidence A). Pneumococcal polysaccharide vaccine is recommended for patients with COPD who are 65 years and older and for patients with COPD who are younger than age 65 with an FEV_1 < 40 percent predicted (Evidence B).
- All patients with COPD benefit from exercise training programs, improving with respect to both exercise tolerance and symptoms of dyspnea and fatigue (Evidence A).
- The long-term administration of oxygen (> 15 h/d) to patients with chronic respiratory failure has been shown to increase survival (Evidence A).

Introduction

The overall approach to managing stable COPD should be characterized by an increase in treatment, depending on the severity of the disease and the clinical status of the patient. Management of COPD is based on an individualized assessment of disease severity and response to various therapies. The classification of severity of stable COPD incorporates an individualized assessment of disease severity and therapeutic response into the management strategy. The severity of airflow limitation provides a general guide to the use of some treatments, but the selection of therapy is predominantly determined by the patient's symptoms and clinical presentation. Treatment also depends on the patient's educational level and willingness to apply the recommended management, on cultural and local practice conditions, and on the availability of medications.

Education

Although patient education is generally regarded as an essential component of care for any chronic disease, assessment of the value of education in COPD may be difficult because of the relatively long time required to achieve improvements in objective measurements of lung function. Patient education alone does not improve exercise performance or lung function[35-38] (Evidence B), but it can play a role in improving skills, ability to cope with illness, and health status.[39] Patient education regarding smoking cessation has the greatest capacity to influence the natural history of COPD (Evidence A). Education also improves patient response to exacerbations[40,41] (Evidence B). Prospective end-of-life discussions can lead to understanding of advance directives and effective therapeutic decisions at the end of life[42] (Evidence B).

Ideally, educational messages should be incorporated into all aspects of care for COPD and may take place in many settings: consultations with physicians or other health care workers, home-care or outreach programs, and comprehensive pulmonary rehabilitation programs. Education should be tailored to the needs and environment of the individual patient, interactive, directed at improving quality of life, simple to follow, practical, and appropriate to the intellectual and social skills of the patient and the caregivers. The topics that seem most appropriate for an education program include the following: smoking cessation; basic information about COPD and pathophysiology of the disease, general approach to therapy and specific aspects of medical treatment, self-management skills, strategies to help minimize dyspnea, advice about when to seek help, self-management and decision making during exacerbations, and advance directives and end-of-life issues.

Pharmacologic Treatments

Pharmacologic therapy is used to prevent and control symptoms (Fig. A1.1), reduce the frequency and severity of exacerbations, improve health status, and improve exercise tolerance. None of the existing medications (Table A1.5) for COPD have been shown to modify the long-term decline in lung function that is the hallmark of this disease [43-46] (Evidence A). However, this should not preclude efforts to use medications to control symptoms.

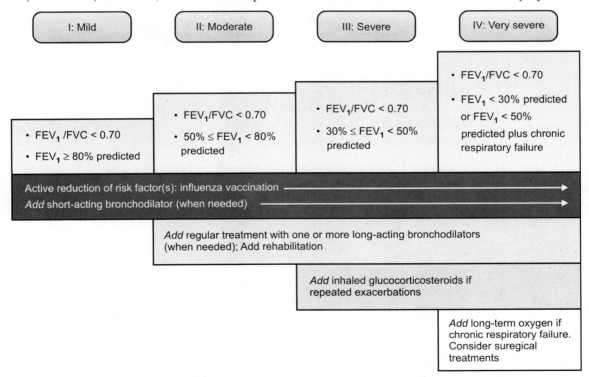

FIGURE A1.1. Therapy at each stage of chronic obstructive pulmonary disease (COPD). Post-bronchodilator FEV$_1$ is recommended for the diagnosis and assessment of severity of COPD

TABLE A1.5. Commonly used formulations of medications used in chronic obstructive pulmonary disease

Medication	Inhaler (µg)	Solution for Nebulizer (mg/ml)	Oral	Vials for Injection (mg)	Duration of Action (h)
β₂-Agonists Short-acting					
Fenoterol	100-200 (MDI)	1	0.5% (syrup)	4-6	
Salbutamol (albuterol)	100, 200 (MDI and DPI)	5	5 mg (pill) 0.24% (syrup)	0.1, 0.5	4-6
Terbutaline	400, 500 (DPI)			0.2, 0.25	4-6
Long-acting					
Formoterol	4.5-12 (MDI and DPI)				12+
Salmeterol	25-50 (MDI and DPI)				12+
Anticholinergics Short-acting					
Ipatropium bromide	20, 40 (MDI)	0.25-0.5			6-8
Oxitropium bromide	100 (MDI)	1.5			7-9
Long-acting					
Tiotropium	18 (DPI)				24+
Combination short-acting β₂-agonists plus anticholinergic in one inhaler					
Fenoterol/ipratropium	200/80 (MDI)	1.25/0.5			6-8
Salbutamol/ipratropium	75/15 (MDI)	0.75/4.5			6-8
Methylxanthines					
Aminophylline			200-600 mg (pill)	240	Variable, up to 24
Theophylline (SR)			100-600 mg (pill)		Variable, up to 24
Inhaled glucocorticosteroids					
Beclomethasone	50-400 (MDI and DPI)	0.2-0.4			
Budesonide	100, 200, 400 (DPI)	0.20, 0.25, 0.5			
Fluticasone	50-500 (MDI and DPI)				
Triamcinolone	100 (MDI)	40		40	
Combination long-acting β₂-agonists plus glucocorticosteroids in one inhaler					
Formoterol/budesonide	4.5/160, 9/320 (DPI)				
Salmeterol/fluticasone	50/100, 250, 500 (DPI) 25/50, 125, 250 (MDI)				
Systemic glucocorticosteroids					
Prednisone			5-60 mg (pill)		
Methylprednisolone			4, 8, 16 mg (pill)		

Definition of abbreviation: DPI = dry powder inhaler; MDI = metered-dose inhaler; SR = slow release.

Bronchodilators

Bronchodilator medications are central to the symptomatic management of COPD (47-50) (Evidence A) (Table A1.6). They are given either on an as-needed basis for relief of persistent or worsening symptoms or on a regular basis to prevent or reduce symptoms. The side effects of bronchodilator therapy are pharmacologically predictable and dose dependent. Adverse effects are less likely, and resolve more rapidly after treatment withdrawal, with inhaled than with oral treatment. When treatment is given by the inhaled route, attention to effective drug delivery and training in inhaler technique are essential.

TABLE A1.6. Bronchodilators in stable chronic obstructive pulmonary disease

- Bronchodilator medications are central to symptom management in COPD.
- Inhaled therapy is preferred.
- The choice among β_2-agonist, anticholinergic, theophylline, or combination therapy depends on availability and individual response in terms of symptom relief and side effects.
- Bronchodilators are prescribed on an as-needed or on a regular basis to prevent or reduce symptoms.
- Long-acting inhaled bronchodilators are more effective and convenient.
- Combining bronchodilators may improve efficacy and decrease the risk of side effects compared to increasing the dose of a single bronchodilator.

Definition of abbreviation: COPD = chronic obstructive pulmonary disease.

Bronchodilator drugs commonly used in treating COPD include β_2-agonists, anticholinergics, and methylxanthines. The choice depends on the availability of the medications and the patient's response. All categories of bronchodilators have been shown to increase exercise capacity in COPD, without necessarily producing significant changes in FEV_1[51-54] (Evidence A).

Regular treatment with long-acting bronchodilators is more effective and convenient than treatment with short-acting bronchodilators[55-58] (Evidence A). Regular use of a long-acting β_2-agonist[56] or a short- or long-acting anticholinergic improves health status.[55-57] Treatment with a long-acting inhaled anticholinergic drug reduces the rate of COPD exacerbations[59] and improves the effectiveness of pulmonary rehabilitation.[60] Theophylline is effective in COPD, but, due to its potential toxicity, inhaled bronchodilators are preferred when available. All studies that have shown efficacy of theophylline in COPD were done with slow-release preparations.

Combining bronchodilators with different mechanisms and durations of action may increase the degree of bronchodilation for equivalent or lesser side effects. A combination of a short-acting $_2$-agonist and an anticholinergic produces greater and more sustained improvements in FEV_1 than either drug alone and does not produce evidence of tachyphylaxis over 90 days of treatment[61-63] (Evidence A).

The combination of a β_2-agonist, an anticholinergic, and/or theophylline may produce additional improvements in lung function[61-67] and health status.[61,68] Increasing the number of drugs usually increases costs, and an equivalent benefit may occur by increasing the dose of one bronchodilator when side effects are not a limiting factor. Detailed assessments of this approach have not been performed.

Dose-response relationships using the FEV_1 as the outcome are relatively flat with all classes of bronchodilators.[47-50] Toxicity is also dose related. Increasing the dose of either a β_2-agonist or an anticholinergic by an order of magnitude, especially when given by a wet nebulizer, appears to provide subjective benefit in acute episodes[69] (Evidence B) but is not necessarily helpful in stable disease[70] (Evidence C).

When treatment is given by the inhaled route, attention to effective drug delivery and training in inhaler technique are essential. The choice of inhaler device will depend on availability, cost, the prescribing physician, and the skills and ability of the patient. Patients with COPD may have more problems in effective coordination and find it harder to use a simple metered-dose inhaler than do healthy volunteers or younger patients with asthma. It is essential to ensure that inhaler technique is correct and to recheck this at each visit.

Glucocorticosteroids

Regular treatment with inhaled glucocorticosteroids does not modify the long-term decline of FEV_1 in patients with COPD.[44-46,71] However, regular treatment with inhaled glucocorticosteroids is appropriate for symptomatic patients with COPD with an $FEV_1 <$ 50 percent predicted (stages III and IV) and repeated exacerbations (e.g. three in the last 3 yr)[72-75] (Evidence A). This treatment has been shown to reduce the frequency of exacerbations and thus improve health status[76] (Evidence A), and withdrawal from treatment with inhaled glucocorticosteroids can lead to exacerbations in some patients.[77] Reanalysis of pooled data from several longer studies of inhaled glucocorticosteroids in COPD suggests that this treatment reduces all-cause mortality,[78] but this conclusion requires confirmation in prospective studies before leading to a change in current treatment recommendations. An inhaled glucocorticosteroid combined with a long-acting β_2-agonist is more effective than the individual components[72,74,75,79,80] (Evidence A). The dose-response relationships and long-term safety of inhaled glucocorticosteroids in COPD are not known.

Long-term treatment with oral glucocorticosteroids is not recommended in COPD (Evidence A). A side effect of long-term treatment with systemic glucocorticosteroids is steroid myopathy[81-83], which contributes to muscle weakness, decreased functionality, and respiratory failure in subjects with advanced COPD.

Other Pharmacologic Treatments

Vaccines

Influenza vaccines can reduce serious illness[84] and death in patients with COPD by approximately 50 percent[85,86] (Evidence A). Vaccines containing killed or live, inactivated viruses are recommended[87] because they are more effective in elderly patients with COPD.[88] The strains are adjusted each year for appropriate effectiveness and should be given once each year.[89] Pneumococcal polysaccharide vaccine is recommended for patients with COPD who are 65 years and older.[90,91] In addition, this vaccine has been shown to reduce the incidence of community-acquired pneumonia in patients with COPD who are younger than 65 years with an $FEV_1 < 40$ percent predicted[92] (Evidence B).

α_1-Antitrypsin Augmentation Therapy

Young patients with severe hereditary α_1-antitrypsin deficiency and established emphysema may be candidates for α_1-antitrypsin augmentation therapy. However, this therapy is very expensive, not available in most countries, and not recommended for patients with COPD that is unrelated to α_1-antitrypsin deficiency (Evidence C).

Antibiotics

Prophylactic, continuous use of antibiotics has been shown to have no effect on the frequency of exacerbations in COPD[93-95], and a study that examined the efficacy of chemoprophylaxis undertaken in the winter months over a period of 5 years concluded that there was no benefit.[96] There is no current evidence that the use of antibiotics, other than for treating infectious exacerbations of COPD and other bacterial infections, is helpful[97,98] (Evidence A).

Mucolytic (Mucokinetic, Mucoregulator) Agents (Ambroxol, Erdosteine, Carbocysteine, Iodinated Glycerol)

The regular use of mucolytics in COPD has been evaluated in a number of long-term studies with controversial results.[99-101] Although a few patients with viscous sputum may benefit from mucolytics[102,103], the overall benefits seem to be very small, and the widespread use of these agents cannot be recommended at present (Evidence D).

Antioxidant Agents

Antioxidants, in particular N-acetylcysteine, have been reported in small studies to reduce the frequency of exacerbations, leading to speculation that these medications could have a role in the treatment of patients with recurrent exacerbations[104-107] (Evidence B). However, a large randomized controlled trial found no effect of N-acetylcysteine on the frequency of exacerbations, except in patients not treated with inhaled glucocorticosteroids.[108]

Immunoregulators (Immunostimulators, Immunomodulators)

Studies using an immunoregulator in COPD show a decrease in the severity and frequency of exacerbations.[109,110] However, additional studies to examine the long-term effects of this therapy are required before its regular use can be recommended.[111]

Antitussives

Cough, although sometimes a troublesome symptom in COPD, has a significant protective role.[112] Thus, the regular use of antitussives is not recommended in stable COPD (Evidence D).

Vasodilators

In patients with COPD, inhaled nitric oxide can worsen gas exchange because of altered hypoxic regulation of ventilation–perfusion balance.[113,114] Therefore, based on the available evidence, nitric oxide is not indicated in stable COPD.

Narcotics (Morphine)

Oral and parenteral opioids are effective for treating dyspnea in patients with advanced COPD disease. There are insufficient data to conclude whether nebulized opioids are effective.[115] However, some clinical studies suggest that morphine used to control dyspnea may have serious adverse effects and its benefits may be limited to a few sensitive subjects.[116-120]

Others

Nedocromil, leukotriene modifiers, and alternative healing methods (e.g. herbal medicine, acupuncture, homeopathy) have not been adequately tested in patients with COPD and thus cannot be recommended at this time.

NONPHARMACOLOGIC TREATMENTS

Rehabilitation

The principal goals of pulmonary rehabilitation are to reduce symptoms, improve quality of life, and increase physical and emotional participation in everyday activities. To accomplish these goals, pulmonary rehabilitation covers a range of nonpulmonary problems that may not be adequately addressed by medical therapy for COPD. Such problems, which especially affect patients with stages II through IV COPD, include exercise deconditioning, relative social isolation, altered mood states (especially depression), muscle wasting, and weight loss.

Although more information is needed on criteria for patient selection for pulmonary rehabilitation programs, patients with COPD at all stages of disease appear to benefit from exercise training programs, improving with respect to both exercise tolerance and symptoms of dyspnea and fatigue[121] (Evidence A). Data suggest that these benefits can be sustained even after a single pulmonary rehabilitation program.[122-124] Benefit does wane after a rehabilitation program ends, but if exercise training is maintained at home, the patient's health status remains above pre-rehabilitation levels (Evidence B). To date, there is no consensus on whether repeated rehabilitation courses enable patients to sustain the benefits gained through the initial course. Benefits have been reported from rehabilitation programs conducted in inpatient, outpatient, and home settings.[125-127]

Ideally, pulmonary rehabilitation should involve several types of health professionals. The components of pulmonary rehabilitation vary widely from program to program, but a comprehensive pulmonary rehabilitation program includes exercise training, nutrition counseling, and education. Baseline and outcome assessments of each participant in a pulmonary rehabilitation program should be made to quantify individual gains and target areas for improvement. Assessments should include the following:

- Detailed history and physical examination
- Measurement of spirometry before and after use of a bronchodilator drug
- Assessment of exercise capacity
- Measurement of health status and impact of breathlessness
- Assessment of inspiratory and expiratory muscle strength and lower limb strength (e.g. quadriceps) in patients who suffer from muscle wasting.

The first two assessments are important for establishing entry suitability and baseline status but are not used in outcome assessment. The last three assessments are baseline and outcome measures.

Oxygen Therapy

The long-term administration of oxygen (> 15 h/d) to patients with chronic respiratory failure has been shown to increase survival.[128,129] It can also have a beneficial impact on hemodynamics, hematologic characteristics, exercise capacity, lung mechanics, and mental state.[130]

Long-term oxygen therapy is generally introduced in patients with stage IV COPD, who have

- Pa_{O_2} at or below 7.3 kPa (55 mm Hg) or Sa_{O_2} at or below 88 percent, with or without hypercapnia (Evidence B), or
- Pa_{O_2} between 7.3 kPa (55 mm Hg) and 8.0 kPa (60 mm Hg), or Sa_{O_2} of 88 percent, if there is evidence of pulmonary hypertension, peripheral edema suggesting congestive cardiac failure, or polycythemia (hematocrit > 55%) (Evidence D).

The primary goal of oxygen therapy is to increase the baseline Pa_{O_2} to at least 8.0 kPa (60 mm Hg) at sea level and rest, and/or produce an Sa_{O_2} of at least 90 percent, which will preserve vital organ function by ensuring adequate delivery of oxygen. A decision about the use of long-term oxygen should be based on the waking Pa_{O_2} values. The prescription should always include the source of supplemental oxygen (gas or liquid), method of delivery, duration of use, and flow rate at rest, during exercise, and during sleep.

Ventilatory Support

Although long-term noninvasive positive-pressure ventilation (NIPPV) cannot be recommended for the routine treatment of patients with chronic respiratory failure due to COPD, the combination of NIPPV with long-term oxygen therapy may be of some use in a selected subset of patients, particularly in those with pronounced daytime hypercapnia.[131]

SURGICAL TREATMENTS

Bullectomy

In carefully selected patients, this procedure is effective in reducing dyspnea and improving lung function[132] (Evidence C). A thoracic CT scan, arterial blood gas measurement, and comprehensive respiratory function tests are essential before making a decision regarding suitability for resection of a bulla.

Lung Volume Reduction Surgery

A large multicenter study of 1,200 patients comparing lung volume reduction surgery with medical treatment has shown that after 4.3 years, patients with upper lobe emphysema and low exercise capacity who received the surgery had a greater survival rate than similar patients who received medical therapy (54 vs. 39.7%).[133] In addition, the surgery patients experienced greater improvements in their maximal work capacity and their health-related quality of life. The advantage of surgery over medical therapy was less significant among patients who had other emphysema distribution or high exercise capacity before treatment. Although the results of this study showed some very positive results of surgery in a select group of patients[17,133], lung volume reduction surgery is an expensive palliative surgical procedure and can be recommended only in carefully selected patients.

Lung Transplantation

In appropriately selected patients with very advanced COPD, lung transplantation has been shown to improve quality of life and functional capacity[134-137] (Evidence C). Criteria for referral for lung transplantation include $FEV_1 < 35$ percent predicted, $Pa_{O2} < 7.3$-8.0 kPa (55-60 mm Hg), $Pa_{CO2} > 6.7$ kPa (50 mm Hg), and secondary pulmonary hypertension.[138,139]

SPECIAL CONSIDERATIONS

Surgery in COPD

Postoperative pulmonary complications are as important and common as postoperative cardiac complications and, consequently, are a key component of the increased risk posed by surgery in patients with COPD. The principal potential factors contributing to the risk include smoking, poor general health status, age, obesity, and COPD severity. A comprehensive definition of postoperative pulmonary complications should include only major pulmonary respiratory complications, namely lung infections, atelectasis, and/or increased airflow obstruction, all potentially resulting in acute respiratory failure and aggravation of underlying COPD.[140-145]

Component 4: Manage Exacerbations

KEY POINTS

- An exacerbation of COPD is defined as an event in the natural course of the disease characterized by a change in the patient's baseline dyspnea, cough, and/or sputum that is beyond normal day-to-day variations, is acute in onset, and may warrant a change in regular medication in a patient with underlying COPD.
- The most common causes of an exacerbation are infection of the tracheobronchial tree and air pollution, but the cause of about one-third of severe exacerbations cannot be identified (Evidence B).
- Inhaled bronchodilators (particularly inhaled β_2-agonists with or without anticholinergics) and oral glucocorticosteroids are effective treatments for exacerbations of COPD (Evidence A).
- Patients experiencing COPD exacerbations with clinical signs of airway infection (e.g. increased sputum purulence) may benefit from antibiotic treatment (Evidence B).
- Noninvasive mechanical ventilation in exacerbations improves respiratory acidosis, increases pH, decreases the need for endotracheal intubation, and reduces Pa_{CO2}, respiratory rate, severity of breathlessness, the length of hospital stay, and mortality (Evidence A).
- Medications and education to help prevent future exacerbations should be considered as part of follow-up, because exacerbations affect the quality of life and prognosis of patients with COPD.

Introduction

COPD is often associated with exacerbations of symptoms.[146-150] An exacerbation of COPD is defined as "an event in the natural course of the disease characterized by a change in the patient's baseline dyspnea, cough, and/or sputum that is beyond normal day-to-day variations, is acute in onset, and may warrant a change in regular medication in a patient with underlying COPD".[151,152] Exacerbations are categorized in terms of either clinical presentation (number of symptoms[199]) and/or heath care resources utilization.[151] The impact of exacerbations is significant and a patient's symptoms and lung function may both take several weeks to recover to the baseline values.[153]

The most common causes of an exacerbation are infection of the tracheobronchial tree and air pollution,[154] but the cause of approximately one-third of severe exacerbations cannot be identified. The role of bacterial infections is controversial, but recent investigations have shown that at least 50 percent of patients have bacteria in high concentrations in their lower airways during exacerbations.[155-157] Development of specific immune responses to the infecting bacterial strains, and the association of neutrophilic inflammation with bacterial exacerbations, also support the bacterial causation of a proportion of exacerbations.[158-161]

DIAGNOSIS AND ASSESSMENT OF SEVERITY

Medical History

Increased breathlessness, the main symptom of an exacerbation, is often accompanied by wheezing and chest tightness, increased cough and sputum, change of the color and/or tenacity of sputum, and fever. Exacerbations may also be accompanied by a number of nonspecific complaints, such as tachycardia and tachypnea, malaise, insomnia, sleepiness, fatigue, depression, and confusion. A decrease in exercise tolerance, fever, and/or new radiologic anomalies suggestive of pulmonary disease may herald a COPD exacerbation. An increase in sputum volume and purulence points to a bacterial cause, as does prior history of chronic sputum production.[148,161]

Assessment of Severity

Assessment of the severity of an exacerbation is based on the patient's medical history before the exacerbation, preexisting comorbidities, symptoms, physical examination, arterial blood gas measurements, and other laboratory tests. Physicians should obtain the results of previous evaluations, where possible, to compare with the current clinical data. Specific information is required on the frequency and severity of attacks of breathlessness and cough, sputum volume and color, and limitation of daily activities. When available, prior arterial blood gas measurements are extremely useful for comparison with those made during the acute episode, as an acute change in these tests is more important than their absolute values. Thus, where possible, physicians should instruct their patients to bring the summary of their last evaluation when they come to the hospital with an exacerbation. In patients with stage IV COPD, the most important sign of a severe exacerbation is a change in the mental status of the patient and this signals a need for immediate evaluation in the hospital.

Spirometry and PEF

Even simple spirometric tests can be difficult for a sick patient to perform properly. These measurements are not accurate during an acute exacerbation; therefore, their routine use is not recommended.

Pulse Oximetry and Arterial Blood Gas Measurement

Pulse oximetry can be used to evaluate a patient's oxygen saturation and need for supplemental oxygen therapy. For patients that require hospitalization, measurement of arterial blood gases is important to assess the severity of an exacerbation. A $Pa_{O_2} < 8.0$ kPa (60 mm Hg) and/or $Sa_{O_2} < 90$ percent with or without $Pa_{CO_2} > 6.7$ kPa (50 mm Hg) when breathing room air indicate respiratory failure. In addition, moderate to severe acidosis (pH < 7.36) plus hypercapnia ($Pa_{CO_2} > 6$-8 kPa, 45-60 mm Hg) in a patient with respiratory failure is an indication for mechanical ventilation.[145,162]

Chest X-ray and ECG

Chest radiographs (posterior/anterior plus lateral) are useful in identifying alternative diagnoses that can mimic the symptoms of an exacerbation. An ECG aids in the diagnosis of right heart hypertrophy, arrhythmias, and ischemic episodes. Pulmonary embolism can be very difficult to distinguish from an exacerbation, especially in advanced COPD, because right ventricular hypertrophy and large pulmonary arteries lead to confusing ECG and radiographic results. A low systolic blood pressure and an inability to increase the Pa_{O_2} above 8.0 kPa (60 mm Hg) despite high-flow oxygen also suggest pulmonary embolism. If there are strong indications that pulmonary embolism has occurred, it is best to treat for this together with the exacerbation.

Other Laboratory Tests

The complete blood count may identify polycythemia (hematocrit > 55%) or suggest bleeding. White blood cell counts are usually not very informative. The presence of purulent sputum during an exacerbation of symptoms is sufficient indication for starting empirical antibiotic treatment.[163] *Streptococcus pneumoniae*, *Hemophilus influenzae*, and *Moraxella catarrhalis* are the most common bacterial pathogens involved in COPD exacerbations. If an infectious exacerbation does not respond to the initial antibiotic treatment, a sputum culture and an antibiogram should be performed.

Biochemical test abnormalities can be associated with an exacerbation and include electrolyte disturbance(s) (e.g. hyponatremia, hypokalemia), poor glucose control, or metabolic acid–base disorder. These abnormalities can also be due to associated comorbid conditions.

DIFFERENTIAL DIAGNOSES

Patients with apparent exacerbations of COPD who do not respond to treatment[153,164] should be reevaluated for other medical conditions that can aggravate symptoms or mimic COPD exacerbations,[102] including pneumonia, congestive heart failure, pneumothorax, pleural effusion, pulmonary embolism, and cardiac arrhythmia. Noncompliance with the prescribed medication regimen can also cause increased symptoms that may be confused with a true exacerbation. Elevated serum levels of brain-type natriuretic peptide, in conjunction with other clinical information, can identify patients with acute dyspnea secondary to congestive heart failure and enable them to be distinguished from patients with COPD exacerbations.[165,166]

Home Management

There is increasing interest in home care for patients with end-stage COPD, although the exact criteria for this approach as opposed to hospital treatment remain uncertain and will vary by health care setting.[167-170]

Bronchodilator Therapy

Home management of COPD exacerbations involves increasing the dose and/or frequency of existing short-acting bronchodilator therapy, preferably with a β_2-agonist (Evidence A). If not already used, an anticholinergic can be added until the symptoms improve (Evidence D).

Glucocorticosteroids

Systemic glucocorticosteroids are beneficial in the management of exacerbations of COPD. They shorten recovery time, improve lung function (FEV_1) and hypoxemia (Pa_{O_2})[171-174] (Evidence A), and may reduce the risk of early relapse, treatment failure, and length of hospital stay.[175] They should be considered in addition to bronchodilators if the patient's baseline FEV_1 is less than 50 percent predicted. A dose of 30 to 40 mg prednisolone per day for 7 to 10 days is recommended.[171,172,176]

Antibiotics

The use of antibiotics in the management of COPD exacerbations is discussed below in Hospital Management.

Hospital Management

The risk of dying of an exacerbation of COPD is closely related to the development of respiratory acidosis, the presence of significant comorbidities, and the need for ventilatory support.[177] Patients lacking these features are not at high risk of dying, but those with severe underlying COPD often require hospitalization in any case. Attempts at managing such patients entirely in the community have met with only limited success,[178] but returning them to their homes with increased social support and a supervised medical care package after initial emergency room assessment has been much more successful.[179] Savings on inpatient expenditures[180] offset the additional costs of maintaining a community-based COPD nursing team. However, detailed cost-benefit analyses of these approaches are awaited.

A range of criteria to consider for hospital assessment/admission for exacerbations of COPD are shown in Table A1.7. Some patients need immediate admission to an intensive care unit (ICU) (Table A1.8). Admission of patients with severe COPD exacerbations to intermediate or special respiratory care units may be appropriate if personnel, skills, and equipment exist to identify and manage acute respiratory failure successfully.

TABLE A1.7. Indications for hospital assessment or admission for exacerbations of chronic obstructive pulmonary disease*

- Marked increase in intensity of symptoms, such as sudden development of resting dyspnea, change in vital signs
- Severe underlying COPD
- Onset of new physical signs (e.g. cyanosis, peripheral edema)
- Failure of exacerbation to respond to initial medical management
- Significant comorbidities
- Frequent exacerbations
- Newly occurring arrhythmias
- Diagnostic uncertainty
- Older age
- Insufficient home support

Definition of abbreviation: COPD = chronic obstructive pulmonary disease.

* Local resources need to be considered.

TABLE A1.8. Indications for intensive care unit admission of patients with exacerbations of chronic obstructive pulmonary disease*

- Severe dyspnea that responds inadequately to initial emergency therapy
- Changes in mental status (confusion, lethargy, coma)
- Persistent or worsening hypoxemia (Pa_{O_2} < 5.3 kPa, 40 mm Hg), and/or severe/worsening hypercapnia (Pa_{CO_2} > 8.0 kPa, 60 mm Hg), and/or severe/worsening respiratory acidosis (pH < 7.25) despite supplemental oxygen and noninvasive ventilation
- Need for invasive mechanical ventilation
- Hemodynamic instability—need for vasopressors

* Local resources need to be considered.

The first actions when a patient reaches the emergency department are to provide supplemental oxygen therapy and to determine whether the exacerbation is life threatening. If so, the patient should be admitted to the ICU immediately. Otherwise, the patient may be managed in the emergency department or hospital (Table A1.9).

TABLE A1.9. Management of severe but not life-threatening exacerbations of chronic obstructive pulmonary disease in the emergency department or the hospital*[176]

- Assess severity of symptoms, blood gases, chest X-ray
- Administer controlled oxygen therapy and repeat arterial blood gas measurement after 30–60 min
- Bronchodilators:
  - Increase doses and/or frequency
  - Combine $_2$-agonists and anticholinergics
  - Use spacers or air-driven nebulizers
  - Consider adding intravenous methylxanthines, if needed
- Add oral or intravenous glucocorticosteroids
- Consider antibiotics (oral or occasionally intravenous) when there are signs of bacterial infection
- Consider noninvasive mechanical ventilation
- At all times:
  - Monitor fluid balance and nutrition
  - Consider subcutaneous heparin
  - Identify and treat associated conditions (e.g., heart failure, arrhythmias)
  - Closely monitor condition of the patient

* Local resources need to be considered.

Controlled Oxygen Therapy

Oxygen therapy is the cornerstone of hospital treatment of COPD exacerbations. Supplemental oxygen should be titrated to improve the patient's hypoxemia. Adequate levels of oxygenation ($Pa_{O_2} > 8.0$ kPa, 60 mm Hg, or $Sa_{O_2} > 90\%$) are easy to achieve in uncomplicated exacerbations, but CO_2 retention can occur insidiously with little change in symptoms. Once oxygen is started, arterial blood gases should be checked 30 to 60 minutes later to ensure satisfactory oxygenation without CO_2 retention or acidosis. Venturi masks (high-flow devices) offer more accurate delivery of controlled oxygen than do nasal prongs but are less likely to be tolerated by the patient.[145]

Bronchodilator Therapy

Short-acting inhaled β_2-agonists are usually the preferred bronchodilators for treatment of exacerbations of COPD[102,145,181] (Evidence A). If a prompt response to these drugs does not occur, the addition of an anticholinergic is recommended, even though evidence concerning the effectiveness of this combination is controversial. Despite its widespread clinical use, the role of methylxanthines in the treatment of exacerbations of COPD remains controversial. Intravenous methylxanthines (theophylline or aminohylline) are currently considered second-line therapy, used when there is inadequate or insufficient response to short-acting bronchodilators[182-186] (Evidence B). Possible beneficial effects in terms of lung function and clinical endpoints are modest and inconsistent, whereas adverse effects are significantly increased.[187,188] There are no clinical studies that have evaluated the use of inhaled long-acting bronchodilators (either β_2-agonists or anticholinergics) with or without inhaled glucocorticosteroids during an acute exacerbation.

Glucocorticosteroids

Oral or intravenous glucocorticosteroids are recommended as an addition to other therapies in the hospital management of exacerbations of COPD[172,173] (Evidence A). The exact dose that should be recommended is not known, but high doses are associated with a significant risk of side effects. Thirty to forty mg of oral prednisolone daily for 7 to 10 days is effective and safe (Evidence C). Prolonged treatment does not result in greater efficacy and increases the risk of side effects.

Antibiotics

On the basis of the current available evidence,[145,10] antibiotics should be given to the following individuals:
- Patients with exacerbations of COPD with the following three cardinal symptoms: increased dyspnea, increased sputum volume, and increased sputum purulence (Evidence B)
- Patients with exacerbations of COPD with two of the cardinal symptoms, if increased purulence of sputum is one of the two symptoms (Evidence C)

- Patients with a severe exacerbation of COPD that requires mechanical ventilation (invasive or noninvasive) (Evidence B)

The infectious agents in COPD exacerbations can be viral or bacterial.[89,189] The predominant bacteria recovered from the lower airways of patients with COPD exacerbations are *H. influenzae*, *S. pneumoniae*, and *M. catarrhalis*.[89,155,156,190] So-called atypical pathogens, such as *Mycoplasma pneumoniae* and *Chlamydia pneumoniae*,[190,191] have been identified in patients with COPD exacerbations, but because of diagnostic limitations the true prevalence of these organisms is not known.

Respiratory Stimulants

Respiratory stimulants are not recommended for acute respiratory failure.[181] Doxapram, a nonspecific but relatively safe respiratory stimulant available in some countries as an intravenous formulation, should be used only when noninvasive intermittent ventilation is not available or not recommended.[192]

Ventilatory Support

The primary objectives of mechanical ventilatory support in patients with COPD exacerbations are to decrease mortality and morbidity and to relieve symptoms. Ventilatory support includes both noninvasive intermittent ventilation using either negative- or positive-pressure devices, and invasive (conventional) mechanical ventilation by orotracheal tube or tracheostomy.

Noninvasive Mechanical Ventilation.

Noninvasive intermittent ventilation (NIV) has been studied in several randomized controlled trials in acute respiratory failure, consistently providing positive results, with success rates of 80 to 85%.[131,1193-195] These studies provide evidence that NIV improves respiratory acidosis (increases pH, and decreases Pa_{CO_2}), and decreases respiratory rate, severity of breathlessness, and length of hospital stay (Evidence A). More importantly, mortality—or its surrogate, intubation rate—is reduced by this intervention.[195-198] However, NIV is not appropriate for all patients, as summarized in Table A1.10.[131]

TABLE A1.10. Indications and relative contraindications for noninvasive intermittent ventilation

Selection criteria
- Moderate to severe dyspnea with use of accessory muscles and paradoxical abdominal motion
- Moderate to severe acidosis (pH ≤ 7.35) and/or hypercapnia (Pa_{CO_2} > 6.0 kPa, 45 mm Hg)[145,193,199-201]
- Respiratory frequency > 25 breaths/min

Exclusion criteria (any may be present)
- Respiratory arrest
- Cardiovascular instability (hypotension, arrhythmias, myocardial infarction)
- Change in mental status; uncooperative patient
- High aspiration risk
- Viscous or copious secretions
- Recent facial or gastroesophageal surgery
- Craniofacial trauma
- Fixed nasopharyngeal abnormalities
- Burns
- Extreme obesity

Invasive Mechanical Ventilation

The indications for initiating invasive mechanical ventilation during exacerbations of COPD are shown in Table A1.11 and include failure of an initial trial of NIV.[202] As experience is being gained with the generalized clinical use of NIV in COPD, several of the indications for invasive mechanical ventilation are being successfully treated with NIV.

TABLE A1.11. Indications for invasive mechanical ventilation

- Unable to tolerate NIV or NIV failure (or exclusion criteria, *see* Table A1.10)
- Severe dyspnea with use of accessory muscles and paradoxical abdominal motion
- Respiratory frequency > 35 breaths/min
- Life-threatening hypoxemia
- Severe acidosis (pH < 7.25) and/or hypercapnia (Pa_{CO_2} > 8.0 kPa, 60 mm Hg)
- Respiratory arrest

(Contd...)

- Worsening in mental status despite optimal therapy
- Cardiovascular complications (hypotension, shock)
- Other complications (metabolic abnormalities, sepsis, pneumonia, pulmonary embolism, barotrauma, massive pleural effusion)

Definition of abbreviation: NIV = noninvasive intermittent ventilation.

The use of invasive ventilation in patients with end-stage COPD is influenced by the likely reversibility of the precipitating event, the patient's wishes, and the availability of intensive care facilities. Major hazards include the risk of ventilator-acquired pneumonia (especially when multiresistant organisms are prevalent), barotrauma, and failure to wean to spontaneous ventilation. Contrary to some opinions, acute mortality among patients with COPD with respiratory failure is lower than mortality among patients ventilated for non-COPD causes.[203] When possible, a clear statement of the patient's own treatment wishes—an advance directive or "living will"—makes these difficult decisions much easier to resolve.

Weaning or discontinuation from mechanical ventilation can be particularly difficult and hazardous in patients with COPD and the best method (pressure support or a T-piece trial) remains a matter of debate.[204-206] In patients with COPD who fail weaning trials, noninvasive ventilation facilitates extubation. It can also prevent reintubation in patients with extubation failure and may reduce mortality.

Other Measures

Further treatments that can be used in the hospital include the following: fluid administration (accurate monitoring of fluid balance is essential); nutrition (supplementary when needed); deep venous thrombosis prophylaxis (mechanical devices, heparins, etc.) in immobilized, polycythemic, or dehydrated patients with or without a history of thromboembolic disease; and sputum clearance (by stimulating coughing and low-volume forced expirations as in home management). Manual or mechanical chest percussion and postural drainage may be beneficial in patients with excessive sputum production or with lobar atelectasis.

Hospital Discharge and Follow-up

Insufficient clinical data exist to establish the optimal duration of hospitalization in individual patients who develop an exacerbation of COPD.[146,207,208] Consensus and limited data support the discharge criteria listed in Table A1.12. Table A1.13 provides items to include in a follow-up assessment 4 to 6 weeks after discharge from the hospital. Thereafter, follow-up is the same as for patients with stable COPD, including supervising smoking cessation, monitoring the effectiveness of each drug treatment, and monitoring changes in spirometric parameters (179). Home visits by a community nurse may permit earlier discharge of patients hospitalized with an exacerbation of COPD, without increasing readmission rates.[102,209-211]

TABLE A1.12. Discharge criteria for patients with exacerbations of chronic obstructive pulmonary disease

- Inhaled β_2-agonist therapy is required no more frequently than every 4 h
- Patient, if previously ambulatory, is able to walk across room
- Patient is able to eat and sleep without frequent awakening by dyspnea
- Patient has been clinically stable for 12-24 h
- Arterial blood gases have been stable for 12-24 h
- Patient (or home caregiver) fully understands correct use of medications
- Follow-up and home care arrangements have been completed (e.g. visiting nurse, oxygen delivery, meal provisions)
- Patient, family, and physician are confident patient can manage successfully at home

TABLE A1.13. Items to assess at follow-up visit 4-6 weeks after discharge from hospital for exacerbations of chronic obstructive pulmonary disease

- Ability to cope in usual environment
- Measurement of FEV_1
- Reassessment of inhaler technique
- Understanding of recommended treatment regimen
- Need for long-term oxygen therapy and/or home nebulizer (for patients with stage IV, very severe COPD)

Definition of abbreviation: COPD = chronic obstructive pulmonary disease.

In patients who are hypoxemic during a COPD exacerbation, arterial blood gases and/or pulse oximetry should be evaluated before hospital discharge and in the following 3 months. If the patient remains hypoxemic, long-term supplemental oxygen therapy may be required.

Opportunities for prevention of future exacerbations should be reviewed before discharge, with particular attention to smoking cessation, current vaccination (influenza, pneumococcal vaccines), knowledge of current therapy including inhaler technique,[212-214] and how to recognize symptoms of exacerbations. Pharmacotherapy known to reduce the number of exacerbations and hospitalizations and delay the time of first/next hospitalization, such as long-acting inhaled bronchodilators, inhaled glucocorticosteroids, and combination inhalers, should be specifically considered. Social problems should be discussed and principal caregivers identified if the patient has a significant persisting disability.

Translating Guideline Recommendations to the Context of (Primary) Care

KEY POINTS

- There is considerable evidence that management of COPD is generally not in accordance with current guidelines. Better dissemination of guidelines and their effective implementation in a variety of health care settings are urgently required.
- In many countries, primary care practitioners treat the vast majority of patients with COPD and may be actively involved in public health campaigns and in bringing messages about reducing exposure to risk factors to both patients and the public.
- Spirometric confirmation is a key component of the diagnosis of COPD and primary care practitioners should have access to high-quality spirometry.
- Older patients frequently have multiple chronic health conditions. Comorbidities can magnify the impact of COPD on a patient's health status, and can complicate the management of COPD.

The recommendations provided in sections 1 through 3 define—from a *disease* perspective—best practices in the diagnosis, monitoring, and treatment of COPD. However, (primary) medical care is based on an engagement with *patients*, and this engagement determines the success or failure of pursuing best practice. For this reason, medical practice requires a translation of disease-specific recommendations to the circumstances of individual patients—with regard to the local communities in which they live, and the health systems from which they receive medical care.

Diagnosis

In pursuing early diagnosis, a policy of identifying patients at high risk of COPD, followed by watchful surveillance of these patients, is advised.

Respiratory Symptoms

Of the chronic symptoms characteristic of COPD (dyspnea, cough, sputum production), dyspnea is the symptom that interferes most with a patient's daily life and health status. When taking the medical history of the patient, it is therefore important to explore the impact of dyspnea and other symptoms on daily activities, work, and social activities, and provide treatment accordingly.

Spirometry

High-quality spirometry in primary care is possible[215,216], provided that good skills training and an ongoing quality assurance program are provided. An alternative is to ensure that high-quality spirometry is available in the community—for example, within the primary care practice itself, in a primary care laboratory, or in a hospital setting, depending on the structure of the local health care system.[217] Ongoing collaboration between primary care and respiratory care also helps assure quality control.

Comorbidities

Older patients frequently have multiple chronic health conditions and the severity of comorbid conditions and their impact on a patient's health status will vary between patients and in the same patient over time. Comorbidities for patients with COPD may include the following: other smoking-related diseases, such as ischemic heart disease and lung cancer; conditions that arise as a complication of a specific preexisting disease, such as pulmonary hypertension and consequent heart failure; coexisting chronic conditions with unrelated pathogenesis related to aging, such as bowel or prostate cancer, depression, diabetes mellitus, Parkinson's disease, dementia, and arthritis; or acute illnesses that may have a more severe impact in patients with a given chronic disease. For example, upper respiratory tract infections are the most frequent health problem in all age groups, but they may have a more severe impact or require different treatment in patients with COPD.

Reducing Exposure to Risk Factors

Reduction of total personal exposure to tobacco smoke, occupational dusts and chemicals, and indoor and outdoor air pollutants, including smoke from cooking over biomass-fueled fires, is an important goal to prevent the onset and progression of COPD. In many health care systems, primary care practitioners may be actively involved in public health campaigns and can play an important part in bringing messages about reducing exposure to risk factors to patients and the public.

Primary care practitioners can also play a very important role in reinforcing the dangers of passive smoking and the importance of implementing smoke-free work environments.

Smoking cessation is the most effective intervention to reduce the risk of developing COPD, and simple smoking cessation advice from health care professionals has been shown to make patients more likely to stop smoking. Primary care practitioners often have many contacts with a patient over time, which provides the opportunity to discuss smoking cessation, enhance motivation for quitting, and identify the need for supportive pharmacologic treatment. It is very important to align the advice given by individual practitioners with public health campaigns to send a coherent message to the public.

Implementation of COPD Guidelines

GOLD national leaders play an essential role in the dissemination of information about prevention, early diagnosis, and management of COPD in health systems around the world. A major GOLD program activity that has helped to bring together health care teams at the local level is World COPD Day, held annually on the third Wednesday in November. GOLD national leaders, often in concert with local physicians, nurses, and health care planners, have hosted many types of activities to raise awareness of COPD. WONCA (the World Organization of Family Doctors) is also an active collaborator in organizing World COPD Day activities. Increased participation of a wide variety of health care professionals in World COPD Day activities in many countries would help to increase awareness of COPD.

GOLD is a partner organization in the World Health Organization's GARD with the goal to raise awareness of the burden of chronic respiratory diseases in all countries of the world, and to disseminate and implement recommendations from international guidelines.

Although awareness and dissemination of guidelines are important goals, the actual implementation of a comprehensive care system in which to coordinate the management of COPD will be important to pursue. Evidence is increasing that a chronic disease management program for patients with COPD that incorporates a variety of interventions, includes pulmonary rehabilitation, and is implemented by primary care reduces hospital admissions and bed days. Key elements are patient participation and information sharing among health care providers.[218]

THE 2008 UPDATE

The Gold Science Committee was established in 2002 to review published research on COPD management and prevention, to evaluate the impact of this research on recommendations in the GOLD documents related to management and prevention, and to post yearly updates on the GOLD website. The first update of the 2006 report included the impact of publications from July 1, 2006 through June 30, 2007; this second update includes the impact of publications from July 1, 2007 through June 30, 2008. This update refers to published literature between July 1, 2007 and June 30, 2008. A 2009 update is under process.

Some new issues presented in the 2008 update include the following points:

1. Some significant extrapulmonary effects and important co-morbidities that may contribute to the severity of the diseases in individual patients have been emphasized.
2. In definition of COPD, the phrase "preventable and treatable" has been incorporated following the ATS/ERS recommendations to recognize the need to present a positive outlook for patients, to encourage the health care community to take a more active role in developing programs for COPD prevention, and to stimulate effective management programs to treat those with the diseases.
3. "Stage 0: At Risk," has been omitted as it not necessary that they do not necessarily progress on to Stage I. Nevertheless, the importance of the public health message that chronic cough and sputum are not normal is unchanged.
4. The spirometric classification of severity continues to recommend use of the fixed ratio, post-bronchodilator $FEV_1/FVC < 0.7$, to define airflow limitation. Using the fixed ratio (FEV_1/FVC) is particularly problematic in milder patients who are elderly as the normal process of aging affects lung volumes.
5. It is estimated that about 15 to 25 percent of adults aged 40 years and older may have airflow limitation classified as Stage I : Mild COPD or higher. Evidence is also provided that the prevalence of COPD (Stage I : Mild COPD and higher) is appreciably higher smokers and ex-smokers than in nonsmokers, in those over 40 years than those under 40, and higher in men than in women. New information on COPD morbidity and mortality is provided.
6. Although cigarette smoke is the most commonly encountered risk factor for COPD, other risk factor should be taken into account like occupational dusts and chemicals, and indoor air pollution from biomass cooking and heating in poorly ventilated dwellings – the latter especially among women in developing countries. Avoidance of these factors will help in preventing COPD.
7. Management of COPD continues to be presented in four components and all components have been updated based on recently published literature. Throughout the document, it is emphasized that the overall approach to managing stable COPD should be individualized to address symptoms and improve quality of life.

8. The COPD exacerbation had been defined as: "an event in the natural course of the disease characterized by a change in the patients baseline dyspnea, cough, and/or sputum that is beyond normal day-to-day variations, is acute in onset and may warrant a change in regular medication in a patient with underlying COPD".

9. The new update has also emphasized the necessity of the health care providers required to assure that COPD is diagnosed accurately, and that individuals who have COPD are treated effectively. The identification of effective health care teams will dependent on the local health care system, and much work remains to identify how best to build these health care teams. A chapter on COPD implementation programs and issues for clinical practice has been included but it remains a field that requires considerable attention.

REFERENCES

1. Soriano JB, Visick GT, Muellerova H, Payvandi N, Hansell AL. Patterns of comorbidities in newly diagnosed COPD and asthma in primary care. Chest 2005;128:2099–2107.

2. Agusti AG. Systemic effects of chronic obstructive pulmonary disease. Proc Am Thorac Soc 2005;2:367-70.

3. Johannessen A, Lehmann S, Omenaas ER, Eide GE, Bakke PS, Gulsvik A. Post-bronchodilator spirometry reference values in adults and implications for disease management. Am J Respir Crit Care Med 2006;173:1316-25.

4. Fairall LR, Zwarenstein M, Bateman ED, Bachmann M, Lombard C, Majara BP, Joubert G, English RG, Bheekie A, van Rensburg D, et al. Effect of educational outreach to nurses on tuberculosis case detection and primary care of respiratory illness: Pragmatic cluster randomised controlled trial. BMJ 2005;331:750-54.

5. de Valliere S, Barker RD. Residual lung damage after completion of treatment for multidrug-resistant tuberculosis. Int J Tuberc Lung Dis 2004;8:767–71.

6. Bateman ED, Feldman C, O'Brien J, Plit M, Joubert JR. Guideline for the management of chronic obstructive pulmonary disease (COPD): 2004 revision. S Afr Med J 2004;94:559-75.

7. Georgopoulas D, Anthonisen NR. Symptoms and signs of COPD. In: Cherniack NS. Chronic obstructive pulmonary disease. Toronto, ON, Canada: WB Saunders 1991;357-63.

8. Schols AM, Soeters PB, Dingemans AM, Mostert R, Frantzen PJ, Wouters EF. Prevalence and characteristics of nutritional depletion in patients with stable COPD eligible for pulmonary rehabilitation. Am Rev Respir Dis 1993;147:1151-56.

9. Calverley PMA. Neuropsychological deficits in chronic obstructive pulmonary disease. Monaldi Arch Chest Dis 1996;51:5-6.

10. Holguin F, Folch E, Redd SC, Mannino DM. Comorbidity and mortality in COPD-related hospitalizations in the United States, 1979 to 2001. Chest 2005;128:2005-11.

11. Kesten S, Chapman KR. Physician perceptions and management of COPD. Chest 1993;104:254-58.

12. Loveridge B, West P, Kryger MH, Anthonisen NR. Alteration in breathing pattern with progression of chronic obstructive pulmonary disease. Am Rev Respir Dis 1986;134:930–934.

13. Pellegrino R, Viegi G, Brusasco V, Crapo RO, Burgos F, Casaburi R, Coates A, van der Grinten CP, Gustafsson P, Hankinson J, et al. Interpretative strategies for lung function tests. Eur Respir J 2005;26:948-68.

14. Hardie JA, Buist AS, Vollmer WM, Ellingsen I, Bakke PS, Morkve O. Risk of over-diagnosis of COPD in asymptomatic elderly never-smokers. Eur Respir J 2002;20:1117-22.

15. Burge PS, Calverley PM, Jones PW, Spencer S, Anderson JA. Prednisolone response in patients with chronic obstructive pulmonary disease: Results from the ISOLDE study. Thorax 2003;58:654-58.

16. Calverley PM, Burge PS, Spencer S, Anderson JA, Jones PW. Bronchodilator reversibility testing in chronic obstructive pulmonary disease. Thorax 2003;58:659-64.

17. Fishman A, Martinez F, Naunheim K, Piantadosi S, Wise R, Ries A, Weinmann G, Wood DE. A randomized trial comparing lung-volume-reduction surgery with medical therapy for severe emphysema. N Engl J Med 2003;348:2059-73.

18. Wilson DH, Wakefield MA, Steven ID, Rohrsheim RA, Esterman AJ, Graham NM. "Sick of smoking": Evaluation of a targeted minimal smoking cessation intervention in general practice. Med J Aust 1990;152:518-21.

19. Britton J, Knox A. Helping people to stop smoking: The new smoking cessation guidelines. Thorax 1999;54:1-2.

20. Fiore MC, Bailey WC, Cohen SJ, Dorfman SF, Fox BJ, Goldstein MG, Gritz E, Hasselblad V, Heyman RB, Jaen CR, et al.; The Tobacco Use and Dependence Clinical Practice Guideline Panel, Staff, and Consortium Representatives. A clinical practice guideline for treating tobacco use and dependence: A US Public Health Service report. JAMA 2000;28:3244-54.

21. American Medical Association. Guidelines for the diagnosis and treatment of nicotine dependence: How to help patients stop smoking. Washington, DC: American Medical Association 1994.

22. Glynn TJ, Manley MW. How to help your patients stop smoking: A National Cancer Institute manual for physicians. Bethesda, MD: US Department of Health and Human Services, Public Health Service, National Institutes of Health, National Cancer Institute 1990.

23. Glynn TJ, Manley MW, Pechacek TF. Physician-initiated smoking cessation program: The National Cancer Institute trials. Prog Clin Biol Res 1990;339:11-25.

24. Fiore MC, Bailey WC, Cohen SJ. Smoking cessation: Information for specialists. Rockville, MD: US Department of Health and Human Services, Public Health Service, Agency for Health Care Policy and Research, and Centers for Disease Control and Prevention 1996.

25. Lancaster T, Stead L, Silagy C, Sowden A. Effectiveness of interventions to help people stop smoking: Findings from the Cochrane Library. BMJ 2000;321:355-58.

26. Tashkin D, Kanner R, Bailey W, Buist S, Anderson P, Nides M, Gonzales D, Dozier G, Patel MK, Jamerson B. Smoking cessation in patients with chronic obstructive pulmonary disease: A double-blind, placebo-controlled, randomised trial. Lancet 2001; 357:1571-75.

27. Jorenby DE, Leischow SJ, Nides MA, Rennard SI, Johnston JA, Hughes AR, Smith SS, Muramoto ML, Daughton DM, Doan K, *et al*. A controlled trial of sustained-release bupropion, a nicotine patch, or both for smoking cessation. N Engl J Med 1999;340:685-91.

28. Jorenby DE, Hays JT, Rigotti NA, Axoulay S, Watsky EJ, Williams KE, Billing CB, Gong J, Reeves KR. Varenicline Phase 3 Study Group. Efficacy of varenicline, an alpha4beta2 nicotinic acetylcholine receptor partial agonist, vs placebo or sustained-release bupropion for smoking cessation: A randomized controlled trial. *JAMA* 2006;296:56–63.

29. Nides M, Oncken C, Gonzales D, Rennard S, Watsky EJ, Anziano R, Reeves KR. Smoking cessation with varenicline, a selective alpha4beta2 nicotinic receptor partial agonist: Results from a 7-week, randomized, placebo- and bupropion-controlled trial with 1-year follow-up. Arch Intern Med 2006;166:1561-68.

30. Tonstad S, Tonnesen P, Hajek P, Williams KE, Billing CB, Reeves KR, Varenicline Phase 3 Study Group. Effect of maintenance therapy with varenicline on smoking cessation: A randomized controlled trial. JAMA 2006;296:64-71.

31. Chapman RS, Xingzhou H, Blair AE, Lan Q. Improvement in household stoves and risk of chronic obstructive pulmonary disease in Xuanwei, China: Retrospective cohort study. BMJ 2005;331:1050.

32. Ghambarian MH, Feenstra TL, Zwanikken P, Kalinina AM. Can prevention be improved? Proposal for an integrated intervention strategy. Prev Med 2004;39: 337-43.

33. Nichter M. Introducing tobacco cessation in developing countries: An overview of Quit Tobacco International. Tob Control 2006;15:12-17.

34. Ackermann-Liebrich U, Leuenberger P, Schwartz J, Schindler C, Monn C, Bolognini G, Bongard JP, Brändli O, Domenighetti G. Elsasser S, et al. Lung function and long term exposure to air pollutants in Switzerland. Study on Air Pollution and Lung Diseases in Adults (SAPALDIA) team. Am J Respir Crit Care Med 1997;155:122-29.

35. Reis AL. Response to bronchodilators. In: Clausen J (Ed). Pulmonary function testing: Guidelines and controversies. New York: Academic Press 1982.

36. Janelli LM, Scherer YK, Schmieder LE. Can a pulmonary health teaching program alter patients' ability to cope with COPD? Rehabil Nurs 1991;16:199–202.

37. Ashikaga T, Vacek PM, Lewis SO. Evaluation of a community-based education program for individuals with chronic obstructive pulmonary disease. J Rehabil 1980;46:23–27.

38. Toshima MT, Kaplan RM, Ries AL. Experimental evaluation of rehabilitation in chronic obstructive pulmonary disease: Short-term effects on exercise endurance and health status. *Health Psychol* 1990;9:237-52.

39. Celli BR. Pulmonary rehabilitation in patients with COPD. *Am J Respir Crit Care Med* 1995;152:861–64.

40. Stewart MA. Effective physician-patient communication and health outcomes: A review. *CMAJ* 1995;152: 1423-33.

41. Clark NM, Nothwehr F, Gong M, Evans D, Maiman LA, Hurwitz ME, Roloff D, Mellins RD. Physician-patient partnership in managing chronic illness. Acad Med 1995;70:957-59.

42. Heffner JE, Fahy B, Hilling L, Barbieri C. Outcomes of advance directive education of pulmonary rehabilitation patients. Am J Respir Crit Care Med 1997;155:1055–1059.

43. Anthonisen NR, Connett JE, Kiley JP, Altose MD, Bailey WC, Buist AS, Conway WA Jr, Enright PL, Kanner RE, O'Hara P, et al. Effects of smoking intervention and the use of an inhaled anticholinergic bronchodilator on the rate of decline of FEV_1. The Lung Health Study. JAMA 1994;272:1497-1505.

44. Pauwels RA, Lofdahl CG, Laitinen LA, Schouten JP, Postma DS, Pride NB, Ohlsson SV. Long-term treatment with inhaled budesonide in persons with mild chronic obstructive pulmonary disease who continue smoking. European Respiratory Society Study on Chronic Obstructive Pulmonary Disease. N Engl J Med 1999; 340:1948-53.

45. Vestbo J, Sorensen T, Lange P, Brix A, Torre P, Viskum K. Long-term effect of inhaled budesonide in mild and moderate chronic obstructive pulmonary disease: A randomised controlled trial. Lancet 1999;353:1819-23.

46. Burge PS, Calverley PM, Jones PW, Spencer S, Anderson JA, Maslen TK. Randomised, double blind, placebo controlled study of fluticasone propionate in patients with moderate to severe chronic obstructive pulmonary disease: the ISOLDE trial. BMJ 2000; 320:1297-1303.

47. Vathenen AS, Britton JR, Ebden P, Cookson JB, Wharrad HJ, Tattersfield AE. High-dose inhaled albuterol in severe chronic airflow limitation. Am Rev Respir Dis 1988;138:850-55.

48. Gross NJ, Petty TL, Friedman M, Skorodin MS, Silvers GW, Donohue JF. Dose response to ipratropium as a nebulized solution in patients with chronic obstructive pulmonary disease: A three-center study. Am Rev Respir *Dis* 1989;139:1188-91.

49. Chrystyn H, Mulley BA, Peake MD. Dose response relation to oral theophylline in severe chronic obstructive airways disease. BMJ 1988;297:1506-10.

50. Higgins BG, Powell RM, Cooper S, Tattersfield AE. Effect of salbutamol and ipratropium bromide on airway calibre and bronchial reactivity in asthma and chronic bronchitis. Eur Respir J 1991;4:415-20.

51. Ikeda A, Nishimura K, Koyama H, Izumi T. Bronchodilating effects of combined therapy with clinical dosages of ipratropium bromide and salbutamol for stable COPD: Comparison with ipratropium bromide alone. Chest 1995;107:401-05.

52. Guyatt GH, Townsend M, Pugsley SO, Keller JL, Short HD, Taylor DW, Newhouse MT. Bronchodilators in chronic air-flow limitation: Effects on airway function, exercise capacity, and quality of life. Am Rev Respir Dis 1987;135:1069-74.

53. Man WD, Mustfa N, Nikoletou D, Kaul S, Hart N, Rafferty GF, Donaldson N, Polkey MI, Moxham J. Effect of salmeterol on respiratory muscle activity during exercise in poorly reversible COPD. Thorax 2004;59:471-76.

54. O'Donnell DE, Fluge T, Gerken F, Hamilton A, Webb K, Aguilaniu B, Make B, Magnussen H. Effects of tiotropium on lung hyperinflation, dyspnoea and exercise tolerance in COPD. Eur Respir J 2004;23:832-40.

55. Vincken W, van Noord JA, Greefhorst AP, Bantje TA, Kesten S, Korducki L, Cornelissen PJ. Improved health outcomes in patients with COPD during 1 yr's treatment with tiotropium. Eur Respir J 2002;19:209-16.

56. Mahler DA, Donohue JF, Barbee RA, Goldman MD, Gross NJ, Wisniewski ME, Yancey SW, Zakes BA, Rickard KA, Anderson WH. Efficacy of salmeterol xinafoate in the treatment of COPD. Chest 1999;115:957-65.

57. Dahl R, Greefhorst LA, Nowak D, Nonikov V, Byrne AM, Thomson MH, Till D, Della Cioppa G. Inhaled formoterol dry powder versus ipratropium bromide in chronic obstructive pulmonary disease. Am J Respir Crit Care Med 2001;164:778-84.

58. Oostenbrink JB, Rutten-van Molken MP, Al MJ, Van Noord JA, Vincken W. One-year cost-effectiveness of tiotropium versus ipratropium to treat chronic obstructive pulmonary disease. Eur Respir J 2004; 23:241-49.

59. Niewoehner DE, Rice K, Cote C, Paulson D, Cooper JA Jr, Korducki L, Cassino C, Kesten S. Prevention of exacerbations of chronic obstructive pulmonary disease with tiotropium, a once-daily inhaled anticholinergic bronchodilator: A randomized trial. Ann Intern Med 2005;143:317-26.

60. Casaburi R, Kukafka D, Cooper CB, Witek TJ Jr, Kesten S. Improvement in exercise tolerance with the combination of tiotropium and pulmonary rehabilitation in patients with COPD. Chest 2005;127:809-17.

61. COMBIVENT Inhalation Aerosol Study Group. In chronic obstructive pulmonary disease, a combination of ipratropium and albuterol is more effective than either agent alone: An 85-day multicenter trial. Chest 1994;105:1411-19.

62. COMBIVENT Inhalation Solution Study Group. Routine nebulized ipratropium and albuterol together are better than either alone in COPD. *Chest* 1997;112:1514-21.

63. Gross N, Tashkin D, Miller R, Oren J, Coleman W, Linberg S. Inhalation by nebulization of albuterol-ipratropium combination (Dey combination) is superior to either agent alone in the treatment of chronic obstructive pulmonary disease. Dey Combination Solution Study Group. Respiration (Herrlisheim) 1998;65:354-62.

64. Taylor DR, Buick B, Kinney C, Lowry RC, McDevitt DG. The efficacy of orally administered theophylline, inhaled salbutamol, and a combination of the two as chronic therapy in the management of chronic bronchitis with reversible air-flow obstruction. Am Rev Respir Dis 1985;131:747-51.

65. van Noord JA, de Munck DR, Bantje TA, Hop WC, Akveld ML, Bommer AM. Long-term treatment of chronic obstructive pulmonary disease with salmeterol and the additive effect of ipratropium. Eur Respir J 2000;15:878-85.

66. ZuWallack RL, Mahler DA, Reilly D, Church N, Emmett A, Rickard K, Knobil K. Salmeterol plus theophylline combination therapy in the treatment of COPD. Chest 2001;119:1661-70.

67. Bellia V, Foresi A, Bianco S, Grassi V, Olivieri D, Bensi G, Volonte M. Efficacy and safety of oxitropium bromide, theophylline and their combination in COPD patients: A double-blind, randomized, multicentre study (BREATH trial). Respir Med 2002;96:881-89.

68. Guyatt GH, Berman LB, Townsend M, Pugsley SO, Chambers LW. A measure of quality of life for clinical trials in chronic lung disease. Thorax 1987;42:773-78.

69. O'Driscoll BR, Kay EA, Taylor RJ, Weatherby H, Chetty MC, Bernstein A. A long-term prospective assessment of home nebulizer treatment. Respir Med 1992;86:317-25.

70. Jenkins SC, Heaton RW, Fulton TJ, Moxham J. Comparison of domiciliary nebulized salbutamol and salbutamol from a metered-dose inhaler in stable chronic airflow limitation. Chest 1987;91:804-07.

71. The Lung Health Study Research Group. Effect of inhaled triamcinolone on the decline in pulmonary function in chronic obstructive pulmonary disease: Lung Health Study II. N Engl J Med 2000;343:1902-09.

72. Mahler DA, Wire P, Horstman D, Chang CN, Yates J, Fischer T, Shah T. Effectiveness of fluticasone propionate and salmeterol combination delivered via the Diskus device in the treatment of chronic obstructive pulmonary disease. Am J Respir Crit Care Med 2002;166:1084-91.

73. Jones PW, Willits LR, Burge PS, Calverley PM. Disease severity and the effect of fluticasone propionate on chronic obstructive pulmonary disease exacerbations. Eur Respir J 2003;21:68-73.

74. Calverley P, Pauwels R, Vestbo J, Jones P, Pride N, Gulsvik A, Anderson J, Maden C. Combined salmeterol and fluticasone in the treatment of chronic obstructive pulmonary disease: A randomised controlled trial. Lancet 2003;361:449-56.

75. Szafranski W, Cukier A, Ramirez A, Menga G, Sansores R, Nahabedian S, Peterson S, Olsson H. Efficacy and safety of budesonide/formoterol in the management of chronic obstructive pulmonary disease. Eur Respir J 2003;21:74-81.

76. Spencer S, Calverley PM, Burge PS, Jones PW. Impact of preventing exacerbations on deterioration of health status in COPD. Eur Respir J 2004;23:698-702.

77. van der Valk P, Monninkhof E, van der Palen J, Zielhuis G, van Herwaarden C. Effect of discontinuation of inhaled corticosteroids in patients with chronic obstructive pulmonary disease: the COPE study. Am J Respir Crit Care Med 2002;166:1358–63.

78. Sin DD, Wu L, Anderson JA, Anthonisen NR, Buist AS, Burge PS, Calverley PM, Connett JE, Lindmark B, Pauwels RA, et al. Inhaled corticosteroids and mortality in chronic obstructive pulmonary disease. Thorax 2005;60:992-97.

79. Hanania NA, Darken P, Horstman D, Reisner C, Lee B, Davis S, Shah T. The efficacy and safety of fluticasone propionate (250 microg)/salmeterol (50 microg) combined in the Diskus inhaler for the treatment of COPD. Chest 2003;124:834-43.

80. Calverley PM, Boonsawat W, Cseke Z, Zhong N, Peterson S, Olsson H. Maintenance therapy with budesonide and formoterol in chronic obstructive pulmonary disease. Eur Respir J 2003;22:912-19.

81. Decramer M, de Bock V, Dom R. Functional and histologic picture of steroid-induced myopathy in chronic obstructive pulmonary disease. Am J Respir Crit Care Med 1996;153:1958-64.

82. Decramer M, Lacquet LM, Fagard R, Rogiers P. Corticosteroids contribute to muscle weakness in chronic airflow obstruction. Am J Respir Crit Care Med 1994;150:11-16.

83. Decramer M, Stas KJ. Corticosteroid-induced myopathy involving respiratory muscles in patients with chronic obstructive pulmonary disease or asthma. Am Rev Respir Dis 1992;146:800-02.

84. Wongsurakiat P, Maranetra KN, Wasi C, Kositanont U, Dejsomritrutai W, Charoenratanakul S. Acute respiratory illness in patients with COPD and the effectiveness of influenza vaccination: A randomized controlled study. Chest 2004;125:2011-20.

85. Nichol KL, Margolis KL, Wuorenma J, Von Sternberg T. The efficacy and cost effectiveness of vaccination against influenza among elderly persons living in the community. N Engl J Med 1994;331:778-84.

86. Wongsurakiat P, Lertakyamanee J, Maranetra KN, Jongriratanakul S, Sangkaew S. Economic evaluation of influenza vaccination in Thai chronic obstructive pulmonary disease patients. J Med Assoc Thai 2003;86:497-508.

87. Edwards KM, Dupont WD, Westrich MK, Plummer WD Jr, Palmer PS, Wright PF. A randomized controlled trial of cold-adapted and inactivated vaccines for the prevention of influenza A disease. J Infect Dis 1994;169:68-76.

88. Hak E, van Essen GA, Buskens E, Stalman W, de Melker RA. Is immunising all patients with chronic lung disease in the community against influenza cost effective? Evidence from a general practice based clinical prospective cohort study in Utrecht, The Netherlands. J Epidemiol Community Health 1998;52:120-25.

89. Woodhead M, Blasi F, Ewig S, Huchon G, Ieven M, Ortqvist A. Schaberg T, Torres A, van der Heijden G, Verheij TJ. Guidelines for the management of adult lower respiratory tract infections. Eur Respir J 2005;26:1138-80.

90. Jackson LA, Neuzil KM, Yu O, Benson P, Barlow WE, Adams AL, Hanson CA, Mahoney LD, Shay DK, Thompson WW. Effectiveness of pneumococcal polysaccharide vaccine in older adults. N Engl J Med 2003;348:1747-55.

91. Advisory Committee on Immunization Practices. Prevention of pneumococcal disease: Recommendations

of the Advisory Committee on Immunization Practices (ACIP). MMWR Morb Mortal Wkly Rep 1997;46(RR-08):1-24.

92. Alfageme I, Vazaque R, Reyes N, Munoz J, Fernandez A, Hernandez M, Merino M, Perez J, Lima J. Clinical efficacy of anti-pneumococcal vaccination in patients with COPD. Thorax 2006;61:189-95.

93. Francis RS, May JR, Spicer CC. Chemotherapy of bronchitis: Influence of penicillin and tetracycline administered daily, or intermittently for exacerbations. BMJ 1961;2:979-85.

94. Francis RS, Spicer CC. Chemotherapy in chronic bronchitis: Influence of daily penicillin and teracycline on exacerbations and their cost: A report to the research committee of the British Tuberculosis Association by their Chronic Bronchitis subcommittee. BMJ 1960;1:297-03.

95. Medical Research Council. Value of chemoprophylaxis and chemotherapy in early chronic bronchitis: A report to the Medical Research Council by their Working Party on trials of chemotherapy in early chronic bronchitis. BMJ 1966;1(5499):1317-22.

96. Johnston RN, McNeill RS, Smith DH, Dempster MB, Nairn JR, Purvis MS, Watson JM, Ward FG. Five-year winter chemoprophylaxis for chronic bronchitis. BMJ 1969;4:265-69.

97. Isada CM, Stoller JK. Chronic bronchitis: The role of antibiotics. In: Niederman MS, Sarosi GA, Glassroth J (Eds). Respiratory infections: A scientific basis for management. London: WB Saunders 1994;621-33.

98. Siafakas NM, Bouros D. Management of acute exacerbation of chronic obstructive pulmonary disease. In: Postma DS, Siafakas NM. Management of chronic obstructive pulmonary disease. Sheffield, UK: ERS Monograph 1998;264-77.

99. Allegra L, Cordaro CI, Grassi C. Prevention of acute exacerbations of chronic obstructive bronchitis with carbocysteine lysine salt monohydrate: A multicenter, double-blind, placebo-controlled trial. Respiration (Herrlisheim) 1996;63:174-80.

100. Guyatt GH, Townsend M, Kazim F, Newhouse MT. A controlled trial of ambroxol in chronic bronchitis. Chest 1987;92:618-20.

101. Petty TL. The National Mucolytic Study: Results of a randomized, double-blind, placebo-controlled study of iodinated glycerol in chronic obstructive bronchitis. Chest 1990;97:75-83.

102. Siafakas NM, Vermeire P, Pride NB, Paoletti P, Gibson J, Howard P, Yernault JC, Decramer M, Higenbottam T, Postma DS, *et al*. Optimal assessment and management of chronic obstructive pulmonary disease (COPD). The European Respiratory Society Task Force. Eur Respir J 1995;8:1398-1420.

103. American Thoracic Society. Standards for the diagnosis and care of patients with chronic obstructive pulmonary disease (COPD) and asthma. Am Rev Respir Dis 1987;136:225-44.

104. Hansen NC, Skriver A, Brorsen-Riis L, Balslov S, Evald T, Maltbaek N, Gunnersen G, Garsdal P, Sander P, Pedersen JZ, et al. Orally administered N-acetylcysteine may improve general well-being in patients with mild chronic bronchitis. Respir Med 1994;88:531-35.

105. British Thoracic Society Research Committee. Oral N-acetylcysteine and exacerbation rates in patients with chronic bronchitis and severe airways obstruction. Thorax 1985;40:832-35.

106. Boman G, Backer U, Larsson S, Melander B, Wahlander L. Oral acetylcysteine reduces exacerbation rate in chronic bronchitis: Report of a trial organized by the Swedish Society for Pulmonary Diseases. Eur J Respir Dis 1983;64:405-15.

107. Rasmussen JB, Glennow C. Reduction in days of illness after long-term treatment with N-acetylcysteine controlled-release tablets in patients with chronic bronchitis. Eur Respir J 1988;1:351-55.

108. Decramer M, Rutten-van Molken M, Dekhuijzen PN, Troosters T, van Herwaarden C, Pellegrino R, van Schayck CP, Olivieri D, Del Donno M, De Backer W, et al. Effects of N-acetylcysteine on outcomes in chronic obstructive pulmonary disease (Bronchitis Randomized on NAC Cost-Utility Study, BRONCUS): A randomised placebo-controlled trial. Lancet 2005;365:1552-60.

109. Collet JP, Shapiro P, Ernst P, Renzi T, Ducruet T, Robinson A. Effects of an immunostimulating agent on acute exacerbations and hospitalizations in patients with chronic obstructive pulmonary disease. The PARI-IS Study Steering Committee and Research Group (Prevention of Acute Respiratory Infection by an Immunostimulant). Am J Respir Crit Care Med 1997;156:1719-24.

110. Li J, Zheng JP, Yuan JP, Zeng GQ, Zhong NS, Lin CY. Protective effect of a bacterial extract against acute exacerbation in patients with chronic bronchitis accompanied by chronic obstructive pulmonary disease. Chin Med J (Engl) 2004;117:828-34.

111. Anthonisen NR. OM-8BV for COPD. Am J Respir Crit Care Med 1997;156:1713-14.

112. Irwin RS, Boulet LP, Cloutier MM, Fuller R, Gold PM, Hoffstein V, Ing AJ, McCool FD, O'Byrne P, Poe RH, et al. Managing cough as a defense mechanism and as a symptom: A consensus panel report of the American College of Chest Physicians. *Chest* 1998;114(2 Suppl Managing):133S–181S.

113. Barbera JA, Roger N, Roca J, Rovira I, Higenbottam TW, Rodriguez-Roisin R. Worsening of pulmonary gas exchange with nitric oxide inhalation in chronic obstructive pulmonary disease. Lancet 1996;347:436-40.

114. Jones AT, Evans TW. NO: COPD and beyond. Thorax 1997;52:S16–S21.

115. Jennings AL, Davies AN, Higgins JP, Gibbs JS, Broadley KE. A systematic review of the use of opioids in the management of dyspnoea. Thorax 2002;57:939-44.

116. Eiser N, Denman WT, West C, Luce P. Oral diamorphine: Lack of effect on dyspnoea and exercise tolerance in the "pink puffer" syndrome. Eur Respir J 1991;4:926-31.

117. Young IH, Daviskas E, Keena VA. Effect of low dose nebulised morphine on exercise endurance in patients with chronic lung disease. Thorax 1989;44:387-90.

118. Woodcock AA, Gross ER, Gellert A, Shah S, Johnson M, Geddes DM. Effects of dihydrocodeine, alcohol, and caffeine on breathlessness and exercise tolerance in patients with chronic obstructive lung disease and normal blood gases. N Engl J Med 1981;305:1611-16.

119. Rice KL, Kronenberg RS, Hedemark LL, Niewoehner DE. Effects of chronic administration of codeine and promethazine on breathlessness and exercise tolerance in patients with chronic airflow obstruction. Br J Dis Chest 1987;81:287-92.

120. Poole PJ, Veale AG, Black PN. The effect of sustained-release morphine on breathlessness and quality of life in severe chronic obstructive pulmonary disease. Am J Respir Crit Care Med 1998;157:1877-80.

121. Nici L, Donner C, Wouters E, Zuwallack R. ATS/ERS Pulmonary Rehabilitation Writing Committee. American Thoracic Society/European Respiratory Society statement on pulmonary rehabilitation. Am J Respir Crit Care Med 2006;173:1390-1413.

122. Foglio K, Bianchi L, Bruletti G, Battista L, Pagani M, Ambrosino N. Long-term effectiveness of pulmonary rehabilitation in patients with chronic airway obstruction. Eur Respir J 1999;13:125-32.

123. Young P, Dewse M, Fergusson W, Kolbe J. Improvements in outcomes for chronic obstructive pulmonary disease (COPD) attributable to a hospital-based respiratory rehabilitation programme. Aust N Z J Med 1999;29:59-65.

124. Griffiths TL, Burr ML, Campbell IA, Lewis-Jenkins V, Mullins J, Shiels K, Turner-Lawlor PJ, Payne N, Newcombe RG, Ionescu AA, et al. Results at 1 year of outpatient multidisciplinary pulmonary rehabilitation: a randomised controlled trial. Lancet 2000;355:362-68.

125. Goldstein RS, Gort EH, Stubbing D, Avendano MA, Guyatt GH. Randomised controlled trial of respiratory rehabilitation. Lancet 1994;344:1394-97.

126. Wijkstra PJ, Van Altena R, Kraan J, Otten V, Postma DS, Koeter GH. Quality of life in patients with chronic obstructive pulmonary disease improves after rehabilitation at home. Eur Respir J 1994;7:269-73.

127. McGavin CR, Gupta SP, Lloyd EL, McHardy GJ. Physical rehabilitation for the chronic bronchitic: Results of a controlled trial of exercises in the home. Thorax 1977;32:307-11.

128. Nocturnal Oxygen Therapy Trial Group. Continuous or nocturnal oxygen therapy in hypoxemic chronic obstructive lung disease: a clinical trial. Ann Intern Med 1980;93:391-98.

129. Report of the Medical Research Council Working Party. Long term domiciliary oxygen therapy in chronic hypoxic cor pulmonale complicating chronic bronchitis and emphysema. Lancet 1981;1:681-86.

130. Tarpy SP, Celli BR. Long-term oxygen therapy. N Engl J Med 1995;333:710-14.

131. Clinical indications for noninvasive positive pressure ventilation in chronic respiratory failure due to restrictive lung disease, COPD, and nocturnal hypoventilation consensus conference report. Chest 1999;116:521-34.

132. Mehran RJ, Deslauriers J. Indications for surgery and patient work-up for bullectomy. Chest Surg Clin N Am 1995;5:717-34.

133. Naunheim KS. Wood DE, Mohsenifar Z, Sternberg AL, Criner GJ, DeCamp MM, Deschamps CC, Martinez FJ, Sciurba FC, Tonascia J, et al. Long-term follow-up of patients receiving lung-volume-reduction surgery versus medical therapy for severe emphysema by the National Emphysema Treatment Trial Research Group. Ann Thorac Surg 2006;82:431-43.

134. Trulock EP. Lung transplantation. Am J Respir Crit Care Med 1997;155:789-18.

135. Theodore J, Lewiston N. Lung transplantation comes of age. N Engl J Med 1990;322:772-74.

136. Hosenpud JD, Bennett LE, Keck BM, Fiol B, Boucek MM, Novick RJ. The Registry of the International Society for Heart and Lung Transplantation: Fifteenth official report—1998. J Heart Lung Transplant 1998;17:656-68.

137. Annual report of the US Scientific Registry for Transplant Recipients and the Organ Procurement and Transplantation Network. Transplant data: 1988–1994. Washington, DC: Division of Transplantation, Health Resources and Services Administraion, US Department of Health and Human Services; 1995.

138. Hosenpud JD, Bennett LE, Keck BM, Edwards EB, Novick RJ. Effect of diagnosis on survival benefit of lung transplantation for end-stage lung disease. Lancet 1998;351:24-27.

139. Maurer JR, Frost AE, Estenne M, Higenbottam T, Glanville AR. International guidelines for the selection of lung transplant candidates. The International Society for Heart and Lung Transplantation, the American Thoracic Society, the American Society of Transplant Physicians, the European Respiratory Society. Transplantation 1998;66:951-56.

140. Smetana GW. Preoperative pulmonary evaluation. N Engl J Med 1999;340:937-44.

141. Trayner E Jr, Celli BR. Postoperative pulmonary complications. Med Clin North Am 2001;85:1129-39.

142. Weisman IM. Cardiopulmonary exercise testing in the preoperative assessment for lung resection surgery. Semin Thorac Cardiovasc Surg 2001;13:116-25.

143. Bolliger CT, Perruchoud AP. Functional evaluation of the lung resection candidate. Eur Respir J 1998;11:198-12.

144. Schuurmans MM, Diacon AH, Bolliger CT. Functional evaluation before lung resection. Clin Chest Med 2002;23:159-72.

145. Celli BR, MacNee W. Standards for the diagnosis and treatment of patients with COPD: A summary of the ATS/ERS position paper. Eur Respir J 2004;23:932-46.

146. Regueiro CR, Hamel MB, Davis RB, Desbiens N, Connors AF Jr, Phillips RS. A comparison of generalist and pulmonologist care for patients hospitalized with severe chronic obstructive pulmonary disease: Resource intensity, hospital costs, and survival. SUPPORT Investigators (Study to Understand Prognoses and Preferences for Outcomes and Risks of Treatment). Am J Med 1998;105:366-72.

147. Gibson PG, Wlodarczyk JH, Wilson AJ, Sprogis A. Severe exacerbation of chronic obstructive airways disease: Health resource use in general practice and hospital. J Qual Clin Pract 1998;18:125-33.

148. Anthonisen NR, Manfreda J, Warren CP, Hershfield ES, Harding GK, Nelson NA. Antibiotic therapy in exacerbations of chronic obstructive pulmonary disease. Ann Intern Med 1987;106:196-204.

149. Warren PM, Flenley DC, Millar JS, Avery A. Respiratory failure revisited: Acute exacerbations of chronic bronchitis between 1961–68 and 1970–76. Lancet 1980;1:467-70.

150. Gunen H, Hacievliyagil SS, Kosar F, Mutlu LC, Gulbas G, Pehlivan E, Sahin I, Kizkin O. Factors affecting survival of hospitalised patients with COPD. Eur Respir J 2005;26:234-41.

151. Rodriguez-Roisin R. Toward a consensus definition for COPD exacerbations. Chest 2000;117(5, Suppl 2):398S-401S.

152. Burge S, Wedzicha JA. COPD exacerbations: Definitions and classifications. Eur Respir J Suppl 2003;41:46s–53s.

153. Seemungal TA, Donaldson GC, Bhowmik A, Jeffries DJ, Wedzicha JA. Time course and recovery of exacerbations in patients with chronic obstructive pulmonary disease. Am J Respir Crit Care Med 2000;161:1608-13.

154. White AJ, Gompertz S, Stockley RA. Chronic obstructive pulmonary disease 6: The aetiology of exacerbations of chronic obstructive pulmonary disease. Thorax 2003;58:73-80.

155. Monso E, Ruiz J, Rosell A, Manterola J, Fiz J, Morera J, Ausina V. Bacterial infection in chronic obstructive pulmonary disease: A study of stable and exacerbated outpatients using the protected specimen brush. Am J Respir Crit Care Med 1995;152:1316-20.

156. Pela R, Marchesani F, Agostinelli C, Staccioli D, Cecarini L, Bassotti C, Sanguinetti CM. Airways microbial flora in COPD patients in stable clinical conditions and during exacerbations: A bronchoscopic investigation. Monaldi Arch Chest Dis 1998;53:262-67.

157. Sethi S, Evans N, Grant BJ, Murphy TF. New strains of bacteria and exacerbations of chronic obstructive pulmonary disease. N Engl J Med 2002;347:465-71.

158. Sethi S, Wrona C, Grant BJ, Murphy TF. Strain-specific immune response to *Haemophilus influenzae* in chronic obstructive pulmonary disease. Am J Respir Crit Care Med 2004;169:448-53.

159. Sethi S, Muscarella K, Evans N, Klingman KL, Grant BJ, Murphy TF. Airway inflammation and etiology of acute exacerbations of chronic bronchitis. Chest 2000;118:1557-65.

160. White AJ, Gompertz S, Bayley DL, Hill SL, O'Brien C, Unsal I, Stockley RA. Resolution of bronchial inflammation is related to bacterial eradication following treatment of exacerbations of chronic bronchitis. Thorax 2003;58:680-85.

161. Murphy TF, Brauer AL, Grant BJ, Sethi S. *Moraxella catarrhalis* in chronic obstructive pulmonary disease: burden of disease and immune response. Am J Respir Crit Care Med 2005;172:195-99.

162. Emerman CL, Connors AF, Lukens TW, Effron D, May ME. Relationship between arterial blood gases and spirometry in acute exacerbations of chronic obstructive pulmonary disease. Ann Emerg Med 1989;18:523-27.

163. Al-Fayez SF, Salleh M, Ardawi M. Azahran FM. Effects of sheesha and cigarette smoking on pulmonary function of Saudi males and females. Trop Geogr Med 1988;40:115-23.

164. Adams SJM, Luther M. Antibiotics are associated with lower relapse rates in outpatients with acute exacerbations of chronic obstructive pulmonary disease. Chest 2000;117:1345-52.

165. Mueller C, Laule-Kiliam K, Frana B, Rodriguez D, Rudez J, Swcholer A, Buser P, Pfisterer M, Perruchoud AP. The use of B-natriuretic peptide in the managment of elderly patients with acute dyspnea. J Intern Med 2005;258:77-85.

166. Richards AM, Nicholls MG, Epiner EA, Lainchbury JD, Troughton RW, Elliott J, Framton C, Turner J, Crozier IG, Yandle TG. B-type natriuretic peptide and ejectrion fraction for prognosis after myocardial infarction. Circulation 2003;107:2786.

167. Davies L, Wilkinson M, Bonner S, Calverley PM, Angus RM. "Hospital at home" versus hospital care in patients with exacerbations of chronic obstructive pulmonary disease: Prospective randomised controlled trial. BMJ 2000;321:1265-68.

168. Ojoo JC, Moon T, McGlone S, Martin K, Gardiner ED, Greenstone MA, Morice AH. Patients' and carers' preferences in two models of care for acute exacerbations of COPD: Results of a randomised controlled trial. Thorax 2002;57:167-69.

169. Skwarska E, Cohen G, Skwarski KM, Lamb C, Bushell D, Parker S, MacNee W. Randomized controlled trial of supported discharge in patients with exacerbations of chronic obstructive pulmonary disease. Thorax 2000;55:907-12.

170. Hernandez C, Casas A, Escarrabill J, Alonso J, Puig-Junoy J, Farrero E, Vilagut G, Collvinent B, Rodriguez-Roisin R, Roca J, et al. Home hospitalisation of exacerbated chronic obstructive pulmonary disease patients. Eur Respir J 2003;21:58-67.

171. Thompson WH, Nielson CP, Carvalho P, Charan NB, Crowley JJ. Controlled trial of oral prednisone in outpatients with acute COPD exacerbation. Am J Respir Crit Care Med 1996;154:407-12.

172. Davies L, Angus RM, Calverley PM. Oral corticosteroids in patients admitted to hospital with exacerbations of chronic obstructive pulmonary disease: A prospective randomised controlled trial. Lancet 1999;354:456-60.

173. Niewoehner DE, Erbland ML, Deupree RH, Collins D, Gross NJ, Light RW, Anderson P, Morgan NA. Effect of systemic glucocorticoids on exacerbations of chronic obstructive pulmonary disease. Department of Veterans Affairs Cooperative Study Group. N Engl J Med 1999;340:1941-47.

174. Maltais F, Ostinelli J, Bourbeau J, Tonnel AB, Jacquemet N, Haddon J, Rouleau M, Boukhana M, Martinot JB, Duroux P. Comparison of nebulized budesonide and oral prednisolone with placebo in the treatment of acute exacerbations of chronic obstructive pulmonary disease: a randomized controlled trial. Am J Respir Crit Care Med 2002;165:698-03.

175. Aaron SD, Vandemheen KL, Hebert P, Dales R, Stiell IG, Ahuja J, Dickinson G, Brison R, Rowe BH, Dreyer J, et al. Outpatient oral prednisone after emergency treatment of chronic obstructive pulmonary disease. N Engl J Med 2003;348:2618–2625.

176. Rodriguez-Roisin R. COPD exacerbations. 5: Management. Thorax 2006;61:535-44.

177. Connors AF, Jr., Dawson NV, Thomas C, Harrell FE, Jr, Desbiens N, Fulkerson WJ, Kussin P, Bellamy P, Goldman L, Knaus WA. Outcomes following acute exacerbation of severe chronic obstructive lung disease. The SUPPORT investigators (Study to Understand Prognoses and Preferences for Outcomes and Risks of Treatments). Am J Respir Crit Care Med 1996;154:959-67.

178. Shepperd S, Harwood D, Gray A, Vessey M, Morgan P. Randomised controlled trial comparing hospital at home care with inpatient hospital care. II: Cost minimisation analysis. BMJ 1998;316:1791-96.

179. Gravil JH, Al-Rawas OA, Cotton MM, Flanigan U, Irwin A, Stevenson RD. Home treatment of exacerbations of chronic obstructive pulmonary disease by an acute respiratory assessment service. Lancet 1998;351:1853-55.

180. Soderstrom L, Tousignant P, Kaufman T. The health and cost effects of substituting home care for inpatient acute care: a review of the evidence. CMAJ 1999;160:1151-55.

181. National Institute for Clinical Excellence (NICE). Chronic obstructive pulmonary disease: National clinical guideline on management of chronic obstructive pulmonary disease in adults in primary and secondary care. Thorax 2004;59:1-232.

182. Barbera JA, Reyes A, Roca J, Montserrat JM, Wagner PD, Rodriguez-Roisin R. Effect of intravenously administered aminophylline on ventilation/perfusion inequality during recovery from exacerbations of chronic obstructive pulmonary disease. Am Rev Respir Dis 1992;145:1328-33.

183. Mahon JL, Laupacis A, Hodder RV, McKim DA, Paterson NA, Wood TE, Donner A. Theophylline for irreversible chronic airflow limitation: a randomized study comparing n of 1 trials to standard practice. Chest 1999;115:38-48.

184. Lloberes P, Ramis L, Montserrat JM, Serra J, Campistol J, Picado C, Agusti-Vidal A. Effect of three different bronchodilators during an exacerbation of chronic obstructive pulmonary disease. Eur Respir J 1988;1:536-39.

185. Murciano D, Aubier M, Lecocguic Y, Pariente R. Effects of theophylline on diaphragmatic strength and fatigue in patients with chronic obstructive pulmonary disease. N Engl J Med 1984;311:349-53.

186. Emerman CL, Connors AF, Lukens TW, May ME, Effron D. Theophylline concentrations in patients with acute exacerbation of COPD. Am J Emerg Med 1990;8:289-92.

187. Barr RG, Rowe BH, Camargo CA Jr. Methylxanthines for exacerbations of chronic obstructive pulmonary disease: Meta-analysis of randomised trials. BMJ 2003;327:643.

188. Duffy N, Walker P, Diamantea F, Calverley PM, Davies L. Intravenous aminophylline in patients admitted to hospital with non-acidotic exacerbations of chronic obstructive pulmonary disease: A prospective randomised controlled trial. Thorax 2005;60:713-17.

189. Seemungal T, Harper-Owen R, Bhowmik A, Moric I, Sanderson G, Message S, Maccallum P, Meade TW, Jeffries DJ, Johnston SL, et al. Respiratory viruses, symptoms, and inflammatory markers in acute exacerbations and stable chronic obstructive pulmonary disease. Am J Respir Crit Care Med 2001;164:1618-23.

190. Blasi F, Damato S, Cosentini R, Tarsia P, Raccanelli R, Centanni S, Allegra L. Chlamydia pneumoniae and chronic bronchitis: Association with severity and bacterial clearance following treatment. Thorax 2002;57:672-76.

191. Seemungal TA, Wedzicha JA, MacCallum PK, Johnston SL, Lambert PA. Chlamydia pneumoniae and COPD exacerbation. Thorax 2002;57:1087-88.

192. Greenstone M, Lasserson TJ. Doxapram for ventilatory failure due to exacerbations of chronic obstructive pulmonary disease. Cochrane Database Syst Rev 2003;1:CD000223.

193. Lightowler JV, Wedzicha JA, Elliott MW, Ram FS. Non-invasive positive pressure ventilation to treat respiratory failure resulting from exacerbations of chronic obstructive pulmonary disease: Cochrane systematic review and meta-analysis. BMJ 2003;326:185.

194. Meyer TJ, Hill NS. Noninvasive positive pressure ventilation to treat respiratory failure. Ann Intern Med 1994;120:760-70.

195. Brochard L, Mancebo J, Wysocki M, Lofaso F, Conti G, Rauss A, Simonneau G, Benito S, Gasparetto A, Lemaire F. Noninvasive ventilation for acute exacerbations of chronic obstructive pulmonary disease. N Engl J Med 1995;333:817-22.

196. Kramer N, Meyer TJ, Meharg J, Cece RD, Hill NS. Randomized, prospective trial of noninvasive positive pressure ventilation in acute respiratory failure. Am J Respir Crit Care Med 1995;151:1799-1806.

197. Bott J, Carroll MP, Conway JH, Keilty SE, Ward EM, Brown AM, Paul EA, Elliott MW, Godfrey RC, Wedzicha JA, et al. Randomised controlled trial of nasal ventilation in acute ventilatory failure due to chronic obstructive airways disease. Lancet 1993;341:1555-57.

198. Plant PK, Owen JL, Elliott MW. Early use of non-invasive ventilation for acute exacerbations of chronic obstructive pulmonary disease on general respiratory wards: A multicentre randomised controlled trial. Lancet 2000;355:1931-35.

199. Esteban A, Anzueto A, Alia I, Gordo F, Apezteguia C, Palizas F, Cide D, Goldwaser R, Soto L, Bugedo G, et al. How is mechanical ventilation employed in the intensive care unit? An international utilization review. Am J Respir Crit Care Med 2000;161:1450-58.

200. International Consensus Conferences in Intensive Care Medicine. Noninvasive positive pressure ventilation in acute respiratory failure. Am J Respir Crit Care Med 2001;163:283-91.

201. Plant PK, Owen JL, Elliott MW. Non-invasive ventilation in acute exacerbations of chronic obstructive pulmonary disease: Long term survival and predictors of in-hospital outcome. Thorax 2001;56:708-12.

202. Conti G, Antonelli M, Navalesi P, Rocco M, Bufi M, Spadetta G, Meduri GU. Noninvasive vs. conventional mechanical ventilation in patients with chronic obstructive pulmonary disease after failure of medical treatment in the ward: A randomized trial. Intensive Care Med 2002;28:1701-07.

203. Esteban A, Anzueto A, Frutos F, Alia I, Brochard L, Stewart TE, Benito S, Epstein SK, Apezteguia C, Nightingale P, et al. Characteristics and outcomes in adult patients receiving mechanical ventilation: a 28-day international study. JAMA 2002;287:345-55.

204. Esteban A, Frutos F, Tobin MJ, Alia I, Solsona JF, Valverdu I, Fernandez R, de la Cal MA, Benito S, Tomas R, et al. A comparison of four methods of weaning patients from mechanical ventilation. Spanish Lung Failure Collaborative Group. N Engl J Med 1995;332:345-50.

205. Brochard L, Rauss A, Benito S, Conti G, Mancebo J, Rekik N, Gasparetto A, Lemaire F. Comparison of three methods of gradual withdrawal from ventilatory support during weaning from mechanical ventilation. Am J Respir Crit Care Med 1994;150:896-03.

206. Hilbert G, Gruson D, Portel L, Gbikpi-Benissan G, Cardinaud JP. Noninvasive pressure support ventilation in COPD patients with postextubation hypercapnic respiratory insufficiency. Eur Respir J 1998;11:1349-53.

207. Kessler R, Faller M, Fourgaut G, Mennecier B, Weitzenblum E. Predictive factors of hospitalization for acute exacerbation in a series of 64 patients with chronic obstructive pulmonary disease. Am J Respir Crit Care Med 1999;159:158-64.

208. Mushlin AI, Black ER, Connolly CA, Buonaccorso KM, Eberly SW. The necessary length of hospital stay for chronic pulmonary disease. JAMA 1991;266:80-83.

209. Cotton MM, Bucknall CE, Dagg KD, Johnson MK, MacGregor G, Stewart C, Stevenson RD. Early discharge for patients with exacerbations of chronic obstructive pulmonary disease: A randomized controlled trial. Thorax 2000;55:902-06.

210. Hughes SL, Weaver FM, Giobbie-Hurder A, Manheim L, Henderson W, Kubal JD, Ulasevich A, Cummings J. Effectiveness of team-managed home-based primary care: A randomized multicenter trial. JAMA 2000;284:2877-85.

211. Hermiz O, Comino E, Marks G, Daffurn K, Wilson S, Harris M. Randomised controlled trial of home based care of patients with chronic obstructive pulmonary disease. BMJ 2002;325:938.

212. Jindal SK, Aggarwal AN, Chaudhry K, Chhabra SK, D'Souza GA, Gupta D, Katiyar SK, Kumar R, Shah B,

Vijayan VK. A multicentric study on epidemiology of chronic obstructive pulmonary disease and its relationship with tobacco smoking and environmental tobacco smoke exposure. Indian J Chest Dis Allied Sci 2006;48:23-29.

213. Stoller JK, Lange PA. Inpatient management of chronic obstructive pulmonary disease. Respir Care Clin N Am 1998;4:425-38.

214. Peach H, Pathy MS. Follow-up study of disability among elderly patients discharged from hospital with exacerbations of chronic bronchitis. Thorax 1981;36:585-89.

215. Eaton T, Withy S, Garrett JE, Mercer J, Whitlock RM, Rea HH. Spirometry in primary care practice: The importance of quality assurance and the impact of spirometry workshops. Chest 1999;116:416-23.

216. Schermer TR, Jacobs JE, Chavannes NH, Hartman J, Folgering HT, Bottema BJ, van Weel C. Validity of spirometric testing in a general practice population of patients with chronic obstructive pulmonary disease (COPD). Thorax 2003;58:861-66.

217. Schermer T, Eaton T, Pauwels R, van Weel C. Spirometry in primary care: Is it good enough to face demands like World COPD Day? Eur Respir J 2003;22:725-27.

218. Rea H, McAuley S, Stewart A, Lamont C, Roseman P, Didsbury P. A chronic disease management programme can reduce days in hospital for patients with chronic obstructive pulmonary disease. Intern Med J 2004;34:608-14.

There are over 40 different guidelines from different countries on diagnosis and management of Chronic Obstructive Pulmonary Disease (COPD). The guidelines formulated by the Global Initiative for Chronic Obstructive Lung Disease (GOLD) are perhaps the most popular and global in nature. The need to formulate a different set of guidelines for India was felt because of the differences in risk factors, disease prevalence and pattern, and above all, the different overall health-care infrastructure. Moreover, a large burden of tuberculosis, which is an important cause of cough, adds to the difficulties of diagnosis and management.

These guidelines have been developed at the initiative of WHO (India) under the WHO-Government of India Biennium (2002-2003) program. A consensus workshop was held in December 2002 with representative participation from several national professional bodies, medical colleges, general health sector, and other institutes. The recommendations were subsequently compiled and reviewed by the participants and other experts.

The guidelines essentially incorporate general GOLD recommendations. The major alterations include a greater stress on clinical criteria, exclusion of diagnosis of tuberculosis, and a three-tier approach at different levels of health care, especially the primary and secondary care levels. It is hoped that the recommendations will help the physicians of all hues to effectively manage COPD.

Introduction

Chronic Obstructive Pulmonary Disease (COPD) is a common clinical problem. It is also known by various other names, such as Chronic Obstructive Lung Disease (COLD), Chronic Obstructive Airway Disease (COAD), Chronic Airflow Obstruction (CAO), Chronic Airway (or Airflow) Limitation (CAL), or simply as Chronic Bronchitis and Emphysema.

COPD, which includes chronic bronchitis and emphysema, is a progressive disease characterized by airflow limitation/obstruction that is either not reversible at all or only partially reversible. It is generally difficult to separate out the two conditions (chronic bronchitis and emphysema), hence these are grouped together as COPD.[1-4] COPD does not include asthma in which the airflow obstruction is largely reversible. The airflow obstruction in COPD is associated with abnormal inflammatory response of the lungs to chronic inhalational exposure from smokes, dusts and other air pollutants.

COPD manifests as chronic cough with or without sputum production. To define COPD, the presence of these symptoms for more than three months of a year for at least two consecutive years is considered essential. It may or may not be accompanied with progressive breathlessness. The disease progresses with time ultimately leading to respiratory disability and death.

Acute exacerbations of COPD occur whenever there is an episode of infection or some other complication. There is worsening of symptoms, deterioration of clinical condition and impairment of lung function during the period of exacerbation.

Epidemiology and Risk Factors

COPD is primarily a disease of the adult. The prevalence of COPD reported in different population based studies from India is highly variable (Table A2.1).[5-16]

TABLE A2.1: Prevalence of COPD and its smoking association in various population studies from India

	Population	COPD prevalence (%)		Smoker: Nonsmoker ratio
		Men	Women	M:F Ratio	
Wig (1964)[6]	Rural Delhi	3.36	2.54	1.3	2.0
Sikand (1966)[7]	Delhi	7.0	4.3	1.6	2.5
Viswanathan (1966)[8]	Patna	2.12	1.33	1.6	
Bhattacharya (1975)[9]	Rural UP	6.67	4.48	1.6	
Radha (1977)[10]	New Delhi	8.1	4.6	1.8	1.8
Thiruvengadam (1977)[11]	Madras	1.9	1.2	1.6	10.2
Viswanathan (1977)[12]	Delhi Rural	4.7	3.5	1.3	9.6
	Urban	8.0	4.3	1.9	4.0
Charan (1977)[13]	Rural Punjab	2.28	1.63	1.4	
Malik (1986)[14]	N.India Rural	9.4	4.9	1.9	5.5
	Urban	3.7	1.6	2.3	7.0
Jindal (1993)[15]	N.India Rural	6.2	3.9	1.6	
	Urban	4.2	1.6	2.6	9.6
Ray (1995)[16]	South India	4.08	2.55	1.6	1.6

The prevalence rates in male subjects of 2.12 to 9.4 percent in studies reported from North are generally higher than 1.4 to 4.08 percent reported from South India. The respective range for female subjects vary from 1.33 to 4.9 percent from North and from 2.55 to 2.7 percent from South India. For epidemiological assessment, the rounded-off median prevalence rates were assessed as 5 percent for male and 2.7 percent for female subjects of over 30 years of age.

The disease is distinctly more common in males. The male to female ratio had varied from 1.32:1 to 2.6:1 in different studies with a median ratio of 1.6:1.

COPD results from chronic inhalational exposure to various smokes, noxious particles and gases.

Tobacco Smoke

Tobacco smoke, which is a mixture of over 4000 chemical constituents, is the most important cause. Amongst males, tobacco smoking is responsible for more than 80 percent of patients.[5,17] Both cigarette and 'bidi' smoking are equally responsible.[18] Pipe and 'hookah' smoking are also important in causing COPD. There is no reliable information on smoking associated COPD in women in whom the overall prevalence of smoking is very low. Besides active tobacco smoking, exposure to smoking from others, i.e. passive smoking, better termed as Environmental Tobacco Smoke (ETS) exposure, may also play a contributory role especially in nonsmoker individuals including women.[19,20]

Solid Fuel Combustion

The smoke from combustion of solid fuels such as dried dung, wood and crop residue used for cooking and heating, especially in villages, semi urban and slum areas, is an important cause of pollution of the indoor air. It is responsible for a large number of COPD in the rural inhabitants in general and women in particular.[20-23]

Air Pollution

Exhausts from vehicles and industrial units; dusts, fumes and smoke from burning of crop residues in the field constitute important sources of air pollution. Chronic exposure to polluted air is an important cause of chronic respiratory diseases such as the COPD.[24-27]

Pathogenesis and Pathophysiology

Although cigarette smoking is the most important cause of COPD, only 10 to 15 percent of long-term smokers develop clinically significant COPD, and approximately half will never develop any symptomatic physiological deficit.[28] Why the normal, protective inflammatory response becomes an exaggerated, harmful one in only some smokers is poorly understood, and the precise mechanisms underlying the development of this disorder remain largely unknown. Presumably the inflammation caused by cigarette smoking interacts with other host or environmental factors to produce excess decline in lung function that results in COPD.

It is believed that inhaled noxious particles and gases result in lung inflammation, induce tissue destruction, and impair defense mechanisms that serve to limit or repair this damage. This damage leads to the mucous hypersecretion, airway narrowing and fibrosis, destruction of lung parenchyma and vascular changes. In turn, these pathological changes lead to airflow limitation and other physiological abnormalities characteristic of COPD. It is characterized by an increase in neutrophils, macrophages and T-lymphocytes in various parts of the lung. These activated inflammatory cells release a variety of chemical mediators, many of which (e.g. leukotreine B4, interleukin-8, and tumour necrosis factor) are capable of damaging lung structures and/or sustaining neutrophilic inflammation. In addition to inflammation, two other processes thought to be important in the pathogenesis of COPD are an imbalance of proteinases and antiproteinases in the lung, and oxidative stress.[29-31] Although both these processes may themselves result from ongoing inflammation, they can also arise from genetic (e.g. alpha-1 antitrypsin deficiency) or environmental (e.g. oxidant compounds in cigarette smoke) factors.

The peripheral airways are the major site of airways obstruction in patients of COPD. The structural changes in the airway wall, as well as airway edema and mucus hypersecretion contribute to airway narrowing. The irreversible component of airflow limitation is primarily due to remodelling of the smaller airways; lung parenchymal destruction may also play a role. In advanced COPD, peripheral airways obstruction, parenchymal destruction, and pulmonary vascular abnormalities reduce the lung's capacity for gas exchange, producing hypoxemia and, later on, hypercapnia. Ventilation-perfusion mismatch is the dominant mechanism of hypoxemia in COPD.

How to Diagnose COPD?

Suspecting COPD

COPD can be suspected in most patients on the basis of symptoms and signs.[32] Alternate diagnosis such as bronchial asthma, pulmonary tuberculosis, bronchiectasis, malignancies and other chronic lung diseases may require exclusion. Investigations would be required to confirm the diagnosis.

Clinical History

Diagnosis is considered in any individual who presents with characteristic symptoms and presence of one or more risk factors. The important clinical indicators are as follows:

1. Chronic cough: Present on most days for at least 3 months in a year for 2 or more consecutive years.[33] Cough may be either present throughout the day or only intermittently. Cough is sometimes nocturnal in nature.
2. Chronic sputum production: Cough may or may not be associated with production of mucoid or mucopurulent sputum. Both cough and sputum productions are characteristically more in the early morning, on waking up.
3. Breathlessness (dyspnea): Dyspnea may not be present initially, but develops later in the course. It is progressive over the time. Dyspnea is worse on exercise and during acute exacerbations.
4. Acute exacerbations: There are repeated episodes of acute bronchitis causing worsening of symptoms. Most patients would seek medical help only during these episodes of worsening.
5. Risk factors: History of tobacco smoking is present in most male patients. Nonsmoker patients (especially women) are significantly exposed to other risk factors such as the combustion of solid fuels or occupational exposures to dusts and fumes.

Physical Examination

Though an important component of clinical assessment, physical examination is rarely diagnostic in COPD.[34] Physical signs of airflow limitation are rarely present until significant impairment of lung function has occurred. However, certain findings on clinical examination point towards the diagnosis of COPD.[35]

The chest examination may reveal signs of emphysema such as the barrel shape (increased anteroposterior diameter, more horizontally set ribs, prominent sternal angle and wide subcostal angle). Due to the elevation of sternum, the distance between the suprasternal notch and the cricoid cartilage is reduced from the normal 3 and 4 finger breadths. The patient may use accessory muscles of respiration.

Chest percussion will reveal findings of hyperinflation with obliteration of cardiac dullness and downward displaced upper border of liver dullness. Elsewhere, the note will be hyperresonant. Breath sounds will have a prolonged expiratory phase with a uniformly diminished intensity. Fine inspiratory crepitations and rhonchi are commonly heard. Forced expiratory time (FET) will be prolonged to more than 6 seconds and patient may have pursed lip breathing.[36]

The physical findings may change in the presence of complications.

Alternate Diagnosis

Asthma is generally excluded on the basis of history. It is usually present from childhood and is characterized by episodes of breathlessness and wheezing with asymptomatic periods in between. Rhonchi are more prominent and extensive on physical examination. More importantly, there is greater variability and reversibility of symptoms, physical signs and tests of airway obstruction in asthma than COPD.

Diseases such as tuberculosis and bronchiectasis are common causes of chronic cough in this country. They are usually not confused with COPD. Physical findings of fibrocavitary disease support a diagnosis of tuberculosis. Sputum is purulent and greater in amount in patients with bronchiectasis. Coarse crepitations and finger clubbing are generally present.

Any chronic lung disease can occasionally pose a problem in differential diagnosis. Whenever, there is confusion, investigations will help.

Presence of Complications

i. Chronic cor pulmonale: Almost all cases of COPD will progress to chronic cor pulmonale in due course of time. It is detected from the presence of signs suggestive of pulmonary hypertension and right ventricular enlargement and/or failure, such as a loud second heart sound, parasternal heave and raised jugular venous pressure (JVP).
ii. Respiratory failure: Chronic respiratory failure results from disease progression. It is suspected from the presence of tachypnea, cyanosis, flapping tremors, and altered sensorium.
iii. Chest infections, such as pneumonias.
iv. Pneumothorax.

Investigations

Investigations are required for exclusion of an alternate diagnosis, confirmation of diagnosis of COPD, assessment of severity of disease and diagnosis of complications.

Excluding Alternate Diagnosis

It is especially important to exclude tuberculosis in all patients having chronic cough. Examine sputum smears for acid-fast bacilli (AFB), at least thrice.

Chest radiograph will help to identify alternate diseases such as fibrocavitary tuberculosis, bronchiectasis, lung tumors and detect complications such as chronic cor pulmonale, pneumothorax or bronchopneumonia.

Additional tests such as the spirometry may be carried out where physician feels the diagnosis of asthma is under consideration. Bronchodilator reversibility testing is useful to help rule out a diagnosis of asthma and to establish patient's best attainable lung function. PEFR with reversibility may be substituted for FEV_1 when spirometry is not available.

In situation when patient is not responding to adequate and properly prescribed therapy or if there is a doubt of an alternate diagnosis such as asthma, glucocorticoid reversibility test with 2 week of oral corticosteroids should be attempted (by a specialist at the secondary care center with facilities for spirometry).[37] Criteria for reversibility are an increase in FEV_1 of 200 ml and 15 percent above baseline.

Confirming the Diagnosis

Spirometry remains the gold standard for confirmation and staging of COPD. Patients should be referred for spirometry if diagnosis is doubtful. Spirometry is used to measure the forced vital capacity (FVC), i.e. maximal volume of air forcibly exhaled from the point of maximal inhalation; the volume of air exhaled during the first second of this maneuver (FEV_1), and the ratio of these two measurements (FEV1/FVC). The presence of a postbronchodilator $FEV_1 <$ 80 percent of the predicted value in combination with a FEV_1/FVC < 70 percent confirms the presence of airflow limitation that is not fully reversible. Predicted values of different spirometric parameters are available as normograms and Tables drawn from different prediction equations.

Staging Severity of COPD

Assessment of severity is based on the degree of the spirometric abnormality. Based on the results of spirometry, COPD can be categorized into four stages: At risk, Mild, Moderate and Severe (Table A2.2).

TABLE A2.2: Staging of COPD based on spirometry

At risk	Normal spirometry, chronic symptoms
Mild	FEV_1/ FVC < 70% FEV_1 > 80% predicted
Moderate	FEV_1/ FVC < 70% FEV_1 30 - 80% predicted
Severe	FEV_1/ FVC < 70% FEV_1 < 30% predicted

If spirometry is not available, both staging of the disease and follow-up of patients should be done on the basis of severity of symptoms/level of disability/6 minute walk test and/or peak expiratory flow (PEF) (Table A2.3).[38-40]

Although spirometry is the gold standard for staging, PEF can serve as a good substitute if spirometry is not available. Six minute walking test is performed by measuring distance covered in 6 minutes when patient walks at his/her own speed (under physician supervision). This is a simple test, which can be performed at the primary care level. Measurement of arterial blood gases/pulse oximetry in patients with severe COPD is desirable although severity of respiratory failure may

TABLE A2.3: Staging of COPD based on symptoms, signs, 6 minute walk test and peak expiratory flow rate

	Symptoms (cough and sputum)	Signs	6 minute walk test	PEF (optional)
At risk	No dyspnea, hypersecretion +			
Mild	Dyspnea on unaccustomed activity or climbing two flight of stairs	Mild hyperinflation	> 200 m	50-70%
Moderate	Dyspnea on accustomed activity	Moderate hyperinflation	100-200 m	30-50%
Severe	Dyspnea at rest	Near absence of breath sounds, respiratory failure, polycythemia, CCF	< 100 m	< 30%

be assessed by symptoms of hypercapnia (bounding pulse, warm extremities, flaps and tremulousness) and hypoxia (tremors, restlessness, mental obtundation and cyanosis.

Treatment of Patient with Stable COPD

The important components of managing patients with stable COPD include (a) minimization of risk factors, (b) pharmacotherapy appropriate to the disease severity and (c) supportive nonpharmacological measures (such as patient education and rehabilitation).

Assess the risk factors and other complications and manage accordingly. Advise and help to quit smoking.[41] Similar attempts should be made to minimize other risk factors (Table A2.4).

TABLE A2.4: Treatment guidelines depending upon severity of COPD	
Mild COPD	Short acting bronchodilators, when needed.
Moderate COPD	Regular treatment with one/more bronchodilators. Pulmonary rehabilitation.
Severe COPD	As in moderate COPD, plus inhaled corticosteroids, Treatment of complications.

Assess the disease severity on an individual basis by taking into account the patient's symptoms, airflow limitations, frequency and severity of exacerbations, complications, respiratory failure, co-morbidities, and general health status. Start treatment depending upon the severity of the disease. None of the existing medication for COPD has been shown to modify the long-term decline in lung function.[42] Therefore, pharmacotherapy for COPD is used only to decrease symptoms and complications. Patient education is necessary to improve skills, ability to cope with illness and the health status. Health education is particularly effective for sustained smoking cessation. In addition, appropriate information about the nature of the disease, instructions on how to use different medications and inhalers, and clues to recognize symptoms of exacerbation are mandatory.

Smoking Cessation

Smoking cessation is the most important and effective step.[43,44] Follow the standard guidelines for helping patients with COPD to quit smoking (Tables A2.5 and A2.6).

TABLE A2.5: Guidelines for physicians on tobacco cessation
Follow the 5A Strategy
• ASK (about tobacco use)
• ASSESS (the status and severity of use)
• ADVISE (to stop)
• ASSIST (in smoking cessation)
• ARRANGE (follow-up program)
Details of advice for the patient
• Review your tobacco use. Accept that smoking is a problem and harmful for your health
• Make a decision and determination to quit. Don't be over confident that you can quit any time you like
• Share your decision with family, friends, doctor. Accept their help
• Fix a quit date. Don't postpone
• Remove ashtrays and other objects that are reminders to the habit
• Keep away from trigger situations
• Adopt healthy life-style such as relaxation, exercise, plenty of water, fruits, vegetables and avoid tea/coffee/alcohol
• Take help from family, friends and doctor

Reduction in Other Risk Factors

General measures aimed at reducing risk of COPD include the following: (1) avoiding open burning of crop residue, (2) use of water to suppress dust and (3) wearing masks at work place in areas of dust generation.

Specific measures such as the use of smokeless 'chullahs' should be aimed at reducing risk associated with solid fuel combustion and ETS exposure.

Substitution of solid fuels with LPG or electricity is the best approach. The "kitchen" at home should at least be located outside the living and sleeping areas. Kitchens should be adequately ventilated by providing 'chimneys', exhaust pipes and/or fans.

TABLE A2.6: First few steps of quitting tobacco smoking

a. To reduce quantity
  i. Change to nonpreferred brand
  ii. Keep a record of the amount and frequency of tobacco use
  iii. Decrease the number of puffs when smoking
  iv. Leave large stubs
  v. Don't inhale deeply.
b. To deal with triggers when you have an urge to smoke (Trigger coping)
  i. For extra-ordinary urge to take tobacco, try alternatives (chewing gum, toffee, peppermint, cardamom)
  ii. Increase your water intake
  iii. Breathe deeply and quietly
  iv. Do some other work to engage your mind and to keep your mind off tobacco
  v. Delay the act of smoking—count till 100 and think of pleasant situations.
c. Once you quit
  i. Learn to say "no" to tobacco offers from others
  ii. Don't take even a single puff
  iii. Try to remain in smoke free areas
  iv. Avoid company of smokers and even tobacco chewers
  v. Make a group of people who have quit tobacco—share their experiences
  vi. Collect the money saved from each pack of cigarette or "paan masaala". Buy a gift for your loved ones with that money
  vii. Try alternate ways to deal with mental stress and tension, such as relaxation, deep breathing, listening to music
  viii. Remember there can be some withdrawal symptoms after quitting, such as headache, irritability, lack of concentration, etc. **But** bear with them. These are temporary and disappear in a few days.

Even if you fail in quitting smoking
• Don't get disheartened—Try again
• Seek help of those who have quit smoking
• Seek professional help and medical advice.

Exposure to products of solid fuel combustion can be minimized by the use of smokeless 'chullahs', reducing the duration of stay in the kitchen or place of fuel use, and by covering nose and mouth with a thin cloth near the source of combustion.

Exposure to ETS can be reduced by stopping/minimizing indoor smoking, especially in front of children, and by adequate ventilation in the living rooms.

Drug treatment

A. Bronchodilators
   Bronchodilator medication is central to the symptomatic management of COPD.[45] Inhaled drugs are preferred to oral preparations.[46] However, the choice of drugs depends on the availability of medications and patient's affordability (Table A2.7).

TABLE A2.7: Commonly used bronchodilator drugs in India

Drugs	Metered dose/dry powder inhalers (ug/dose)	Oral
Beta agonists		
Salbutamol	100-200	2-4 mg tid/qid
Terbutaline	250-500	2.5-5 mg tid
Salmeterol	25-50	
Formeterol	6-12	
Bambuterol		10-20 mg/day
Anticholinergics		
Ipratropium	40-80	
Tiotropium	18	
Methyxanthines		
Aminophyllins		225-450 mg/day
Theophyllins		200-600 mg/day

Short acting bronchodilators can be used 'as-needed' to relieve intermittent or worsening symptoms, and on regular basis to prevent or reduce persistent symptoms.[47] Stepwise treatment should be recommended. In general, nebulized therapy for stable patients is not appropriate unless it has been shown to be better than conventional dose therapy.[48-50]

Regular treatment with short-acting bronchodilators is cheaper but less convenient than treatment with long-acting bronchodilators[51,52]. The long acting inhaled beta agonist salmeterol has been shown to improve health status significantly in doses of 50 µg twice daily. Similar data for short acting beta agonists are not available. Use of inhaled tiotropium (an anticholinergic) once daily also improves symptoms and health status.[53]

Combining drugs with different mechanisms and durations of action may increase the degree of bronchodilatation for equivalent or lesser side effects. A combination of a short-acting beta agonist and the anticholinergic drug ipratropium in stable COPD produces greater and more sustained improvements in FEV_1 than either alone and does not produce evidence of tachyphylaxis.[54]

The addition of oral theophylline should normally be considered only if inhaled treatments have failed to provide adequate relief. Sustained release preparations are better.[55] All studies that have shown efficacy of theophylline in COPD were done with slow-release preparations.

Addition of theophylline to β_2-agonists or anticholinergics may produce additional improvements in lung function and health status[56,57]. However, combination of salbutamol with theophylline in a single Tablet is not recommended.

B. Corticosteroids

Inhaled corticosteroids do not change the rate of decline in lung function, but can increase postbronchodilator FEV_1, reduce the number of exacerbations, and slow the rate of decline in health status.[58-61]

Regular treatment with inhaled glucocorticosteroids should be prescribed for symptomatic patients with COPD with a documented spirometric response to glucocorticosteroids or for those with $FEV_1 < 50$ percent predicted and repeated exacerbations requiring treatment with antibiotics or oral glucocorticoids.[62-65] Long-term treatment is required in such patients; in fact, withdrawal of inhaled corticosteroids can lead to increase in symptoms and exacerbation rate.

Chronic treatment with systemic glucocorticosteroids should be avoided because of unfavorable benefit-to-risk ratio.

C. Role of other drugs

The use of antibiotics other than treating infectious exacerbations of COPD and other bacterial infections is not recommended.[66] Although a few patients with viscous sputum may benefit from mucolytic agents (such as ambroxol, carbocysteine, iodinated glycerol, etc.) the overall benefit seems to be very small.[67]

Cough, although sometimes a troublesome symptom in COPD, has a significant protective role. Hence, the regular use of antitussives should be discouraged in stable COPD.

The use of respiratory stimulants like doxapram, almitrine bismesylate are not recommended for regular use in stable patients. Sedatives and narcotics should be avoided in patients with COPD because of their respiratory depressant effects and potential to worsen hypercapnia.

Malnutrition (both under nutrition and over nutrition) should be managed appropriately.[68,69] Nutritional supplements can increase fat free mass and muscle strength. A diet rich in proteins and fats, but low in carbohydrates, is preferred.

Currently available prophylactic vaccines for influenza are not recommended for routine use, as insufficient information is available on serotypes prevalent in India. They may, however, be administered to the selected patients (especially the elderly). Similarly, routine administration of pneumococcal vaccine is not recommended.[70] Immuno-modulatory drugs may also have a moderate protective role in reducing infective exacerbations.[71]

Pulmonary Rehabilitation

Pulmonary rehabilitation is a multidimensional continuum of services directed to persons with pulmonary disease and their families, usually by an interdisciplinary team of specialists, with the goal of achieving and maintaining the individual's maximum level of independence and functioning in the community.

Goals of pulmonary rehabilitation are (a) to reduce symptoms, disability and handicap, and (b) to improve functional independence. It should comprise of physical training program, disease education, and nutritional, psychological, social and behavioral intervention (including smoking cessation).[72] The program should be tailored to individual functional needs and capacity, and should be targeted especially to patients with coexisting locomotor or cognitive impairment, and to those with associated cardiac disease. Clinicians, physiotherapists, dieticians, occupation therapists, social workers, nurses and pulmonary function technicians should be involved in rehabilitation programs. Optimum medical management should continue along with the rehabilitation process.

Management of Acute Exacerbations

Exacerbation of COPD is defined as "a sustained worsening of the patient's condition, from the stable state and beyond normal day-to-day variations, that is acute in onset and necessitates a change in regular medication".[73]

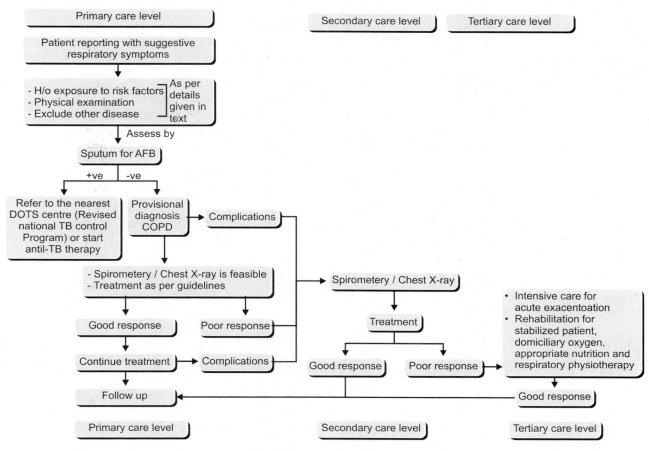

FIGURE A2.1: COPD algorithm

Patient Assessment

The symptoms of an exacerbation are increased breathlessness often accompanied by wheezing, increased cough and sputum, change of the color or tenacity of sputum, and fever.

The common causes of an exacerbation are infection of the tracheobronchial tree and air pollution.[74-76] The cause of approximately one-third of severe exacerbations cannot be identified. Conditions that may mimic an acute exacerbation include pneumonia, congestive heart failure, pneuomothorax, pleural effusion, pulmonary embolism, and arrhythmias. These conditions should be ruled out by clinical examination and investigations.

The assessment of severity of acute worsening is based on the patient's medical history before the exacerbation, symptoms, physical examination, lung function tests, arterial blood gas measurements, and other laboratory tests. The medical history should cover the period of worsening since the new symptoms have been present, the frequency and severity of breathlessness and coughing attacks, sputum volume and color, limitation of daily activities, any previous episodes/exacerbations, hospitalization, and the present treatment regimen.

Treatment of Acute Exacerbations

Bronchodilators are the cornerstone of managing exacerbations of COPD. Patients need to increase the dose and/or frequency of existing bronchodilator therapy. New drugs, which patient is not taking at the time of worsening, may be added. Short-acting bronchodilators should ideally be administered using inhalers (preferably with spacers). In a severe case, nebulizers may be used for drug administration. In situations where these drugs are not available, parenteral aminophylline can be used with due attention to its toxicity. Aminophylline dose should be appropriately modified in elderly patients, those in congestive cardiac failure or having liver cirrhosis, and those already taking oral methylxanthines, cimetidine, ciprofloxacin or erythromycin.

Antibiotics should be used when symptoms of breathlessness and cough are increased and sputum is purulent and increased in volume.[77,78] The choice of antibiotic depends on the affordability of the patient, the severity of exacerbation and the bacterial spectrum.[79] Amoxycillin, doxycycline, cotrimoxazole, flouroquinolones or a second generation macrolide/cephalosporin are used as the first choice. For severe exacerbations higher-grade antibiotics, such as coamoxiclav or a fourth generation cephalosporin can be used.

Systemic glucocorticoids should be used in acute exacerbations. They shorten recovery time and help to restore lung function more quickly.[80-82] A dose of 40 mg oral prednisolone per day (or equivalent) for 5 to 10 days is recommended. Carefully look for tuberculosis by sputum examination and chest radiograph before starting corticosteroids.

Controlled oxygen therapy can be administered at low flow rates (preferably with a Venturi mask) with monitoring for features of CO_2 retention.[83] Chest physiotherapy, inhaled corticosteroids and mucolytic agents are generally not useful in the management of acute exacerbations.

Patients with the following features should be hospitalized for further management:
- Marked increase in intensity of symptoms, such as sudden development of resting dyspnea
- Onset of new physical signs (e.g. cyanosis, drowsiness, confusion, flaps, peripheral edema)
- Failure of exacerbation to respond to initial medical management
- Significant comorbidities such as diabetes or associated cardiac disease
- Newly occurring arrhythmias
- Diagnostic uncertainty.

Disease Progression and Prognosis

Physiological changes characteristic of the disease include mucus hypersecretion, ciliary dysfunction, airflow limitation, pulmonary hyperinflation, gas exchange abnormalities, pulmonary hypertension and cor pulmonale, and they usually develop in this order over the course of disease. Pulmonary hypertension develops late in the course of COPD. It is the major cardiovascular complication of COPD and is associated with a poor prognosis.

No drug treatment has been shown to alter the natural history of COPD. Smoking cessation is the only intervention that can arrest the rapid decline in lung function. Domiciliary oxygen therapy is the only other treatment known to improve prognosis in patients of COPD with hypoxemia.

The best guide to the progression of COPD is the change in FEV_1 over time. FEV_1 declines with normal aging at about 30 ml/year and this increases to an average of 45 ml/year in smokers.[84] However, the individual susceptibility to cigarette smoking is very wide. Stopping smoking produces only small improvements in FEV_1, but the subsequent fall in FEV_1 progressively slows to the nonsmoker rate of about 30 ml/year.

Depending of disease severity, the five-year mortality rate of patients with COPD varies from 40 to 70 percent.[85] The three major causes of death have been identified as COPD itself, lung cancer, and cardiovascular disease. The age and the degree of airways obstruction, as reflected by FEV_1, are the most commonly recognized prognostic factors.

WHO-INDIA GUIDELINES FOR MANAGEMENT OF COPD

A Practical Approach at Different Levels of Care

A. Primary care Level (Primary health centers, dispensaries, general practice clinics)

Facilities for diagnosis at the primary health care centers are generally few. Diagnosis can however be made with the help of a good history and physical examination following the algorithm shown in Figure A2.1.

Sputum examination for AFB should be done as per RNTCP guidelines which recommend this investigation in any patient with chronic cough because the disease (pulmonary tuberculosis) is rather common. If the sputum is negative, a provisional diagnosis of COPD can be made and treatment given depending on the disease severity, classified as per Table A2.2.

Mild COPD
a. Advice on smoking cessation (Tables A2.5 and A2.6) and reduction of exposures to other risk factors (for all stages).
b. Drug therapy: Salbutamol or terbutaline (inhalational): 2 to 4 inhalation/day on "as and when needed" basis.

Moderate COPD
a. Start with oral theophylline—300-600 mg per day.
b. Inhalational ipratropium or tiotropium on regular basis.
c. Inhalational salmeterol or formeterol—twice daily.
d. Salbutamol or terbutaline inhalation on "as and when needed" basis.

Severe COPD
a. Treatment steps (a to d) as above.
b. In the presence of infective complications: A short course of oral antibiotics amoxycillin, quinolones (levofloxacin or gatifloxacin), macrolides (azithromycin/clarithromycin/roxithromycin) or oral first/second generation cephalosporin (cephalexin, cefadroxil). If response is not good, refer to a secondary care level center.

B. **Secondary care level (district level hospitals and clinics)**
a. Chest radiograph and sputum examination should be done to look for complications such as pneumonias, pneumothorax, chronic cor pulmonale, etc.
b. Treat infective exacerbation with a course of antibiotic (as above). Higher grade antibiotics may be required.
c. Confirm diagnosis and severity of COPD with the help of spirometry.
d. Institute drug treatment as at primary care level.
e. Consider addition of inhaled corticosteroids (beclomethasone, fluticasone or budesonide), if COPD is severe. Add long-term inhaled corticosteroid therapy, only if the patient shows good response to a trial of inhaled corticosteroids administered for about six weeks. A patient who shows frequent exacerbations can also be advised long-term inhaled steroid treatment.

   If the patient does not show good response to treatment, refer to a tertiary care level center. Faulty technique is perhaps the important cause of failure of response to inhalational therapy. It is therefore important to properly explain and let the patient practice inhalation technique in your presence.

C. **Tertiary care level (medical colleges, large corporate, institutional and specialty hospitals)**
It is important for a tertiary care center to establish facilities for specialty advice and intensive respiratory care. This should include assisted ventilation and all other steps of acute care such as the monitoring of vital parameters, blood gas assessment, maintenance of blood pressure, fluids, electrolytes, nutrition and general organ functions.

At a tertiary care center, acute exacerbation should be handled followed by stabilization and rehabilitation therapy.

Respiratory rehabilitation: Advice on respiratory rehabilitation is important at all levels of care. Advice on smoking cessation and avoidance of risk factors is an essential component of respiratory rehabilitation. Guidelines on advice to quit smoking are listed in Tables A2.5 and A2.6.

Rehabilitation at secondary and tertiary care level centers should include advice on nutrition, maintenance bronchodilators and inhalational corticosteroids, prophylactic vaccines and domiciliary oxygen.

Once the patient is stabilized, he should be sent back to the primary care doctor with appropriate briefing and advice on follow up management.

REFERENCES

1. American Thoracic Society. Standards for the diagnosis and care of patients with chronic obstructive pulmonary disease. Am J Respir Crit Care Med 1995;152(5 Pt 2):S77-S121.
2. British Thoracic Society. Guidelines for the management of chronic obstructive pulmonary disease. Thorax 1997;52(Suppl 5):S1-S28.
3. Global Initiative for Chronic Obstructive Lung Disease. Global strategy for the diagnosis, management and prevention of chronic obstructive lung disease. NHLBI/WHO workshop report. Bethesda, National Heart, Lung and Blood Institute 2001;2701:1-100.
4. Siafakas NM, Vermeire P, Pride NB, Paoletti P, Gibson J, Howard P, et al. Optimal assessment and management of chronic obstructive pulmonary disease (COPD). The European Respiratory Society Task Force. Eur Respir J 1995;8:1398-1420.
5. Jindal SK, Aggarwal AN, Gupta D. A review of population studies from India to estimate national burden of chronic obstructive pulmonary disease and its association with smoking. Indian J Chest Dis Allied Sci 2001;43:139-47.
6. Wig KL, Guleria JS, Bhasin RC, Holmes E (Jr), Vasudeva YL, Singh H. Certain clinical and epidemiological patterns of chronic obstructive lung disease as seen in Northern India. Indian J Chest Dis 1964;6:183-94.
7. Sikand BK, Pamra SP, Mathur GP. Chronic bronchitis in Delhi as revealed by mass survey. Indian J Tuberc 1966;13:94-101.
8. Viswanathan R. Epidemiology of chronic bronchitis: Morbidity survey in Patna urban area. Indian J Med Res 1966;54:105-11.
9. Bhattacharya SN, Bhatnagar JK, Kumar S, Jain PC. Chronic bronchitis in rural population. Indian J Chest Dis 1975;17:1-7.
10. Radha TG, Gupta GK, Singh A, Mathur N. Chronic bronchitis in an urban locality of New Delhi: An epidemiological survey. Indian J Med Res 1977;66:273-95.
11. Thiruvengadam KV, Raghva TP, Bhardwaj KV. Survey of prevalence of chronic bronchitis in Madras city. In Viswanathan R, Jaggi OP (Ed): Advances in Chronic Obstructive Lung Disease. Delhi: Asthma and Bronchitis Foundation of India 1977;59-69.
12. Vishwanathan R, Singh K. Chronic bronchitis and asthma in urban and rural Delhi. In Viswanathan R, Jaggi OP (Eds): Advances in chronic obstructive lung disease. Delhi: Asthma and Bronchitis Foundation of India 1977;44-58.

13. Charan NB. Chronic bronchitis in North India, Punjab. In Viswanathan R, Jaggi OP (Eds): Advances in Chronic Obstructive Lung Disease. Delhi: Asthma and Bronchitis Foundation of India 1977;92-102.

14. Malik SK. Profile of chronic bronchitis in North India: The PGI experience (1972-1985). Lung India 1986;4: 89-100.

15. Jindal SK. A field study on follow up at 10 years of prevalence of chronic obstructive pulmonary disease and peak expiratory flow rate. Indian J Med Res (B) 1993;98:20-26.

16. Ray D, Abel R, Selvaraj KG. A 5-year prospective epidemiological study of chronic obstructive pulmonary disease in rural South India. Indian J Med Res 1995;101:238-44.

17. US Surgeon General. The health consequences of smoking. Chronic obstructive lung disease. US Department of Health and Human Resources: Washington, DC 1984;84-502-05.

18. Khan MM, Tandon SN, Khan MT, Pandey US, Idris MZ. A comparative study of effects of cigarette and bidi smoking on respiratory function tests. J Environ Biol 2002;23:89-93.

19. Jaakkola MS, Jaakkola JJ. Effects of environmental tobacco smoke on the respiratory health of adults. Scand J Work Environ Health 2002;28 Suppl 2:52-70.

20. Smith KR. National burden of disease in India from domestic air pollution. Proc Natl Acad Sci 2000;24: 13286-93.

21. Pandey MR. Domestic smoke pollution and chronic bronchitis in a rural community of the Hill Region of Nepal. Thorax 1984;39:337-39.

22. Behera D, Jindal SK. Respiratory symptoms in Indian women using domestic cooking fuels. Chest 1991;100: 385-88.

23. Perez-Padilla R, Regalado U, Vedal S, et al. Exposure to biomass smoke and chronic airway disease in Mexican women. Am J Respir Crit Care Med 1996;154: 701-06.

24. Becklake MR. Occupational exposures: Evidence for a causal association with chronic obstructive pulmonary disease. Am Rev Respir Dis 1989;140(3 Pt 2):S85-S91.

25. Oxman AD, Muir DC, Shannon HS, Stock SR, Hnizdo E, Lange HJ. Occupational dust exposure and chronic obstructive pulmonary disease: A systematic overview: of the evidence. Am Rev Respir Dis 1993;148:38-48.

26. Sunyer J. Urban air pollution and chronic obstructive pulmonary disease: a review. Eur Respir J 2001;17: 1024-33.

27. Karakatsani A, Andreadaki S, Katsouyanni K, Dimitroulis I, Trichopoulos D, Benetou V, et al. Air pollution in relation to manifestations of chronic pulmonary disease: A nested case-control study in Athens, Greece. Eur J Epidemiol 2003;18:45-53.

28. Tashkin DP, Detels R, Simmons M, Liu H, Coulsen AH, Sayre J, et al. The UCLA population study of chronic obstructive respiratory disease: Impact of air pollution and smoking on annual change in FEV1. Am J Respir Crit Care Med 1994;149:1209-17.

29. Laurell CB, Eriksson S. The electrophoretic alpha-1 globulin pattern of serum in alpha-1 antitrypsin deficiency. Scand J Clin Lab Invest 1963;15:132-40.

30. Dekhuijzen PN, Aben KK, Dekker I, Aarts LP, Wielders PL, van Herwaarden CL, et al. Increased exhalation of hydrogen peroxide in patients with stable and unstable chronic obstructive pulmonary disease. Am J Respir Crit Care Med 1996;154:813-16.

31. Repine JE, Bast A, Lankhorst I. Oxidative stress in chronic obstructive pulmonary disease. Am J Respir Crit Care Med 1997;156:341-57.

32. Georgopoulos D, Anthonisen NR. Symptoms and signs of COPD. In Cherniack NS (Ed): Chronic obstructive pulmonary disease. Toronto: WB Saunders, 1991; 357-63.

33. Medical Research Council. Definition and classification of chronic bronchitis for clinical and epidemiological purposes. A report to the Medical Council by their committee on the aetiology of chronic bronchitis. Lancet 1965;1:775-80.

34. Badgett RG, Tanaka DJ, Hunt DK, Jelley MJ, Feinberg LE, Steiner JF, et al. Can moderate chronic obstructive pulmonary disease be diagnosed by historical and physical findings alone? Am J Med 1993;94:188-96.

35. Campbell EJ. Physical signs of diffuse airways obstruction and lung distention. Thorax 1969;24:1-3.

36. Lal S, Ferguson AD, Campbell EJM. Forced expiratory time: a simple test for airways obstruction. Br Med J 1964;1:814-17.

37. Weir DC, Gove RI, Robertson AS, Burge PS. Corticosteroid trials in non-asthmatic airflow obstruction: Comparison of oral prednisolone and inhaled beclomethasone dipropionate. Thorax 1990;45:112-17.

38. Butland RJ, Pang J, Gross ER, Woodcock AA, Geddes DM. Two-, Six-, and twelve-minute walking tests in respiratory disease. Br Med J 1982;284:1607-08.

39. Gerald LB, Sanderson B, Redden D, Bailey WC. Chronic obstructive pulmonary disease stage and 6-minute walk outcome. J Cardiopulm Rehabil 2001;21:296-99.

40. Kelly CA, Gibson GJ. Relation between FEV1 and peak expiratory flow in patients with chronic obstructive pulmonary disease. Thorax 1988;43:335-36.

41. The Tobacco Use and Dependence Clinical Practice Guideline Panel Staff and Consortium Representatives. A clinical practice guideline for treating tobacco use and dependence. JAMA 2000;28:3244-54.

42. Nishimura K, Tsukino M. Clinical course and prognosis of patients with chronic obstructive pulmonary disease. Curr Opin Pulm Med 2000;6:127-32.

43. Anthonisen NR, Connett JE, Kiley JP, et al. Effects of smoking intervention and the use of an inhaled anticholinergic bronchodilator on the rate of decline of FEV1. The Lung Health Study. JAMA 1994;272:1497-1505.

44. Tashkin D, Kanner R, Bailey W, Buist S, Anderson P, Nides M, et al. Smoking cessation in patients with chronic obstructive pulmonary disease: a double-blind, placebo-controlled, randomised trial. Lancet 2001;357: 1571-75.

45. Manning HL. Bronchodilator therapy in chronic obstructive pulmonary disease. Curr Opin Pulm Med 2000;6:99-103.

46. Shim CS, Williams MH. Bronchodilator response to oral aminophylline and terbutaline versus aerosol albuterol in patients with chronic obstructive pulmonary disease. Am J Med 1983;75:697-701.

47. Ram FSF, Sestini P. Regular inhaled short acting β_2 agonists for the management of stable chronic obstructive pulmonary disease: Cochrane systematic review and meta-analysis. Thorax 2003;58:580-84.

48. O'Driscoll BR, Kay EA, Taylor RJ, Weatherby H, Chetty MCP, Bernstein A. A long-term prospective assessment of home nebulizer treatment. Respir Med 1992;86:317.

49. British Thoracic Society Nebulizer Project Group. Nebulizer therapy. Guidelines. Thorax 1997;52 Suppl 2:S4-S24.

50. Boe J, Dennis JH, O'Driscoll BR, Bauer TT, Carone M, Dautzenberg B, et al. European Respiratory Society Guidelines on the use of nebulizers. Eur Respir J 2001;18:228-42.

51. Dahl R, Greefhorst LA, Nowak D, Nonikov V, Byrne AM, Thomson MH, et al. Inhaled formoterol dry powder versus ipratropium bromide in chronic obstructive pulmonary disease. Am J Respir Crit Care Med 2001;164:778-84.

52. Vincken W, van Noord JA, Greefhorst AP, Bantje TA, Kesten S, Korducki L, et al. Improved health outcomes in patients with COPD during 1 yr's treatment with tiotropium. Eur Respir J 2002;19:209-16.

53. van Noord JA, Bantje TA, Eland ME, Korducki L, Cornelissen PJ. A randomised controlled comparison of tiotropium and ipratropium in the treatment of chronic obstructive pulmonary disease. The Dutch Tiotropium Study Group. Thorax 2000,55:289-94.

54. Combivent Inhalation Aerosol Study Group. In chronic obstructive pulmonary disease, a combination of ipratropium and albuterol is more effective than either agent alone. Chest 1994:105:1411-19.

55. Weinberger M, Hendeles L. Slow release theophylline. Rationale and basis for product selection. New Engl J Med 1983;308:760-64.

56. ZuWallack RL, Mahler DA, Reilly D, Church N, Emmett A, Rickard K, et al. Salmeterol plus theophylline combination therapy in the treatment of COPD. Chest 2001;119:1661-70.

57. Bellia V, Foresi A, Bianco S, Grassi V, Olivieri D, Bensi G, et al. Efficacy and safety of oxitropium bromide, theophylline and their combination in COPD patients: A double-blind, randomized, multicentre study (BREATH Trial). Respir Med 2002;96:881-89.

58. Pauwels RA, Lofdahl CG, Laitinen LA, Schouten JP, Postma DS, Pride NB, et al. Long-term treatment with inhaled budesonide in persons with mild chronic obstructive pulmonary disease who continue smoking. European Respiratory Society Study on Chronic Obstructive Pulmonary Disease. N Engl J Med 1999; 340:1948-53.

59. Vestbo J, Sorensen T, Lange P, Brix A, Torre P, Viskum K. Long-term effect of inhaled budesonide in mild and moderate chronic obstructive pulmonary disease: A randomised controlled trial. Lancet 1999; 353:1819-23.

60. Burge PS, Calverley PM, Jones PW, Spencer S, Anderson JA, Maslen TK. Randomised, double blind, placebo controlled study of fluticasone propionate in patients with moderate to severe chronic obstructive pulmonary disease: The ISOLDE trial. BMJ 2000;320: 1297-303.

61. The Lung Health Study Research Group. Effect of inhaled triamcinolone on the decline in pulmonary function in chronic obstructive pulmonary disease: Lung Health Study II. N Engl J Med 2000; 343:1902-09.

62. Calverley P, Pauwels R, Vestbo J, Jones P, Pride N, Gulsvik A, et al. Combined salmeterol and fluticasone in the treatment of chronic obstructive pulmonary disease: A randomised controlled trial. Lancet 2003; 361:449-56.

63. Szafranski W, Cukier A, Ramirez A, Menga G, Sansores R, Nahabedian S, et al. Efficacy and safety of budesonide/formoterol in the management of chronic obstructive pulmonary disease. Eur Respir J 2003;21: 74-81.

64. Jones PW, Willits LR, Burge PS, Calverley PM. Disease severity and the effect of fluticasone propionate on chronic obstructive pulmonary disease exacerbations. Eur Respir J 2003; 21:68-73.

65. Mahler DA, Wire P, Horstman D, Chang CN, Yates J, Fischer T, et al. Effectiveness of fluticasone propionate and salmeterol combination delivered via the Diskus device in the treatment of chronic obstructive pulmonary disease. Am J Respir Crit Care Med 2002;166: 1084-91.

66. Johnston RN, McNeill RS, Smith DH, Dempster MB, Nairn JR, Purvis MS, et al. Five-year winter chemoprophylaxis for chronic bronchitis. Br Med J 1969;4:265-69.

67. Poole PJ, Black PN. Mucolytic agents for chronic bronchitis or chronic obstructive pulmonary disease. Cochrane Database Syst Rev 2000;2:CD001287.

68. Wilson DO, Rogers SM, Sanders MH, Pennock BE, Reilly JJ. Nutritional intervention in malnourished patients with emphysema. Am Rev Rspir Dis 1986;134:672-77.

69. Schols AMWJ. Nutrition in chronic obstructive pulmonary disease. Curr Opin Pulm Med 2000;6: 110-15.

70. Williams JH Jr., Moser KM. Pneumococcal vaccine and patients with chronic lung disease. Ann Intern Med 1986;104:106-09.

71. Collet JP, Shapiro P, Ernst P, Renzi T, Ducruet T, Robinson A. Effects of an immunostimulating agent on acute exacerbations and hospitalizations in patients with chronic obstructive pulmonary disease. Am J Respir Crit Care Med 1997;156:1719-24.

72. British Thoracic Society Standards of Care Subcommittee on Pulmonary Rehabilitation. Pulmonary rehabilitation. Thorax 2001;56:827-34.

73. Rodriguez-Roisin R. Toward a consensus definition for COPD exacerbations. Chest 2000, 117:398S-401S.

74. Wilson R. The role of infection in COPD. Chest 1998;113:242S-248S.

75. Anderson HR, Spix C, Medina S, Schouten JP, Castellsague J, Rossi G, et al. Air pollution and daily admissions for chronic obstructive pulmonary disease in 6 European cities: results from the APHEA project. Eur Respir J 1997;10:1064-71.

76. White AJ, Gompertz S, Stockley RA. The aetiology of exacerbations of chronic obstructive pulmonary disease. Thorax 2003;58:73-80.

77. Anthonisen NR, Manfreda J, Warren CP, Hershfield ES, Harding GK, Nelson NA. Antibiotic therapy in exacerbations of chronic obstructive pulmonary disease. Ann Intern Med 1987; 106:196-204.

78. Saint S, Bent S, Vittinghoff E, Grady D. Antibiotics in chronic obstructive pulmonary disease exacerbations: A meta-analysis. JAMA 1995;273:957-60.

79. Niederman MS. Antibiotic therapies of exacerbations of chronic bronchitis. Semin Respir Infect 2000;15: 59-70.

80. Thompson WH, Nielson CP, Carvalho P, Charan NB, Crowley JJ. Controlled trial of oral prednisone in outpatients with acute COPD exacerbation. Am J Respir Crit Care Med 1996;154:407-12.

81. Davies L, Angus RM, Calverley PM. Oral corticosteroids in patients admitted to hospital with exacerbations of chronic obstructive pulmonary disease: A prospective randomized controlled trial. Lancet 1999; 354:456-60.

82. Niewoehner DE, Erbland ML, Deupree RH, Collins D, Gross NJ, Light RW, et al. Effect of systemic glucocorticoids on exacerbations of chronic obstructive pulmonary disease. Department of Veterans Affairs Cooperative Study Group. N Engl J Med 1999;340: 1941-47.

83. Dunn WF, Nelson SB, Hubmayr RD. Oxygen induced hypercarbia in obstructive pulmonary disease. Am Rev Respir Dis 1991;144:526-30.

84. Fletcher C, Peto R. The natural history of chronic airflow obstruction. BMJ 1977;1:1645-48.

85. Nishimura K, Tsukino M. Clinical course and prognosis of patients with chronic obstructive pulmonary disease. Curr Opin Pulm Med 2000;6:127-32.

Chapter
17

Respiratory Failure

DEFINITION

Respiratory failure is the body's inability to clear itself of carbon dioxide and to provide sufficient oxygen for its own metabolic needs. Thus, it can be defined as "*a condition in which arterial PaO_2 is below the range of normal values (excluding right to left intracardiac shunts) and/or arterial $PaCO_2$ is above the range of normal values (excluding respiratory compensation for metabolic alkalosis)*". The normal range of variation from the mean value at a given age and certain altitude is ± 5 mm Hg for both PaO_2 and $PaCO_2$. The range of normal values is important since both age and altitude affect them. At birth, PaO_2 is approximately 65 mm Hg which rises to mid-80s within the first two years of life and thereafter, more slowly to the mid-90s. This value remains stable till about the age of 30 or 40 years, when it begins to decline that reaches about 75 mm Hg at the age of 75. On the contrary, $PaCO_2$ does not vary with age except during the first few days of life, when it increases from about 30 to the normal value of 40 mm Hg. Both PaO_2 and $PaCO_2$ decreases in normal persons as they ascend in altitude. It is suggested that a PaO_2 of < 60 mm Hg at rest at sea level or a $PaCO_2$ level of > 49 mm Hg should be used to define respiratory failure. The definition and diagnosis of respiratory failure depends on the measurements of the values of PaO_2 and $PaCO_2$. Thus, respiratory failure is a laboratory, and not a clinical diagnosis (diagnosis based on clinical features is too late). Two types of respiratory failure are generally recognized: type I or hypoxic respiratory failure and type II or hypercapnic respiratory failure.[1] In type I respiratory failure the PaO_2 is low, but the $PaCO_2$, is normal or low; and in type II failure, the alveolar ventilation is not adequate and the PaO_2 is low with raised $PaCO_2$.

Respiratory failure may be *acute* as in drug overdoses or *chronic* with permanent blood gas abnormalities as in COPD.

ETIOPATHOGENESIS

The respiratory system consists of two parts: the gas exchanging organs (the lungs); and the ventilatory pump, which brings fresh air into the lungs and expels alveolar gas. The latter consists of the chest wall (rib cage, and abdomen), the muscles that displace the chest wall (diaphragm, inspiratory and expiratory muscles), and the respiratory centers with intervening neural connections. Respiratory failure can result from failure of either of the two main components of the respiratory system, or by any of the subcomponents of ventilatory pump. Failure in the gas exchanging unit usually results in hypoxemia and that due to pump failure results in hypercapnia. Thus, respiratory failure can be due to: Failure of the gas exchange in the lungs, Inadequate central respiratory drive. Failure of the respiratory muscles to generate force in spite of adequate central output, and a mechanical defect in the chest wall components of the pump[1-3] (Fig. 17.1).

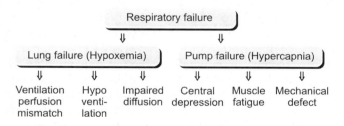

FIGURE 17.1: The underlying mechanisms of respiratory failure

Although one can divide respiratory failure into the main two components of lung failure and pump failure, interactions between them are common. Lung disease can overload the muscles because of abnormalities in the pulmonary mechanics or can decrease energy supply because of hypoxia. Similarly, pump failure, although, in principle, can exist in isolation, in most instances they probably occur in combination. There is increasing evidence that overloaded and failing respiratory muscles result in afferent feedback at the spinal level of higher, which diminishes firing frequency of inspiratory motor neurons or decreases central respiratory drive. Some important causes of respiratory failure are summarized in Table 17.1.

TABLE 17.1: Causes of respiratory failure[4-16]

Lung failure	Pump failure
Chronic bronchitis and emphysema	(a) *Central causes*
Pulmonary edema	Drug overdose
Interstitial fibrosis	Poisoning
Bronchial asthma	Disorders of brainstem
Pneumothorax	Sleep apnea syndrome
Pulmonary embolism	Obesity
Pneumoconiosis	(b) *Neuromuscular disorders*
Acute respiratory distress syndrome	Myasthenia gravis
Bronchiectasis	Poliomyelitis
Obesity	Myopathies
Lymphangitis carcinomatosis	Polyneuropathy
Advanced pulmonary TB	Porphyria
	Cervical cord injury
	Spinal muscular atrophies
	Motor neuron disease
	LGB syndrome
	(c) *Chest wall disorders*
	Crushed chest injury
	Kyphoscoliosis

Arterial hypoxia can be caused by five different physiologic abnormalities: *hypoventilation, impaired diffusion, ventilation-perfusion mismatching, right-to-left shunting,* and *breathing air or gas mixture with a low PO_2.* Two or more of these can coexist in patients with respiratory disease. The contribution of each mechanism can be inferred from results of routine blood gas analysis, and when the subject breathes 100 percent oxygen. Of these, pathologic hypoxia from breathing low O_2 occurs in smoke filled rooms or in mines when CO or methane dilutes oxygen or in which oxygen is consumed as by fire. Pure hypoventilation is caused by either severe parenchymal or airways disease or by pump failure. The alveolar-arterial PO_2 difference is not increased in pure hypoventilation. Most commonly, hypoventilation is found in association with other disturbances of gas exchange. When these coexist they can be recognized by the fact that the decrease in arterial PO_2 is more than that can be accounted for by the increase in arterial PCO_2 and that the alveolar-arterial PO_2 difference is increased. Oxygen uptake is not limited by diffusion in healthy subjects except when they breathe air or gas mixtures

containing a low PO_2 as in high altitude or possibly during heavy exercise. Even when abnormalities of diffusion exist, because of adequate transit time of RBC in pulmonary capillaries, their contribution to hypoxia is negligible. Increased mismatching of ventilation and perfusion is by far the most common cause of arterial hypoxia encountered in clinical practice. Virtually all forms of lung diseases are associated with a detectable ventilation-perfusion abnormality. Right-to-left shunts of blood in, around, or distal to the lungs is another cause of hypoxemia. It is not possible to differentiate arterial hypoxia caused by ventilation-perfusion abnormality from right-to-left shunts while the subject is breathing ambient air. For that, the subject should breathe 100 percent oxygen and then the arterial PO_2 is measured. While inhalation of 100 percent oxygen corrects ventilation-perfusion abnormalities, the same is not true for the shunt abnormality. An increased (above normal) alveolar-arterial PO_2 difference signifies the presence of an excessive right-to-left shunt. Thus in summary, the important causes of clinically encountered hypoxia are mainly due to three physiological abnormalities: hypoventilation, ventilation-perfusion mismatch, and right-to-left shunt (diffusion abnormalities do not contribute significantly, and inhalation of low oxygen is typical of certain obvious situations). Because arterial PO_2 and PCO_2 change in opposite directions by nearly the same amount during hypoventilation, the contribution of hypoventilation to the patient's arterial hypoxia can be readily assessed. For example, if PaO_2 is 50 mm Hg, and $PaCO_2$ is 80 mm Hg in a 30 year old patient, both the values have changed from their normal values by the same amount ($90 - 50 = 40$ for PaO_2 and $80 - 40 = 40$ for $PaCO_2$), and pure hypoventilation is present. In contrast, if PaO_2 is 30 mm Hg and $PaCO_2$ is 80 mm Hg in the same patient, the change of $PaCO_2$ from normal does not account for the entire change in PaO_2, so that hypoventilation plus either ventilation-perfusion abnormality or shunt must be present. These can be differentiated by inhalation of 100 percent oxygen.

Identification of the underlying pathophysiologic mechanisms of respiratory failure is important, because therapeutic considerations are different for different processes. Hypoventilation implies failure of neural or neuromuscular control of breathing and is treated by vigorous efforts to improve alveolar ventilation. When these are unsuccessful, intubation and mechanical ventilation will be necessary. Ventilation-perfusion mismatch usually denotes a disorder involving airways (secretions, oedema, bronchospasm), so that distribution of inspired air to affected regions is decreased more than the blood flow to these areas and the aim of treatment there is to relieve bronchial obstruction by suction, bronchodilators and anti-inflammatory drugs. Right-to-left shunts or perfusion of non-ventilated regions, nearly always indicate the closure of terminal respiratory units by micro- or macroatelectasis or the filling of these units by blood, oedema fluids, or pus. Treatment is then aimed at controlling these problems.[17-21]

Decreases in cardiac output have a secondary pathophysiologic consequence in patients with lung disease. Similarly, factors affecting oxygen delivery to the tissues like red blood cells and factors affecting oxygen loading and unloading are also important while considering respiratory failure.

Respiratory failure is still an important complication of chronic obstructive pulmonary disease (COPD) and hospitalization with an acute episode being a poor prognostic marker. However, other comorbid conditions, especially cardiovascular disease, are equally powerful predictors of mortality. The physiological basis of acute respiratory failure in COPD is now clear. Significant ventilation/perfusion mismatching with a relative increase in the physiological dead space leads to hypercapnia and hence acidosis. This is largely the result of a shift to a rapid shallow breathing pattern and a rise in the dead space/tidal volume ratio of each breath. This breathing pattern results from adaptive physiological responses which lessen the risk of respiratory muscle fatigue and minimize breathlessness.[16]

Changes in lung mechanics are thought to be the major determinants of the physiological abnormalities that characterize hypercapnic respiratory failure. In practice, a subject would need to increase their ventilation very substantially to overcome the wasted ventilation in high ventilation/perfusion ratio units, but their inability to do so despite the respiratory stimulus that a rising CO_2 tension provides, has been the subject of much debate.[22] One useful analysis has been provided by Moxham,[23] who placed the respiratory muscle pump in the central role, being affected to some extent by the load that it has to overcome, e.g. the expiratory airflow limitation seen in severe COPD, but also by its own capacity to generate pressure, which is significantly reduced by the respiratory muscle shortening that accompanies pulmonary hyperinflation. This is a common and important finding in acute exacerbations of COPD. The drive to the respiratory muscles is itself influenced by chemoreceptor and mechanical receptor inputs and also modulated by sleep. However, sleep structure is probably poor in most episodes of respiratory failure, as in stable disease,[24] and sleep related hypoventilation, therefore, plays a smaller role than would be the case in other chronic respiratory conditions.

There has been much debate about whether respiratory muscle fatigue is the precipitating factor in patients who develop acute respiratory failure. Respiratory muscle fatigue is an important physiological concept, which was initially thought to exist as a chronic state. Fatigue reflects the results of severe loading of the respiratory muscles and their inability to develop the appropriate force or tension to overcome this loading.[25] Characteristically, this process is relieved by rest and much of the benefit of positive pressure ventilation in stable hypercapnic COPD was initially believed to be due to reduction in the degree of chronic fatigue. However, the physiological indices which were believed to reflect the onset of respiratory muscle fatigue have proven to be less robust than initially envisaged. Thus changes in the ratio of the high to low electromyogram power spectrum can be induced by acute respiratory loading and resolve when the load is removed, at least in healthy subjects. Similar problems exist for other indices such as the maximum relaxation rate of the diaphragm, which had been proposed as a specific test to predict the onset of respiratory muscle fatigue. The demonstration in patients with stable COPD that the reduced ability of the diaphragm to develop pressure was a consequence not of fatigue but of geometric factors related to chronic hyperinflation[26] led to significant reevaluation of the role of muscle fatigue in acute respiratory failure. It is now seen more as a "limit condition" than a chronic state. Patients approaching the fatigue threshold usually adopt breathing strategies which reduce the chance of this highly deleterious state occurring.

Initial observations in stable patients showed that their respiratory drive, as assessed by mouth occlusion pressure, was high but that there was a difference in the breathing pattern of patients who showed a high CO_2 tension when stable and those that did not.[27] The former tended to exhibit a more rapid shallow breathing pattern and this was investigated subsequently by workers in Italy who found that the tidal volume was inversely related to CO_2 tension as was the maximum pleural pressure that the subjects could develop.[28] When the patients were categorized by the intensity of their reported breathlessness using the Medical Research Council dyspnea scale, those patients using the greatest amount of pleural pressure as a percentage of the maximum were the most breathless and were also the individuals with the shortest inspiratory time and the most rapid breathing pattern.

CLINICAL ASSESSMENT

One should become suspicious in the clinical setting when a patient is at high risk for acute respiratory failure. Patients with COPD having any acute illness superimposed on the chronic disease process are more likely to develop acute respiratory failure.[29-31] Similarly, there are certain situations when chances of acute respiratory distress syndrome are very high. These conditions include sepsis syndrome, aspiration of gastric contents, massive emergency transfusions of > 10 units of blood in 12 hours, trauma with lung contusion, and multiple major fractures.

When there is a concomitant disease process, diagnosis of respiratory failure by blood gas analysis becomes easier. However, when the patient presents primarily with central nervous system or cardiovascular symptoms or signs, the appropriate diagnosis becomes difficult. Clinical evidence of hypoxia is best appreciated by observing central cyanosis. However, the sign is very unreliable, particularly during the early stages, since a great deal of intra- and interobserver variation exists in finding out the presence of cyanosis. Polycythemia may be present in subjects with chronic hypoxia. Hypoxia affects central nervous system the most at an early stage and is manifested by restlessness, and irritability, impaired intellectual function, and clouding of consciousness. This may progress to convulsions, "coma and death". Acute hypoxia is well tolerated by chronically hypoxic patients than a previously healthy individual. Ventilation may be increased through the stimulation of carotid receptor, but severe hypoxia leads to suppression of ventilation. Cardiac rate and output are increased by hypoxia and peripheral vasodilatation occurs. Cardiac arrhythmias may occur and these may be exaggerated by concurrent administration of digitalis or theophylline or hypokalemia due to diuretic therapy. Pulmonary arteries constrict in response to hypoxia which may progress to cor pulmonale in chronic cases.

The clinical effects of hypercapnia are variable. Changes in $PaCO_2$ are more important than the actual level. Thus while a level of 70 mm Hg in a COPD patient with chronic respiratory failure may be well tolerated, an acute rise to this level will prove fatal. Hypercapnia results in cerebral vasodilatation, increased cerebral blood flow and increased CSF pressure. Clinical features include drowsiness, altered sleep pattern, headache, flapping tremor, coma, cerebral edema, and papilledema. Muscle twitching and hyperreflexia are also possible. Peripheral vasodilatation occurs as a result of direct effect on the smooth muscle but vasoconstriction is also possible because of sympathetic stimulation. The clinical effect depends on the balance between the two. Sympathetic stimulation will result in tachycardia, and sweating. Vasodilatation will result in high bounding pulse, with warm peripheries. In severe hypercapnia, hypotension can occur due to intense vasodilatation.

Recently, respiratory muscle fatigue is gaining increasing attention as a cause of respiratory failure. This can be suspected from three clinical manifestations: (i) rapid shallow breathing, important but nonspecific; (ii) paradoxical abdominal movements and (iii) respiratory alternans. Paradoxical abdominal motion reflects asynchronous movements of the rib cage (intercostal muscles) and abdomen (diaphragm). Respiratory alternans is the phenomenon of a patient's breathing almost entirely with the diaphragm for a short time, then switching to breathing almost entirely with the rib cage muscles, and alternating back and forth between the two patterns. These are accompanied by characteristic electromyographic patterns.[30-32]

Thus, a combination of history with particular emphasis on the patient's clinical situation, the physical examination which includes pulmonary, cardiac, and central nervous system assessments and evaluation of tissue perfusion and organ function, arterial blood gas measurements, the chest radiograph, and other laboratory examinations that help to determine the presence of generalized or localized inflammation and the status of organ function is necessary for the full assessment of respiratory failure.

MANAGEMENT

The aim of management of respiratory failure is to maintain adequate airways, to ensure adequate alveolar ventilation and oxygen with treatment of the underlying primary cause.[33-39] Treatment of the primary cause will depend upon the etiology, as for example, antibiotics for pneumonia, bronchodilators and anti-inflammatory drugs for bronchial asthma and so on. Physiotherapy for removal of secretions from the airways, and encouragement of coughing whenever possible will ensure adequate and patent airways.[38]

The aim of oxygen therapy is to maintain adequate PaO_2 without producing serious side effects or oxygen toxicities. The basic principles are discussed briefly in the previous chapter for treatment of COPD. In previously healthy acutely hypoxemic persons the aim is to alleviate hypoxemic symptomatology and to maintain PaO_2 as normal as possible, whereas that for a patient with COPD with chronic hypoxia, this should be maintained at 60 mm Hg to avoid carbon dioxide retention.

Oxygen can be delivered to the patient with a variety of devices. The choice of a particular device depends on the FiO_2 required, ability of the patient to cooperate, the ease and comfort of the patient to tolerate, and the adequacy of desired blood gas levels. The source of oxygen can be obtained from wall systems, cylinders, liquid systems, concentrators or enrichers. Most often the gas requires humidification.

The oxygen delivery devices include the *low flow oxygen delivery devices* and the *high flow delivery devices.* The most common method of oxygen administration involves the use of low flow devices in which the actual concentration of oxygen received by the patient varies with changes in the respiratory pattern. The device delivers a set flow of 100 percent oxygen, which is then mixed with room air as the patient inhales. The amount of air entrained, which varies with the patient's minute ventilation, will affect the final concentration delivered. Various low flow devices include nasal cannula or nasal prong, simple; face mask, non-rebreathing mask, and partial rebreathing mask, oxygen conserving cannula, transtracheal catheter, tracheostomy collar, and tracheostomy T-bar. Of these *nasal cannulas* are simple and widely used. This can be used even in a restless patient, it is relatively comfortable and acceptable, and the patient can talk, eat, and move about in bed. The disadvantage of the method is that high flow rates of > 4 L/min may dry the nasal mucosa and cause pain in the frontal sinuses, ulcerations around nose, lips, and ear may develop due to pressure or reaction to plastic or rubber. The major disadvantage of nasal cannulas is the variability in the inspired oxygen fraction with change in minute ventilation of the patient which can present considerable problems in the management of patients who are oxygen-sensitive. Roughly, each liter increment increases FiO_2 approximately 3 to 4 percent, and humidification is not necessary for flow rates < 3 L/min. New designs are now available which have cannula built into eye glass frame or headband. Use of *simple face mask* can achieve oxygen concentrations of 35 to 50 percent with flow rates of 6 to 12 liters. The disadvantages are the lack of patient tolerance as it is quite uncomfortable since a tight seal must be maintained between the face and the mask. The mask may produce pressure necrosis, hampers heat radiation from face, and needs to be removed while eating, drinking or talking. In adult patients, at least 5 L/min flow is required to prevent accumulation of expired air in the mask with subsequent increase in inspired CO_2. High concentrations of oxygen can be delivered through *non-rebreathing masks.* Oxygen flows into the bag, (which

serves as the reservoir) and mask during inhalation; one valve prevents expired air from flowing back into the bag, and two others prevent inspiration of room air into the mask. Concentrations of 60 to 90 percent can be achieved using flow rates of 10 to 15 L/min. The disadvantages are the same as those for a simple mask. *Partial rebreathing mask* is similar to non-rebreathing mask, except concentrations of only 40 to 60 percent can be achieved. In this mask, all the three valves are removed allowing some dilution of inhaled oxygen by exhaled gas decreasing FiO_2 The high flow devices Include *Venturi masks* or *air entrainment masks.* The advantages of this mask are that it can deliver precise concentrations of oxygen, it is of light weight, and can deliver a wide range of concentrations of oxygen from 24 to 50 percent. The mask is particularly helpful to provide low, constant oxygen concentrations to patients of COPD with carbon dioxide retention. The disadvantage of the mask is that the patient may not tolerate it and the mask has to be removed during eating, drinking, and talking. New devices for oxygen delivery are available now with the aim of lowering the oxygen flow requirements, with both financial benefits and patient convenience and therefore better compliance. These include reservoir type cannulas, transtracheal cannulas, and intermittent demand flow systems.

Potential Hazards of Oxygen Therapy

While beneficial in the treatment of hypoxia in the acute and chronic settings, oxygen therapy is not without potential problems.[36,37] These include combustion (fire hazards), ventilatory depression particularly in chronic hypoxia in COPD, and oxygen toxicity. Oxygen toxicity depends upon a number of variables including degree of pulmonary dysfunction, metabolic and nutritional status, and prior exposure to other compounds capable of causing oxidant damage. End organ damage from hyperoxia depends on both the concentration of oxygen administered and the pressure used during administered. Prolonged exposure to hyperbaric oxygen causes central nervous system toxicity and produce pulmonary edema. Normobaric hyperoxic exposure results in lung damage as the predominant manifestation of toxicity. Although the exact mechanism of oxygen induced lung injury is unknown, the most acceptable hypothesis is that oxygen produces lung cell damage as a result of the production of activated oxygen species or free radicals. These include superoxide anion, hydrogen peroxide, and hydroxyl radicals, and singlet oxygen. These oxygen species are produced by single-electron transfers to molecular oxygen and are thought to be formed in large quantities during hyperoxic exposure. Then, they produce destructive chain reactions that lead to cell injury. These radicals react with the polyunsaturated fatty acid side chains of membrane lipids to initiate the process of lipid peroxidation. The lipid peroxides so formed act as powerful enzyme inhibitors resulting in damages to cell proteins. Oxygen radicals also directly damage nucleic acids with DNA destruction and cell death.

The administration of high inspired oxygen to adults with acute respiratory failure results in direct pulmonary damage and loss of lung function. Changes begin to occur rapidly both at the cellular and whole-lung level. Normal human beings breathing 100 percent oxygen only for 6 hours exhibit a 50 percent decrease in tracheal mucus flow. Alveolar macrophage function also appears to be altered during hyperoxic exposure. When normal individuals are exposed to 100 percent inspired oxygen, during the first 6 hours no measurable changes are found in lung function. However, tracheobronchitis, associated with a nonproductive cough and substernal chest pain does occur during this period. Vital capacity decreases during the next 12 to 24 hours with decreasing lung compliance, widening alveolar-arterial oxygen tension difference and decreasing exercise PaO_2, occurring between 24 to 30 hours of exposure. Diffusion capacity decreases by 30 to 72 hours of exposure. Toxicity from low-flow supplemental oxygen in patients who received as little as 24 to 28 percent inspired oxygen for a period of months as in chronic respiratory failure due to COPD, has been reported to produce both proliferative and fibrotic changes in the lungs. However, the value of supplemental oxygen therapy in these patients with chronic respiratory insufficiency far outweighs any of the minor cell changes that have been reported.

The clinical manifestations of oxygen toxicity include cough, substernal chest pain, nausea, vomiting, paresthesia, nasal stuffiness, sore throat and malaise. The later stages affect the alveolar-capillary gas exchange units, and surfactant inactivation, leading to acute respiratory distress syndrome. Replacement of nitrogen may lead on to absorption collapse. In neonates, retrolental fibroplasia and bronchopulmonary dysplasia are additional complications.

Although a safe limit of oxygen has not been established, as a general principle, the lowest possible inspired oxygen concentration that maintain tissue oxygen should always be administered. Concentrations above 50 to 60 percent are potentially toxic and who exhibit inadequate oxygenation at these concentrations, other therapeutic measures to achieve this goal should be considered. No specific pharmacological agent is recommended at present to be used for protection from oxidant lung damage. The use of bacterial endotoxins, superoxide dismutase and vitamin E has shown promise in experimental animals, but they are not yet recommended for human use.

Mechanical Ventilation

Mechanical ventilation is the most widely used supportive technique in intensive care units.[40] Several forms of external support for respiration have long been described to assist the failing ventilatory pump, and access to lower airways through tracheostomy or endotracheal tubes had constituted a major advance in the management of patients with respiratory distress. More recently, however, new "noninvasive" ventilation (NIV) techniques, using patient/ventilator interfaces in the form of facial masks, have been designed.

The reasons for promoting NIV include a better understanding of the role of ventilatory pump failure in the indications for mechanical ventilation, the development of ventilatory modalities able to work in synchrony with the patient, and the extensive recognition of complications associated with endotracheal intubation and standard mechanical ventilation.

I. NONINVASIVE POSITIVE PRESSURE VENTILATION[41-48]

Since the early 1990s there has been much clinical and academic interest in the use of noninvasive positive pressure ventilation (NPPV). There is more evidence to direct the application of this therapy than perhaps any other respiratory care modality. NPPV for the treatment of patients suffering acute respiratory failure (ARF) has been reviewed extensively and has been the topic of several consensus conferences. The British Thoracic Society has published guidelines for the use of NPPV for ARF. A prospective survey for 3 weeks in 42 intensive care units (ICUs) found that NPPV was used as first-line therapy with 16 percent of mechanically ventilated patients. The percentage of patients receiving NPPV ranged from 0 (in 8 ICUs) to 67 percent (in one ICU). In that survey NPPV was never used with patients in coma but was used with 14 percent of patients suffering hypoxemic respiratory failure, 27 percent of patients suffering pulmonary edema, and 50 percent of patients suffering hypercapnic respiratory failure. Endotracheal intubation was eventually performed in 40 percent of the patients who received NPPV (i.e. a 60% success rate).

NIV has been used primarily for patients with acute hypercapnic ventilatory failure, and especially for acute exacerbation of chronic obstructive pulmonary disease.

In this population, the use of NIV is associated with a marked reduction in the need for endotracheal intubation, a decrease in complication rate, a reduced duration of hospital stay and a substantial reduction in hospital mortality. Similar benefits have also been demonstrated in patients with asphyxic forms of acute cardiogenic pulmonary edema. In patients with primarily hypoxemic forms of respiratory failure, the level of success of NIV is more variable, but major benefits have also been demonstrated in selected populations with no contraindications such as multiple organ failure, loss of consciousness or hemodynamic instability.

One important factor in success seems to be the early delivery of noninvasive ventilation during the course of respiratory failure. Noninvasive ventilation allows many of the complications associated with mechanical ventilation to be avoided, especially the occurrence of nosocomial infections. The current use of noninvasive ventilation is growing up, and is becoming a major therapeutic tool in the intensive care unit.

Without mechanical support for respiration, many patients would die within hours to days due to acute hypoxemic and hypercapnic respiratory failure. Observational, physiological and case/control studies form a large body of evidence demonstrating that noninvasive ventilation (NIV) can be used in many situations to decrease a patient's dyspnea and work of breathing, improve gas exchange and ultimately avoid the need for endotracheal intubation (ETI).[49-51] Randomized controlled trials have confirmed this and helped delineate when NIV should be used as a first-line treatment. Studies conducted outside the context of clinical trials are also of great importance in ensuring that the results of these trials can be obtained in real life.[52-54] Indeed, the success of NIV may follow a learning curve, and early results may not be as good as those obtained later. In addition, it must be clear to clinicians that NIV is a complementary technique and cannot replace ETI in all instances.

In theory, the modes and settings for the delivery of NIV could be very similar to those for traditional mechanical ventilation through an endotracheal tube or tracheotomy cannula. In practice, because the circumstances of ventilation are different, the population of patients more selected and the equipment available sometimes more limited, this is not the case. In addition, leaks are a quasiconstant feature of NIV.[55,56] NIV is usually delivered in the form of assisted ventilation, in which every breath is supported by the ventilator. Rarely, controlled mechanical ventilation is used.

Acute Exacerbation of Chronic Respiratory Failure

Patients with hypercapnic forms of acute respiratory failure are most likely to benefit from NIV.[49-51] Their respiratory muscles become unable to generate adequate alveolar ventilation despite large pressure swings because of the presence of severe abnormalities in respiratory mechanics (intrinsic positive end-expiratory pressure (PEEP) and high inspiratory resistances). Stimulation of the respiratory centers and the large negative intrathoracic pressure swings generated do not permit compensation for these abnormalities; rapid shallow breathing ensues, associated with carbon dioxide retention and respiratory acidosis, and a risk of respiratory muscle fatigue. Dyspnea, right ventricular failure and encephalopathy characterize the severe acute exacerbation. Delivery of NIV allows the patient to take deeper breaths with less effort. NIV at two levels of pressure (pressure support and PEEP) delivers a positive inspiratory pressure swing in synchrony with the patient's inspiratory effort. A low level of pressure during expiration counterbalances the effects of dynamic hyperinflation, which result in a positive residual alveolar pressure at the end of expiration. The combination of the two levels of pressure has the greatest efficacy in reducing patient effort. NIV can reverse the clinical abnormalities related to hypoxemia, hypercapnia and acidosis.

Early NIV to prevent further deterioration must become an important part of the first-line therapy of acute exacerbation of COPD. A very low arterial blood pH, marked alteration in mental status when NIV is started, and the presence of comorbid conditions or a high severity score characterize patients who experience NIV failure. The presence of several of these factors seems to indicate that late delivery of NIV during the course of the exacerbation reduces the likelihood of success. Every effort should be made to deliver NIV early, and close monitoring is therefore in order when NIV is started late. In addition, a recent randomized controlled trial indicates that the efficacy of NIV diminishes when this therapy is applied late in the course of the exacerbation.

Negative Pressure Ventilation

Nowadays, the technique of negative pressure ventilation is only available in very few centers in the world. It should be mentioned, however, that negative pressure ventilation was the first mode of delivering noninvasive ventilation, before positive pressure ventilation became the rule in the 1950s.[57,58] Its efficacy in the treatment of acute exacerbations of COPD may be superior, in experienced hands, to a traditional approach with invasive mechanical ventilation, and similar to noninvasive ventilation *via* a face mask.[59,60]

Helium-oxygen Mixture

The use of a helium-oxygen mixture during NIV seems very promising for further reducing dyspnoea and work of breathing in patients with COPD.[61,62] Several randomized controlled trials are in progress to test the hypothesis that this gas mixture could increase the success rate of this technique.

Cardiogenic Pulmonary Edema

Continuous positive airway pressure (CPAP) has the ability, by raising intrathoracic pressure, to decrease shunting and improve arterial oxygenation and dyspnea in patients with acute cardiogenic pulmonary oedema. CPAP can both lessen the work of breathing substantially and improve cardiovascular function by decreasing the left ventricular afterload in nonpreload-dependent patients. Pressure support plus PEEP induces similar pathophysiological benefits.

Most patients with cardiogenic pulmonary edema improve rapidly with medical therapy. A few, however, develop acute asphyxic respiratory distress and require ventilatory support until the medical treatment starts to work. This may be particularly common in elderly patients with heart disease and patients with concomitant chronic lung disease. Several NIV modalities have been tried successfully, the goal being to avoid ETI.

Continuous Positive Airway Pressure or Pressure Support Plus Positive End-expiratory Pressure

Randomized trials comparing either CPAP or pressure support plus PEEP to standard medical therapy found similar results with the two techniques in terms of improvement in arterial blood gas levels and respiratory frequency. Both CPAP and pressure support plus PEEP significantly reduced the ETI rate.

Hypoxemic Respiratory Failure

Positive pressure ventilation was reintroduced during the first half of the twentieth century, for support of patients requiring general anesthesia for surgery, especially thoracic procedures. When the earliest case series of patients with adult respiratory distress syndrome were reported in the late 1960s, positive pressure ventilation was used with increasing frequency for nonsurgical patients with acute respiratory failure of various causes, including obstructive airways disease and severe pneumonia. NIV was proposed, in the early 1990s, for treating these patients, but initial studies have not all been successful. More recently, new trials with careful selection of patients have demonstrated clear benefits of NIV.

A subject of considerable controversy has been the role of NPPV with patients who have hypoxemia but not hypercapnia. In a randomized controlled trial of continuous positive airway pressure (CPAP) via face mask with patients suffering acute hypoxemic respiratory failure it is reported that, despite early physiologic improvement, CPAP neither reduced the need for intubation not improved outcomes such as survival. However, 5 randomized controlled trials have reported success with NPPV for acute hypoxemic respiratory failure. In a randomized controlled trial of NPPV for acute hypoxemic respiratory failure. It was reported that NPPV benefited several outcome variables. However, patients were randomized to NPPV or intubation and invasive ventilation. That study design is different than other NPPV studies. The more conventional design is to randomize patients to NPPV or conventional medical therapy, with intubation being an outcome variable. When patients in the control group are intubated per study protocol, it prompts the question of whether intubation was indeed mandatory in all patients in the control group. Moreover, the study included patients with a variety of diagnoses, making it difficult to apply the study findings to individual patients presenting with hypoxemic respiratory failure.

The success of noninvasive ventilation is dependent on various clinical aspects and the organization of care, but also on a lot of technical issues. Far from being details, they can make a large difference. They include the patient/ventilator interface, type of humidifier and ventilator used and its capabilities for triggering and pressurization. The general care of the patient is different from that for a patient receiving invasive ventilation, and will thus potentially greatly influence the success of the technique. There is now a good evidence base for the use of noninvasive ventilation in numerous different conditions and settings; however, it remains a complementary therapy to invasive ventilation and clinicians need to be aware of the contraindications.

II. INVASIVE VENTILATION

If adequate respiratory effort cannot be maintained by the above measures and alveolar hypoventilation becomes the critical factor for survival, the use of mechanical ventilation becomes necessary.[63-68] Thus, the indications for mechanical ventilation are: (i) inadequate alveolar ventilation (rise in $PaCO_2$ and acidosis), (ii) inadequate lung expansion, (iii) inadequate muscle strength, (iv) excessive work of breathing, (v) inadequate drive to breathe, and (vi) severe hypoxemia. In some postoperative cases, prophylactic mechanical ventilation may be useful. Mechanical ventilation is used to adjust alveolar ventilation, to improve ventilation-perfusion relationships, to improve oxygenation, and to decrease the work of breathing. This is usually instituted for the management of four broad categories of disorders: (a) respiratory failure with normal lungs (i.e. neuromuscular disease), (b) diseases causing carbon dioxide retention (e.g. COPD), (c) diseases causing hypoxemia with or without elevated pulmonary artery wedge pressures (e.g. adult respiratory syndrome or cardiogenic pulmonary edema), and (d) progressive respiratory fatigue. Mechanical ventilators are of two broad categories according to the pressure applied to the chest: *Negative pressure ventilators,* which are no more in use, and *Positive-pressure ventilators* which are the major device for assistance in the therapy of severe respiratory failure. These devices are further classified into three types according to their cycling mechanisms as time-cycled, pressure-cycled, or volume-cycled. Some of them are piston-driven, some use a bellows, and some are compressor-driven. Many of these ventilators are equipped with many monitoring facilities and many external features such as gas mixers, intermittent mandatory ventilation, continuous positive airway pressure devices, and humidifiers, etc. Time-cycled ventilators are governed by a predetermined timing mechanism that ends inspiration. Pressure-cycled ventilators terminate inspiration when a predetermined pressure is reached. This peak pressure and time in which it is reached, markedly influence the volume achieved. Thus, changes in airway resistance and pulmonary compliance significantly influence the volumes generated. Volume-cycled ventilators are the most widely used of all mechanical ventilators. Inspiration ends when a predetermined volume is delivered to the patient, regardless of changes in airway resistance or pulmonary compliance. If very high pressures are generated and they exceed the preset limiting pressure, excess volume will be vented to the outside air, decreasing the effective tidal volume. These ventilators are expensive. They have some degree of versatility and may be used for most modes of ventilation.

Various modes of ventilation that are used include: Assisted Intermittent Positive Pressure Ventilation (IPPV); Controlled IPPV; Intermittent Mandatory Ventilation or (IMV) and Positive End-Expiratory Pressure Ventilation (PEEP). In IPPV, the patient's initial breath is followed by a ventilator-derived breath, which is limited either by a preset volume or pressure. This mode has been used as a primary mode to ventilate patients, although its major application is during the process of weaning. Because of lower intrathoracic pressures, cardiovascular side effects are less. The respiratory rate is set by the patient, which has the advantage of adjustment for PCO_2. Muscle disuse is decreased by active inspiration. However, in tachypneic patients, this mode becomes ineffectual, requiring the use of sedation or paralysis. In controlled IPPV, the patient is ventilated in a preset volume, which is delivered to the patient provided excessive pressure or leaks are not generated. This mode is indicated in apneic patients. When the patient starts to breathe on his own, IMV is more beneficial which provides for improved synchronization and less carbon dioxide retention. IMV is also being used now frequently as a ventilatory mode although it was initially introduced as a means of weaning. This consists of a combination of both spontaneous respiration and mandatory (controlled) breaths. Stacking or superimposition of a mandatory ventilator breath on a spontaneous exhalation may result in the generation of higher peak airway pressures with barotrauma. This can be prevented by the use of synchronization of mandatory breaths with the initiation of spontaneous respiration. PEEP is used to increase functional residual capacity and to improve ventilation-perfusion relationships. It may also be protective in instances in which volume overload or elevated hydrostatic pressures are operative as in cardiogenic pulmonary edema. All the mentioned modes of ventilation, including spontaneous ventilation, may be used with PEEP. The cardiovascular effects of PEEP are the limitations for its use. However, it is the most common mode used for the management of ARDS. Various other modes of ventilation include; pressure control ventilation (PCV), pressure-control with inverse-ratio ventilation (PCIRV), airway pressure release ventilation (APRV), high frequency positive-pressure ventilation (HPPPV), high-frequency jet ventilation (HJV), and high-frequency oscillation (HFO).

Besides the modes of ventilation, their adjuncts, including tracheal tubes, ventilator circuits, humidifiers and nebulizers, bacterial filters, and alarms are important in successful management of the patient. Although tubes have complications, they can be used for 10 to 14 days before tracheostomy is needed to be considered. Circuits must be chosen carefully and monitored for disconnections and leaks, and for their resistance to breathing and their compromise of delivered gas volumes. Infection remains a major problem with mechanical ventilation.

Of the many modes discussed, IMV and assist-control are being used increasingly to achieve the goals of mechanical ventilation. IMV is most widely used in USA, and is the ventilatory mode of choice in patients with severe underlying lung disease, perhaps ARDS, and who are breathing rapidly and shallowly. These patients may not be maintainable on assist-control, but some may be ventilated successfully on IMV without a great deal of sedation. The second potential use of IMV is in the COPD patients who have air trapping. Barotrauma is less likely to develop in patients with IMV than in those with assist-control. Assist-control is the method of choice for resting the patient who is acutely ill in respiratory failure. Weaning from mechanical ventilation is the process of switching a patient from mechanical to spontaneous ventilation. This process can be either the simple act of discontinuing ventilatory support or the gradual withdrawal of one mode of ventilation and its progressive replacement by another. However, this weaning process is not that simple. The usual protocol of weaning includes an improvement in the primary respiratory process, adequate oxygenation on a FiO_2 of 0.5 or less, ventilatory needs are manageable, minute ventilation < 10 L/min (for a $PaCO_2$ of 40 mm Hg), ventilatory mechanics adequate for needs (VC > 10 ml/kg, MIF > 20 cm H_2O, MVV is more than 2 times the resting minute ventilation requirements), and elimination or minimum use of respiratory depressants.

CHRONIC RESPIRATORY FAILURE

The traditional approach to the management of chronic respiratory failure due to COPD has included supplemental oxygen, and rehabilitation, the beneficial effects of which have been demonstrated. While these continue to be important, three new approaches have been suggested to manage these patients. The first is the, reduction of afterload and resting of the respiratory muscles by mechanical means such as continuous positive airway pressure and assisted ventilation. These modalities may be capable of improving ventilation, exercise function, and of relieving dyspnea. The second approach is the enhancement of respiratory contractility and reversal of possible muscle fatigue by pharmacological means. Although the role of drugs in achieving these goals remains controversial, theophylline has been found to improve respiratory muscle function. Finally lung transplantation has a role to play in the management of some patients with chronic respiratory failure.

Exacerbations of chronic obstructive pulmonary disease (COPD) cause morbidity, hospital admissions, and mortality, and strongly influence health-related quality of life. Some patients are prone to frequent exacerbations, which are associated with considerable physiologic deterioration and increased airway inflammation. About half of COPD exacerbations are caused or triggered primarily by bacterial and viral infections (colds, especially from rhinovirus), but air pollution can contribute to the beginning of an exacerbation. Type 1 exacerbations involve increased dyspnea, sputum volume, and sputum purulence; Type 2 exacerbations involve any two of the latter symptoms, and Type 3 exacerbations involve one of those symptoms combined with cough, wheeze, or symptoms of an upper respiratory tract infection. Exacerbations are more common than previously believed (2.5-3 exacerbations per year); many exacerbations are treated in the community and not associated with hospital admission. We found that about half of exacerbations were unreported by the patients, despite considerable encouragement to do so, and, instead, were only diagnosed from patients' diary cards. COPD patients are accustomed to frequent symptom changes, and this may explain their tendency to underreport exacerbations. COPD patients tend to be anxious and depressed about the disease and some might not seek treatment. At the beginning of an exacerbation physiologic changes such as decreases in peak flow and forced expiratory volume in the first second (FEV_1) are usually small and therefore are not useful in predicting exacerbations, but larger decreases in peak flow are associated with dyspnea and the presence of symptomatic upper-respiratory viral infection. More pronounced physiologic changes during exacerbation are related to longer exacerbation recovery time. Dyspnea, common colds, sore throat, and cough increase significantly during prodrome, indicating that respiratory viruses are important exacerbation triggers. However, the prodrome is relatively short and not useful in predicting onset. As colds are associated with longer and more severe exacerbations, a COPD patient who develops a cold should be considered for early therapy. Physiologic recovery after an exacerbation is often incomplete, which decreases health-related quality of life and resistance to future exacerbations, so it is important to identify COPD patients who suffer frequent exacerbations and to convince them to take precautions to minimize the risk of colds and other exacerbation triggers. Exacerbation frequency may vary with the severity of the COPD. Exacerbation frequency may or may not increase with the severity of the COPD. As the COPD progresses, exacerbations tend to have more symptoms and take longer to recover from. Twenty-five to fifty percent of COPD patients suffer lower airway bacteria colonization, which is related to the severity of COPD and cigarette smoking and which begins a cycle of epithelial cell damage, impaired mucociliary clearance, mucus hypersecretion, increased submucosal vascular leakage, and inflammatory cell infiltration. Elevated sputum interleukin-8 levels are associated with higher bacterial load and faster FEV_1 decline; the bacteria increase airway inflammation in the stable patient, which may accelerate disease progression. A 2 week course of oral corticosteroids is as beneficial as an 8 week course, with fewer adverse effects, and might extend the time until the next exacerbation. Antibiotics have some efficacy in treating exacerbations. Exacerbation frequency increases with progressive airflow obstruction; so patients with chronic respiratory failure are particularly susceptible to exacerbation.

As mentioned, respiratory failure is still an important complication of chronic obstructive pulmonary disease (COPD) and hospitalization with an acute episode being a poor prognostic marker. However, other comorbid conditions, especially cardiovascular disease, are equally powerful predictors of mortality. The physiological basis of acute respiratory failure in COPD is now clear. Significant ventilation/perfusion mismatching with a relative increase in the physiological dead space leads to hypercapnia and hence acidosis. This is largely the result of a shift to a rapid shallow breathing pattern and a rise in the dead space/tidal volume ratio of each breath. This breathing pattern results from adaptive physiological responses which lessen the risk of respiratory muscle fatigue and minimize breathlessness. Treatment is directed at reducing the mechanical load applied to each breath, correcting specific precipitating factors, e.g. bacterial infection, and maintaining gas exchange. Both bronchodilators and oral corticosteroids can improve spirometric results in exacerbations of COPD and should be routinely offered to patients with respiratory failure. Controlled oxygen is still not always prescribed appropriately and high inspired oxygen concentrations can lead to severe acidosis by either worsening ventilation/ perfusion mismatching and/or inducing a degree of hypoventilation. Ventilatory support using noninvasive ventilation has revolutionized the approach to these patients. Acute respiratory failure due to chronic obstructive pulmonary disease remains a common medical emergency that can be effectively managed. More attention should be focused on the prevention of these episodes and identifying the factors which cause early relapse.

CHRONIC NEUROMUSCULAR DISEASE

Chronic neuromuscular diseases may affect all major respiratory muscle groups including inspiratory, expiratory, and bulbar, and respiratory complications are the major cause of morbidity and mortality. Untreated, many of these diseases lead inexorably to hypercapnic respiratory failure, precipitated in some cases by chronic aspiration and secretion retention or pneumonia, related to impairment of cough and swallowing mechanisms. Many measures are helpful including inhibition of salivation, cough-assist techniques, devices to enhance communication, and physical therapy. In addition, ventilatory assistance is an important part of disease management for patients with advanced neuromuscular disease. Because of its comfort, convenience, and portability advantages, noninvasive positive pressure ventilation (NPPV) has become the modality of first choice for most patients. Patients to receive NPPV should be selected using consensus guidelines, and initiation should be gradual to maximize the chances for success. Attention should be paid to individual preferences for interfaces and early identification of cough impairment that necessitates the use of cough-assist devices. For patients considered unsuitable for noninvasive ventilation, invasive mechanical ventilation should be considered, but only after a frank but compassionate discussion between the patient, family, physician, and other caregivers.

STATUS ASTHMATICUS

Status asthmaticus is a life-threatening episode of asthma that is refractory to usual therapy.[69] Recent studies report an increase in the severity and mortality associated with asthma. In the airways, inflammatory cell infiltration and activation and cytokine generation produce airway injury and edema, bronchoconstriction and mucus plugging. The key pathophysiological consequence of severe airflow obstruction is dynamic hyperinflation. The resulting hypoxemia, tachypnea together with increased metabolic demands on the muscles of respiration may lead to respiratory muscle failure. The management of status asthmaticus involves intensive pharmacological therapy particularly with beta-adrenoceptor agonists (beta-agonists) and corticosteroids. Salbutamol is the most commonly used beta2-selective inhaled bronchodilator in the US. Epinephrine (adrenaline) or terbutaline, administered subcutaneously, have not been shown to provide greater broncho-dilatation compared with inhaled beta-agonists. Corticosteroids such as methylprednisolone should be administered early. Aerosolized corticosteroids are not recommended for patients with status asthmaticus. Inhaled anticholinergic agents may be useful in patients refractory to inhaled beta-agonists and corticosteroids. In patients requiring mechanical ventilation, the strategy aims to avoid dynamic hyperinflation by enhancing expiratory time to allow complete exhalation. Complications of dynamic inflation are hypotension and barotrauma. Sedation with opioids, benzodiazepines or propofol is required to facilitate ventilator synchrony but neuromuscular blockade should be avoided as myopathy has been a reported complication. Overall, in the management of patients with status asthmaticus, the challenge to the pulmonary/critical care clinician is to provide optimal pharmacological and ventilatory support and avoid the adverse consequences of dynamic hyperinflation.

POST-TRAUMATIC RESPIRATORY FAILURE

Acute respiratory distress syndrome (ARDS) is a severe and common complication of major trauma. The most important early management principle is to identify the inciting event and remove the ongoing insult aggressively. It is important to immediately resuscitate the patients and prepare them for a complex and difficult hospitalization. Avoiding secondary insults is the cornerstone of supportive care, and this is based primarily on aggressive immune surveillance, full nutrition, and unrelenting oxygen delivery. The use of aggressive immune surveillance, nutritional support, and fluid management is critical to support ventilator management for oxygenation and ventilation. In general, although essential, the ventilator has great potential for harm in patients who are compromised seriously with ARDS. Physicians must establish reasonable therapeutic goals based on oxygen delivery rather than arbitrary normal values of blood gas measurement. The impact of the ventilator should be limited with regard to respiratory pressure, tidal volume, inspired oxygen, and levels of expiratory end-expiratory pressure. Use of pulmonary toilet, including therapeutic bronchoscopy; patient positioning, including intermittent prone positioning, and recruitment maneuvers are useful therapeutic complements for maintaining functional residual capacity and decreasing shunt. Overall, ARDS represents a clear indication that the patient is failing to meet the demands of their stress and without prompt attention likely will die. It is a challenge and an opportunity to identify the underlying situation and to manage the patient while not causing additional harm as the patient's intrinsic resources can bring about the healing necessary to recover from the situation of extremis.

TUBERCULOSIS AND RESPIRATORY FAILURE

Acute respiratory failure is more common in miliary tuberculosis than in tuberculous bronchopneumonia and also has a worse prognosis. Chronic hypercapnic respiratory failure is frequent after both spinal tuberculosis and surgical treatments for pulmonary tuberculosis. It may develop insidiously or present acutely, for instance, during a chest infection. Hypoventilation appears during REM sleep before non-REM sleep or wakefulness and is readily treatable with noninvasive ventilation. The prognosis is good even if initially tracheostomy ventilation is required temporarily.

FLAIL CHEST

Flail chest occurs when a series of adjacent ribs are fractured in at least 2 places, anteriorly and posteriorly.[70] This section of the chest wall becomes unstable and it moves inwards during spontaneous inspiration. The physiological impact of a flail chest depends on multiple factors, including the size of the flail segment, the intrathoracic pressure generated during spontaneous ventilation, and the associated damage to the lung and chest wall. Treatment varies with the severity of the physiologic impairment attributable to the flail segment itself. Immediate surgical fixation may decrease morbidity, but conservative treatment with positive pressure ventilation is preferred when multiple injuries to the intrathoracic organs are present.

POISONING

Organophosphates may cause serious life-threatening conditions, such as an initial acute cholinergic crisis and intermediate syndrome.[71] Each of these conditions has a potential for respiratory failure requiring ventilatory support. For this reason, it is very important to recognize them early, especially to institute appropriate management. The diagnosis of organophosphate poisoning is based essentially on a clinical assessment, followed by laboratory examinations. Sometimes the diagnosis may be difficult. It is to be emphasized about the importance of early and accurate diagnosis for the appropriate management of acute organophosphate poisoning.

REFERENCES

1. Murray JF. Pathophysiology of respiratory failure. Respir Care 1983;28:531.
2. Murray JF. The Normal Lung: The basis for diagnosis and treatment of pulmonary disease. WB Saunders Co.: Philadelphia, 1976.

3. Murray JF. Respiration. In Smith LH, Thier SO (Eds): Pathophysiology. Tlie biological principles of disease. WB Saunders Co. Philadelphia 1981;l051.

4. Perrin C, Unterborn JN, Ambrosio CD, Hill NS. Pulmonary complications of chronic neuromuscular diseases and their management. Muscle Nerve 2004; 29:5-27.

5. Kelly BJ, Luce JM. The diagnosis and management of neuromuscular disease causing respiratory failure. Chest 1991;99:1485.

6. Macklem PT. The respiratory muscles; vital pump. Chest 1980;78:753.

7. Olshaker JS. Submersion. Emerg Med Clin North Am 2004;22:357-67.

8. Michaels AJ. Management of post traumatic respiratory failure. Crit Care Clin 2004;20:83-99.

9. Enkhbaatar P, Traber DL. Pathophysiology of acute lung injury in combined burn and smoke inhalation injury. Clin Sci (Lond). 2004;107:137-43.

10. Shneerson JM. Respiratory failure in tuberculosis: A modern perspective. Clin Med 2004;4:72-76.

11. Hudson LD. Causes of the adult respiratory distress syndrome—Clinical recognition. Clin Chest Med 1982;3:195.

12. Brun-Buisson C, Minelli C, Bertolini G, Brazzi L, Pimentel J, Lewandowski K, Bion J, Romand JA, Villar J, Thorsteinsson A, Damas P, Armaganidis A, Lemaire F, Group AS. Epidemiology and outcome of acute lung injury in European intensive care units. Results from the ALIVE study. Intensive Care Med 2004;30:524.

13. Lu Y, Song Z, Zhou X, Zhu D, Yang X, Bai C, Sun B. A 12-months clinical survey of incidence and outcome of acute respiratory distress syndrome in Shangai intensive care units. Intensive Care Med 2004. (http://dx.doi.org/10.1007/s00134-004-2479-y).

14. Gomersall CD, Joynt GM, Lam P, Li T, Yap F, Lam D, Buckley TA, Sung JJ, Hui DS, Antonio GE, Ahuja AT, Leung P. Short-term outcome of critically ill patients with severe acute respiratory syndrome. Intensive Care Med 2004;30:381-87.

15. Wedzicha JA, Donaldson GC. Exacerbations of chronic obstructive pulmonary disease. Respir Care. 2003;48:1204-13; discussion 1213-15.

16. Calverley PM. Respiratory failure in chronic obstructive pulmonary disease. Eur Respir J Suppl 2003;47:26s-30s.

17. West JB. Ventilation-perfusion inequality and overall gas exchange in computer models of lung. Respir Physiol 1969;7:88.

18. Davidson FF, Glazier JB, Murray JF. The components of the alveolar-arterial tension difference in normal subjects and in patients with pneumonia and obstructive lung disease. Am J Med 1972;52:754.

19. 32nd Annual Aspen Conference: Chronic respiratory failure. Cherniack RM (Guest Editor). Chest 1990;97 (Suppl):112S.

20. Finch CA, Lenfant C. Oxygen transport in man. N Engl J Med 1972;286:407.

21. Ward M, Macklem FT. The act of breathing and how it fails. Chest 1990;97 Suppl:36S.

22. Roussos C, Koutsoukou A. Respiratory failure. Eur Respir J 2003;22:Suppl 47,3s-14s.

23. Moxham J. Respiratory failure: Definitions and causes In Wetherall DA, Ledingham JM, Warrell D (Eds): Oxford Textbook of Medicine, Oxford, Oxford University Press 1996;2901-6.

24. Calverley PM, Brezinova V, Douglas NJ, Catterall JR, Flenley DC. The effect of oxygenation on sleep quality in chronic bronchitis and emphysema. Am Rev Respir Dis 1982;126:206-10.

25. Roussos C, Bellemare F, Moxham J. Respiratory muscle fatigue In Roussos C (Ed): The Thorax New York, NY, Marcel Dekker, 1995;1405-62.

26. Similowski T, Yan S, Gauthier AP, Macklem PT, Bellemare FM. Contractile properties of the human diaphragm during chronic hyperinflation. New Engl J Med 1991;325:917-23.

27. Scano G, Spinelli A, Duranti R, et al. Carbon dioxide responsiveness in COPD patients with and without chronic hypercapnia. Eur Respir J 1995;8:78-85.

28. Gorini M, Misuri G, Corrado A, et al. Breathing pattern and carbon dioxide retention in severe chronic obstructive pulmonary disease. Thorax 1996;51:677-83.

29. Hudson LD. Evaluation of the patient with acute respiratory failure. Respir Care 1983;28:542.

30. Cohen CA, Zagelbaum G, Gross D, Roussos C, Macklem PT. Clinical manifestations of respiratory muscle fatigue. Am J Med 1982;73:308.

31. Ashutosh K, Gilbert R, Auchicloss JH Jr, Peppi HLBI. National Conference of Oxygen Therapy. Chest 1984; 86:234.

32. Campbell EJ, Baker D, Crites D. Asynchronous breathing movements in patients with chronic obstructive disease. Chest 1975;67:553.

33. Demers RR. Oxygen delivery systems for use in acute respiratory failure. Respir Care 1983;28:553.

34. Campbell E, Baker MD, Cretes-Silver P. Subjective effects of humidification of oxygen for delivery by nasal cannula: A prospective study, Chest 1988;93:289-93.

35. Massaro D. Oxygen: Toxicity and tolerance. Hasp Pract 1986;15:95.

36. Jenkinson SG. Oxygen toxicity in acute respiratory failure. Respir Care 1983;28:614.

37. Bone RC. Treatment of respiratory failure due to advanced chronic lung disease. Arch Int Med 1980;140:1018.

38. Pierson DJ. Respiratory therapy techniques. In Kelly WN (Ed): Textbook of Internal Medicine. JB Lippincott: Philadelphia 1989;2009.

39. Schumaker GL, Epstein SK. Managing acute respiratory failure during exacerbation of chronic obstructive pulmonary disease. Respir Care 2004;49:766-82.

40. Brochard L. Mechanical ventilation: Invasive versus noninvasive. Eur Respir J 2003; 22:31S-37S.

41. Ewans TW. International Consensus Conferences in Intensive Care Medicine: Noninvasive positive pressure

ventilation in acute respiratory failure. Organised jointly by the American Thoracic Society, the European Respiratory Society, the European Society of Intensive Care Medicine, and the Societe de Reanimation de Langue Francaise, and approved by the ATS Board of Directors, December 2000. Intensive Care Med 2001;27: 166-78.

42. L Her E, Duquesne F, Girou E, de Rosiere XD, Le Conte P, Renault S, Allamy JP, Boles JM. Noninvasive continuous positive airway pressure in elderly cardiogenic pulmonary edema patients. Intensive Care Med 2004;30:882-88.

43. Squadrone E, Frigerio P, Fogliati C, Gregoretti C, Conti G, Antonelli M, Costa R, Baiardi P, Navalesi P. Noninvasive vs invasive ventilation in COPD patients with severe acute respiratory failure deemed to require ventilatory assistance. Intensive Care Med 2004;30:1303-10.

44. Keenan SP, Sinuff T, Cook DJ, Hill NS. Does noninvasive positive pressure ventilation improve outcome in acute hypoxemic respiratory failure? A systematic review. Crit Care Med 2004;32:2516-23.

45. Scala R, Bartolucci S, Naldi M, Rossi M, Elliott MW. Comorbidity and acute decompensations of COPD requiring non-invasive positive-pressure ventilation. Intensive Care Med 2004;30:1747-54.

46. Hill NS. Noninvasive ventilation for chronic obstructive pulmonary disease. Respir Care 2004;49:72-87; Discussion 87-89.

47. Ram FS, Picot J, Lightowler J, Wedzicha JA. Noninvasive positive pressure ventilation for treatment of respiratory failure due to exacerbations of chronic obstructive pulmonary disease. Cochrane Database Syst Rev 2004;(3):CD004104.

48. Hess DR. The evidence for noninvasive positive-pressure ventilation in the care of patients in acute respiratory failure: A systematic review of the literature. Respir Care 2004;49:810-29.

49. Mehta S, Hill NS. Noninvasive ventilation. Am J Respir Crit Care Med 2001;163:540-77.

50. Peter JV, Moran JL, Phillips-Hughes J, Warn D. Noninvasive ventilation in acute respiratory failure—A meta-analysis update. Crit Care Med 2002;30:555-62.

51. Lightowler JV, Wedzicha JA, Elliott MW, Ram FS. Noninvasive positive pressure ventilation to treat respiratory failure resulting from exacerbations of chronic obstructive pulmonary disease: Cochrane systematic review and meta-analysis. BMJ 2003;326:185-87.

52. Carlucci A, Richard J-C, Wysocki M, Lepage E, Brochard L, and the Société de Réanimation de Langue Française Collaborative Group on Mechanical Ventilation. Noninvasive versus conventional mechanical ventilation. An epidemiological survey. Am J Respir Crit Care Med 2001;163:874-80.

53. Nourdine K, Combes P, Carton MJ, Beuret P, Cannamela A, Ducreux JC. Does noninvasive ventilation reduce the ICU nosocomial infection risk? A prospective clinical survey. Intensive Care Med 1999;25:567-73.

54. Girou E, Schortgen F, Delclaux C, et al. Association of noninvasive ventilation with nosocomial infections and survival in critically ill patients. JAMA 2000;284:2361-67.

55. Carrey Z, Gottfried SB, Levy RD. Ventilatory muscle support in respiratory failure with nasal positive pressure ventilation. Chest 1990;97:150-58.

56. Lellouche F, Maggiore SM, Deye N, et al. Effect of the humidification device on the work of breathing during noninvasive ventilation. Intensive Care Med 2002;28:1582-89.

57. Drinker P, Shaw L. An apparatus for the prolonged administration of artificial respiration. J Clin Invest 1929;7:229.

58. Drinker P, McKhann C. The iron lung. First practical means of respiratory support. JAMA 1986;225:1476-80.

59. Corrado A, Gorini M, Ginanni R, et al. Negative pressure ventilation versus conventional mechanical ventilation in the treatment of acute respiratory failure in COPD patients. Eur Respir J 1998;12:519-25.

60. Corrado A, Confalonieri M, Marchese S, et al. Iron lung vs mask ventilation in the treatment of acute on chronic respiratory failure in COPD patients: A multicenter study. Chest 2002;121:189-95.

61. Jolliet P, Tassaux D, Thouret JM, Chevrolet JC. Beneficial effects of helium: Oxygen versus air: Oxygen noninvasive pressure support in patients with decompensated chronic obstructive pulmonary disease. Crit Care Med 1999;27:2422-29.

62. Jaber S, Fodil R, Carlucci A, et al. Noninvasive ventilation with helium-oxygen in acute exacerbations of chronic obstructive pulmonary disease. Am J Respir Crit Care Med 2000;161:1191–1200.

63. Pierson DJ. Indications for mechanical ventilation in acute respiratory failure. Respir Care 1983;28:570.

64. Hubmayer RD, Abel MD, Physiologic approach to mechanical ventilation. Crit Care Med 1990;18:103.

65. MacIntyre NR. New forms of mechanical ventilation in the adult. Clin Chest Med 1988;9:47.

66. Slutsky AS. Nonconventional methods of ventilation. Am Rev Respir Dis 1988;138:175.

67. Grum CM, Chauncey JB. Conventional mechanical ventilation. Clin Chest Med 1988;9:37.

68. Weisman IM, Rinaldo JE, Rogers RM, Sanders MH. Intermittent mandatory ventilation. Am Rev Respir Dis 1983;127:641.

69. Shapiro JM. Management of respiratory failure in status asthmaticus. Am J Respir Med 2002;1:409-16.

70. Davignon K, Kwo J, Bigatello LM. Pathophysiology and management of the flail chest. Minerva Anestesiol 2004;70:193-99.

71. Aygun D. Diagnosis in an acute organophosphate poisoning: Report of three interesting cases and review of the literature. Eur J Emerg Med 2004;11:55-58.

Chapter
18

Cor Pulmonale

DEFINITION

The definition of "cor pulmonale" varies and there is presently no consensual definition. Forty years ago an expert committee of the World Health Organization defined cor pulmonale as "enlargement (dilatation and/or hypertrophy) of the right ventricle due to increased right ventricular afterload from intrinsic pulmonary diseases including pulmonary circulation, or inadequate function of the chest bellows or inadequate ventilatory drive from the respiratory centers; when right heart abnormalities secondary to left heart failure or congenital heart disease are excluded".[1] Right heart failure need not be present, although this is a clinical manifestation of the overloaded right ventricle that precedes the clinically unrecognizable cor pulmonale. Cor pulmonale is usually chronic except in rare instances of massive pulmonary thromboembolism. This pathological definition is in fact of limited value in clinical practice. It has been proposed to replace the term "hypertrophy" by "alteration in the structure and function of the right ventricle". It has also been proposed to define clinically cor pulmonale by the presence of edema in patients with respiratory failure. Finally, as pulmonary arterial hypertension is "the sine qua non" of cor pulmonale,[2] some suggested that the best definition of cor pulmonale is—"pulmonary arterial hypertension resulting from diseases affecting the structure and/or the function of the lungs; pulmonary arterial hypertension results in right ventricular enlargement (hypertrophy and/or dilatation) and may lead with time to right heart failure".[3]

A new diagnostic classification of pulmonary hypertension was developed by a group of experts in 1998.[4] Cor pulmonale corresponds to the third part of that classification (pulmonary hypertension associated with disorders of the respiratory system and/or hypoxemia) and must be distinguished from pulmonary venous hypertension, and also from primary pulmonary hypertension, and from thromboembolic pulmonary hyper-

TABLE 18.1: New diagnostic classification of pulmonary hypertension[4]

Pulmonary hypertension associated with disorders of the respiratory system and/or hypoxemia
- Chronic obstructive pulmonary disease
- Interstitial lung disease
- Sleep disordered breathing
- Alveolar hypoventilation disorders
- Chronic exposure to high altitude
- Neonatal lung disease
- Alveolar capillary dysplasia
- Others

Pulmonary hypertension caused by chronic thrombotic and/or embolic disease
- Thromboembolic obstruction of proximal pulmonary arteries
  Obstruction of distal pulmonary arteries
  - Pulmonary embolism (thrombus, tumor, ova and/or parasites, foreign material)
  - *In situ* thrombosis
  - Sickle cell disease

Pulmonary hypertension caused by disorders directly affecting the pulmonary vasculature
- Inflammatory
  - Schistosomiasis
  - Sarcoidosis
  - Other
- Pulmonary capillary hemangiomatosis

tension, although most authors include the later as an important component (Table 18.1).

Pulmonary hypertension complicating chronic respiratory disease is generally defined by the presence of a resting mean pulmonary artery pressure (PAP) > 20 mm Hg. This is slightly different from the definition of primary pulmonary hypertension (PAP > 25 mm Hg).[4] In young (< 50 years) healthy subjects PAP is most often between 10 to 15 mm Hg. With aging there is a slight increase in PAP, by about 1 mm Hg/10 years. A resting PAP > 20 mm Hg is always abnormal. In the "natural history" of COPD, pulmonary hypertension is often preceded by an abnormally large increase in PAP during exercise, defined by a pressure > 30 mm Hg for a mild level of steady state exercise. The term "exercising" pulmonary hypertension has been used by some authors, but the term "pulmonary hypertension" should be reserved for resting pulmonary hypertension.

Incidence and Prevalence

The incidence and prevalence of cor pulmonale is difficult to establish because not all cases can be adequately diagnosed clinically during life. It is estimated that about 5 to 10 percent of all organic heart diseases are due to cor pulmonale. Cor pulmonale is a common type of heart disease, as a result of its close association with COPD which has emerged in recent years as a leading cause of disability and death.[5] But there are in fact very few data about the incidence and prevalence of cor pulmonale. The main reason is that right heart catheterization cannot be performed on a large scale in patients at risk. An alternative approach is the use of non-invasive methods, particularly Doppler echocardiography. It should be possible to investigate large groups of respiratory patients with echo Doppler within the next few years. A UK study performed in Sheffield[6] has tried to determine the prevalence of patients at risk of developing pulmonary hypertension and cor pulmonale—that is, patients with hypoxemic lung disease. In the study population, aged 45 years, an estimated 0.3 percent had both an arterial oxygen tension (PaO_2) < 7.3 kPa (55 mm Hg) and a forced expiratory volume in one second (FEV_1) < 50 percent of the predicted value. For England and Wales this could represent 60,000 subjects at risk of pulmonary hypertension and eligible for long-term oxygen therapy. In an autopsy study from UK, it was reported that 40 percent of patients with chronic bronchitis and emphysema had anatomic evidence of cor pulmonale. Chronic cor pulmonale occurs more commonly in male smokers, between the ages of 50 to 60 years of age. The incidence in women is increasing, because of increased smoking by them. In developing countries, cor pulmonale in nonsmoking women is reported to be due to exposure to domestic cooking fuels. The mortality related to cor pulmonale is also difficult to assess. There are data about the mortality resulting from chronic lung disease[5,7] but the precise role of secondary pulmonary hypertension in this mortality. Pulmonary hypertension is a complication, among others, of advanced COPD and it is not possible to separate it from its causative diseases.

ETIOLOGY

The possible causes of cor pulmonale have been shown in Table 18.2.[3,8-27] Of these, the most important cause is the chronic obstructive pulmonary disease.

TABLE 18.2: Common etiologies of cor pulmonale

I. Chronic cor pulmonale
   (a) *Hypoxic vasoconstriction*
       Chronic bronchitis and emphysema
       Cystic fibrosis
       Bronchiolitis obliterans
       Irreversible phase of bronchial asthma
       Hypoventilation
       Obesity
       Sleep apnea syndrome
       Obesity–hypoventilation syndrome (formerly "Pickwickian syndrome")
       Respiratory muscle diseases
       Chest wall abnormalities
       High altitude dwellers
       Neuromuscular diseases: (amyotrophic lateral sclerosis, myopathy, bilateral diaphragmatic paralysis, etc.)
       Kyphoscoliosis
       Thoracoplasty
   (b) *Pulmonary vascular diseases*
       Pulmonary thromboembolism
       Embolism by parasitic ova (Schistosomiasis), tumor
       Primary pulmonary hypertension
       Intrinsic pulmonary venous disease (veno-occlusive disease)
       Pulmonary vasculitis due to systemic diseases (collagen vascular diseases)
       Drugs and chemicals (crotalaria, aminorex or fenfluramine)
   (c) *Diminished vascular cross-sectional area*
       Emphysema
       Bronchiectasis
       Cystic fibrosis
       Sequelae of pulmonary tuberculosis
       Sarcoidosis
       Interstitial fibrosis
       Pneumoconiosis
       Drug related lung diseases
       Extrinsic allergic alveolitis
       Connective tissue diseases
II. Acute cor pulmonale
    Massive pulmonary thromboembolism
    Infections causing acute exacerbation of cor pulmonale due to COPD
III. Reversible cor pulmonale
     Upper airways obstruction
     (Adenoids, polyps, papillomas, foreign body)
IV. Cor pulmonale in children
    Congenital diaphragmatic hernia
    Chronic lung disease of prematurity
    Pneumonitis
    Reactive airway disease
    Cystic fibrosis

COPD is the major cause of chronic respiratory insufficiency and cor pulmonale, and it probably accounts for 80 to 90 percent of the cases. COPD includes chronic obstructive bronchitis and emphysema which are often associated. Among the restrictive lung diseases kyphoscoliosis, idiopathic pulmonary fibrosis, and pneumoconiosis are the main causes of cor pulmonale. Among the etiologies of respiratory insufficiency of "central" origin the obesity–hypoventilation syndrome (formerly "Pickwickian syndrome") is a relatively frequent cause of cor pulmonale. Cor pulmonale in children is most often due to congenital diaphragmatic hernia, chronic lung disease of prematurity, pneumonitis, reactive airway disease, or cystic fibrosis.[17]

PATHOGENESIS

The underlying basic pathophysiology of cor pulmonale due to all the causes is an increase in the pulmonary vascular resistance and pulmonary hypertension. Mechanisms causing these changes include hypoxia (most important factor), acidosis with hypercapnia, occlusion or destruction of vascular bed with diminished cross-sectional area of the pulmonary circulation, and increased blood viscosity due to polycythemia.[27-44]

The factors leading to an increased PVR in chronic respiratory disease are numerous but alveolar hypoxia is by far the most predominant[2] at least in COPD, kyphoscoliosis, and the obesity–hypoventilation syndrome. Two distinct mechanisms of action of alveolar hypoxia must be considered: acute hypoxia causes pulmonary vasoconstriction, and chronic long-standing hypoxia induces structural changes in the pulmonary vascular bed (pulmonary vascular remodelling).

Hypoxic pulmonary vasoconstriction (HPV) has been known since the studies in 1946 of Von Euler and Liljestrand on the cat. HPV explains the rise of PVR and PAP observed in humans, and in almost all species of mammals, during acute hypoxia. This vasoconstriction is localized in the small precapillary arteries. Its precise mechanism is not fully understood. The clinical situations which bear the closest analogy with acute hypoxic challenges are probably exacerbations of COPD leading to acute respiratory failure, and the sleep related episodes of worsening hypoxemia.[3]

Pulmonary hypertension is generally observed in respiratory patients exhibiting pronounced chronic hypoxemia (PaO_2 < 55-60 mm Hg). It is accepted that chronic alveolar hypoxia leads to remodelling of the pulmonary vascular bed (hypertrophy of the muscular media of the small pulmonary arteries, muscularization of pulmonary arterioles, and intimal fibrosis) comparable to that observed in natives living at high altitude. This remodelling leads to elevation of PVR and to pulmonary hypertension. In fact the remodelling of the pulmonary vessels may be observed early in nonhypoxemic COPD patients with mild disease severity.

Furthermore, other functional factors must be considered, namely hypercapnic acidosis and hyperviscosity caused by polycythemia, but their role seems small when compared to that of alveolar hypoxia. In idiopathic pulmonary fibrosis the increase of PVR is caused by anatomical factors: loss of pulmonary vascular bed or compression of arterioles and capillaries by the fibrosing process.

Pulmonary hypertension increases the work of the right ventricle, which leads more or less rapidly to right ventricular enlargement (associating hypertrophy and dilatation) which can result in ventricular dysfunction (systolic, diastolic). Later, right heart failure (RHF) characterized by the presence of peripheral edema can be observed, at least in some respiratory patients. The interval between the onset of pulmonary hypertension and the appearance of RHF is not known and may vary from one patient to another. There is a relation between the severity of pulmonary hypertension and the development of RHF.

Humans encounter hypoxia throughout their lives. This occurs by destiny in utero, through disease, and by desire, in their quest for altitude. Hypoxic pulmonary vasoconstriction (HPV) is a widely conserved, homeostatic, vasomotor response of resistance pulmonary arteries to alveolar hypoxia. HPV mediates ventilation-perfusion matching and, by reducing shunt fraction, optimizes systemic PO_2. HPV is intrinsic to the lung, and, although modulated by the endothelium, the core mechanism is in the smooth muscle cell (SMC). The Redox Theory for the mechanism of HPV proposes the coordinated action of a redox sensor (the proximal mitochondrial electron transport chain) that generates a diffusible mediator [a reactive O_2 species (ROS)] that regulates an effector protein [voltage-gated potassium (K(v) and calcium channels]. A similar mechanism for regulating O_2 uptake/distribution is partially recapitulated in simpler organisms and in the other specialized mammalian O_2-sensitive tissues, including the carotid body and ductus arteriosus. Inhibition of O_2-sensitive K(v) channels, particularly K(v) 1.5 and K(v) 2.1, depolarizes pulmonary artery SMCs, activating voltage-gated Ca^{2+} channels and causing Ca^{2+} influx and vasoconstriction. Downstream of this pathway, there is important regulation of the contractile apparatus' sensitivity to calcium by rho kinase. Controversy remains as to whether hypoxia decreases or increases ROS and which electron transport chain complex generates the ROS (I and/or III). Possible roles for cyclic adenosine diphosphate ribose and an unidentified endothelial constricting factor are also proposed by some groups. Modulation of HPV has therapeutic relevance to cor pulmonale, high-altitude pulmonary edema, and sleep apnea. HPV is clinically exploited in single-lung anesthesia, and its mechanisms intersect with those of pulmonary arterial hypertension.[30]

Pulmonary artery adventitial fibroblasts (FBPA) may play a central role in lung vascular remodeling under conditions of hypoxia and inflammation, the result being pulmonary hypertension and cor pulmonale. In cultured human FBPA, both angiotensin II (Ang II) and hypoxia promoted cell cycle progression and cell proliferation and suppressed apoptosis. These effects were further enhanced when both stimuli were applied simultaneously. Hypoxia elevated the expression of hypoxia-inducible factor 1 alpha (HIF-1alpha) and increased the expression of genes regulated by the hypoxia-responsive element (HRE). Up-regulation of both angiotensin-converting enzyme (ACE) and Ang II receptor type 1 (AT1) was also observed. Exogenous Ang II further increased HIF/HRE-dependent signaling in FBPA, whereas suppression of the autocrine ACE-Ang II-AT1 loop with inhibitors of ACE, AT1, and phosphatidy-linositol 3-kinase (PI3K) reduced the proliferative response to both hypoxia and exogenous Ang II. Overexpression of HIF-1alpha by transient transfection caused the same proliferative effect and up-regulation of AT1 expression that were observed under hypoxic conditions. In contrast, small interfering RNA targeting HIF-1alpha inhibited hypoxia-induced ACE and AT1 expression. Studies indicate that the ACE-Ang II-AT1 system serves as a positive feedback loop and fosters FBPA proliferation under hypoxic conditions, with the PI3K-HIF-HRE axis as the central effector pathway. This pathway may thus facilitate vascular remodeling under hypoxic conditions.[31]

The recent observation of an increase during hypertrophy and a decrease in failure may suggest a role of oxidative stress in the pathogenesis of right ventricular dysfunction.[39]

The pulmonary circulation is interposed on the blood return to the left ventricle and is such an efficient, low resistance system that the right ventricle is hardly necessary under normal circumstances. Blood is propelled by a milking movement as the ventricle moves from a high compliance diastolic pressure volume slope to a low compliance systolic slope. Physiologically, flow through the pulmonary circulation (right ventricular function) depends largely on the left ventricle and the breathing movements. Thus, an increase in the force of left ventricular contraction causes, through the common ventricular septum, an augmented right ventricular ejection; left atrial pressure is reduced and facilitates pulmonary blood flow; systemic venous pressure rises with rising inflow to aid venous return; ventricular interdependence in the cardiac fossa results in lowered

right ventricular pressure and improved venous return as the left heart shrinks. Respiratory movements facilitate pulmonary blood flow by aspirating blood into the thorax on inspiration and then propelling it forward by the positive pressure of exhalation acting on a valve system. While volume overloads are well tolerated, the pressure loads not. The load that causes the right ventricular changes of cor pulmonale is not understood, but pulmonary hypertension, external pressure, and geometrical changes in the cardiac fossa possibly contribute to this.[9,10]

The mechanisms by which patients with COPD retain salt and water are not completely understood. Several abnormalities have been found including reduced renal blood flow with relatively preserved glomerular filtration rate and elevated levels of renin, aldosterone, arginine vasopressin and atrial natriuretic peptide. Generally, these abnormalities worsen with the severity of COPD and are most marked during the edematous phases. Cardiac output is remarkably normal, suggesting that "cor pulmonale" is not primarily a cardiac disorder but rather a condition of volume overload due to activation of sodium-retaining mechanisms. The stimulus for this activation could be underfilling of the arterial system (reduced effective circulating volume) secondary to a fall in total peripheral vascular resistance. The latter is caused by hypercapnia-induced dilation of the precapillary sphincters. Apparently, the massive sodium retention by the kidney is not able to restore the circulating volume and a vicious cycle ensues ultimately leading to a clinical picture which resembles right-sided heart failure. Predictably, only blockade of the effects of carbon dioxide at the level of the precapillary sphincters would be able to halt this process.[44]

The normal pulmonary circulation is low in resistance and highly distensible. This low-pressure, low-resistance, circulation transmits the entire cardiac output without much change in pressure because the pulmonary arteries are thin-walled with little resting muscular tone, there is negligible response in terms of capacity, distensibility, or resistance to flow to autonomic nervous stimulation in the adult (vasomotor control), and many small arterioles and capillaries are nonperfused at rest, but can be recruited when needed to expand the pulmonary vascular bed causing a decrease in pulmonary vascular resistance, and there is no humoral counterpart of the renin-angiotensin system that is capable of evoking sustained pulmonary hypertension.

Normal mean pulmonary artery pressure is 13 ± 4 mm Hg in a young adult and less than 18 mm Hg in 80 percent of subjects of all ages. Pulmonary artery pressure of greater than 20 mm Hg signifies pulmonary hypertension as stated above. Blood flow through the pulmonary capillaries is achieved by a pressure drop of only 5 to 9 mm Hg (pulmonary artery to left atrial pressure) compared to 90 mm Hg for the systemic circuit. Accordingly, the normal pulmonary vascular resistance is 10 to 20 times less than systemic vascular resistance.

Pulmonary Hypertension

As stated above pulmonary hypertension is the "sine qua non" of cor pulmonale. Accordingly, the mechanisms of cor pulmonale are first those of pulmonary hypertension. In chronic respiratory diseases pulmonary hypertension results from increased pulmonary vascular resistance (PVR) whereas cardiac output and pulmonary "capillary" wedge pressure are normal; pulmonary hypertension is said to be precapillary.

It is generally agreed that the decrease in extent of the pulmonary vascular bed is generally insufficient to play a predominant role in the pathogenesis of pulmonary hypertension unless the reduction is extreme. The effective cross-sectional area of the pulmonary vascular bed must be reduced by more than 50 percent before any change in pulmonary artery pressure can be detected at rest, although exercise will increase the pressure at lower levels of increased blood flow. Experiments in dogs have shown that more than two-thirds of the lungs had to be ablated before pulmonary artery pressures approach hypertensive levels. Obliterative vascular diseases increases pulmonary vascular resistance by vascular occlusion, while diffuse interstitial and parenchymal diseases act primarily by compressing and obliterating small vessels. However, arteriolar constriction is the predominant cause of pulmonary hypertension.

Hypoxia

The most common cause of pulmonary arteriolar constriction is alveolar hypoxia. Although the mechanism is not clear, it is believed that this is accomplished by (i) mediator release such as histamine from the mast cells in the pulmonary parenchyma, and (ii) a direct effect of hypoxia on pulmonary arterial smooth muscle. Other influences may enhance hypoxic vasoconstrictor like extrapulmonary reflexes operating by way of systemic arterial chemoreceptors. Nonetheless, intrapulmonary local effects of hypoxia generally predominate. The degree of hypoxic vasoconstriction primarily depends upon the alveolar oxygen tension. When the PAO_2 is about 55 mm Hg, pulmonary artery pressure rises sharply. When the pulmonary artery pressure is more than 40 mm Hg, arterial saturation is most likely less than 75 percent. There is great individual variation in the hypoxic pressure response. A usual sequel of hypoxia is the hypertrophy of pulmonary arterial smooth muscle which extends further towards the alveoli. It seems that these hypertrophied muscles are hyperactive. This hyperreactivity also shows individual and species variation, suggesting that there is also a genetic predisposition for this. Hypoxic vasoconstriction in regions of lung with poor ventilation diverts blood from the hypoxic region to the better ventilated areas in an attempt to maximize net arterial oxygenation. Moreover, the phenomenon of "recruitment", prevents further pulmonary hypertension due to localized hypoxia. Generalized hypoxia causes generalized hypoxic vasoconstriction and the development of pulmonary hypertension.

The hypoxic vasoconstriction is enhanced by acidosis and blunted by alkalosis. In addition, acidosis has a direct pressure effect on the pulmonary circulation. Increased PCO_2 in blood seems to exert no direct molecular effect, but operates by way of increasing the hydrogen ion concentration which it induces. Hypercapnia plays an extracirculatory role in cor pulmonale by dilating cerebral vessels, causing disturbances in central nervous system, and if extreme, depresses the ventilation. Other side effects are due to increased sympathetic activity. Heart failure due to cor pulmonale is invariably associated with carbon dioxide retention even with interstitial fibrosis.

Other Factors

As mentioned, reduction of cross-sectional area *per se* may not be important for the causation of pulmonary hypertension itself unless extreme. However, with any condition of increased cardiac output, heart rate, blood volume, or direct effects of acidosis and/or hypoxia on the myocardium may contribute to pulmonary hypertension. Increased blood flow during exercise will generate high pulmonary artery pressure and the effects of hypoxia and acidosis will be exaggerated. Chronic hypoxia results in secondary polycythemia with increased viscosity which is increased rapidly after the hematocrit value exceeds 55 percent, further raising pulmonary vascular resistance and also decreasing cerebral function. If left ventricular dysfunction/failure is superimposed on an already compromised vascular bed, the pressure in the pulmonary artery will rise further. Once established, pulmonary hypertension becomes self perpetuating.

Certain pulmonary arterial diseases are more effective in eliciting pulmonary hypertension in man. One such group in which the lung interstitium is involved includes scleroderma, sarcoidosis, fibrosing alveolitis, pulmonary arteritis, lymphangitis carcinomatosis, and obliterative pulmonary vascular disease, typified by multiple pulmonary emboli to the lungs. Much more uncommon are the obliterative vascular diseases such as primary pulmonary hypertension and pulmonary arteritis. In these obliterative disorders, pulmonary arterial hypertension may reach or surpass systemic blood pressure levels while left atrial pressure and cardiac output remain at normal or low levels. Veno-occlusive disease is a rare disease of the veins which presents with pulmonary hypertension and pulmonary edema. Sickle cell disease can cause cor pulmonale due to multiple episodes of pulmonary infarctions from local pulmonary sickling or from thromboembolism. Rarely, cirrhosis of the liver is associated with pulmonary hypertension although it is commonly associated with pulmonary vasodilatation.

Episodic hypoxia is associated with sleep apnea syndrome and COPD, which may also lead to cor pulmonale. Like the fall in oxygen saturation during sleep apnea, the rise in pulmonary artery pressure is precipitous when the airway is obstructed; when it is open fresh air is drawn in as oxygen saturation is raised and the change is less dramatic.

The lung volume changes in respiratory diseases may have an important effect in further increasing pulmonary hypertension. When lung volume increases, there is lengthening and narrowing of the alveolar vessels, which are exposed to the alveolar pressures. These vessels are compressed because the alveolar pressure rises more than the intrapleural pressure around the heart. Vascular resistance also rises when regional volumes decrease below normal FRC due to narrowing of extra-alveolar vessels similar to the way the small airways narrow as the outward tension of the lung structures diminishes. Since most disease causing lung volume changes also cause hypoxia, individual effects on the pulmonary circulation becomes difficult to establish. Positive end expiratory pressure (PEEP) is known to cause right ventricular insufficiency. In hyperinflated obstructive lung diseases a condition like "auto-PEEP" is created which may further compromise right heart function.

The raised mean pulmonary arterial pressure is not the only factor causing cor pulmonale and right heart failure in patients with COPD or restrictive lung disease. This is observed from people living in high altitudes with chronic hypoxia who have high pulmonary artery pressure, but without right heart failure. Similarly many patients with congenital heart disease, but no pulmonary heart disease can sustain very high pulmonary pressures without failure. It seems, therefore, some other factors

other than pulmonary hypertension, could be raising right ventricular afterload. It is likely that external impedance to right ventricular function may be present in the cardiac fossa. Right heart enlargement relative to the size of the fossa is opposed by the tensing of the pleural surfaces when lung volumes are increased. This may be the dynamic stresses during the beating of the right ventricle. There may also be locally higher static pressures and thus, a reduction in the pressure gradient for venous return. It is important that enlargement of the lower lobes, which form the cardiac fossa, is an early response to COPD. This could explain the right ventricular failure during times of exacerbated airflow obstruction. However, there are some observations which may not explain this phenomenon.

Other pathogenetic mechanisms suggested for the right heart failure are hypoxic myocardial damage, and raised cardiac output associated with chronic hypoxia.

Hemodynamic Consequences of Cor Pulmonale

The hemodynamic changes in cor pulmonale depend on the cause and duration of the lung disease. In patients with multiple pulmonary embolism and primary pulmonary hypertension, pulmonary artery pressures are more likely to reach systemic levels than that due to COPD. Patients with diffuse interstitial lung disease tend to have moderate levels of pulmonary arterial pressures until late in the course of the disease with ventilation-perfusion abnormality when the levels may reach 60 to 80 mm Hg.

The cardiac output is normal at rest except late in the course of the disease, when it is low. In cor pulmonale associated with hypoxia, the cardiac output is at the upper limit of normal or supranormal. Recovery from heart failure brings back the cardiac output towards normal. Exercise increases the cardiac output. The left atrial pressure is almost consistently normal in cor pulmonale except in association with left heart failure or an increase in circulating lung volume.

The thin walled right ventricle is better able to handle an increase in volume load than to meet an increased pressure load. Thus, a chronic pressure load (after load) due to pulmonary artery hypertension is the primary cause of right ventricular failure. Small increases in pulmonary artery pressure may result in large increases in right ventricular work. Pulmonary hypertension at rest indicates advanced disease. Response of the right ventricle to pulmonary hypertension depends on the acuteness and severity of the pressure load. Acute cor pulmonale is manifested with ventricular dilatation and failure without hypertrophy. Chronic cor pulmonale, on the other hand, is associated with a more slowly progressive hypertrophic response. Like left heart failure, failure of the right heart is associated with an expanded circulating blood volume; but in contrast to left ventricular failure, in which the pulmonary blood volume may comprise a disproportionately large fraction of the total blood volume, the fraction is approximately 10 percent of the total as in normal. Increased blood cell mass may not present, particularly if chronic infection or malnutrition complicate the underlying pulmonary disease.[41-44]

Different stages of the sequence of events from pulmonary hypertension to right heart failure are characterized by particular hemodynamic features and are as follows:

1. Before the stage of cor pulmonale, the cardiac output is normal at rest and increases normally during exercise. The right ventricular end-diastolic pressures remain normal all throughout. Pulmonary hypertension may vary according to the cardiac output and level of hypoxemia.

2. The stage of cor pulmonale, is characterized by high filling pressures. Pulmonary arterial pressure may increase considerably or remains unchanged, depending on the level of cardiac output and degree of hypoxia.

3. During the stage of right ventricular failure, the end-diastolic pressure is abnormally high, and the cardiac output, which may be normal at rest, fails to increase normally during exercise. Systemic venous congestion becomes manifest and, the circulating plasma volume increases like other types of heart failure. Both circulating plasma volume and lung water decreases as the failure improves.

Left Ventricle in Cor Pulmonale

Left ventricular failure is detrimental to the existing cor pulmonale. It increases pulmonary blood volume and promotes the accumulation of extravascular water; pulmonary compliance is reduced and airway resistance is increased. These changes increase the work of breathing and disturb the gas exchange. Although experimental data suggest that hypertrophy and failure of the right ventricle can lead to disorders in left ventricular performance, their relevance to human situations has not been fully established. Most observers have failed to find evidence of abnormal left ventricular function in cor pulmonale. Whenever it is found, some other cause needs be sought. In elderly people, some independent disease of the left ventricle is the likely cause. Although some explain that the enlarged right ventricle compromises left ventricular performance due to the hypertrophied interventricular septum, the view is taken with some skepticism. Other explanations given for the dysfunction is the wide swings in transpulmonary pressure in obstructive lung disease, which can reduce left ventricular filling and increase left ventricular afterload. It seems that cor pulmonale is not etiologically related to left ventricular dysfunction.[45-49] The left heart may be involved due to the basic underlying cause of cor pulmonale like sarcoidosis, and in elderly persons hypertension and arteriosclerosis are often the underlying etiologies. However, when the left ventricle is already dysfunctional, further derangement can be possible by the direct effect of hypoxia and acidosis on the myocardium. On the other hand, in patients with cor pulmonale due to advanced lung disease, left ventricular failure may precipitate a life-threatening crisis.

PATHOLOGY

The media of the muscular pulmonary arteries is usually normal or atrophic.[50] The outstanding changes observed in hypoxic cor pulmonale include musculoelastic proliferation of the intima of muscular arteries due to active deposition of longitudinal muscle, fibrosis, and elastosis. These changes extend distally to arterioles. In the larger vessels, the new muscle is longitudinal. In arterioles, it is circular but sometimes, in addition, there is longitudinal muscle. In these arterioles, a medial coat of circular smooth muscle bounded by a new internal elastic lamina usually develops, while there is deposition of longitudinal muscle and fibrosis in the intima. Development of multiple tubes in the lumen of arterioles is extensive in a number of these cases. These features are distinctive of hypoxemia and obstructive airway disease. Changes continue till death. The conspicuous longitudinal muscle may be attributable to stretching of vessels around the distorted terminal airways. Usually there is no correlation between quantitative pathological findings and arterial blood gas tensions, pulmonary artery pressure or hematocrit. These changes are clearly different from those found in pure hypoxia as in natives of high altitude. In the latter, in the muscular pulmonary arteries (80-500 μm in diameter), there is little or no hypertrophy of the medial coat and in the intima very occasional bands of longitudinal muscles have been observed. The predominant changes are in the peripheral portions of the arterial tree. There is muscularization of arterioles (less than 80 μm). In cor pulmonale due to hypoxia and obstructive lung disease, the predominant changes are in the intima.

CLINICAL FEATURES

The diagnosis of cor pulmonale is not often made until significant right ventricular hypertrophy or overt right ventricular failure is present. Cor pulmonale should be considered in any patient with pulmonary hypertension and particularly so, with chronic hypoxemia. The symptoms are mainly those of the progression of the underlying disorder. Heart failure occurs insidiously, causing further impairment of lung function and frequently misinterpreted as worsening of the underlying lung disease. Episodes of leg edema, atypical chest pain, exertional dyspnea, exercised-induced cyanosis in the periphery, prior respiratory failure, and excessive daytime sleepiness are nonspecific but important historical clues suggesting the possibility of cor pulmonale.

Some predisposing conditions are more likely to be recognized easily than others. Diffuse pulmonary lesions are easily recognized than are disturbances that cause alveolar hypoventilation. COPD may be overlooked for years. It is not uncommon for an elderly patient to be admitted for evidence of heart failure attributable to arteriosclerotic heart disease until the blood gas shows hypoxia with hypercapnia with pulmonary hypertension and cor pulmonale.

General physical examination will reveal distended neck veins, peripheral edema, and cyanosis. Edema in cor pulmonale may not necessarily be due to overt heart failure. The other mechanisms of edema are hypoxia, hypercarbia, and increased systemic venous pressure. Primary pulmonary hypertension *per se* does not cause edema, although the total body water is increased. However, if the pulmonary artery pressure is excessively high, as in primary pulmonary hypertension, edema formation can occur. Decreased clearance of aldosterone from the passively congested liver contributes to salt retention. Hypercarbia stimulates plasma renin activity and increases the plasma aldosterone and antidiuretic hormone levels. Hypoxia, when severe (PaO_2 between 30-45 mm Hg), decreases urine formation by affecting the kidneys. Other mechanisms of edema formation are increased systemic capillary hydrostatic pressure due to increased systemic venous pressure and blood volume, and due to a direct effect of hypoxia on peripheral tissue.

Signs and symptoms suggestive of heart failure like dyspnea, orthopnea, edema, hepatomegaly, and raised jugular venous pressure (JVP) can also occur due to COPD without right heart failure. However, the raised JVP is present in both phases of respiration in right heart failure, whereas it is observed during inspiration only in COPD. The hepatomegaly is tender in heart failure and nontender in COPD.

The apical impulse and the right ventricular lift are often not palpable. The second heart sound may be palpated in the pulmonary area. The earliest sign of pulmonary hypertension is an accentuated pulmonic component of the second heart sound. A right ventricular S_3 gallop is heard in the epigastrium along the sternum. Other heart sounds are best heard in the epigastrium. With advanced pulmonary hypertension, characteristic diastolic (pulmonary valvular insufficiency) and pansystolic (tricuspid insufficiency, increases during inspiration) murmurs are heard along with a systolic ejection sound. Right ventricular failure is usually precipitated by some acute episode like pneumonia.

Associated clinical features of the underlying basic disease with those of hypoxemia and hypercarbia and polycythemia will be present.

Cor pulmonale due to restricted vascular bed and occlusive vascular diseases including primary pulmonary hypertension is manifested by strikingly high pulmonary arterial pressure associated with a low cardiac output. Mild hypoxemia is the rule. Tachypnoea, which persists even during sleep is the rule, particularly with multiple pulmonary emboli. Chest pain is common. Enlargement of right ventricle in its pure form is manifested in these disorders. Prominent "a" and "v" waves appear in the JVP. Other features described above are typically heard without any modification because there is no underlying COPD.

The clinical signs of cor pulmonale are relatively insensitive[51] and some of them (signs related to an increased jugular venous pressure) are often obscured by hyperinflation of the chest[52] which is present in a number of COPD patients. Furthermore, the clinical signs occur late, being observed at an advanced stage of the disease far after the development of pulmonary hypertension. Peripheral (ankle) edema is the best sign of right heart failure but it is not specific and can arise from other causes; in some patients with pulmonary hypertension, it does not occur at all. A murmur of tricuspid regurgitation, suggesting right ventricular dilatation, is a very late sign in respiratory patients. Accentuation of the pulmonary component of the second heart sound is only observed in patients with severe pulmonary hypertension.

Radiology

The chest radiograms are not sensitive indicators of enlargement of the right ventricle. Detection may be difficult in the vertical heart of emphysema. The classic evidence of radiographic evidence of right ventricular enlargement will be evident (crossing the right vertebral border) in pulmonary emboli, scleroderma, etc. where hyperinflation of the lungs does not coexist. However, existence of pulmonary hypertension will be obvious in the film. This is manifested by enlargement of the outflow tract of the right ventricle, the main pulmonary arteries, and their central branches, in association with attenuated peripheral branches of the pulmonary arterial tree. Enlargement of the pulmonary artery is considered to exist when the diameter of the right descending pulmonary artery is greater than 16 mm and the left descending pulmonary artery is greater than 18 mm, although the true sensitivity and specificity of these measurements are not known.

Associated features of underlying lung disease will be evident with any precipitating cause like pneumonia. In pure hyperventilation syndrome, the lungs may be normal.[52,53]

In acute cor pulmonale, particularly due to massive pulmonary thromboembolism, CT scan is an important diagnostic clue.[54,55]

Electrocardiogram

The diagnostic value of electrocardiogram (ECG) in cor pulmonale depends upon the underlying pulmonary or ventilatory disorder, levels of pulmonary artery pressure, pulmonary vascular resistance, rotation and displacement of the heart by hyperinflated lungs, arterial PO_2, myocardial ischaemia, and associated electrolyte imbalances. It is quite reliable, if pulmonary hypertension is due to pulmonary vascular or interstitial lung diseases rather than when COPD is present. These features may also be seen in patients with alveolar hypoventilation with normal lungs,[3,56-58] but the changes are not that striking because the level of pulmonary hypertension is not generally high. The "suggestive" indices of pulmonary hypertension (right ventricular enlargement) include: p-pulmonale in leads II, III, AVF, S,Q_3, or $S_r S_2$-S_3 patterns, right axis deviation, R:S ratios in V_6 of 1.0, rSR' pattern in the right precordial leads, and partial or complete right bundle branch block. Dominant R or R' in lead V_i or V_3R in association with inverted T waves in the right precordial leads in combination with "suggestive" criteria, are more definite indices.

Because of the hyperinflated lungs and episodic elevation of the pulmonary artery pressure in COPD, characteristic patterns of right ventricular hypertrophy are uncommon. This is because of rotation and displacement of heart, and widened distance between the electrodes and the cardiac surface. P-pulmonale reflects more of the effects of hyperinflation on the position of heart than of the effect of pulmonary hypertension on the right ventricle. Presence of distinct right ventricular enlargement in the presence of COPD indicates a severe degree of cardiomegaly. Because of these difficulties, only about 1/3rd of the patients with COPD show ECG evidence of right ventricular hypertrophy during life in autopsy proved cases of cor pulmonale.

The ECG patterns may also change according to the degree of hypoxia. As the PaO_2 decreases to below 70 mm Hg, changes in T wave, mean electrical axis and S-T segments occur, which reverse back to normal as the oxygenation improves. The traditional changes of right ventricular hypertrophy occur late in the course of COPD. When classic changes are absent, diagnosis is based on the combination of rS in V_s to V_6; right axis deviation, qR in aVR; and "p pulmonale". Arrhythmias are not frequent in uncomplicated cor pulmonale. When present, they are mostly supraventricular and transient. Hypoxemia, hypokalemia, digitalis, theophylline, or beta agonists may predispose to arrhythmias. The usual types are atrial tachycardia, nodal rhythm, and wandering pace makers. Much less common are atrial flutters and fibrillations. Ventricular arrhythmias are rare and are associated with high mortality.

The detection of right ventricular hypertrophy by electrocardiography has a high specificity but a very low sensitivity. A normal ECG does not exclude the presence of pulmonary hypertension, particularly in COPD patients. Similarly, the radiological signs of pulmonary hypertension (increased width of the right descending pulmonary artery) are poorly sensitive and the radiological appearance of a dilated right ventricle is a very late (and inconsistent) sign.

Other Investigations

Echocardiogram and ultrasound examination are not sensitive enough to determine the right ventricular size. Quantitative first pass radionuclide angiocardiography and Thallium 201 myocardial imaging are helpful in the noninvasive evaluation of right ventricular function and myocardial thickness respectively. Right sided heart catheterization is helpful in directly measuring the pulmonary artery pressure and pulmonary artery wedge pressure. It helps in differentiating cor pulmonale from left ventricular failure. In the former, the pulmonary artery diastolic pressure is significantly higher than wedge pressure, whereas in the latter the difference is smaller. Measurement of pulmonary artery pressure at rest and exercise is possible with this technique.

The noninvasive diagnosis of pulmonary hypertension is presently based on echocardiography. Continuous wave Doppler echocardiography allows the calculation of the transtricuspid pressure gradient from the peak velocity of the tricuspid regurgitant jet, by applying the Bernouilli equation. Assuming a right atrial pressure of 5 mm Hg, it is thus possible to calculate right ventricular systolic pressure (right atrial pressure + transtricuspid pressure gradient) which is identical to pulmonary artery systolic pressure. It is also possible to estimate the diastolic pulmonary artery pressure by summing the right atrial pressure and the end diastolic pressure gradient between the pulmonary artery and the right ventricle. Pulsed wave Doppler echocardiography, also based on the measurement of flow velocity, allows an indirect estimation of pulmonary artery systolic pressure. However, hyperinflation makes echocardiography difficult in many COPD patients and a reliable examination cannot be obtained in more than 60 to 80 percent of the cases. The good correlations that have been observed in cardiac patients between PAP estimated from echo data and pressures measured invasively have not always been confirmed in COPD patients[7] and a mean error of the estimate, for PAP, of about 10 mm Hg has been reported.[59,60]

Two dimensional echocardiography is used to measure right ventricular dimensions and the right ventricular wall thickness, making it possible to assess the presence of right ventricular hypertrophy and/or dilatation. However, magnetic resonance imaging (MRI) is probably the best method for measuring right ventricular dimensions because it produces the best images of the right ventricle. In COPD patients good correlations have been noted between right ventricular free wall volume measured by MRI and PAP. MRI is also a good method for detecting changes in right ventricular function, but it is expensive and available only in specialized centers.

Radionuclide ventriculography allows the measurement of right ventricular ejection fraction (RVEF). An RVEF < 40 to 45 percent is considered abnormal, but RVEF is not a good index of right ventricular function; it gives only an estimate of the systolic function and is afterload dependent, decreasing when PAP and PVR increase.[61] Accordingly, the decreased RVEF observed in many COPD patients is caused primarily by increased afterload conditions and is not an indicator of "true" right ventricular dysfunction.

MANAGEMENT

Reduction of pulmonary hypertension is the primary goal of therapy. The approach varies with the cause and the state of the disease. Since hypoxia is the main underlying disturbance, correction of this abnormality is of primary importance. However, little improvement is expected when anatomic lesions, such as healed multiple emboli or destruction of the pulmonary vascular bed are the causes of pulmonary hypertension. The principles and methods of oxygen administration are discussed earlier. In COPD, low-flow oxygen relieves the hypoxemic effects with prompt decrease in pulmonary pressure. Continued oxygen therapy for weeks to months brings about a gradual decline, presumably by reducing the pulmonary vascular smooth muscle hypertrophy. Patients of restrictive lung diseases may get some benefit from oxygen therapy.

Diuretics are important adjuncts in managing cor pulmonale in heart failure. The treatment of RHF involves diuretics (most often fursemide (furosemide) and oxygen therapy.[62,63] There is excess accumulation of water in the body including the lungs, which compromises pulmonary gas exchange. Even in the absence of heart failure, diuretics are beneficial by reducing the excess water load. They must be given with great caution because of the possibility of volume depletion with diminished cardiac output, and hypokalemic metabolic alkalosis, which diminishes the effectiveness of the carbon dioxide stimulus on the respiratory centers. Renal excretion of bicarbonates is compromised by excess diuretic therapy due to depletion of potassium and chloride. Therefore, strict monitoring of these parameters is essential while using diuretics, particularly when salt restriction is done in cardiac failure.

Use of digitalis in cor pulmonale with heart failure is controversial, although some advocate its use to support the failing right ventricle. However, it seems that digitalis does not do any good. Moreover, in the presence of hypoxia and electrolyte imbalances, cardiotoxicity of digitalis is enhanced. Digitalis is used only in the case of an associated left heart failure or in the case of arrhythmia.

Phlebotomy may reduce the pulmonary artery pressure and pulmonary resistance when the hematocrit's are more than 55 to 60 percent. The right ventricular function is probably also improved. Its beneficial effect is by the way of a reduction in blood viscosity. Phlebotomy should be done cautiously, taking only small volumes of 200 to 300 ml at a time. It must be remembered that increased hematocrit is a compensatory phenomenon for improved oxygen carriage.

The treatment of pulmonary hypertension includes vasodilators and LTOT. Pulmonary hypertension is generally mild to moderate in COPD and the necessity for treating a mild hypertension has been questioned. An argument in favor of treatment is that pulmonary hypertension, even when modest during a stable period of the disease, may worsen, particularly during acute exacerbations, and these acute increases in PAP can contribute to the development of RHF. The best argument in favor of treatment is that LTOT, which is prescribed to very hypoxemic respiratory patients, has favorable pulmonary hemodynamic effects.

Experience with vasodilator therapy has come from the treatment of primary and severe pulmonary hypertension. There are very few selective pulmonary vasodilators. At present, inhaled nitric oxide cannot be administered for long periods because of toxicological reasons. Prostacyclin, bosentan, and sildenafil, which are effective in treating patients with primary pulmonary hypertension, do not seem appropriate for COPD patients and there is, at present, no justification for the long-term use of vasodilators in these patients.

One of the aims of LTOT in COPD patients is to attenuate the development of pulmonary hypertension and to reduce the frequency of episodes of RHF. Since alveolar hypoxia is the major determinant of the rise of PVR and PAP, it is logical to treat with LTOT hypoxemic COPD patients exhibiting pulmonary hypertension. The NOTT (nocturnal oxygen therapy trial)[64] and Medical Research Council[65] multicenter studies have shown that LTOT improve[64] or at least stabilizes[65] pulmonary hypertension. LTOT has also been shown to reverse the progression of pulmonary hypertension in COPD patients.[66] However, PAP rarely returns to normal. The longer the period of LTOT (> 16 hours/day) the better the hemodynamic results. At present LTOT is the best treatment for pulmonary hypertension in COPD patients. In the future, this treatment may combine LTOT and specific vasodilators.

While treating cor pulmonale, the underlying disease should be treated vigorously. For COPD, bronchodilators, removal of secretions and treatment of acute precipitating event like infections are important.

Prognosis

The prognosis of cor pulmonale depends upon the underlying pulmonary disease or disorder.[68] Patients with COPD have potentially reversible pulmonary hypertension because of hypoxia, which if corrected; right ventricular failure can be improved. Even with repeated episodes of right ventricular failure, some patients have long survival times. With anatomic restrictions of the vascular bed, pulmonary hypertension becomes sustained, initially only on exercise, and subsequently even at rest. Once right ventricular failure occurs, the prognosis is poor. In alveolar hypoventilation, the prognosis depends on the degree of improvement of the blood gas abnormalities prior to the development of nonreversible changes in vessel walls. The occurrence of documented RHF (peripheral edema) was classically an indicator of poor prognosis in respiratory patients. In fact it is now accepted that a prolonged survival (* 10 years) can be observed after the first episode of peripheral edema. The prevalence of clinical RHF has greatly decreased with the application of long-term oxygen therapy (LTOT), with a resulting improvement in prognosis.

The level of PAP is a good indicator of prognosis in COPD[60,68] but also in various categories of chronic respiratory disease such as idiopathic pulmonary fibrosis and sequelae of pulmonary tuberculosis.[68] The prognosis is worse in COPD patients with pulmonary hypertension when compared to similar patients without pulmonary hypertension.[60] In COPD patients with a mild degree of pulmonary hypertension (20-35 mm Hg) the five year survival rate is about 50 percent.[60,68] The prognosis is particularly poor for patients with severe pulmonary hypertension.[68] LTOT greatly improves the survival of hypoxemic COPD patients[64,65] and, accordingly, the prognosis of pulmonary hypertension is improved by LTOT, which could partly be explained by the reduction of RHF episodes with LTOT. Of interest, PAP is still an excellent prognostic indicator in COPD patients receiving LTOT, probably because it is a good marker of both the duration and the severity of alveolar hypoxia in these patients.

REFERENCES

1. Anon. World Health Organization. Chronic cor pulmonale. Report of an expert committee. Circulation 1963;27:594-615.
2. Fishman AP. Chronic cor pulmonale. Am Rev Respir Dis 1978;114:775-94.
3. Weitzenblum E. Chronic cor pulmonale. Am Heart J 2003;89(2):225-30.
4. Rich S (Ed). Primary pulmonary hypertension: Executive summary from the World Symposium—Primary Pulmonary Hypertension 1998. Available from the World Health Organization. URL: http://www.who.int/ncd/cvd/pph.html. Report of an expert panel on primary pulmonary hypertension", with presentation of the new diagnostic classification of pulmonary hypertension.
5. Pauwels RA, Buist AS, Calverley PMA, et al. On behalf of the GOLD Scientific Committee. Global strategy for the diagnosis, management, and prevention of chronic

obstructive pulmonary disease. NHLBI/WHO global initiative for chronic obstructive lung disease (GOLD) workshop summary. Report of a very recent consensus workshop organised by National Heart, Lung, and Blood Institute and the World Health Organization on the definition, classification of severity, burden, and management of COPD. Am J Respir Crit Care Med 2001;163:1256-76.

6. Williams BT, Nicholl JP. Prevalence of hypoxaemic chronic obstructive lung disease with reference to long-term oxygen therapy. Lancet 1985;i:369-72.

7. Ringbaek T, Seersholm N, Viskum K. Standardised mortality rates in females and males with COPD and asthma. Eur Respir J 2005;25:891-95.

8. Ross JC, Newman JH. Chronic cor pulmonale. Textbook of cardiology. Hurst 1986;55:120.

9. Butler J. The heart is not always in good hands. Chest 1990;97:453-60. Comment in: Chest 1990;98:1312.

10. Murray JF, Nadel JA. WB Saunders Company 1988; 58:1410.

11. McGinn S, White PD. Acute cor pulmonale resulting from pulmonary embolism, its clinical recognition. JAMA 1935;104:1473.

12. Ferrer MI. Cor pulmonale (pulmonary heart disease): Present day status. Am Heart J 1975;89:657.

13. Toure NO, Diao M, Kane A, Diop IB, Sarr M, Ba SA, Diouf SM. Chronic cor pulmonale: A study of 34 cases in the Dakar University Hospital Center Cardiology Department. Dakar Med 2000;45:108-12.

14. Venance SL, Koopman WJ, Miskie BA, Hegele RA, Hahn AF. Rigid spine muscular dystrophy due to SEPN1 mutation presenting as cor pulmonale. Neurology 2005;64:395-96.

15. Khattar RS, Fox DJ, Alty JE, Arora A. Pulmonary artery dissection: An emerging cardiovascular complication in surviving patients with chronic pulmonary hypertension. Heart 2005;91:142-45.

16. Aderaye G. Causes and clinical characteristics of chronic cor-pulmonale in Ethiopia. East Afr Med J 2004;81:202-06.

17. Geggel RL. Conditions leading to pediatric cardiology consultation in a tertiary academic hospital. Pediatrics. 2004;114:e409-17.

18. Winter RB. A tale of two brothers: Ultra-long-term follow-up of juvenile idiopathic scoliosis. J Spinal Disord Tech 2004;17:446-50.

19. Engelmann L. Right ventricular function in ARDS and mechanical respiration. Internist (Berl). 2004;45:1147-54.

20. Kirk V, Kahn A, Brouillette RT. Diagnostic approach to obstructive sleep apnea in children. Sleep Med Rev 1998;2:255-69.

21. Nakamura H, Adachi H, Sudoh A, Yagyu H, Kishi K, Oh-ishi S, Kusama H, Hashimoto T, Matsuoka T. Subacute cor pulmonale due to tumor embolism. Intern Med 2004;43:420-22.

22. Bergofsky EN. Respiratory failure in disorders of thoracic cage. Am Rev Respir Dis 1979;119:643.

23. Enson Y, Thomas HS III, Bosken CH, et al. Pulmonary hypertension in interstitial lung disease: Relation of vascular resistance to abnormal lung structure. Trans Assoc Am Phys 1975;88:248.

24. Enson Y. Pulmonary heart disease: Relation of pulmonary hypertension to abnormal lung structure and function. Bull NY Acad Med 1977;53:551.

25. Segel N, Kay JM, Bayley TJ, Paton A. Pulmonary hypertension with hepatic cirrhosis. Br Heart J 1968;30:575.

26. Editorial. Pulmonary veno-oclusive disease. Br Med J 1972;3:369.

27. Bohr DF. The pulmonary hypoxic response: State of the field. Chest 1977;71:244.

28. Mansencal N, Lavergne T, Bordachar P, Abergel E, Le Heuzey JY, Hidden F, Guize L. Chronic cor pulmonale: A rare complication of undiagnosed pacemaker lead endocarditis. Int J Cardiol 2004;96:119-20.

29. Krick S, Hanze J, Eul B, Savai R, Seay U, Grimminger F, Lohmeyer J, Klepetko W, Seeger W, Rose F. Hypoxia-driven proliferation of human pulmonary artery fibroblasts: Cross-talk between HIF-1alpha and an autocrine angiotensin system. FASEB J 2005;19:857-59.

30. Moudgil R, Michelakis ED, Archer SL. Hypoxic pulmonary vasoconstriction. J Appl Physiol 2005; 98:390-403.

31. Molthen RC, Karau KL, Dawson CA. Quantitative models of the rat pulmonary arterial tree morphometry applied to hypoxia-induced arterial remodeling. J Appl Physiol 2004;97:2372-84.

32. Harvey RM, Enson Y, Ferrer MI. A reconsideration of the origin of pulmonary hypertension. Chest 1971;59:82.

33. 30th Annual Aspen Conference: Pulmonary circulation and pulmonary hypertension. Chest 1988;93(Suppl): 80S.

34. Verbitskii ON, Buturov IV, Purkh TIu, Mohamed Fadi Fanari, Paraska VI. Hemodynamics, blood gas composition and viscosity in patients with chronic obstructive bronchitis complicated by chronic cor pulmonale. Probl Tuberk Bolezn Legk 2004;42-45.

35. Burrows B. Arterial oxygenation and pulmonary hemodynamics in patients with chronic airways obstruction. Am Rev RespirDis 1974;110(Suppl):64.

36. Lloyd TC. Respiratory system compliance as seen from the cardiac fossa. J Appl Physiol 1982;53:57.

37. Butler J. The heart in good hands. Circulation 1983; 67:1163.

38. Craven KD, Wood LDH. Extrapericardial and esophageal pressures with positive end expiratory pressure in dogs. J Appl Physiol 51:798.

39. Farahmand F, Hill MF, Singal PK. Antioxidant and oxidative stress changes in experimental cor pulmonale. Mol Cell Biochem. 2004;260:21-29.

40. Bacakoglu F, Atasever A, Ozhan MH, Gurgun C, Ozkilic H, Guzelant A. Plasma and bronchoalveolar lavage fluid levels of endothelin-1 in patients with chronic obstruc-

tive pulmonary disease and pulmonary hypertension. Respiration 2003;70:594-99.

41. Campbell EJM. The cause of oedema in cor pulmonale. Lancet 1960;1:1184.

42. Samet P, Fritts HW Jr, Fishman AP. The blood volume in heart disease. Medicine 1957;36:211.

43. de Leeuw PW, Dees A. Fluid homeostasis in chronic obstructive lung disease. Eur Respir J Suppl 2003; 46:33s-40s.

44. Fishman AP, Maxwell MH, Crowder CE, Morales P. Kidney function in cor pulmonale. Circulation 1951; 3:703.

45. Fishman AP. The left ventricle in "chronic bronchitis and emphysema". N Engl J Med 1971;285:402.

46. Murphy ML, Adamson J, Hutcheson F. Left ventricular hypertrophy in patients with chronic bronchitis and emphysema. Ann Intern Med 1974;81:307.

47. Khaja F, Parjker JO. Right and left ventricular performance in chronic obstructive lung disease. Am Heart J 1971;82:319.

48. Frank MJ, Weisse AB, Moschos CB, Levinson GE. Left ventricular function, metabolism, and blood flow in chronic cor pulmonale. Circulation 1973;47:798.

49. Mathay RA, Berger HO. Cardiovascular function in cor pulmonale. Clin Chest Med 1983;4:269.

50. Wilkinson M, Langhorne CA, Heath D, Barer GR, Howard P. A pathophysiologic study of 10 cases of hypoxic cor pulmonale. Q J Med 1988;66:65.

51. MacNee W. Pathophysiology of cor pulmonale in chronic obstructive pulmonary disease. Am J Respir Crit Care Med 1994;150:833-52;1158-68.

52. Chang CH. The normal roentgenographic measurement in right descending pulmonary artery in 1058 cases. Am J Roentgenol 1962;87:929.

53. Mathay RA, Schwarz MI, Ellis JH. Pulmonary artery hypertension in chronic obstructive pulmonary disease: Chest radiographic assessment. Invest Radiol 1981;16:95.

54. Collomb D, Paramelle PJ, Calaque O, Bosson JL, Vanzetto G, Barnoud D, Pison C, Coulomb M, Ferretti G. Severity assessment of acute pulmonary embolism: Evaluation using helical CT. Eur Radiol 2003;13:1508-14.

55. Ferretti GR, Collomb D, Ravey JN, Vanzetto G, Coulomb M, Bricault I. Severity assessment of acute pulmonary embolism: Role of CT angiography. Semin Roentgenol 2005;40:25-32.

56. Hudson LD, Kurt TL, Petty TL, Genton E. Arrhythmias associated with acute espiratory failure in patients with chronic airway obstruction. Chest 1973;63:661.

57. Kleiger RE, Senior RM. Long-term electrocardiographic monitoring of ambulatory patients with chronic airway obstruction. Chest 1974;65:483.

58. Padmavati S, Raizada V. Electrocardiogram in chronic cor pulmonale. Br Heart J 1975;34:648.

59. Vozniuk VV. Instrumental diagnostics of pulmonary hypertension in patients with chronic pulmonary heart. Lik Sprava 2004;(3-4):34-39.

60. Tramarin R, Torbicki A, Marchandise B, et al. Doppler echocardiographic evaluation of pulmonary artery pressure in chronic obstructive pulmonary disease. A European multicenter study. Eur Heart J 1991;12:103-11.

61. Brent BN, Berger HJ, Matthay RA, et al. Physiologic correlates of right ventricular ejection fraction in chronic obstructive pulmonary disease: A combined radionuclide and hemodynamic study. Am J Cardiol 1982; 50:255-62.

62. Nobel MIM, Trenchcard D, Guz A. The value of diuretics in respiratory failure. Lancet 1966;2:257.

63. Stark RD, Finnegan P, Bishop JM. Long-term domiciliary oxygen in chronic bronchitis with pulmonary hypertension. Br Med J 1973;3:467.

64. Nocturnal Oxygen Therapy Trial Group. Continuous or nocturnal oxygen therapy in hypoxemic chronic obstructive lung disease. Ann Intern Med 1980;93:391-98.

65. Medical Research Council Working Party. Long-term domiciliary oxygen therapy in chronic hypoxic cor pulmonale complicating chronic bronchitis and emphysema. Lancet 1981;i:681.

66. Weitzenblum E, Sautegeau A, Ehrhart M, et al. Long-term oxygen therapy can reverse the progression of pulmonary hypertension in patients with chronic obstructive pulmonary disease. Am Rev Respir Dis 1985;131:493-98.

67. Stevens PM, Terplan M, Knowles JH. Prognosis of cor pulmonale. N Engl Med 1963;269:1289.

68. Bishop JM, Cross KW. Physiological variables and mortality in patients with various categories of chronic respiratory disease. Bull Eur Physiopathol Respir 1984;20:495-500.

Pulmonary Embolism

The true incidence of clinically significant pulmonary embolism is not known because of difficulties in diagnosis during life. Even, it is difficult to assess the reliable estimate at autopsy because of seasonal variation in incidence, disappearance of emboli due to thrombolysis, large variation in the size of emboli, and the difficulty in differentiating embolization vs *in situ* formed thrombi. It is demonstrated that the major source of pulmonary emboli is from thrombi arising in deep veins of the lower extremities. Reports from USA suggest that about five million patients each year suffer an episode of venous thrombosis; 10 percent of these have a pulmonary embolic event and approximately 300,000 hospitalizations are due to venous thromboembolism with 50,000 deaths per year due to this.[1,2] More recent data shows venous thromboembolism is the third most common cardiovascular disease after acute ischemic syndromes and shock. Venous thromboembolism is a potentially life-threatening disease with > 200,000 first lifetime cases reported each year in the United States.[3] In the United States, pulmonary embolism occurs in approximately 600,000 patients each year.[4] Fatalities in the United States from pulmonary embolism are estimated at 100,000 to 200,000 persons per year[5] with about 60,000 deaths. In France, fatal pulmonary embolism is estimated at 100,000 to 200,000 cases yearly.[4] However, reports from UK, suggest a much less incidence of pulmonary embolism. About only 0.6 percent of all deaths are primarily due to pulmonary embolism as evidenced from autopsy studies, and this is the primary mode of death in only 0.4 percent of all hospitalized patients.[6] In Italy, as many as 50,000 new cases per year occur with an overall short-term case fatality of 11.4 percent.[7] Recently Stein and Henry has reported the prevalence of acute pulmonary embolism to be 1 percent in hospitalized patients in a General hospital and the same was observed in 14.6 percent of the autopsy cases. In the clinical cases it was estimated to cause or contribute to death in 0.2 percent of cases and the figure was 37.3 percent in autopsy cases. The diagnosis was unsuspected in 70 percent of the cases and was detected only at autopsy. Most of these cases had advanced associated disease. In most cases (92%) death from pulmonary embolism occurred within 2.5 hours.[8]

ETIOLOGY

(A) THROMBOEMBOLISM

More than 90 percent of all pulmonary emboli originate from lower extremity deep vein thrombosis. Occasionally other sites may give rise to such emboli. Veins draining into the internal iliac system of veins, prostatic and uterine veins are rare sources. Since they are small veins, the emboli are small. Thrombi may also arise in the renal vein, right cardiac chambers (infarction, ventricular or atrial dilatation, atrial fibrillation, tricuspid and pulmonary valves in the presence of valvular endocarditis), the left ventricle following myocardial infarction, and upper extremities (trauma, intravascular catheters, intravenous drug abuse). Deep vein thrombosis is a common event, occurring in 20 to 50 percent of patients undergoing surgery or with other risk factors such as myocardial infarction, or prolonged bed rest. Thrombosis developing in association with these risk factors is predominantly limited to the calf veins and is clinically silent. Approximately 20 percent of patients developing deep vein thrombosis will have proximal thrombosis, the majority in association with calf vein thrombosis, but may be isolated in about a third of cases.

All venous thrombi of the lower extremities are not equally prone to give rise to embolism. The location of the thrombus is of critical importance. Thrombi that are confined to the calf pose limited risk, whereas those extend into or arise in, the popliteal veins and above are prone to give rise to clinically significant pulmonary thromboembolism because of their large size.[2]

Virchow provided the pathogenetic basis of venous thrombosis. The triad of venous stasis, intimal injury and disordered coagulation properties of the blood constitute the basis of thrombus formation. Stasis alone or alterations of coagulation properties alone do not give rise to venous thrombosis. Stasis and coagulation changes are important for this. Venous thrombosis usually originates as a platelet nidus in the region of venous valves in the lower extremities, the site of turbulence. Elaboration of thrombogenic material from this platelet focus, if not swept away lead to the formation of a red thrombus. The thrombus grows by accretion of platelets and fibrin. The growth is either interrupted by detachment or by total occlusion of the vessel. At any time after formation, the thrombus can be detached from the venous wall as an embolus. On the otherhand, the thrombus undergoes dissolution by endogenous thrombolytic activities. If complete dissolution does not occur, it gets organized and incorporated into the venous wall. Since most thrombi occur near venous valves, organization leads to incompetence of the valve and becomes a potential for venous stasis.[2,9-12]

Although stasis and intimal injury are more important, it is believed that a state of hypercoagulability exists in patients who develop venous thrombosis. Several such markers have recently been identified. These include deficiencies of antithrombin III, of protein C, of protein S, and the presence of a lupus anticoagulant. Rarely, abnormalities in plasminogen, production of tissue plasminogen activator (excess of plasminogen activator inhibitor 1), or the excessive production of tPA inhibitor have been associated with venous thrombosis.[13,14] However, only 10 to 15 percent of patients with venous thrombosis demonstrate these abnormalities. A search for these factors is necessary in patients with a strong family history of thrombosis or recurrent thrombosis without apparent cause. Even in these cases, another associated factor known to precipitate thrombus formation is present.[2,15-23]

Other risk factors for increased thromboembolism include[2,24-27] immobilization, trauma, heart disease, malignancy, pregnancy and puerperium, and estrogen therapy. Fractures of femur and tibia, and burn predispose to pulmonary embolism more frequently than other types of trauma. Leg amputation, hip, pelvic, and spinal surgery are more prone to produce thromboembolic episodes. Heart disease is an important risk factor irrespective of etiology. Congestive failure and arrhythmias are important contributory factors. Thrombophlebitis migrans is commonly associated with pancreatic malignancy followed by that of the bronchus, genitourinary tract, colon, stomach, and breast, the reported incidence of thromboembolic disease in pregnancy varies from 1:200 to 1:600. Such events are frequent in older, multi-

parous women in the last trimester and the incidence is increased further by cesarian section. However, fatalities are rare. Estrogen-containing oral contraceptive agents increase the chances of venous thrombosis, the rise being proportionate to the estrogen content. Other rare conditions reported to increase the risk of thromboembolism include: obesity, chronic obstructive pulmonary disease, ulcerative colitis, diabetes mellitus, Cushing's syndrome, Behçet's syndrome, homocystinuria, polycythemia vera, thrombocythemia, paroxysmal nocturnal hemoglobinuria, and Gram-negative sepsis.

Various risk factors associated with venous thromboembolism are shown in Table 19.1 and various hypercoagulable states predisposed to this condition are shown in Table 19.2.

TABLE 19:1. Risk factors for development of venous thrombo-embolism-possible contributing factors for pathogenesis[28,29]

	Hypercoagulability	Stasis	Trauma/injury to the vessel wall
Previous venous thromboembolism	√	√	√
Major surgery		√	
Cancer	√	√	
Obesity		√	
Trauma		√	
Fracture (hip/leg)		√	√
Pregnancy	√	√	
Myocardial infarction		√	
Congestive heart failure		√	
Stroke	√		
Estrogen therapy		√	
Prolonged immobilization		√	
Burns		√	

TABLE 19.2: Inherited and acquired hypercoagulable states[30-32]

Variable	Prevalence in general population (%)	Prevalence in patients with venous thrombo-embolism (%)
Protein C deficiency	0.1-0.3	2-5
Protein S deficiency	0.3	2
Antithrombin III deficiency	0.5	1
Factor V Leiden	4-6	20-25
Prothrombin G-A20210 gene variant		
↑ Factor XI (> 90th percentile)	10	19
↑ Factor VIII (> 1500 IU/L)	11	25
Hyperhomocystinemia	5	12

In a large series of 988 consecutive patients,[7] in whom a diagnosis of pulmonary embolism was made, the following conditions were associated with the clinical conditions preceding the embolic episode and are shown in Table 19.3.

TABLE 19.3: Clinical conditions preceding the embolic episodes

Clinical condition	% of patients
Apparently primary	40.3
After surgery	36.7
Heart disease	11.6
After trauma	6.1
Neoplasms	4.3
Systemic diseases (collagen diseases, generalized venous anomalies)	1.0

According to the Prospective Investigation of Pulmonary Embolism Diagnosis (PIPED) study, the risk factors for pulmonary embolism were the same for women and men, except that women using oral contraceptives had an increased risk of pulmonary embolism following surgery.[33] However, when all risk factors when considered simultaneously, male sex, surgery within 3 months, immobilization, and history of thrombophlebitis were each associated with the presence of pulmonary embolism and there was an increased risk for men compared to women.

PATHOLOGY[34]

The incidence of pulmonary thromboembolism peaks in spring and autumn, possibly related to weather conditions. Because of endogenous thrombolytic properties, a considerable percentage of emboli disappear prior to morphologic investigations. Similarly, differences in the size of thromboemboli influences the clinical effects and mortality and also for the evaluation at autopsy. While large emboli in the pulmonary trunk or main pulmonary arteries will be obvious, those in the lobar and segmental arteries will not be visible unless these are cut regularly and systematically. Thus, grossly recognizable emboli in routine autopsies of adult patients vary widely from 15 to 30 percent. Microscopic examination greatly increases the number of observed recent and old emboli to 52 to 64 percent and according to some reports the figure may be as high as 90 percent when more blocks of lung tissues are studied, and occasional post-thrombotic lesions are included. While primary thrombi are more common in the upper lobes of the lungs, both large and small thromboemboli are more numerous in the lower lobes and on the right side because of distribution of blood supply.

In a large autopsy series of 583 cases, the point of origin of thromboemboli could only be demonstrated in 53 percent of cases. Eighty-six percent of these 286 cases had one or more thromboses in the territory of inferior vena cava, more frequently at the level of femoral and iliac veins[35] the other localizations were; inferior vena cava + right heart or superior vena cava 8.06 percent; right heart 3.15 percent; and superior vena cava 2.79 percent. Usually there will be multiple than single localizations in the pulmonary vascular bed.[36]

The thromboembolic episode can be *Acute* or *Chronic*. Acute embolization obstructing the pulmonary trunk and/or both main pulmonary arteries can cause sudden death. Additional thrombi may be present in the right side of the heart. Sometimes, unilateral obstruction of a main pulmonary artery may be fatal. However, since pulmonary emboli are usually multiple and often bilateral, it is likely that in these circumstances the embolic attack is preceded by thromboembolism affecting the contralateral lung.

Complete or near complete obstruction of a large pulmonary artery may be due to a single thromboembolism arising from a large systemic vein, or by several smaller emboli, or by folding or twisting of an embolus. It is also possible that a saddle shaped embolus may be arrested at the bifurcation of the pulmonary trunk or at a more distant peripheral ramification, which may fail to completely occlude the vessel and some blood flow is maintained. Thus, survival is possible with a saddle shaped embolus even if the thromboembolism is massive. Similarly, V-shaped or Y-shaped clots may allow residual blood flow.

A fresh thromboembolus is a cast of the vein in which it originates, and therefore is cylindrical shape with blunt ends and a smooth surface, sometimes showing the impression of the venous valves. It is usually dry and friable in contrast to a postmortem clot which is usually moist, structureless, and rubbery, and that can be removed as a ramifying cast from the pulmonary arterial tree. The embolus contains pale lines of Zahn on its dark red cut exposed surface and these lines represent layers of platelets and fibrin alternating with layers of RBC. Since an embolus is forced into a pulmonary artery, the vessel is usually dilated at that area and therefore, the wall is thinner than normal. If the patient survives the initial insult several processes determine the fate of a thromboembolus. One of these is endogenous *thrombolysis* by enzymatic activity. Other processes include *fragmentation, organization, canalization,* and formation of *bands and webs*.

Thrombotic lesions in muscular pulmonary arteries are not unusual in routine autopsies. However, they are usually small in number. They can be numerous and in that event they will produce pulmonary hypertension. It was presumed earlier that patients with unexplained pulmonary hypertension who have thrombotic lesions in their muscular pulmonary arteries suffered from thromboembolic pulmonary hypertension.[36] In these cases there will be no recognizable source of embolus in systemic veins nor there will be a history suggestive of thromboembolism. However, "silent recurrent thromboembolism" cannot be excluded. To produce sustained pulmonary hypertension by microembolism, the number of small emboli has to be extraordinarily large. Such small emboli can be formed due to mechanical fragmentation of a large embolus.

NATURAL HISTORY AND HEMODYNAMIC CONSEQUENCES

Acute massive pulmonary embolism often leads to death within an hour of the event, often too soon to make a diagnosis or institution of therapy. Patients who die from pulmonary embolism, 75 to 90 percent do so within one hour.[9,11] In other types, the consequences may be divided into respiratory, and hemodynamic. The *respiratory consequences*[37,38] following pulmonary embolism include creation of an alveolar dead space,[37] pneumoconstriction,[38] hypoxemia,[39-44] and hyperventilation.[45] Later, regional loss of surfactant[46-48] and pulmonary infarction occur.

Although complete occlusion is possible, some blood flow occurs distally by the action of the endogenous thrombolytic system within hours of embolism.[49] Total or partial occlusion leads to an absence or diminished blood flow respectively, while the ventilation continues. Thus a region of high $\dot{V}/\dot{Q}$ will be present.

A second immediate consequence is the pneumoconstriction in lung zones with proximal obstruction. This results from very low levels of carbon dioxide. Although this phenomenon is demonstrated in experimental animals, in human situations this does not occur, because the patient soon breaths the high carbon dioxide containing tracheal dead space air into these alveolar zones.

Hypoxemia is a frequent finding in acute pulmonary embolism. Several mechanisms are responsible for this. One common one is a reduction in cardiac output due to acute right ventricular decompensation resulting in a wide arteriovenous oxygen difference. $\dot{V}/\dot{Q}$ mismatch is the second contributor. Low $\dot{V}/\dot{Q}$ zones can be produced acutely by embolism, which results from hyperperfusion in the remaining open vascular bed. That is, blood is diverted from the obstructed zones to perfused zones, but ventilation may not increase proportionately. Other factors include low mixed venous PO_2, shunting, and diffusion limitation. All of these potential mechanisms are magnified as the extent of embolic obstruction increases.

The other event following pulmonary embolism is hyperventilation due to an increase in respiratory rate and a modest increase in depth. Thus hyperventilation tries to increase arterial oxygen. In the vast majority of patients, this increase in ventilation leads to hypocapnia. Rarely, with massive embolism, hypercapnia may occur despite substantial increase in minute ventilation. The

mechanism of hyperventilation in pulmonary embolism remains controversial and it is suggested that it is a response due to stimulation of J receptors, although other potential factors may be responsible.

In some patients, depletion of local alveolar surfactant occurs resulting in atelectasis and edema. It occurs approximately 24 hours after total pulmonary occlusion. This appears due to a failure of the circulation (due to obstruction) to deliver the basic components for surfactant synthesis by type II alveolar cells.

Various syndromes of acute pulmonary embolism are:
- Pulmonary infarction/hemorrhage
- Massive pulmonary embolism/acute cor pulmonale
- Acute unexplained dyspnea.

I. Pulmonary Infarction[34,50-52]

It is defined as the necrosis of lung tissue distal to the site of embolic obstruction. This can occur with thromboembolic obstruction of a medium-sized pulmonary artery. Occlusion of a main pulmonary artery or that of a small-caliber elastic or muscular artery rarely causes it. Pulmonary infarction is uncommon in the absence of passive congestion. This has been shown both experimentally also, wherein embolism of a healthy lung does not cause true infarction, that is, necrosis of the alveolar wall. Some authors have described this as the "incomplete pulmonary infarction"—intra-alveolar hemorrhage without necrosis of the alveolar walls. This is the most common finding in the first two days of infarction. After 2 days, necrosis of the alveolar wall begins and leads to true pulmonary infarction, which leads to an organized healed scar. Incomplete infarction causes a radiological shadow that disappears completely in 2 to 4 days, which is consistent with the resolution of the intra-alveolar hemorrhage instead of organization of the lesion. In patients with healthy lungs, the infarction remains incomplete and resolves, and the pulmonary infiltrates disappears. However, in patients with congestive heart failure, the infarction goes on to necrosis, resulting in true pulmonary infarction with a scar and persistent radiological findings. Pulmonary infarction is a sequelae of submassive embolism with obstruction of subsegmental branches of the pulmonary circulation as opposed to obstruction of the central pulmonary circulation. It was noted long ago that ligation of the main right pulmonary artery does not lead to pulmonary infarction.

The infarction is uncommon because of peculiar blood supply of the lungs. Unlike other tissues (cerebral and myocardium), pulmonary infarction is a quite uncommon sequel of pulmonary occlusion. About less than one-third of such patients develop infarction. The reasons for this are due to the different sources of oxygen supply to the lungs. The lung is supplied blood by three sources: the airways, the pulmonary artery, and the bronchopulmonary connections. Nutrient supply comes from both the bronchial and pulmonary blood. The bronchial arteries have extensive connections at the capillary level with pulmonary circulation, which can prevent serious damage to the lung tissue deprived of pulmonary blood flow. Finally studies have suggested that reflux flow from pulmonary venous side or even from the left atrium[53] may be an additional source of oxygen and nutrient. In patients with underlying lung disease and compromised cardiovascular function with reduced cardiac output or shock, development of infarction is more common. Thus, pulmonary infarction is unlikely unless there is an impaired general cardiovascular circulation, particularly an inadequate bronchial circulation or an impediment to the pulmonary venous outflow. Patients with heart disease, particularly mitral stenosis, and terminally ill, are more prone to develop infarction as discussed above. Pulmonary infarction is very uncommon in individuals younger than 40 years of age. Another sequel of thromboembolism[34] may be pulmonary hemorrhage. Infarction or necrosis of lung tissue is not always an inevitable result of an inadequate blood supply. A mild transient ischemia of lung tissue may result in marked dilatation of capillaries, arterioles, and venules with an increased vascular permeability with leakage of fluid and RBC as the endothelium of these vessels are very susceptible to hypoxia. A septic infarct, due to an infected embolus or to an infectious process in the lung is grayish white in color due to lysis of RBC and accumulation of WBC in contrast to the dark red color of a thromboembolic infarct.[34] The septic infarct may produce a lung abscess.

Hemodynamic consequences[54-58] The central abnormality is a reduction in the cross-sectional area of the pulmonary vascular bed. This reduction will increase pulmonary vascular resistance and an increment in the right ventricular afterload, which if severe, will result in right ventricular failure. Since the reserve in the pulmonary vascular bed is enormous, these consequences are noticed once there is a substantial loss of more than 50 percent. Other factors that are responsible for the increase in vascular resistance include the potential role of humoral and reflex mechanisms. Release of vasoactive amines (serotonin and thromboxane A_2) from platelet coatings of emboli has been demonstrated in experimental animal, the effect of which can be blocked by inhibitors of these amines. These neurohumoral factors can cause vasoconstriction and bronchoconstriction. The final fact or that contribute to the hemodynamic consequences is the prior cardiorespiratory status of the patient. A patient

with extensive lung disease or with an already elevated pulmonary pressure, will tolerate poorly even to small emboli. As right ventricular afterload increases, other consequences follow. As the cardiac output falls, the pulmonary arterial pressure may fall, even though the pulmonary vascular resistance is raised.

II. Massive Pulmonary Embolism/ Acute Cor Pulmonale

Massive, Central pulmonary embolism leads to shock, and collapse accompanied by dilatation of the pulmonary artery and the right heart chambers. Engorgement of neck veins occurs as a direct evidence of increased venous pressure resulting from failure of the right side of the heart. This condition is distinguished from chronic cor pulmonale due to progressive enlargement of the right side of the heart secondary to various pulmonary diseases. The condition of acute cor pulmonale is physiologically similar to the clamping of the main left artery in experimental animals, which increases the main pulmonary artery pressure. The systemic blood pressure remains normal until the occlusion is more than 50 percent.

Typical ECG changes reflect $S_1Q_3T_3$ pattern, which reverts back to normal once the recovery occurs.

The hemodynamic and angiographic correlates of acute cor pulmonale usually reveals that the pulmonary artery systolic pressure does not exceed 50 to 60 mm Hg, unless there is preexisting heart disease even in patients with massive pulmonary embolism. Right atrial pressure usually remains between 10 to 22 mm Hg. Cardiac index is usually normal. The right ventricle can generate pressure up to 50 to 60 mm Hg. At that point the right ventricle dilates and the right ventricular end diastolic pressure and the mean right atrial pressure increases. Right ventricular stroke volume decreases, cardiac output decreases, and hypotension develop. As the degree of embolic obstruction decreases, right heart pressure return to near normal levels. The consequences are summarized below:

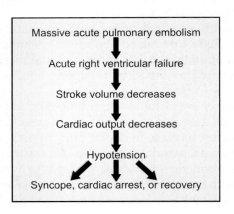

Acute Unexplained Dyspnea

Pulmonary infarction is seen in about 50 to 60 percent of cases and the syndrome of acute cor pulmonale is present in an additional 10 to 15 percent of cases. In the absence of these two syndromes, a sizable number will present with acute unexplained dyspnea. Pulmonary angiography demonstrates submassive pulmonary embolism that is not sufficient to cause acute cor pulmonale but is sufficient to cause dyspnea. Tachypnea and tachycardia are usually present. There may be evidence of deep vein thrombosis. The chest radiology and ECG are usually normal. The differential diagnosis is congestive heart failure or pneumonia, which can easily be recognized. The condition may also be confused with hyperventilation. However, the key laboratory finding is arterial blood gas analysis which will reveal hypoxemia and hypocapnia, which will distinguish the condition from hyperventilation.

LONG-TERM SEQUELA[59-65]

When thrombi remain confined to calf veins, with-holding treatment does not increase morbidity, mortality, or recurrence during the first 6 months of follow-up. However, some studies suggest that, symptomatic calf vein thrombosis may recur unless treated. Above-knee acute venous thrombosis gradually returns to normal after treatment, over a period of 1 year as evidenced by normal impedance plethysmography over 90 percent of cases.

The overall prognosis of patients who survive the first episode of pulmonary embolism is also good. In dogs, the resolution rate of pulmonary emboli is extremely rapid and complete restoration of the pulmonary vascular bed is the rule. Although in humans, the thrombolytic system is not as potent as that in dogs, resolution is the rule, although somewhat slower. Data from the National Institutes of Health (USA) clinical trials of thrombolytic agents suggest that, with heparin therapy alone, embolic resolution proceeded rather rapidly during the first two weeks after embolic episode. At five days after initiation of therapy, 36 percent of the scan defects had resolved; by day 14, 52 percent; at 3 months, 73 percent; and at 1 year, 76 percent. These resolution rates are similar to those obtained with treatment regimens that included various durations of intravenous streptokinase or urokinase infusions before heparin was instituted. Although several other reports have indicated that significant long-term residuals are quite uncommon leading to pulmonary hypertension or cor pulmonale, repeated embolism will result in significant hemodynamic changes resulting in cor pulmonale and heart failure.

CLINICAL FEATURES

The symptoms, signs, and prognosis of pulmonary thromboembolism depend on the size and number of emboli, the patient's cardiopulmonary status, the rate at which clot fragmentation and lysis occurs and whether there is a source from which further embolism can continue. Of patients who die from pulmonary embolism, 75 to 90 percent die within the first few hours after the embolic episode. It means that most embolic deaths occur so rapidly that neither appropriate diagnostic nor therapeutic measures can be instituted. It has also been observed that when death occurs beyond the first few hours, it is due to a recurrent embolic event. The clinical diagnosis of embolism is unreliable and a high degree of suspicion is necessary to suggest the possibility.[56] Acute massive pulmonary embolism in a previously healthy patient can result in acute cor pulmonale with right heart failure. The degree of pulmonary hypertension in this situation correlates well with the extent of vascular occlusion on angiography.

The proportion of pulmonary embolism increases progressively with age, and reaches the peak in the seventh decade.[66] The sex distribution has been controversial. Associated risk factors as described above will be present in varying proportion of cases. The main symptoms and signs of pulmonary embolism can be classified into three syndromes: (a) Pulmonary infarction with acute pleuritic chest pain, dyspnea, hemoptysis, and pleural rub: (b) acute cor pulmonale with sudden development of dyspnea, cyanosis, right ventricular failure, and hypotension; and (c) unexplained dyspnea.[67] About 95 percent of patients with documented pulmonary embolism will have clinical findings consistent with one of the above three syndromes.[68] However, these findings are not sensitive enough in the presence of chronic obstructive lung disease and congestive heart failure. Therefore, they have a low accuracy in confirming or excluding pulmonary embolism. The classic triad of dyspnea, pleuritic chest pain, and hemoptysis is present in about 20 percent of the patients only with major pulmonary embolism. The most consistent findings however is a sudden onset of dyspnea, and chest pain. These two symptoms along with tachypnea may be present in as much as 97 percent of patients who have no previous cardiopulmonary disease. According to Palla, et al[65] the first two symptoms will be present in as much as 52 percent of patients with proved pulmonary embolism. Other symptoms include anxiety, and impending doom. In massive embolism, syncope or near-syncope may occur. Physical findings are also nonspecific and are not sensitive. The most common findings are tachycardia and tachypnea. A low-grade fever, rarely exceeding 38.5°C, is common. Localized rhonchi, and crepitations due to surfactant loss may be heard. Pulmonary hypertension rarely develops in classical pulmonary embolism, but if it occurs, findings of that condition will be detected. They include right ventricular tap, raised jugular venous pulse, and increased pulmonary component of S_2, right ventricular S_3, split second sound, hepatomegaly, and edema. Findings of associated deep vein thrombosis like redness, tenderness, and swelling may be present. Most often they are absent.

Chronic pulmonary embolism (CPE) is a relatively rare phenomenon and occurs in less than 2 percent of patients following pulmonary embolism. It is due to a failure of the emboli to resolve which may be due to the deficiencies of the coagulation inhibitors discussed above. Embolization from the previously organized thrombi that are resistant to resolution may be another cause of CPE. When this leads to pulmonary hypertension, a syndrome of progressive respiratory deterioration with pulmonary hypertension and right ventricular dysfunction occur. The majority of these patients have a previous history of pulmonary embolism or venous thrombosis. These may go unnoticed. Patients usually complain of exertional dyspnea progressing to severe respiratory and cardiac failure. There may be recurrent episodes of thrombophlebitis.

The signs and symptoms of pulmonary embolism are shown in Table 19.4.[66,69]

TABLE 19.4: Signs and symptoms of acute pulmonary embolism

	Incidence (%)
Symptoms	
Breathlessness	84
Chest pain	74-83
Apprehension	59-63
Cough	50
Hemoptysis	30
Sweating	27
Syncope	13
Signs	
Tachypnea (rate > 16/min)	92
Crepitation	58
Accentuated P_2	53
Tachycardia (rate > 100/min)	44
Temperature (> 37.5°C)	43
Phlebitis	32

DIAGNOSIS

Pulmonary embolism recurs after an initial episode in about 8 percent of cases treated with anticoagulation therapy, but may reach 30 percent in untreated patients.[70,71] Establishing or ruling out the diagnosis is difficult due to lack of specificity of clinical findings and of most biological and imaging tests.[72-74] For patients with cardiac or pulmonary disease, clinical findings suggestive of pulmonary embolism are frequently misleading because the same can often be related to an underlying disease. In this particular group of patients, exclusion pulmonary embolism is of primary importance because recurrence can be severe due to deranged cardiac or respiratory status.[75] Despite some advances in clinical diagnosis, a delay in the diagnosis is still the main source of mortality from pulmonary embolism. An autopsy series has indicated that pulmonary embolism remains undiagnosed at death in as many as 40 to 70 percent of patients.[76]

CHEST RADIOGRAPHY

Although some reports suggest that there is no definite radiological feature of pulmonary embolism, others report an abnormality in more than 80 percent of cases.[77-80] The abnormalities include enlargement of descending pulmonary arteries (66.6%), elevation of diaphragmatic domes (62%), enlargement of heart shadow (55.8%), pruning of peripheral vessels, presence of densities and atelectasis, small effusions (50.9%) and infarctions.[78] These may be nonspecific and of little diagnostic help except ruling out other causes. Loss of surfactant is responsible for atelectasis and raised hemidiaphragm and pulmonary infiltrates. The enlargement of descending pulmonary artery (sausage like enlargement) is a frequent sign due to acute occlusion of a vessel and exclusion of a part of the vascular bed from pulmonary blood flow resulting in an increase in the pulmonary vascular resistance. The increased pulmonary artery pressure causes dilatation of a vascular section above the obstruction. Infarctions, if present are typically pleural based. Other pulmonary densities may appear as opacities in the costophrenic angle and are known as "Hampton hump".[80] Avascular lung zones (*Westermark sign*) may suggest the diagnosis. This is due to pulmonary hyperluscency caused by marked reduction in blood content of pulmonary vessels. Although considered almost typical of pulmonary embolism, this sign is present in only ~10 percent of cases. Patients with infarction will present with a "wedge-shaped shadow". In patients without infarction, anemia or oligemia of the lung area corresponding to the embolized arterial branch is noted. In case of larger emboli, a whole lobe or an entire lung may be anemic. These areas of decreased vascularity have been termed as *Westermark sign*. The radiographic appearance of an infarct is a shadow or density corresponding to the lung segment involved. The shadow is always in contact with one or more pleural surfaces. The cardiac margin of the consolidation is sharp in outline, and convex or hump-shaped ("Hampton hump"). At this early stage, the infarction is hemorrhagic or incomplete. In patients without heart disease, the incomplete infarction may heal without scarring. In patients with pulmonary congestion, the infarction passes through a healing phase leading to scar formation. As the healing occurs, the infarction may produce a sharp, dense line, which is a linear shadow confused with platelike atelectasis. On the other hand, chest skiagram may be completely normal in spite of extensive embolism. However, these findings of pleural effusion, pleural-based opacity, elevated hemidiaphragm, atelectasis, and consolidation are nonspecific.

In a recent study of 196 cases of which 96 were proved to be pulmonary embolism by pulmonary angiography, Donnomaria, et al[81] have reported that history of previous pulmonary embolism, presence of immobilization, thrombophlebitis, enlarged descending pulmonary artery, enlarged right heart, pulmonary infarction, *Westermark sign*, elevated diaphragm, and hypoxemia have 2.8 to 15 times increased chance to be having pulmonary embolism than those having not these symptoms or signs.

ECG

The ECG findings are abnormal in vast majority of cases, although they may be nonspecific. About 21 ECG signs have been described with pulmonary embolism. Sinus tachycardia and ST segment depression are the most common findings.[82] Only with severe right ventricular overload, classic findings of pulmonary embolism are seen. They include S_1Q_3 pattern, right axis deviation, and ST changes in lead III (inversion) indicative of ischemia (now known as $S_1Q_3T_3$ pattern). Other changes include T-wave inversion in V_1-V_2, late R in aVR, and PR displacement. ST depression and T-wave inversion in V_1-V_2 are associated with severity of embolism and have a good correlation with umber of un-perfused lung segments on perfusion lung scans. Some ECG changes may be due to myocardial ischemia of the right ventricle because of pressure overload and humoral factors, such as histamine, or catecholamine release. ECG is useful to rule out other differential diagnoses like acute pericarditis and myocardial infarction. Another finding in ECG is the incomplete bundle branch block. These changes can revert back to normal on recovery. The appearance of a new $S_1Q_3T_3$ or a new right bundle branch block is quite specific for acute pulmonary embolism.

ARTERIAL BLOOD GASES

In patients with pulmonary embolism the arterial oxygen concentration (PaO_2) is usually low in the range of less than 80 mm Hg. Hypocapnia is another characteristic finding because of hyperventilation. In about 15 percent of cases the PaO_2 may have values more than 80 mmHg.[83-85] However, in these cases the $PaCO_2$ will still be low. In patients with COPD and chronic CO_2 retention, a drop in both PaO_2 and $PaCO_2$ should raise the suspicion of pulmonary embolism.[84] In the follow-up of patients with pulmonary embolism, measurement of PaO_2 and $P(a-A)$ O_2 and ($PACO_2$-$PaCO_2$) are helpful which will show improvement and have good correlation with perfusion scans.

LUNG SCANS

Perfusion lung scans are helpful in establishing or excluding the diagnosis reasonably short of a pulmonary angiogram.[86-90] However, the V/Q scans are not fully diagnostic.[91] The PIOPED (prospective Investigation of Pulmonary Embolism Diagnosis) has described three patterns of V/Q abnormalities. They are shown in Table 19.5.

TABLE 19.5: Interpretation of ventilation-perfusion scans[91]

I. **Normal V/Q scan** (Pulmonary embolism excluded)
II. **High probability scans** (indicative of pulmonary embolism in 87%)
>/= 2 large segmental mismatches, or
>/= 2 large segmental matches > ventilation defect, or
1 large and >/= moderate mismatches or
>/= 4 moderate mismatches
III. **Low probability scan** (can correctly exclude pulmonary embolism in 86%)
Nonsegmental defects
1 moderate mismatch with normal chest skiagram
Any perfusion defect < chest skiagram defect
</= 4 large or moderate matching defects (and </= 3 segments in one lung region) </= ventilation defect and > skiagram defect, or > 3 small segmental defects with normal chest skiagram
IV. **Intermediate or indeterminate interpretation** (Pulmonary embolism will be present in 21-30% of cases)

If a normal perfusion scan is obtained, the diagnostic interpretation is same as that of a normal angiogram. Embolic suspects with normal perfusion scans have excellent outcomes. However, a small embolus in the distant small peripheral branch may be missed on such a scan and angiogram. If the perfusion scan is abnormal showing one or more defects, the interpretation should be made with the chest X-ray. If there are radiographic infiltrates in the same area as that of the scan, the perfusion defects become nondiagnostic. Secondly, if the perfusion defects are subsegmental in size, the scan also becomes nondiagnostic. On the other hand, if the perfusion defects are large in size or segmental in size, ventilation scans are to be carried out further. If the ventilation scan is normal ($\dot{V}/\dot{Q}$ mismatch), the likelihood of embolism is nearly 90 percent, and most clinicians will not go for further pulmonary angiography. On the other hand, if the ventilation scan shows poor entry or exit of the radioactive gas from such areas, the scan becomes nondiagnostic. There are considerable variations among institutions, regarding which scan to do first, and what substance to use for such scanning.

PULMONARY ANGIOGRAPHY

Although scans are very useful, the only definitive procedure for making the diagnosis of acute embolic disease is pulmonary angiography.[90,92,93] However, this is an invasive procedure and in experienced hands is associated with complications particularly in an acute condition like pulmonary embolism. On the contrary, it is demonstrated that the procedure is safe in experienced hands even in the presence of severe pulmonary hypertension. Moreover, use of ionic contrast media and limiting the procedure by injecting abnormal areas only using the scan as a guide, safety can be enhanced. The frequency of major complications has been reported to be about 1.3 percent. These include death, respiratory distress requiring cardiopulmonary resuscitation or intubation, renal failure requiring dialysis, or bleeding requiring a transfusion of 2 or more units of blood. These risks are independent of the magnitude of pulmonary artery pressure and are similar to those without pulmonary embolism. The complications are however more in those referred from medical intensive care units than from elsewhere. Renal complications are more frequent in elderly patients than among young subjects.[94,95] Finding of constant intraluminal filling defects in several films or a sharp cutoffs in vessels greater than 2.5 mm in diameter are definite criteria of diagnosing pulmonary embolism. Reduced perfusion, peripheral pruning (a well-visualized artery with a paucity of small branches in comparison to similar sized arteries in other parts of the lung), oligemia, and loss of filling of small vessels are nonspecific. Other abnormalities include asymmetrical filling, prolongation of the arterial phase, and bilateral lower lobe delay are seen in some patients, but are nonspecific. *Digital subtraction angiography* has the potential advantage of allowing more peripheral injections of lesser contrast volumes. Although the frequency of pulmonary embolism is very low following a normal angiogram, there is a real and measurable rate of clinically important pulmonary embolism over the subsequent 12 months, and that is higher than reported in the general population.[96]

Stein, et al[97] have described a strategy for diagnosis of patients with suspected acute pulmonary embolism based on clinical evaluation, lung scans, and noninvasive tests for deep venous thrombosis.

Recently, experimental and clinical studies have described the ability of pulmonary intravascular ultrasound to diagnose both acute and chronic pulmonary embolism.[98,99] The course and fate of embolus can also be followed by these methods. Other noninvasive techniques that have been suggested to refine the accuracy of patient exclusion include the evaluation of D-dimer test,[100,101] and thrombin-antithrombin complexes.[102,103] If these are normal, they are highly suggestive for the absence of pulmonary embolism.[100-103]

D-DIMER TEST

Initially, elevated levels of fibrin split products (FSPs) were considered to be suggestive of pulmonary embolism. These tests were of high sensitivity, but low specificity, and therefore were not useful clinically. These tests were sensitive to fibrinogen and its degradation products, and thus were not specific for fibrin derivatives. Newer tests involving an immunoassay using monoclonal antibodies to specifically measure cross-linked fibrin derivatives in plasma are specific for d-dimer and other larger cross-linked fibrin derivatives. Two types of tests are available for this estimation: enzyme-linked immunosorbent (ELISA) assay and the rapid latex agglutination test. The advantage of the latex agglutination test is that it can be performed rapidly, whereas the standard ELISA test for d-dimer requires several hours. The sensitivity of d-dimer by ELISA test greatly exceeds that of the rapid latex agglutination test; 100 percent vs 73 percent. The negative predictive value of a normal d-dimer test result is greater in patients with a low clinical probability of venous thromboembolism.

ECHOCARDIOGRAPHY

Echocardiography is one of the tests to evaluate patients with suspected pulmonary embolism. Right ventricular dilatation and paradoxical septal motion are noted on echocardiography in patients with pulmonary embolism. M-mode echocardiography is a good modality to detect these changes. Doppler echocardiography will further enhance the detection of abnormalities. In critically ill patients, bedside transesophageal echocardiography will help in identifying a number of abnormalities.

Various echocardiographic findings that can be observed in acute pulmonary embolism include:

Abnormality	Percentage
Dilatation of right pulmonary artery	77
Dilated right ventricle	75
↓E/F slope of mitral valve	50
↓Left ventricular dimension	42
Abnormal intraventricular septal motion	40
Embolus in right pulmonary artery	10
Thrombus in right atrium or right ventricle	4
Normal echocardiogram	19

Echocardiography is a noninvasive test and can be performed at the bedside of critically ill patients. It is valuable in the evaluation of patients suspected of acute pulmonary embolism. A normal echocardiogram finding does not exclude the presence of pulmonary embolism. But findings of the above-mentioned abnormalities can lead to further diagnostic evaluations. Transesophageal echocardiography detection of emboli in the central pulmonary circulation may prove to be highly specific for pulmonary embolism, although the sensitivity of this finding and its validation by pulmonary angiography remain to be determined. The detection of thrombus in the right heart is a clear indication of treatment. Further, evaluation of right ventricular size and contractility are useful indicators of hemodynamic severity of pulmonary embolism. Some investigators suggest that right ventricular hypokinesia is an indication for thrombolytic treatment, and echocardiography is a good modality to detect this abnormality.

Palla, et al[65] have suggested a flow chart for clinical practice in diagnosing pulmonary embolism. All patients with unexplained dyspnea or chest pain should undergo perfusion lung scintigraphy. This is the most important step to improve the detection and treatment of this condition. These two alone has a sensitivity of 97 percent and a specificity of 10 percent. If within 1 hour, no invasive test is possible, then arterial blood gas analysis, electrocardiogram, and chest X-ray should be obtained. They will increase the specificity to 24 percent. If still perfusion scans are not available (within 24 hours), high probability suspicion with clinical data and other noninvasive tests will enhance the specificity to 92 percent. However, at any of these three levels of suspicion, if available, perfusion lung scintigraphy should be carried out.

OTHER TECHNIQUES

Some other tests under investigations for diagnosing pulmonary embolism include, radiolabeled platelets, angioscopy, chest computed tomography scanning with contrast, and perhaps magnetic resonance imaging. Transthoracic parenchymal sonography of the lung in patients with pulmonary embolism (PE) will show characteristic multiple, hypoechoic, pleural-based, wedge-shaped or rounded parenchymal lesions, which generally are well-demarcated from the surrounding tissue that are observed in cases of PE.[104,105]

Spiral CT (SCT)

Spiral CT (SCT) is a cost-effective strategy in the diagnosis of pulmonary embolism, However, the specificity and sensitivity of SCT have been shown to vary widely when compared to angiography or a "gold standard" obtained with ventilation/perfusion scintigraphy.[106-109] The clinical validity of a negative SCT is similar to that of angiography.[110-114] However, systematic review of sensitivity and specificity of SCT showed that the use of SCT in the diagnosis of pulmonary embolism has not yet been adequately evaluated.[115] A recent report suggests that the rate of recurrence after a negative spiral CT angiographic finding varied between 1.8 percent and 4.9 percent. The authors concluded that SCT angiography can be used confidently to rule out significant pulmonary embolism, and further investigations may not be necessary.[115]

Chest CT scanning (CT angiography) offers many advantages in the diagnosis of pulmonary embolism. It directly identifies the pulmonary embolus as an intraluminal filling defect within a pulmonary artery. It is in direct contrast to the detection of pulmonary embolism without infarction by plain radiograph where the main evidence of pulmonary embolism is the appearance of an avascular area. The advantage over V/Q scan and pulmonary angiography is the ability to identify other conditions that may have symptom and signs suggestive of pulmonary embolism, like congestive cardiac failure, pulmonary fibrosis, pneumonia, chest trauma, malignancy, pleural disease, and postoperative changes in the lungs. However, this may lead to unnecessary work up of relatively benign conditions. The greatest advantage is that the test can be done quickly in critically ill patients. The ideal circumstance for chest CT scanning in diagnosing pulmonary embolism is in critically ill patients with shock and/or acute cor pulmonale. A normal CT scan in this situation essentially rules out central pulmonary embolism as the cause of the patient's signs and symptoms (Fig. 19.1 to 19.4).

However, a normal CT scan does not rule out pulmonary embolism, especially if the emboli are limited to the subsegmental arteries. This is one of the greatest limitations of the test.

DVT

Since a clear relationship has been established between pulmonary embolism and deep vein thrombosis, looking for DVT now has been integrated into the diagnostic algorithms for patients with suspected pulmonary embolism.[116-127] The prevalence of DVT in patients with confirmed pulmonary embolism is subject to discrepancies that are mostly due to the procedure employed to diagnose pulmonary embolism and DVT. Compression duplex ultrasonography (CDUS) is a safe tool that is used routinely in patients with suspected venous thromboembolism. Among patients with confirmed pulmonary embolism, 15 to 50 percent presented with a DVT that was diagnosed by CDUS. The sensitivity decreases in asymptomatic patients and is weak for the detection of pelvic DVT (from the external iliac vein to the inferior vena cava). Contrast venography, a more invasive test, detected DVT in 70 to 80 percent of cases with confirmed pulmonary embolism. As for CDUS, the exploration of pelvic veins by venography is imperfect.

In some studies, magnetic resonance angiography (MRA) has been evaluated for the diagnosis of lower limb DVT. In patients with clinically suspected DVT, MRA seemed to be accurate, showing a 95 to 100 percent sensitivity and 80 to 100 percent specificity for the detection of DVT. Furthermore, in 25 patients with femoroiliocaval venous thrombosis, MRA demonstrated 100 percent sensitivity and 98.5 percent specificity compared with contrast venography. Among patients with negative findings on CDUS, a substantial proportion of the DVTs that are responsible for pulmonary embolism, originates in the pelvic veins. MRA disclosed pelvic DVT in about a third of cases when the traditional investigations were negative. The common iliac vein is the commonest site followed by Internal iliac veins (hypogastric).

Establishing a diagnosis of deep venous thrombosis, is a significant contribution to the suspicion of pulmonary embolism in appropriate clinical setting. Negative studies of the leg veins could rule out the diagnosis of embolism in an embolic suspect because most emboli originate from them.[128-132] However, about a third of the patients with acute embolism may have negative venous studies. There are three techniques that have been useful in the diagnosis of deep venous thrombosis of the lower extremities. They are contrast venography,[128] impedance plethysmography,[129] and radiofibrinogen leg scanning.[130] There are difficulties in interpreting these test results. However, it has been suggested that the combination of impedance plethysmography,[133] and radiofibrinogen leg scanning is an excellent noninvasive diagnostic approach for the detection of deep vein thrombosis in the lower extremities. If both tests are negative, venous thrombosis is excluded. If equivocal results are obtained, venography will be necessary. Serial impedance plethysmography over a two-week period is equally useful. Using venography as the gold standard, impedance plethysmography has an overall sensitivity of 93 percent and specificity of 95 percent for the diagnosis of proximal, occlusive deep vein thrombosis.[134] However, recently ultrasound is the preferred noninvasive test for deep vein thrombosis, because of higher sensitivity and specificity compared to impedance plethysmography.[135-138]

Palla, et al[65] have suggested a flow chart for clinical practice in diagnosing pulmonary embolism (see above). All patients with otherwise unexplained dyspnea or chest pain should undergo lung scintigraphy. This is the most important step to improve the detection and treatment of pulmonary embolism. Stein, et al[139] reported that asymmetry of the calves of 1 cm or more is abnormal although such asymmetry did not distinguish between patients with pulmonary embolism and those without pulmonary embolism. However, when considered in proper perspective with other nonspecific signs and symptoms in patients with suspected acute pulmonary embolism, the presence of such a sign should call attention to a possibility of pulmonary embolism and more noninvasive tests are needed. In recent years, more sonograms are performed compared to fewer angiograms and venograms compared to investigations in earlier years. Henschke, et al[140] recommend that better diagnostic screening approaches with more explicit guidelines need to be developed that take into account the local disease prevalence and hospital diagnostic and practice patterns. Other helpful tests that may provide important clues to the diagnosis, but are not routinely used.[141,142]

Outcome of pulmonary embolism. The natural history of untreated pulmonary embolism is well documented in earlier years when angiography was not in use and before the universal use of anticoagulants.[143,144] Hermann, et al[144] from autopsy studies reported a mortality of 37 percent from the initial pulmonary embolism. The frequency of recurrent pulmonary embolism in their series was 36 percent which were fatal, and nonfatal recurrent embolism was observed in 21 percent of patients. Barritt and Jordan[143] reported a mortality of 26 percent among untreated patients, although some of them might be having recurrent pulmonary embolism. In a recent report, Stein, et al concluded that mild untreated pulmonary embolism carries a lower immediate mortality (5%) from recurrent pulmonary embolism than overt embolism described in

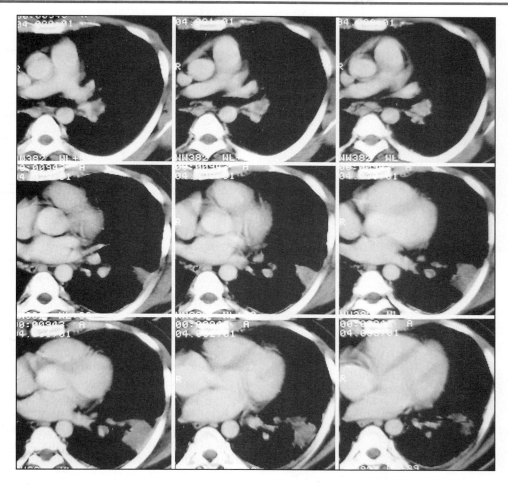

FIGURE 19.1: CT Chest - Hypodense thrombus in left segmental pulomonary artery and classical distal wedge shaped pleural based lesion-pulmonary infarct

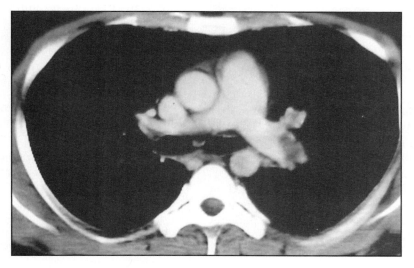

FIGURE 19.2: CT Chest - Left main pulmonary artery embolism

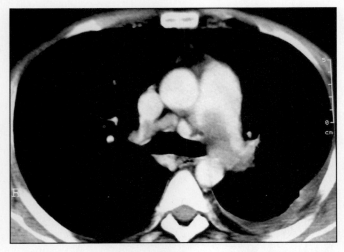

FIGURE 19.3: CT Chest - Thrombus in left main pulmonary artery

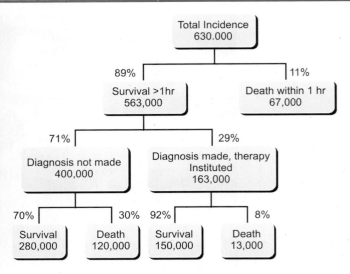

TREATMENT

Because of the high mortality rate (30-35%) in patients with untreated acute pulmonary embolism, therapy should be initiated when pulmonary embolism is seriously considered. The diagnosis can be confirmed by a positive pulmonary angiogram or chest CT finding or a high-probability ventilation/perfusion ($\dot{V}/\dot{Q}$) scan result. Echocardiographic evidence of intracardiac thrombus or thrombus in the central pulmonary arteries with echocardiographic evidence of right ventricular dilatation also confirms the diagnosis of pulmonary embolism. Deep venous thrombosis can be confirmed by venography, compression ultrasonography, or impedance plethysmography. Table 19.6 shows when to treat or not to treat venous thromboembolism.[148]

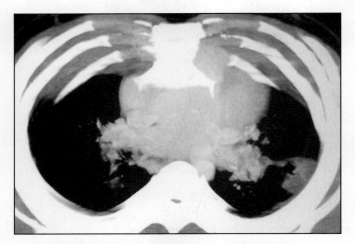

FIGURE 19.4: SSD reconstruction CT showing thrombus in left segmental pulmonary artery with distal wedge shaped pulmonary infarct

prior decade.[145] Nonfatal recurrent pulmonary embolism occurred in 5 percent. This lower mortality in mild pulmonary embolism is comparable to the fatal pulmonary embolism in untreated patients with subtle deep venous thrombosis, about 5 percent.[146]

The outcome of pulmonary embolism, if treated, is quite promising. Of an estimated 200,000 deaths per year in the United States, only 13,000 (6%) occur in patients who have received treatment. The vast majority of patients (94%) who die of pulmonary embolism do not receive treatment because the diagnosis is not made.[147] This is summarized as follows:

TABLE 19.6: When to treat or to withhold therapy for pulmonary embolism

Treat for venous thromboembolism
- Positive pulmonary angiogram, positive CT scan of chest, or high probability V/Q scan
- Echocardiac evidence of intracardiac thrombus
- Echocardiographic evidence of clot in main pulmonary artery, right pulmonary artery, or left pulmonary artery, and right ventricular dilatation
- Diagnosis of DVT by venography, compression ultrasonography, or impedance plethysmography

To withhold therapy
- Normal pulmonary angiogram or normal perfusion scan findings
- Low clinical probability of pulmonary embolism plus
  — Normal d-dimer, or
  — Normal compression ultrasound of legs, or
  — Indeterminate V/Q scan, or
  — Normal chest CT findings

The treatment of pulmonary embolism consists of:
- Thrombolytic therapy
- Anticoagulant therapy
- Surgery.

Each of these modalities has their own indications.

Thrombolytic Therapy[59,60,149]

This is not needed when the acute embolism is minor or even in massive pulmonary embolism (more than 50 percent obstruction of pulmonary arterial bed on angiography) unless there is considerable hemodynamic embarrassment. These patients do well with heparin alone, which reduces the chances of further embolism. Natural thrombolytic processes will remove thrombus from the circulation. Thrombolytic therapy neither improves early mortality nor improves long-term clinical results, although minor abnormalities of pulmonary function due to capillary damage in the form of reduced diffusing capacity, is less. However, such minor abnormalities are otherwise not important. The indications of thrombolytic therapy are (i) sustained hypotension, (ii) peripheral circulatory failure, (iii) poor urine flow, (iv) severe hypoxia and (v) possibly echocardiographic evidence of right ventricular dysfunction. Streptokinase, urokinase, and tissue plasminogen activator are the usual thrombolytic agents. Following a loading dose of about 250,000 units of streptokinase over a period of 1/2 hour to neutralize anti-bodies from previous streptococcal infection, a constant infusion of 100,000 units per hour is administered for 48 to 72 hours. Urokinase has the advantage of directly activating plasminogen to plasmin without prior forma-tion of a urokinase-plasminogen complex. However, the drug is more expensive and less widely available. Recombinant human tissue-type plasminogen activator (rt-PA) have been used in a dose of 100 mg given over 2 hours or reduced dose of bolus rt-PA can be given in a dose of 0.6 mg/kg with a maximum of 50 mg over 15 minutes.[150,151] Some attention is being paid recently on the use of bolus and accelerated thrombolysis both in experimental animals and clinical use in myocardial infarction and pulmonary embolism.[152,153] The time window for administering thrombolytic therapy appears to be at least 14 days after symptoms or signs of pulmonary embolism. However it has been shown that patients receiving such therapy 6 to 14 days after embolism do as good as those receiving such therapy 0-5 days after pulmonary embolism.[150,151,154,155] Bleeding episodes both fatal and nonfatal are important side effects of thrombolytic therapy. The drugs act by selec-tively lysing fibrin. Following completion of thrombolytic therapy, heparin should only be started without a loading dose 4 hours later or when the thrombin time has fallen to less than twice of the normal value. The disadvantages of thrombolytic therapy include the high cost and potential of bleeding complications. Moreover, these drugs are dangerous within the first week of major trauma or surgery. The FDA, USA has approved the following regimens of thrombolytic therapy. They are shown in Table 19.7. The fourth ACCP Consensus Conference on Antithrombotic therapy, 1995 has appro-ved the same.[156] The conference has also given guidelines for anticoagulation.

TABLE 19.7: Recommended dosage of thrombolytic agents[156,167]

Stop heparin infusion: Start thrombolytic infusion when APTT or thrombin time (TT) is equal or < 1.5 times control.

Streptokinase: 250,000 IU as a loading dose over 30 minutes followed by 100,000 IU/hour for 24 hours (pulmonary embolism, 48-72 hours deep venous thrombosis).

Urokinase: 4,400 IU/kg as a loading dose over 10 minutes, followed by 4,400 IU/kg /hour for 12 hours (pulmonary embolism; 24-48 hours deep venous thrombosis).

rt-PA: 100 mg (56 million IU) as a continuous peripheral intravenous infusion administered over 2 hours. The drug has recently been used in a reduced dosage (see above).

After terminating thrombolytic infusion, restart heparin infusion without a loading dose or with a small loading dose when APTT or TT equal or < 1.5 times control.

All the three drugs are used in a fixed or weight adjusted doses. Therefore there is no need to obtain laboratory tests during therapy since no dose adjustment is needed. Locally administered rt-PA through pulmo-nary artery has no advantage over systemically adminis-tered drug. Recently, a new thrombolytic agent, saruplase has been tried in small number of patients which showed a fast and highly significant hemodynamic and angio-graphic improvement.[158] Patients with high clinical suspicion of pulmonary embolism and a high-probability ventilation-perfusion scan can receive thrombolytic therapy without angiographic confirmation of the diagnosis. However, angiography should be performed in non-high-probability scans prior to administration of thrombolytic therapy. None of these regimens require concomitant heparin therapy, which is an usual approach to thrombolysis in myocardial infarction. At the conclusion of thrombolytic infusion, a partial thromboplastin time (PTT) should be obtained. If the test result is less than 80 seconds, heparin therapy can be initiated or resumed as a continuous infusion, without a loading dose. If it exceeds 80 seconds, the test should be repeated after 4 hours.[157] Some other practical aspects of thrombolytic therapy include to take a careful neurological history of transient ischemic attacks, headache etc. to exclude patients of possible bleed. Before starting therapy, blood cross matching should be made with Arrangement of immediate availability of blood for transfusion. Initiation of therapy should be started during daylight. Physical handling of the patient should be minimal and drawing of blood during the period of thrombolytic therapy should be avoided as far as possible. Concomitant heparin should not be administered and the guidelines outlined above should be followed. Although it has been suggested that direct delivery of standard doses of thrombolytic agents into the pulmonary artery is no more efficacious than systemic delivery,[159] recent experimental studies using animal models suggest that placing an infusion catheter into the pulmonary artery and infusing less than 20 percent of systemic doses of urokinase, will enhance the thrombolysis by a combination of mechanical and pharmacological action.[84]

Anticoagulant Therapy

Anticoagulant therapy is to be instituted as soon as a diagnosis of pulmonary embolism is strongly suspected.[160] Intravenous bolus heparin in a dose of 10,000 IU should be given in an average sized adult (except when the patient is on thrombolytic therapy, see above). The object of heparin therapy is to give enough doses to prevent recurrent thrombosis and embolism while avoiding hemorrhagic complications. However, early recurrence can develop in spite of heparin therapy under two circumstances: (i) residual venous thrombi can detach while in their early, fragile, nonorganized phase; and (ii) retention of some embolic material in the right atrium and/or right ventricle is common, which serve as potential sources of recurrences. Despite these limitations, heparin is the most efficacious therapy available. It exerts an immediate and substantial antithrombotic effect. Its major action is to alter the conformation of antithrombin 3, thereby allowing this inhibitor to combine with, and more effectively inactivating thrombin (factor 2A) and factor 10A. Its effect on platelet is less striking and thus is maximally active in the presence of antithrombin 3. Both intermittent therapy (usually four hourly) and continuous infusions have been used. Recently the later is being used more often because of less hemorrhagic complications. The usual dose is about 1250 units per hour by infusion, after the loading dose of 10,000 units. The hemorrhagic complications occur in about 5 to 20 percent of cases. However, with proper monitoring of the dose by clotting tests will avoid these. The commonly used ones include activated partial thromboplastin time, thrombin time, and Lee-White clotting time. The aim is to maintain a plasma level of heparin at 0.3 to 0.4 units/ml. The most convenient one is the bedside determination of clotting time. For optimal effects the activated partial thromboplastin time should be maintained at 1.5 to 2.5 times the control value. The most important complicating factors responsible for bleeding complications include age over 60 years, uraemia, a preexisting hemorrhagic defect, severe hypertension, recent surgery, previous gastrointestinal hemorrhage, and major pulmonary embolism. Dose of heparin is another important risk factor. The recommended duration of heparin therapy is 7 to 10 days with oral anticoagulants overlapping which is continued for a variable period.

Continuation of anticoagulation therapy beyond 7 to 10 days is necessary to prevent recurrent venous thrombosis. This is conveniently achieved by oral warfarin sodium although low dose subcutaneous heparin therapy will serve the same purpose. Coumarin drugs act by inhibiting the synthesis of vitamin K dependent clotting factors 2, 7, 9, and 10. An effective antithrombotic state takes several days to develop because of slow fall in some coagulation factors. The dose is 5 to 10 mg warfarin sodium daily depending on age, body mass and hepatic status, from the second day of heparin therapy. Prothrombin time is measured after few hours after stopping heparin therapy. Further dose **of** warfarin is adjusted on the basis of daily prothrombin time measurements. Once stable at 1.5 to 2.5 times the control value, such measurements can be made at weekly to monthly intervals. The duration of anticoagulation is determined by the risk of recurrence. With short-term risk factors, like immobilization and surgery, 1 to 3 months of therapy is recommended. In those having persistent risk factors or recurrent thromboembolism therapy may be continued indefinitely.

Monitoring of Oral Anticoagulant Therapy

Earlier, prothrombin time was utilized in monitoring the intensity of oral anticoagulant therapy. The goal was to reduce prothrombin time to 20 percent of normal activity. The prothrombin time was prolonged to 30 to 35 seconds, with a normal control of 14 to 16 seconds. This corresponds to a prothrombin time ratio, PTR (patient/control) of 1.9 to 2.5. The usual goal used to be a PTR of 1.5 to 2.5 times control. However, because of variability in the sensitivity of thromboplastin used for determining the prothrombin time, as a result of different sources in different countries, it was recommended that all PTRs are to be reported as International Normalized Ratio (INR).

The obtained PTR is converted to an INR by increasing the PTR to the power of the sensitivity (International Sensitivity Index, ISI) of the thromboplastin that was used in the test. Thus;

INR = (Observed PTR) [ISI]

If an ISI of 1 is used, then INR = PTR.

In clinical practice, the targeted goal is for an INR of 2.0 to 3.0.[161]

These drugs are not without serious side effects. The most serious and important complication of all the above drugs is bleeding. Careful monitoring of the above parameters during surgery, and avoidance of invasive procedures during such therapy minimizes risk. Streptokinase can produce allergic reactions that can be managed with hydrocortisone or promethazine. Antiplatelet drugs and antithrombin drugs should not be given simultaneously with streptokinase. There are some case reports of reperfusion pulmonary edema following thrombolytic therapy. Less common side effects of heparin include thrombocytopenia and osteopenia. Protamine sulfate is the antidote for heparin. Warfarin may cause skin necrosis. Anticoagulation therapy during pregnancy is complicated by spontaneous abortion and embryopathy.

Recently, low molecular weight derivatives of heparin have become available for clinical use. These are fractions of commercial heparin produced by controlled depolymerization of unfractionated heparin, with a mean molecular weight of 4000 to 5000 daltons. They have antifactor Xa activity similar to that of heparin, but have little effect on aPTT and thrombin clotting time. The advantages of these substances are many over unfractionated or conventional heparin. Their pharmacokinetics is more predictable and the elimination half-life is longer than standard heparin. They can be administered in fixed doses and do not require laboratory monitoring. Further, there are other limitations of unfractionated heparin. Heparin binds to plasma resulting in poor availability at low doses, dose response is variable, there is a possibility of heparin resistance, heparin/antithrombin III complex is unable to access thrombin bound to fibrin and factor Xa bound to platelets, and heparin impairs platelet function which contributes to its effect on hemostasis. These limitations of heparin are not shared by the low molecular weight heparins. Therefore, they are excellent candidates for the treatment of venous thromboembolism. The efficacy and safety of low molecular weight heparin have been proved in prospective randomized trials in submassive pulmonary embolism. The dose used is 160 IU/kg. They also can be used for prophylaxis of thromboembolism when given once or twice daily without laboratory monitoring. They

produce less bleeding than unfractionated heparin for an equivalent antithrombotic effect.[162-165]

Several antithrombin III-independent thrombin inhibitors are now available.[166] These include hirudin, hirudin fragments (hirugen, hirulog), and small molecular weight peptides including argatroban, the chloromethylketone inhibitor, D-phe-pro-argCH2CL (PPACK), and their derivatives. Recently two antithrombin-independent factor Xa inhibitors are also available-a tick anticoagulant peptide (TPA) and a leech anticoagulant peptide (Antistasin). These drugs are not yet available foe extensive clinical use in pulmonary thromboembolism.[167]

SURGERY[168-170]

In massive embolism producing sufficient cardiopulmonary compromise, besides thrombolytic therapy and heparin, two other options are available. One is the placement of a filter in the inferior vena cava to prevent recurrence, or acute pulmonary embolectomy. Although attractive, few patients will qualify for the later procedure and the mortality is very high.

Various inferior vena cava interruption procedures include ligation, suture grid, suture plication, stapler plication, and various transvenously inserted intraluminal filters. However the role of caval interruption procedures remain controversial. Most currently preferred method is the insertion of a Greenfield filter. The expertise of the operator is more important than the choice of the device being used.

Selected patients with chronic pulmonary embolism and symptoms of severe respiratory insufficiency, hypoxemia, and pulmonary hypertension with proximal pulmonary obstruction and adequate bronchial circulation, and with minimally impaired right ventricular function are appropriate candidates for surgical embolectomy. However, patients having this syndrome but distal pulmonary emboli in small arterial branches with patent proximal vessels are generally not suitable for surgical embolectomy. Similarly patients with severe right ventricular failure, massive obesity, severe coronary artery disease, and renal insufficiency are not suitable candidates. Such patients may be considered for heart-lung transplantation. Long-term follow-up of patients with operable pulmonary emboli show favorable cardiorespiratory changes.

Pulmonary thromboendarterectomy results in restoration of normal or near-normal pulmonary hemodynamic, when it is complicated by chronic thromboembolic pulmonary hypertension (CTEPH), even in the presence of severe pulmonary hypertension or right-sided heart failure.[171,172] The risk of recurrence is low, since patients generally have preoperative placement of an inferior vena cava filter and are treated indefinitely with oral anticoagulants once surgery has been performed.[173] In experienced centers, the mortality has been ≤ 5 percent.[171,172] Continuous intravenous epoprostenol (prostacycline) has been used as a "medical bridge" to stabilize such patients prior to surgery.[174,175]

PROPHYLAXIS

Several effective and safe prophylactic modalities are now available. These methods may prevent the development of deep venous thrombosis or may prevent extension of calf thrombi upwards. The important thing is to identify the persons who are at increased risk. There are strong associations between thromboembolism and increasing age over 40 years, bed rest for longer than 4 days, major surgery or trauma, disseminated malignancy, recent myocardial infarction, recent stroke, oral contraceptives, and previous thromboembolism.[176,177] Various forms of prophylaxis that can be used include application of intermittent venous compression pneumatic devices of different types to the lower extremities, passive compression stockings, and active movement of the lower extremities against the bed. The other prophylactic options include "low-dose" heparin therapy and warfarin sodium. The low-dose heparin therapy is an effective and safe approach to prophylaxis when the patient is in the low or moderate risk of developing deep venous thrombosis. The standard regimen consists of 5000 units of heparin subcutaneously every 8 to 12 hours starting at the time of risk (2 hours before surgery) and continuing till the patient is ambulatory. The risk is minimum even in surgical patients, although it is increased in prostatic surgery. Low molecular weight heparin can also be used for this purpose.[178] Some studies indicate that warfarin in small doses of 1 to 2 mg before surgery, may be useful in high-risk patients. Hip replacement and hip fractures are more often associated with proximal thrombosis. These patients are frequently given prophylactic heparin or warfarin. A number of other agents including aspirin, sulfinpyrazone, and dextran have been suggested for venous prophylaxis, although adequate clinical data on their efficacy is lacking. In a study of 900 patients, it was concluded that six months of prophylactic oral anticoagulation (warfarin or dicumarol) after a first episode of venous thromboembolism led to a lower recurrence rate than did treatment lasting for six weeks.[179]

Standard treatment for proximal deep vein thrombosis has been infusion of unfractionated heparin administered during a hospital admission of approximately 5 to 7 days. With the advent of low-molecular-weight heparin (LMWH), outpatient heparin treatment has become feasible because of more predictable anticoagulant response and administration via subcutaneous injection.[180] A Canadian randomized clinical trial established the safety and efficacy of treating acute proximal DVT with enoxaparin, a LMWH, administered primarily at home relative to unfractionated heparin administered in the hospital.[181] Retrospective replication of the Canadian study in a US routine care setting found similar clinical and economic outcomes.[182] Initial anticoagulant therapy of intravenous unfractionated heparin administered in the hospital or subcutaneous LMWH (enoxaparin) administered primarily at home, followed by warfarin therapy for at least 3 months (target International Normalization Ration, INR), no statistically significant differences were observed in the number of recurrent venous thromboembolic events or bleeding events.

Because the risk of hemorrhage rises exponentially with rising values of the international normalized ratio (INR)[183-185] experts agree that the dose of warfarin sodium should be decreased when the INR exceeds 4 or 5.[186,187] However, there is no consensus on warfarin dose reductions for asymptomatic INRs that are only slightly supratherapeutic. For example, consider a patient with a target INR of 2.5 who presents with an asymptomatic INR in the range of 3.2 to 3.4. Some experts would continue the current dose[187-190] while others would reduce the weekly warfarin dose by 2 to 4 percent,[191] 5 to 15 percent[192-194] or 13 to 18 percent.[195] How these opposing strategies affect the subsequent INR is unknown.

Determining the treatment patterns for mild INR elevations and associated follow-up INRs and risk of hemorrhage is important and timely. First, mild elevations may preceed greater INRs with a higher risk of hemorrhage. Second, because the INR is > 5 only 1 percent of the time[196] most iatrogenic hemorrhages occur at INRs < 5.[183-185] Third, as patient self-monitoring[197] grows in popularity, it will be important to have validated protocols that can guide self-dosing.

Some protocols[187] advocate that the warfarin dose need not be reduced for isolated, asymptomatic INRs of ≤ 3.4. A recent report suggest that same warfarin dose can be maintained in asymptomatic patients with an INR of 3.3, and reducing the dose for patients who have a greater INR or an increased risk of hemorrhage. Warfarin dose reductions > 20 percent should be avoided for mildly elevated INRs.[198]

Thrombosis of the superior vena cava (SVC) is an uncommon cause of SVC syndrome.[199] Rarely, pulmonary embolism with the SVC syndrome has been observed at autopsy.[200,201] There are also occasional case reports in living patients.[202,203] In addition, one case of pulmonary embolism due to brachiocephalic vein thrombosis has been reported.[204] In view of the frequent use of central venous access lines, and the known association of such instrumentation with thrombosis,[205-207] it would seem that thrombotic involvement of the brachiocephalic veins and SVC should be diagnosed more frequently than is generally believed. In a recent report[208] the authors evaluated the frequency of diagnosis and the characteristics of thromboembolic disease involving the brachiocephalic vein and SVC in a community/teaching hospital to test the hypothesis that such disease merits consideration, particularly in patients with cancer and in those with central venous access lines. Thromboembolic disease of the brachiocephalic veins or SVC was diagnosed in 23 of 34,567 hospitalized 20 years old. Two of 23 patients (8.7%) had pulmonary embolism. Cancer was present in 17 of 23 patients (74%), and 15 of 23 patients (65%) had central venous access lines. Edema of the arm, face, or neck was present in 21 of 23 patients (91%). Pain or discomfort was present 15 of 23 patients (65%).

Isolated brachiocephalic vein and SVC thrombosis occur in a sufficient number of hospitalized patients to merit consideration of the diagnosis in patients who have cancer, central venous access lines, or both. The signs and symptoms of brachiocephalic vein thrombosis have features in common with SVC syndrome as well as with upper extremity deep venous thrombosis. In a patient with appropriate clinical findings, venography or other imaging may be indicated.

(B) NONTHROMBOTIC PULMONARY EMBOLISM

Substances arising from extravascular sources may rarely cause pulmonary embolism. These include fat embolism, tumor embolism, air embolism, and amniotic fluid or placental trophoblastic tissue embolism.

Fat Embolism

Trauma-related fat embolism is defined by the blockage of blood vessels from fat globules that are usually released from traumatic or iatrogenic injury to the long bones. Fat embolism develops in nearly all patients with bone fractures or during orthopedic procedures.[209,210] Rarely, fat embolism may occur in other nontrauma-related pathologic conditions such as pancreatitis and sickle cell disease. Fat embolism is usually asymptomatic, but in the minority of the patients symptoms and signs develop as a result of dysfunction of several organs,

notably of the lungs, brain, and skin, in which case the term *fat embolism syndrome* (FES) is reserved. FES most commonly is associated with long bone and pelvic fractures, and is more frequent in closed, rather than open, fractures. Patients with long-bone fractures have a 1 to 20 percent chance of acquiring the syndrome. However, the true incidence of FES is rather unknown because mild cases may be unnoticed. Although the incidence of fat embolism syndrome remains uncertain, the incidence after long bone fracture may range from less than 5 percent to 35 percent[211] and may be as high as 40 percent as reported during the Korean War.[1] This wide variation in the incidence of the condition probably results from difference in the criteria used for its diagnosis and the difference in the study population. The presence or absence of associated injuries of the head, chest, or abdomen, or the number of fractures may affect the incidence. In the prospective study of Chan, et al the incidence was 8.75 percent with single fractured shaft of the femur or tibia, but increased to 35 percent in patients with multiple fractures.[212] Opening the fracture promptly and evacuation of hematoma will reduce the incidence of fat embolism syndrome.[213]

The pathogenesis of FES remains controversial, and several theories have been proposed.[214] The lung is the most frequently affected organ, but reported incidence of pulmonary fat embolism varies considerably between different series. It is reported that some degree of pulmonary fat embolism regularly follows long-bone injury. The clinical syndrome, however, is reported to develop between 0.5 percent and 2 percent following fractures of the long bones (particularly the shafts of femurs and the tibias), reaching 5 to 10 percent after multiple fractures including the pelvis with occasional visualization of fat droplets in veins by imaging techniques.

It is believed that the organ dysfunction in FES is the result of the direct entry of depot fat globules from disrupted tissue into the bloodstream, or of the production of toxic intermediaries of plasma-derived fat such as chylomicrons or infused lipids.[210,214] The 24 to 72 hrs delay in syndrome appearance after the insult indicates the production of toxic intermediaries as the predominant pathogenetic mechanism. Fracture of the proximal segment of the femoral shaft, just cranial to the isthmus, is the commonest cause of fat embolism syndrome. At this location there are many venous sinusoids within the marrow with large capillaries that do not have any wall musculature. This structural peculiarity is responsible for large quantity of marrow fat release into the venous circulation from this location. Following osseous trauma, neutral fat may enter into the circulation from injured long bones and are lodged in the pulmonary circulation.[215] Although neutral fat is harmless, hydrolysis to fatty acids by pulmonary lipase are highly toxic to the lungs and cause hemorrhage and pulmonary edema. A complex interaction of marrowfat embolized to pulmonary capillaries along with platelets, leukocytes and free fatty acid lead onto pulmonary capillary leak with flooding of alveolar spaces. Histopathological changes are same as those observed in ARDS. The only difference is the presence of massive amounts of fat in the pulmonary tissues and cells as demonstrated by specific stains for neutral fat. There is a latent period of few hours to several days from the time of trauma to the onset of adult respiratory distress syndrome type of manifestation because of the chemical phase. Release of various vasoactive substances or mediators by local aggregation of platelets and leukocytes contribute further to the capillary leak syndrome. Further evidence of local inflammatory changes come from the bronchoalveolar lavage findings.[216]

Fat embolism occurs in nearly all patients (> 90%) with bone fractures during orthopedic prosthesis procedures and rarely in other pathologic conditions.[217,218] Although fat emboli can virtually reach any organ in the body, the results of the embolic shower are most often evident in the lungs, brain, and skin as discussed above. Approximately 3 to 4 percent will acquire the classical triad of the fat embolism syndrome (FES), which consists of respiratory distress, cerebral abnormalities, and petechial hemorrhages, while the rest of the patients will remain asymptomatic.[217,219] Clinically severe cases make up 10 to 20 percent of all patients in whom the diagnosis can be made,[217,219] and have been associated with mortality rates as high as 20 percent in some series.[222] Diagnosis is crucial; it is mainly based on clinical criteria and may be masked by associated pathology especially in the multitrauma victim. Imaging plays a key role in the differential diagnosis and assists in the recognition of FES. The full-blown picture is termed as the fat embolism syndrome. This must be distinguished from fat embolism often found at autopsy, which is of doubtful significance in the absence of the syndrome.[211] The fat embolism syndrome is a serious but uncommon clinical disorder observed mainly in subjects with serious traumatic injuries. The syndrome manifests primarily as:[220]

- Respiratory failure with bilateral pulmonary infiltrates
- Cerebral disturbances
- Petechial rash.

The spectrum of clinical presentations ranges from minor symptoms and signs to respiratory failure and even death. Classically the full-blown picture develops within 24 to 72 hrs after the initial insult (trauma or orthopedic operation) and consists of fever, hypoxemia, delirium, lipuria, and petechiae. Affected patients present with a classic triad of hypoxemia, neurological abnormalities, and a petechial rash. Respiratory system dysfunction occurs frequently, and its severity may vary ranging from mild, manifested only with dyspnea and/or tachypnea, to severe, characterized by symptoms and signs indistinguishable from ARDS. It has been shown that approximately 50 percent of patients with FES caused by long-bone fractures acquire severe hypoxemia and require mechanical ventilation. Neurologic abnormalities, consisting of altered levels of consciousness, seizures, or focal deficits, develop in the majority of patients with FES and often occur after the development of respiratory system dysfunction.[221,222] The characteristic petechial rash is usually observed on the head, neck, anterior thorax, subconjunctiva, and axillae.[223] One or the other of the above classical triad may be missing. Laboratory tests including the detection of fat globules in the urine and blood or measurements of serum lipase activity are useful but have poor sensitivity and specificity. Arterial hypoxemia with wide alveolar-arterial oxygen gradient following major bone fracture seems to be the most sensitive and accurate indicator for a suspicion of fat embolism syndrome and should be done early after admission and frequently during the next few days in all patients with significant bony trauma.[224] An objective scoring system has been suggested by Schonfeld and colleagues[225] based on seven parameters: petechiae, diffuse alveolar infiltrates, hypoxemia, confusion, fever above 38°C, tachycardia (heart rate > 120/min), and tachypnea (respiratory rate > 30/min). A score of 5 or more is considered as diagnostic of the syndrome. However, the score is not useful in the presence of concomitant major cerebral, thoracic, or abdominal injuries that may give rise to false positive scores. Cytological analysis of blood drawn from a pulmonary artery floatation catheter has recently been used as a useful method to diagnose fat embolism syndrome.[229] It is also possible to study bronchoalveolar lavage fluid for fat globules in patients suspected to have this syndrome.

Clinical diagnosis of cerebral FES can be aided by noting the presence of respiratory failure, hypoxemia, and cutaneous petechiae. The radiologic differential diagnosis includes lung contusion, pulmonary edema, and aspiration. Cerebral CT scan results are usually negative, while MRI, especially diffusion-weighted MRI, is more sensitive.[227-229] Mild cases of respiratory system dysfunction may be associated with normal chest radiographic findings, and this may complicate the interpretation of symptoms and signs reflecting the lung function. BAL has been proposed to detect fat droplets in alveolar macrophages as a means to diagnose FES.[230-232] However, the invasive nature of the procedure limits the usefulness of this technique. In addition, the diagnostic criteria vary considerably between studies while the sensitivity and specificity are unknown. The diagnostic value of noninvasive methods, like induced sputum, have not been evaluated and compared with BAL.

Malagari, et al[233] reported the high-resolution CT (HRCT) findings of the lungs in patients with mild FES. They observed that in these patients HRCT revealed bilateral ground-glass opacities and thickening of the interlobular septa, whereas in some cases centrilobular nodular opacities were present. In most patients, chest radiographic findings were reported normal. The clinical significance of these findings, however, is not clear. FES is a clinical diagnosis; currently, it is not known to what extent high-cost diagnostic tests such as HRCT may improve the accuracy of the clinical examination. Although the authors suggest that HRCT in mild cases of FES may aid in diagnosis prior to development of clinical manifestations, the design of their study does not permit firm conclusions regarding the clinical value of HRCT. HRCT was performed in patients in whom a clinical diagnosis of FES had been made. This precludes any statement as far as the diagnostic role of HRCT is concerned. Furthermore, the specificity and sensitivity of HRCT is not known. At present, the existing data in the literature do not support the routine use of HRCT as a tool to diagnose the respiratory system dysfunction in FES. Further studies with appropriate designs are needed to resolve this issue. Even in the current era of high technology, FES is one of the few pathologic entities that are diagnosed based on readily available clinical criteria. Nevertheless, the study of Malagari, et al[233] may serve as a useful framework to further assess the role of HRCT in diagnosing mild cases of FES. Resolution of the abnormalities occurred within 16.4 days (range, 7 to 25 days). Until the appropriate studies are available, careful clinical examination remains the "gold standard" for diagnosing FES.

The prognosis of fat embolism syndrome varies between 14 to 35 percent. Several studies claim corticosteroids to be effective therapy.[234,235] However, these claims are controversial. Supportive therapy like ventilatory support will be required for respiratory failure.

Tumor emboli occur in over 2 percent of cases in patients dying from solid tumors. Clinical evidence of pulmonary embolism during life is difficult to recognize. Unexplained dyspnea in the absence of obvious chest abnormalities may be a diagnostic clue. Tumors implicated in giving rise to such emboli include carcinoma of breast, stomach, colon, cervix, liver, and choriocarcinomas and hypernephromas.

Air embolism may result from injection of large volumes of air during faulty cannulation of neck veins, and insufflation of fallopian tubes or from intrauterine manipulations. While small amounts are harmless, large volumes may cause mechanical obstruction to pulmonary flow and death. Massive air embolism from CVP line removal particularly following lung transplant may be a problem during clinical practice although these occur rarely.[236-238] Lung transplant patients can generate an enormous negative intrathoracic pressure when the diseased lung is replaced with a normal lung. Treatment of air embolism consists of prompt intervention by manually occluding the tract while turning the patient to the left side with the head down. Intubation with positive airway ventilation to reverse the transthoracic pressure gradient to prevent further air aspiration should be tried, although this may not be always adequate. The mortality of massive air embolism is about 50 percent.[239] Right to left shunting may occur resulting in coronary embolism leading to ventricular fibrillation, or in cerebral embolism resulting in stroke. The problem therefore should be prevented. Care should be taken to avoid air embolism both during line insertion and removal. A trained person should carry out the procedure. The central line needs to be removed with patient in the Trendelenburg position and with the use of an occlusive dressing. If the catheter is large, the tract should be closed with sutures.

PROGNOSIS OF PTE

Although pulmonary thromboembolism (PTE) is associated with high morbidity and mortality rates all over the world, its epidemiology remains unclear. The acute and recurrent nature of the disease, its variable and nonspecific clinical picture, and the difficulty in establishing an accurate diagnosis, even when sophisticated laboratory techniques are used, keep its real incidence unknown and make it difficult to determine if it is the main cause of death or just a co-morbidity or even an incidental finding.[240-242] The most accurate information about incidence, origin of the thrombi, probable causes of thrombosis, and significance of PTE is provided by

`**1216**  Textbook of Pulmonary Medicine`

studies of unselected autopsies performed in general hospitals using rigid and systematic techniques.[244-246] Even though PTE risk factors are widely known,[243,244,247,248] the factors that influence the development of acute episodes of the disease remain unclear. In a recent study from a series of autopsies carried out in a tertiary general medical school (São Paulo, Brazil), the potential PTE prognostic factors was developed using a mathematical model to predict the risk for fatal and nonfatal PTE.[249] The autopsy rate was 50.2 percent, and PTE prevalence was 10.6 percent. In 212 cases, PTE was the main cause of death (fatal PTE). The independent variables selected by the regression significance criteria that were more likely to be associated with fatal PTE were age (odds ratio [OR], 1.02; 95% confidence interval [CI], 1.00 to 1.03), trauma (OR, 8.5; 95% CI, 2.20 to 32.81), right-sided cardiac thrombi (OR, 1.96; 95% CI, 1.02 to 3.77), pelvic vein thrombi (OR, 3.46; 95% CI, 1.19 to 10.05); those most likely to be associated with nonfatal PTE were systemic arterial hypertension (OR, 0.51; 95% CI, 0.33 to 0.80), pneumonia (OR, 0.46; 95% CI, 0.30 to 0.71), and sepsis (OR, 0.16; 95% CI, 0.06 to 0.40). The results obtained from the application of the equation in the 512 cases studied using logistic regression analysis suggest the range in which logit p > 0.336 favors the occurrence of fatal PTE, logit p < - 1.142 favors nonfatal PTE, and logit P with intermediate values is not conclusive. The cross-validation prediction misclassification rate was 25.6 percent, meaning that the prediction equation correctly classified the majority of the cases (74.4%).

Although the usefulness of this method in everyday medical practice needs to be confirmed by a prospective study, for the time being the results suggest that concerning prevention, diagnosis, and treatment of PTE, strict attention should be given to those patients presenting the variables that are significant in the logistic regression model.

Whether or not early deaths are considered or not to be related to a recurrent PE, the rate of recurrence after a negative spiral CT angiographic finding varied between 1.8 percent and 4.9 percent. Spiral CT angiography can be used confidently to rule out significant PE, and may prevent further investigations and unnecessary treatment in an inpatient population with cardiac and/or respiratory diseases.[250]

REFERENCES

1. Goldhaber SZ. Thrombolysis for pulmonary embolism. Prog Cardiovasc Dis 1991;34:113-34.
2. Moser KM. Venous thromboembolism. Am Rev Respir Dis 1990;141:235-49.
3. Silverstein MD, Heit JA, Mohr DN, et al. Trends in the incidence of deep vein thrombosis and pulmonary embolism: A 25-year population-based study. Arch Intern Med 1998;158:585-93.
4. Hirsh J, Hoak J. Management of deep vein thrombosis and pulmonary embolism: A statement for healthcare professionals: Council on thrombosis (in consultation with the Council on Cardiovascular Radiology), American Heart Association. Circulation 1996;93: 2212-25.
5. Anderson FA, wheeler HB, Goldberg RJ, et al. A population based perspective of the hospital incidence and case-fatality rates of deep vein thrombosis and pulmonary embolism: The Worcester DVT study. Arch Intern Med 1991;151:933-38.
6. Benatar Sr, Immelman EJ, Jeffery P. Pulmonary embolism. Br J Dis Chest 1986;80:313.
7. Giuntini C, Di Ricco G, Marini C, Mellilo E, Palla A. Epidemiology of pulmonary thromboembolism. Chest 1995;107:S3-S9.
8. Stein PD, Henry JW. Prevalence of acute pulmonary embolism among patients in a general hospital and at autopsy. Chest 1995;108:978-81.
9. Bell WR, Simon TL. Current status of pulmonary thromboembolic disease: Pathophysiology, diagnosis, prevention, and treatment. Am Heart J 1982;103:239-62.
10. Coon WW. Venous thromboembolism. Prevalence, risk factors, and prevention. Clin Chest Med 1984;5:391-40.
11. Dalen JE, Alpert JS. Natural history of pulmonary embolism. Progr Cardiovasc Dis 1975;17:259-70.
12. Goldhaber SJ, Hennekens CH. Time trends in hospital mortality and diagnosis of pulmonary embolism. Am Heart J 1982;104:305-06.
13. Heijboer H, Brandjes DPM, Buller HR, et al. Deficiency of coagulation-inhibiting and fibrinolytic proteins in outpatients with deep vein thrombosis. N Engl J Med 1990;323:1512-16.
14. Tabernero MD, Estelles A, Vicente V, et al. Incidence of plasminogen activator inhibitor in patients with deep venous thrombosis and/or pulmonary embolism. Thromb Res 1989;56:565-70.
15. Egeberg O. Inherited antithrombin deficiency causing thrombophilia. Thrombo Haemostat 1965;13:516-19.
16. Marciniak F. Familial thrombosis due to antithrombin III deficiency. Blood 1974;43:209-14.
17. Griffin JH, Evatt B, Zimmerman TS, et al. Deficiency of protein C in congenital thrombotic disease. J Clin Invest 1981;68:1370-73.
18. Esmon CT. Protein C. Biochemistry, physiology and clinical implications. Blood 1983;62:1155-62.
19. Comp PC, Esmon CT. Recurrent venous thrombo-embolism in patients with a partial deficiency of protein S. N Engl J Med 1984;311:1525-28.
20. Elias M, Eldor A. Thromboembolism in patients with the lupus type circulating anticoagulant. Arch Intern Med 1984;144:510-15.

21. Aoki N, Moroi M, Sakata N, et al. Abnormal plasminogen: A hereditary molecular abnormality found in a patient with recurrent thrombosis. J Clin Invest 1978;61:1186-89.

22. Nilson IM, Ljunger H, Tengborn L. Two different mechanisms in patients with venous thrombosis and defective fibrinolysis: Low concentration of plasminogen activator or increased concentration of plasminogen activator inhibitor. Br Med J 1985;290:1453-66.

23. Johanson K, Hedner V, Nilsson IM. A family with thromboembolic disease associated with deficient fibrinolytic activity in vessel wall. Acta Med Scand 1978;203:477-81.

24. National Institute of Health Concensus conference. Prevention of venous thrombosis and pulmonary embolism. JAMA 1986;256:744-48.

25. Venous thrombosis clinical study group. Small doses of subcutaneous heparin in the prevention of deep vein thrombosis after elective hip operations. Br J Surg 1975;62:348-52.

26. Manucci PM, Citterio LA, Panajotopoulus N. Low dose heparin and deep vein thrombosis after total hip replacement. Thromb Haemost 1976;36:157-64.

27. Shackford SR, Moser KM. Deep venous thrombosis and pulmonary embolism in pregnancy. J Respir Dis 1988;9:17-24.

28. Dalen JE. Pulmonary embolism: What have we learned since Virchow? Natural history, pathophysiology, and diagnosis. Chest 2002;122:1440-56.

29. Anderson FA, Wheeler HB, Goldberg RJ, et al. Physician practice in the prevention of venous thromboembolism. Ann Intern Med 1991;115:591-95.

30. Thomas DP, Roberts HR. Hypercoagulability in venous and arterial thrombosis. Ann Intern Med 1997;126:638-44.

31. Dahlback B. Inherited thrombophilia: Resistance to protein C as a pathogenic factor for venous thromboembolism. Blood 1995;85:607-14.

32. Margaglione M, Brancaccio V, Giuliani N, et al. Increased risk for venous thrombosis in carriers of the prothrombin $\gamma \to \alpha$ gene variant. Ann Intern Med 1998;129:89-93.

33. Qinn DA, Taylor TB, Terrin ML, et al. A prospective investigation of pulmonary embolism in women and men. JAMA 1992;268:1689-96.

34. Wagenvoort CA. Pathology of pulmonary thromboembolism. Chest 1995;107:S10-S17.

35. Morpurgo M, Schmid C. Clinicopathological correlations in pulmonary embolism: A posterior evaluation. Prog Respir Res 1980;13:8-15.

36. Hatano S, Strasser T. Primary pulmonary hypertension: Report on a WHO meeting. World Health Organization: Geneva 1975.

37. Burki NK. The dead space to tidal volume ratio in the diagnosis of pulmonary embolism. Am Rev Respir Dis 1986;133:679-85.

38. Severinghaus JW, Swanson EW, Finley J, et al. Unilateral hypoventilation produced by occlusion of one pulmonary artery. J Appl Physiol 1961;16:53-60.

39. Dantzaker DR, Wagner PD, Tornabene VW, Alazraki ND, West JP. Gas exchange after thromboembolism in dogs. Circulation 1978;42:92-103.

40. Stein M, Forkner CE, Robin ED, Wessler S. Gas exchange after autologous pulmonary embolism in dogs. J Appl Physiol 1961;16:488-92.

41. D'Alonzo GE, Bower JS, Deltart P, Dantzker DR. The mechanisms of abnormal gas exchange in massive pulmonary embolism. Case report. Am Rev Respir Dis 1983;128:170-72.

42. Levy SE, Simmons DH. Mechanism of arterial hypoxemia following pulmonary thromboembolism in dogs. Cir Res 1978;42:92-103.

43. Mamer G, Castaing D, Guenard H. Determinants of hypoxaemia during the acute phase of pulmonary embolism in humans. Am Rev Respir Dis 1985;132;332-38.

44. Herve P, Petitpretz P, Simonneau G, Salmeron S, Laine JF, Duroux P. The mechanisms of abnormal gas exchange in acute massive pulmonary embolism. Am Rev Respir Dis 1983;128(6):1101-02.

45. Boochama D, Curley W, Al-Dossary S, Elgundi S. Refractory hypocapnia complicating massive pulmonary embolism. Am Rev Respir Dis 1988;138:466-68.

46. Chernick V, Hodson WA, Greenfiield LJ. Effect of chronic pulmonary artery ligation on pulmonary mechanics and surfactant. J Appl Physiol 1966;21:1315-19.

47. Finely TH, Swensen EW, Clements JA, et al. Changes in mechanical property, appearance, and surface activity of extracts of one lung following occlusion of its pulmonary artery in dogs. Physiologist 1960;3:56-72.

48. Finely TH, Tooley WH, Swensen EW. Pulmonary surface tension in experimental atelectasis. Am Rev Respir Dis 1964;89:372-78.

49. James SW, Minh VD, Minteer MA, Moser KM. Rapid resolution of a pulmonary embolus in man. West J Med 1978;128:60-64.

50. Freiman D, Wessler S, Lerztman W. Experimental pulmonary embolism with serum induced aged in vivo. Am J Pathol 1962;39:95-104.

51. Tsao MS, Schraufnagel D, Wong NS. Pathogenesis of pulmonary infarction. Am J Med 1982;72:599-608.

52. Parker BM, Smith JR. Pulmonary embolism and infarction. Am J Med 1958;24:402-27.

53. Butler J, Kowalski TF, Willoughby S, Lakshminarayan S. Preventing infarctions after pulmonary artery occlusion. Clin Res 1989;37:163A.

54. McIntyre KM, Sasahara AA. Determinants of right ventricular function and haemodynamics after pulmonary embolism. Chest 1974;65:534-43.

55. Vlahakes GJ, Turley K, Hoffman JIE. The pathophysiology of failure in acute right ventricular

hypertension. Haemodynamics and biochemical correlations. Circulation 1981;63:87-95.

56. Dalen JE, Haynes FW, Hopper FG Jr, et al. Cardio-vascular responses to experimental pulmonary embolism. Am J Cardiol 1967;20:3-9.

57. McGoon MD, VanHoutte PM. Aggregating platelets contract isolated canine pulmonary arteries by releasing 5-hydroxytryptamine. J Clin Invest 1984;74:828-33.

58. Laks MM, Juratsch MS, Garver D, Biagell L, Criley M. Acute pulmonary hypertension produced by distension of the main pulmonary artery in conscious dog. Chest 1975;68:807-13.

59. National Heart, Lung, and Blood Institute. Urokinase pulmonary embolism trial: Phase I results. JAMA 1970;214:2163-72.

60. National Heart, Lung, and Blood Institute. Urokinase-streptokinase embolism trial: Phase II results. JAMA 1974;229:1606-13.

61. Hall RJC, Sutton GC, Kerr IH. Long-term prognosis of treated acute massive pulmonary embolism. Br Heart J. 1977;39:1128-34.

62. Hall R. Difficulties in the treatment of acute pulmonary embolism. Thorax 1985;40:729-33.

63. Dalen JD, Vanes JS, Brooks HL, et al. Resolution rate of pulmonary embolism in man. N Engl J Med 1969;280:1194-97.

64. Paraskos JA, Adelstein SJ, Smith RE, et al. Late prognosis of acute pulmonary embolism. N Engl J Med 1973;289:55-58.

65. Palla A, Petruzzeli S, Donnamaria V, Giuntini C. The role of suspicion in the diagnosis of pulmonary embolism. Chest 1995;107:21S-24S.

66. Manganelli D, Palla A, Donnamaria V, Giuntini C. Clinical features of pulmonary embolism. Doubts and certainties. Chest 1995;107:25S-32S.

67. Sharma GVRK, Sasahara AA. Diagnosis and treatment of pulmonary embolism. Med Clin North Am 1979;63:239-50.

68. Dalen JE. The clinical diagnosis of acute pulmonary embolism. Geneva: WHO/ISFC Task Force on Pulmonary Embolism, 1991.

69. Stein PD, Willis PW, deMets DL. History and physical examination in acute pulmonary embolism in patients without preexisting cardiac or pulmonary disease. Am J Cardiol 1981;47:218-23.

70. Quinn DA, Thompson BT, Terrin MI, et al. A prospective investigation of pulmonary embolism in women and men. JAMA 1992;268:1989-96.

71. Carson JL, Kelly MA, Duff A, et al. The clinical course of pulmonary embolism. N Engl J Med 1992;326:1240-45.

72. Goldhaber SZ. Pulmonary embolism. N Engl J Med 1998;339:93-104.

73. Perrier A, Bounameaux H, Morabia A, et al. Diagnosis of pulmonary embolism by a decision analysis based strategy including clinical probability. D-dimer levels and ultrasonography: A management study. Arch Intern Med 1996;156:531-36.

74. Ferretti GR, Bosson JL, Bullaz PD. Acute pulmonary embolism: Role of helical CT in 164 patients with intermediate probability at ventilation-perfusion scintigraphy and normal results at duplex ultrasound of the legs. Radiology 1997;205:453-58.

75. Carson JL, Terrin MI, Duff A, et al. Pulmonary embolism and mortality in patients with COPD. Chest 1996;110:1212-19.

76. Rubinstein I, Murray D, Hoffstein V. Fatal pulmonary embolism in hospitalized patients. Arch Intern Med 1988;148:1425-26.

77. Hilder FJ, Ormond RS. Accuracy of the clinical diagnosis of pulmonary embolism. JAMA 1967;202:567-70.

78. Greenspan RH, Ravin CE, Polansky SM, et al. Accuracy of chest radiograph in diagnosis of pulmonary embolism. Invest Radiol 1982;17:539-43.

79. Figley NM, Gerdes AJ, Ricketts HJ. Radiographic aspects of pulmonary embolism. Semin Roentgenol 1967;2:389-405.

80. Homptom AO, Castelman B. Correlation of post-mortem chest teleroentgenogram with autopsy findings with special reference to pulmonary embolism and infarction. Am J Radiol 1940;43:305-26.

81. Donnamaria V, Palla A, Petruzzelli S, et al. A way to select on clinical grounds patients with high risk for pulmonary embolism. A retrospective analysis of Nested case control study. Respiration 1995;62:201-04.

82. Petruzzelli S, Palla A, Pearaccini F, et al. Routine electrocardiography in screening for pulmonary embolism. Respiration 1986;50:233-43.

83. Urokinase Pulmonary Embolism Trial. Circulation 1973;47(Suppl 2):86-90.

84. Menzoian JO, Williams LF. Is pulmonary angiography essential for the diagnosis of acute pulmonary embolism? Am J Surg 1979;137:543-48.

85. Palla A, Donnamaria V, Petruzzelli S, et al. Follow up of pulmonary perfusion recovery after embolism. J Nucl Med 1986;30:23-28.

86. Hull R, Hirsh J, Carter CJ, et al. Pulmonary angiography, ventilation lung scanning and venography for clinically suspected pulmonary embolism with abnormal scans. Ann Intern Med 1983;98:891-99.

87. Moser KM. Pulmonary embolism. State of the art. Am Rev Respir Dis 1977;115:829-51.

88. Mercandetti AJ, Kipper MS, Moser KM. Influence of ventilation and perfusion scans on therapeutic decision making and outcome in pulmonary embolism. West J Med 1985;142:208-13.

89. Ramanna L, Alderson PO, Waxman AD, et al. Regional comparison of technitium -99m DTPA aerosol and radioactive gas ventilation (xenon and crypton) studies in patients with suspected pulmonary embolism. J Nucl Med 1986;27:1391-96.

90. The PISA-PED Investigators: Invasive and noninvasive diagnosis of pulmonary embolism. Preliminary results of the prospective investigative study of acute

pulmonary embolism diagnosis (PISA-PED). Chest 1995;107:33S-38S.

91. A collaborative study by the PIOPED Investigators: Value of the ventilation/perfusion scan in acute pulmonary embolism results of the prospective investigation of pulmonary embolism diagnosis (PIOPED). JAMA 1990;263:2753-59.

92. Dalen JE, Brooks HL, Johnson LW, et al. Pulmonary angiography in acute pulmonary embolism: Indications, techniques, and results in 367 patients. Am Heart J 1971;81:175-85.

93. Perlmutt LM, Braun SD, Newman GE, et al. Pulmonary arteriography in the high risk patient. Radiology 1982;162:187-89.

94. Stein PD, Gottschalk A, Saltzman HA, Terrin ML. Diagnosis of pulmonary embolism in the elderly. J Am Coll Cardiol 1991;18:1452-57.

95. PIOPED investigators. Value of the ventilation perfusion scan in acute pulmonary embolism: Result of the Prospective Investigation Of Pulmonary embolism diagnosis (PIOPED). JAMA 1990;263:2753-59.

96. Henry JW, Relyea B, Stein PD. Continuing risk of thromboemboli among patients with normal pulmonary angiograms. Chest 1995;107:1375-78.

97. Stein PD, Hull RD, Saltzman HA, Pineo G. Strategy for diagnosis of patients with suspected acute pulmonary embolism. Chest 1993;103:1553-59.

98. Porter TR, Mohanty PK, Pandian NG. Intravascular ultrasound imaging of pulmonary arteries. Methodology, clinical applications, and future potential. Chest 1994;106:1551-57.

99. Kumar R, Katz S, Tutar A, et al. A new method to diagnose acute pulmonary thromboembolism: Intravascular ultrasound. Circulation 1990;82:359-62.

100. Bounameaux H, Cirafici P, de Moerloose P, et al. Measurement of D-dimer in plasma as diagnostic aid in suspected pulmonary embolism. Lancet 1991;1:196-200.

101. Goldhaber SZ, Simons GR, Elliott CG, et al. Quantitative plasma D-dimer levels among patients undergoing pulmonary angiography for suspected pulmonary embolism. JAMA. 1993;270:2819-22.

102. Leitha T, Speiser W, Dudczak R. Pulmonary embolism: Efficacy of D-dimer and thrombin-antithrombin III complex determinations as screening tests before lung scanning. Chest 1991;100:1536-41.

103. Palla A, Pazzagli M, Manganelli D, et al. Clinical, anamnestic and coagulation data in patients with suspected or confirmed pulmonary embolism. Respiration 1994;61:93-98.

104. Reissig A, Heyne JP, Kroegel C. Sonography of lung and pleura in pulmonary embolism: Sonomorphologic characterization and comparison with spiral CT scanning. Chest 2001;120,1977-1983.

105. Mathis G, Bitschnau R, Gehmacher O, et al. Chest ultrasound in diagnosis of pulmonary embolism in comparison to helical CT. Ultraschall Med 1999;20, 54-59.

106. Remy-Jardin M, Remy J, Wattinne L, et al. Central pulmonary thromboembolism: Diagnosis with helical volumetric CT with the single-breath-hold technique: Comparison with pulmonary angiography. Radiology 1992;185:381-87.

107. Garg K, Welsh CH, Feyerabend AJ, et al. Pulmonary embolism: diagnosis with spiral CT and ventilation-perfusion scanning: Correlation with pulmonary angiographic results or clinical outcome. Radiology 1998;208:201-08.

108. Mayo JR, Remy-Jardin M, Muller ML. Pulmonary embolism: Prospective comparison of spiral helical CT with ventilation-perfusion scintigraphy. Radiology 1997;205:445-52.

109. Remy-Jardin M, Remy J, Deschildre F, et al. Diagnosis of pulmonary embolism with spiral CT: Comparison with pulmonary angiography. Radiology 1996;200:699-706.

110. Rathbun SW, Raskob GE, Whittset TL. Sensitivity and specificity of helical computed tomography in the diagnosis of pulmonary embolism: A systematic review. Arch Intern Med 2000;132:227-32.

111. Lomis NN, Yoon HC, Moran AG, et al. Clinical outcome of patients after a negative spiral CT pulmonary arteriogram in the evaluation of acute pulmonary embolism. J Vasc Interv Radiol 1999;10:707-12.

112. Goodman LR, Lipchik RJ, Kuzo RS, et al. Subsequent pulmonary embolism risk after a negative helical CT pulmonary angiogram: Prospective comparison with scintigraphy. Radiology 2000;215:535-42.

113. Garg K, Sieler H, Welsh CH, et al. Clinical validity of helical CT being interpreted as negative for pulmonary embolism: Implications for patient treatment. AJR Am J Roentgenol 1999;172:1627-31.

114. Henry JW, Relyea B, Stein PD. Continued risk of thromboemboli in patients with normal pulmonary angiogram. Chest 1995;107:1375-78.

115. Bourriot K, Couffinhal T, Bernard V, Montaudon M, Bonnet J, Laurent F. Clinical outcome after a negative spiral CT pulmonary angiographic findings in an inpatient population from cardiology or pneumology ward. Chest 2003;123:359-65.

116. Tapson VF, Carroll BA, Davidson BL, et al. The diagnostic approach to acute venous thromboembolism: Clinical practice guidelines: American Thoracic Society. Am J Respir Crit Care Med 1999;160:1043-66.

117. Wells PS, Lensing AW, Davidson BL, et al. Accuracy of ultrasound for the diagnosis of deep venous thromboembolism in asymptomatic patients after orthopaedic surgery: A meta-analysis. Ann Intern Med 1995;122:47-53.

118. Lensing AW, Doris CI, McGrath FP, et al. A comparison of compression ultrasound with color Doppler ultrasound for the diagnosis of symptomless postoperative deep vein thrombosis. Arch Intern Med 1997;157:765-68.

119. Girard P, Musset D, Parent F, et al. High prevalence of detectable deep venous thrombosis in patients with acute pulmonary embolism. Chest 1999;116:903-08.

120. Evans AJ, Sostman HD, Witty LA, et al. Detection of deep venous thrombosis: Prospective comparison of MR imaging and sonography. J Magn Reson Imaging 1996;6:44-51.

121. Foster SA, Holland GA, Lotke PA, et al. Prospective comparison of MR venography with standard contrast venography for patient with lower extremity joint replacement (abstract). Radiology 1994;193:323.

122. Carpenter JP, Holland GA, Baum RA, et al. Magnetic resonance venography for the detection of deep venous thrombosis: Comparison with contrast venography and duplex Doppler ultrasonography. J Vasc Surg 1993;18:734-41.

123. Laissy JP, Cinqualbre A, Loshkajian A, et al. Assessment of deep venous thrombosis in the lower limb and pelvis. MR venography versus duplex Doppler sonography. AJR Am J Roentgenol 1996;167:971-75.

124. Evans AJ, Sostman HD, Knelson MH, et al. ARRS Executive Council Award: Detection of deep vein thrombosis: Prospective comparison of MR imaging with contrast venography. AJR Am J Roentgenol 1993;161:131-39.

125. Spritzer CE, Norconk JJ, Sostman HD, et al. Detection of deep venous thrombosis by magnetic resonance imaging. Chest 1993;104:54-60.

126. Dupas B, el Kouri D, Curtet C, et al. Angiomagnetic resonance imaging of iliofemorocaval venous thrombosis. Lancet 1995;346:17-19.

127. Stern JP, Abehsera M, Grenet D, et al. Detection of pelvic vein thrombosis by magnetic resonance angiography in patients with acute pulmonary embolism and normal lower limb compression ultrasonography. Chest 2002;122:115-21.

128. Rabinov K, Paulin S. Roentgen diagnosis of venous thrombosis in the leg. Arch Surg 1972;104:134-39.

129. Hull R, Taylor DW, Hirsch J, et al. Impedance plethysmography: The relation between venous filling and sensitivity and specificity for proximal vein thrombosis. Circulation 1978;58:896-906.

130. Kakkar VV, Corrigan TP. Detection of deep thrombosis: Survey and current status. Prog Cardiovasc Dis 1974;17:207-13.

131. Hull R, Hirsh J, Sakett DL, et al. Clinical validity of a negative venogram in patients with suspected venous thrombosis. Circulation 1981;64:622-25.

132. Hull R, Hirsh J, Sackett DL, et al. Replacement of venography in suspected venous thrombosis by impedance plethysmography and 125-I fibrinogen scanning: A less invasive approach. Ann Intern Med 1981;94:12.

133. Akers SM, Bartter T, Pratter MR. Impedance plethysmography. It's the clinical outcome that counts. Chest 1994;106:1317-18.

134. Wheeler HB, Anderson FA Jr. Impedance plethysmography. In Kempezinski RF, Yao JST (Eds): Practical noninvasive vascular diagnosis. New York. Yearbook Medical Publishers 1982;277-304.

135. Anderson DR, Lensing AWA, Wells PS, Levine MN, Weitz JI, Hirsh J. Limitations of impedance plethysmography in the diagnosis of clinically suspected deep vein thrombosis. Ann Intern Med 1993;118:25-30.

136. Verstraete M. The diagnosis and treatment of deep vein thrombosis. N Engl J Med 1993;329:1418-19.

137. Lensing AWA, Prandoni P, Brandjes D, Huisman PM, et al. Detection of deep vein thrombosis by real time-b mode ultrasonography. N Engl J Med 1989;320:342-46.

138. Becker DM, Philbrick JT, Abbitt PL. Real time ultrasonography for the diagnosis of lower extremity deep venous thrombosis. Arch Intern Med 1989;149:1731-34.

139. Stein PD, Henry JW, Gopalkrishnan D, Relyea B. Asymmetry of the calves in the assessment of patients with suspected acute pulmonary embolism. Chest 1995;107:936-39.

140. Henschke CI, Mateescu I, Yankelevitz DF. Changing practice patterns in the workup of pulmonary embolism. Chest 1995;107:940-45.

141. Ginsberg JS, Bill-Edwards PA, Demers C, Donovan D, Panju A. D-dimer in patients with clinically suspected pulmonary embolism. Chest 1993;104:1679-84.

142. Patil S, Henry JW, Rubenfire N, Stein PD. Neural network in the diagnosis of acute pulmonary embolism. Chest 1993;104:1685-89.

143. Barritt DW, Jordan SC. Anticoagulant drugs in the treatment of pulmonary embolism: A controlled trial. Lancet 1960;1:1309-12.

144. Hermann RE, Davis JH, Holden DW. Pulmonary embolism: A clinical and pathologic study with emphasis on the effect of prophylactic therapy with anticoagulants. Am J Surg 1961;102:19-28.

145. Stein PD, Henry JW, Relyea B. Untreated patients with pulmonary embolism. Outcome, Clinical, and laboratory assessment. Chest 1995;107:931-35.

146. Collins R, Scrimgeour A, Yusuf S, et al. Reduction in fatal pulmonary embolism and venous thrombosis by perioperative administration of subcutaneous heparin. N Engl J Med 1988;318:1162-73.

147. Dalen JE, Alpert JS. Natural history of pulmonary embolism. Prog Cardiovasc Dis 1975;17:259-70.

148. Dalen JE. Pulmonary embolism: What have we learned since Virchow? Treatment and prevention. Chest 2002;122:1801-17.

149. Tapson VF, Gurbel PA, Witty LA, Pieper KS, Stack RS. Pharmacomechanical thrombolysis of experimental pulmonary emboli. Rapid low-dose intraembolic therapy. Chest 1994;106:1558-62.

150. Sors H, Pacouret G, Azarian R, Meyer G, et al. Hemodynamic effects of bolus vs 2-h infusion of Alteplase in acute massive pulmonary embolism -A randomized controlled multicenter trial. Chest 1994;106:712-17.

151. Goldhaber SZ, Agnelli G, Levine ML. Reduced dose bolus alteplase vs conventional alteplase infusion for pulmonary embolism thrombolysis: An international multicenter randomized trial. Chest 1994;106:718-24.

152. Goldhaber SZ. Bolus and accelerated thrombolysis. Experimental observations and clinical management of myocardial infarction and pulmonary embolism. Chest 1995;107:889-91.

153. Perwitt RM, Gu S, Schick U, Ducas J. Intravenous administration of recombinant tissue plasminogen activator. Optimizing the rate of coronary thrombolysis. Chest 1995;107:1146-51.

154. Goldhaber SZ, Feldstein ML, Sors H. Two trials of reduced bolus alteplase in the treatment of pulmonary embolism—An overview. Chest 1994;106:725-26.

155. Stein PD, Hull RD. Relative risks of anticoagulant treatment of acute pulmonary based on an angiographic diagnosis vs a ventilation/perfusion scan diagnosis. Chest 1994;106:727-30.

156. Hyers TM, Hull RD, Weg JG. Antithrombotic therapy for venous thrombolic disease. Chest 1995;105 (Suppl) 335S-351S.

157. Goldhaber SZ. Contemporary pulmonary embolism thrombolysis. Chest 1995;107:45S-51S.

158. Pacouret G, Charbonnier B, Barnes S. Rapid haemodynamic improvement following infusion of saruplase in massive pulmonary embolism. (Abstract). Chest 1995;108(Suppl):125S.

159. Verstraete M, Miller GAH, Bounameaux H, et al. Intravenous and intrapulmonary recombinant tissue type plasminogen activator in the treatment of acute massive pulmonary embolism. Circulation 1988;77:353-60.

160. Clagett GP, Anderson FA, Heit J, Levine MN, Wheeler HB. Prevention of venous thromboembolism. Chest 1995;108(Suppl):312S-34S.

161. Hirsch J, Deykin D, Poller I, et al. Therapeutic range for oral anticoagulant therapy. Chest 1986;89:11S-15S.

162. Prandoni P, Lensing AWA, Buller H, et al. Comparison of subcutaneous low-molecular-weight heparin with intravenous standard heparin in proximal deep vein thrombosis. Lancet 1992;339:441-45.

163. Hull RD, Raskob GE, Pineo G, et al. Subcutaneous low-molecular weight heparin in the treatment of proximal vein thrombosis. N Engl J Med 1992;326:975-82.

164. Thery C, Simmonneau G, Meyer O, et al. Randomized trial of subcutaneous low-molecular weight heparin CY 216 (Fraxiparin) compared with intravenous unfractionated heparin in the treatment of submassive pulmonary embolism. Circulation 1992;85:1380-89.

165. Agnelli G. Anticoagulation in the prevention and treatment of pulmonary embolism. Chest 1995;107:39S-44S.

166. Neeper MP, Waxman L, Smith DE, et al. Characterization of recombinant tick anticoagulant peptide. J Biol Chem 1990;265:17746-52.

167. Nutt EM, Gasic T, Rodkey J, et al. The amino acid sequence of antistatin. J Biol Chem 1988;263:10162-67.

168. Cross FS, Mowlem A. A survey of current status of pulmonary embolectomy for massive pulmonary embolism. Circulation 1974;50:236-44

169. Chittwood WR, Lyerly HK, Sabiston DC. Surgical management of chronic pulmonary embolism. Ann Surg 1985;201:11-26.

170. Simmonneau G, Azarian R, Brenot F, Dartevelle PG, et al. Surgical management of unresolved pulmonary embolism. A personal series of 72 patients. Chest 1995;107:52S-55S.

171. Fedullo PF, Auger WR, Kerr KM, et al. Chronic thromboembolic pulmonary hypertension. N Engl J Med 2001;345:1465-72.

172. Jamieson SW, Kapelanski DP. Pulmonary endarterectomy. Curr Prob Surg 2000;37:165-252.

173. Archibald CJ, Auger WR, Fedullo PF, et al. Long-term outcome after pulmonary endarterectomy. Am J Respir Crit Care Med 1999;160:523-28.

174. Kerr KM, Rubin LJ. Epoprostenol therapy as a bridge to pulmonary endarterectomy for chronic thromboembolic pulmonary hypertension. Chest 2003;123:319-20.

175. Nagaya N, Sasaki N, Ando M, et al. Prostacycline therapy before pulmonary thromboendarterectomy in patients with thromboembolic pulmonary hypertension. Chest 2003;123:338-43.

176. Anderson FA Jr, Wheeler WB, Goldberg RJ. The prevalence of risk factors for venous thromboembolism among hospital patients. Arch Intern Med 1992;152:1660-64.

177. Kean MG, Ingenito EP, Goldhaber SZ. Utilization of venous thromboembolism prophylaxis in the medical intensive care unit. Chest 1994;106:13-14.

178. Agnelli G. Anticoagulation in the prevention and treatment of pulmonary embolism. Chest 1995;107:39S-44S.

179. Schulman S, Rhedin AS, Lindmarker P, et al. A comparison of six weeks with six months of oral anticoagulant therapy after a first episode of venous thromboembolism. N Engl J Med 1995;332:1661-65.

180. Ginsberg JS. Management of venous thromboembolism. N Engl J Med 1996;33:1816-28.

181. Levine M, Gent M, Hirsh J, et al. A comparison of low molecular weight heparin administered primarily at home with unfractionated heparin administered in the hospital for proximal deep vein thrombosis. N Engl J Med 1996;334:677-81.

182. Spyropoulos AC, Hurley JS, Ciesla GN, de Lissovoy G. Management of acute proximal deep vein thrombosis. Pharmacoeconomic evaluation of outpatient treatment with Enoxaparin vs inpatient treatment with unfractionated heparin. Chest 2002;122:108-14.

183. Fihn, SD, Callahan CM, Martin DC, et al. The risk for and severity of bleeding complications in elderly

patients treated with warfarin: The National Consortium of Anticoagulation Clinics. Ann Intern Med 1996; 124,970-79.

184. The Stroke Prevention in Reversible Ischemia Trial (SPIRIT) Study Group. A randomized trial of anticoagulants vs aspirin after cerebral ischemia of presumed arterial origin. Ann Neurol 1997;42,857-65.

185. Hylek EM, Singer DE. Risk factors for intracranial hemorrhage in outpatients taking warfarin. Ann Intern Med 1994;120,897-902.

186. Ansell J, Hirsh J, Dalen J, et al. Managing oral anticoagulant therapy. Chest 2001;119,22S-38S.

187. Gage BF, Fihn SD, White RH. Management and dosing of warfarin therapy. Am J Med 2000;109,481-88.

188. Vadher BD, Patterson DL, Leaning MS. Validation of an algorithm for oral anticoagulant dosing and appointment scheduling. Clin Lab Haematol 1995;17,339-45.

189. Waterman AD, Milligan PE, Banet GA, et al. Establishing and running an effective telephone-based anticoagulation service. J Vasc Nurs 2001;19,126-34.

190. Swenson CN, Fundak G. Observational cohort study of switching warfarin sodium products in a managed care organization. Am J Health Syst Pharm 2000;57,452-55.

191. Ryan PJ, Gilbert M, Rose PE. Computer control of anticoagulant dose for therapeutic management. BMJ 1989;299,1207-09.

192. Triplett DA. Current recommendations for warfarin therapy: Use and monitoring. WB Saunders: Philadelphia, PA 1998.

193. Horton JD, Bushwick BM. Warfarin therapy: Evolving strategies in anticoagulation. Am Fam Physician 1999;59,635-46.

194. Dalere GM, Coleman RW, Lum BL. A graphic nomogram for warfarin dosage adjustment. Pharmacotherapy 1999;19,461-67.

195. Britt RP, James AH, Raskino CL, et al. Factors affecting the precision of warfarin treatment. J Clin Pathol 1992;45,1003-06.

196. Vadher B, Patterson DL, Leaning M. Evaluation of a decision support system for initiation and control of oral anticoagulation in a randomised trial. BMJ 1997;314, 1252-56.

197. Sawicki PT. A structured teaching and self-management program for patients receiving oral anticoagulation: A randomized controlled trial; Working Group for the Study of Patient Self-Management of Oral Anticoagulation. JAMA 1999;281,145-50.

198. Banet GA, Waterman AD, Milligan PE, Gatchel SK, Gage BF. Warfarin dose reduction vs watchful waiting for mild elevations in the International Normalized Ratio. Chest 2003;123:499-503.

199. Gucalp R, Dutcher J. Oncologic emergencies. In Braunwald E, Fauci AS, Kasper DL (Eds): Harrison's principles of internal medicine (15th edn). McGraw-Hill: New York, NY 2001;642-50.

200. Maddox AM, Valdivieso M, Lukeman J, et al. Superior vena cava obstruction in small cell bronchogenic carcinoma: Clinical parameters and survival. Cancer 1983;52,2165-72.

201. Ryan JA, Abel RM, Abbott WM, et al. Catheter complications in total parenteral nutrition: A prospective study of 200 consecutive patients. N Engl J Med 1974;290,757-61.

202. Kwong T, Leonidas JC, Ilowite NT. Asymptomatic superior vena cava thrombosis and pulmonary embolism in an adolescent with SLE and antiphospholipid antibodies. Clin Exp Rheum 1994;12,215-17.

203. Goldstein MF, Nestico P, Olshan AR, et al. Superior vena cava thrombosis and pulmonary embolus: association with right atrial mural thrombus. Arch Intern Med 1982;142,1726-28.

204. Black MD, French GJ, Rasuli P, et al. Upper extremity deep venous thrombosis: Underdiagnosed and potentially lethal. Chest 1993;103,1887-90.

205. Prandoni P, Polistena P, Bernardi E, et al. Upper-extremity deep vein thrombosis: Risk factors, diagnosis, and complications. Arch Intern Med 1997;157,57-62.

206. Torosian MH, Meranze S, Mullen JL, et al. Central venous access with occlusive superior central venous thrombosis. Ann Surg 1986;203,30-33.

207. Haire WD, Lieberman RP, Edney J, et al. Hickman catheter-induced thoracic vein thrombosis: Frequency and long-term sequelae in patients recovering from high-dose chemotherapy and marrow transplantation. Cancer 1990;66,900-08.

208. Otten TR, Stein PD, Patel KC, Mustafa S, Silbergleit A. Thromboembolic disease involving the superior vena cava and brachiocephalic veins. Chest 2003;123:809-12.

209. Bulger EM, Smith DG, Maier RV, et al. Fat embolism syndrome: A 10-year review. Arch Surg 19997;132, 435-39.

210. Johnson MJ, Lucas GL. Fat embolism syndrome Orthopedics 1996;19,41-48;discussion 48-99.

211. Chastre J. The fat embolism syndrome. Pulmonary Perspective 1991;8:1-4.

212. Chan KM, Tham KT, Chow YN, et al. Posttraumatic fat embolism. It's clinical and subclinical presentation. J Trauma 1984;24:45-49.

213. Tenduis HT, Nijsten MW, Klasen HS, Binnendijk B. Fat embolism in patients with an isolated fracture of the femoral shaft. J Trauma 1988;28:383-90.

214. Muller C, Rahn BA, Pfister U, et al. The incidence, pathogenesis, diagnosis, and treatment of fat embolism. Orthop Rev 1994;23,107-17.

215. Peltier F, Leonard P. Fat embolism. A perspective. Clin Orthop 1988;232:263-70.

216. Chastre J, Fagon JY, Soler P, et al. Bronchoalveolar lavage for rapid diagnosis of fat embolism syndrome in trauma patients. Ann Intern Med 1990;113:583-88.

217. Levy DL. The fat embolism syndrome: A review. Clin Orthop 1990;261,281-86.

218. Aoki, N, Soma, K, Shinedo, M, et al. Evaluation of potential fat emboli during placement of intramedullary nails after orthopedic fractures. Chest 1998;3,178-81.

219. Mudd KL, Hunt A, Matherly RC, et al. Analysis of pulmonary fat embolism in blunt force fatalities. J Trauma 2000;48,711-15.

220. Gurd AR. Fat embolism: An aid to diagnosis. J Bone Joint Surg 1970;52B:732-37.

221. Jacobson DM, Terrence CF, Reinmuth OM. The neurologic manifestations of fat embolism. Neurology 1986;36,847-51.

222. Morioka T, Yagi H. Brain function in patients with cerebral fat embolism evaluated using somatosensory and brain-stem auditory evoked potentials. J Neurol 1989;236,415-17.

223. Georgopoulos D, Bouros D. Fat embolism syndrome. Clinical examination is still the preferable diagnostic method. Chest 2003;123:982-83.

224. Fabian TC, Hoots AV, Stanford DS, Patterson CR, Mangiante EC. Fat embolism syndrome. Prospective evaluation in 92 fracture patients. Crit Care Med 1990;18:42-46.

225. Schonfeld SA, Ploysongsang Y, Dilisio R, et al. Fat embolism prophylaxis with corticosteroids. A prospective study in high risk patients. Ann Intern Med 1983;99:438-43.

226. Masson GR, Ruggieri J. Pulmonary microvascular cytology. A new diagnostic application of the pulmonary artery catheter. Chest 1985;88:908-14.

227. Stoeger A, Daniaux M, Felber S, et al. MRI findings in cerebral fat embolism Eur Radiol 1998;8,1590-93.

228. Yoshida A, Okada Y, Nagata Y, et al. Assessment of cerebral fat embolism by magnetic resonance imaging in the acute stage. J Trauma 1996;40,437-40.

229. Parizel PM, Demey HE, Veeckmans G, et al. Early diagnosis of cerebral fat embolism syndrome by diffusion-weighted MRI (starfield pattern) Stroke 2001;32,2942-49.

230. Mimoz O, Edouard A, Beydon L, et al. Contribution of bronchoalveolar lavage to the diagnosis of post-traumatic pulmonary fat embolism. Intensive Care Med 1995;21,973-80.

231. Roger N, Xaubet A, Agusti C, et al. Role of broncho-alveolar lavage in the diagnosis of fat embolism syndrome. Eur Respir J 1995;8,1275-80.

232. Chastre J, Fagon JY, Soler P, et al. Bronchoalveolar lavage for rapid diagnosis of the fat embolism syndrome in trauma patients. Ann Intern Med 1990;113,583-88.

233. Malagari K, Economopoulos N, Stoupis C, et al. High-Resolution CT Findings in Mild Pulmonary Fat Embolism. Chest 2003;123:1196-1201.

234. Ashbug GD, Petty TL. The use of corticosteroids in the treatment of respiratory failure associated with massive fat embolism. Surg Gynecol Obstet 1966;123:493-500.

235. Moylan JA, Trirnubaun M, Katz A, et al. Fat emboli syndrome. J Trauma 1976;16:341-47.

236. Mennim P, Coyle CF, Taylor JD. Venous air embolism associated with removal of central venous catheter. BMJ 1992;305:171-72.

237. Phifer TJ, Bridges M, Conrad SA. The residual central venous catheter tract: An occult source of lethal air embolism. J Trauma 1991;31:1558-60.

238. McCarthy PM, Wang N, Birchfield F, Mehta AC. Air embolism in single-lung transplant patients after central venous catheter removal. Chest 1995;107:1178-79.

239. Kashuk JL, Penn I. Air embolism after central venous catheterization. Surg Gynecol Obstet 1984;159:249-52.

240. PIOPED Investigators. Value of the ventilation/perfusion scan in acute pulmonary embolism: Results of the prospective investigation of pulmonary embolism diagnosis (PIOPED). JAMA 1990;26:2753-59.

241. Alpert JS, Dalen JE. Epidemiology and natural history of venous thromboembolism. Prog Cardiovasc Dis 1994;36,417-22.

242. Moser KM, Fedullo PF, LitteJohn JK, et al. Frequent asymptomatic pulmonary embolism in patients with deep venous thrombosis. JAMA 1994;271,223-25.

243. Giuntini C, Di Ricco G, Marini C, et al. Epidemiology of pulmonary embolism. Chest 1995;107(Suppl),3S-9S.

244. Freiman DG, Suyemoto J, Wessler S. Frequency of pulmonary thromboembolism in man. N Engl J Med 1965;272,1278-80.

245. Karwinski B, Svendsen E. Comparison of clinical and postmortem diagnosis of pulmonary embolism. J Clin Pathol 1989;42,135-39.

246. Saeger W, Genzkow M. Venous thromboses and pulmonary embolisms in post-mortem series: Probable causes by correlations of clinical data and basic diseases. Pathol Res Pract 1994;190,394-99.

247. Coon WW. Risk factors in pulmonary embolism. Surg Gynecol Obstet 1976;143,385-90.

248. Cioff G, Pozzoli M, Forni G, et al. Systemic thromboembolism in chronic heart failure: A prospective study in 406 patients. Eur Heart J 1996;17,1381-89.

249. Yoo HYB, Sérgio de Paiva AR, de Arruda Silveira LV, Queluz TT. Logistic regression analysis of potential prognostic factors for pulmonary thromboembolism Chest 2003;123:813-21.

250. Bourriot K, Couffinhal T, Bernard V, Montaudon M, Bonnet J, Laurent F. Clinical outcome after a negative spiral CT pulmonary angiographic finding in an inpatient population from cardiology and pneumology wards. Chest 2003;123:359-65.

Acute Respiratory Distress Syndrome

INTRODUCTION

The acute (previously adult) respiratory distress syndrome (ARDS) is a dramatic clinical catastrophe resulting from acute lung injury due to a large number of unrelated massive insults, both pulmonary and extrapulmonary. Although the causes are many, and often varying, the final common pathway is injury of the gas exchange interface and acute respiratory failure. These insults result in impaired lung mechanics including lung compliance, abnormal gas exchange, and intrapulmonary shunting. However, ARDS is not only an acute lung injury, but represents a syndrome in which there is a derangement of the whole body homeostasis in which the liver, kidney, gut, blood, and endocrine organs participate in the damage and are, indeed recipients of the damaging responses.

DEFINITION

Although sudden lung collapse was known to military physicians during the war casualties at the time of World War I, the entity with its clinical features and pathophysiology was first described by Ashbaugh et al[1] in 1967, but the name ARDS was reported in 1971. There are a number of synonyms used in the past for ARDS, which imply the underlying pathophysiologic mechanism of the condition. They include: shock lung, non-cardiogenic pulmonary edema, traumatic wet lung, Da Nang lung, pump lung, capillary leak syndrome, blast lung, adult hyaline membrane disease, stiff lung syndrome, and respirator lung. The current name, ARDS was given due to its many similarities in clinical features and pathophysiology with the infant respiratory distress syndrome. Surfactant deficiencies are present in both, but are due to consequences of diffuse lung injury in ARDS, and are primary disorders (quantity and quality) in the other. Besides, many other different cellular and biochemical events occur in ARDS.

There is a great deal of confusion regarding the terminology of ARDS. Earlier it was decided that the name "acute" rather than "adult" respiratory distress syndrome should be used since the later term is a misnomer. In fact, in the original description of the condition, one of the 12 patients described was 11 years of age[1] and subsequently it was reported and seen that the disorder is not confined to the adults only. Confusion over the term was created because of the description and name given as "adult" in 1971 by the same group.[2] However, subsequently it was admitted by one of the original investigators that it was a mistake.[3] Secondly, it was recognized that the clinical spectrum of the disorder included a spectrum of radiographic and arterial blood gas abnormalities and the cutoff point for any definition of ARDS would be arbitrary. Therefore, the recent American-European Consensus Conference on ARDS[4] has recommended the use of the term "**Acute Lung Injury (ALI)**" instead of ARDS to explain such a wide spectrum of this continuum of pathologic processes. It was felt by the Committee that the term ARDS should be reserved for the most severe end of the spectrum. Thus, all patients of ARDS have ALI, but not all patients of ALI have ARDS. The Committee recommends that ALI be defined as:

"A syndrome of inflammation and increased permeability that is associated with a constellation of clinical, radiologic, and physiologic abnormalities that can not be explained by, but may coexist with, left atrial or pulmonary capillary hypertension."

Patients with hypoxemia and pulmonary infiltrates caused by volume overload and/or heart failure (left atrial hypertension) are not considered to have ALI or ARDS, although the abnormalities are similar. Nonetheless, such patients may also have ARDS in addition to hydrostatic edema. Mechanical ventilator support was not considered a requirement in defining ALI or ARDS because of differing practices of treatment

TABLE 20.1: Criteria for acute lung injury (ALI) and acute respiratory distress syndrome (ARDS)[4]

Disease	Timing	Oxygenation	Chest radiograph	Pulmonary artery wedge pressure
ALI criteria	Acute onset	PaO_2/FiO_2 300 mm Hg or less regardless of PEEP level	Bilateral infiltrates	18 mm Hg or < when measured. No clinical evidence of left atrial hypertension
ARDS criteria	Acute onset	PaO_2/FiO_2 200 mm Hg or less regardless of PEEP level	Bilateral infiltrates	18 mm Hg or < when measured. No clinical evidence of left atrial hypertension

and varying decision of the mode of treatment both by the patient and the physician. It was also recognized in the conference that it may sometimes be desirable to exclude nonmechanically ventilated patients to allow for better assessment of pulmonary parameters. Finally, the committee recognized that since ALI and ARDS are not specific diseases, any definitions would be compromised by the necessity of imposing somewhat arbitrary threshold limits.

It must be recognized that ALI and ARDS are:
- Acute in onset and persistent, lasting for days to weeks
- Associated with one or more known risk factors
- Characterized by arterial hypoxemia resistant to oxygen therapy alone
- Associated with diffuse radiological infiltrates.

Chronic lung diseases such as interstitial pulmonary fibrosis, sarcoidosis, and others that would technically meet the criteria except the chronicity, are excluded by the above definition. The specific recommended criteria for ALI and ARDS are shown in Table 20.1.

Schuster[5] in 1995 has proposed the following criteria for acute lung injury (ALI) and acute respiratory distress syndrome (ARDS).

Acute lung injury: Any significant deterioration in lung function due to characteristic pathologic abnormalities in the lungs' normal underlying structure or architecture.

ARDS A specific form of injury with diverse causes, characterized pathologically by diffuse alveolar damage, and pathophysiologically by a breakdown in both the barrier and gas exchange functions of the lung, resulting in proteinaceous alveolar edema and hypoxemia.

Unfortunately, both the above definitions have problem of the inclusion of pathological descriptions, which is not useful in a clinical setting, although they include the underlying disturbances. However, they have well described clinical counter parts.

EPIDEMIOLOGY

Data from USA reveal that approximately 150,000 cases occur annually making ARDS more common than lung cancer. More than half of this number dies. This condition is tragic in the sense that many of the victims are young and previously healthy. On the other hand, about 15,000 to 30,000 cases occur in a year in UK[6-11] although these figures are challenged and they may be overestimates. Data from many other countries is not available, even if the entity is well recognized and encountered all over the world. The published mortality rate of patients with ARDS varies from 10 percent to as high as 90 percent. The difficulty in determining the incidence and outcome of ARDS is largely because of heterogeneity and use of different definitions for the underlying disease processes, no uniformity in the definition of ARDS, no uniformity in the form of therapy, and the failure to define the population within which patients with ARDS are identified.[9]

ETIOLOGY

There are a number of different unrelated causes, which can lead on to ARDS.[12-17] These are shown in Table 20.2. Although the causes are many, few specific clinical conditions are associated with a high risk of ARDS. The major ones are sepsis syndrome (septic shock), aspiration of gastric contents, massive emergency blood transfusions (> 10 units of blood in 12 hours), trauma with lung contusion, multiple major fractures particularly pelvis fractures and long bones, major burns, cardiopulmonary bypass, intensive care unit pneumonias, and disseminated intravascular coagulation. In one study, if any one of these conditions is present, 34 percent developed ARDS. Patient's likelihood of developing ARDS is increased as the number of risk factors or conditions increase. Another study reported similar risk factors, but a lower incidence of the complications. Recently the concept of sepsis syndrome has emerged as a major clinical entity for the highest risk of development of ARDS.[15] However, most patients with sepsis syndrome will not be having no evidence of an infectious pathogen,

TABLE 20.2: Conditions associated with ARDS

Sepsis	Burn
Aspiration of gastric contents	Drug overdoses. Heroin, methadone
Trauma	acetylsalicylic acid, propoxyphene,
Diffuse pneumonia	ethchlorvynol.
Viral, bacterial, fungal, mycoplasma,	Drug idiosyncrasy
Legionnaires', pneumocystis,	Head injury
miliary tuberculosis	High altitude
Near drowning	Paraquat toxicity
Multiple transfusions	Irritant gases (NO_2, Cl_2, SO_2, NH_3)
Cardiopulmonary bypass	Smoke inhalation
Fat embolism	Oxygen toxicity
Pancreatitis	Thrombotic thrombocytopenic purpura
Disseminated intravascular coagulation	Leukemia
Eclampsia	Reperfusion injury
Lung contusion	Radiation
Venous air embolism	Neurogenic

the term systemic inflammatory response syndrome (SIRS) has been used to a multi-organ response to an inflammatory insult.[16,18] The incidence of ARDS varies from 25 to 42 percent in this condition and appears to increase when sustained hypotension is present as part of this syndrome.[14, 17-19] This is being described in more detail below.

The major categories of risks identified by the subcommittee of the American-European Consensus Conference on ARDS are as follows:[4]

I. Direct injury
1. Aspiration
2. Diffuse pulmonary infections (bacterial, viral, pneumocystis)
3. Infections and others
4. Near-drowning
5. Toxic inhalation
6. Lung contusion.

II. Indirect injury
1. Sepsis syndrome, with or without clinically significant hypotension (systolic blood pressure of 90 mm Hg or less), with or without evidence of infection outside the lung. This syndrome can be described as having both signs of systemic inflammation (SIRS, i.e. abnormalities of body temperature, heart rate, respiratory rate, and white blood cell count) and signs of organ system dysfunction including, but not limited to, pulmonary, hepatic, renal, central nervous, and cardiovascular systems.
2. Severe nonthoracic trauma
1. Clinical description
2. Scoring systems such as the injury severity score (ISS) or APACHE II/III (see below)
3. Treatment interventions such as the treatment intervention scoring system (TISS)

3. Hypertransfusion for emergency resuscitation
4. Cardiopulmonary bypass (rare).

Although there was controversy regarding diffuse lung infections, the consensus was that pulmonary infection like *Pneumocystis carinii* pneumonia should be considered ALI/ARDS when the physiologic criteria described above are met.

All patients with sudden respiratory distress do not have ARDS. Similarly all forms of noncardiogenic pulmonary edema are not ARDS, nor all diffuse alveolar infiltrates represent this condition.

PATHOGENESIS OF ARDS

Acute lung injury results from injury to both the lung endothelium and epithelium.[3,4] However, it is possible that clinical lung dysfunction sufficient to cause respiratory failure may result from injury to either of the two that is not possible to distinguish. Both cellular and humoral factors take part in producing acute lung injury. Pulmonary capillary endothelial injury is an integral and key aspect in the pathogenesis of ARDS. Pathogenesis of lung injury essentially consists of two pathways:

(i) The direct effects of an insult on the lung cells, and
(ii) The indirect result of an acute systemic inflammatory response.

The inflammatory response includes both cellular and humoral components.[4] The cellular components responsible for this reaction include neutrophils, macrophages/monocytes, and lymphocytes. Various cellular events that may play a role include adhesion, chemotaxis,/chemokinesis, and activation. These processes include the expression of cell adhesion molecules like selectins and integrins. Events in the inflammatory response include many changes in the plasma independent of the cellular events. These include a number of processes such as complement activation, alterations in the coagulation and fibrinolysis, and kinin systems. Various mediators generated by cells include cytokins, lipid mediators, arachidonic acid metabolites, tumor necrosis factor, oxidants, proteases, nitric oxide, growth factors, neuropeptides, platelet, and endothelial factors. Other mediators include interleukins such as IL-1, IL-6, and IL-8. The inflammatory response also includes induction of protein synthesis such as activation of NFkB, an early step in the production of cytokines.[20-38] These factors are generally considered to be responsible for cell injury, defects in surfactant balance, V/Q mismatch, etc. typical of ARDS.[3,4]

It is also demonstrated that both a qualitative and quantitative surfactant abnormality exists in patients who die of ARDS, along with reduced compliance of the whole, fresh, excised human lungs compared with normal control subjects. These observations have led on to the "surfactant hypotheses" in the pathogenesis of ARDS.[3,39-44] This hypothesis suggests that following a variety of lung insults, alveoli become flooded with proteolytic and/or exudative substances, which result in surfactant damage which in turn leads to alveolar instability and which in turn results in an increase in hydrostatic forces favoring pulmonary edema. Thus a vicious cycle is set in. Interestingly, all the above describe events can attack the surfactant system of the lung resulting in high surface tension pulmonary edema and damage and necrosis of the gas exchanging interface.

It is important to emphasize the fact that ARDS is an inflammatory pulmonary edema, which is different from other forms of permeability pulmonary edema, such as high altitude, postictal, and drug associated pulmonary edema, where inflammation and damage and destruction at the air-blood interface is not present.

Although various cells take part in lung injury neutrophils are the key ones and are described below.

NEUTROPHILS

Both clinical and experimental data have proved a primary or contributing role for neutrophils in ARDS in most, but not all, cases.[3,4, 45-48] Their importance is proved by the fact that the quantity of neutrophils is increased in the lungs of patients with ARDS, neutrophils from the blood of patients with this condition is found to be activated, and a wide variety of neutrophil activators and primers (neutrophil elastase, and oxidants) are present in the blood and lung lavage of patients with ARDS. Furthermore, addition of stimulated neutrophils damage cultured lung endothelial cells and isolated perfused lungs, which are blocked by addition of inhibitors of toxic products of neutrophils. Morphological

studies have demonstrated deposition and aggregation of neutrophils in the pulmonary vasculature in animals with acute lung injury. It has also been observed that neutrophil depletion prevents ARDS-like injury after injection of neutrophil activators, in animal models, although ARDS can occur in clinically neutropenic patients. However, blood levels of neutrophils may not reflect what is going on at the alveolar level. Neutrophils also have useful roles, particularly by way of their bactericidal activity. It has been reported that bactericidal activity, oxygen radical generation, and chemotaxis are deficient in alveolar neutrophils lavaged from lungs of patients with ARDS. This alveolar neutrophil defect increases susceptibility to pulmonary infections.

Neutrophil accumulation follows some potent stimulus. Chemo-attractants released by alveolar macrophages and the activation of the complement cascade causes accumulation of neutrophils. Complement component C5a has been shown to attract and aggregate neutrophils in vivo. The stimulated neutrophils release many products including oxygen free radicals (superoxide anions, hydrogen peroxide, singlet oxygen, and hydroxyl radical), proteases, arachidonic acid metabolites, and platelet-activating factor (acetyl glycerol ether phosphorylcholin, AGEPC). Proteases so released can activate a number of inflammatory pathways such as Hageman factor and its associated intrinsic coagulation pathway, complement sequence, kinin system, and fibrinolysis. Many of these factors are capable of injuring pulmonary interstitium and endothelium. Many of these, also possess neutrophil attractant properties. Adherence of neutrophils is also increased in the presence of hypoxic endothelial injury. Thus a self-perpetuating cycle is produced, resulting in initiation and continuation of inflammation.

COAGULATION PRODUCTS AND LUNG INJURY

Pulmonary intravascular coagulation is an important change observed in acute lung injury.[49-53] Disseminated intravascular coagulation and pulmonary occlusion observed angiographically occur in a substantial number of these patients. Platelet consumption with reduced platelet life span and pulmonary sequestration are other changes observed in ARDS.[54] Histologically, diffuse microvascular occlusion by fibrin and platelet thrombi and leukocyte aggregation are present.[55, 49] Moreover, both the extrinsic and intrinsic coagulation cascades are activated, particularly by endotoxins, Hageman factor, collagen exposed due to endothelial damage, and thromboplastin and proteases from neutrophils. Fibrin degradation product, D antigen, is elevated in these patients.[56,57]

All these observations point to the possibility that coagulation products are either a cause or effect of ARDS. Further studies confirmed that fibrin, FDP, complements and neutrophils are necessary for the development of ARDS. Although platelet is not directly responsible for such reactions following microembolization, vasoactive substances, including arachidonic acid products, and serotonin, released by them, aggravate the existing pulmonary hypertension. Coagulation products have potentials for direct injury to pulmonary vascular endothelium. The role of such coagulation products in inducing injury comes further from observation that blockade of reticuloendothelial system, which normally clears these substances by the way of secreting fibronectin, amplifies the effects.[58]

ARACHIDONIC ACID PRODUCTS[59-64]

All types of insult that injures the lung can stimulate endogenous production of arachidonic acid metabolites. Neutrophils, endothelial cells, and platelets are all capable of producing these metabolites. These products are potent bronchoconstrictors. Prostaglandins (PGE_2, PGF_2, PGH_2), thromboxanes (TXA_2), and leukotrienes cause vasoconstriction, alter vascular permeability, and are chemoattractants for neutrophils. All these changes are pathognomonic of ARDS. Their inhibitors can effectively block increased pulmonary vascular resistance in acute lung injury due to these substances, particularly the first two. This increase in vascular resistance alters Starling's forces in such a way to encourage net transudation of fluid from the capillary to the interstitium and alveoli. Increased vascular permeability is induced by leukotrienes C_4, D_4, and E_4 possibly by direct action on the vessel wall. Leukotriene B_4 also stimulates enzyme release and superoxide generation in human neutrophils. Decreased pulmonary compliance in ARDS is due to pulmonary edema as a result of increased vascular permeability or may represent active constriction of airways.

Other mediators, such as tumor necrosis factor, and cytokines, such as the interleukins, are also important in the pathogenesis of ARDS. The other mechanisms of endothelial cell damage involve tight adherence interactions between neutrophils, participation of iron for neutrophil-mediated killing of endothelial cells, and participation of endothelial-cell derived xanthine oxidase (XO).

SURFACTANT (See above)

As originally thought, surfactant deficiency may be an important pathogenetic factor in ARDS, like that in infants with respiratory distress syndrome. However, subsequently it was believed that this is an effect, not a cause of ARDS. Recently, renewed interest has been created in the potential role of surfactants in this condition. Surfactant is damaged **in** these patients. Abnormally aggregated and inactive surfactant occurs in bronchoalveolar lavage fluid from patients with this condition. The functional impairment of surfactant is exaggerated by a quantitative deficiency of the substance due to damage to type 2 pneumocytes early in the course of ARDS. In the original description of ARDS, it was noted that high minimum surface tension values of greater than 20 dyne/cm in lung extracts from 2 of the 12 patients. Subsequent studies showed that, phospholipid concentrations in bronchoalveolar lavage samples from patients with ARDS were normal or even high, with low levels of dipalmitoylphosphatidylcholine and phosphatidyl glycerol. Animal studies have confirmed these data.

Other events: Most patients at risk to develop ARDS do so within 72 hours of exposure to risk factors, a period in which inflammatory mechanisms are initiated and cascade to the point of increasing permeability to plasma proteins. These changes then proceed to involve multiple organs. Numerous markers have been proposed to recognize early injury including C5a, coagulation factor 8, and FDP, all of which may be elevated in ARDS. Platelets, polymorphs, and fibronectin may be decreased in the circulating blood heralding the onset of ARDS. Angiotensin converting enzyme, elastase, and neutrophil endopeptidase, once considered as markers, may not be as promising because of lack of sensitivity and specificity. Intrapulmonary markers, including leukotrienes D4, elastase, and chemotactic factors may be promising.

SEPSIS AND ACUTE LUNG INJURY

Recently, the concept of sepsis syndrome has emerged as a major clinical scenario with the highest risk of developing ARDS.[65,66] However, many patients with sepsis syndrome will have no evidence of an infectious pathogen. Therefore the term systemic inflammatory response syndrome (SIRS) has been used to refer to a multi-organ response to an inflammatory insult. This term also can result from a noninfectious insult although infection is the most important cause for the same, and the most important among them are the Gram-negative organisms. The mortality is to the extent of 30 to 50 percent reflecting the frequent development of acute lung injury and nonpulmonary organ failure.[67-70]

There are a lot of confusion regarding the use of various terms related to sepsis and its consequences.

However, a recent consensus conference has tried to identify different spectrums of the process. For the purpose of clinical diagnosis, sepsis is generally referred to as sepsis syndrome to avoid the confusion that infection is always the cause, although it is so most often. Sepsis syndrome is diagnosed when fever and other abnormalities of vital signs are present along with abnormalities of one or more organ systems that are not the site of infection or trauma. Various nomenclatures used to define the problems are shown in Table 20.3.[65,71]

TABLE 20.3: Definition of sepsis and the SIRS

I. Systemic inflammatory response syndrome (SIRS)
At least two of the following:

Temperature	> 38° C
Heart rate	> 90/min
Respiratory rate	> 20/min
WBC counts	12,000/mm³

II. Severe systemic inflammatory response syndrome (SIRS)
SIRS with related organ failure
III. Sepsis
SIRS with infection
IV. Severe sepsis
Severe SIRS with infection
(Presence of hypotension, i.e. systolic pressure less than 90 mm Hg, or a systemic manifestation of peripheral hypoperfusion, such as lactic acidosis, oliguria, or acute alteration of mental status)
V. Septic shock
Presence of hypotension not responding to 500 ml of intravenous fluid challenge plus manifestations of peripheral hypo perfusion

The mortality associated with SIRS without organ failure is approximately 10 to 15 percent.[72] It has been suggested that the phrase sepsis syndrome should be reserved for patients with an identifiable locus of infection. However, in the seriously ill patient this may not be easy always.

The Systemic inflammatory response syndrome (SIRS) is mediated by macrophage-derived cytokines that target end-organ receptors.[71] In response to infection or injury, a number of cytokines, which includes tumor-necrosis factor, IL-1, IL-6, and IL-8, are produced locally. These compounds stimulate release of secondary mediators derived from arachidonic acid such as prostaglandin 1₂, thromboxane A₂, prostaglandin E₂, and platelet activating factor (PAF); vasoactive peptides such as bradykinin, angiotensin, and vasoactive intestinal peptide; amines like histamine and serotonin; and a number of complement-derived products. These agents are useful under normal circumstances and the cytokine response is regulated by an intricate network of mediators that keep the initial inflammatory response in check by

down regulating production and countering the effects of cytokines already produced. However, when the body finds it impossible to reestablish homeostasis, all control is lost, and a massive systemic reaction begins. These mediators directly influence cardiovascular, hemodynamic and coagulation mechanisms. Endothelial damage is potentially life threatening and makes blood vessels permeable to water and solutes, resulting in pulmonary edema, peripheral edema, weight gain, and development of shock. Unless the inflammatory reaction is brought under control, multiple organ failure ensues with a greater risk of mortality. SIRS is a continuous process characterized by a generalized activation of the inflammatory response involving organs remote from the initial insult. Rangel-Frausto et al[73] in a recent study have observed that there is a continuum from SIRS to shock as well as a progressive increase in mortality as the number of above clinical signs increase.

Many pathophysiologic derangements are associated with Gram-negative sepsis, which result from the release of endotoxin, the lipopolysaccharide component of the bacterial cell walls. Release of endotoxin into the blood stream initiates a complex interaction between cellular and humoral mediators.[74] The importance of activated neutrophils has been well recognized as the critical mediator in sepsis syndrome and, particularly, in acute lung injury. Sequestration of neutrophils in various organs including lungs, followed by extracellular release of reactive oxygen intermediates and potent lytic enzymes, are believed to be primary events in the genesis of multi-organ failure. A critical first stage in this complex sequence of events is the adhesion of neutrophils to endothelium. The adhesion phenomenon is a multistage process, which results from expression of adhesion molecules on both endothelial cells and polymorphonuclear leukocytes or PMN.[75-79] Three main families of adhesion molecules are known to be responsible for adhesion, penetration of the vessel wall, and trans-endothelial migration into the tissue;[75,77] the immunoglobulin superfamily (IGSF, e.g. vascular cell adhesion molecule 1 [VCSM-1]; intracellular adhesion molecule 1 [ICAM-1]), the integrin family, and the selectins (E-selectin = endothelial leukocyte adhesion molecule [ELAM-1]; L-selectin = leukocyte endothelial cell adhesion molecule [LECAM]; P-selectin = granule membrane protein 140 [GMP-140]). Initial interactions of leukocytes and the endothelium are mediated by members of selectin family inducing (loose) contact with endothelium, followed by firm adhesion requiring members of the integrin and immunoglobulin family.[77,78,80] Leukocyte beta-2 integrins (CD11/CD18) are essential for PMN adhesion and subsequent trans-endothelial migration and interact with intercellular adhesion molecules 1 and 2. However, under physiologic conditions of flow selectins are expressed and engaged to induce leukocyte rolling along the endothelial surface.

Along with these inflammatory process brought about by various mediators, abnormalities in the vasoregulation and coagulation develops in sepsis.[71] The inflammatory mediators are mechanically important at the onset of sepsis, which usually begins with a nidus of infection or injury. Endotoxin, enterotoxin, or other stimuli prompts macrophages and other inflammatory cells to release cytokines, PAF, and eicosanoids and stimulates B and T cell products. The initial event in this type of reaction is the release of endotoxin.[81] The circulating endotoxin then prompts the release of TNF-alfa, IL-1, IL-6, IL-8, and PAF. All these agents affect the endothelium and when combine together may have different effects than their individual effect.[82] These inflammatory mediators may continue to circulate until they become inactive, or they may reach the capillaries and cause endothelial damage, which if sufficient, may cause organ failure at that site. Once organ failure occurs, local release of mediators may be extensive. If endothelium cannot repair itself, additional mediators are released into the circulation and further remote damage will occur. Different mixes of mediators may be seen at each site and are responsible for site-specific damage. This way, a pattern of multiple and progressive symptoms and signs that are pathologically related develop, which is termed as multiple organ dysfunction syndrome (MODS).

Endothelium derived relaxing factor and endothelin-1 are released from the endothelium and exert regulatory effects counterbalancing each other. Production of these mediators may be reduced in patients with sepsis. Increased production of some mediators and decreased production of others alters the body homeostasis. The length of illness is important because this alters the mix of mediators decreasing the synthesis of some cytokines, and down-regulating relevant receptors or generating inhibitors. All these lead on to a state of metabolic disorder in which the body has no control over its own inflammatory response.[83]

PATHOLOGY[1,84-88]

Even if the etiological factors of ARDS are extremely diverse including those of pulmonary and extra-pulmonary causes, the pathological features are remarkably similar. The first description of pathology in ARDS is available from the lungs of seven patients who died out of the 12 patients first described by Ashbaugh et al.[1] Although that was too simple a description of the pathology in this condition, they represent the overall change in the lungs of the patients having ARDS. All these seven patients demonstrated remarkably consistent pathologic findings with hyaline membrane formation and inflammatory cellular debris. Since that classic description the gradual evolution of pathology has been identified. Four stages of the development can be recognized from histological studies. These stages are:
- Phase of insult, or initiation
- Early progressive phase
- Late progressive phase
- Late resolving stage (recovery phase).

The phases 2 and 3 are also known as the fibroproliferative phase.

In the first phase, the onset clearly must follow an insult to either the lung epithelium (aspiration or inhalation injuries), or damage to the pulmonary vascular endothelium (blood-borne injuries). Lesions in this stage include interstitial edema, fibrin thrombi in small vessels, platelet and leukocyte aggregations, few hyaline membranes, free alveolar edema, and red blood cell extravasation. Type I pneumocytes are injured more than the type II cells and the epithelial injury is most marked at the thinnest portions of the membrane where most gas exchange occurs. Gross examination will reveal non-homogenous areas of petechial hemorrhage, hyperemia, and congestive atelectasis or alveolar collapse.[89-91]

The microscopic hallmark of the second phase is the formation of hyaline membrane around the alveolar duct. There will be associated marked capillary congestion and interstitial edema. These changes are most marked within the first 4 to 5 days of injury.[90,92] Macroscopically, there will be wide spread hemorrhagic and lobar consolidation. The lung becomes dark red, airless, and indurated like a consistency of liver. Copious edema fluid is often expressed from cut surfaces. If no resolution occurs, the consolidation persists with progressive fibrosis. The lungs may look gray, with gross evidence of abscess, purulent bronchitis, and thromboembolic are observed at autopsy.

In the third stage, hyaline membranes, edema, and vascular congestion are decreased in extent and severity.[89,90,93,94] Localized interstitial fibrosis around the alveolar duct is the most prominent finding. These changes may be due to oxygen radical injury. Regeneration of type II pneumocytes is recognizable. Decreased capillary number accompanies interstitial thickening. These processes develop over a course measured in days in contrast to those over years in idiopathic pulmonary fibrosis. The onset of this phase heralds a poor outcome. The major sequel of ARDS is the severe interstitial and intra-alveolar fibrosis, especially fibrosis centered on alveolar ducts. These appear to be the principal cause of death in most of the patients. Increased collagen content of the lungs of all patients who survived for more than 12 days was demonstrated by measuring the hydroxyproline contents of the lungs. Therefore prevention of acute pulmonary fibrosis is essential for improving survival. The pulmonary vasculature is altered. Capillary obliteration may lead on to pulmonary hypertension.[95]

The final resolving stage is heralded by a gradual improvement in the respiratory function, presumably due to lysis of the interstitial fibrosis by alveolar macrophages.[96,97]

The first description of the condition by Asbaugh et al[1] had shown the focal nature of the lesion. The whole excised human lungs from patients dying of ARDS indicated that the acute lung injury was partly focal in nature. This allows some possibility of maintaining adequate oxygenation through the remaining functional lung units with ventilatory support. Subsequent studies using computed tomography scans confirmed the focal nature of the lung injury in ARDS.[88] The uninjured or partially injured regions of the lungs allow for survival and the most injured zones must regenerate to re-establish the air-blood interface.

Thus the pathological changes of diffuse alveolar damage can be summarized as:[98,99]
1. Alveolar epithelial cell necrosis
2. Inflammatory cell infiltration
3. Proteinaceous alveolar and interstitial edema
4. Alveolar hyaline membranes
5. Type II pneumocyte proliferation, later
6. Varying degrees of intra-alveolar and interstitial fibrosis (occurs late).

PHYSIOLOGICAL ABNORMALITIES

With the damage of vascular endothelium, exudation of fluid occurs into the alveoli and interstitium due to disturbed Starling's forces. As alveolar filling with edema fluid occurs, the surface forces are increased causing collapse.[100,101] Surfactant abnormalities further aggravate the situation. The surfactant becomes inactive, aggregated, oxidized and nonfunctional. This results in a stiff lung with low compliance.[102]

Profound arterial hypoxemia, a diagnostic hallmark of the condition results due to an increase in the right-to-left shunt and ventilation-perfusion mismatch, with the first one being the predominant mechanism.[9,89,103-110] The shunt results from blood flow through areas of alveolar edema and atelectasis. Many also have low $\dot{V}/\dot{Q}$ regions, in spite of a high FiO_2. This $\dot{V}/\dot{Q}$ mismatch interferes with carbon dioxide elimination as it causes an increased alveolar-arterial oxygen difference. Regions of high $\dot{V}/\dot{Q}$ result in an increased physiological dead space. Unless minute ventilation increases, there will be increased $PACO_2$.

The mechanism of hypoxia can be summarized as:[5]

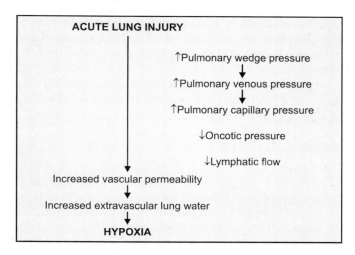

Other mechanical changes include reduced lung volumes and reduced compliance (stiff lung).[111] The lung volumes are reduced due to fluid filled alveoli, which occupy small volume than air filled alveoli, atelectasis, alveolar compression by interstitial edema, and increased surface tension.[112] Substantial reduction of surfactant activity further leads to loss of lung volume. Preferential obliteration of air spaces occurs in the dependent areas of the lungs as is shown by computed tomography.[113] This process is partly due to consolidation and is also influenced by redistribution of edema fluid within the lungs. It may also be due to the compressive effect of the overlying edematous tissue.[114] In spite of a considerable increase in lung weight, the transverse thoracic area as assessed by computed tomography is similar to that in normal subjects. This implies that gas volume, but not the lung volume is decreased.[115] Dynamic breath-to-breath variation in the degree of this dependent atelectasis has been demonstrated.[116] The clinical consequences of all these are decreased accessible alveolar volume and a substantial fall in pulmonary compliance (the total static lung compliance may be less than 10 ml/cm H_2O). Further, the stiff noncompliant lungs are due to a combination of active bronchoconstriction, and edema of the alveoli and interstitium.[117-119] This change in compliance will require high peak pressures for delivering an adequate tidal volume.

All the above factors lead on to arterial hypoxemia secondary to widespread intrapulmonary shunting, and increased work of breathing. This hypoxemia is resistant to conventional oxygen therapy and only ventilatory support may be able to correct the hypoxemia. Although pulmonary vascular micro-emboli contribute to acute lung injury, hypercarbia secondary to increased physiological dead space is rarely encountered during the early phase. The $PaCO_2$ is maintained at a lower level because of hyperventilation during the early phase. However, low compliance in established acute lung injury and in patients who proceed to the late fibrotic phase may lead to hypercarbia.

Patients recovering from ARDS demonstrate varying degrees of interstitial fibrosis[120] with main abnormality of a decreased diffusion capacity for carbon monoxide.

CLINICAL FEATURES

The development of characteristic features of ARDS follows usually a gap of 12 to 48 hours after the insult. In the original description of the syndrome, the time from the original insult to full blown ARDS ranged from 1 to 96 hours.[1] However in the compressive study on epidemiology[14] slightly more than 80 percent of ARDS cases had developed within 48 hours of the initial injury and 90 percent by 80 hours following the original insult. The first description of the clinical features of the syndrome still holds good today. The authors had observed at the bedside, the sudden emergence of tachypnoea, obvious respiratory distress with use of accessory muscles of respiration, the presence of diffuse bilateral and usually symmetrical pulmonary infiltrates on chest skiagrams, with a high mortality of nearly 60 percent.[1] The hallmark of ARDS is refractory hypoxemia, which is not improved with conventional oxygen therapy. The important diagnostic features of ARDS are shown in Table 20.4.

TABLE 20.4: Diagnostic features of ARDS

1. Clinical history of insult known to cause ARDS
2. Chronic lung disease, and left ventricular failure to be excluded
3. Must be clinical respiratory distress in the form of
   Tachypnea > 20 breaths/min
   Labored breathing
4. Chest radiographic features of Diffuse pulmonary infiltrates (interstitial/alveolar)
5. Physiological abnormalities
   PaO_2 < 50 mm Hg in spite of FiO_2 > 0.6
   Total respiratory compliance equal to or less than 50 ml/cm H_2O
   Increased shunt fraction and dead space ventilation
   Wedge pressure less than 12 cm H_2O*

* (See above for the Consensus report)

All these features may be present in association with those due to the primary catastrophic event. Sepsis syndrome due to infections is both the main risk factor for ARDS and also the most important complication of ARDS. Retrospective and prospective studies of ARDS have shown that sepsis has been associated in 4 to 50 percent of cases. This has been discussed in detail in the section on pathophysiology. The syndrome is manifested by (i) temperature of > 39°C or < 36°C; (ii) WBC count of < 3000 or > 1200/cmm or with 10 percent band forms of neutrophils; (iii) positive blood culture for commonly accepted pathogens with a known or strongly suspected source for systemic infection; and (iv) gross pus in a closed space. Features indicating a deleterious systemic effect include (i) unexplained metabolic acidosis with a base excess of > 5 mmol (mEq)/L, or (ii) systemic vascular resistance of < 800 dynes/s/cm, or (iii) unexplained hypotension with systolic blood pressure of < 90 mm Hg for more than 2 hours. When two of the above findings indicating possible infection is associated with any one of the features of systemic features, the sepsis syndrome is present. In most of the patients, secondary infection mainly arises from the respiratory tract, whereas intra-abdominal infections are the main source of sepsis syndrome. The predominance respiratory infections in patients of ARDS are expected from the high incidence of colonization and infection due to hospital acquired pathogens in mechanically ventilated patients in the intensive care units. Another factor for increased infection in these patients is due to a reduced clearance mechanism by edema.

As mentioned, ARDS is considered as a disorder of multi-organ failure. Accordingly, derangements in many other body systems will be evident.

Diagnostic criteria for ARDS have been suggested as:[5]

Definitive criteria for the diagnosis of ARDS
- Diffuse (bilateral) alveolar edema
- Increased vascular permeability
- Diffuse alveolar damage pathologically.

Practical criteria for the diagnosis of ARDS
- Radiographic infiltrates consistent with diffuse (bilateral) alveolar edema
- Significantly increased vascular permeability (a 4-5 fold increase over normal value or > 2 Standard deviation from the normal population mean)
- Appropriate clinical setting.

CLINICAL EVALUATION OF ARDS

I. Chest Radiography

The chest radiographs may be normal for some hours after the precipitating event. However, full progression to diffuse, bilateral alveolar infiltrates ordinarily takes place within 4 to 24 hours after the first abnormal radiographic signs appear.[121] Two classic X-ray patterns are often observed: (i) the pulmonary edema pattern, and the (ii) galloping pneumonia pattern.[122] The pulmonary edema pattern has a normal cardiac silhouette, a normal vascular pedicle, and slow clearing. The densities tend to be more peripheral and less gravitationally oriented than those seen in typical heart failure.[123] As alveolar filling progresses, more and more of the lung paren-chyma is involved radiographically, occasionally progressing to a near-total "whiteout" of both lung fields. The second pattern is not common. Occasionally bacterial lobar pneumonia results in the subsequent development of diffuse bilateral symmetrical infiltrations. This may be due to activation of humoral and cellular mechanisms that are involved in the pathogenesis of ARDS (Figs 20.1 to 20.4).

The effects of therapy may influence the radiologic appearance. Aggressive fluid administration will worsen alveolar fluid and diuretic use will limit or reduce it. Mechanical ventilation with PEEP or other modes that increase the mean airway pressure, may reduce regional lung density by increasing lung inflation giving a false appearance of radiographic improvement despite continued severe abnormal gas exchange.[124]

II. Computed Tomography

Computed tomography of the chest had shown that the involvement of lung fields are infect patchy with normal skipping areas, which is not forthcoming in the frontal chest radiograph.[125-127] The degree of lung involvement

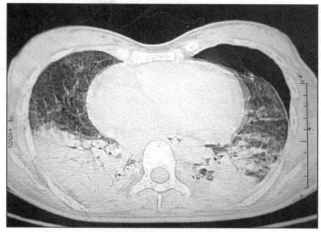

FIGURE 20.2

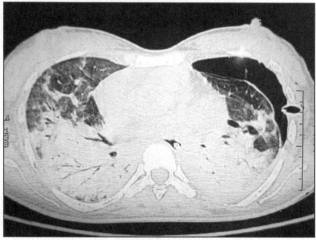

FIGURE 20.3

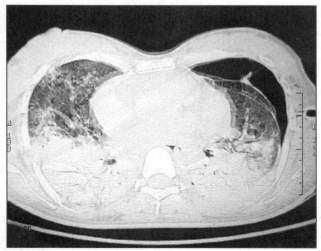

FIGURE 20.4

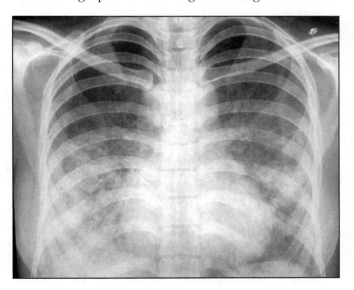

FIGURE 20.1: ARDS

FIGURES 20.2 TO 20.4: CT scan of a patient with ARDS

on computed tomography has a good correlation with the efficiency of gas exchange and the compliance of the lung.[128,129] CT scan also will reveal the presence of barotrauma and the presence of infection such as loculated empyema or lung abscess, which may be missed on plain radiographs.[130] Although, clinically it may not be required for management of a patient of ARDS, with appropriate precaution, clinically indicated CT scan can be undertaken safely in all but the unstable patients.[127]

III. Evaluation of Gas Exchange

Since abnormality is the hallmark of ARDS, laboratory evaluation of this disorder is essential both in the diagnosis, management, and evaluation of response to therapy. The initial arterial blood gas analysis will reveal respiratory alkalosis and varying degrees of hypoxemia. The hallmark is resistant hypoxemia, i.e. little improvement occurs when oxygen is administered by nasal prongs or facemask. This becomes gradually severe. The efficiency of gas exchange at the onset of lung injury as reflected by the ratio of PaO_2 to FiO_2, correlates with outcome.[131] This has been used to develop a lung injury score (see below). The dead-space ventilation is markedly increased in patients with ARDS. Therefore, they need a high rate of minute ventilation to maintain normal or near normal carbon dioxide.[132]

IV. Hemodynamic Monitoring

Although no hemodynamic profile is diagnostic of ARDS, the general importance of invasive monitoring of pulmonary artery occlusion pressure and cardiac output needs no emphasis.[133,134] Pulmonary edema, a high cardiac output, and a low pulmonary artery occlusion pressure are characteristics of ARDS. However, partially treated intravascular volume overload, and the flash pulmonary edema are two clinical conditions that can have similar hemodynamic profiles as that of ARDS, because of the transient nature of the elevated filling pressures that can cause pulmonary edema in these conditions.[135] Similarly, filling pressures can be elevated artifactually by increased intrathoracic pressure or therapeutically by fluid administration for hypotension.[136] Cardiac function can be depressed by acidosis, hypoxia, or depressant factors associated with sepsis.[137] Therefore, hemodynamic monitoring is extremely important in the initial evaluation of ARDS in ruling out cardiogenic pulmonary edema associated with elevated pulmonary artery occlusion pressures usually > 20 mm Hg and its subsequent management.

V. Measurement of Lung Injury

A method of measuring the lung injury has been proposed by Murray et al[138] in a semi quantitative way. This takes into account 4 different parameters; extent of pulmonary infiltration on chest skiagram; degree of hypoxemia; measure of the compliance of the respiratory system; and a PEEP score when the patient is ventilated. This ARDS score has subsequently been proved that the scoring system has valid diagnostic accuracy for identifying patients with ARDS who will follow a complicated course.[139] The components of the lung injury score are shown in Table 20.5.

From the above parameters, the severity of lung injury score can be calculated as follows:

Severity of lung injury Score
No lung injury	0
Mild-to-moderate lung injury	0.1-2.5
Severe lung injury	> 2.5

Other scoring systems used in the intensive care units for managing such patients are the APACHE III (Acute Physiology and Chronic Health Evaluation) systems or the organ system failure index (OSFI).[140-142]

TABLE 20:5. Lung injury score[138]

Components		Value
I. Chest radiography score		
No alveolar consolidation		0
Alveolar consolidation confined to one quadrant		1
Alveolar consolidation confined to two quadrant		2
Alveolar consolidation confined to three quadrant		3
Alveolar consolidation in all four quadrant		4
II. Hypoxemia score		
PaO_2/FiO_2	= or > 300	0
PaO_2/FiO_2	225-299	1
PaO_2/FiO_2	175-224	2
PaO_2/FiO_2	100-174	3
PaO_2/FiO_2	<100	4
III. PEEP score		
PEEP	</= 5cm H_2O	0
PEEP	6-8 cm H_2O	1
PEEP	9-11cm H_2O	2
PEEP	12-14 cm H_2O	3
PEEP	>/= 15cm H_2O	4
IV. Respiratory system compliance score* (if available)		
Compliance	>/= 80 ml/cm H_2O	0
Compliance	60-79 ml/cm H_2O	1
Compliance	40-59 ml/cm H_2O	2
Compliance	20-39 ml/cm H_2O	3
Compliance	< /= 19 ml/cm H_2O	4

The final value is obtained by dividing the aggregate by the number of components used for calculation.
* Static respiratory system compliance (C_{rs}) = $V_T/(P_S$ - total PEEP), where V_T is ventilator expired volume; Total PEEP is applied PEEP plus intrinsic PEEP; and P_S is the inspiratory plateau pressure.

VI. Other Useful Parameters

Other tests that may be useful in assessing lung injury should include the measurements of membrane barrier function and the bronchoalveolar lavage. However, these tests although can be carried out in patients with acute lung injury, they are not required as routine investigations. They may have some research values. The former can be evaluated by measuring the protein content of the alveolar fluid[143-145] or by measuring the flux of radio-labeled proteins from blood to the lung tissue.[146] Extravascular water in the lungs can also be measured by the thermal indocyanine green technique or other methods, which can be performed at the bedside.[147] The amount of extravascular water in lungs of these patients may be as high as three to eight times of the normal limit, which is about 500 ml.[148-150]

Bronchoalveolar lavage can safely be performed in patients with ARDS to search for infecting agents. Normally, the BAL fluid will show a predominance of neutrophils (up to 80% against abnormal of less than 5%). Eosinophilic BAL fluid may have important therapeutic implications since these patients may respond to steroids better.[151]

MANAGEMENT

Patients presenting with ARDS are seriously ill. The main goal of therapy is to (i) maintain adequate gas exchange while maintaining and not compromising hemodynamic stability, and (ii) identification and treatment of the precipitating causes, for example, antibiotics for infections, removal of drugs causing ARDS, and drainage of the abscess; and other supportive therapy.

Reversal of hypoxemia, which is usually severe and resistant to conventional oxygen therapy in ARDS, will require assisted ventilation. The PaO_2 should be maintained at least 50 to 60 mm Hg. The basic principle of oxygenation, i.e. ventilatory support remains the same since the early description of the syndrome 30 years ago. However, the modes of ventilatory support with near physiological means have been refined over the years. The subject has been reviewed extensively.[38,152-155]

MECHANICAL VENTILATION

Since the lung injury is partly focal, at least during the early phases, that allows some possibility of maintaining adequate arterial oxygenation through the remaining functional lung units with mechanical ventilation. The uninjured or partly injured lung allows for survival, the most injured zones must regenerate to re-establish normal gas exchange. Unfortunately, the uninjured lung represents a small proportion for ventilation, it is important to use ventilation strategies, which can minimize damage to these regions. Thus, high tidal volume, high inflation pressures, high PEEP, and oxygen concentration should be avoided if possible. Accordingly newer concepts of ventilation are emerging recently. The patient is to be managed in an Intensive Care Unit. A tracheostomy remains the ideal airway for managing patients who require ventilatory support for more than 1 week. A tracheostomy is much more comfortable than an endotracheal tube, and it allows for better mouth care. It also allows the patient to eat and to talk if the occluding balloon is slightly deflated.

It is important to use the correct type, mode, ideal tidal volume, peak inspiratory pressure, inspiratory-expiratory time ratios, and ideal levels of PEEP to maintain an ideal oxygenation, but at the same time not to compromise with the hemodynamics of the patient. In the conventional approach to respiratory support in patients with acute lung injury, a volume-cycled mechanical ventilator is to be used in the assist-control mode.[155] In this form of ventilatory support, the ventilator delivers all breaths. The breaths are either actuated by the patient's ventilatory effort (assist mode) or by the ventilator (control mode). Intermittent mandatory ventilation could be used as an alternative. With this type, the breaths spontaneously, but a breath is delivered by the ventilator periodically at a rate set previously. The problems with conventional ventilatory support however may be many.

Positive end expiratory pressure (PEEP) ventilation will be required in the successful management of many patients with acute lung injury.[1,156] Mechanical ventilation with PEEP is the standard method of managing these patients. The goal of this therapy is to improve oxygenation while minimizing FiO_2 to avoid oxygen toxicity. Although the safe level of FiO_2 in ARDS is not known, it is probably around 0.5 to 0.6. It does not mean that if necessary, concentrations above these values are not to be given. PEEP therapy improves oxygenation by three mechanisms: (a) it decreases extravascular water; (b) it minimizes ventilation-perfusion mismatch; and (c) it increases the functional residual capacity (FRC). The $\dot{V}/\dot{Q}$ abnormalities, including shunting, are partially corrected at PEEP levels of 5 to 15 cm H_2O due to reopening of the atelectatic alveoli and holding the extra-alveolar pulmonary capillaries open, which are otherwise closed due to edema. The FRC is increased by increasing the gas volume of the partially filled alveoli and by recruitment of previously collapsed alveoli. However, the problem with PEEP therapy is the reduction in cardiac output due to impedance of systemic venous return or decreased left ventricular function. Therefore, even if the PaO_2 can be increased, the ultimate delivery of oxygen will not improve. The application of PEEP may substantially increase peak inspiratory pressure. Barotrauma will then be a major concern. This will manifest in pneumothorax, pneumomediastinum, pulmonary interstitial emphysema, and hemorrhage at the peri-alveolar and perivascular levels. These complications can occur at levels of between 40 to 50 cm of H_2O. Overdistension of the lung in the absence of high peak inspiratory pressure may lead to lung microvascular injury and high permeability pulmonary edema. Pulmonary edema and atelectasis can occur at a peak inspiratory pressure of as low as 30 cm H_2O. Currently most physicians aim at a peak inspiratory pressure of below 50 cm of H_2O. Another problem is the concept of alveolar overdistension or "volotrauma" which may be potential cause for ventilator induced lung damage in patients with acute lung injury. When a high tidal volume, even conventional tidal volume is applied to the small residual component of the functional lung tissue, it may result in pronounced regional overdistension of the remaining functional alveoli.[157-161] Mechanical ventilation might also contribute by improving the surfactant regeneration.[162]

In view of the above difficulties, newer strategies for respiratory support have been evolved. Instead of the earlier recommendation of 12 to 15 ml/kg of tidal volume, it is now recommended that it should be 6 to 10 ml/kg to keep a airway pressure of 40 to 45 cm H_2O. However, since the compliance and airway resistance changes frequently, it may be necessary to change the tidal volume periodically. As an alternative to the peak airway pressure, the plateu pressure and effective static lung compliance have been used to select the best tidal volume. The optimal level of PEEP is controversial. It should be increased by 3 to 5 cm H_2O, to a maximum of 15 cm of water with careful cardiac output monitoring. The goal is to achieve acceptable arterial oxygen saturation of 90 percent or more, with nontoxic FiO_2 values of 0.6 or less with a peak air way pressure of < 40 to 45 cm water.[155,163-165] Ventilatory rates should be such that hypercapnia and respiratory acidosis are avoided. Although with normal lungs the rates can be 8 to 14 per minute, in ARDS this may be more than 20 to 25/min because of increased physiological dead space and smaller lung volumes. These rates are often well tolerated, but there is a potential for excessive gas trapping (auto PEEP), which may create further problem.[166-168] The guidelines for initial and subsequent ventilator settings are recommended in more detail by Kollef et al.[142,155]

NEWER MODES OF VENTILATION

A number of strategies have been developed recently to overcome some of the above problems and for better oxygenation with minimum complications. Some of these strategies will be discussed in brief.

A. Inverse-ratio ventilation. Inverse ratio ventilation is a variation of the conventional ventilation in which the I:E ratio is lengthened by prolonging the inspiratory time to more than half of the respiratory cycle. This can be either volume controlled or pressure controlled inverse ratio ventilation.[169-172] By this, the mean airway pressure is increased but an acceptable peak airway pressure is maintained. Sustained increased inspiratory pressure will affect the nonfunctional lung units more uniformly. The problem of this type of ventilation is that it requires heavy sedation, and neuromuscular blockade. This form of therapy is still considered experimental and should be reserved only in situations where acceptable arterial oxygenation can not be achieved with a PEEP of 15 cm of water or more or when application of PEEP is associated with excessive peak airway pressure.

B. Continuous positive airway pressure ventilation (CPAP) In this form, a predetermined increased airway pressure is maintained throughout the spontaneous respiration.[154] Thus, the effective lung volume is increased. This requires high gas flow and efficient pressure release valves. Mild forms of lung injury can be treated with CPAP alone without requiring intubation. This can be used either through a tightly fitting mask or in conjunction with low frequency mandatory ventilation. The work of breathing is reduced and periodic alveolar distension is avoided by CPAP.

C. Airway pressure release ventilation. This is a variation of inverse ratio ventilation and the system is essentially a CPAP applied intermittently, over which the patient may superimpose spontaneous respiration.[173] This method of ventilation helps in opening and stabilizing collapsed portions of the lung. This is still not used extensively in clinical practice.

D. High-frequency ventilation. In this form, small tidal volumes of 1 to 5 ml/kg are administered at rates of 60 to 3600 cycles per minute.[174-176] Gas is delivered through high-pressure nozzle at frequencies of 1.6 to 10 Hz and the expiration is passive. Potential advantages of this technique are enhanced gas kinetics in the alveoli, and minimal barotrauma. However, studies have shown no important advantage in ARDS over conventional forms of mechanical ventilation.

E. Permissive hypercapnia. This is a recent concept of ventilatory strategy that has been used successfully. This is referred to as controlled hypoventilation with permissive hypercapnia or pressure targeted ventilation.[177-179] In this form, hypoventilation and hypercapnia are allowed in order to avoid unacceptable increase in the peak airway pressure. The respiratory rate and tidal volume (as low as 5 ml/kg) are adjusted to prevent increase in peak airway pressure (limited to 30 cm of water). However, during the process the $PaCO_2$ rises. It has been shown that gradual rise in the $PaCO_2$ values to 100 mm Hg or less are usually tolerated. Marked acidosis (pH of < 7.25) can be corrected with intravenous sodium bicarbonate if necessary. Extracorporeal removal of carbon dioxide can be utilized during the process to correct acidosis, if necessary. Many clinicians now recommend the use of this type of approach in treating ARDS.

F. Extracorporeal gas exchange. Two forms of extracorporeal respiratory support have been evaluated in patients with ARDS. (a) extracorporeal membrane oxygenation; and (b) extracorporeal carbon dioxide removal, which may be total or partial. Although prospective trials have shown no extra-advantage of extracorporeal membrane oxygenation, this is a useful supportive treatment, particularly in selected patients awaiting lung transplantation.[180,181]

G. Intravascular gas exchange. Another important recent advance in the oxygen support system is the development of an intravascular oxygenation device.[182-184] This is a scaled down hollow fiber oxygenator inserted surgically into the vena cava. Oxygen is drawn at subatmospheric pressure to prevent possible air embolism through the device. The gas exchanging membrane is up to 0.5 m^2 in area and is nonthrombogenic. This is capable of exchanging up to 150 ml/min of oxygen and carbon dioxide. However, the role of this device in the treatment of acute lung injury is still to be defined.

OTHER RELATED PROBLEMS OF VENTILATORY MANAGEMENT

1. Positioning of the patient. Posture manipulations have been shown to be beneficial in improving gas exchange.[185-187] The basis of this approach lies in the fact the lung injury is not uniform in ARDS (described previously). Thus by changing the position can improve the distribution of perfusion to ventilated lung regions. Both lateral decubitus positioning and prone positions used periodically are to be attempted in patients not responding to conventional approaches.

Ventilation in the prone position improves "oxygenation" in patients with acute hypoxemic respiratory failure.[187] Overall, prone positioning helps to improve gas exchange in approximately two thirds of the patients with ARDS.[189] In animal models,[190,191] as well as in many patients with ARDS[189] the poorly and/or nonaerated lung units appear to be mainly localized in the dependent regions both in the supine and prone position. The time constant of the dependent collapsed/flooded lung units is such that tidal ventilation distributes preferentially to the "open" nondependent lung units[191] Since the distribution of perfusion is largely gravity-independent, at least under West zonal 3 conditions, the largest proportion of the perfusion goes through the dorsal lung regions, with patients in both the supine and prone positions.[192] As a result, perfusion is largest in the dependent regions with the patient in the supine position and is largest in the nondependent region when the patient is in the prone position, and this remains true in the setting of lung injury[193] Regardless of position, positive-pressure ventilation (i.e. the creation of West zonal conditions 2 or 1) alters the vertical distribution of perfusion, and blood flow tends to be redistributed from the nondependent region to the dependent regions. Positive airway pressure thus tends to reduce the vertical perfusion gradient with the patient in the prone position and tends to amplify the gradient with the patient in the supine position.[194] It follows that with the patient in the supine position the vertical ventilation and perfusion gradients of mechanically ventilated injured lungs vary in opposite direction, promoting ventilation-perfusion mismatch and shunting. In contrast, a larger proportion of perfusion distributes to the well-ventilated nondependent regions (dorsal) and, everything else being equal, a smaller amount of desaturated blood perfuses the poorly and/or nonaerated lung regions with the patient in the prone position. This helps to explain the fact that the ventilation-perfusion relationship is more favorable with patients in the prone position than in the supine position.[190,195]

Additionally and/or alternatively, other factors may contribute to the improved gas exchange afforded by prone positioning. Along the vertical axis, the pleural pressure gradient is smaller with the patient in the prone position than in the supine position.[196] In the dependent regions, the pleural pressure is also comparatively less positive (more negative) with the patient in the prone position rather than in the supine position[197] in large part because in the prone position the heart rests almost entirely on the sternum and exerts significantly less pressure on the lungs and pleural space than in the supine position.[198] These physiologic characteristics of prone positioning help to explain the more uniform vertical distribution of regional lung volume at relaxation and the rise in functional residual capacity that may be observed after turning from the supine position to the prone position.[199] Although a rise in functional residual capacity or recruitment can contribute to the improvement in gas exchange, PaO$_2$ may clearly rise without any demonstrable change in lung volume.[200] Together, these suggest that the improved gas exchange that is observed with the patient in the prone position may be due to the relatively larger perfusion in the dorsal aerating lung regions and/or to recruitment and better aeration of the dependent lung unit. In patients with ARDS, the effect of prone positioning on gas exchange apparently also depends on chest wall compliance[201] suggesting that prone positioning is an important determinant of the regional ventilation/perfusion relationship in paralyzed mechanically ventilated subjects. Which one of the above mechanisms prevails and best explains the effect on gas exchange of prone positioning in a given patient is unknown but could be important in regard to its potential protective effects against ventilator-induced lung injury, and thus to its possible impact on outcome.

The improved physiologic understanding of the effect of prone positioning on the respiratory system and the encouraging preliminary clinical data have made it very tempting to ventilate patients with severe ARDS in the prone position in the recent years. A randomized prospective study[189] has confirmed its safety and efficacy in improving gas exchange but has failed to show an overall reduction in mortality.

Prone positioning has been established as safe in adults.[189] When close attention is paid particularly to the lines, the endotracheal tube, and the secretions that may occasionally enter the endotracheal tube during or shortly after repositioning, the rate of complications is not different in the prone position than in the supine position. Compared to supine positioning, the lesser positive pleural pressure in the dependent thorax regions, the more uniform regional pleural pressure, lung volume, and perfusion observed in the prone position as the potential to limit lung volume loss/trauma due to atelectasis and to distribute the tidal mechanical stress imposed on the vessels and airways more evenly between all lung regions.[202,203]

However it is not clear what population will benefit the most from prone positioning, and the optimal timing for its use (i.e. at what stage of the natural course of ARDS, and how often and for how long should we turn patients to the prone position and keep patients prone).

It is also likely that the best prone ventilatory strategy differs from the best supine ventilatory strategy and that the intensity of abdominal compression that is allowed for the patient in the prone position also may be important. These issues have not been comprehensively addressed so far.[204]

An interesting concept of 'kinetic therapy' has been advocated where patients are nursed in a bed that constantly rotates through 670 each side of horizontal.[205]

2. Fluid management. Even if pulmonary edema in ARDS is due to increased endothelial permeability, intravascular hydrostatic forces may still be important. Clinical studies support that weight loss and fall in the pulmonary artery occlusion pressure are associated with better survival and improved lung functions. Therefore, most authorities recommend that fluid restriction and diuresis, if possible should be undertaken which are consistent with an adequate cardiac out put. It is important to see that hypovolemia is not induced. Central hemodynamic monitoring will be required to determine appropriate fluid management.[155]

3. Enhancing oxygen transport. Besides oxygenation, maintenance of cardiac output will be necessary by ionotropic agents such as dopamine or adrenaline. In septic shock, where vascular resistance is low, pressor agents such as neosynephrine or noradrenaline are helpful in increasing the blood pressure. If the patient is severely hypovolemic, careful administration of fluid might be beneficial. However, the role of such agents remains controversial.[155]

As discussed above, a syndrome of multi-organ failure develops in many patients with ARDS. Therefore, adequate support for all the organ systems is very essential. Complications of management are also common in ARDS. These include barotrauma, nosocomial pneumonia, stress bleeding, etc. Measures should be aimed at preventing these complications, and appropriate management of them is required if they occur. These will affect the ultimate outcome of ARDS.

PHARMACOLOGICAL MANAGEMENT

Over the years after it was recognized that a number of inflammatory mediators, various cells, surfactant abnormalities, importance of sepsis, etc. are responsible for the pathogenesis of ARDS attempts were made to counter the altered pathophysiology in ARDS. A number of substances have been developed, and tried both in experimental animals and in clinical trials. However, they are not yet recommended for routine use in ARDS. These drugs will be discussed in brief in Table 20.6.

TABLE 20.6: Pharamacologic therapy tried in ARDS

Drugs	Comments
Exogenous surfactant	May improve alveolar stability, ? antibacterial and immunological properties[207-209]
Corticosteroids	alters inflammatory response
	Ultimate outcome not changed
	May be beneficial if eosinophilia in BAL
	Some try prednisolone (2-4 mg/kg for 1-2 weeks[87,156,210-215]
Acetylcystein	Scavanger for oxygen free radicals
	No survival benefit[216,217]
Ketoconazol	Potent inhibitor of thromboxane synthesis
	Inhibits leukotrienes biosynthesis
	May prevent ARDS in high risk patients, sepsis or multiple trauma[218,219]
Nitric oxide (inhaled)	Selective pulmonary vasodilator (5-80 ppm)
	Improves arterial oxygenation
	Reduces intrapulmonary shunting[220]
SEPSIS ASSOCIATED ARDS[72,74,221-228]	
Eicosanoids and their inhibitors	
-Ibuprofen,Indomethacin	Prostaglandin inhibitors, improve outcome in experimental sepsis
-Alprostadil	Blocks platelet aggregation, modulates inflammation,
(Prostaglandin E$_1$)	Vasodilator; Improves oxygenation
Pentoxyphylline	Phosphodiesterase inhibitor, inhibits chemotaxis and activation of neutrophils in sepsis
Antiendotoxin and	May help in sepsis induced ARDS
Anticytokines	
(monoclonal antiendotoxins,	
interleukin-1 receptor antagonist,	
monoclonal anti TNF-alpha antibody)	
Antibiotics	Helpful in specific infections

If the patient survives the first few days of critical periods with intensive management, then the goal of management changes to maintain a chronically and critically ill ventilated patient till the lungs start to repair themselves. Most patients of ARDS, who die, do so within the first two weeks of their illness. It may take several weeks and as long as 4 to 8 weeks for those who recover. Management of such patients is very difficult, time-consuming, and expensive. A protocol has been suggested for this.[38] The five points of the protocol (*Bruce-Jenner protocol*) include: I. Exercise (respiratory and whole body); II. Nutrition (to attain anabolism); III. Fluid management; IV. Emotional support; and V. Sleep. For recovery to occur, type II cell proliferation is an essential step. There is some suggestion that corticosteroids can accelerate this process. Nutritional support is essential to be able to provide the building blocks for lung regeneration. It is best to provide nutrition by oral route in order to utilize the gastrointestinal tract and prevent gut atrophy. When this is not possible alimentation via intravenous feeding is required. Usually, critically ill patients with ARDS require 40 to 50 cal/kg to attain anabolism.

The overall mortality of ARDS even in the best of centers is over 50 percent and published mortality rates varies from 10 percent to as high as 90 percent.

Respiratory failure is not the primary cause of death in most of these patients. Rather other complicating factors like sepsis are responsible for most of the mortality. Thus it is reported that respiratory failure is the primary cause of death only in 16 percent of cases, whereas mortality rates for patients with ARDS associated with sepsis, are 80 to 90 percent. Other risk factors include underlying predisposing illness, or multi-organ dysfunction.[228-234] Unfavorable outcome in acute lung injury is related to the degree of inflammatory response at the onset and during the course of ARDS. Patients with higher levels of TNF-alpha, IL-1beta, IL-6, and IL-8 on day 1 of ARDS will have persistent elevation of these inflammatory cytokines over time and these will die. Survivors will have less elevation of plasma elevated cytokines on day 1 and a rapid reduction over time. Plasma IL-1beta and IL-6 levels are consistent and efficient predictors of outcome.[235] A recent international, multicenter, prospective survey in 25 centers (11 in USA and 14 in Europe) comprising of 1426 patients with acute respiratory failure were evaluated for the hospital survival rates.[236] These patients were treated in sophisticated intensive care units by leading critical care specialists using current (from 1991-1992) support and treatment techniques and protocols. Patients who were hypoxic and hypercarbic at the time of entry requiring ventilatory support had a survival of 33.3 percent compared to 63.6 percent in those who were not hypoxic or hypercarbic. Survival rates were higher in patients with acute respiratory failure due to pneumonia (63%) or post shock lung injury (67%). Survival was lower in patients was lower in patients with acute respiratory failure due to sepsis (46%). Severity of lung injury was a major prognostic factor, varying from 18 percent hospital survival rate for those with far advanced lung injury to a survival rate of 67 percent in those with less severe injury. Low survival rates were seen (< 20%) if mechanical ventilator FiO_2 was 0.8 to 1.0; while 50 percent of the patients survived whose FiO_2 was 0.50. Other prognostic factors included level pf peak inspiratory pressure (less than 20 percent if > 50 cm H_2O, and 60 percent if < 30 cm H_2O; and shorter periods of mechanical ventilation (< 48 hours- survival of 38% vs 30% in those requiring the same for more than 2 weeks. Patients with multiorgan failure had higher mortality rates (90%) than those with pulmonary dysfunction alone (55%).

LONG-TERM OUTCOME OF ARDS[237-239]

Patients who survive acute lung injury are usually considered to have no respiratory symptom. However, pulmonary function impairment at one year is seen in about two-thirds of the patients. Various indices of ventilatory parameters used during treatment and the association of sepsis affects the outcome and severity of these abnormalities. Reduced mortality may not be the only goal of modern ARDS treatment. Some survivors of ARDS will have persistent lung function impairment consisting of restrictive or obstructive ventilatory defects, bronchial hyperreactivity, impaired diffusing capacity of the lung for carbon monoxide (DLCO), and a drop in PaO_2 during exercise. Improvement or normalization of pulmonary function may be observed for up to 1 year after hospital discharge, and residual defects thereafter typically consist of an impaired oxygen transfer. This may be explained by fibrosis and microvascular obliteration, which are characteristic pathologic sequels after ARDS.[240,241] Pulmonary function has been studied in survivors of ARDS by several groups at various time intervals, the longest being 9 years, but only three studies describe cardiopulmonary exercise capacity in survivors of ARDS 3 to 24 months after ARDS. Residual obstructive and restrictive defects as well as impaired pulmonary gas exchange remain common after severe ARDS. Cardiopulmonary exercise testing (CEPT) is a very sensitive measure to evaluate residual impairment of lung function after ARDS. Using CPET, reduced pulmonary gas exchange can be detected in many patients with normal D_{LCO}.[242]

REFERENCES

1. Ashbaugh DG, Biglow DB, Petty TL, Levine BE. Acute respiratory distress in adult. Lancet 1967;2:319-23.
2. Petty TL, Ashbaugh DG. The adult respiratory distress syndrome-Clinical features, factors influencing prognosis, and principles of management. Chest 1971;60:233-39.
3. Petty TL. The acute respiratory distress syndrome. Historic perspective. Chest 1994;105:44S-47S.
4. Bernard GR, Artigas A, Brigham KL, et al. The American-European Consensus Conference on ARDS. Definitions, Mechanisms, Relevant Outcomes, and Clinical Trial Coordination. Am J Respir Crit Care Med 1994;149:818-24.
5. Schuster DP. What is acute lung injury? What is ARDS? Chest 1995;107:1721-26.
6. Murray JF and the staff of the division of Lung Diseases, NHLBI. Mechanisms of acute respiratory failure. Am Rev Respir Dis 1977;115:1071-78.
7. Villar J, Slutsky AS. The incidence of the adult respiratory distress syndrome. Am Rev Respir Dis 1989;140:814-16.
8. Webster NR, Cohen AT, Nunn JF. Adult respiratory distress syndrome: How many cases in the UK. Anaesthesia 1988;43:923-26.
9. Thomsen GE, Morris AH, Danino D, Ellsworth J, Wallace GJ. Incidence of the respiratory distress syndrome in Utah. Am Rev Respir Dis 1993;147:A347.
10. Petty TL, Fowler AA. Another look at ARDS. Chest 1982;82:98-104.
11. Fein AM, Lippman M, Holtzman H, Eliraz A, Goldberg SK. The risk factors, incidence, and prognosis of the adult respiratory distress syndrome following septicaemia. Chest 1983;83:40-42.
12. Hudson LD. Causes of the adult respiratory distress syndrome: Clinical recognition. Clin Chest Med 1982;3:195-212.
13. Pepe PE, Potkin RT, Holtman-Reus D, Hudson LD, Carrico CJ. Clinical predictors of the adult respiratory distress syndrome. Am J Surg 1982;144:124.
14. Fowler AA, Hamman RF, Good JT, et al. Adult respiratory distress syndrome: Risk with common predispositions. Ann Intern Med 1983;98:593-97.
15. Bone RC, Fisher CJ Jr, Clemmer TP, et al. Sepsis syndrome: A valid clinical entity: Methyl prednisolone severe sepsis study group. Crit Care Med 1989;17:389-93.
16. Bone RC, Balk RA, Cerra FB, et al. Definitions for sepsis and organ failure and guidelines for the use of innovative therapies in sepsis. Chest 1992;101:1644-55.
17. Montgomery AB, Stager MA, Carrico CJ, Hudson LD. Causes of mortality in patients with adult respiratory distress syndrome. Am Rev Respir Dis 1985;132:485-89.
18. Bone RC, Sibbald WJ, Sprung CL. The ACCP-SCCM consensus conference on sepsis and organ failure. Chest 1992;101:1481-83.

19. The Veterans Administration Systemic Sepsis Study Group. The effects of high dose glucocorticoid therapy on mortality in patients with clinical signs of systemic sepsis. N Engl J Med 1987;317:659-65.

20. Fowler AA, Hyers TM, Fisher BJ, et al. The adult respiratory distress syndrome: Cell population and soluble mediators in the air spaces of patients at high risk. Am Rev Respir Dis 1987;136:1225-31.

21. Maeda J, Ueki N, Hada T, Higashino K. Elevated serum hepatocyte growth factor, scatter factor levels in inflammatory lung disease. Am J Respir Crit Care Med 1995;152:1587-91.

22. Ridings PC, Windsor ACJ, Jutila MA, et al. A dual binding antibody to E- and L-selectin attenuates sepsis induced lung injury. Am J Respir Crit Care Med 1995;152:247-53.

23. Montravers P, Chollet-Martin S, Marmuse JP, et al. Lymphatic release of cytokines during acute lung injury complicating severe pancreatitis. Am J Respir Crit Care Med 1995;152:1527-33.

24. American Thoracic Society. Medical section of the American Lung Association. Future Directions for research on diseases of the lung. Am J Respir Crit care Med 1995;152:1713-35.

25. Bone RC, Balk G, Slotman R, et al. Adult respiratory distress syndrome: Sequence and importance of development of multiple organ failure. Chest 1992;101:320-26.

26. Cochrane CG, Spragg R, Revak SD. Pathogenesis of the adult respiratory distress syndrome: Evidence of oxidant activity in bronchoalveolar lavage fluid. J Clin Invest 1983;71:754-61.

27. Repine JE, Beehler CJ. Neutrophils and adult respiratory distress syndrome: Two interlocking perspectives in 1991. Am rev Respir Dis 1991;144:251-52.

28. Shale DJ. The adult respiratory distress syndrome-20 years on. Thorax 1987;42:641.

29. Stevens JH, Raffin TA. Adult respiratory distress syndrome-I. Aetiology and mechanisms. Postgrad Med J 1984;60:505-13.

30. Bernard GR, Korley V, Chee P, et al. Persistent generation of peptido leukotrienes in patients with adult respiratory distress syndrome. Am Rev Respir Dis 1991;144:263-67.

31. Evans TW. Adult respiratory distress syndrome. Med Int 1989;71:29-44.

32. Hyers TM, Tricomi SM, Dettenmeier PA, Fowler AA. Tumor necrosis factor levels in serum and bronchoalveolar lavage fluid of patients with the adult respiratory syndrome. Am Rev Respir Dis 1991;144:268-71.

33. Repine JE. Scientific perspectives on adult respiratory distress syndrome. Lancet 1992;339:466-69.

34. Rinaldo JE, Christman JW. Mechanisms and mediators of the adult respiratory distress syndrome. Clin Chest Med 1990;11:621-32.

35. Donnelly SC, Haslett C. Cellular mechanisms of acute lung injury: Implications for future treatment in the adult respiratory distress syndrome. Thorax 1992;47:260-63.

36. Suter PM, Suter S, Girardin E, et al. High bronchoalveolar levels of tumor necrosis factor and its inhibitors, interleukin-1, interferon, and elastase, in patients with adult respiratory distress syndrome. After trauma, shock, or sepsis. Am rev Respir Dis 1992;145: 1016-22.

37. Henson PM, Barnes PJ, Banks-Schlegel SP. NHLBI workshop summary: Platelet-activating factor; role in pulmonary injury and dysfunction and blood abnormalities. Am Rev Respir Dis 1992;145:726-31.

38. Weinberger SE. Recent advances in pulmonary medicine (Second of two parts). New Engl J Med 1993; 328:1462-70.

39. Petty TL, Reiss OK, Paul GW, et al. Characteristics of pulmonary surfactant in adult respiratory distress syndrome Associated with trauma and shock. Am Rev Respir Dis 1977;115:531-36.

40. Petty TL, Silvers GK, Paul GW, et al. Abnormalities in lung elastic properties and surfactant function in adult respiratory distress syndrome. Chest 1979;75:571-74.

41. Doyle IR, Nicholas TE, Berstern AD. Serum surfactant protein-A levels in patients with acute cardiogenic pulmonary oedema and adult respiratory distress syndrome. Am J Respir Crit Care Med 1995;152: 307-17.

42. Holm BA, Matalon S. Role of pulmonary surfactant in the development and treatment of adult respiratory distress syndrome. Anaesth Analg 1989;69:805-18.

43. Morton NS. Exogenous surfactant treatment for the adult respiratory distress syndrome? A historical perspective. Thorax 1990;45:825-30.

44. Maunder RJ, Hackman RC, Riffe E, et al. Occurrence of the adult respiratory distress syndrome in neutropaenic patients. Am rev Respir Dis 1986;133: 313-16.

45. Martin TR, Pistorese BP, Hudson LD, Maunder RJ. The function of lung and blood neutrophils in patients with the adult respiratory distress syndrome. Implications for the pathogenesis of lung infections. Am Rev Respir Dis 1991;144:254.

46. Weiss SJ, Young J, LoBuglio AF, Slivka A, Nimeh NF. Role of hydrogen peroxide in neutrophil mediated destruction of cultured endothelial cells. J Clin Invest 1981;68:714-21.

47. Varani J, Fligiel SEG, Till GO, Kunkel RG, Ryan US, Ward PA. Pulmonary endothelial cell killing by human neutrophils. Possible involvement of hydroxyl radical. Lab Invest 1985;53:656-63.

48. Gannon DE, Varani J, Phan SH, Ward JH, Kaplan J, Till GO, Simon RH, Ryan US, Ward PA. Source of iron in neutrophil-mediated killing of endothelial cells. Lab Invest 1987;57:37-44.

49. Salden T. The microembolization syndrome. Microvascular Research 1976;11:221.

50. Carlson RW, Schaeffer RC, Carpio M, Weil MH. Edema fluid and coagulation changes during fulminant pulmonary oedema. Chest 1981;79:43.

51. Bone RC, Francis PB, Pierce AK. Intravascular coagulation associated with adult respiratory distress syndrome. Am J Med 1976;61:585-89.

52. Breene R, Zapol WM, Snider MT, Red SORS, Novelline RA. Early bed side detection of pulmonary vascular occlusion during acute respiratory failure. Am Rev Respir Dis 1981;124:593.

53. Schneider RC, Zapol WM, Carvalho AC. Platelet consumption and sequestration in severe acute respiratory failure. Am Rev Respir Dis 1980;122:445-51.

54. Hyers TM. Pathogenesis of adult respiratory distress syndrome. Current concepts. Semin Respir Med 1981;2:104.

55. Wintrobe MM. Clinical haematology. Lee and Febiger: Philadelphia 1981.

56. Morrison DC, Ulevitch RJ. The effect of bacterial endotoxins on host mediation systems: A Review. Am J Pathol 1978;93:526-617.

57. Haynes JB, Hyers TM, Giclas PC, franks JJ, Pehy TL. Elevated fibrinogen degradation products in the adult respiratory distress syndrome. Am Rev Respir Dis 1980;122:841-47.

58. Rinaldo JE, Rogers RM. Adult respiratory distress syndrome. Changing concepts of lung injury and repair. New Engl J Med 1982;306:900-09.

59. Brigham KL, Ogletree M, Snapper J, Hinson J, Parker R. Prostaglandins and lung injury. Chest 1983;83:705S-72S.

60. Gee MH, Perkowisky SZ, Havill AM, Flynn JT. Role of prostaglandins and leukotrienes in complement initiated lung vascular injury. Chest 1983;83:82S-85S.

61. Garcia-szabo RR, Minnear FL, Bizios R, Johnson A, Malik AB. Role of thromboxane in the pulmonary response to pulmonary microembolization. Chest 1983;83:76S-78S.

62. Brigham KL. Mechanisms of lung injury. Clin Chest Med 1982;3:9-24.

63. Demling RH. Role of prostaglandins in acute pulmonary microvascular injury. Ann NY Acad Sci 1982;384:517-34.

64. Ogletree ML. Pharmacology of prostaglandins in the pulmonary microcirculation. Ann NY Acad Sc 1982;384:191-206.

65. Bone RC, Balk RA, Cerra FB. The ACCP/SCCM Consensus Conference Committee. Definitions for sepsis and organ failure and guidelines for the use of innovative therapies in sepsis. Chest 1992;101:11644-55.

66. Bone RC, Sibbald WJ, Sprung CL. The ACCP/SCCM Consensus Conference on sepsis and organ failure. Chest 1992;101:1481-83.

67. Schumer W. Steroids in the treatment of clinical septic shock. Ann Surg 1976;184:333-41.

68. Sprung CL, Caralis PV, Marcial EH, et al. The effects of high-dose corticosteroids in patients with septic shock. A prospective, controlled study. N Engl J Med 1984;311:1137-43.

69. Bone RC, Fischher CJ, Clemmer TP, Slotman GJ, Metz CA. Early methyl prednisolone treatment for septic syndrome and the adult respiratory distress syndrome. Chest 1987;96:1032-36.

70. Bernard GR, Harris T, Luce JE, et al. High dose corticosteroid in patients with adult respiratory distress syndrome: A randomized double blind trial. N Engl J Med 1987;317:1565-70.

71. Bone RC. SIRS, sepsis, and MODS. Pulmonary Perspectives 1995;12:1-5.

72. Bernard GR. Sepsis trials. Intersection of investigation, regulation, funding and practice. Am J Respir Crit Care Med 1995;152:4-10.

73. Rangel-Frausto MS, Pittet D, Costigan M, Hwang T, Davis CS, Wenzel RP. The natural history of the systemic inflammatory response syndrome (SIRS). JAMA 1995;273:117-23.

74. Manthous CA, Hall JB, Samsel RW. Endotoxin in human diseases. Part 2. Biological effects and clinical evaluation of antiendotoxin therapy. Chest 1993;104:1872-81.

75. Williams TJ, Hellewell PG. Endothelial cell biology. Am Rev Respir Dis 1992;146:S45-S50.

76. Maiscalco MM. Leucocyte and the inflammatory response. Crit Care Med 1993;21:S347.

77. Springer TA. Adhesion receptors of the immune system. Nature 1990;346:425-34.

78. Stoolman LM. Adhesion molecules involved in leucocyte recruitment and lymphocyte recirculation. Chest 1993;103(Suppl):79S-86S.

79. Osborn L. Leucocyte adhesion to endothelium in inflammation. Cell 1990;62:3-6.

80. Lawrence MB, Springer TA. Leukocytes roll on a selectin at physiologic flow rates: Distinction from prerequisite for adhesion through integrins. Cell 1991;65:1-20.

81. Wolff SM. Biological effects of bacterial endotoxins in man. J Infect Dis 1973;128:Suppl:259-64.

82. Orfanos SE, Mavrommati I, Korovesi I, Roussos C. Pulmonary endothelium in acute lung injury: From basic science to the critically ill. Intensive Care Med 2004;30:1702-14.

83. Bone RC. The pathogenesis of sepsis. Ann Intern Med 1991;115:457-69.

84. Lami M, Pallat RJ, Koeniger E, et al. Pathologic features and mechanisms of hypoxemia in adult respiratory distress syndrome. Am Rev Respir Dis 1976;114:267-84.

85. Hallman M, Spragg R, Harrell JH, et al. Evidence of lung surfactant abnormality in respiratory failure. J Clin Invest 1982;70:673-83.

86. Goldstein RH, Fine A. Potential therapeutic initiatives for fibrogenic lung diseases. Chest 1995;108:848-55.

87. Meduri GU, Belenchia JM, Estes RJ, et al. Fibroproliferative phase of ARDS: Clinical findings and effects of corticosteroids. Chest 1991;100:943-52.

88. Gattinoni L, Presenti A. ARDS: The nonhomogenous lungs: Facts and hypothesis. Intensive Crit Care Dig 1987;6:1-4.

89. Bachofen M, Weibel ER. Structural alteration in the adult respiratory distress syndrome. Clin Chest Med 1982;4:79.

90. Hill JP, Ratliff JL, Parrot JC, Lamy M, Fallat RJ, Koeniger E, Yaeger EM, Whitmer G. Pulmonary pathology in acute respiratory insufficiency: Lung biopsy as a diagnostic tool. J Thorac Cardiovasc Surg 1976;71:64-71.

91. Vreim CE, Staub NC. Protein composition of lung fluids in acute alloxan edema in dogs. Am J Physiol 1976;230:376-79.

92. Orell SR. Lung pathology in respiratory distress following shock in the adult. Acta Pathol Microbiol Scand 1971;79:65-76.

93. Pietra GG, Puttner JR,Wust W, Glinz W. The lung after trauma and shock. Fine structure at the alveolar-capillary barrier at autopsies. J Trauma 1982;21:454-62.

94. Pratt PC, Vollmer RT, Shelburne JD, Crapo JD. Pulmonary morphology in a multihospital collaborative extracorporeal membrane oxygenation project. Am J Pathol 1979;94:191-214.

95. Zapol WM, Snider MT. Pulmonary hypertension in severe acute respiratory failure. Chest 1977;71:306-07.

96. Elliot CG, Morris AH, Cenzig M. Pulmonary function and exercise gas exchange in survivors of adult respiratory distress syndrome. Am Rev Respir Dis 1981;123:492.

97. Rotman HH, Lavelle TF, Bimcheff DG, Vanderbelt RJ, Weg JC. Long-term physiologic consequences of the adult respiratory distress syndrome. Chest 1977;72:190.

98. Crouch E. Pathobiology of pulmonary fibrosis. Am J Physiol 1990;3:L159-L184.

99. Katzenstein ALA, Askin FB. Surgical pathology of non-neoplastic lung disease. Philadelphia: WB Saunders 1990;9-57.

100. Dantzker DR. Gas exchange in adult respiratory distress syndrome. Clin Chest Med 1982;3:57-67.

101. Ralph D, Robertson HT. respiratory gas exchange in adult respiratory distress syndrome. Semin Respir Med 1981;2:115.

102. West JB. Respiratory physiology: The essentials: Williams and Wilkins: Baltimore,1979.

103. Teplitz C. The ultrastructural basis for pulmonary pathophysiology following trauma: Pathogenesis of pulmonary oedema. J Trauma 1968;8:700.

104. Case record of the Masschusetts General Hospital. Case No 22-1977. New Engl J Med 1977;296:1279-87.

105. Wallace PG, Spence AA. Adult respiratory distress syndrome. Br Med J 1983;286:1167-68.

106. Staub NC, Nagano H, Pearce ML. Pulmonary oedema in dogs. Especially the sequence of fluid accumulation in the lungs. J Appl Physiol 1967;22:227-40.

107. Iliff ID, Greene RE, Hughes JMB. Effects of interstitial oedema on distribution of ventilation and perfusion in isolated lung. J Appl Physiol 1972;33:462-67.

108. Muir AL, Hall DL, Despas P, Hogg JC. Distribution of blood flow in the lungs in acute pulmonary oedema in dogs. J Appl Physiol 1972;33:763-69.

109. Dantzker DR, Brook CJ, Dehart P, Lynch JP, Weg JG. Ventilation-perfusion distribution in the adult respiratory distress syndrome. Am Rev Respir Dis 1979;120:1039-52.

110. Watson WE. Some observation on dynamic lung compliance during intermittent positive pressure respiration. Br J Anaesth 1962;34:153-57.

111. Pontoppidan H, Geffen B, Lowenstein E. acute respiratory failure in the adult. New Engl J Med 1972;287:690-98.

112. Fein AM, Goldberg SK, Lippmann ML, Fischer R, Morgan L. Adult respiratory distress syndrome. Br J Anaesth 1982;54:723-36.

113. Gattinoni L, Pesenti A, Baglioni S, et al. Inflammatory pulmonary oedema and positive end expiratory pressure: Correlation between imaging and physiologic studies. J Thorac Imaging 1988;3:59-64.

114. Pesenti A, Pelosi P, Gattinoni L. Lung mechanics in ARDS. In Vincent JL (Ed): Update in intensive care and emergency medicine. Berline, Springer. 1990;231-38.

115. Levy P, Andre-Poyaud P, Guigner M, et al. Lung collapse and reopening within ventilatory cycle in adult respiratory distress syndrome (ARDS). [abstract]. Eur Respir J 1990;3(Suppl 10):101S.

116. Swami A, Keogh BF. The pulmonary physician and critical care. The injured lung: Conventional and novel respiratory therapy. Thorax 1992;47:555-62.

117. Snapper JR, Sheller JR. Effects of pulmonary oedema on lung mechanics. Semin Respir Med 1983;4:289.

118. Snapper JR, Ogletree MC, Hutchinson AF, Brigham KA. Meclofenamate prevents increased resistance of the lungs following endotoxemia in unanaesthezied sheep. Am Rev Respir Dis 1981;123:200.

119. Hinson JM, Brigham KL, Hutchinson AP, Snapper JR. Granulocytes participate in the early changes in lung mechanics caused by endotoxaemia. Am Rev Respir Dis 1982;125:275.

120. Zapol WM, Trelstad RL, Coffey JW, Isai I, Salvador RA. Pulmonary fibrosis in severe acute respiratory failure. Am Rev Respir Dis 119:547-54.

121. Aberle DR, Brown K. Radiologic considerations in adult respiratory distress syndrome. Clin Chest Med 1990;11:737-54.

122. Petty TL. Acute respiratory distress syndrome. (ARDS). Dis Mon 1990;36:1-58.

123. Milne EN, Pistolesi M, Miniati M, Giuntini C. The radiologic distribution of cardiogenic and noncardiogenic oedema. Am J Roentgenol 1985;144:879-94.

124. Johnson TH, Altman AR, McCaffree RD. Radiologic considerations in the adult respiratorydistress syn-

drome treated with positive end expiratory pressure (PEEP). Clin Chest Med 1982;3:89-100.

125. Gattinoni L, Presenti A, Torresin A, et al. Adult respiratory distress syndrome profiles by computed tomography. J Thorac Imag 1986;1:25-30.

126. Gattinoni L, Presenti A. Computed tomography scanning in acute respiratory failure. In Zapol WM, Lemaire F (Ed): Adult respiratory distress syndrome. New York: Marcel Dekker 1991;199-221.

127. Maunder RJ, Shuman WP, McHugh JW, Marglin SI, Butler J. Preservation of normal lung regions in the adult respiratory distress syndrome: Analysis by computed tomography. JAMA 1986;255:2463-65.

128. Gattinoni L, Presenti A. Bombino M, et al. Relationships between lung computed tomographic density, gas exchange, and PEEP in acute respiratory failure. Anaesthesiology 1988;69:824-32.

129. Owens EM, Evans TW, Keogh BF, Hansell DM. Computed tomography in established adult respiratory distress syndrome: Correlation with lung injury score. Chest 1994;106:1815-21.

130. Tocino IM, Miller MH, Frederich PR, Bahr AL, Thomas F. CT detection of occult pneumothorax in head trauma. Am J Roentgenol 1984;143:987-90.

131. Bone RC, Maunder R, Slotman G, et al. An early test of survival in patients with the adult respiratory distress syndrome: The PaO$_2$/FiO$_2$ ratio and its differential response to conventional therapy. Chest 1989;96:849-51.

132. Dantzker DR. Gas exchange in acute lung injury. Crit Care Clin 1986;2:527-36.

133. Goldenheim PD, Kazemi H. Cardiopulmonary monitoring of critically ill patients. N Engl J Med 1984; 311:717-20;776-80.

134. Wiedemann HP, Matthay MA, Matthay RA. Cardiovascular-pulmonary monitoring in the intensive care unit. Chest 1984;85:537-49;656-68.

135. Fein A, Grossman RF, Jones JG, et al. The value of oedema fluid protein measurements in patients with pulmonary oedema. Am J Med 1979;67:32-38.

136. Pinsky M, Vincent JL, De Smet JM. Estimating left ventricular filling pressure during positive end expiratory pressure in humans. Am Rev Respir Dis 1991;143:25-31.

137. Parrillo JE, Parker MM, Natanson C, et al. Septic shock in humans: Advances in the pathogenesis, cardiovascular dysfunction, and therapy. Ann Intern Med 1990; 113:227-42.

138. Murray JF, Matthay MA, Luce JM, Flick MR. An expanded definition of the adult respiratory distress syndrome. Am Rev Respir Dis 1988;138:720-23.

139. Heffner JE, Brown LK, Barbieri CA, Harpel KS, Deleo J. Prospective validation of an acute respiratory distress syndrome.predictive score. Am J Respir crit Care Med 1995;152:1518-26.

140. Knaus WA, Wagner DP, draper EA, et al. The APACHE III prognostic system: Risk prediction of hospital mortality for critically ill hospitalized adults. Chest 1991;100:1619-33.

141. Rubin DB, Weiner-Kronish JP, Murray JF, et al. Elevated Von Willebrand factor antigen is an early plasma predictor of acute lung injury in nonpulmonary sepsis syndrome. J Clin Invest 1990;86:474-80.

142. Kollef MH, Wragge T, Pasque C. Determinants of mortality and multiorgan dysfunction in cardiac surgery patients requiring prolonged mechanical ventilation. Chest 1995;107:1395-1401.

143. Sprung CL, Rackow EC, Fein IA, Jacob AI, Isikoff SK. The spectrum of pulmonary oedema: Differentiation of cardiogenic, intermediate, and noncardiogenic forms of pulmonary oedema. Am rev Respir Dis 1981;124:718-22.

144. Idell S, Cohen AB. Bronchoalveolar lavage in patients with adult respiratory distress syndrome. Clin Chest Med 1985;6:459-71.

145. Matthay MA, Wiener-Kronish JP. Intact epithelial barrier function is critical for the resolution of alveolar oedema in humans. Am Rev Respir Dis 1990;142:1250-57.

146. Drake RE, Laine GA. Pulmonary microvascular permeability to fluid and macromolecules. J Appl Physiol 1988;64:487-501.

147. Sivak ED, Wiedemann HP. Clinical measurement of extravascular lung water. Crit Care Clin 1986;2:511-26.

148. Mitchell JP, Schuller D, Calandrino FS, Schuster DP. Improved outcome based on fluid management in critically ill patients requiring pulmonary artery catheterization. Am Rev Respir Dis 1992;145:990-98.

149. Carlile PV, Lowery DD, Gray BA. Effect of PEEP and type of injury on thermal-dye estimation of pulmonary oedema. J Appl Physiol 1986;60:22-31.

150. Wiedmann HP, Matthay MA, Gill CN. Pulmonary endothelial injury and altered lung metabolic function: Early detection of the adult respiratory distress syndrome and possible functional significance. Clin Chest Med 1990;11:723-36.

151. Steinberg KP, Mitchell DR, Maunder RJ, et al. Safety of bronchoalveolar lavage in patients with adult respiratory distress syndrome. Am Rev Respir Dis 1993;148:556-61.

152. Stevens JH, Raffin TA. Adult respiratory distress syndrome-II. Management. Postgrad Med J 1984;60:573-76.

153. Gong H Jr. Positive pressure ventilation in adult respiratory distress syndrome. Clin Chest Med 1982;3:69-88.

154. Swami A, Keogh BF. The injured lung: Conventional and novel respiratory therapy. Thorax 1992;47:555-62.

155. Kollef MH, Schuster DP. The acute respiratory distress syndrome. New Engl J Med 1995332:27-37.

156. Petty TL. A historical perspective of mechanical ventilation. Crit Care Clin 1990;6:489-504.

157. Petereson GW, Baier H. Incidence of pulmonary barotrauma in a medical ICU. Crit Care Med 1983;11:67-69.

158. Woodring JH. Pulmonary interstitial emphysema in the adult respiratory distress syndrome. Crit Care Med 1985;13:786-91.

159. Dreyfuss D, Soler P, Basser G, Sruman G. High inflation pressure pulmonary oedema: Respective effects of high air way pressure, high tidal volume, and positive end expiratory pressure. Am Rev Respir Med 1988;137: 1159-64.

160. Kolobow T, Moretti MP, Fumagalli R, et al. Severe pulmonary function impairment in lung function induced by high peak airway pressure during mechanical ventilation: An experimental study. Am Rev Respir Dis 1987;135:312-15.

161. Tsuno K, Prato P, Kolobow T. Acute lung injury from mechanical ventilation at moderately high airway pressures. J Appl Physiol 1990;69:956-61.

162. Balamugesh T, Kaur S, Majumdar S, Behera D. Surfactant protein-A levels in patients with acute respiratory distress syndrome. Ind J Med Res 2003; 117:129-33.

163. Leatherman JW, Lari RL, Iber C, Ney AL. Tidal volume reduction in ARDS: Effects on cardiac output and arterial oxygenation. Chest 1991;99:1227-31.

164. Kiiski R, Takala J, Kari A, Mulje-Emili J. Effect of tidal volume on gas exchange and oxygen transport in the adult respiratory distress syndrome. Am Rev Respir Dis 1992;146:1131-35.

165. Stoller JK, Kacmarek RM,. Ventilatory strategies in the management of the adult respiratorydistress syndrome. Clin Chest med 1990;11:755-72.

166. Schuster DP. A physiologic approach to initiating, maintaining, and withdrawing mechanical support during acute respiratory failure. Am J Med 1990;88:268-78.

167. Kacmarek RM, Venegas J. Mechanical ventilatory rates and tidal volumes. Respir care 1987;32:466-78.

168. Eberhard I, Guttmann J, Wolf G, et al. Intrinsic PEEP monitored in the ventilated ARDS patients with a mathematical method. J Appl Physiol 1992;73:479-85.

169. Gurevitch MJ, Van dyke J, Young ES, Jackson K. Improved oxygenation and lower peak airway pressure in severe adult respiratory distress syndrome: Treatment with inverse ratio ventilation. Chest 1986;89:211-13.

170. Tharatt RS, Allen RP, Albertson TE. Pressure controlled inverse ratio ventilation in severe adult respiratory failure. Chest 1988;94:755-62.

171. Mercat A, Graini L, Teboul JL, Lenique L, Richard C. Cardiorespiratory effects of pressure controlled ventilation with and without inverse ratio in the adult respiratory distress syndrme. Chest 1993;104:871-75.

172. Gurevitch MJ. Pressure-controlled inverse ratio ventilation. What have you learned? (Editorial) Chest 1993;104:664-65.

173. Garner W, Downs JB, Stock MC, Rasanen J. Airway pressure release ventilation (APRV): A human trial. Chest 1988;94:779-81.

174. Schuster DP, Klain M, Snyder JV. Comparison of high frequency jet ventilation to conventional ventilation during severe acute respiratory failure.in humans. Crit Care Med 1982;10:625-30.

175. Holzapfel L, Robert D, Perrin F, Gaussorgues P, Giudicelli DP. Comparison of high frequency jet ventilation to conventional ventilation in adults with respiratory distress syndrome. Intensive care Med 1987;13:100-05.

176. Carlon GC, Howland WS, Ray C, et al. High frequency jet ventilation: A prospective randomized evaluation. Chest 1983;84:551-59.

177. Hikling KG, Henderson SJ, Jackson R. Low mortality associated with low volume pressure limited ventilation with permissive hypercapnia in severe adult respiratory distress syndrome. Intensive Care Med 1990;16:372-77.

178. Darioli R, Perrett C. Mechanical controlled hypoventilation in status asthmaticus. Am Rev Respir Dis 1984;129:385-87.

179. Gattinoni L, Pesenti A, Mascheroni D, et al. Low frequency positive pressure ventilation with extracorporeal CO_2 removal in severe acute respiratory failure. JAMA 1986;256:881-86.

180. Zapol WM, Snider MT, Hill JD, et al. Extracorporeal membrane oxygenation in severe acute respiratory failure: A randomized prospective study. JAMA 1979;242:2193-96.

181. Evans TW, Keogh BF. Extracorporeal membrane oxygenation: A breath of fresh air or yesterday's treatment? Thorax 1991;46:692-94.

182. Kallis P, Al-saady NM, Bennet D, Treasure T. Clinical use of intravascular oxygenation (letter). Lancet 1991;337:546.

183. Shapiro BA, Peruzzi WT. Intracorporeal respiratory support. A potential supplement to airway pressure therapy? Chest 1993;103:1-2.

184. Conrd SA, Eggerstedt JM, Morris VF, Romero MD. Prolonged intracorporeal support of gas exchange with an intracaval oxygenator. Chest 1993;103:158-61.

185. Piehl MA, Brown RS. Use of extreme position changes in acute respiratory failure. Crit Care Med 1976;4:13-14.

186. Douglas WW, Rehder K, Beynen FM, Sessler AD, Marsh HM. Improved oxygenation in patients with acute respiratory failure: The prone position. Am Rev Respir Dis 1977;115:559-66.

187. Langer M, Mascheroni D, Marcolin R, Gattinoni L. The prone position in ARDS patients.: a clinical study. Chest 1988;94:103-107.

188. Piehl MA, Brown RS. Use of extreme position changes in acute respiratory failure. Crit Care Med 1976;4,13-14.

189. Gattinoni L, Tognoni G, Pesenti A, et al. Effect of prone positioning on the survival of patients with acute respiratory failure. N Engl J Med 2001;345,568-73.

190. Lamm WJ, Graham MM, Albert RK. Mechanism by which the prone position improves oxygenation in acute lung injury. Am J Respir Crit Care Med 1994; 150,184-93.

191. Martynowicz MA, Minor TA, Walters BJ, et al. Regional expansion of oleic acid-injured lungs. Am J Respir Crit Care Med 1999;160,250-58.

192. Glenny RW, Lamm WJ, Albert RK, et al. Gravity is a minor determinant of pulmonary blood flow distribution. J Appl Physiol 1991;71,620-29.

193. Wiener CM, Kirk W, Albert RK. Prone position reverses gravitational distribution of perfusion in dog lungs with oleic acid-induced injury. J Appl Physiol 1990;68, 1386-92.

194. Nyren S, Mure M, Jacobsson H, et al. Pulmonary perfusion is more uniform in the prone than in the supine position: Scintigraphy in healthy humans. J Appl Physiol 1999;86,1135-41.

195. Pappert D, Rossaint R, Slama K, et al. Influence of positioning on ventilation-perfusion relationships in severe adult respiratory distress syndrome. Chest 1994;106,1511-16.

196. Mutoh T, Lamm WJ, Embree LJ, et al. Abdominal distension alters regional pleural pressures and chest wall mechanics in pigs in vivo. J Appl Physiol 1991; 70,2611-18.

197. Mutoh T, Guest RJ, Lamm WJ, et al. Prone position alters the effect of volume overload on regional pleural pressures and improves hypoxemia in pigs in vivo. Am Rev Respir Dis 1992;146,300-06.

198. Albert RK, Hubmayr RD. The prone position eliminates compression of the lungs by the heart. Am J Respir Crit Care Med 2000;161,1660-65.

199. Pelosi P, Croci M, Calappi E, et al. The prone positioning during general anesthesia minimally affects respiratory mechanics while improving functional residual capacity and increasing oxygen tension. Anesth Analg 1995;80,955-60.

200. Albert RK, Leasa D, Sanderson M, et al. The prone position improves arterial oxygenation and reduces shunt in oleic-acid-induced acute lung injury. Am Rev Respir Dis 1987;135,628-33.

201. Pelosi P, Tubiolo D, Mascheroni D, et al. Effects of the prone position on respiratory mechanics and gas exchange during acute lung injury. Am J Respir Crit Care Med 1998;157,387-93.

202. Broccard AF, Shapiro RS, Schmitz LL, et al. Influence of prone position on the extent and distribution of lung injury in a high tidal volume oleic acid model of acute respiratory distress syndrome. Crit Care Med 1997; 25,16-27.

203. Broccard A, Shapiro RS, Schmitz LL, et al. Prone positioning attenuates and redistributes ventilator-induced lung injury in dogs. Crit Care Med 2000;28,295-303.

204. Broccard AF. Prone Position in ARDS. Are we looking at a half-empty or half-full glass? Chest 2003;123: 1334-36.

205. Schlitt HJ, Warner U, Schandelmaier P, et al. (abstract). Eur Respir J 1991;4(Suppl):177.

206. Anzueto A, Baughman R, Guntupalli K, et al. An international, randomized, placebo-controlled trial evaluating the safety and efficacy of aerosolized surfactant in patients with sepsis-induced ARDS. Am J Crit Care Med 1994;149:A567.

207. Lewis JF, Jobe JH. Surfactant and the adult respiratory distress syndrome. Am Rev Respir Dis 1993;147:218 233.

208. Spragg RG, Gillard N, Richman P, et al. Effect of a single dose of porcine surfactant on patients with adult respiratory distress syndrome. Chest 1994;105:195-202.

209. Sibbald WJ, Anderson RR, Reid B, Holliday RI, Driedger AA. Alveolo-capillary permeability in human sepsis ARDS: Effect of high dose corticosteroid therapy. Chest 1981;79:133-42.

210. Sprung CL, Caralis PV, Marcial EH, et al. The effect of high dose corticosteroids in patients with septic shock: A prospective controlled study. New Engl J Med 1984;311:1137-43.

211. Bernard GR, Luce JM, Sprung Cl, et al. High dose corticosteroid in patients with the adult respiratory distress syndrome. New Engl J Med 1987;317:1565-70.

212. Luce JM, Montgomery AB, Marks JD, et al. Ineffective-ness of high dose methylprednisolone in preventing parenchymal lung injury and improving mortality in patients with septic shock. Am rev Respir Dis 1988; 138:62-68.

213. Bone RC, Fisher CJ Jr, Clemmer TP, Slottman GJ, Metz CA. Early methylprednisolone treatment for septic syndrome and the adult respiratory distress syndrome. Chest 1987;92:1032-1036.

214. Hooper RG, Kearle RA. Established ARDS treated with a sustained course of adrenocortical steroids. Chest 1990;97:138-43.

215. Jepsen S, Herlevsen P, Knudsen P, Bud MI, Klausen NO. Anti-oxidant treatment with N-acetylcystein during adult respiratory distress syndrome: A prospective, randomized, placebo-controlled study. Crit Care Med 1992;20:918-23.

216. Suter P, Domenighetti G, Schaller MD, et al. N-acetyl cystein enhances recovery from acute lung injury in man. Chest 1994;105:190-94.

217. Slotman GJ, Burchard KW, D'Arezzo A, Gann DS. Ketoconazole prevents acute respiratory failure in critically ill surgical patients. J Trauma 1988;28:648-54.

218. Yu M, Tomasa G. A double-blind, prospective, randomized trial of ketoconazole, a thromboxane synthatase inhibitor, in the prophylaxis of the adult respiratory distress syndrome. Crit Care Med 1993;21:1635-42.

219. Puybasset L, Rouby JJ, Mourgeon E, et al. Factors influencing cardiopulmonary effects of inhaled nitric oxide in acute respiratory failure. Am J Crit Care Med 1995;152:318-28.

220. Bernard GR, Reines HD, Haluskka PV, et al. Prostacycline and thromboxane A2 formation is increased in human sepsis syndrome: Effects of cyclooxygenase inhibition. Am Rev Respir Dis 1991;144:1095-1101.

221. Houp MT, Jastremeski MS, Clemmer TP, Metz CA, Goris GB. Effect of ibuprofen in patients with severe

sepsis: A randomized, double blind, multicenter study. Crit Care Med 1991;19:1339-47.

222. Bone RC, Slotman G, Maunder R, et al. Randomized, double blind, multicenter study of prostaglandin E1 in patients with adult respiratory distress syndrome. Chest 1989;96:114-19.

223. Ziegler EJ, Fischer CJ Jr, Sprung CL, et al. Treatment of Gram-negative bacteremia and septic shock with HA-1A human monoclonal antibody against endotoxin: A randomized, double blind, placebo-controlled trial. New Engl J Med 1991;324:429-36.

224. Greenman RL, Schein RMH, Martin MA, et al. A controlled clinical trial of E5 murine monoclonal IgM antibody to endotoxin in the treatment of Gram-negative sepsis. JAMA 1991;266:1097-1102.

225. Fisher CJ, Opal SM, Dhainault JF, et al. Influence of an anti-tumor necrosis factor monoclonal antibody on cytokine levels in patients with sepsis. Crit Care Med 1993;21:318-27.

226. Torre D, Minoja G, Maraggia D, et al. Effect of IL-1 beta and recombinant gamma-interferon on septic acute lung injury in mice. Chest 1994;105:1241-45.

227. John RC St, Dorinsky PM. Immunologic therapy for ARDS, septic shock, and multiple organ failure. Chest 1993;103:932-43.

228. Petty TL. Indicators of risk, course, and prognosis in adult respiratory distress syndrome (ARDS). Am Rev Respir Dis 1985;132:471.

229. Rinaldo JE. Letter. Indicators of risk, course, and prognosis in adult respiratory distress syndrome. Am Rev Respir Dis 1986;133:343-44.

230. Fowler AA, Hamman RF, Good JT, et al. Adult respiratory distress syndrome: Risk with common predispositions. Ann Intern Med 1983;98:593-97.

231. Bell RC, Coalson JJ, Smith JD, Johanson WG Jr. Multi-organ system failure and infection in adult respiratory distress syndrome. Ann Intern Med 1983;99:293-98.

232. Montgomery AB, Stager MA, Carrico CJ, Hudson LD. Causes of mortality in patients with adult respiratory distress syndrome. Am Rev Respir Dis 1985;132:485-89.

233. Suchyata MR, Clemmer TP, Elliot CG, Orme JF Jr, Weaver LK. The adult respiratory distress syndrome: A report of survival and modifying factors. Chest 1992;101:1074-79.

234. Steinberg KP, McHuge LG, Hudson LD. Causes of mortality in patients with the adult respiratory distress syndrome.(ARDS): An update. Am Rev Respir Dis 1993;147 (Suppl): A347.

235. Meduri GU, Headley S, Kohler G, et al. Persistent elevation of inflammatory cytokines predicts a poor outcome in ARDS. Plasma IL-1beta and IL-6 levels are consistent and efficient predictors of outcome over time. Chest 1995;107:1062-67.

236. Vasilyev S, Schaap RN, Mortensen JD. Hospital survival rates of patients with acute respiratory failure in modern respiratory intensive care units. An International, multicenter, prospective survey. Chest 1995;107:1083-88.

237. Alberts WM, Priest GR, Moser KM. The outlook for survivors of ARDS. Chest 1983;84:272-74.

238. Ghio AJ, Elliot CG, Crapo RA, Berlin SL, Jensen RL. Impairment after adult respiratory distress syndrome. An evaluation based on American Thoracic Society recommendations. Am Rev Respir Dis 1989;139:1158-62.

239. Elliot CG, Rasmusson BY, Crapo RA, Morris AH, Jens RL. Prediction of pulmonary function abnormalities after adult respiratory distress syndrome. (ARDS). Am Rev Respir Dis 1987;135:634-38.

240. Connell RS, Swank RL, Webb MC. The development of pulmonary ultrastructural lesions during hemor-rhagic shock. J Trauma 1975;15,116-29.

241. Lakshminarayan S, Stanford RE, Petty TL. Prognosis after recovery from adult respiratory distress syndrome. Am Rev Respir Dis 1976;113,7-16.

242. Neff TA, Stocker R, Frey H, Stein S, Russi EW. Long-term assessment of lung function in survivors of severe ARDS. Chest 2003;123:845-53.

Chapter
21

Interstitial Lung Diseases

DEFINITION

Interstitial lung disease, or more appropriately interstitial fibrosis is a chronic progressive inflammatory disorder characterized by both inflammation and fibrosis of lung parenchyma and is associated with a wide variety of clinical situations (more than 150 clinicopathological entities) with progressive damage to the alveolar wall.[1,2] Many acute and chronic lung disorders with variable degrees of pulmonary inflammation and fibrosis are collectively referred to as interstitial lung diseases (ILDs) or diffuse parenchymal lung diseases. Idiopathic pulmonary fibrosis (IPF) or cryptogenic fibrosing alveolitis (CFA) is one of the several ILDs. The term interstitial is a misnomer, since the disease not only affects the interstitium, but also involves all the cellular and biochemical components of the alveolar wall extending into the alveolar space as well. Most often the terminal bronchioles and small vessels are also involved in the inflammatory process.[3-5]

It was first described by Sandoz in 1907, but was recognized as a clinical entity by Hamman and Rich in 1935[6,7] in four patients manifested by dyspnea with a rapidly downhill course and death within 6 months due to cor pulmonale or respiratory failure. However, the fulminant form is rare, and majority of patients pursue a more chronic and protracted course lasting for few years.[8,9] Systematic study of the disease entity started with availability of lung biopsy specimens. Liebow was the first to critically examine the pathologic features of interstitial pneumonias and divided them into five groups based on specific histologic criteria.[10] Subsequently other investigators lumped then into a single entity using a variety of terms, including diffuse interstitial fibrosis, diffuse fibrosing alveolitis, cryptogenic fibrosing alveolitis, classical interstitial pneumonitis-fibrosis, diffuse interstitial pneumonitis and interstitial pulmonary fibrosis.[11-17] Recently, in the European countries, the term cryptogenic fibrosing alveolitis is often used,[18] whereas in USA, the entity is called as interstitial pulmonary fibrosis (IPF). The term Hamman-Rich syndrome is still used for the rapidly progressive forms of the disease.

ETIOLOGY

Although a number of causes/etiological agents are known to cause interstitial lung disease, in more than 70 percent of this heterogeneous group of disease have no known cause (idiopathic). Some of the important known causes that can produce interstitial lung disease are shown in Table 21.1.

TABLE 21.1: Causes of interstitial lung disease[19-26]

1. Idiopathic	ARDS
2. Hypersensitivity pneumonitis	Inhalation injury (toxic gas)
3. Infections	Drug (bleomycin, nitrofurantoin,
Fungal (histoplasmosis, coccidioidomycosis)	amiodarone, etc.)
Viral, Tuberculosis, Nocardiosis	Left ventricular failure
Lyme disease, Legionnaires' disease	Chronic aspiration
Mycoplasma infections	Lymphangitis carcinomatosis
Pneumocystis carinii	Organic antigens
4. Collagen vascular diseases	Pneumoconioses
Systemic lupus erythematosus	Sarcoidosis
Rheumatoid arthritis	Histiocytosis X
Progressive systemic sclerosis	Oxygen toxicity, radiation
Polymyositis	Idiopathic pulmonary hemosiderosis
Mixed connective tissue disease	Lymphangioleiomyomatosis

Idiopathic pulmonary fibrosis will be discussed as a prototype of ILDs.

IDIOPATHIC PULMONARY FIBROSIS

Definition

In 2000, an International consensus statement defines the diagnosis, evaluation, and management of patients with IPF.[27,28] This was a collaborative effort from the American Thoracic Society, European Respiratory Society, and the American College of Chest physicians. IPF, according to this committee is defined as "a specific form of chronic fibrosing interstitial pneumonia limited to the lung and associated with the histologic appearance of usual interstitial pneumonia (UIP) on surgical (thoracoscopic or open) lung biopsy. The etiology is unknown". Definite diagnostic criteria are defined (see below).

Epidemiology

Although the exact incidence and prevalence of the disease is not known, patients with this disease comprised about 15 percent of a pulmonary physician's practice.[29] Recent epidemiological studies indicate that it is at least ten times more common than the original estimates.[30] It is true that death certificates and state mortality data are neither sensitive nor accurate for describing the occurrence of interstitial lung disease.[29] Mortality from cryptogenic fibrosing alveolitis continues to increase in many countries including England, Wales, Australia and Canada. Data from seven different countries have confirmed this.[31] In an analysis of mortality data from England and Wales it is reported that death from this disease has increased approximately two-fold or more between 1979 and 1988.[32] It is estimated that about more than 10,000 hospital admissions in USA each year are due to this disease, particularly the idiopathic variety. A prevalence of as low as 3 per 100,000 in USA[2] and as high as 29 per 100,000 in the state of New Mexico[33] has been reported. A recent report describes pulmonary fibrosis mortality in the United States from 1979 through 1991 by analyzing death certificate reports compiled by the National Centre for Health Statistics.[34] This is about 0.4 percent of all deaths. Among men, age-adjusted mortality rates increased from 48.6 per 1,000,000 in 1979 to 50.9 per 1,000,000 in 1991 and, among women, these rates increased from 21.4 to 27.2 respectively. Among both men and women, rates were higher in older age strata than in younger age strata. Age-adjusted mortality rates were consistently higher among whites and people of races other than blacks. The frequency with which pulmonary fibrosis was listed as the underlying cause of death increased from 40 percent in 1979 to 56 percent in 1991. Incidence of IPF is estimated to be 10.7 cases per 100,000 per year for males and 7.4 cases per 100,000 per year for females.[34] The mortality rate for IPF was estimated to be 3.3 in men and 2.5 in women, with an overall rate of 3.0 in both sexes in Japan.[35] In England and Wales, the annual number of deaths due to CFA has doubled between 1979 and 1988.[36] The mean length of survival from the time of diagnosis varied between 28.2 months and 5 years.[37,38]

In India, the entity was earlier considered to be a rare disease. Therefore, published data on the subject in Indian literature is few. In 1979, Jindal et al.[39] published their data in 61 cases seen over a period of five years. Subsequently a number of other publications described various other aspects of the disease.[40-49] However, the scenario is different now and the disease is not all that rare or uncommon. This increase may be a true reflection of the increase in the incidence or may be apparent because of increased awareness of the condition or because of increased diagnostic facilities available now like high-resolution CT or transbronchial lung biopsy through fiber-optic bronchoscopy. The first one appears to be more likely.

Males are more commonly affected than females.[30,35,50-53] IPF patients are more often middle-aged with a range of 40 to 70 years. More than two-thirds of patients are over the age of 60 years at the time of presentation with a mean age of diagnosis of 66 years.[15,16,30,50,51,53-56] The incidence increases as the age increases. Whereas the prevalence of the disease is 2.7 per 100,000 between the age group of 35 to 44 years, the prevalence is more than 175 per 100,000 for persons above the age of 75 years.[33] The disease is uncommon in children.[57,58]

Interstitial pulmonary fibrosis has no definite geographic distribution and has been reported from all over the world from both rural and urban areas. There is no predilection for any race or ethnicity although age-adjusted mortality rates are higher among whites and lower in blacks.[38] There is a great variability in the mortality from the disease, possibly because of the effect of differences in occupational or environmental exposures.[38]

Risk Factors for IPF

Epidemiologic studies show that cigarette smoking, antidepressant use, gastroesophageal reflux, and occupational dust exposure are potential risk factors for IPF. Patients with IPF are often middle aged, usually between 40 years and 70 years of age. The incidence of the disease increases with age. Certain life-style modifying factors like diabetes mellitus are also thought to be predisposing factors for idiopathic pulmonary fibrosis.

Smoking

Although the exact cause of IPF is not clear, certain potential factors for the development of the disease have been identified. In case control studies, cigarette smoking has been identified as a potential risk factor with the odds ratio (OR) from various parts of the world ranging from 1.6 to 2.9 for the development of IPF for ever-smokers.[35,50,59,60] The risk increases as the number of pack years of smoking increases. One case-control study has suggested an association between intake of antidepressants and the risk of development of IPF.[61] Chronic aspiration due to gastroesophageal reflux has also been implicated in the development of pulmonary fibrosis.[62]

Genetics

There is some evidence that there is a genetic susceptibility to interstitial lung disease and idiopathic pulmonary fibrosis (IPF) in particular,[63-69] although no specific genetic marker has been identified.[70] A subset of patients with IPF clearly has a familial form of the disease-familial idiopathic interstitial fibrosis (FIPF). Familial form of the disease is defined as at least two members of a primary biological family (parent, child, sibling) having clinical features of IPF that are confirmed histologically.[70,71] Although the genetic mode of transmission is not known, it seems likely that it is autosomal dominant with variable penetrance.[69] Males and females are equally affected. Search for the "fibrotic genes" responsible for susceptibility in the major histocompatibility complex, has found locations in human chromosome 6. Even, if there has been no clear association with human leucocyte antigen (HLA) an increased incidence of HLA-B15, HLA-B8, HLA-B12 HLA-Dr2 and Dw6 have been reported in patients with IPF.[65,72-74] However, most cases familial association can be difficult to establish since environmental factors tend to cluster around families as well. Several investigators have reported an association between IPF and a1-antitrypsin inhibition (Pi) alleles present on chromosome 14.[75-77] In a recent study, the familial form in Finland has been found to be 3.3 to 3.7 percent of all Finnish cases of IPF.[78] Geographic clustering of multiplex families gives a prevalence of 5.9/million for familial form of the disease.

Environmental Factors

Various environmental exposures in rural or agricultural areas and in urban and industrial settings have been linked to the development of IPF, when a defined pneumoconiosis was not present.[27,35,38,50]

The most consistent association has been with exposure to wood dust and metal dust. The risk increases with the number of years of exposure.[79] Dust containing steel, brass, lead and pinewood, are most specifically linked. A casual relationship has been reported between IPF and exposure to high concentrations of welding fumes.[80] Exposure to solvents[81] and atopy[82] are also blamed. The diagnosis, of course, was mainly based on clinical features rather than on HRCT or biopsy. In a case control study from 16 different centers involving 248 cases, it was confirmed that increased risk is associated with dusty environment.[83] Several occupational factors adjusted for age and smoking in conditional multivariate logistic regression analyses showed significant association with IPF: farming (OR = 1.6; livestock, OR = 2.7; hairdressing OR = 4.4; metal dust, OR = 2.0; raising birds, OR = 4.7; stone cutting/polishing, OR = 3.9; and vegetable dust/animal dust, OR = 4.7. Interaction was detected between smoking and exposure to livestock and farming.

Bronchoalveolar lavage studies in toxic gas exposed subjects in Bhopal gas tragedy had revealed that there was a subclinical alveolitis characterized by accumulation of macrophages in the lower respiratory tract, especially in severely exposed subjects.[84] Further studies after varying periods of times have suggested that persisting clinical, roentgenographic and ventilatory abnormalities, as well as macrophage-neutrophil alveolitis along with abnormally elevated fibrinonectin levels in a proportion of subjects can lead on to lung fibrosis in these subjects exposed to toxic gas during Bhopal gas tragedy.[85] Restrictive type of ventilatory defect has been described in women exposed to cooking fuels during cooking.[86] A type of interstitial lung disease, known as "Gujjar Lung" is described from Kashmir valley, India.[87]

Infections

Numerous viruses have been implicated and viral triggers to the immunopathogenic mechanism in IPF have long been sought, although a definite evidence of a viral etiology is not clear.[88,89] There are some evidences for an association between Epstein-Barr Virus (EBV) infection and IPF and EBV viral capsid antigen has been demonstrated in lung tissue.[90-93] Although Japanese and Italian workers found an increased prevalence of antibodies to hepatitis C virus in patients with IPF, the same has not been found in British studies. A higher incidence of EBV, influenza, CMV and hepatitis C infection has been reported in these patients.[27] Italian patients with IPF showed an increased prevalence (~ 13%) of HCV infection and viral replication, but the prevalence of anti-HCV antibodies does not differ from other lung diseases.[94,95] Other agents like parainfluenza

1 virus, HIV-1, measles virus, parainfluenza-3 virus, herpes virus, mycoplasma, and Legionnaires' disease have also been implicated as potential contributors to the pathogenesis IPF. Recently a TT virus infection has also been implicated as a contributor.[96]

PATHOGENESIS

Several cellular and biochemical processes occur in interstitial lung disease, although the precise stimulus for this is not known.[97] Possibly viral, genetic, immune, and environmental factors play a role as initiating or contributing factors. Regardless of etiology, the parenchymal abnormalities follow a similar progression of inflammation involving the alveolar walls, adjacent air spaces, and laying down of an excess of connective tissue. The entire process from injury to fibrosis can be very rapid or more gradual depending on the type of injury/tissue reaction.

In all of these processes, activation of macrophages is the central event. These cells are activated by many ways via surface Fc receptors. In idiopathic type, both local and circulating immune complexes induce the activation. Alveolar wall B-lymphocytes produce antibodies to antigens, which may be some component of the alveolar wall erroneously recognized as foreign, or some other exogenous antigen. The activated macrophages produce fibronectin, chemoattractants, and many other substances that are injurious to cell. Fibronectin is an important regulator of cell adherence and chemotactic for fibroblasts. This also enhances fibroblast replication. Neutrophils attracted to the site of injury, produce a number of potentially damaging substances. These include platelet-derived growth factor, oxygen radicals, and elastase. There is an increased endothelial cell-neutrophil adherence. The damage to endothelial cells involves the formation of H_2O_2 and the participation of iron. In addition, endothelial cell-derived xanthine oxidase appears to participate in the process of cell injury. Activation of xanthine oxidase within endothelial cells can also be achieved by interaction of these cells with three chemotactic peptides: C5a, tumor necrosis factor (TNF)-α, and N'-formyl-Met-Leu-Phe. Recently, interferon is recognized as an important mediator of pulmonary fibrosis.[98,99] Cytokines play an important role in lung injury. Such injury can also be produced by intra-alveolar deposition of immune complexes consisting of IgG. Platelet-derived growth factor (PDGF) is released spontaneously by alveolar macrophages in idiopathic pulmonary fibrosis. The c-sis, a proto-oncogene encoding for β-chain of PDGF is up regulated in lavage fluid cells.[100,101] This factor causes fibroblast proliferation. Recently, it has been also recognized that mast cells play

important role in lying of fibroblasts.[102] Anti-collagen antibodies have been identified in patients of IPF and may be useful as clinical markers for activity and may perpetuate the lung tissue inflammation.[103] It is unclear if the autoimmunity of the collagen participates in the pathogenesis of IPF or the presence of the antibody just an epiphenomenon. Interleukin-8 may play a role in neutrophilic alveolitis, particularly during the subacute phase of IPF.[104]

Both major basic protein and eosinophilic cationic protein have been found in bronchoalveolar lavage fluid from these patients. Activated macrophages also produce oxidants, proteases, collagenase, and growth factors, in addition to their production by neutrophils. Such mediators modulate fibroblast growth and collagen deposition resulting in fibrosis.

Thus, idiopathic pulmonary fibrosis is thought to arise as a response to persistent lung injury and inflammation.[105] The early response to injury to the alveolar epithelium and/or the vascular endothelium results in the influx of neutrophils to the interstitium and airspaces, which may persist.[106] Support for immunologically mediated injury comes from the fact that there is a phase of mononuclear cell abundance in which the recruitment of monocytes/macrophages and lymphocytes in the lungs occurs, presumably in response to an as yet unidentified antigen or immunological target. These cells are thought to release fibrogenic cytokines such as tumor necrosis factor alpha, transforming growth factors alpha and beta, and eicosanoids such as leukotrienes B4 and C4 in addition to other factors mentioned above, which recruit and activate fibroblasts and stimulate deposition of connective tissue.[107] Major steps in the pathogenesis of IPF, as was thought earlier, have been shown in Figure 21.1.[108]

Oxidant/antioxidant imbalance in the lower respiratory tract has been proposed as the mechanism of lung injury in a number of inflammatory lung conditions including IPF.[109] An increased oxidant burden in the lungs in IPF is thought to arise from the accumulation of inflammatory cells in the lower respiratory tract.[2] including activated alveolar macrophages and neutrophil, which show an exaggerated release of oxygen radicals.[110] Oxidants have been implicated in the epithelial injury, which is characteristic of this condition. Studies have also shown that increased amounts of reactive oxygen intermediates (ROI) are spontaneously released by inflammatory cells in the lungs of patients with IPF.[111] These react with the excessive amounts of myeloperoxidases present in the epithelial lining fluid of patients with IPF to form the highly toxic hypohalide ion.[112] Although the mechanisms responsible for

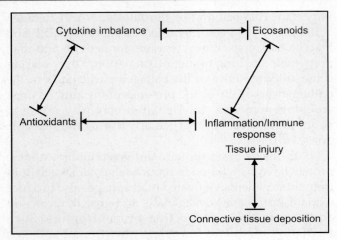

FIGURE 21.1: Schematic representation of pathogenesis of IPF

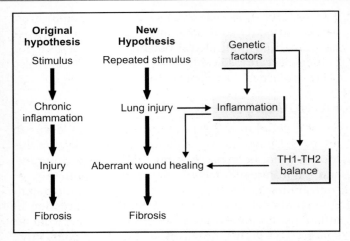

FIGURE 21.2: Pathogenesis of idiopathic pulmonary fibrosis

increased release of ROIs are not known, it is possible that immune complexes may be involved.[113,114] Other potential oxidants, which may be involved in the tissue injury of IPF are the nitrogen centered radicals. In addition to direct tissue injury, oxidants may also up regulate cytokine production possibly through activation of the transcriptional factor for cytokine genes NFκB[115] and thus promote fibrosis through enhanced release of cytokines. More recent reports indicate an increased oxidant burden and antioxidant, e.g. glutathione (GSH), deficiency in the lower respiratory tract to play a role in the progression of IPF.[116,117]

Understanding various mechanisms of development of IPF is important to understand because treatment strategies will be thus categorized whether one tries to treat (i) the inflammatory/immune responses or tissue injury (ii) treatment for subsequent release of eicosanoids and cytokines or (iii) treatment for subsequent deposition of connective tissue deposition.

In certain other diseases causing interstitial lung disease, like sarcoidosis, and hypersensitivity pneumonitis, lymphocytes are the predominant immune effector cells that are recruited in response to lymphocyte activating factor (IL-1) and chemotactic factor released by activated macrophages. There is a change in the helper: suppressor T lymphocyte subset.

Serum cytokeratin 19-fragment (CYFRA) is elevated in some nonmalignant respiratory diseases, especially in IPF. The value of serum CYFRA would reflect the severity of lung injury in nonmalignant respiratory diseases and might be related to the prognosis in patients with IPF.

Although the exact march of events leading to the development of IPF are not very clear, more and more reports elucidate the role of various inflammatory mediators, cytokines, growth factors, alterations in the surfactant properties, coagulation parameters, genetic abnormalities, abnormal regulation of apoptosis and microsatellite instabilty.[118-162]

In the past, the primary focus was on the inflammatory component leading on to IPF as is depicted in Figure 21.1. The role of various inflammatory cells and mediators in the injury to the alveoli that characterizes IPF and the contribution of the inflammatory process to the fibrosis have been highlighted earlier. According to this original hypothesis, IPF was viewed as a smoldering inflammatory response that ultimately led to chronic lung injury with subsequent fibrosis. More recently, the role of fibrogenesis *per se* has emerged as an important component of the pathogenesis of the disease. IPF is thought to be as a result of aberrant wound healing following repeated episodes of acute lung injury due to a still-unidentified stimulus. Figure 21.2 depicts the recent concept of pathogenesis of IPF.[35,163] Newer insight suggests that idiopathic pulmonary fibrosis results from sequential acute lung injury. The resultant wound healing response to this injury culminates in pulmonary fibrosis. Several interacting factors that modify this fibrotic response include the genetic background of the patient, the predominant inflammatory phenotype (Th1 or Th2), and environmental inflammatory triggers like smoke, viral infection, and respirable toxins.

PATHOLOGY

Irrespective of the etiology of interstitial lung disease, the histological changes are similar and consist of varying degrees of parenchymal infiltration with inflammatory cells and interstitial edema, denuded basement membrane, desquamated alveolar epithelial cells, proliferation of type II pneumocytes, disruption of basement membrane, endothelial cell damage, and proliferation of fibroblasts with varying degrees of interstitial and intra-alveolar fibrosis.[164] These changes vary in proportion at different stages of the disease.[165] Rindfleisch recognized smooth muscle proliferation in the lung under pathologic circumstances as early as 1872 in a study of brown indurations and in the next year, von Buhl used the term muscular cirrhosis.[166] In recent years smooth muscle proliferation in pulmonary fibrotic lesions is considered to be one of the important pathologic features of idiopathic pulmonary fibrosis or usual interstitial pneumonia.[165,167,168] Some authors have graded the smooth muscle proliferation into 3 grades in a semi-quantitative manner: Grade 1- less than several smooth muscle cells in pulmonary fibrotic changes; Grade 2-intermediate between Grade 1 and 2; Grade 3- diffuse smooth muscle cell proliferation forming bundles or nodular growth.[169] In some areas, the lumen of terminal bronchioles is occluded with inflammatory process, bronchiolitis obliterans. Varying degrees of vasculitis affecting the capillaries and small to medium size vessels occur in interstitial lung diseases particularly associated with collagen vascular diseases. In IPF, there is disturbance of extracellular matrix protein deposition resulting from fibroblast activation and proliferation. The structural and functional features of the fibrillar collagens I and III in the interstitium are altered and there is an inappropriate accumulation in the fibrotic lung.[170-173] Collagen VI, which forms a microfibrillar meshwork and serve as an anchoring element between collagen I and III fibrils and basement membrane and as a cell binding substrate, is also expressed increasingly in the fibrotic lung.[174]

Three broad patterns of histological changes in interstitial fibrosis have been described.[175-177] (i) A cellular pattern characterized by increased number of macrophages and lymphocytes in the intra-alveolar space, particularly in the early stages of the disease. This pattern has been termed as "desquamative interstitial pneumonia" (DIP). Hyperplastic type II cells line the alveolar wall. Lymphocytes and occasional eosinophils infiltrate the alveolar septa. There may be slight increase in the mesenchymal cells, but fibrosis is distinctly uncommon at this stage. (ii) The other pattern is a mixed cellular-fibrotic pattern, termed as "usual interstitial pneumonitis" (UIP). This is characterized by intense interstitial inflammation composed of lymphocytes, eosinophils, monocytes, and plasma cells. Thickening of the alveolar wall due to increased number of mesenchymal cells is a characteristic feature in this stage. The intra-alveolar space may contain proteinaceous debris, and early honeycombing may be present in some areas. Thus, the mixed cellular-fibrotic pattern is heterogeneous histological change with areas of inflammation inter-

mixed with areas of fibrosis. (iii) The end-stage, or honeycomb pattern is characterized by replacement of the pulmonary parenchyma by irregular cysts of 1.0 to 2.5 mm in size. The alveolar septa are thick and lined by metaplastic alveolar epithelial cells. The distribution of honeycombing is also heterogeneous. The changes may not be uniform. Different changes may be present in the same lobe or even in the same area in a patchy manner. These histological patterns are important for prognosis and response to corticosteroid therapy. More cellular is the histology, better is the prognosis and greater is the response to corticosteroids.

A scoring system for the lung biopsies in idiopathic pulmonary fibrosis has been suggested. A qualitative assessment on the basis of overall cellularity and fibrosis is made on a scale from 0 to 5. In addition, 15 specific histopathological features that are divided into three sections, inflammatory/exudative changes, fibrotic/ reparative changes, and airway alterations are scored in a semi-quantitative fashion. It is suggested that this scoring points should be used in reporting the disease activity in interstitial pulmonary fibrosis.[165]

Thus, the pathology of IPF may be summarized as follows: in the development of IPF after injury, there is disruption of the alveolar epithelial surface with leakage of serum contents into the alveolar lumen, and this is followed by the collection of inflammatory and immune effector cells as discussed above within the interstitium, i.e. active cellularity. This is followed by organization of the intra-alveolar exudate and apposition of the alveolar walls. Alterations in the connective tissue matrix occur, and this may progress to interstitial fibrosis.[170,178]

The gross histologic findings of IPF range from a normal appearance in early cases to diffuse honeycombing in the later stages of the disease process. The involvement is usually heterogenous and worse in the lower lobes. A subpleural, peripheral, and paraseptal distribution of fibrosis is often seen. Areas of mildly involved or even normal pulmonary parenchyma may be interspersed throughout a background of extensive fibrosis and honeycombing.

Liebow was the first to describe the pathological features of interstitial pneumonias and divided them into five major groups based on specific histologic criteria.[10] They were as follows: usual interstitial pneumonia (UIP); Desquamative interstitial pneumonia (DIP); bronchiolitis obliterans with interstitial pneumonia (BIP); lymphoid interstitial pneumonia (LIP); and giant cell interstitial pneumonia (GIP). However, the original description of BIP, is now known as bronchiolitis obliterans-organizing pneumonia (BOOP) is a well accepted and distinct clinical entity, predominantly being an intraluminal rather than interstitial disease both pathologically as well as radiologically (patchy air space opacities). Lymphoid interstitial pneumonia, once rare, has become significant because of its association with acquired immune deficiency syndrome (AIDS), and giant-cell interstitial pneumonia (GIP) has been shown to represent the pathologic counterpart of hard-metal pneumoconiosis.[179] Some investigators still believe that DIP and UIP are the spectrum of the same disease, with DIP representing the early or cellular stage of the disease.

However, the current classification of interstitial pneumonias includes four clinicopathologically distinct and easily separable variants.[180,181] These are shown in Table 21.2. *However, the International Consensus Statement clarifies that UIP is the histopathological pattern that identifies patients with IPF (27). The other types are excluded from the group of patients with IPF.*

<table>
<tr><td colspan="1">TABLE 21.2: Pathologic classification of idiopathic pulmonary fibrosis[181]</td></tr>
</table>

Usual interstitial pneumonia (UIP)
Desquamative interstitial pneumonia (DIP) or respiratory bronchiolitis associated interstitial lung disease (RBILD)
Acute interstitial pneumonia (AIP) or Hamman-Rich syndrome
Nonspecific interstitial pneumonia (NSIP)

Usual Interstitial Pneumonia (UIP)

The histologic hallmark and main diagnostic criterion is a heterogenous appearance with a patchy, nonuniform, and variable distribution of interstitial changes. This appearance is usually appreciated under low power of the microscope. The histological features are typically described as *temporal and spatial heterogeneity*. Temporal heterogeneity refers to the combination of lesions at different stages. Spatial heterogeneity refers to the nonuniform involvement at a microscopic level. The *temporal and spatial heterogeneity* are unique for UIP. These changes include alternating areas of normal lung, interstitial inflammation, fibrosis, and honey combing. These histological changes affect the peripheral, subpleural parenchyma most severely. The interstitial inflammation is usually patchy and consists of alveolar septal infiltration by lymphocytes and plasma cells, and associated with hyperplasia of Type II pneumocytes. The fibrotic zones mainly consist of eosinophilic collagen with few associated inflammatory or stromal cells. This collagen deposition results in thickening of the alveolar septae and forms patchy scars. The fibrotic zones are mainly composed of dense collagen along with scattered foci of proliferating fibroblasts ("fibroblastic foci"), which

are again a very characteristic feature of UIP. Although most of the fibrotic zones are composed of old relatively acellular collagen bundles, small aggregates of actively proliferating myofibroblasts and fibroblasts, which are termed as "fibroblast foci". These are characterized by spindle-shaped cells present within lightly staining, myxoid-appearing matrix, and are arranged with their long axis parallel to the long axis of the alveolar septae. Electron microscopy shows that these foci represent the organization of prior foci of acute lung injury and active collagen synthesis. These fibroblastic foci contain proteoglycans versican and decoran, integrin, vinculin, and tenescin. Although fibroblast foci are not pathognomonic for UIP, they are essential features of diagnosis of UIP. They indicate that fibrosis is ongoing.[182]

Areas of honeycomb changes consist of cystic fibrotic air spaces that are lined by bronchiolar epithelium and filled with mucin. The enlarged airspaces may be empty or may contain inspissated mucin mixed with hystiocytes, neutrophils, and other inflammatory cells. Honeycomb changes are due to scarring and architectural restructuring following lung injury. Thus, it is not specific to UIP. The pathogenesis is due to alveolar collapse and reorganization. It is irreversible and referred to as "end-stage lung". Smooth muscle hyperplasia is commonly seen in areas of fibrosis and honeycomb changes. Presence of changes at different stage probably indicates an ongoing or recurring lung injury.

Inflammation is usually mild and may consist of small lymphocytes, scattered plasma cells, and neutrophils and eosinophils. The presence of severe inflammation should suggest some other diagnosis. Intraalveolar accumulation of macrophages is a common, nonspecific finding in IPF.

Desquamative Interstitial Pneumonia (DIP) or Respiratory Bronchiolitis Associated Interstitial Lung Disease (RBILD)

Lung biopsy reveals a uniform, diffuse, intra-alveolar macrophage accumulation, which is the most striking feature of DIP.[182-186] The macrophage may diffuse throughout the lung parenchyma, but most often accentuated around respiratory bronchioles. The macrophages are evenly dispersed within the alveolar space and the cells contain an eccentric nucleus and abundant, lightly pigmented cytoplasm. These cells were originally thought to represent exfoliated epithelial cells or "desquamated" from the alveolar septa. Thus, the name DIP is a misnomer. There is little fibrotic change with only mild to moderate thickening of alveolar walls. In contrast to UIP, DIP is homogenous there is no scarring fibrosis or lung remodeling of the lung architecture. Fibroblastic foci are absent or very minimal and inconspicuous. Whatever fibrous tissues are present, they appear to be of the same age. Interstitial inflammation is usually mild and consists of lymphocytes and few plasma cells.

Respiratory bronchiolitis-associated interstitial pneumonia is a clinical syndrome often described with DIP.[182,187-189] It is defined by the presence of pigmented macrophages within the lumen of respiratory bronchioles. The changes are patchy and have a bronchocentric or peribronchial distribution. Respiratory bronchioles, alveolar ducts, and peribronchiolar alveolar spaces contain clusters of these pigmented cells which are dusty brown in color, accompanied by a patchy submucosal and peribronchiolar infiltration of lymphocytes and histiocytes. Peribronchiolar fibrosis is seen which extends into the contiguous alveolar septa, which in turn are lined by hyperplastic type II pneumocytes and cuboidal bronchiolar-type epithelium. RBILD and DIP represent different ends of a spectrum of the same disease.

Acute Interstitial Pneumonia or Hamman-Rich Syndrome (AIP)

Lung biopsies from patients with AIP typically show histological features similar to those of the exudative, proliferative, and/or fibrotic phases of diffuse alveolar damage or acute respiratory distress syndrome.[181,182,190,191] Although AIP is characterized by diffuse interstitial fibrosis, it differs from other interstitial pneumonias in that the fibrosis is active, consisting of proliferating fibroblasts, and myofibroblasts with minimal collagen deposition. The changes are temporarily uniform and appear relatively acute reflecting the reaction to lung injury several weeks back. They resemble the organizing stage of diffuse alveolar damage. Fibroblast proliferation occurs within a myxomatous-appearing stromal background within thickened alveolar septa. The appearance resembles fibroblast foci of UIP except that the process is too diffuse rather than focal. Diffuse epithelial necrosis and alveolar collapse occurs. If the process is prolonged, honeycombing may appear. They differ from those seen in UIP in the way that the walls of the airspaces are lined by fibroblasts as well as collagen and are lined by alveolar rather than bronchiolar epithelium. Rapid development of honeycomb changes occurs as a result of partial or complete collapse of some alveoli and enlargement of others or as result of ventilator therapy for such patients. Other changes include hyaline membrane within alveolar spaces, small arterial thrombi,

and squamous metaplasia with cytological atypia in bronchiolar epithelium.

Nonspecific Interstitial Pneumonia (NSIP)

Katzenstein and Fiorelli.[180,182] described this as a specific and separate entity. NSIP is characterized by the presence of varying degrees of inflammation and fibrosis within the alveolar walls, but it lacks more specific changes as seen in UIP, DIP, or AIP. Mostly, changes consist of a mixture of inflammation with minimal fibrosis or a mixture of both inflammation and fibrosis. The process may be patchy with intervening areas of unaffected lung, but the changes are temporally uniform and thus, appear to have occurred over a single, relatively narrow time span. This temporal homogeneity contrasts sharply with heterogeneity characteristic of UIP.[182]

About half of the cases of NSIP predominantly consist of interstitial inflammation with little or no fibrosis. The inflammatory cells are mainly plasma cells and lymphocytes with the former being the predominant cell type. Hyperplasia of alveolar pneumocytes is often present. In another 40 percent of cases, there is an equal mixture of inflammation and fibrosis. These cases may, sometimes be difficult to distinguish from UIP. But the main differentiating feature is the uniformity of distribution in contrast to heterogeneity in UIP and presence of honeycombing. In the remaining 10 percent of cases, interstitial collagen deposition with minimal inflammation is present. Other accompanying features may be the presence of foci of intraluminal organization characteristic of BOOP, but these foci are always small and inconspicuous. Patchy intraalveolar macrophage accumulation occurs in about a third of cases and they are always an admixture of lymphoid cells and they are patchy in distribution. Lymphoid hyperplasia is seen in about a fourth of cases. Rarely, poorly formed, nonnecrotizing granulomas accompany these changes.

The main pathological differentiating features are shown in Table 21.3.

CLINICAL FEATURES[192]

The common age of presentation is between 40 to 60 years, although rarely the disease can occur in infants a few months old or after the age of 80 years.[97,193] Most reports indicate that both sexes are affected equally, perhaps with a slight male predominance. Report from India suggest that the usual age is between 30 to 60 years although, this can occur in young persons below the age of 20 years, i.e. in about 10 percent of cases.[25] In this series there was a predominance of females, possibly because the report

TABLE 21:3. Differentiating pathological features of idiopathic interstitial pneumonias[182]

Features	UIP	DIP/RBILD	AIP	NSIP
Temporal appearance	Heterogenous	Uniform	Uniform	Uniform
Interstitial inflammation	Scanty	Scanty	Scanty	Usually prominent
Collagen fibrosis	Present, Patchy	Variable, Diffuse (DIP), or local, and mild (RBILD)	Absent	Variable, Diffuse
Fibroblast proliferation	Fibroblast foci are prominent	No	Diffuse	Occasional, diffuse, or rare fibroblast foci
BOOP	No	No	No	Occasional, Focal
Microscopic honey-comb changes	Yes	No	No	Rare
Intra-alveolar macrophage accumulation	Occasional, Focal	Yes, Diffuse (DIP), or peribronchiolar (RBILD)	No	Occasional, Patchy
Hyaline membranes	No	No	Occasional, Focal	No

included cases of ILD secondary to collagen vascular diseases. The usual chief complaint is dyspnea and dry cough.[194-196] This begins as exertional dyspnea with an insidious onset. The cough is generally unproductive. Constitutional symptoms including arthralgias, myalgias, malaise, fever, and weight loss occur in about 50 percent of the cases. Rarely, the onset or worsening may be heralded by a flue-like illness. A most characteristic physical finding is the frequency of finger clubbing, present in about 25 to 60 percent of cases.[97,195,197] This may precede the chest symptoms by several years. Incidence of finger clubbing is more frequent in males than females and in patients who have lesser grades of honey combing and higher grades of smooth muscle proliferation in the pulmonary fibrotic changes.[169] Cyanosis is a late feature of the disease. Examination of the chest reveals diminished lung volumes with characteristic fine "Velcro" crackles over the lower lung zones.[198] With progression of the disease, rales extend towards the upper lung zones. These are dry, fine, end-inspiratory crepitations, which alter with change in posture (increase on bending forwards). Cor pulmonale is a very late feature.[197,199]

Extrapulmonary manifestations are unusual, but weight loss, malaise, and fatigue may be noted. Fever is rare and its presence suggests an alternate diagnosis. Symptoms and signs of connective tissue disorder like joint pains, swelling, musculoskeletal pain, weakness, fatigue, fever, photosensitivity, Raynaud's phenomenon, pleuritis, dry eyes, dry mouth etc. should be clearly elicitated.

Studies from North India revealed the following clinical presentation:[39]

Duration of illness

less than 6 months	24.6%
6 to 12 months	20.4%
1 to 3 years	30.4%
3 to 5 years	24.6%

Clinical symptoms

Dyspnea	100%
Dry cough	65.6%
Joint pains	7.1%
Raynaud's phenomenon	3.6%

Clinical signs

Clubbing	57.1%
Cyanosis	59%
Dry crackles	100%

Bronchoalveolar cell carcinoma may complicate some cases. There is an increased incidence of bronchoalveolar cell carcinoma in patients with interstitial fibrosis.[200,201] The increased risk of lung cancer in these patients occurs as a result of the occurrence of atypical or dysplastic epithelial changes in fibrosis which progresses to invasive malignancy, and p53 mutations that occur frequently and substantially in IPF.[202] Recent reports indicate that in about 7.5 percent of cases of lung cancer are associated with IPF and lung cancer is more frequent in elderly male smokers. Most lung cancers in IPF arise in peripheral areas involving fibrosis and squamous cell carcinoma is the predominant cell type (46%). The incidence of multiple lung cancer is also significantly higher.[203,204]

Chest Radiography

The chest radiograph is more useful, although not specific. Virtually all patients will have an abnormal chest radiograph at the time of presentation,[27,163, 197] however, very rarely some cases may present with normal chest skiagram. The most common abnormality consists of bilateral lower zone infiltrates, with reduced lung volumes. Ground glass appearance, nodular infiltrates, reticular, and reticulo-nodular shadows are other abnormalities, which are more prominent in the periphery of the lungs.[205] The involvement may proceed to affect the middle and upper lobes with shrinkage of lung volumes. Confluent alveolar opacities are rarely seen and if present, may suggest DIP or BOOP.[205,206] Patients with combined emphysema and IPF may have preserved or increased lung volumes and may have upper lobe oligemia. The sensitivity and specificity of chest radiograph in the diagnosis of IPF vary from 48 to 87 percent. End stage lung disease is characterized by cystic changes measuring 0.5 to 1 cm, suggestive of honeycombing. These changes reflect cystic dilatation of the distal air spaces due to progressive fibrosis. Decreased parenchymal compliance may lead to traction bronchiectasis, which is visible as thickened and dilated airways. Changes of pulmonary hypertension with cor pulmonale may be seen in advanced cases. Pleural involvement, lymphadenopathy, and parenchymal densities are uncommon in idiopathic pulmonary fibrosis. Whenever such a change is present, it suggests another interstitial process or the presence of a complication like pneumonia or malignancy.

High Resolution CT Scanning (HRCT)

Computed tomography,[27,163,207-211] particularly high-resolution thin section computed tomography (HRCT) has revolutionized the diagnostic evaluation of the patient with IPF. The technique allows detailed evaluation of the lung parenchyma by using 1- to 2-mm-thick slices, with a reconstruction algorithm that maximizes spatial resolution. HRCT is useful in differentiating idiopathic pulmonary fibrosis from other interstitial processes, the detection of disease in its early stage when radiographic changes are minimal or normal, to identify associated emphysema, and to determine the site and extent of the disease.[207,212,213] HRCT is now recognized as a sensitive means of identifying disease in IPF.[214-216] The HRCT findings include a predominant involvement of the lower zones, predominantly peripheral, usually subpleural reticular pattern with areas of haziness (ground glass opacity) or air space opacification. In areas of more severe involvement, there is often traction bronchiectasis. Honeycombing may also be present. A characteristic crescent of abnormality affecting the periphery of the lung over the lower zones posteriorly has been demonstrated with CT scanning. Serial studies show that as the disease progresses, the crescent extends anteriorly and centripetally towards the hilum. Different studies have shown that the appearance of the HRCT scans can predict histological patterns made evident in open lung biopsy specimens. Both reticular and honeycombing patterns correlate with fibrosis, whereas a ground glass pattern identifies zones of alveolar and interstitial inflammation.[217-219] In fact in patients with IPF the cell population in the bronchoalveolar lavage fluid is not homogeneous and seems to be related to the characteristics of the abnormalities on the HRCT scan present in the lavaged lobe.[220]

HRCT increases the level of diagnostic confidence compared with chest radiograph. The diagnostic accuracy for UIP is nearer to 90 percent, when reported by an experienced observer.[27] Scleroderma, rheumatoid arthritis and asbestosis may present with similar CT findings. These conditions are differentiated from UIP by the presence of parenchymal bands of fibrosis and pleural plaques. Patients with hypersensitivity pneumonitis of the subacute and chronic variety may have similar findings, but often lack the bibasilar predominance seen in IPF. Further, the presence of centrilobular nodules, middle and upper lobe predominance and the absence of honeycombing favor hypersensitive pneumonitis over IPF.[221] Sarcoidosis and BOOP may also resemble IPF. HRCT has also been proposed as a technique to assess the activity of IPF. Ground glass opacity usually represents alveolitis. When this finding is associated with reticular linings, and traction bronchiectasis, it always indicates lung fibrosis.[222,223] Patients with honeycombing or with predominant reticular pattern usually do not respond to therapy. HRCT is also being used increasingly for the quantitative assessment of disease extent, which has good physiological correlations.[224,225] For detection of early or mild infiltrative lung disease, HRCT is clearly more sensitive than plain chest radiograph. However, a normal HRCT cannot be used to exclude ILD, particularly in its early stages.[209] Features that can differentiate UIP from other types of interstitial lung diseases are shown in Table 21.4 (Figs 21.3 to 21.22).

TABLE 21.4: HRCT features to differentiate UIP and others

UIP	Not UIP
Basal predominance	Upper or midzone predominance
Peripheral predominance	Peribronchovascular
Honeycombing	Nonhoneycomb cysts
	Prominent ground glass attenuation
	Nodules or micronodules

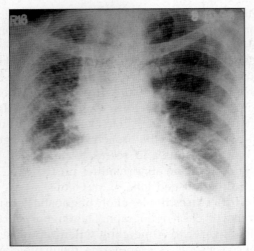

FIGURE 21.3: Interstitial lung disease. Note reticular shodows honeycombing and loss of lung volume

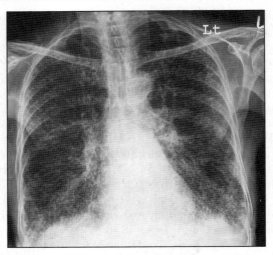

FIGURE 21.4: Reticular shadows in a case of ILD

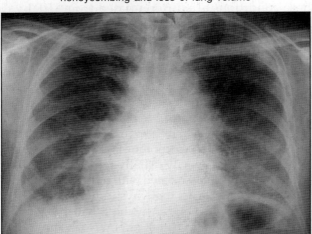

FIGURE 21.5: IPF. Note the reticular shadows and loss of lung volume

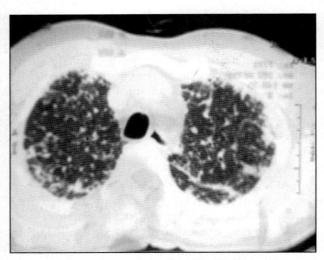

FIGURE 21.6: CT scan of chest in a case of ILD

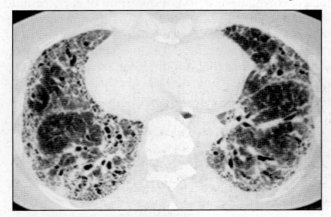

FIGURE 21.7: HRCT Chest - Basal region showing multiple, tiny radiolucent lesions with definitive walls and patchy ground glass haziness – Honeycombing

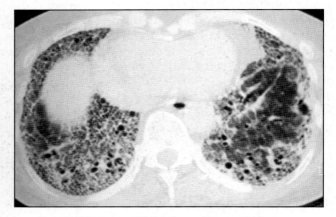

FIGURE 21.8: HRCT Chest - Honeycombing

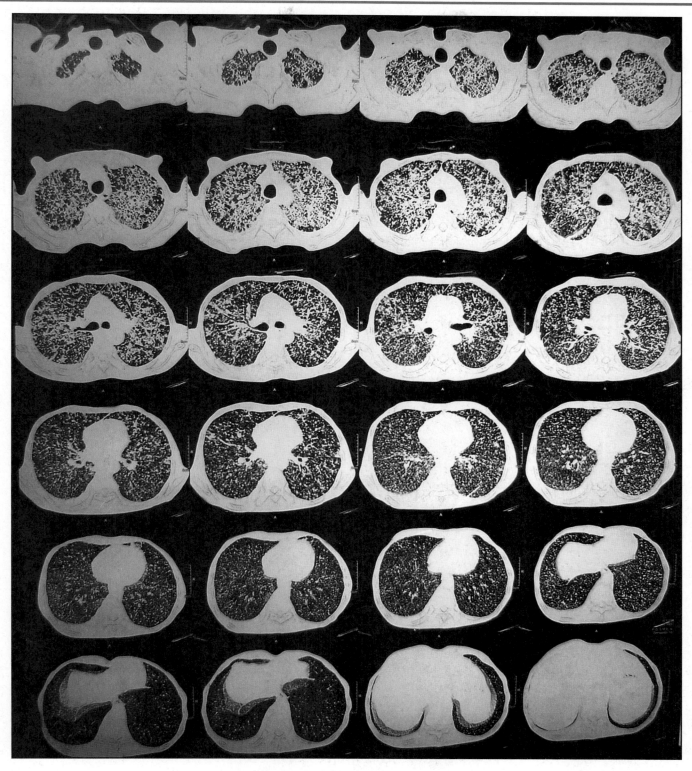

FIGURE 21.9: HRCT of chest showing interstitial, nodular opacities with honeycombing

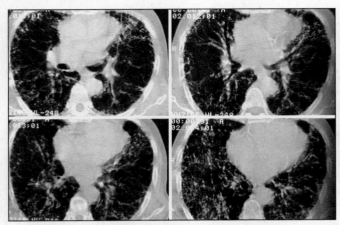

FIGURE 21.10: CT Chest - Interlobular septal thickening, irregular lung and fibrosis

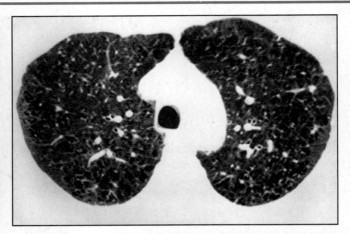

FIGURE 21.11: HRCT Chest - Multiple radiolucencies of varying size and shape

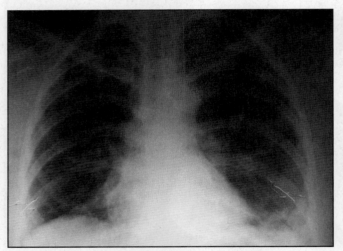

FIGURE 21.12: CXR of a case of nonspecific ILD

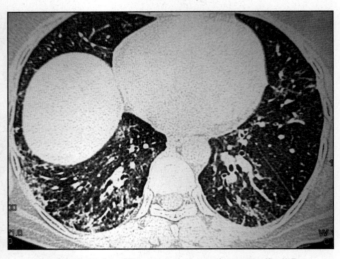

FIGURE 21.13: CT scan in a case of nonspecific ILD

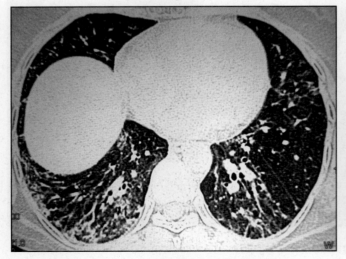

FIGURE 21.14: CT scan in a case of nonspecific ILD

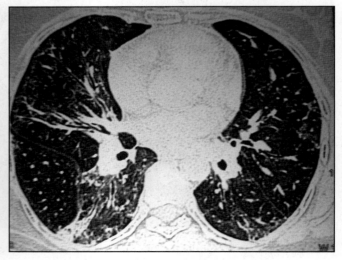

FIGURE 21.15: CT scan in a case of nonspecific ILD

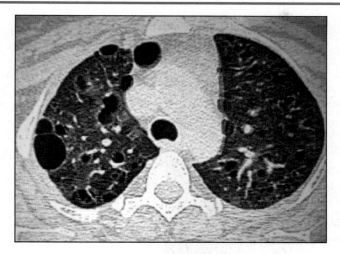

FIGURE 21.16: A case of lymphangioleiomyomatosis

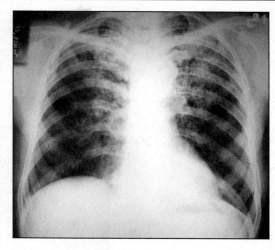

FIGURE 21.17: CXR of a case of diffuse alveolar hemorrhage

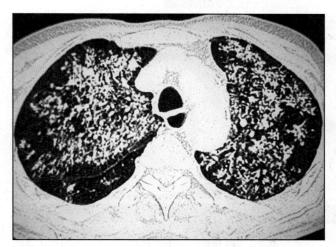

FIGURE 21.18: CT scan of the previous patient - A case of diffuse alveolar hemorrhage

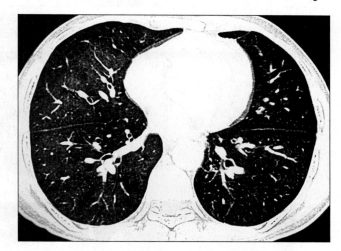

FIGURE 21.19: Idiopathic pulmonary hemorrhage

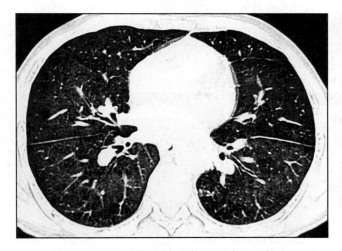

FIGURE 21.20: Idiopathic pulmonary hemorrhage

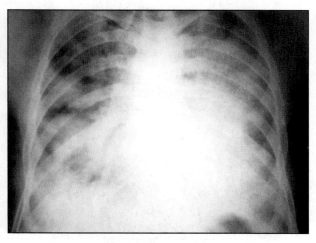

FIGURE 21.21A

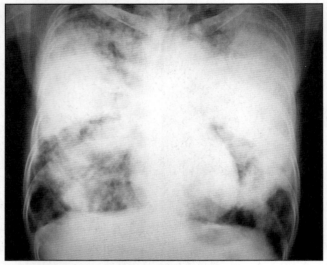

FIGURE 21.21B

FIGURE 21.21A and B: CXR in a case of pulmonary alveolar proteinosis

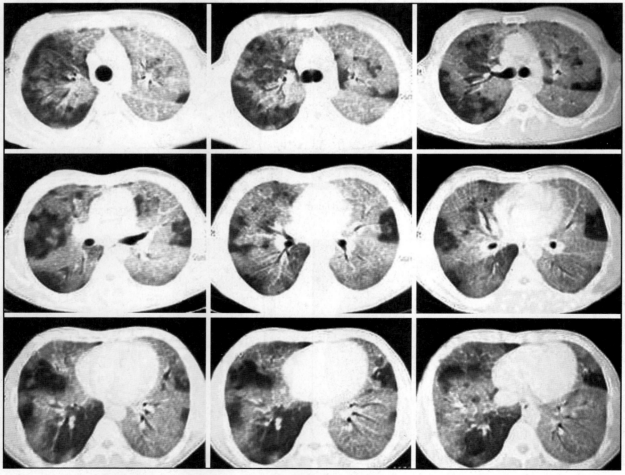

FIGURE 21.22: CT scan of the chest in a case of pulmonary alveolor proteinosis

Other Imaging Techniques

Nuclear scintigraphic scanning with Gallium 67 has been used to stage the disease activity. The radionuclide is predominantly concentrated in activated macrophages and to a lesser extent in neutrophils. The ^{67}Ga index, a visual measure of the extent, intensity and texture of ^{67}Ga uptake in the lungs, correlates well with the interstitial and alveolar cellularity in open lung biopsy specimens and with the cell population in BAL cell counts. Positron emission tomography imaging using technetium-99mDTPA (diethylenetriamine-pentaacetic acid) has been used to measure lung permeability, which shows that the lung leakiness is increased in idiopathic pulmonary fibrosis.[226-228] This is useful to evaluate disease activity and clinical course of the disease. MRI has very little in the diagnosis of IPF because of the extreme inhomogeneity of the disease.[229]

Pulmonary Function Testing

Pulmonary function tests in early disease may be normal, but lung volumes are reduced as in a restrictive process. Both FEV_1 and FVC are reduced with FEV_1 and FVC ratio being normal or increased due to elevated airflow rates because of the increased static elastic recoil. But, spirometric values do not correlate well with the histological changes or the subsequent clinical course. However, a marked reduction in FVC is associated with pulmonary hypertension and a reduced two-year survival.

All the lung volumes (TLC, functional residual capacity (FRC), and residual volume (RV) are reduced at some point in the course of the disease.[230] Early in the course of the disease and more commonly in patients with associated COPD, the lung volumes may be normal. The values are higher in smokers compared to non-smokers having IPF. The pressure volume curve is shifted downwards and to the right due to a stiff, poorly compliant lung. This test may be abnormal at the early stage of the disease. As the disease progresses, the lung compliance decreases and lung volumes fall.[231-237] In smokers, however the changes are opposite.

Patients with IPF are tachypneic and have more rapid shallow breaths as the disease progresses. Therefore the work of breathing increases.[238-239] The rapid breath is due to altered mechanical reflexes because of the increased elastic load and/or vagal mechanisms, since no definite chemical basis for the hyperventilation has been identified.[240-247] The flow rates like FEV_1 and FVC are reduced because of the reduction of the lung volumes with a maintained FEV_1/FVC ratio or may be increased.

However, as the static elastic recoil is increased, flow rates when compared to lung volumes are often increased. Functional and pathological changes of small airways disease has been described, but COPD has been seen exclusively among smokers with IPF.

Patients with ILD usually demonstrate an elevated minute ventilation for a given work rate during exercise.[248] Tidal volume is less during exercise and respiratory frequency is greater than normal humans. Tidal volume is also reduced in proportion to their decreased vital capacity.[249,250] Normal individuals increase their minute ventilation by increasing the tidal volume (VT) rather than the respiratory rate in contrast to IPF, where the respiratory rate is increased. A part of this increase is due to an increase in the dead space ventilation (VD). The ratio of VD/VT is increased at rest and is maintained or decreased with exercise. The ratio is increased either due to scleroderma, chronic pulmonary embolism or associated emphysema. Ventilatory stress is greater in these patients. Because of abnormal ventilatory mechanics, the maximal ventilatory capacity is significantly less than in normal individuals.[250-252] Impaired maximal exercise performance is a very prominent feature and is thought primarily due to respiratory (ventilatory mechanics or gas exchange or both) dysfunction.[253] The maximal breathing capacity is quite normal. However, it does not predict the extent or severity of the disease and the changes over time does not accurately predict the clinical course or response to therapy, although a recent study had shown that it correlated with the desquamation and the total pathology scores, whereas the TLC and FVC correlated with the cellularity factor score.[254] A reduction below 50 percent, however, is associated with pulmonary hypertension and widened P(A-a)O_2 with exercise.

The diffusing capacity for carbon monoxide corrected for hemoglobin is reduced and may become so quite early in the course of the disease and may precede abnormalities in lung volumes. The reduction in the DLCO is probably caused by a contraction of the pulmonary capillary volume and by ventilation perfusion abnormalities. The resting PaO_2 is normal in most cases, or it may reveal mild hypoxemia with alkalosis, although hypoxemia is usual with advanced disease. With exercise, the PaO_2 decreases and the P(A-a)O_2 widens with demonstration of a significant drop in arterial oxygen saturation.[255-257] The major cause of hypoxemia is ventilation-perfusion mismatching, and impairment of diffusion is a less common cause, and so also anatomic shunting. The gas measurements with exercise are the most sensitive tests of the overall process of idiopathic pulmonary fibrosis. These correlate well with the histologic changes and clinical course of the disease. Resting hypoxemia is associated with extensive fibrosis, pulmonary hypertension, and poor prognosis. Hematocrit values may be elevated as a result of chronic hypoxia.[258] During exercise, 20 to 30 percent of the exercise-induced widening of the $P(A-a)O_2$ may be caused by some impairment of oxygen diffusion. The abnormalities identified at rest do not accurately predict the magnitude of the abnormalities that may be seen with exercise. Although these abnormalities can be assessed by oximetry saturation, the changes may not be appreciated. Formal cardiopulmonary exercise testing is more sensitive than resting physiologic testing in the detection of abnormalities in oxygen transfer. Thus, exercise gas exchange has been a more sensitive index.

Elevation of pulmonary artery pressure rarely occurs in IPF at rest. But, during exercise pulmonary hypertension is commonly seen even in early stages of the disease. When the VC is less than 50 percent or the DLCO is less than 45 percent of the predicted value, pulmonary hypertension at rest can be expected.[27] In advanced IPF, clinical evidence of pulmonary hypertension can be present. The mean pulmonary artery pressure at rest ranges between 23 and 28 mm Hg and rarely exceeds 40 mm Hg. Patients having a resting pressure of greater than 30 mm Hg will have a poor prognosis. The exact cause of pulmonary hypertension is unknown. The pulmonary artery wedge pressure remains normal in IPF. Cor pulmonale is a late sequelae. Oxygen therapy at rest and during exercise improves pulmonary hemodynamics and likely improves exercise capacity and prognosis. Role of pulmonary vasodilator therapy is controversial in IPF.

IPF patients having a daytime oxygen saturation of less than 90 percent and/or having a history of snoring during sleep, develop sleep disturbances during sleep. They have reduced REM sleep. Severe hypoxemia can develop during sleep even in the absence of these abnormalities. The tachypnea even continues during sleep because of the active reflexes even during sleep. Thus, oxygen therapy during sleep improves prognosis.[27]

Various pulmonary function abnormalities as seen in interstitial fibrosis are shown in Table 21.5.

Bronchoalveolar Lavage

Bronchoalveolar lavage (BAL) has been used extensively in the diagnostic evaluation of interstitial fibrosis.[259] It is a safe repeatable, and minimally invasive method of sampling inflammatory cells of the lungs.[260] Analysis of the cellular constituents retrieved from BAL fluid could provide information regarding the inflammatory activity

TABLE 21.5: Pulmonary function changes in interstitial fibrosis

Parameters	Abnormality
Respiratory rate (f)	Increased
Tidal volume (V_T)	Decreased
Minute ventilation (V_I)	Increased
Maximal ventilatory capacity	Decreased
Vital capacity (VC)	Decreased
Forced expiratory volume (FEV_1)	Decreased
FEV_1/VC percentage	Normal or increased
Total lung capacity (TLC)	Decreased
Functional residual capacity (FRC)	Decreased
Residual volume (RV)	Decreased
Diffusing capacity (DLCO)	Decreased
Exercise capacity	Decreased
PaO_2	Decreased
$P(A-a)O_2$	Increased

*Most of the parameters even may be normal during early stages at rest, they become abnormal on exercise.

of the disease and therefore the prognosis.[261-269] Bronchoalveolar lavage is usually performed on the middle lobe or lingula in patients with IPF, although some authors prefer the right lower lobe as IPF predominantly affects the bases of the lung.[264,265]). However, a major concern related to the use of BAL in IPF is whether lavaging one lobe is representative of the interstitial lung disorder, based on the presumption that the inflammatory process is uniform throughout the lung parenchyma and Gallium-67 scans and open lung biopsies had shown nonhomogeneity of lung involvement. Thus, the results obtained with BAL may misrepresent the degree of underlying interstitial inflammation by sampling a relatively noninvolved area.[270] The differential cell counts in BAL specimens correlate well with the histological changes in open lung biopsy and may be helpful in predicting the response to treatment. The total cell count is increased, so also the macrophages, neutrophils, and lymphocytes compared to normal individuals. Eosinophils are present in varying proportions. The percentage of neutrophils and lymphocytes are increased in different conditions (see chapter on diagnostic methods). The role of differential cellular analysis and T-lymphocyte subsets in BAL for diagnostic and prognostic purposes in interstitial lung disease remains controversial. A predominantly neutrophilic type of response is common in idiopathic pulmonary fibrosis and a lymphocytic type in sarcoidosis. Lymphocytosis correlates with alveolar septal inflammation and a relative absence of honeycombing. There is no correlation, however, between any histological abnormality and neutrophil or eosinophil counts. An increase in the percentage of lymphocytes is associated with improvement after treatment with steroids.[271] However, the mere presence of BAL lymphocytosis is nonspecific. In addition to sarcoidosis and hypersensitivity pneumonitis, other diseases such as berylliosis, radiation pneumonitis, tuberculosis, opportunistic lung infections especially *Pneumocystis carinii* infection, and IPF have also been associated with increased T-lymphocytes.[272] Total proteins, and immunoglobulins (IgG, IgA, IgM) are also increased in BAL fluid. Abnormalities in the phospholipid components of the pulmonary surfactant are also present in idiopathic pulmonary fibrosis. These abnormalities have been correlated with the clinical course of the disease. Many other biochemical parameters have been described to be useful in the diagnosis.[273] Recently, a validated computer program based on the polychotomous logistic regression model has been developed which can be used to predict the diagnosis for an arbitrary patient with information provided by bronchoalveolar lavage fluid analysis, which is thought to be of diagnostic value in patients suspected of having interstitial lung disease.[271]

Bronchoalveolar lavage has been useful in elucidating the pathogenetic mechanisms in IPF that elucidate the key effector cells during the inflammatory response in IPF. Increase in polymorphonuclear neutrophils, neutrophil products, eosinophils and their products, macrophages and their products, cytokines, growth factors and immune complexes have been noted in the BAL fluid. The exact value of BAL however, has limitations in IPF except in specific situations like malignancy, infections, eosinophilic pneumonia, pulmonary histiocytosis X, some occupational dust exposures, etc. An increase in the neutrophils in excess of 5 percent has been noted in 70 to 90 percent of patients with IPF. An increase in eosinophils (> 5%) is apparent in 40 to 60 percent of cases and lymphocytes can be seen in 10 to 20 percent of cases with IPF. However, these findings are nonspecific and are seen in a wide variety of clinical conditions. A lone increase in lymphocytes is seen in less than 10 percent of cases of IPF and should suggest an alternative diagnosis. A neutrophilic type of BAL is present in fibrosing processes like IPF, ILDs associated with rheumatological conditions, asbestosis, or fibrotic sarcoidosis. A BAL lymphocytosis is found in sarcoidosis, nonspecific interstitial pneumonia, and drug induced lung disease. The value in clinical monitoring of the disease progression is limited. Increases in the percentages of neutrophils or eosinophils or both have been associated with a worse prognosis as reported by some studies. BAL lymphocytosis, seen in less than 20 percent of cases of IPF has been associated with a more cellular lung biopsy, less honeycombing, and a greater responsiveness to corticosteroids.

Laboratory and Serological Tests

Routine laboratory tests are not much help in the diagnosis IPF except to rule out certain conditions. Polycythemia is rare despite the presence of hypoxemia. An elevated ESR and hypergammaglobulinemia are frequent, but less specific. Antinuclear antibodies (ANAs) or rheumatoid factor positivity may be seen in 10 to 20 percent of patients with IPF, but the titers are rarely high. The presence of high titers (> 1:160) would suggest the presence of a connective tissue disease.[274-276]

Lung Biopsy[277,278]

For the confirmation of diagnosis, an open lung biopsy is essential. Transbronchial lung biopsy (TBLB) which is relatively safe, and easy has the disadvantage of sampling error and smaller tissue samples which may not be adequate to stage the activity of disease. Open lung biopsy allows larger samples, which is helpful to distinguish between active inflammation and end-stage fibrosis, which is important to decide about the use of corticosteroids and immunosuppressive drugs. TBLB is helpful in many situations when one demonstrates granuloma (sarcoidosis/hypersensitivity pneumonitis/berylliosis); infection, malignancy (lymphangitic and bronchoalveolar cell carcinoma), eosinophilic pneumonia and histiocytosis X. When none of these features are present only interstitial fibrosis may be demonstrated. The positivity rate of TBLB varies from series to series and depends upon the expertise of the bronchoscopist, number of specimens collected, site of biopsy, and the ability of the pathologist to pick up abnormality in a small piece of specimen.[279] Open lung biopsy via a limited thoracotomy is a relatively safe procedure with little morbidity and less than 0.5 percent mortality. Biopsy specimens should be taken at least from two sites, an upper lobe and a lower lobe site, and should include both abnormal and normal looking areas.[280] Thoracoscopy-guided lung biopsy is being used increasingly.[281-283] Results are being comparable to that with open lung biopsy with additional advantage of a significant reduction in perioperative morbidity and length of hospital stay, and the lung specimens obtained provide equivalent specimen volume and diagnostic accuracy.

Surgical lung biopsy, either open thoracotomy or preferentially by video-assisted thoracoscopy (VAT), provides the best tissue samples to distinguish different histological patterns of interstitial lung disease as described above. This procedure is to be adopted for all suspected cases of IPF, provided that there is no surgical contraindication. This is more important in suspected cases of IPF where the clinical or CT findings are not typical of IPF. However, the cost and risk to the patient are to be balanced with that of clinical benefit to the patient. Increased risk of complications is more often seen in patients who are above 70 years or more of age, extreme obesity, concomitant cardiac disease or gross impairment of pulmonary functions. VATS lung biopsy has the advantage of less morbidity; less prolonged chest tube drainage, and reduced length of hospital stay compared with open lung biopsy.[284-286] Some clinicians believe that transbronchial lung biopsy (TBLB) may be enough for the diagnosis of IPF. But, the tissue sample so obtained is not sufficient to make a confirmed diagnosis of UIP,[287,288] although it may be helpful in excluding this conditions by identifying another cause for the ILD (Figs 21.23 to 21.26).

DIAGNOSTIC APPROACH

Every effort should be made to make a histological diagnosis either by transbronchial lung biopsy/open lung biopsy/or thoracoscopy guided lung biopsy.[289] However, always this may not be possible and one can settle with a clinical diagnosis supported by HRCT. Progressive breathlessness with dry cough in a middle aged person with clubbing, with evidence of reduced lung volumes and presence of dry, Velcro, end-inspiratory crackles at lung bases, which are position dependent are highly suggestive of interstitial fibrosis. Typical radiological and HRCT findings along with a restrictive type of ventilatory defect and reduced DLCO along with hypoxemia either at rest or on exercise are almost enough to make a clinical diagnosis. Although histological proof is the only way of a definite diagnosis, because of reduced lung functions and hypoxemia this may not be feasible in some cases and in those cases clinical diagnosis is good enough. The next step is to establish the possible etiology. Collagen vascular diseases, drug induced lung diseases, and infections may be apparent

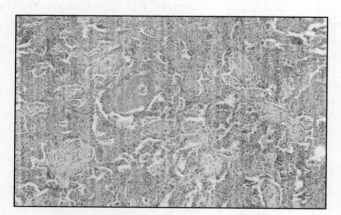

FIGURE 21.23: H&E stain, 50X, COP with fibrosing polyps

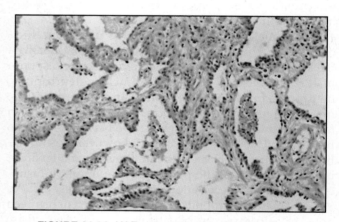

FIGURE 21.24: H&E stain, 50X, interstitial fibrosis with NSIP pattern in open lung biopsy

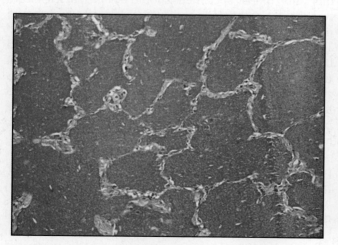

FIGURE 21.25: Histopathology of the lungs in a case of pulmonary alveolar proteinosis

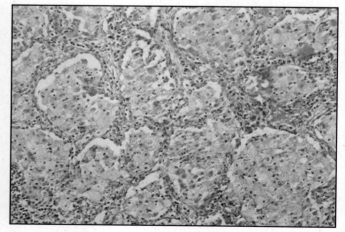

FIGURE 21.26: H&E, 200X, air spaces filled with pigmented macrophages in a case of DIP

from clinical and other appropriate investigations. When no etiology can be found out, the label of idiopathic interstitial lung disease can be applied. Interstitial lung diseases can be classified either as *acute syndromes* like infectious (virtually any); allergic-hypersensitivity pneumonitis, nitrofurantoin, eosinophilic pneumonia; toxic-drugs, radiation, fumes; hemodynamic-interstitial oedema either cardiogenic or ARDS; and idiopathic which may be acute interstitial pneumonitis, and bronchiolitis obliterans with organizing pneumonia (BOOP); and *chronic syndromes* like: fibrotic-idiopathic, radiation, pneumoconioses, drugs and BOOP; granulomatous-sarcoidosis, hypersensitivity pneumonitis, berylliosis, talc, eosinophilic, infectious; neoplastic-alveolar cell carcinoma, lymphangitic carcinomatosis, lymphoma; and infiltrative-aspiration, alveolar proteinosis, amyloidosis, and many others. Another way the etiology can be grouped as (i) collagen vascular/connective tissue diseases; (ii) inhalation causes; (iii) granulomatous diseases; (iv) some specific entities, (v) inherited causes; and (vi) idiopathic pulmonary fibrosis.

Contrasting clinical features of the idiopathic interstitial pneumonias are shown in Table 21.6.

Although histopathological confirmation is ideal to make a definite diagnosis of IPF, open or videoassisted thoracoscopic surgical lung biopsy is performed in only a minority of patients with chronic ILD as most clinicians believe that findings on lung biopsy will hardly change proposed treatment plan.[285] In the United Kingdom, transbronchial or open lung biopsies in IPF are performed only in 33 percent and 7.5 percent of patients respectively.[287] Clinical practice in the United States and other countries is almost similar to this approach and they rely largely on clinical and radiological features to make the diagnosis of IPF.[291,292] In most clinical series describing patients with presumed IPF, open or thoraco-

scopic lung biopsy is performed only in a minority of patients, and many of these reports include patients with connective tissue disease or occupational exposures known to be associated with ILD. Most studies show that expert observers will make a confident CT diagnosis of UIP in only about two-thirds of patients with histologic UIP, thus missing about a third of cases of UIP being missed by this approach.[27]

In the absence of a surgical lung biopsy, the diagnosis of IPF remains uncertain. However, the International Consensus Statement has laid down the following criteria in the immunocompetent adult. The presence of all of the following major diagnostic criteria as well as at least three of the four minor criteria increases the likelihood of a correct clinical diagnosis of IPF.[27]

Major Criteria

- Exclusion of other known causes of ILD, such as certain drug toxicities, environmental exposures, and connective tissue disorders.
- Abnormal pulmonary function tests that include evidence of a restrictive pattern (reduced VC often with an increased FEV1/FVC ratio) and impaired gas exchange (increased AaPO$_2$ with rest or exercise or decreased DLCO).
- Bibasilar, reticular abnormalities with minimal ground glass opacities on HRCT scans.
- Transbronchial lung biopsy or bronchoalveolar lavage (BAL) showing no features to support an alternative diagnosis.

Minor Criteria

- Age > 50 years
- Insidious onset of otherwise unexplained dyspnea on exertion

TABLE 21.6: Clinical features of different interstitial pneumonias[182,208,290]					
Features	UIP	DIP	RBILD	AIP	NSIP
Mean age (yr)	57	42	36	49	49
Onset	Insidious	Insidious	Insidious	Acute	Subacute, Insidious
Imaging features	Reticular abnormality, honeycombing, Basal, peripheral predominance, Often patchy	Ground glass attenuation, Cyst ±, Basal, peripheral predominance	Centrilobular nodules, ground glass attenuation	Diffuse alveolar opacities	Ground glass abnormality, Bilateral patchy opacities, Reticular abnormality, Basal, peripheral predominance
Mortality (Mean survival)	68% (5-6yrs)	27% (12 yrs)	0%	62% (1-2 mon)	11% (17 mon)
Response to steroids	Poor	Good	Good	Poor	Good
Complete recovery possible?	No	Yes	Yes	Yes	Yes

UIP—Usual interstitial pneumonia; DIP—Desquamative interstitial pneumonia; RBILD—Respiratory bronchiolitis interstitial lung disease; AIP—Acute interstitial pneumonia; NSIP—nonspecific interstitial pneumonia.

- Duration of illness > 3 months
- Bibasilar, inspiratory crepitations (dry or Velcro type in quality).

APPROACH TO MANAGEMENT

Before deciding about any form of treatment, the diagnosis should be reasonably confirmed.[293] All patients should be evaluated for collagen vascular disease, drug-induced lung disease, and pneumoconiosis through history, physical examination, and serological tests. Fiber-optic bronchoscopy should also be performed in all patients which will allow exclusion of granulomatous diseases, neoplasm, infection, and specific disease entities like pulmonary alveolar proteinosis, and histiocytosis X (see above for diagnostic evaluation). Next, one should establish the stage of disease—cellular or fibrotic. Disease progression is also important to establish, since a fibrotic reaction related to some past injury, but without progression will be present in about 10 to 15 percent of cases. Recognition of this group is important to avoid unnecessary treatment. Progressive disease is identified by progression of dyspnea, advancing radiological changes, or deterioration in pulmonary function tests. The criteria for significant changes in pulmonary function tests are a decrease in 10 percent in vital capacity, an increase in the $P(A-a)O_2$ at rest of 5 mm Hg while breathing room air, and a decrease in DLCO of 20 percent.[193] In UK, physicians generally consider IPF as a clinical diagnosis and do not initiate treatment in up to half of patients at presentation.[294]

Idiopathic pulmonary fibrosis has the highest mortality of all the diffuse lung diseases. Mortality rates from the disease almost doubled in England and Wales between 1979 and 1988,[295] an increase that was not due to differences in the way the diagnosis was made. This rate of increase continued till 1992.[296] Fifty percent of patients with the disease die within four to five years of their diagnosis. Patients with a new diagnosis have a much shorter median survival than patients with preexisting disease—three years as compared to nine years.[297] IPF progresses relentlessly and in an insidious manner that may be difficult to detect using parameters like clinical, radiological or spirometric methods. Spontaneous remission does not occur. In earlier clinical studies, the clinical course of IPF was quite variable, with a mean survival ranging from 4 to 6 years after the time of diagnosis. However, more recent clinical reports with better-defined cases of IPF have identified a much shorter survival, with mean survival ranging from 2 to 4 years (5-year survival range, 30-50%).[197,298-300]

The response to therapy in idiopathic pulmonary fibrosis is inconsistent. However, the subset of patients who will respond well to therapy and have improved survival include:[300-305]
- Patients with disease of less than 1 year duration
- Younger age of the patient (< 50 years of age)
- Female sex
- Shorter symptomatic period (< 1 year) with less dyspnea
- Relatively preserved lung functions
- Presence of ground glass and reticular opacities on HRCT
- Bronchoalveolar lavage fluid showing lymphocyte count of more than 5 percent (20-25%), neutrophils of less than 10 percent, and eosinophil count of less than 5 percent
- A history of current cigarette smoking at the time of diagnosis
- Open lung biopsy showing more inflammation (cellularity, exudation) than fibrosis. While patients with interstitial fibrosis due to systemic lupus erythematosus, Sjögren's syndrome, polymyositis-dermatomyositis, and mixed connective tissue disease respond well to cyclophosphamide therapy, those with rheumatoid arthritis and scleroderma respond very poorly or refractory to such therapy
- CRP scoring (clinical, radiological, and physiological scoring) as developed by King, et al.
- Histological types other than UIP
- A beneficial response or stable disease 3 to 6 months after initial corticosteroid therapy.

Factors that affect the likelihood of progressive disease include the following:[300,301]
- Male gender
- Moderate to severe dyspnea with exertion
- Extensive smoking history (the greater the number of pack-years, the worse is the prognosis)
- Moderate to severe loss of lung function at presentation as assessed by DLCO and gas exchange with exercise
- Neutrophilia or eosinophilia on BAL fluid analysis
- Mixed ground glass and reticular pattern of interstitial opacities or predominance of reticular or honeycombing on HRCT
- Histological features of UIP on lung biopsy
- Failure to respond to a three months trial of high-dose corticosteroids.

The concept of treatment of IPF has been based of the presumption that inflammation leads to injury and fibrosis. Although the initial emphasis was on inflammation primarily, altered fibrogenesis has been the new thought for the pathogenesis of IPF. However, to date most treatment strategies have been based on eliminating or suppressing the inflammatory component. No pharmacologic therapy has equivocally been proved to halt or alter the course of inflammation. Little progress has been made to reverse the fibrotic progress. However, the current therapeutic approach for the management of IPF can be divided into the following:[27,28,163, 306-311]

1. Anti-inflammatory drugs (corticosteroids, newer anti-inflammatory drugs like TGF-beta).
2. Immunosuppressive/cytotoxic drugs (azathioprine, cyclophosphamide, chlorambucil, methotraxate).
3. Antifibrotic drugs (cholchicine, D-penicillamine, pirfenidone).
4. Immunomodulators (interferon gamma-1b).
5. Experimental (cytokine inhibitors, growth factor inhibitors, antiproteases, antioxidants, surfactant, regulation of white cell traffic, gene therapy)
6. Lung transplantation.
7. Supportive therapy.

Only a small number of patients (< 20%) respond to any form of therapy. Although the prognosis of those who respond to therapy is better than that of nonresponders, it is likely that this reflects the fact that these individuals are in an earlier phase of the evolution of their disease or they are a unique subset of patients. There is a wide variation in the natural history of the disease among individual subjects. Despite some success in therapy, the lung disease in most patients eventually worsens.

Anti-inflammatory Agents

*Corticosteroid*s. Corticosteroids are the most commonly and widely used drugs for the treatment of IPF, although no prospective, randomized, double-blind, placebo-controlled trials has evaluated the efficacy of corticosteroids in the treatment of IPF. The standard therapeutic approach is high-dose corticosteroids.[312] The response rate and extent of improvement vary from patient to patient and about 10 to 30 percent of these patients will have measurable improvement in pulmonary function tests, whereas up to 40 percent respond on the basis of subjective or undefined assessment criteria. Responses are usually transient and partial. Cures are achieved only in very few patients. Even among responders, relapses or progression of the disease after an initial response suggests prolonged therapy. Patients, who respond to steroids, do so by two weeks with maximal improvement between 1 to 3 months.

The standard dose is prednisolone or prednisone, 1 to 2 mg/kg of body weight or 40 to 100 mg daily for 2 to 4 months, with a subsequent taper, then tapering the

dose to maintain the lowest that showed stabilization of symptoms and lung function.[313] After 3 months of therapy objective clinical parameters like dyspnea score, physiological studies, chest radiographs, HRCT are required to monitor response as only objective responses are not adequate because of placebo effector mood-elevation effects of corticosteroids. Maintenance corticosteroid therapy is to be reserved for patients showing stabilization or objective improvement. Corticosteroid-responsive patients are maintained on prednisolone chronically, sometimes indefinitely, but in a gradually tapering dose. Relapse or deterioration needs escalation of the dose or addition of an immunosuppressive agent. The dose and rate of taper should be guided by clinical and physiological parameters. Prolonged treatment for 1 to 2 years, and sometimes indefinitely, is reasonable in patients with unequivocal response. Chronic low-dose prednisolone in a dose of 15 to 20 mg every alternate day may be adequate. High-dose intravenous "pulse" methyl prednisolone (1-2 gm once a week or biweekly) has been used, but has no proven advantage.

Immunosupressants

Azathioprine and cyclophosphamide. Immunosuppressive or cytotoxic therapy is usually tried when the patient is not responding to corticosteroids or when too much steroid is required to suppress symptoms or patients at high risk of steroid complications (age > 70 years, poorly controlled diabetes mellitus or hypertension, severe osteoporosis or peptic ulcer disease) Good response has been observed in small number of patients.

Azathioprine has been used with success in few patients.[314] The drug can be used as an addition to the corticosteroid. No definite recommendation of the drug is possible because of lack of proper controlled clinical trial in adequate number of cases. Azathioprine with low dose prednisolone may be more effective in improving survival than prednisolone alone. Azathioprine is converted to mercaptopurine, which affects RNA and DNA synthesis. In general cellular immunity is suppressed to a greater extent than humoral immunity. However, the usual dose given is 2 mg/kg orally as a single dose and not to exceed 200 mg/day. Since the degree of leukopenia does not correlate with clinical efficacy, the dose need not be adjusted according to WBC count except for maintaining the count above 4000/cmm. An appreciable response may not be observed until the patient has received 3 to 6 months of therapy. Gastrointestinal side effects, including nausea, vomiting, and diarrhea are the most common side effects. Hepatic, and hematological side effects are also possible. The drug is teratogenic.

Cyclophosphamide is a commonly used steroid sparing agent in the treatment of IPF. It is most often used as a second-line therapy like azathioprine, when condition is deteriorating despite corticosteroid therapy. It is also being used increasingly as a first line drug in those who have contraindication of corticosteroids. The drug may be beneficial along with low dose corticosteroid. It is metabolized into the active form by the P-450 system of enzymes into its active form. These metabolites decrease the lymphocyte number and function and may also have anti-inflammatory effects. Cyclophosphamide is usually administered orally as a once a day therapy. The starting dose is 25 to 50 mg/day; the dose is gradually increased by 25 mg increments, aiming to reduce and maintain the WBC count between 4000 and 7,000/cmm. The WBC count should be measured twice weekly for the first 6 to 12 weeks and then at least monthly thereafter. The dose should not be increased beyond 150 to 200 mg/day as beneficial effects are not observed beyond these doses. Beneficial therapy is not expected till about 3 to 6 months after initial treatment. Forced diuresis, with at least 8 glasses of water daily, and monthly monitoring of red blood cells in the urine is recommended to detect hemorrhagic cystitis, which is a known side effect of cyclophosphamide.

Intravenous cyclophosphamide therapy has been used occasionally in patients with progressive disease. A dose of 2 mg/kg is given over 30 to 60 minutes, once daily for 3 to 5 days and, then the oral therapy follows. Long-term intermittent (pulse 0 intravenous cyclophosphamide is advocated by some). But, long-term experience is lacking. An escalating regimen of cyclophosphamide is used with an intravenous dose of 500 mg, which is increased by 100 to 200 mg every two weeks, provided that the total WBC counts is above 3000/cmm. The maximum single administered dose is 1000 to 1800 mg depending upon the body size.

The common side effects are; reduction in all hematological cell counts, increased risk of infection, hemorrhagic cystitis, infertility, teratogenicity, and gastrointestinal side effects and an increase in the risk of development of future cancer.

Cyclo Sporine

Cyclo sporine has been recently suggested as an antifibrotic agent for the treatment of IPF, but experience with this drug is limited. A specific role of cyclosporine has been suggested for patients awaiting lung transplantation. The drug exerts its action through suppression of T cells. There is no apparent myelosuppression with the use of cyclosporine. Although the optimal dose is unknown, it is usually given in a daily dose of 5 to 10 mg/kg for the first three to nine months. The dose may be adjusted to maintain a blood level of 100 to 200 ng/ml. Maintenance therapy should be continued at the lowest dose associated with stabilization of disease activity, usually 3 to 5 mg/kg per day. The major side effects are renal dysfunction, tremor, hirsutism, hypertension, and gum hyperplasia.

Methotrexate is an immunosuppressant and antineoplastic drug. Clinical experience of use of this drug for the treatment of IPF is limited, although it has been used in sarcoidosis. It inhibits replication and function of T lymphocytes and possibly B-lymphocytes. It can be administered orally or intramuscularly. The dose is 7.5 mg once weekly. The dose is then gradually increased at interments of 2.5 mg every two weeks until a weekly dose of 15 mg is reached. A trial of methotrexate therapy should be at least for 4 to 6 months to assess efficacy. Liver function tests and WBC count should be monitored.

Chlorambucil has been used by some as a substitute for cyclophosphamide in the treatment of IPF. It may cause gastrointestinal and bone marrow toxicities and may induce neoplasia including leukemias. Given its toxicity profile and lack of data as therapy in IPF, this drug cannot be recommended for the treatment of IPF.

Renewed interest has been shown in view of the recent understanding the pathogenesis of the disease. As depicted in Figures 21.1 and 21.2, the strategy of treatment of the use of drugs is to attack at various steps. These include cytokine inhibitors, growth factor inhibitors, antifibrotic agents, antiproteases, newer anti-inflammatory agents (diphosphonates), antioxidants, surfactant, regulation of white cell traffic, and gene therapy.[108,315]

Anti-fibrotic Drugs

Colchicine inhibits collagen formation and modulates the extracellular matrix *in vitro* and in animal models. It blocks the release of fibronectin and alveolar-derived growth factors involved in fibroblast proliferation. The benefits of colchicine in the treatment of IPF are not substantial. The drug acts by arrest of cell division, inhibition of granulocyte migration, and inhibition of release of several proteins from cells. It also interferes with secretion of collagen from fibroblasts and may increase collagen degradation by enhancing the action of collagenase. A dose of 0.6 mg orally is given once or twice daily as tolerated. The drug is quite well tolerated and side effects may be nausea, vomiting, abdominal pain, and diarrhea.

Penicillamine. Several animal studies suggest a possible role for penicillamine in the treatment of fibrotic lung disorders. The drug may improve the DLCO, but not other pulmonary function parameters. Experience of the drug in the treatment of IPF is limited. Along with prednisolone the drug is more effective compared to prednisolone alone or prednisolone plus azathioprine. The drug acts by inhibiting collagen synthesis, by interfering with collagen cross linkage and suppression of T cell function. The recommended dose is 125 to 250 mg given orally as a single dose. After four to eight weeks, the dose is increased weekly to a final dose of 500 mg/day. Daily dose of 1000 mg may be used if tolerated. The effect is not appreciated before three to six months. Side effects include nausea, vomiting, diarrhoea, dyspepsia, anorexia, transient loss of taste for sweet and salt, cutaneous lesions, hematological toxicities, (leukopenia, aplastic anemia, granulocytopenia), renal toxicity (reversible proteinuria, hematuria, nephritic syndrome), myasthenia gravis, and bronchoalveolitis.

Interferon gamma 1b. Animal models suggest that interferon gamma can inhibit the proliferation of fibroblasts and reduce collagen synthesis. These observations prompted a trial in which 18 patients with IPF who were nonresponsive to corticosteroid, who were randomized to treatment with prednisolone alone or to prednisolone (7.5 mg/day) plus interferon gamma 1b (200 mcg administered subcutaneously three times per week). The patients treated with interferon gamma had significantly better total lung capacity and oxygenation after 12 months of treatment. The drug has side effects like fever, chills, and muscle pain, which subside with time.

Other antifibrotic agents include *interferon beta*, *relaxin* (increases procollagenase), *pirfenidone*, *halfuginone* (inhibits collagen synthesis), *suramin* (profibrotic cytokine inhibition), and *prostaglandin E2* (inhibits collagen production).

Other Novel Therapeutic Approaches

Although not in clinical use, the diversity of pathogenetic mechanisms have led to speculations/development of agents that can block some of those pathways leading to IPF. Some of these novel therapeutic approaches include endothelin I inhibitors, inflammatory response modifiers like inhibition of interleukin-1, interleukin-4 and interleukin-13 and the pluripotent transferring growth factor beta-1. Other agents include antiproteases, surfactant replacement, interference with leukocyte retention, and gene therapy. Possible strategies for antioxidants include delivery of antioxidant enzymes to the lung parenchyma or promotion of increasing the genetic expression of antioxidant enzymes. *Glutathione, taurine* and *niacin* inhibit the development of experimental fibrosis. High-dose *N-acetylcysteine*, a glutathione precursor has been suggested as a maintenance immunosuppressive therapy in patients with IPF. Surfactant proteins A and D and some of the lipid components of surfactant have some important anti-inflammatory properties, which can be used as potential therapeutic agents in IPF. Another potential strategy is the interference with the process of leukocyte retention in the lung. As leukocyte adhesion molecules play an important role in the process, antibodies to such adhesion molecules can help to prevent collagen deposition. Although, no specific genetic defect has been found, gene therapy might be of help to target specific sites in the pathogenetic sequence of this disease. One might devise gene therapy to inhibit the effects of specific growth factors or cytokines.

There is not sufficient evidence that any treatment improves survival or quality of life of patients with IPF. However, there is always potential for a positive outcome that has encouraged clinicians to treat IPF. In view of the above all poor prognosis of these patients, many experts recommend that treatment be initiated in all patients with IPF who do not have contraindications. However, the International Consensus Committee recommends that therapy is not indicated in all cases of IPF.[27] The committee recommends that:

- The potential benefit of any treatment protocol for an individual patient with IPF may be outweighed by increased risk for treatment-related complications, in view of the limited success of current treatment.
- Such risky group includes those above 70 years of age, extreme obesity, concomitant major illness such as cardiac disease, diabetes mellitus, osteoporosis, severe impairment in pulmonary function, end-stage honeycomb lung on radiography.
- The treatment should start early in the course of the disease before irreversible fibrosis develops. Thus, the best time to start therapy is at the first identification of clinical or physiological evidence of impairment or documentation of decline in lung function.

Further, the Committee has recommended the following combined therapy of corticosteroid and azathioprine or cyclophosphamide for those patients who are adequately informed about the drugs and who possess feature consistent with a more likely favorable outcome.

- *Corticosteroid* therapy should consist of prednisone or prednisolone or equivalent at a dose of 0.5 mg/kg of lean body weight per day for 4 weeks; 0.25 mg/kg of lean body weight per day for 8 weeks, and then tapered to 0.125 mg/kg of ideal body weight daily or 0.25 mg/kg of lean body weight every other day as initial therapy; and

- *Azathioprine* is to be given at a dose of 2 to 3 mg/kg lean body weight per day to a maximum dose of 150 mg per day orally. Dosing should begin at 25 to 50 mg/day and increased gradually, by 25 mg increments, every 7 to 14 days until the maximum dose is reached.

or

- *Cyclophosphamide* at 2 mg/kg lean body weight per day to a maximum of 150 mg/day orally. Dosing should begin at 25 to 50 mg/day and increased gradually, by 25 mg increments, every 7 to 14 days until the maximum dose is reached.

(*Lean body weight is calculated as the ideal weight expected for a patient of his age, sex, and height*)

It is very essential that the side effects of all the above drugs be monitored strictly with proper instructions to the patient. Particular care should be taken for azathioprine and cyclophosphamide by measuring the WBC counts and platelet counts. If the WBC count is less than 4000/cmm and the platelet count is < 1,00,000/cmm, then the drugs are to be stopped and weekly monitoring required. The dose is to be stopped till the counts improve. Further, hepatocellular function should be monitored. If the enzyme levels are more than three times the normal value, the drugs are to be stopped and resumed slowly only when they are normal. Forced diuresis is to be ensured by drinking sufficient water (at least 8 glasses a day) and monthly monitoring of urine for red blood cells to detect hemorrhagic cystitis due to cyclophosphamide.

Duration of Therapy

Objective response to therapy may not be apparent till the patient receives therapy for at least three months. Thus, in the absence of complications, or adverse effects of the drugs, combined therapy should be continued for at least 6 months. At that time, repeat objective assessments should be performed to determine the response to therapy (as discussed below).

Six Months after Onset of Therapy

- If the patient is worse, the therapy should be stopped over changed. The steroid should be continued at the present dose and the cytotoxic drug is to be changed to the other one. Alternative therapy or lung transplantation may also be considered.

- If the patient improves, or stable, the combined therapy should be continued, using the same doses of the drugs.

Twelve Months after Therapy

- If the patient is worse, the therapy should be stopped over changed. The steroid should be continued at the present dose and the cytotoxic drug is to be changed to the other one. Alternative therapy or lung transplantation may also be considered.

- If the patient improves, or stable, the combined therapy should be continued, using the same doses of the drugs.

More than Eighteen Months after Therapy

- Therapy should be individualized on the basis of clinical response and tolerance of the patient to the therapy. The therapy should be continued indefinitely only in individuals with objective evidence of continued improvement or stabilization.

There is no standard approach to stage IPF clinically or pathologically. IPF is a progressive form of interstitial lung disease and the extent and rate of progression varies from patient to patient. Subjective improvement may occur in patients (almost in 70%) in response to therapy, which should not be the lone factor in determining whether treatment is to be continued or not. Improvement in physiologic abnormalities occur in about 20 to 30 percent of patients who are treated, Changes in pulmonary function parameters are used by some to assess "responders" or "nonresponders". However, this is not uniform. Increases of only 10 to 15 percent from the pretreatment baseline even in single parameters like VC or DLCO have been taken as favorable response by some clinicians. Radiologic assessment is not very helpful either. However, some investigators believe that at least a stabilization of the lesions is a good indicator of response to therapy. It is also possible that while some parameters may show improvement, others do not. A Clinical, Radiological and Physiological Scoring (CRP) scoring system has been advocated by some investigators as a very useful adjunct.[314, 316,317] This scoring system included different clinical variables like age, smoking status, dyspnea, clubbing, extent of interstitial opacities, presence of pulmonary hypertension on chest radiograph, spirometry, lung volumes, diffusion capacity, resting alveolar-arterial oxygen difference, and exercise oxygen saturation. This CRP scoring system correlates with the extent and severity of the important histopathologic features of IPF like cellularity, fibrosis, and the granulation/

connective tissue deposition. These findings suggest that a defined scoring system might be the best in staging the extent of IPF and helpful in monitoring the clinical course.

The International Consensus Committee defines response into the following three categories:[27]

1. Favorable or improved response
2. Stable or presumed favorable response
3. Failure to response to therapy.

The detailed parameters are shown in Table 21.7.

Lung Transplantation

Lastly, one may consider heart-lung transplantation in patients with severe disease unresponsive to other therapy (see lung transplantation for details in subsequent chapter). Currently, single lung transplantation is the preferred surgical operation. Transplantation should be considered for patients who experience progressive physiologic deterioration, despite optimal medical management.[318-322] Unless specific contraindications exist, patients with progressive severe functional impairment, oxygen dependency, and a deteriorating course should be listed for lung transplantation. Relative contraindications to lung transplantation are unstable or inadequate psychological profile/stability, significant extrapulmonary disorder like liver, renal or cardiac dysfunction that may negatively influence survival. Many limit transplants to those below the age of 60 years.

Successful transplantation improves arterial oxygen tension and there may not be need for supplemental oxygenation, increase in lung volumes and diffusion capacity, and pulmonary hypertension and right ventricular dysfunction improves. The five years survival after transplantation also improves to 50 to 60 percent. The overall quality of life improves in transplant recipients.[323,324]

Symptomatic Treatment

Patients should be under a pulmonary rehalitation program. Since dyspnea is one of the main disabling symptoms, exercise should not be discouraged. For motivated patients, a combination of exercise training, education, and psychosocial support may help although unlikely will improve lung function. With improved exercise tolerance and decreased symptoms of breathlessness, the quality of life will improve.[325] Daily walks or a stationary bicycle are excellent routine exercises.

Severe hypoxemia (PaO_2 less than 55 mm Hg at rest or during exercise, should be managed by supplemental oxygen. Supplemental oxygen during exercise will improve performance.[325,326] Higher flows can be used in contrast to COPD without the fear of CO_2 retention.

Another distressing symptom is the severe paroxysms of cough. A number of antitussive are available, and anyone can be used. Sometimes they may not be effective. Oral codein is one of the best drugs. Opioids have been

TABLE 21.7: International consensus committee criteria of response to therapy

Favorable or improved response	Stable or presumed favorably response	Failure to response

Two or more of the following documented on two visits over a 3 to 6 month period:
• A decrease in symptoms, specifically increase in the level of exertion required before the patient must stop because of breathlessness or the decline in the frequency or severity of cough
• Reduction of parenchymal abnormalities on chest radiograph or HRCT
• Physiologic improvement defined by two or more of the following:
  • $\geq$ 10% increase in TLC or VC (or at least 200 ml change)
  • $\geq$ 15% increase in single-breath DLCO (or at least 3 ml/min/mm Hg)
  • An improvement or normalization of oxygen saturation ($\geq$ 4 percentage point increase in the measured saturation) or PO_2 ($\geq$ 4 mm Hg increase from the previous measurement) achieved during a formal cardiopulmonary exercise test
	Two or more of the following documented on two visits over a 3 to 6 months period:
	• 10% change in TLC or VC or < 200 ml change
	• < 15% change in single-breath DLCO or < 3 ml/min/mm Hg
	• No change in oxygen saturation (< 4% increase) or PO_2 (< 4 mm Hg increase) achieved during a formal cardiopulmonary exercise test
		After 6 months of treatment:
		• An increase in symptoms, specifically dyspnea or cough
		• Increase in opacity on chest radiograph or HRCT, specifically development of honeycombing or signs of pulmonary hypertension
		• Physiologic deterioration in two or more of the following:
		  • $\geq$ 10% decrease in TLC or VC (or at least 200 ml change)
		  • $\geq$ 15% decrease in single-breath DLCO (or at least 3 ml/min/mm Hg)
		• Worsening or greater fall of oxygen saturation ($\geq$ 4 percentage point decrease in the measured saturation) or rise in the $AaPO_2$ at rest or during a formal cardiopulmonary exercise test ($\geq$ 4 mm Hg increase from the previous measurement)

used for dyspnea, but success has not been uniform. Vasodilators are not effective in patients developing pulmonary hypertension during the late phase of the disease.

PROGNOSIS

Idiopathic pulmonary fibrosis is a progressive disease with poor prognosis. Patients with a cellular pattern on open lung biopsy have a median survival of 10 to 12 years, whereas those with a more fibrotic pattern have a mean survival of only 5 to 6 years. Clinical studies indicate that the medium time from diagnosis to death is 3 to 5 years.[327-329] Those with an associated connective tissue disorder appear to have a less aggressive form of the disease.[329] With steroid treatment, which is the traditional form of therapy, produces an objective response in only 10 to 20 percent of cases.[1] In those who respond to corticosteroids, the treatment has shown only a modest influence on the fatal course of the disease.[1,327,331]

BRONCHIOLITIS OBLITERANS WITH ORGANIZING PNEUMONIA (BOOP)[331-342]

Bronchiolitis obliterans with organizing pneumonia (BOOP) is a distinct clinicopathological syndrome, which is being increasingly recognized during the past decade. The entity has been recognized more and more in association with an increased number of conditions.[332-349] The condition was recognized in 1985 when Epler et al used this term.[332] They analyzed 2500 reports of open lung biopsies and searched for this condition in which they found 57 cases with histological reports showing both bronchiolitis obliterans and organizing pneumonia, and 10 cases of bronchiolitis alone without parenchymal involvement. Of these 57 cases of BOOP, 50 were idiopathic and the remaining 7 were associated with some underlying cause. Since then the cause is unending. In fact, this must be distinguished from conditions like IPF and UIP, as the condition has a much better prognosis. The condition is not a new lesion and was known earlier under various names as bronchiolitis interstitial pneumonia (BIP), COP, and so on.

The terms bronchiolitis, bronchiolitis obliterans and bronchiolitis obliterans with organizing pneumonia are often the sources of confusion, but they are distinct clinical entities. *Bronchiolitis* refers simply to inflammation of small airways. *Bronchiolitis obliterans* is a pure airway disease due to their impingement on bronchiolar lumens by concentric inflammatory constriction or by endobronchiolar inflammatory granulation tissue. This

rare disorder of small airways has constrictive, stenotic, and scarred bronchiolitis without intraluminal plugs or polyps.[332, 350-356] This is characterized by obstructive defect on pulmonary function testing with a normal or hyperinflated chest on skiagram. The response to treatment is poor. The entity may be associated with rheumatoid arthritis, other collagen vascular diseases, graft versus host disease in bone marrow transplantation, chronic rejection in lung transplantation, following penicillamine or gold therapy, virus infections, toxic fume inhalation, or aspiration. But *BOOP* is a focal or diffuse, bronchiolar and infiltrative interstitial disease. Histopathologically, it consists of buds of granulation tissue, which plugs within lumens of small airways (respiratory bronchioles and alveolar ducts) accompanied by interstitial inflammation, with extension of organization into the alveoli (organizing pneumonia).[350-356] *It is defined pathogenically by the presence of granulation tissue buds in the distal air spaces progressing from fibrin exudates to loose collagen containing fibroblasts.* The lesions occur predominantly within the alveolar space but are often associated with buds of granulation tissue occupying the bronchiolar lumen (bronchiolitis obliterans). The involvement of the bronchioles may sometimes be missed in biopsy samples, and the term "cryptogenic organizing pneumonitis (COP)" is used to describe the condition.[350-352] Interstitial mononuclear cell infiltrate and accumulation of foam cells in the alveolar spaces are also frequently observed.

Most cases of BOOP are idiopathic, but this syndrome may be associated with many different conditions, particularly infections, collagen vascular diseases and drugs (Table 21.8). Some conditions like organizing infections, organizing diffuse alveolar damage, exposure to toxic gases and fumes, extrinsic allergic alveolitis, organizing eosinophilic pneumonia, Wegener's granulomatosis, bronchiectasis, and tissue reactions around abscesses, infarcts and tumors may show the histopathological pattern of BOOP in biopsy specimens, often in addition to their condition-specific histological lesions without the typical clinical presentation of BOOP syndrome. These conditions should not be misdiagnosed as the clinicopathological entity of BOOP.[333]

Pathogenesis and Pathology

BOOP is a distinct clinicopathologic entity within the spectrum of ILD that is unrelated to IPF.[357-360] This inflammatory lung disease is related to the inflammatory pathway rather than the fibrosing pathway that occurs with UIP or IPF. BOOP is characterized by polypoidal connective tissue masses composed of myxoid fibroblastic tissue resembling granulation tissue filling the

TABLE 21.8: Causes of BOOP[332-349]

Idiopathic BOOP
- Rapidly progressive BOOP
- Focal nodular BOOP

Postinfectious BOOP
- Chlamydia, Legioneel, Mycoplasma, Coxiella, Nocardia, Pseudomonas, Serratia, Staphylococcus, Group B Streptococcus, *Streptococcus pneumoniae*
- Adenovirus, Cytomegalovirus, Herpes virus, Influenza virus, Parainfluenza virus
- Malaria, Pneumocystis
- Cryptococcus, Penicillium

Drug induced BOOP
- Antibiotics (Amphotericin B, minocycline, cephalosporins, sulfasalazine, nitrofurantoin, sulfamethoxypyridazine)
- Bleomycin
- Methotrexate
- Busulphan
- Gold
- Amiodarone
- Illicit use of cocaine
- L-tryptophan
- Phenytoin
- Carbamazepine
- Ticlopidine hydrochloride
- 5-aminosalicylic acid
- Acebutolol
- Acramin
- Hexamethonium
- Interferon alpha
- Mesalazine
- Nilutamide
- Paraquat
- Sotalol

- Tacrolimus
- Vinabarbital-apobarbital

Collagen vascular disorders-associated BOOP
- Lupus erythematosus
- Rheumatoid arthritis
- Sjögren's syndrome, sweet syndrome
- Polymyositis-dermatomyositis
- Scleroderma, PSS
- Ankylosing spondylitis
- Polymyalgia rheumatica
- Behçet's syndrome

Immunological disorder associated-BOOP
- Human immunodeficiency virus infection
- Common variable immunodeficiency syndrome
- Essential mixed cryoglobulinemia

Organ transplantation associated-BOOP
- Bone marrow, lung and heart transplantation

Radiotherapy induced BOOP

Environmental exposure and toxins
- Textile printing dye
- Penicillium mold dust
- House fire

Miscellaneous conditions associated with BOOP
- Inflammatory Bowel Disease (Ulcerative colitis)
- Malignancies, Lymphoma
- T-cell chronic lymphocytic leukemia
- Myelodysplastic syndrome
- Interstitial cystitis
- Chronic thyroids
- Alcoholic cirrhosis
- Seasonal syndrome with cholecystitis
- Primary biliary cirrhosis
- Coronary artery bypass graft surgery

lumens of terminal respiratory bronchioles. They extend in a continuous fashion into alveolar ducts and alveoli that represent organizing pneumonia. Other histological features include central clusters of mononuclear inflammatory cells found in the intraluminal polyps. These polyps appear to float freely within a bronchiole or are focally attached to the wall. Chronic inflammation is present in the walls of the surrounding alveoli with reactive type II cells, increased foamy macrophages in the alveoli, and preserved lung architecture. There newly formed fibromyxoid tissue in BOOP and UIP, but in BOOP it can be completely reversed with corticosteroid therapy, but in UIP this tissue participates in the remodeling and destruction of interstitium. There is abundant capillarization in the fibromyxoid lesions in the airways in BOOP compared with minimal vascularization in UIP. Possibly, vascular growth factors in BOOP result in normal apoptosis (programmed cell death), but not in UIP. Apoptic activity is more in the fibromyxoid tissue of BOOP compared to UIP, which helps in the resolution process in the former.

CLINICAL FEATURES

Both sexes are equally affected and the usual age is between 50 and 60 years with a range from 20 to 80 years. Occasional cases in adolescents are reported. No predisposing factor has been identified, except the associated conditions as shown in Table 21.8. BOOP is not related to smoking. Most patients are nonsmokers or ex-smokers. Some investigators haver reported seasonal cases. The patient will present with a subacute influenza-like illness followed by cough, dyspnea, which may be rapidly progressive, and constitutional symptoms. Hemoptysis can occur rarely. The clinical findings will be the same as in other ILDs. Clubbing is distinctly uncommon in BOOP in contrast to IPF, and can occur in about 10 percent of cases.

There will be a restrictive type of ventilatory defect of mild to moderate degree with reduced DLCO and moderate to severe hypoxemia. Transfer coefficient may be normal. Obstructive features are uncommon in contrast to bronchiolitis obliterans, except if the patient is an incidental smoker. The hypoxemia is due to shunting.

Standard chest radiographs are characterized by widespread, bilateral patchy and inhomogeneous alveolar infiltrates, which may be migratory, the severity of which correlates with clinical status and extent of histopathological changes. Reticulonodular pattern is seen in less than 20 percent of cases. The HRCT demonstrates multifocal and confluent bilateral hazy densities that indicate airspace consolidation, nodular densities, or organizing pneumonia, and bronchial wall thickening. These changes are predominantly present in the periphery.[361,362] Three main imaging patterns are seen in BOOP. The most frequent and typical imaging profile is of multiple patchy alveolar opacities with a peripheral and bilateral distribution. Their size is variable, ranging from few centimeters to a whole lobe. These opacities may migrate. On the CT scan the density of the opacities varies from ground glass to consolidation, air bronchogram may be present in consolidated areas. The differential diagnosis of such radiological features is with those of chronic eosinophilic pneumonia, primary low-grade pulmonary lymphoma and bronchioalveolar cell carcinoma. The second pattern on radiology is less characteristic and present with diffuse bilateral infiltration associated with interstitial opacities and small alveolar opacities superimposed on them. Sometimes the peripheral opacities may be in the form of a triangle with the base towards the mediastinum. Two types of radiological opacities are also described. The first extends in a radial manner along the line of the bronchi towards the pleura and the second occurs in a subpleural location with no relation to the bronchi. The third pattern may be as a colitary focal lesion associated with a more chronic illness. It usually occurs in the upper lobes and may cavitate, possibly representing a nonresolving pneumonia. Other less common findings will be crescentic opacities surrounding the areas of ground glass attenuation, multiple or cavitary nodules or masses, pneumatoceles, peripheral irregular subpleural tags, and bronchiolar dilatation. Pleural effusions are uncommon (Figs 21.27 and 21.28).

Bronchoalveolar lavage will demonstrate a mixed cellularity with the most consistent increase being seen in the percentage of lymphocytes (20-40%), and also neutrophils and eosinophils. A high lymphocyte count may indicate a good response to treatment and increase in neutrophils or eosinophils without a concurrent increase in lymphocytes may predict a poor response. The lymphocyte CD4/CD8 ratio is decreased.

While HRCT may be strongly suggestive of BOOP, the diagnosis must be established by open or thoracoscopic lung biopsy to get sufficient specimen.

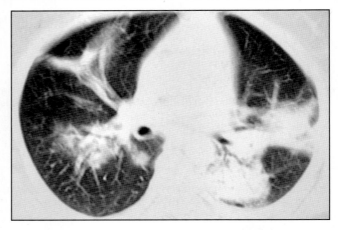

FIGURE 21.27: CT Chest - Pneumonic form of BOOP

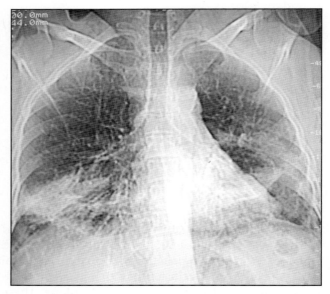

FIGURE 21.28: CXR - Nonresolving consolidation in both basal region – BOOP

Treatment

Idiopathic BOOP should be strongly considered in the differential diagnosis of a critically ill patient with rapidly progressive infiltrates and worsening hypoxia in whom no etiology has been found by a thorough diagnostic evaluation. An aggressive diagnostic approach is indicated since this can be a progressive, life threatening disease. Definitive histological diagnosis is important since BOOP is a steroid-responsive disease with a 65 to 80 percent complete response rate. Treatment is indicated in symptomatic and progressive disease. The treatment of choice is prednisolone in a dose of 1 mg/kg/day for 1 to 3 months followed by 40 mg/day for three months, and then 10 to 20 mg/day for the remainder

1 year.[333,334,362] Alternate-day-scheduling is also possible. A shorter, 6 months period of treatment is sufficient in certain cases. Although other drugs like erythromycin, inhaled triamcinolone, and cyclophosphamide have been used in this condition, but their efficacy has not been confirmed.

The prognosis of BOOP is generally good in most patients, better than that for IPF. However, it may be a lethal disease in a few patients. Risk factors for an unfavorable outcome may include interstitial opacities on radiography, lack of lymphocytosis in BAL fluid, and features of usual interstitial pneumonitis in biopsy specimens.[363]

HISTIOCYTOSIS X

Histiocytosis X is a rare disease and is Langerhans' cell granulomatous interstitial lung disease of unknown etiology.[364-376] It occurs almost exclusively in young smokers between the ages of 20 to 40 years. The entity is otherwise known as Langerhans' cell granulomatosis or Eosinophilic granuloma of the lung. The patient typically present with dry cough and exertional dyspnea, weight loss, fever and fatigue. Chest pain is very common and is due to either because of granulomatous rib erosion or pneumothorax, which occurs in about a forth of patients. Occasionally there may be associated diabetes insipidus because of hypothalamic involvement. About a fourth of patients will be asymptomatic and medical attention is only drawn because of an abnormal pulmonary function test.

Physical examination is by and large normal. Inspiratory crepitations are present in only a minority of patients. Clubbing is also rare and is a late manifestation. Eosinophilia is not a feature of this disease. Pulmonary function test may show obstructive, restrictive, or mixed patterns. Diffusion capacity is reduced in symptomatic patients.[373-375] In late-stage or progressive disease, air trapping and hyperinflation of the chest occurs. This is not correlated with smoking, rather as a result of granulomatous inflammation and is replaced by bullae and cysts. Typically, chest radiography will show mid- and upper-zone nodular opacities and cysts. The lung volumes are either normal or increased in contrast to idiopathic interstitial fibrosis. The costophrenic angles are spared (Fig. 21.29). High resolution CT is quite helpful and characteristic HRCT findings consist of marked profusion of cystic shadows with few nodules. The presence of upper lobe micronodules and cysts are virtually pathognomonic of pulmonary histiocytosis X. Serial HRCT will show a sequence of progression of the disease with nodular opacities,

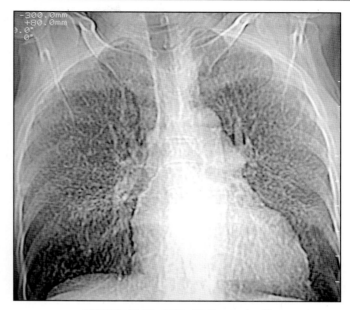

FIGURE 21.29: CXR - Histiocytosis - X

cavitation of nodules, thick-walled cysts, confluent cysts, and honey combing.[374,375]

Histopathological examination of the tissue remains the definitive diagnostic test. Most often, open lung biopsy will be necessary for a satisfactory tissue. The pathologic hallmark of this disorder is nodular histiocytic inflammation centered round the airways in a classic "stellate" appearance with involvement of adjacent airspaces.[369-372] The alveolar septae, terminal airways, and the perivascular interstitium are involved. Langerhans' cells are found in clusters in the nodules, with eosinophils, plasma cells, and occasionally multinucleated giant cells. Langerhans cells have distinct features on light microscopy, but the characteristic features are revealed under electron microscope. This demonstrates small, rodlike, intracytoplasmic inclusions, called X bodies, or Birbeck granules, which are pathognomonic of histiocytosis X. Tissue immunostaining for S-100 protein distinguishes this cell from other histiocytes. Although Langerhans' cells may be found in other conditions like idiopathic interstitial fibrosis, they are sparse and occasional, whereas in this condition they are in plenty, occurs in clusters and found diffusely. These cells also express CD1 antigen (OKT6). The findings of more than 5 percent of CD1-positive cells in BAL is a useful test to reliably identify patients with pulmonary histiocytosis X. Fewer cells can be found in other interstitial fibrosis cases. Fibroblast infiltration is another important feature and is mediated by platelet-derived growth factor.

TABLE 21.9: Causes of hypersensitivity pneumonitis[385-387]

Condition	Exposure	Antigen
Farmer's lung	Moldy hay	Micropolyspora faeni
		Thermoactinomyces vulgaris
Mushroom workers lung	Mushroom compost	Thermophilic actinomycetes
Humidifier lung	Water	Thermophilic actinomycetes
		B.subtilis, *B.cereus*
Bagassosis	Moldy sugar cane	Thermophilic actinomycetes
Washing powder lung	Detergent	*B.subtilis* enzyme
Maltworker's lung	Malt	Aspergillus clavatus
Cheese worker's lung	Moldy cheese rind	Penicillium casei
Maple bark stripper's disease	Wood bark	Cryptostroma corticale
Sequoiosis	Red wood dust	Graphium pullulans
		Aureobasidium pullulans
Suberosis	Moldy cork	Penicillium frequentans
Dry rot lung	Rotten wood	Merulius lacrymans
Bird fancier's lung	Bird droppings, feathers	Avian protein, blood
Rat handler's lung	Rat	Urine, serum, pellets
Wheat weevil lung	Infested flour	Wheat weevil
Pituitary snuff taker's lung	Pituitary snuff	Porcine and bovine pituitary protein
Furrier's lung	Fur industry	Animal fur
Isocyanate lung	Foam factory	TDI, MDI
Pauli's reagent lung	Factory workers	Pauli's reagent
Vineyard sprayer's lung	Bordeaux mixture	Copper sulfate
Hard metal disease	Industry	Cobalt
Cromolyn sodium lung	Drug factory	Cromolyn sodium
Sauna lung	Water	Lake water?
New Guinea lung	Habitat	Hut thatch?
Ramin lung	Wood workers	Ramin wood
Insecticide lung	Workers	Pyrethrum
Amiodarone lung	Therapy	Amiodarone
Summer type hypersensitivity pneumonitis	Residence (Japan)	Trichosporon cutaneum

The clinical course is unpredictable, although a large percentage of cases will have a stable, persistent disease. Many may have a progressive disease. Extremes of age, constitutional symptoms, advanced radiologic changes at presentation, low DLCO, and continued smoking, are poor prognostic indicators. Corticosteroids may be helpful in symptomatic cases. However, their role is not exactly defined. These patients have an increased risk of developing lung cancer because of heavy smoking.[376]

HYPERSENSITIVITY PNEUMONITIS

Hypersensitivity pneumonitis is an immunological lung disease caused by repeated and prolonged inhalation of organic antigen.[377-379] Other alternatives terms for the disease include extrinsic allergic alveolitis, and according to the specific occupations in which it occurs, like farmer's lung, bird Fancier's lung, and bagassosis etc. It is a relatively uncommon disease, even in subjects, known exposed to heavy antigens. The incidence of the disease in farming population is estimated to be 4 to 85 cases per thousand exposed. The difficulty arises partly because of the nonspecificity of the symptoms and partly, because of nonspecificity of serological tests.[380-384]

Various organic antigens known to cause hypersensitivity pneumonitis are shown in Table 21.9.

PATHOGENESIS

The pathogenesis of hypersensitivity pneumonitis involves the following stages: (i) repetitive exposure to the particular antigen; (ii) immunologic sensitization of the host to the antigen; and (iii) immune mediated damage of the lung tissue determined by host susceptibility. The disease only occurs in individuals who are exposed to the antigen repeatedly, often daily, over a prolonged period of time. Single or sporadic exposure does not cause disease. The small, particulate antigens, 1 to 3 mm in diameter reach the alveoli, which withstand degradation by lysosomal enzymes. Lung injury involves both immunologic and nonimmunologic pathways. Immunologic damage is mediated by immune-complex or Type III and cellular hypersensitivity or Type IV reactions. Nonimmune factors include alternate complement (C_3) activation and genetic predisposition.

In support of the immune complex-mediated injury, precipitating antibodies are demonstrated in the serum and bronchoalveolar lavage (BAL) fluid of these patients. C_{1q} and C_3 are also present in the BAL fluid of the affected individuals. Immunofluorescent analysis has also demonstrated antibody and complement in histological sections of lung tissue. Clinically, the delayed onset of symptoms after 4 to 6 hours after exposure to antigen, further suggests the immune complex-mediated or Arthus type of response. However, the vasculitis component of the reaction is not seen on histology.

Involvement of delayed type hypersensitivity reaction is apparent from the fact that mononuclear cell infiltration and granuloma formation are more frequent in hypersensitivity pneumonitis. Peripheral blood and BAL fluid lymphocytes from these patients proliferate in response to antigen, another characteristic feature of the cell-mediated reaction. These cells undergo blast transformation and produce migration inhibition factor (MIF).

It has been suggested and shown both clinically and experimentally that, following exposure to antigen there is a rapid and heavy accumulation of neutrophils early in the reaction which is cleared by about the 8th day, followed by a rapid increase in the number of lymphocytes. The percentage of T-lymphocytes is very high, often as high as 60 to 70 percent. The number of suppressor/cytotoxic cells is usually well above 40 percent of the total lymphocytes. Chemotactic factors released by activated lymphocytes attract monocytes, which lead to granuloma formation. It is suggested that while early inflammatory injury is immunecomplex-mediated, abnormalities in T cell function are important in the initiation and development of hypersensitivity pneumonitis.[388]

Early neutrophilic alveolitis appears to be due to activation of the alternative pathway of complement. The initial response to antigen, although primarily of neutrophilic and lymphocytic in origin, other cell types like eosinophils, B-lymphocytes, basophils, and mast cells may also be important.

The inhaled antigen that initiates the immune reaction is first taken up by macrophages, which may destroy or modify the antigen or may present it to specific T-lymphocytes. These activated macrophages are capable of secreting IL-1 and display antigens on the cell surface. The T-lymphocytes respond by secreting lymphokines including IL-2. Both IL-1 and IL-2 are chemoattractants for lymphocytes and more of these cells are recruited to the site of inflammation, leading on to granuloma formation and fibrosis. A number of pro-inflammatory cytokines have been found to help for the development of hypersensitivity pneumonitis.[389]

Certain risk factors are associated with the development of hypersensitivity pneumonitis since, not all subjects exposed to antigen develop disease. About 50 percent of the nonatopic individuals, if exposed heavily to suitable antigens, will demonstrate Arthus reaction. But only 5 to 15 percent of them develop the disease. Thus immunologic reactivity of the subject is an important determinant. Earlier evidence suggested that genetic and immunologic responsiveness determined by HLA types might play a role in the development of hypersensitivity pneumonitis, particularly in farmer's lung and pigeon breeder's lung disease. However, this finding has not been consistently demonstrated. Similarly role of P_1 erythrocyte antigen has been suggested, but discarded later. It is interesting to note that most patients of hypersensitivity pneumonitis are nonsmokers. It is suggested that since smoking is associated with increased macrophages, activation of these cells enhance the ability of the lung to clear antigens and thus decrease the inflammatory response. Intensity of exposure of antigen is another important determinant of disease. A farmer working with a moderate exposure of moldy hay may inhale as many as 750,000 spores per minute. About half of the nonatopic individuals will develop an Arthus type of reaction if heavily exposed. Hypersensitivity to avian antigens causes two types of syndromes. Intermittent heavy exposure produces acute hypersensitivity pneumonitis and mild, persistent challenges favor chronic disease.

PATHOLOGY

Extrapulmonary involvement is rare in hypersensitivity pneumonitis. The lungs are the organs predominantly affected by the disease. Morphological features include alveolitis in the early stage, luminal and mural granuloma formation, intra-alveolar bud formation, bronchiolitis, and interstitial fibrosis. Involvement of pulmonary vessels is very rare.

In the early stages (*acute stage*), the alveolar wall is infiltrated with neutrophils, lymphocytes, plasma cells and macrophages. The alveoli may contain inflammatory exudates mixed with inflammatory cells. Atypical lymphocytes, called the "hand mirror" cells are seen sometimes. In the *subacute stage*, granuloma formation is typical. These are noncaseating. However, unlike in sarcoidosis, the granulomas are small, ill defined, loosely arranged, and have a high content of neutrophils. They are scattered throughout the lung fields. The granulomas appear about three weeks after exposure and resolve within a year. Intraalveolar prominences due to fibroblasts, myofibroblasts, and macrophages, called intraalveolar buds, are seen in about two-thirds of the patients. Bronchiolitis is due to involvement of terminal and respiratory bronchioles. In the *chronic stage*, the granulomatous alveolitis is replaced by interstitial fibrosis.

CLINICAL FEATURES

Farmer's lung disease will be discussed as a prototype of hypersensitivity pneumonitis. This is the best-known and best studied amongst all the forms of hypersensitivity pneumonitis. The disease is caused by exposure to moldy dusts generated by the thrashing of wet hay and handling of straw and other decomposing vegetable material. Hay, stored in the bins of a farm, if damp and wet, generates heat and humidity. These conditions are favorable to the growth of thermophilic microorganisms. The organisms which include *Micropolyspora faeni, Thermoactinomycetes vulgaris, Thermoactinomycetes candidus, Micropolyspora* and others, when enter the respiratory tract of the previously sensitized individuals, initiate alveolar inflammation. Any farmer working with moldy hay or any such matter is a potential victim. The majority of the patients are in the age group of 20 to 70 years of age group. The disease is common in poor farming communities where the handling of the hay is mostly manual. The disease is common in the agricultural areas of the world being more so in cold and humid regions. Because of damp weather, autumn and winter are the seasons with the highest incidence of the disease. The incidence varies from region to region because of the difference in climatic conditions and farming practices.[390]

The disease is usually has three stages. Classical symptoms of *acute* hypersensitivity pneumonitis include cough, fever, tightness of chest, malaise, body ache, arthralgia, anorexia, dyspnea, headache, and chills. The symptoms appear 4 to 8 hours after exposure to the antigen and subside within 24 hours. These symptoms are usually ignored by the patient as mild flue or cold. *Subacute* cases may have symptoms continued for longer. *Chronic* cases develop gradually increasing dyspnea and fatigue with progressive impaired lung functions. Weight loss may be prominent. Physical examination may reveal fever, tachycardia, and tachypnea in the early stages. Clubbing is uncommon. Bibasilar crepitations are usual. Chronic cases may be complicated by cor pulmonale.

INVESTIGATIONS

Leucocytosis is common in the early stages, with white blood cell counts in the range of 20,000 to 30,000/cmm with neutrophilic excess. Eosinophilia is rare. Serum immunoglobulins are increased in a polyclonal fashion except for IgE, which is usually normal.

Chest radiograph may be normal in acute stages, but more typically shows nodular and interstitial patterns of opacities. They may coalesce during acute episodes and may be confused with alveolar infiltrates of other causes like infective pneumonias and pulmonary edema. With chronic disease and prolonged antigen exposure, the changes are more suggestive of interstitial fibrosis, and honeycombing. The changes are more prominent in the upper lung fields. Pleural effusion, and lymphadenopathy are uncommon.

Precipitating antibodies to one or more thermophilic actinomycetes are positive in most patients (90%). These antibodies are usually of the IgG and IgM class. However, the prevalence of serum antibodies in antigen-exposed populations is much higher than the prevalence of the disease. These antibodies can be positive up to 10 to 20 percent of asymptomatic farmers. Thus the positive test is an evidence of exposure, but not that of the disease. The titre, also does not correlate with the presence of disease. On the other hand, serum antibodies may be negative in cases of farmer's lung disease. Skin tests are not very helpful.

Symptomatic patients in acute stages will show restrictive pattern of abnormalities on lung function studies. The vital capacity, FEV_1, total lung capacity, and diffusing capacity are decreased 4 to 6 hours after exposure, which gradually return to normal levels gradually after few hours. In chronic cases, these changes become permanent without any reversibility. Lung compliance is decreased. It is postulated that hyaluronic acid, due to its pronounced ability to immobilize water may be of importance in the development of pulmonary function abnormality. Its presence in the BAL fluid may be useful in distinguishing symptomatic subjects from those with asymptomatic alveolitis.[391] Hypoxemia may be present on exercise. The alveolar-arterial difference is wide, and is further decreased on exercise. Nonspecific bronchial hyperreactivity may be observed in some cases. Since pulmonary function tests may be normal, challenge with suspected antigen is done in some laboratories, although this not recommended as a routine.

Bronchoalveolar lavage is useful in the diagnosis of farmer's lung disease by demonstration of an excess of lymphocytes, which may account for up to 80 percent of the lavaged cells.[392,393] Most of the cells are of the suppressor/cytotoxic (CD8+) lymphocytes. The ratio of the CD4+/CD8+ lymphocytes in the lavaged cells is decreased. These findings differentiate other lymphocytic type of BAL fluid as in sarcoidosis and berylliosis, which show predominant helper/inducer (CD4+) lymphocytes. Neutrophils are increased in acute situations only. Noncellular components also show abnormalities in the form of increased total proteins, albumin, IgG, IgM, IgA, and complements. Thus a lymphocytic type of alveolitis is typical of farmer's lung disease.

A lung biopsy is not necessary to diagnose farmer's lung disease in most cases. Pertinent history of exposure, with clinical, radiologic, and serologic studies consistent with the diagnosis, is often enough. However, the biopsy will be necessary if another diagnosis is seriously being considered.

Differential diagnosis of acute farmer's lung disease includes viral and mycoplasmal illnesses, bacterial and fungal infections like miliary tuberculosis, acute histoplasmosis, coccidioidomycosis, occupational disorders, and immune-mediated drug reactions. Chronic form of the disease may be confused with other forms of interstitial pulmonary fibrosis.

TREATMENT

In most cases, avoidance of exposure to antigen is essential to prevent deterioration of lung function. Other than antigen avoidance, treatment is mainly supportive. In acute stages, administration of steroids for 2 to 4 weeks produces resolution of clinical, functional, and radiological findings. Steroids may not be helpful in chronic cases, although in a few cases lung function deterioration might be prevented. Prevention can be achieved by wearing facemask during exposure and by thoroughly drying hay before storage.

DRUG-INDUCED ALVEOLITIS

A number of drugs are known to cause interstitial lung disease (Table 21.10). The number is ever increasing. There are various mechanisms by which they cause this reaction. Of these only three, bleomycin, amiodarone, and nitrofurantoin will be discussed as prototypes.

The clinical features of drug-induced alveolitis consist of slowly increasing breathlessness with dry cough, as they are in any other interstitial lung disease. Basilar end-inspiratory dry crepitations are usual. Radiographic features will show diffuse patchy infiltrates. The only characteristic finding is perhaps a raised eosinophil counts in the peripheral blood and in bronchoalveolar lavage. Lung function changes include a decreased diffusion capacity and restrictive type of ventilatory defect. Because of the nonspecificity of the symptoms and other laboratory parameters, it is

TABLE 21.10: Drugs causing alveolitis[394-397]

Antineoplastic drugs	Antibiotics and anti-inflammatory drugs
Bleomycin	Nitrofurantoin
Mitomycin	Sulfonamides
Busulfan	Penicillins
Chlorambucil	PAS
Cyclophosphamide	Sulfasalazine
Methotrexate	Penicillamine
Comustine	Gold
Cardiovascular drugs	*Miscellaneous drugs*
Amiodarone	Phenytoin
Procainamide	Carbamazepine
Quinidine	Amitriptyline
Methyldopa	Imipramine
Hydralazine	Chlorpropamide
Cromoglycate	

often difficult to differentiate the drug-induced alveolitis from that due to lung involvement because of the underlying disease for which the drug is being used. A high degree of suspicion and if feasible, lung biopsy, and bronchoalveolar lavage may be necessary. BAL studies have shown a lymphocytic type of alveolitis, either pure or associated with neutrophilic, eosinophilic or a combination of these cells. Inverted CD4/CD8 lymphocyte is a characteristic feature.[394,398] In amiodarone-associated pneumonitis, two different patterns of BAL fluid values are observed;[398,399] one with no abnormality in lymphocyte counts and the other one similar to those described above with other drugs. The findings closely resemble to those obtained in patients with hypersensitivity pneumonitis due to inhalation of organic dust and suggest that an underlying immunologic cell-mediated mechanism may play a role in amiodarone-induced pulmonary disease.[399]

Bleomycin lung toxicity is related to the generation of toxic oxygen radicals within the lung by the bleomycin-iron complex. High concentrations of oxygen increase the toxicity in human subjects. Depletion of iron decreases the pulmonary toxicity. Because lung cells are exposed to oxygen relative to other cells, and because some lung cells are deficient in bleomycin hydrolase, which inactivates bleomycin, pulmonary tissue is the common site for such toxicity. Moreover, bleomycin is known to cause proliferation of fibroblasts with increased formation of collagen. The incidence of pulmonary fibrosis is between 5 to 10 percent of the patients. The toxicity is both age and dose related. There is a gradual fall in lung function as the duration and dose of the drug used is increased. Serial monitoring of transfer factor is important to detect early changes of lung damage. Rarely, an acute allergic type of reaction with fever and eosinophilia is seen.

The urinary antiseptic *nitrofurantoin* is known to cause acute hypersensitivity reactions. It is manifested by an acute illness with cough, dyspnea, and other signs of acute hypersensitivity reaction. Pleural effusion and vasculitis changes may occur. The more serious type of lung toxicity is however, the development of progressive pulmonary fibrosis. The drug undergoes cyclic reduction/oxidation within the cell in a fashion similar to paraquat. Under anaerobic conditions, nitrofurantoin forms an anion-free radical and under aerobic conditions it reoxidises to the parent compound, releasing a free electron and generating toxic oxygen radicals. The mechanism of the later is different from that by bleomycin, although cells are damaged in a similar fashion.

Amiodarone is a relatively new and potent anti-arrhythmic drug with a high incidence of serious and potentially fatal lung reactions. The adverse drug reaction results from both direct toxic effects of the drug and indirect toxic effects related to activation of inflammatory or immune mechanisms. The reaction is associated with a marked increase in both neutrophils and lymphocytes in the BAL fluid of the patients. There is particularly a specific increase in the T-suppressor/cytotoxic lymphocytes (CD8+ cells), similar to other hypersensitivity pneumonitis. Other drugs like gold, methotrexate, and nitrofurantoin possibly act in this fashion also. Macrophage accumulation and hyperplasia of Type II pneumocytes are prominent features on histology. Amiodarone-pulmonary toxicity occurs in about 13 percent of patients receiving the drug and is usually associated with other toxic manifestations of the drug like corneal deposits. Lung function changes occur in still higher percentage of cases. Because of the potential serious toxicity, the drug should only be used in resistant arrhythmias at the lowest doses with serial monitoring of diffusing capacity.

RADIATION PNEUMONITIS[400-402]

Irradiation (X-rays) damages DNA either directly by ionization or indirectly by producing ions in the surroundings water which then attack DNA. Irradiation of the water molecules in a cell will generate unstable ion pairs, H_2O^+ and electron. These will form hydrogen ions and free hydroxyl radicals. Further reactions will produce other toxic species including H_2O_2. Presence of oxygen facilitates these reactions. The pulmonary vascular endothelial cells and Type II pneumocytes are the cells principally affected by radiation. There is no adverse effect up to a dose of 600 cGy. The risk however, increases thereafter, with damage in about 30 percent with a single dose of 800 cGy and in 80 percent with a dose of 1000 cGy. Spacing with smaller fractions reduces the chances of pulmonary toxicity.

Histologically radiation injury to the lungs can be divided into three stages: (i) a latent period only with histological changes of congestion and intra-alveolar edema; (ii) acute pneumonitis with organization of edema into collagen fibrils and thickening of alveolar septa, and the (iii) late phase of pneumonitis involving repair and proliferation of septal and alveolar cells with reconstruction. Pneumonitis then merges into radiation fibrosis.

Lung damage commonly follows with mediastinal irradiation for lymphoma, breast cancer, bronchogenic carcinoma, and radioiodine therapy for thyroid carcinoma for lung metastasis. With use of modern techniques like megavoltage radiotherapy, electron beam therapy, and high-energy linear transfer radiotherapy, radiation pneumonitis is uncommon since these beams are directed to the site of malignancy with minimum scatter.

The condition usually presents between one and three months after treatment, although it may occur earlier or later. Radiation syndromes of the lung have been divided into 2 clinical phases: acute pneumonitis, and later appearing fibrosis. The injury is more likely to be radiological than clinical. About 50 percent of the patients will show radiological change, and only about 5 to 10 percent will manifest clinically. The signs and symptoms include dyspnea, cough, and pleuritic chest pain depending upon the extent of damage. Usually the symptoms subside with time. Very rarely the disease become progressive and the chronic effects are apparent after 6 to 12 months of radiation.

There is a no definite treatment for radiation pneumonitis. Some experimental drugs like ACE inhibitor captopril, and penicillamine are shown to be helpful in experimental animals. Role of steroids in preventing and treating the condition is controversial.

REFERENCES

1. Turner-Warwick M, Burrows B, Johnson A. Cryptogenic fibrosing alveolitis: Clinical features and their influence on survival. Thorax 1980;35:171-80.
2. Crystal RG, Bitterman PB, Rennard SI, Hance AG, Keough BA. Interstitial lung disease of unknown cause: Disorders characterized by chronic inflammation of the lower respiratory tract. N Engl J Med 1984;310:154-66; 235-44.
3. Tierney LM Jr. Idiopathic pulmonary fibrosis. Semin Respir Med 1991;12:229.
4. Schwarz MI. Idiopathic pulmonary fibrosis. West Med J 1988;149:199-203.
5. Interstitial lung disease. Chest 1986;89(Suppl):146S.

6. Hamman L, Rich AR. Fulminating diffuse interstitial fibrosis of the lungs. Trans Am Clin Climatol Assoc 1935;51:154-63.

7. Hamman L, Rich AR. Acute diffuse interstitial fibrosis of the lungs. Bull Johns Hopkins Hosp 1944;74:177.

8. Olson J, Colby TV, Elliot CG. Hamman-Rich syndrome revisited. Mayo Clin Proc 1990;65:1538-48.

9. Schwarz MI. Diffuse pulmonary infiltrates and respiratory failure following 2 weeks of dyspnea in a 45-year-old woman. Chest 1993;104:927-29.

10. Liebow AA. Definition and classification of interstitial pneumonias in human pathology. Prog Respir Res 1975;8:1-31.

11. Scadding JG, Hinson KFW. Diffuse fibrosing alveolitis (diffuse interstitial fibrosis of the lung): Correlation of histology at biopsy with prognosis. Thorax 1967;22:291-304.

12. Stack BH, Choo Kang YF, Heard BF. The prognosis of cryptogenic fibrosing alveolitis. Thorax 1972;27:535-42.

13. Cherniack RM, Colby TV, Fint A, et al. Correlation of structure and function in idiopathic pulmonary fibrosis. Am J Respir Crit Care Med 1995;151:1180-88.

14. Crystal RG, Fulmer JD, Roberts WC, Moss Ml, Line BR, Reynolds HY. Idiopathic pulmonary fibrosis: Clinical, histologic, radiographic, physiologic, scintigraphic, cytologic, and biochemical aspects. Ann Intern Med 1976;85:769-88.

15. Winterbauer RH, Hammar SP, Hallman KO, et al. Diffuse interstitial pneumonitis. Clinicopathologic correlation in 20 patients treated with prednisolone/azathioprine. Am J Med 1978;65:661-72.

16. Turner-Warwick M, Burrows B, Johnson A. Cryptogenic fibrosing alveolitis: clinical features and their influence on survival. Thorax 1980;35:171-80.

17. Fishman AP. UIP, DIP and all that. N Engl J Med 1978;298:843-44.

18. Scadding JB. Fibrosing alveolitis. Br Med J 1964;2:686.

19. Groen H, Postma DS, Kallenberg CGM. Interstitial lung disease and myositis in a patient with simultaneously occurring sarcoidosis and scleroderma. Chest 1993;104:1298-1300.

20. Ameilli J, Brechot JM, Brochard P, Capron F, Dore MF. Occupational hypersensitivity pneumonitis in a smelter exposed to zinc fumes. Chest 1992;101:862-63.

21. Dalabhanga Y, Constantopoulos SH, Galanpoulou V, Zerva L, Moutsopoulos HM. Alveolitis correlates with clinical pulmonary involvement in primary Sjögren's syndrome. Chest 1991;99:1394-97.

22. Hatron PY, Wallaert B, Gosset D, et al. Subclinical lung inflammation in primary Sjögren's syndrome. Arthritis Rheum 1987;30:1226-31.

23. Wallaert B, Prin L, Hatron PV, Ramon P, Tonnel AB, Voisin C. Lymphocytic subpopulations in bronchoalveolar lavage in Sjögren's syndrome. Chest 1987;92:1025-31.

24. Wade JF III, King TE Jr. Dyspnoea, cough, and interstitial lung disease in a 32-year-old smoker. Chest 1994;105:265-67.

25. Schauble TL. Lymphocytic alveolitis in a crematorium worker. Chest 1994;105:617-19.

26. Drobisky WR, Russler SK, Tapper MA, Knox KK, Ash RC. Interstitial pneumonitis associated with human herpes virus-6 infection after bone marrow transplantation. Lancet 1991;338:147.

27. International Consensus Statement. Idiopathic Pulmonary Fibrosis: Diagnosis and treatment. Am J Respir Crit Care Med 2000;161:646-64.

28. Crystal RG, Bitterman PB, Mossman B, et al. NHLBI Workshop Summary: Future research directions in idiopathic pulmonary fibrosis. Am J Respir Crit Care Med 2002;166:236-46.

29. Coultas DB, Hughes MP. Accuracy of mortality data for interstitial lung diseases in New Mexico, USA. Thorax 1996;51:717-20.

30. Coultas DB. Epidemiology of idiopathic pulmonary fibrosis. Semin Respir Med 1993;14:181-96.

31. Hubbard R, Johnston I, Coultas DB, Britton J. Mortality rates from cryptogenic fibrosing alveolitis in seven countries. Thorax 1996;51:711-16.

32. Johnston I, Britton J, Kinnear W, Logan R. Rising mortality from cryptogenic fibrosing alveolitis. Br Med J 1990;301:1017-21.

33. Coultas DB, Zumwalt RE, Black WC, Sobonya RE. The epidemiology of interstitial lung diseases. Am J Respir Crit Care Med 1994;150:967-72.

34. Mannino DM, Etzel RA, Parrish RG. Pulmonary fibrosis deaths in the United States, 1979-1991: An analysis of multiple cause mortality data. Am J Respir Crit Care Med 1996;153:1548-52.

35. Iwai K, Mori T, Yamada N, Yamaguchi M, Hosoda Y. Idiopathic pulmonary fibrosis: Epidemiologic approaches to occupational exposure. Am J Respir Crit Care Med 1994;150:670-75.

36. Panos RJ, Motenson R, Nicoli SA, King Jr TE. Clinical deterioration in patients with idiopathic pulmonary fibrosis: Causes and assessment. Am J Med 1990;88:396-404.

37. Schwartz DA, Helmers RA, Galvin JR, et al. Determinants of survival in patients with idiopathic pulmonary fibrosis. Am J Respir Crit Care Med 1994;149:450-54.

38. Scott J, Johnston I, Britton J. What causes cryptogenic fibrosing alveolitis? A case control study of environmental exposure to dust. Br Med J 1990;301:1015-17.

39. Jindal SK, Malik SK, Deodhar SD, Sharma BK. Fibrosing alveolitis. A report of 61 cases seen over the past five years. Ind J Chest Dis All Sc 1979;19:174-79.

40. Sharma SK, Pande JN, Verma K, Guleria JS. Bronchoalveolar fluid (BALF) analysis in interstitial lung diseases: A 7 years experience. Ind J Chest Dis All Sc 1989;31:187-96.

41. Kalra L, Verma K, Pande JN, Guleria JS. Diagnostic significance of bronchoalveolar lavage fluid analysis in bilateral diffuse lung diseases. Ind J Med Res 1984;79: 697-703.

42. Kalra S, D'Souza G, Bhusnurmath B, Jindal SK. Transbronchial lung biopsy in diffuse lung disease: A study of 28 cases. Ind J Chest Dis 1989;31:265-70.

43. Behera D, D'Souza G, Rajwanshi A, Jindal SK. Bronchoalveolar cellular in patients with idiopathic pulmonary fibrosis and sarcoidosis. Ind J Chest Dis All Sc 1990;32:107-10.

44. Gupta R, Kulpati DDS, Hira HS, Chauhan MR. Evaluation of bronchoalveolar lavage (BAL) in diffuse infiltrative lung diseases. Ind J Chest Dis All Sc 1985;27:207-10.

45. Potdar PV, Jain K, Prabhakaran L, Kamat SR. Value of bronchoalveolar lavage in interstitial lung diseases. J Asso Phys India 1989;27:444-47.

46. Malhotra NJ, Kher A, Uthup S, Mohan PV, Bharucha BA, Pathare AV. Idiopathic hemosiderosis. Ind J Chest Dis 1995;37:175-78.

47. Marwaha RK, Garewal G, Kumar V, Sarkar B, Malik N. Microcytic hypochromic anaemia in idiopathic hemosiderosis. Ind Peditr 1994;31:1101-07.

48. Nair N, Jindal SK. Idiopathic pulmonary hemosiderosis. Ind J Chest Dis 1993;35:35-40.

49. Suri JC, Goel A, Bhatia A, Kaushik PC. Evaluation of unguided transbronchial biopsy in the diagnosis of pulmonary disease: Its safety and efficacy as an outpatient procedure. Ind J Chest Dis All Sc 1992;34:57-64.

50. Hubbard R, Lewis R, Richards K, Johnston I, Britton J. Occupational exposure to metal or wood dust and aetiology of cryptogenic fibrosing alveolitis. Lancet 1996;347:284-89.

51. Mannino DM, Etzel RL, Parrish RG. Pulmonary fibrosis deaths in the United States, 1979-1991: An analysis of multiple causes mortality data. Am J Respir Crit Care Med 1996;153:1548-52.

52. Johnston ID, Prescott AR, Chaimers JC, et al. British Thoracic Society study of cryptogenic fibrosing alveolitis: Current presentation and initial management. Thorax 1997;52:38-44.

53. Rudd RM, Haslam PI, Turner Warwick M. Cryptogenic fibrosing alveolitis relationships of pulmonary physiology and bronchoalveolar lavage to treatment and prognosis. Am Rev Respir Dis 1981;124:1-8.

54. Watters LC, Schwartz MI, Cherniack RM, Waldron JA, et al. Idiopathic pulmonary fibrosis. Am Rev Respir Dis 1987;135:696-705.

55. Carrington CB, Gaensler EA, Coutu RE, Fitzgerald MX, Gupta RG. Natural history and treated course of usual and desquamative interstitial pneumonias. New Engl J Med 1978;298:801-09.

56. Raghu G. Interstitial lung disease: A diagnostic approach: Are CT scan and lung biopsy indicated in every patient? Am J Respir Crit Care Med 1995;151:909-14.

57. Fan LL, Kozinetz CA, Wojtczak HA, Chatfield BA, Cohen AH, Rothenberg SS. Diagnostic value of transbronchial, thoracoscopic, and open lung biopsy in immunocompetent children with chronic interstitial lung disease. J Pediatr 10997;131:565-69.

58. Fan LL, Kozinetz CA. Factors influencing survival in children with chronic intertstitial lung disease. Am J Respir Crit Care Med 1997;156:939-42.

59. Baumgartner KI, Samet J, Sudley CA, Colby TV, Waldron JA and the collaborating centers. Cigarette smoking: A risk factor for idiopathic pulmonary fibrosis. Am J Respir Crit Care Med 1997;155:242-48.

60. Nagai S, Hoshino Y, Hayashi M, Ito I. Smoking-related interstitial lung diseases. Curr Opin Pulm Med 2000;6:415-19.

61. Hubbard R, Venn A, Smith C, Cooper M, Johnston I, Britton J. Exposure to commonly prescribed drugs and the etiology of cryptogenic fibrosing alveolitis: A case control study. Am J Respir Crit Care Med 1998;157:743-47.

62. Tobin RW, Pope CE 2nd, Pellegrini CA, Emond MJ, Sillery J, Raghu G. Increased prevalence of gastroesophageal reflux in patients with idiopathic pulmonary fibrosis. Am J Respir Crit Care Med 1998;158:1804-08.

63. Hughes EW. Familial incidence of diffuse interstitial fibrosis. Postgrad Med J 1965;41:150-52.

64. Verleden GM, du Bois RM, Bouros D, et al. Genetic predisposition and pathogenetic mechanisms of interstitial lung diseases of unknown origin. Eur Respir J 2001; 32(suppl):17S-29S.

65. Watters LC. Genetic aspects of idiopathic pulmonary fibrosis and hypersensitive pneumonitis. Semin Respir Med 1986;7:317-25.

66. Raghu G. Genetic susceptibility to pulmonary fibrosis. Pulmonary Perspectives 1995;12:5-8.

67. Ellis RH. Familial incidence of diffuse interstitial fibrosis. Postgrad Med J 1965;41:150-52.

68. Murphy A, O'Sullivan BJ. Familial fibrosing alveolitis. Isr J Med Sc 1981;150;204-09.

69. Bitterman PB, Rennard SI, Keogh BA, Wewers MD, Adelberg S, Crystal RG. Familial idiopathic pulmonary fibrosis. Evidence of lung inflammation in unaffected family members. N Engl J Med 1986;314:1343-47.

70. Raghu G, Mageto YN. Genetic predisposition of interstitial lung diseases. In TE King Jr and MI Schwarz (Eds): Interstitial lung disease (3rd edn), BC Dekker, Hamilton, ON, Canada 1998;119-34.

71. Rosenberg DM. Inherited forms of interstitial lung disease. Clin Chest Med 1982;3:635-41.

72. Turton CWG, Morris LM, Lawler SD, Turner-Warwick M. HLA in cryptogenic fibrosing alveolitis. Lancet 1978;I:507-08.

73. Fulmer JD, Sposovska MS, von Gal ER, Crystal RG, Mittal KK. Distribution of HLA antigens in idiopathic pulmonary fibrosis. Am Rev Respir Dis 1978;118:141-47.

74. Libby DM, Gibofsky A, Fotino M, Waters SJ, Smith JP. Immunogenetics and clinical findings in IPF associated with the B cell alloantigen HLA-DR2. Am Rev Respir Dis 1983;127:618-22.

75. Geddes DM, Brewerton DA, Webley M, et al. Alpha-I-antitrypsin phenotypes in fibrosing alveolitis and rheumatoid arthritis. Lancet 1977;ii:1049-51.

76. Musk AW, Zilko PJ, Manners P, Kay PH, Kamboh MI. Genetic studies in familial fibrosing alveolitis possible linkage with immunoglobulin allotypes (Gm). Chest 1986;89:206-10.

77. Hubbard R, Baoku Y, Kaishekar N, Britton J, Johnston I. Alpha-1-antitrypsin phenotypes in patients with cryptogenic fibrosing alveolitis: A case control study. Eur Respir J 1997;10:2881-83.

78. Hodgson U, Laitinen T, Tukiainen P. Nationwide prevalence of sporadic and familial idiopathic pulmonary fibrosis: Evidence of founder effect among multiplex families in Finland. Thorax 2002;57:338-42.

79. Kim KA, Park CY, Lim Y, Lee KH. Recent advances in particulate-induced pulmonary fibrosis: For the application of possible strategy experimentally and clinically. Curr drug targets 2000;1:297-307.

80. Buerke U, Schneider J, Rosler J, Woitowitz HJ. Interstitial pulmonary fibrosis after severe exposure to welding fumes. Am J Ind Med 2002;41:259-68.

81. Billings CG, Howard P. Hypothesis: Exposure to solvents may cause fibrosing alveolitis. Eur Respir J 1994;7:1172-76.

82. Marsh P, Johnston I, Britton J. Atopy as a risk factor for cryptogenic fibrosing alveolitis. Respir Med 1994;88:369-71.

83. Baumgartner KB, Samet JM, Coultas DB, Stidley CA, et al. Occupational and environmental risk factors for idiopathic pulmonary fibrosis: A multicentre case-control study. Am J Epidemiol 2000;152:307-15.

84. Vijayan VK, Pandey VP, Shankaran K, Mehrotra Y, Darbari BS, Misra NP. Bronchoalveolar lavage study in victims of toxic gas leak in Bhopal. Ind J Med Res 1989;90:407-14.

85. Vijayan VK, Sankaran K, Sharma SK, Misra NP. Chronic lung inflammation in victims of toxic gas leak at Bhopal. Resp Med 1995;89:105-11.

86. Behera D, Jindal SK, Malhotra H. Ventilatory function in women exposed to different cooking fuels. Respiration 1994;61:89-92.

87. Raison A, Andeejani AM, Mobiereek A, AI-Rikabi AC. High resolution computed tomography findings in a pathologically proven case of Gujjar lung. Clin Radio 2000;55:155-56.

88. Jakab GJ. Sequential viral infections, bacterial super-infections, and fibrogenesis. Am Rev Respir Dis 1990;142:374-79.

89. Egan JJ, Woodcock AA, Stewart JP. Viruses and idiopathic pulmonary fibrosis. Eur Respir J 1997;10:1433-37.

90. Vergnon JM, Vincent M, deThé G, Mornex JF, Weynants P, Brune J. Cryptogenic fibrosing alveolitis and Epstein-Barr virus: An association. Lancet 1984;2:768-71.

91. Egan JJ, Stewart JP, Hasleton PS, Arrand JR, Carroll KB, Woodcock AA. Epstein-Barr virus replication within pulmonary epithelial cells in cryptogenic fibrosing alveolitis. Thorax 1995;50:1234-39.

92. Lok SS, Stewart JP, Kelly BG, Hasleton PS, Egan JJ. Epstein-Barr virus and p53 in idiopathic pulmonary fibrosis. Respir Med 2001;95:787-91.

93. Tsukamoto K, Hayakawa H, Sato A, Chida K, Nakumura H, Miura K. Involvement of Epstein-Barr virus latent membrane protein 1 in disease progression in patients with idiopathic pulmonary fibrosis. Thorax 200;55:958-61.

94. Meliconi R, Andreone P, Fasano L, et al. Incidence of hepatitis C virus infection in Italian patients with idiopathic pulmonary fibrosis. Thorax 1996;51:315-17.

95. Manganelli P, Salaffi F, Pesci A. Article in Italian, quoted in Pub Med search, Viral infection and IPF. Recent Prog Med 2002;93:322-26.

96. Bando M, Ohno S, Oshikawa K, et al. Infection of TT virus in patients with idiopathic pulmonary fibrosis. Respir Med 2001;95:935-42.

97. Proceedings of the fourth annual Chicago Lung Conference: Interstitial lung diseases. Chest 1991;100:230-54.

98. Amaya M, Shilubo S, Fuji N, Oguma K, Abe S. Oligo-2',5'-adenylate synthetics in pulmonary sarcoidosis and idiopathic pulmonary fibrosis. Chest 1994;105:496-500.

99. Robinson BW, Rose AH. Pulmonary interferon production in patients with fibrosing alveolitis. Thorax 1990;45:105-08.

100. Martinet Y, Rom WN, Grotendorst GR, et al. Exaggerated spontaneous release of platelet-derived growth factor by alveolar macrophages from patients with idiopathic pulmonary fibrosis. N Engl J Med 1987;317:202-09.

101. Chiu IM, Reddy EP, Givol D, et al. Nucleotide sequence analysis identifies the human c-sis proto oncogene as a structural gene for platelet-derived growth factor. Cell 1984;37:1213-29.

102. Pesci A, Bertorelli G, Gabrieli M, Olivieri D. Mast cells in fibrotic lung disorders. Chest 1993;103:989-96.

103. Nakos G, Adams A, Andriopoulos N. Antibodies to collagen in patients with idiopathic pulmonary fibrosis. Chest 1993;103:1051-58.

104. Nakamura H, Fujishima H, Waki Y, et al. Priming of alveolar macrophages for interleukin-8 production in patients with idiopathic pulmonary fibrosis. Am J Respir Crit Care Med 1995;152:1579-86.

105. Crystal RG, Ferrans VJ, Basset F. Biologic bases of pulmonary fibrosis. In Crystal RG, West JB (Eds): The Lung: Scientific foundations, New York: Raven Press 1991;2031-46.

106. Strieter RM, Lukacks NW, Standiford TJ, Kunkel SL. Cytokines and lung inflammation: Mechanisms of neutrophil recruitment to the lungs. Thorax 1993;48:765-69.

107. Gauldie J, Jordan M, Cox G. Cytokines and pulmonary fibrosis. Thorax 1993;48:931-35.

108. Phan SH. New strategies for treatment of pulmonary fibrosis. Thorax 1995;50:415-21.

109. MacNee W, Rahman I. Oxidant/antioxidants in idiopathic pulmonary fibrosis. Thorax 1995;50(Suppl 1):S53-S58.

110. Canti AM, North SL, Fells GA, Hubbard RC, Crystal RG. Oxidant mediated epithelial injury in idiopathic pulmonary fibrosis. J Clin Lab Invest 1987;79:1665-73.

111. Phan SH, Cannon DE, Ward PA, Karmiol S. Mechanisms of xanthine/xanthin oxidase conversion in endothelial cells: Evidence for role for elastase. Am J Respir Cell Mol Biol 1992;6:270-78.

112. Strausz J, Muller-Quernheim J, Steppling H, Ferlinz R. Oxygen radical production by alveolar inflammatory cells in idiopathic pulmonary fibrosis. Am Rev Respir Dis 1990;141:124-28.

113. Dreisen RB, Schwartz MI, Theophilapoulos AN, Stranford RE. Circulating immune complexes in idiopathic interstitial pneumonias. N Engl J Med 1978;298:353-57.

114. Hunninghake GW, Gadek JE, Lawley TJ, Crystal SG. Mechanisms of neutrophil accumulation in the lungs of patients with idiopathic pulmonary fibrosis. J Clin Invest 1981;68:259-69.

115. Schreck R, Rieber P, Baeuerle PA. Reactive oxygen intermediates as apparently used messengers in the activation of NFKB transcription factors and HIV. EMBO J 1991;10:2247-58.

116. Beeh KM, Beier J, Haas IC, Kornamann O, Micke P, Buhl R. Glutathione deficiency in the lower respiratory tract in patients with idiopathic pulmonary fibrosis. Eur Respir J 2002;19:1119-23.

117. Montaldo C, Cannas E, Ledda M, Rosetti L, Congiu L, Atzori L. Bronchoalveolar glutathione and nitrite/nitrate in idiopathic pulmonary fibrosis and sarcoidosis. Sarcoidosis Vasc Diffuse Lung Dis 2002;19:54-58.

118. Aarbiou J, Rabe KF, Hiemstra PS. Role of defensins in inflammatory lung disease. Ann Med 2002;34:96-101.

119. Mukae H, Iiboshi H, Nakazato M, et al. Raised plasma concentrations of alpha-defensin in patients with idiopathic pulmonary fibrosis. Thorax 2002;57:623-28.

120. Schaaf B, Wieghorst A, Aries SP, Dalhoff K, Braun J. Neutrophil inflammation and activation in bronchiec-tasis: Comparison with pneumonia and idiopathic pulmonary fibrosis. Respiration 2000;87:52-9.

121. Nagase T, Uozumi N, Ishii S, et al. A pivotal role of cytosolic phospholipase α_2 in bleomycin-induced pulmonary fibrosis. Nat Med 2002;8:480-84.

122. Yang Y, Fujita J, Bandoh S, et al. Detection of anti-vimentin antibody in sera of patients with idiopathic pulmonary fibrosis and nonspecific interstitial pneumonia. Clin Exp Immunol 2002;128:169-74.

123. Shimizudani N, Murata H, Keino H, et al. Conserved CDR3 region of T cell receptor BV gene in lymphocytes from bronchoalveolar lavage fluid of patients with idiopathic pulmonary fibrosis. Clin Exp Immunol 2002;129:140-49.

124. Kaneko Y, Kuwano K, Kunitake R, Kawasaki M, Hagimoto N, Hara N. B7-1, B7-2 and class II MHC molecules in idiopathic pulmonary fibrosis and bronchiolitis obliterans – Organizing pneumonia. Eur Respir J 2000;15:49-55.

125. Taylor ML, Noble PW, White B, Wise R, Liu MC, Bochner BS. Extensive surface phenotyping of alveolar macrophages in interstitial lung disease. Clin Immunol 2000;94:33-41.

126. Greene KE, King TE Jr, Kuroki Y, et al. Serum surfactant proteins-A, and – D as biomarkers in idiopathic pulmonary fibrosis. Eur Respir J 2002;19:439-46.

127. Dohmoto K, Hojo S, Fujita J, et al. Circulating broncho-epithelial cells expressing mRNA for surfactant protein A in patients with pulmonary fibrosis. Respir Med 2000;94:475-81.

128. Takashashi H, Fujishima T, Koba H, et al. Serum surfactants A, and D as prognostic factors for idiopathic pulmonary fibrosis and their relationship to disease extent. Am J Respir Crit Care Med 2000;162:1109-14.

129. Kuwano K, Maeyama T, Inoshim I, et al. Increased levels of soluble Fas ligand are correlated with disease activity in patients with fibrosing lung diseases. Respirology 2002;7:15-21.

130. Reichenberger F, Schauer J, Kellner K, Sack U, Stiehl P, Winkler J. Different expression of endothelin in the bronchoalveolar lavage in patients with pulmonary diseases. Lung 2001;179:163-74.

131. Satoh H, Ishikawa H, Yamashita YT, Ohtsuka M, Sekizawa K. Serum Lewis X-I antigen in lung adeno-carcinoma and idiopathic pulmonary fibrosis. Thorax 2002;57:263-66.

132. Lasky JA, Brody AR. Interstitial fibrosis and growth factors. Environ Health Perspect 2000;108(Suppl 4):751-62.

133. Meyer KC, Cardoni A, Xiang ZZ. Vascular endothelial growth factor in bronchoalveolar lavage from normal subjects and in patients with diffuse parenchymal lung disease. J Lab Clin Med 2000;135:332-38.

134. Obayashi Y, Fujita J, Nishiyama T, et al. Role of carbohydrate antigens sialyl Lewis (a) (CA19-9) in bronchoalveolar lavage in patients with pulmonary fibrosis. Respiration 2000;67:146-52.

135. Warshamana GS, Pociask DA, Fisher KJ, Liu JY, Sime PJ, Brody AR. Titration of non-replicating adenovirus as a vector for transducing active TGF-beta1 gene expression causing inflammation and fibrogenesis in the lungs of C57BL/6 mice. Int J Exp Pathol 2003;83:183-202.

136. Pala L, Giannini S, Rosi E, et al. Direct measurement of IGF-I and IGFBP-3 in bronchoalveolar lavage fluid from idiopathic pulmonary fibrosis. J Endocrinol Invest 2001;24:856-64.

137. Hutyrova B, Pantelidis P, Drabek J, et al. Interleukin-1 gene cluster polymorphisms in sarcoidosis and idiopathic pulmonary fibrosis. Am J Respir Crit Care Med 2002;165:148-51.

138. Cao B, Guo Z, Zhu Y, Xu W. The potential role of PDGF, IGF-1, TGF-beta expression in idiopathic pulmonary fibrosis. Chin Med J 2000;113:776-82.

139. Keane MP, Belperio JA, Burdick MD, Lynch JP, Fishbein MC, Strieter RM. ENA-78 is an important angiogenic factor in idiopathic pulmonary fibrosis. Am J Respir Crit Care Med 2001;164:2239-42.

140. Pan LH, Yamauchi K, Uzuki M, et al. Type II alveolar epithelial cells and interstitial fibroblasts express connective tissue growth factor in IPF. Eur Respir J 2001;17:1220-27.

141. Bloor CA, Knight RA, Kedia RK, Spiteri MA, Allen JT. Differential mRNA expression of insulin-like growth factor 1 splice variants in patients with idiopathic pulmonary fibrosis and sarcoidosis. Am J Respir Crit Care Med 2001;164:265-72.

142. Krein PM, Winston BW. Roles for insulin-like growth factor I and transforming growth factor-beta in fibrosing lung disease. Chest 2002;122(Suppl 6):289S-293S.

143. Liu JY, Brody AR. Increased TGF-beta 1 in the lungs of asbestos-exposed rats and mice: Reduced expression in TNF-alpha receptor knockout mice. J Environ Pathol Toxicol Oncol 2001;20:97-108.

144. Pantelidis P, Fanning GC, Wells AU, Welsh KI, du Bois RM. Analysis of tumor necrosis factor-alpha, lymphotoxin-alpha, tumor necrosis factor receptor II, interleukin-6 polymorphisms in patients with idiopathic pulmonary fibrosis. Am J Respir Crit Care Med 2001;163:1432-36.

145. Ramos C, Montano M, Garcia-Alvarez J, Ruiz V, Uhal BD, Selman M, Pardo A. Fibroblasts from idiopathic pulmonary fibrosis and normal lung differ in growth rate, apoptosis, and tissue inhibitor of metalloproteinases expression. Am J Respir Cell Mol Biol 2001;24:591-98.

146. Maeyama T, Kuwano K, Kawasaki M, et al. Upregulation of Fas-signalling molecules in lung epithelial cells from patients with idiopathic pulmonary fibrosis. Eur Respir J 2001;17:180-89.

147. Mori M, Kida H, Morishita H, et al. Microsatellite instability in transforming growth factor-beta 1 type II receptor gene in alveolar lining epithelial cells of idiopathic pulmonary fibrosis. Am J Respir Cell Mol Biol 2001;24:398-404.

148. Freeburn RW, Kendall H, Dobson L, Egan J, Simler NJ, Millar AB. The 3' untranslated region of tumor necrosis factor-alpha is highly conserved in idiopathic pulmonary fibrosis. Eur Cytokine Netw 2001;12:33-38.

149. Barbas-Filho JV, Ferreira MA, Sesso A, Kairalla RA, Carvalho CR, Capellozi VL. Evidence of type II pneumocyte apoptosis in the pathogenesis of idiopathic pulmonary fibrosis (IPF)/usual interstitial pneumonia (UIP). J Clin Pathol 2001;54:132-38.

150. van den Blink B, Jansen HM, Peppelenbosch MP. Idiopathic pulmonary fibrosis: Molecular mechanisms and possible therapeutic strategies. Arch Immunol Ther Exp 2000;48:539-45.

151. Shimizu Y, Dobashi K, Iizuka K, et al. Contribution of small GTPase Rho and its target protein rock in murine model of lung fibrosis. Am J respir Crit Care Med 2001;163:210-17.

152. Taniguchi H, Katoh S, Kadota J, et al. Interleukin 5 and granulocyte-macrophage colony-stimulating factor levels in bronchoalveolar lavage fluid in interstitial lung disease. Eur Respir J 2000;16:959-64.

153. Suga M, Iyonaga K, Okamoto T, Gushima Y, Miyakawa H, Akaike T, Ando M. Characteristic elevation of matrix metalloproteinase activity in idiopathic interstitial pneumonias. Am J Respir Crit Care Med 2000;162:1949-56.

154. Yasui H, Gabazza EC, Taguchi O, et al. Decreased protein C activation in associated with abnormal collagen turnover in the intra-alveolar space of patients with interstitial lung disease. Clin Appl Thromb Hemost 2000;6:202-05.

155. Fujii M, Hayakawa H, Urano T, et al. Relevance of tissue factor and tissue factor pathway inhibitor to hypercoagulable state in the lungs of patients with idiopathic pulmonary fibrosis. Thromb Res 2000;99:111-17.

156. Liu L, li Z, Yu R. Increased activity of protein kinase C in alveolar macrophages in idiopathic pulmonary fibrosis. Chin Med J 2001;114:321-23.

157. Gunther A, Mosavi P, Ruppert P, et al. Enhanced tissue factor pathway activity and fibrin turnover in alveolar compartment of patients with interstitial lung disease. Thromb Haemostat 2000;83:853-60.

158. Vasilakis DA, Sourvinos G, Spandidos DA, Siafakas NM, Bouros D. Frequent genetic alterations at the microsatellite level in cytology of sputum samples of patients with idiopathic pulmonary fibrosis. Am J Respir Crit Care Med 2000;162:1115-19.

159. Selman M, Ruiz V, Cabrera S, Segura L, Ramirez R, Barrios R, Pardo S. TIMP-1,-2,-3, and -4 in idiopathic pulmonary fibrosis. A prevailing nondegradative lung microenvironment? Am J Physiol Lung Cell Mol Physiol 2000;279:L562-74.

160. Dobashi N, Fujita J, Ohtsuki Y, et al. Circulating cytokeratin 8: Anti-cytokeratin 8 antibody immune complexes in sera of patients with pulmonary fibrosis. Respiration 2000;67:397-401.

161. Dobashi N, Fujita J, Murota M, et al. Elevation of anti-cytokeratin 18 antibody and circulating cytokeratin 18: Anti-cytokeratin 18 antibody immune complex in sera of patients with idiopathic pulmonary fibrosis. Lung 2000;178:171-79.

162. Inage M, Nakamura H, Kato S, et al. Levels of cytokeratin 19 fragments in bronchoalveolar lavage fluid correlate to the intensity of neutrophil and eosinophil-alveolitis patients with idiopathic pulmonary fibrosis. Respir Med 2000;94:155-60.

163. Gross TJ, Hunninghake GW. Idiopathic pulmonary fibrosis. N Engl J Med 2001;345:517-25.

164. Kawanami O, Ferrans VJ, Crystal RG. Structure of alveolar epithelial cells in patients with fibrotic lung disorders. Lab Invest 1982;46:39-53.

165. Cherniack RM, Colby TV, Flint A, et al. Quantitative assessment of lung pathology in Idiopathic pulmonary fibrosis. Am Rev Respir Dis 1991;144:892-900.

166. Liebow AA, Loring WE, Felton WL. The musculature of the lungs in chronic pulmonary disease. Am J Pathol 1953;29:855-911.

167. Carrington CB, Gaensler EA, Coutu RE, FitzGerald MX, Gupta RG. Natural history and treated course of usual and desquamative interstitial pneumonia. N Engl J Med 1978;298:801-09.

168. Colby TV, Lombard C, Yousem SA, Kitaichi M. Usual interstitial pneumonia. In Atlas of pulmonary surgical pathology; Philadelphia: WB Saunders 1991;242-46.

169. Kanematsu T, Kitaichi M, Nishimura K, Nagai S, Izumi T. Clubbing of fingers and smooth muscle proliferation in fibrotic changes in the lung in patients with idiopathic pulmonary fibrosis. Chest 1994;105:339-42.

170. Kuhn C III, Boldt J, King TE Jr, Crouch E, Vartio T, McDonald JA. An immunohistochemical study of architectural remodelling and connective tissue synthesis in pulmonary fibrosis. Am Rev Respir Dis 1989;140:1693-1703.

171. Madri JA, Furthmayer H. Collagen polymorphism in the lung: An immunohistochemical study of pulmonary fibrosis. Hum Pathol 1980;11:333-66.

172. Raghu G, Striker LJ, Hudson LD, Striker GE. Extracellular matrix in normal ad fibrotic human lungs. Am Rev Respir Dis 985;131:281-89.

173. Spurzem JR. Function at the junction: Dynamic interactions between lung cells and extracellular matrix. Thorax 1996;51:956-58.

174. Specks U, Nerlich A, Colby TV, Wiest I, Timpl R. Increased expression of type VI collagen in lung fibrosis. Am J Respir Crit Care Med 1995;151:1956-64.

175. Fishman AP. UIP, DIP and all that. N Engl J Med 1978;298:843.

176. Cantin A, Crystal RG. Interstitial pathology: An overview of the chronic interstitial lung disorders. Int Arch Allergy Appl Immunol 1985;76(Suppl 1):83.

177. Leibow AA, Steer A, Billingley JG. Desquamative interstitial pneumonia. Am J Med 1965;39:369.

178. Burkhardt A. Alveolitis and collapse in the pathogenesis of pulmonary fibrosis. Am Rev Respir Dis 1989;140:513-24.

179. Katzenstein ALA. Katzenstein and Askin's surgical pathology of nonneoplastic lung diseases. WB Saunders: Philadelphia 1997.

180. Katzenstein ALA, Fiorelli RF. Nonspecific interstitial pneumonia/fibrosis. Histologic features and clinical significance. Am J Surg Pathol 1994;18:136-47.

181. Katzenstein ALA, Myers, Mazur MT. Acute interstitial pneumonia: A clinicopathologic, ultrastructural, and cell kinetic study. Am J Surg Pathol 1986;10:256-67.

182. Katzenstein ALA, Myers. Idiopathic pulmonary fibrosis. Clinical relevance of pathological classification. Am J Respir Crit Care Med 1998;157:1301-15.

183. Liebow AA, Steer A, Billingsley JG. Desquamative interstitial pneumonia. Am J Med 1965;39:369-404.

184. Vedal S, Welsh EV, Miller RR, Mueller NL. Desquamative interstitial pneumonia computed tomographic findings before and after treatment with corticosteroids. Chest 1988;93:215-17.

185. Hartman TE, Primack SL, Kang EY, et al. Disease progression in usual interstitial pneumonia compared with desquamative interstitial pneumonia. Assessment with serial CT. Chest 1996;110:378-82.

186. Hartman TE, Primack SL, Swensen SJ, et al. Desquamative interstitial pneumonia: Thin section CT findings in 22 patients. Radiology 1993;187:787-90.

187. Yousem SA, Colby TV, Gaensler EA. Respiratory bronchiolitis associated interstitial lung disease and its relationship to desquamative interstitial pneumonia. Mayo Clin Proc 1989;64:1373-80.

188. Myers JL. Respiratory bronchiolitis associated interstitial lung disease. In GR Epler (Ed): Diseases of the bronchioles, Ravena Press: New York 1994;297-305.

189. Meyers JL, Veal CF, Shin MS, Katzenstin ALA. Respiratory bronchiolitis causing interstitial lung disease: A clinicopathologic study of six cases. Am Rev Respir Dis 1987;135:880-84.

190. Askin FB. Acute interstitial pneumonia: Histopathologic patterns of acute lung injury and Hamman-Rich syndrome revisited (Editorial comments). Radiology 1993;188:620-21.

191. Primack SL, Hartman TE, Ikezoe J, Akira M, Sakatani M, Muller NL. Acute interstitial pneumonia: Radiographic and CT findings in nine patients. Radiology 1993;188:817-20.

192. Crystal RG, Fulmer JD, Roberts WC, et al. Idiopathic pulmonary fibrosis: Clinical, histologic, radiographic, physiologic, scintigraphic, cytologic, and biochemical aspects. Ann Intern Med 1976;85:769.

193. Schroeder SA, Shannon DC, Mark EJ. Cellular interstitial pneumonitis in infants. A clinicopathologic study. Chest 1992;101:1065-69.

194. Michalson JE, Aguayo SM, Roman J. Idiopathic pulmonary fibrosis: A practical approach for diagnosis and management. Chest 2000;118:788-94.

195. Turner-Warwick MB, Burrows B, Johnson A. Cryptogenic fibrosing alveolitis: clinical features and their influence on survival. Thorax 1980;35:171-180.

196. Crystal RG, Fulmer JD, Roberts WC, Moss Ml, Line BR, Reynolds HY. Idiopathic pulmonary fibrosis: Clinical, histologic, radiographic, physiologic, scintigraphic, cytologic, and biochemical aspects. Ann intern Med 1976;85: 769-88.

197. Johnston IDA, Prescott RJ, Chalmers JC, Rudd RM. The Fibrosing Alveolitis Subcommittee of the Research Committee of the British Thoracic Society. British Thoracic Society Study of cryptogenic fibrosing alveolitis: Current presentation and initial management. Thorax 1997;52:38-44.

198. Baughman RP, Shipley RT, Loudon RG, Lower EE. Crackles in interstitial lung disease. Comparison of sarcoidosis and fibrosing alveolitis. Chest 1991;100:96.

199. Panos RJ, Mortenson R, Niccoli SA, King TE Jr. Clinical deterioration in patients with idiopathic pulmonary fibrosis: Causes and assessment. Am J Med 1990;88: 396-404.

200. Jones AW. Alveolar cell carcinoma occurring in idiopathic interstitial fibrosis. Br J Dis Chest 1970;64:78.

201. Turner-Warwick M, Lebowitz M, Burrows B, Johnson A. Cryptogenic fibrosing alveolitis and lung cancer. Thorax 1980;35:496.

202. Oshikawa K, Sugiyama Y. Serum anti-p53 antibodies from patients with idiopathic pulmonary fibrosis with lung cancer. Respir Med 2000;94:1085-91.

203. Kawasaki H, Nagai K, Yokose T, et al. Clinicopathological characteristics of surgically resected lung cancer associated with idiopathic pulmonary fibrosis. J Surg Oncol 2001;76:53-57.

204. Park J, Kim DS, Shim TS, et al. Lung cancer in patients with idiopathic pulmonary fibrosis. Eur Respir J 2001;17:1216-19.

205. Guerry-Force ML, Mueller NI, Wright JL, et al. A comparison of bronchiolitis obliterans with organizing pneumonia, usual interstitial pneumonia, and small airways disease. Am Rev Respir Dis 1987;135:705-12.

206. Feigin DS, Friedman PJ. Chest radiography in desquamative interstitial pneumonia: A review of 37 patients. Am J Roentgenol 1980;134:91-99.

207. Bergin CJ, Muller NL. CT in the diagnosis of interstitial lung disease. Am J Radiol 1985;145:505.

208. Lynch DA. High-resolution CT of Idiopathic Interstitial Pneumonias. Radiol Clin North Am 2001;39:1153-70.

209. Orens JB, Kazerooni EA, Martinez FJ, et al. The sensitivity of high-resolution CT in detecting idiopathic pulmonary fibrosis proved by open lung biopsy: A prospective study. Chest 1995;108:109-15.

210. Wells AU, Hansell DM, Rubens MB, Cullinan P, Black CM, du Bois RM. The predictive value of appearances on thin-section computed tomography in fibrosing alveolitis. Am Rev Respir Dis 1993;148:1076-82.

211. Wells AU, Rubens MB, du Bois RM, Hansell DM. Serial CT in fibrosing alveolitis: Prognostic significance of the initial pattern. Am J Rontgenol 1993;161:1159-65.

212. Grenier P, Valeyte D, Cluzel P, et al. Chronic diffuse interstitial lung disease: Diagnostic value of chest radiography and high resolution CT. Radiology 1991;179:123-32.

213. Webb WR, Stein MG, Finkheiner WE, et al. Normal and diseased isolated lungs: High resolution CT. Radiology 1988;166:81.

214. Wells AU, Hansell DM, Rubens MB, et al. The predictive value of appearances on thin section computed tomography in fibrosing alveolitis. Am Rev Respir Dis 1993;148:1076-82.

215. Hiwatari N, Shimura S, Takishima T. Pulmonary emphysema followed by pulmonary fibrosis of unknown cause. Respiration 1993;60:354-58.

216. Doherty MJ, Pearson MG, O'Grady EA, Pellegrini V, Calverley PM. Cryptogenic fibrosing alveolitis with preserved lung volume. Thorax 1997;52:998-1002.

217. Muller NL, Miller RR, Webb WR, Evans KG, Ostrow DN. Fibrosing alveolitis: CT-pathologic correlation. Radiology 1986;160:585-88.

218. Muller NL, Stables CA, Miller RR, et al. Disease activity in idiopathic pulmonary fibrosis: CT and pathologic correlation. Radiology 1987;165:731-34.

219. Nishimura K, Litaichi M, Izumi T, et al. Usual interstitial pneumonia: Histological correlation with high resolution CT. Radiology 1992;182:337-42.

220. Augusti C, Xaubet A, Luburich P, Ayuso MC, Roca J, Rodriguez-Roisin R. Computed tomography guided bronchoalveolar lavage in idiopathic pulmonary fibrosis. Thorax 1996;51:841-45.

221. Lynch DA, Newell JD, Logan PM, King TE Jr, Muller NL. Can CT distinguish idiopathic pulmonary fibrosis from hypersensitivity pneumonitis? Am J Roentgenol 1995;165:807-11.

222. Muller N, Staples C, Miller R, Vedal S, Thurlbeck W, Ostrow D. Disease activity in idiopathic pulmonary fibrosis: CT and pathologic correlation. Radiology 1987;165:731-34.

223. Remi-Jardin M, Giraud F, Remy J, Copin MC, Gosselin B, Duhamel A. Importance of ground glass attenuation in chronic diffuse lung diseases: Pathologic-CT correlation. Radiology 1993;189:693-98.

224. Staples C, Muller N, Vedal S, et al. Usual interstitial pneumonia: Correlation of CT with clinical, functional and radiographic findings. Radiology 1987;162:377-81.

225. Xaubet A, Agusti C, Luburich P, et al. Pulmonary function tests and CT scan in the management of

idiopathic pulmonary fibrosis. Am J Respir Crit Care Med 1998;158:431-36.

226. Labrune S, Chinet T, Collignon MA, Barritault L, Huchon GJ. Mechanisms of epithelial lung clearance of DTPA in diffuse fibrosing alveolitis. Eur Respir J 1994;7:651-56.

227. Pantin CF, Valind SO, Sweatman M, et al. Measures of the inflammatory response in cryptogenic fibrosing alveolitis. Am rev Respir Dis 1988;138:1234-41.

228. Yeh SH, Liu RS, Wu LC, Peng NJ, Lu JY. 99Tcm-HMPAO and 99cm-DTPA radioaerosol clearance measurements in idiopathic pulmonary fibrosis. Nucl Med Commun 1995;16:140-44.

229. Primack SL, Mayo JR, Hartman TE, Miller RR, Muller NL. MRI of infiltrative lung disease: Comparison with pathologic findings. J Comput assist Tomogr 1994;18:233-38.

230. Wells AU, Hansell DM, Rubens JB, et al. Functional impairment in lone cryptogenic fibrosing alveolitis and fibrosing alveolitis associated with systemic sclerosis: A comparison. Am J Respir Crit Care Med 1997;155:1657-64.

231. Ostraw D, Cherniack RM. Resistance to airflow in patients with diffuse interstitial lung disease. Am Rev Respir Dis 1973;198:205-10.

232. Englert M, Yernault JC, deCoster A, Clummeeck N. Diffusing properties and elastic properties in interstitial diseases of the lung. Prog Respi Res 1975;8:177-85.

233. Yernault JC, Adelonghe M, deCoster A, Englert M. Pulmonary mechanisms in diffuse fibrosing alveolitis. Bull Physiopathol Respir 1975;11:231-44.

234. Gibson GJ, Pride NB. Lung distensibility: The static pressure-volume curve of the lungs and its use in clinical assessment. Br J Dis Chest 1976;70:143-83.

235. Gibson GJ, Pride NB. Pulmonary mechanics in fibrosing alveolitis: The effect of lung shrinkage. Am Rev Respir Dis 1977;116:137-47.

236. Gibson GJ, Pride NB, Davis J, Schroter RC. Exponential description of the static pressure-volume curve of normal and diseased lungs. Am Rev Respir Dis 1979;120:789-811.

237. Fulmer JD, Roberts WC, von Gal ER, Crystal RG. Morphologic-physiologic correlates of the severity of fibrosis and degree of cellularity in idiopathic pulmonary fibrosis. J Clin Invest 1979;63:665-76.

238. Kornbluth RS, Turino GM. Respiratory control in diffuse interstitial lung disease and disease of the pulmonary vasculature. Clin Chest Med 1980;1:91-102.

239. Renzi G, Milic-Emil J, Grassino AE. The pattern of breathing in diffuse lung fibrosis. Bull Eur Physiopathol Resp 1982;18:461-72.

240. Lourenco RV, Turino GM, Davidson LAG, Fishman AP. The regulation of ventilation in diffuse pulmonary fibrosis. Am J Med 1965;38:199-216.

241. Bradeley GW, Crawford R. Regulation of breathing during exercise in normal subjects and in chronic lung diseases. Clin Sci Mol Med 1976;51:575-82.

242. Patton JMS, Freedman S. The ventilatory response to CO_2 of patients with diffuse pulmonary infiltration or fibrosis. Clin Sci 1972;43:55-69.

243. VanMeerhaeghe A, Scano G, Sergyseils R, Bran M, DeCoster A. Respiratory drive and ventilatory pattern during exercise in interstitial lung disease. Bull Eur Physiopathol Respir 1981;17:18-26.

244. Savory J, Dhingra S, Anthonisen NR. Role of vagal airway reflexes in control of ventilation in pulmonary fibrosis. Clin Sci 1981;61:781-84.

245. Dimarco AF, Kelsen SG, Cherniack NS, Gothe B. Occlusion pressure and breathing pattern in patients with interstitial lung disease. Am Rev Respir Dis 1983;127:425-30.

246. Burton JG, Killian WK, Jones NL. Pattern of breathing during exercise in patients with intertstitial lung disease. Thorax 1983;38:778-84.

247. Renzi G, Milic-Emil J, Grassino AE. Breathing pattern in sarcoidosis and idiopathic pulmonary fibrosis. Ann Ny Acad Sci 1986;465:482-90.

248. Spiro SG, Dowdeswell IRG, Clark TJH. An analysis of submaximal exercise responses in patients with sarcoidosis and fibrosing alveolitis. Br J Dis Chest 1981;75:169-80.

249. Gowda K, Zintel T, McPerland C, Orchard R, Gallagher CC. Diagnostic value of maximal exercise tidal volume. Chest 1990;98:1351-54.

250. Jones NL, Rebuck AS. Tidal volume during exercise in patients with diffuse fibrosing alveolitis. Bull Eur Physiopath Respir 1979;15:321-27.

251. Bye PTP, Anderson SD, Woolcock AJ, Young IH, Alison JA. Bicycle endurance performance of patients with interstitial lung disease breathing air and oxygen. Am Rev Respir Dis 1982;126:1005-12.

252. Burdon JGW, Killian KJ, Jones NJ. Pattern of breathing during exercise in patients with interstitial lung disease. Thorax 1983;38:778-84.

253. Marciniuk DD, Watts RE, Gallagher CG. Dead space loading and exercise limitation in patients with interstitial lung disease. Chest 1994;105:183-89.

254. Cherniack RM, Colby TV, Flint A, et al. Correlation of structure and function in idiopathic pulmonary fibrosis. Am J Respir Crit Care Med 1995;151:1180-88.

255. Kelley MA, Daniele RP. Exercise testing in interstitial lung disease. Clin Chest Med 1984;5:145-56.

256. Denison D, Al-Hillawi H, Turton C. Lung function in interstitial lung disease. Sem Respir Med 1984;6:40-54.

257. Augusti AGN, Roca J, Rodrigues-Roisin R, Xaubet A, Augusti-Videl A. Different patterns of gas exchange response to exercise in asbestosis and idiopathic pulmonary fibrosis. Eur Respir J 1988;1:510-16.

258. Padilla RP, Salas J, Carrillo G, Selman M, Chapela R. Prevalence of high hematocrits in patients with interstitial lung disease in Mexico city. Chest 1992;101;1691-93.

259. The BAL cooperative group steering committee. Bronchoalveolar lavage constituents in healthy

individuals, idiopathic pulmonary fibrosis, and selected comparison groups. Am Rev Respir Dis 1990;141 (Suppl) S192.

260. Hunninghake GW, Gadek JE, Kawanami O, Ferrans VJ, Crystal RG. Inflammatory and immune processes in the human lung in health and disease: evaluation by bronchoalveolar lavage. Am J Pathol 1979;97:149-206.

261. Davis GS, Brody AR, Craighead JE. Analysis of air space and interstitial mononuclear cell population in human diffuse interstitial lung disease. Am Rev Respir Dis 1978;118:7-15.

262. Haslam PL. Bronchoalveolar lavage in interstitial lung disease. Sem Respir Med 1984;6:55-70.

263. Haslam PL. Cryptogenic fibrosing alveolitis: Pathogenetic mechanisms and therapeutic approaches. Eur Respir J 1990;3:355-57.

264. Haslam PL, Turton CWG, Lukoszek A, Collins JV, Salsbury AJ, Turner-Warwick M. Bronchoalveolar lavage fluid cell counts in cryptogenic fibrosing alveolitis and their relation to therapy. Thorax 1980;35:328-39.

265. Rudd RM, Haslam PL, Turner-Warwick M. Cryptogenic fibrosing alveolitis. Relationship of pulmonary physiology and bronchoalveolar lavage to response to treatment and prognosis. Am Rev Respir Dis 1981;124:1-8.

266. Peterson MW, Monik M, Hunninghake GW. Prognostic role of eosinophils in pulmonary fibrosis. Chest 1987; 92:51-56.

267. Watters LC, Schwartz MI, Cherniack RM, et al. Idiopathic pulmonary fibrosis. Pretreatment bronchoalveolar lavage cellular constituents and their relationships with lung histopathology and clinical response to therapy. Am Rev Respir Dis 1987;135:696-704.

268. Schwartz DA, Van Fossen DS, Davis CS, et al. Determinants of progression in idiopathic pulmonary fibrosis. Am J Respir Crit Care Med 1994;149:444-49.

269. Schwartz DA, Helmer Ra, Dayton CS, Merchant RK, Hunninghake GW. Determinants of bronchoalveolar lavage cellularity in idiopathic pulmonary fibrosis. J Appl Physiol 1991;71:1688-93.

270. Scwrtz DA, Helmer RA, Calvin JR, et al. Determinants of survival in idiopathic pulmonary fibrosis. Am J Respir Crit Care Med 1994;149:450-54.

271. Drent M, van Nierop MAMF, Gerritsen FA, Wouters EFM, Mulder PGH. A computer program using BALF-analysis results as a diagnostic tool in interstitial lung diseases. Am J Respir Crit Care Med 1996;153:736-41.

272. Davis GS. Bronchoalveolar lavage in interstitial lung diseases. Semin Respir Med 1994;15:37-60.

273. Perez-Arellano JL, Pedraz MJ, Fuertes A, De la Cruz JL, de Buitrago JMG, Jimenez A. Laminin fragment P1 is increased in the lower respiratory tract of patients with diffuse interstitial lung diseases. Chest 1993;104; 1163-69.

274. Dreisin RB, Schwartz MI, Theofilopoulos AN, Stanford RE. Circulating immunecomplexes in the idiopathic interstitial pneumonia. N Engl J Med 1978;298:353-57.

275. Gottlieb AJ, Spiers H, Tierstein AS, Siltzbach LE. Serological factors in idiopathic diffuse interstitial pulmonary fibrosis. Am J Med 1965;39:405-10.

276. Haslam P, Turner-Warwick M, Lukoszek A. Antinuclear antibody and lymphocyte response to nuclear antigens in patients with lung disease. Clin Exp Immunol 1975;20:379-95.

277. Katzenstein ALA, Myers JL. Idiopathic pulmonary fibrosis: To biopsy or not to biopsy. Am J Respir Crit Care Med 2001;164:185-86.

278. Hunninghake GW, Zimmerman MB, Schwartz DA, et al. Utility of a lung biopsy for the diagnosis of idiopathic pulmonary fibrosis. Am J respir Crit Care Med 2001;164:193-96.

279. Raghu G. Interstitial lung disease: A diagnostic approach. Are CT scan and lung biopsy indicated in every patient? Am J Respir Crit Care Med 1995;151:909-14.

280. Gaensler Ea. Open and closed lung biopsy. In Sackner MA (Ed): Diagnostic techniques in pulmonary disease 1981;16: Marcel Dekker: New York 579-622.

281. Dijkman JH, van der Meer JWM, Bakker W, et al. Transpleural lung biopsy by the thoracoscopic route in patients with diffuse interstitial lung disease. Chest 1982;82:76-83.

282. Hartman DL, Mylet D, Gaither JG, et al. Comparison of thoracoscopic lung biopsy with open lung biopsy in diffuse interstitial lung disorders. Am Rev Respir Dis 1992;145:A750.

283. Bensard DD, McIntyre RC, Simon JS, et al. Comparison of video thoracoscopic lung biopsy with open lung biopsy in the diagnosis of interstitial lung diseases. Chest 1993;103:765-70.

284. Carnochan FM, Walker WS, Cameron EW. Efficacy of videoassisted thoracoscopic lung biopsy: An historical comparison with open lung biopsy. Thorax 1994;49: 361-63.

285. Bensard DD, McIntyre RC Jr, Waring BJ, Simon JS. Comparison of videothoracoscopic lung biopsy to open lung biopsy in the diagnosis of interstitial lung disease. Chest 1993;103:765-70.

286. Ferson PF, Landreneau RJ, Dowling RD, et al. Comparison of open versus thoracoscopic lung biopsy for diffuse infiltrative pulmonary disease. J Thorac Cardiovasc Surg 1993;106:194-96.

287. Johnston ID, Gomm SA, Kalra S, Woodcock AA, Evans CC, Hind CR. The management of cryptogenic fibrosing alveolitis in three regions of the United Kingdom. Eur Respir J 1993;6:891-93.

288. Raghu G. Interstitial lung disease: A diagnostic approach: Are CT scan and lung biopsy indicated in every patient? Chest 1995;151:909-14.

289. Raghu G, Mageto YN, Lokhart D, Schmidt RA, Wood DE, Godwin JD. The accuracy of the clinical diagnosis

of new onset idiopathic pulmonary fibrosis and other interstitial lung disease. Chest 1999;116:1168-74.

290. Park JS, Lee KS, Kim JS, Park CS, Suh YL, Choi DL, Kim KJ. Nonspecific interstitial pneumonia with fibrosis: Radiographic and CT findings in seven patients. Radiology 1995;195:645-48.

291. Smith CM, Moser KM. Management of interstitial lung disease state-of-the-art. Chest 1989;95:676-78.

292. Mapel DW, Samet JM, Coultas DB. Corticosteroids and the treatment of idiopathic pulmonary fibrosis. Chest 1996;110:1058-67.

293. Crystal RG, Gadek JE, Ferrans VJ, et al. Interstitial lung disease: Current concepts of pathogenesis, staging, and therapy. Am J Med 1981;70:542.

294. Johnston IDA, Presscott RJ, Chalmers JC, Rudd RM. Fibrosing Alveolitis Subcommittee of the Research Committee of the British Thoracic Society. British Thoracic Society study of cryptogenic fibrosing alveolitis: Current presentation and initial management. Thorax 1997;52:38-44.

295. Johnson I, Britton J, Kinnear W, Logan R. Rising mortality from cryptogenic fibrosing alveolitis. BMJ 1990;301:1017-21.

296. Hubbard R, Johnson I, Coultas DB, Britton J. Mortality rates from cryptogenic fibrosing alveolitis in seven countries. Thorax 1996;51:711-16.

297. Hubbard R, Johnson I, Britton J. Survival in patients with cryptogenic fibrosing alveolitis: A population based cohort study. Chest 1998;113:396-400.

298. Mapel DW, Hunt WC, Utton R, Baumgartner KB, Samet JM, Coultas DB. Idiopathic pulmonary fibrosis: Survival in population based and hospital based cohorts. Thorax 1998;53:469-76.

299. Bjoraker JA, Ryu JH, Edwin MK, et al. Prognostic significance of histopathologic subsets in idiopathic pulmonary fibrosis. Am J Respir Crit Care Med 1998;157:199-203.

300. Brown K, King TE Jr. Recent advances in interstitial lung disease. In Bone RC, Petty TL (Eds): 1995 Year Book of Pulmonary Disease, Mosby Year Book: St. Louis 1995.

301. Gay SE, Kazerooni EA, Toews GB, Lynch JP 3rd, Gross BH, Cascade PN, Spizarny DL, Fint A, Schork MA, Whyte RI, Popovich J, Hyzy R, Martinez FJ, et al. Idiopathic pulmonary fibrosis: Predicting response to therapy and survival. Am J Respir Crit Care Med 1998;157:1063-72.

302. van Oortegem K, Wallaert B, Marquette CH, Roman P, Perez T, Lafitte JJ, Tonnel AB, et al. Determination of response to immunosuppressive therapy in idiopathic pulmonary fibrosis. Eur Respir J 1994;7:1950-57.

303. Schwartz DA, Helmers RA, Galvin JR, Van Fossen DS, Frees KL, Dayton CS, Burmeister LF, Hunninghake GW, et al. Determination of survival in idiopathic pulmonary fibrosis. Am J respir Crit Care Med 1994;149:450-54.

304. Lee JS, Im JG, Ahm JM, Kim YM, Han MC, et al. Fibrosing alveolitis: Prognostic implications of ground-glass attenuation at high-resolution CT. Radiology 1992;184:451-54.

305. Wells AU, Hansell DM, Rubens MB, et al. The predictive value of appearances On thin-section computed tomography in fibrosing alveolitis. Am Rev Respir Dis 1993;148:1076.

306. Hunninghke CW, Kalica AR. Approaches to the treatment of pulmonary fibrosis. Am J Respir Crit Care Med 1995;151:915-18.

307. Ziesche R, Hofbouer E, Wittmann K, Petkov V, Block LH. A preliminary study of long-term treatment with interferon gamma 1b and low dose prednisolone in patients with idiopathic pulmonary fibrosis. New Engl J Med 1999;341:1264-69.

308. du Bois RM. Interferon gamma 1b for the treatment of idiopathic pulmonary fibrosis. New Engl J Med 1999;341:1302-04.

309. Selman M. From anti-inflammatory drugs through antifibrotic agents to lung transplantation. A long road of research, clinical attempts, and failures in the treatment of idiopathic pulmonary fibrosis. Chest 2002;122:759-61.

310. Behera D, Gupta D, Jindal SK. Response to steroid therapy in patients of idiopathic pulmonary fibrosis: A retrospective analysis. Indian J Chest Dis Allied Sci 1998;40:163-69.

311. Balamugesh T, Behera D. Idiopathic pulmonary fibrosis. J Assoc Physicians India 2007;55:363-70.

312. Raghu G, Depaso WJ, Cain K, et al. Azathioprine combined with prednisone in the treatment of idiopathic pulmonary fibrosis: A prospective double-blind, randomized, placebo-controlled clinical trial. Am Rev Respir Dis 1991;144:291.

313. Kaltreider HB. Interstitial lung disease—Selective aspects. Pulmonary Perspectives 1993;10:6-8.

314. Waters LC, King TE Jr, Schwartz MI, Waldron JA, Stanford RE, Cherniack RM. A clinical, radiographic, and physiologic scoring system for the longitudinal assessment of patients with idiopathic pulmonary fibrosis. Am Rev Respir Dis 1986;133:97-103.

315. King TE Jr, Tooze JA, Schwartz MI, Brown KR, Cherniack RM. Predicting survival in idiopathic pulmonary fibrosis. Scoring system and survival model. Am J Respir Crit Care Med 2001;164:1171-81.

316. Waters LC, Schwartz MI, Cherniack RM, Waldron JA, Dunn TL, Stanford RE, King TE Jr. Idiopathic pulmonary fibrosis: Pretreatment bronchoalveolar lavage cellular constituents and their relationship with lung histopathology and response to therapy. Am Rev Respir Dis 1987;135:696-704.

317. American Thoracic Society. Lung transplantation. Am Rev Respir Dis 1993;147:772-76.

318. American Thoracic Society. International guidelines for the selection of lung transplant candidates. Am J Respir Crit Care Med 1998;158:335-39.

319. Meyers BF, Lynch JP, Trulock EP, et al. Single vs bilateral lung transplantation for idiopathic pulmonary fibrosis: A ten year institutional experience. Thorac Cardiovasc Surg 2000; 120:99-107.

320. Trulock EP. Lung transplantation. Am J Respir Crit Care Med 1997;155:789-818.

321. Mogulkoc N, Brutsche MH, Bishop PW, et al. Pulmonary function in idiopathic pulmonary fibrosis and referral for lung transplantation. Am J Respir Crit Care Med 2001;164:103-08.

322. Lanuza DM, Lefaiver Ca, Farcas GA. Research on the quality of life of lung transplant candidates and recipients: An integrative review. Heart Lung 2000,29:180-95.

323. Stavem K, Bjortuft O, Lund MB, et al. Health-related quality of life in lung transplant candidates and recipients. Respiration 2000;67:159-65.

324. Mahler DA. Pulmonary rehabilitation. Chest 1998;113: 263S-268S.

325. Schreiner R, Mortenson R, Ikle D, King TE Jr. Interstitial lung disease in the elderly: In D Mahler (Ed): Pulmonary disease in the elderly. Marcel Dekker, New York, 1993;339-85.

326. Stack BHR, Chao-Kang YEJ, Heard BE. The prognosis of cryptogenic fibrosing alveolitis. Thorax 1972;27:535-42.

327. Carrington CB, Gaensler EA, Coutu RE, Fitzerald MX, Gupta RA. Natural history and treated course of usual and desquamative intestinal pneumonia. N Engl J Med 1978;298:801-09.

328. Turner-Warwick M, Burrows SB, Johnson A. Cryptogenic fibrosing alveolitis: Clinical features and their effects on survival. Thorax 1980;35:171-80.

329. Augustini C, Xzubet A, Roca J, Agustini AGN, Rodriguez-Roisin R. Interstitial fibrosis with and without associated collagen vascular disease: Results of a 2 year follow up. Thorax 1992;47:1035-40.

330. Meir-Sydow J, Rust M, Dronenberger H. Diagnosis and therapy in idiopathic pulmonary fibrosis. Allergol Immunopathol 1980;8(Suppl): 101-09.

331. Epler GR, Colby TV, McLoud TC, Carrington CB, Gaensler EA. Bronchiolitis obliterans organizing pneumonia. N Engl J Med 1985;312:152-58.

332. Epler GR. Bronchiolitis obliterans organizing pneumonia. Arch Intern Med 2001;161:158-64.

333. Cordier JF. Organizing pneumonia. Thorax 2000:55: 318-28.

334. King TE Jr, Mortenson RL. Cryptogenic organizing pneumonitis. The North American Experience. Chest 1992;102:8S-13S.

335. Mokhtari M, Basch PB, Tietjen PA, Stover DE. Bronchiolitis obliterans organizing pneumonia in cancer: A case series. Respir Med 2002;96:280-86.

336. Chan ED, Kalayanamit T, Lynch DA, Tuder R, Arndt P, Winn R. *Mycoplasma pneumoniae*-associated bronchio-litis causing severe restrictive lung disease in adults: Report of three cases and literature review. Chest 1999;115:1188-94.

337. Stey C, Truninger K, Marti D, Vogt P, Medici TC. Bronchiolitis obliterans organizing pneumonia associated with polymyalgia rheumatica. Eur Respir J 1999;13:926-29.

338. Barron FA, Hermanne JP, Dowlati A, et al. Bronchiolitis obliterans organizing pneumonia and ulcerative colitis after bone marrow transplantation. Bone Marrow Transplant 1998;21:951-54.

339. Epler GR. Heterogeneity of bronchiolitis obliterans organizing pneumonia. Curr Opin Pulm Med 1998;4: 93-97.

340. Camus P, Nemery B. A novel cause of bronchiolitis obliterans organizing pneumonia: Exposure to paint aerosols in textile workshops. Eur Respir J 1998;11: 259-62.

341. Rencken I, Patton WL, Brasch RC. Airway obstruction in paediatric patients: From croup to BOOP. Radiol Clin North Am 1998;36:175-87.

342. Ward F, Rog J. Bronchiolitis obliterans organizing pneumonia mimicking community acquired pneumonia. J Am Board Fam Pract 1998;11:41-45.

343. Worthy SA, Flint JD, Muller NL. Pulmonary complications after bone marrow transplantation: High resolution CT and pathologic findings. Radiographics 1997;17:1359-71.

344. Mahajan L, Kay M, Wyllie R, Steffen R, Goldfarb J. Ulcerative colitis presenting with bronchiolitis obliterans organizing pneumonia in a pediatric patient. Am J Gastroenterol 1997;92:2123-34.

345. Nemery B, Bast A, Behr J, et al. Interstitial lung disease induced by exogenous agents: Factors governing susceptibility. Eur Respir J 2001;(suppl 32):30S-42S.

346. Angle P, Thomas P, Chiu B, Freedman J. Bronchiolitis obliterans with organizing pneumonia and cold agglutinin disease associated with phenytoin hypersensitivity syndrome. Chest 1997;112:1697-99.

347. Yale SH, Adlakha A, Sebo TJ, Ryu JH. Bronchiolitis obliterans organizing pneumonia caused by *Plasmodium vivax* malaria. Chest 1993;104:1294-96.

348. Domingo JA, Calvo JIP, Carretero JA, Ferrando J, Cay A, Civeira F. Bronchiolitis obliterans organizing pneumonia, an unusual cause of solitary pulmonary nodule. Chest 1993;103:1621-23.

349. Colby TV. Pathologic aspects of bronchiolitis obliterans organizing pneumonia. Chest 1992;102:38S-40S.

350. Geddes DM. BOOP and COP. Thorax 1991;46:545-47.

351. Costabel U, Teschler H, Schoenfield B, et al. BOOP in Europe. Chest 1992;102:14S-20S.

352. Katzenstein ALA, Myers JL, Prophet WD, Corley LS, Shin MS. Bronchiolitis obliterans and usual interstitial pneumonia: A comparative clinicopathological study. Am J Surg Pathol 1986;106:373-81.

353. Costabel U, Guzman J. BOOP: What is old what is new? Eur Respir J 1991;4:771-3.

354. duBois RM, Geddes DM. Obliterative bronchiolitis, cryptogenic organizing pneumonitis, and bronchiolitis obliterans or bronchiolitis obliterans organizing pneumonia: three names for two different conditions. Eur Respir J 1991;4:774-75.

355. Oikonomou A, Hansell DM. Organizing pneumonia: The many morphological faces. Eur Radiol 2002:12:1486-96.

356. Guerry-Force ML, Muller NL, Wright JL, et al. A comparison of bronchiolitis obliterans organizing pneumonia, usual interstitial pneumonia and small airway disease. Am Rev Respir Dis 1987;135:705-12.

357. Cordier JF, Loire R, Brune J. Idiopathic bronchiolitis obliterans organizing pneumonia. definition of characteristic clinical profiles in a series of 16 patients. Chest 1989;96:999-1004.

358. Izumi T, Kitaichi M, Nishimura K, Nagai S. Bronchiolitis obliterans organizing pneumonia. Clinical features and differential diagnosis. Chest 1992;102:715-19.

359. Yamamoto M, Ina Y, kitaichi M, Harasawa M, Tamura M. Clinical feature of BOOP in Japan. Chest 1992; 102:21S-25S.

360. Mroz BJ, Sexauer WP, Meade A, Balsara G. Hemoptysis as the presenting symptom in bronchiolitis obliterans organizing pneumonia. Chest 1997;111:1775-78.

361. Chandler PW, Shin MS, Friedman SE, Myers JL, Katzenstein ALA. Radiographic manifestations of bronchiolitis obliterans organizing pneumonia.AJR 1986;147:899-906.

362. Lee KS, Kulinig P, Hartman TE, Muller NL. Cryptogenic organizing pneumonia: CT finding in 43 patients. AJR 1994;162:543-46.

363. Costabel U, Guzman J, Teschler H. Bronchiolitis obliterans organizing pneumonia: Outcome. Thorax 1995;50(Suppl):S59-S64.

364. Crauseman RS, Jennings CA, Tuder RM, Ackerson LM, Irvin CG, King TE Jr. Pulmonary histiocytosis X: Pulmonary function and exercise pathophysiology. Am J Respir Crit Care Med 1996;153:426-35.

365. Davidson AR. Eosinophilic granuloma of the lung. Br J Dis Chest 1976;70:125-28.

366. Basset F, Corrin B, Spencer H, et al. Pulmonary histiocytosis X. Am Rev Respir Dis 1978;118:811-20.

367. Friedman PJ, Liebow AA, Sokoloff J. Eosinophilic granuloma of lung. Medicine 1981;60:385-96.

368. Auld D. Pathology of the eosinophilic granuloma of lung. Arch Pathol 1959;63:113:31.

369. Colby TV, Lombard C. Histiocytosis X in the lung. Hum Pathol 1983;14:847-56.

370. Auerswald U, Barth J, Magnussen H. Value of CD-1 positive cells in bronchoalveolar lavage fluid for the diagnosis of pulmonary histiocytosis X. Lung 1991; 169:305-09.

371. Webber D, Tron V, Askin F, Askin F, Churge A. S-100 stains of eosinophilic granuloma of lung. Am J Clin Pathol 1985;84;447-53.

372. Uebelhoer M, Bewig B, Kriepe H, Nowak D, Magnussen H, Barth J. Modulation of fibroblast activity in histiocytosis X by platelet-derived growth factor. Chest 1995;107:701-05.

373. Schonfeld N, Frank W, Wenig S, et al. Clinical and radiologic features, lung functions and therapeutic results in pulmonary histiocytosis X, Respiration 1993;60:38-44.

374. Kulwiec EL, Lynch DA, Aguyao SM, Schwarz M, King TE Jr. Imaging in pulmonary histiocytosis X. Radiographics 1992;12:515-26.

375. Lacronique J, Roth C, Battesti P, Basset JP, Chretien J. Chest radiological features of pulmonary histiocytosis X: A report based on 50 adult cases. Thorax 1982;37: 104-09.

376. Sadoun D, Veylet R, Valeyre D, et al. Bronchogenic carcinoma in patients with pulmonary histiocytosis X. Chest 1992;101:1610-13.

377. Salvaggio JE. Recent advances in pathogenesis of allergic alveolitis. Clin Exper Allergy 1990;20:137-44.

378. Fink JN. Hypersensitivity pneumonitis. J Allergy Clin Immunol 1984;74:1-9.

379. Fink JN. Clinical features of hypersensitivity pneumonitis. Chest 1986;89(Suppl)1935.

380. Shillito JE. Hypersensitivity pneumonitis. Semin Respir Med 1991;12:196.

381. Pepys J, Jenkins P, Festenstein G, et al. Farmer's lung. Thermophilic actinomyceytes as a source of "farmers' lung hay" antigen. Lancet 1963;2:607.

382. Salvagio JE. Diagnosis and management of hypersensitivity pneumonitis. Hosp Pract 1990;15:93.

383. Sharma OP. Hypersensitivity pneumonitis. Dis Month 1991;37:419.

384. Ando M, Arima K, Yoneda R, Tamura M. Japanese summer-type hypersensitivity pneumonitis. Geographic distribution, home environment, and clinical characteristics of 621 cases. Am Rev Respir Dis 1991;144:765.

385. de Castro FR, Carrillo T, Castillo R, Blanco C, Diaz F, Cuevas M. Relationship between characteristics of exposure to pigeon antigens. Clinical manifestations and humoral immune response. Chest 1993;103:1059-63.

386. Hamagami S, Miyagawa T, Ochi T, Tsuyuguchi I, Kishimoto S. A raised level of soluble CD8 in bronchoalveolar lavage fluid in summer-type hypersensitivity pneumonitis in Japan. Chest 1992;101:1044-49.

387. Yoshida K, Suga M, Yamasaki M, et al. Hypersensitivity pneumonitis induced by a smut fungus *Ustilago esculenta*. Thorax 1996;51:650-51.

388. Schuyler M, Gott K, Edwards B, Nikula KJ. Experimental hypersensitivity pneumonitis: Effect of Thy1.2+ and CD8+ cell depletion. Am J Respir Crit Care Med 1995; 151:1834-42.

389. Denis M. Pro-inflammatory cytokines in hypersensitivity pneumonitis. Am J Respir Crit Care Med 1995;151:164-69.

390. Gaur SN, Gangwar M, Khan ZU, Jain SK, Randhawa HS. Farmer's lung disease in North-Western India. Ind J Chest Dis All Sc 1992;34:49-56.

391. Larsson K, Eklund A, Malmberg P, Bjermer L, Lundren R, Belin L. Hyaluronic acid (Hyaluronan) in BAL fluid

distinguishes farmers with allergic alveolitis from farmers with asymptomatic alveolitis. Chest 1992; 101:109-14.

392. Laviolette M, Cormier Y, Loiseau A, et al. Broncho-alveolar mast cells in normal farmers and subjects with farmer's lung. Diagnostic, prognostic, and physiologic significance. Am Rev Respir Dis 1991;144:855.

393. Larson K, Eklund A, Malmberg P, Belin L. Alterations in bronchoalveolar lavage fluid but not in lung function and bronchial responsiveness in swine confinement workers. Chest 1992;101:767-74.

394. Akoun GM, Cadranel JL, Milleron BJ, D'Ortho MPF, Mayaud CM. Bronchoalveolar lavage cell data in 19 patients with drug associated pneumonitis (except amiodarone). Chest 1991;99:98-104.

395. Cooper JAD Jr, White DA, Mathay RA. Drug induced pulmonary disease. Part II. Non-cytotoxic drugs. Am Rev Respir Dis 1986;133:488-505.

396. Crestani B, Jaccard A, Israel-Biet D, et al. Chlorambucil-associated pneumonitis. Chest 1994;105:634-36.

397. Hamadeh MA, Atkinson J, Smith LJ. Sulfasalazine-induced pulmonary disease. Chest 1992;101:1033-37.

398. Cooper JAD Jr, White DA, Mathay RA. Drug induced pulmonary disease. Part I. Cytotoxic drugs. Am Rev Respir Dis 1986;133:321-40.

399. Akoun GM, Cadranel JL, Milleron BJ, D'Ortho MPF, Mayaud CM. Bronchoalveolar lavage cell data in amiodarone-associated pneumonitis: Evaluation in 22 patients. Chest 1991;99:1177-82.

400. Gross N. Pulmonary effects of radiation therapy. Ann Intern Med 1977;86:81.

401. Withers HR. Biological basis for radiation therapy for cancer 1992;339:156.

402. Maasilta P. Radiation-induced lung injury. From the chest physician's point of view. Lung Cancer 1991; 7:367.

Chapter 22

Lung Cancer

EPIDEMIOLOGY

Lung cancer is the most common malignancy in men all over the world and is the commonest cause of cancer mortality of males in more than 35 countries. In females, it is the sixth leading cancer, and after excluding the sex related malignancies (cervix, breast), it is becoming the leading cause of cancer mortality in them, and even may soon bypass that in men.[1-4] This trend is due to increased incidence of smoking in women in the past few years. Lung cancer is expected to surpass gastric cancer as the most common tumor in the near future. It is estimated that there were 660,500 new cases of lung cancer in 1980. The distribution of these cases are shown in Table 22.1 countrywide.[1]

TABLE 22.1: World wide annual lung cancer incidence in 1980[1]

| Country | New cases per year (X 1000) | | |
	Males	Females	Total
Europe	180.3	34.1	214.4
USA	91.7	39.1	130.8
USSR (past)	63.5	14.6	78.1
China	43.6	22.7	66.3
Latin America	32.0	9.1	41.1
Japan	17.8	6.6	24.4
Africa	7.4	1.9	9.3
Australia/New Zealand	5.5	1.4	6.9
Other Asian countries	71.8	17.4	89.2
Developed countries	358.8	95.8	454.6
Developing countries	154.8	51.1	205.9
World (total)	513.6	146.9	660.5

Some of the increases compared to that prior to 1950, are probably due to improved diagnosis but changes more recently reflect the incidence trend. In 1980, it was estimated as causing 15.8 percent of all new cancer cases in males varying between 4.5 percent in Africa to 23.3 percent in Europe. In females, lung cancer is rarer, but whereas the increase between 1975 and 1980 was 10.1 percent in males, the same was 16 percent in females. The situation is different in 1985. Ignoring the non-melanoma skin cancers, lung cancer was estimated to be the most common cancer in men in the world around 1985 comprising 17.6 percent of all new cancers in men and 5.8 percent of those in women. In men there were about 667,000 incident cases in 1985, and 219,000 in women.[5] The age adjusted mortality trends in 14 countries shows that the increase is universal, at rates between 1 to 5 percent a year. Although the overall mortalities are less in females, marked increases are seen in some countries, like Canada, Denmark, and USA.

Lung cancer is particularly common in men in North America, Europe, and Oceania. The highest incidence rates currently observed in men are in the Maori population of New Zeland. Details of the incidences are shown in Table 22.2.

Trends in mortality from lung cancer in Europe, during the last decade showed that overall mortality from this cancer showed no systematic pattern in Northern and Central Europe, but a modest decline started at younger ages in several countries.[7] In southern Europe, lung cancer mortality started from lower values, but is still rising, and only in Italy is some flattening of rates at relatively high levels becoming apparent in middle age (35-64 years). The average change in lung cancer rates in Southern Europe over the last decade for males was + 24 percent for all ages and + 22 percent in middle age. The upward trends were even more substantial in Eastern European countries (+ 32% in middle age), which now have the highest lung cancer rates in young and middle-aged males. Over the last few last decades, female lung cancer rates have risen in all European countries, but only in Denmark and Britain are overall rates now over 20/100,000. The difference in prevalence and mortality of lung cancer in different regions is most probably related to the smoking habit. These trends are similar to that of the smoking prevalence of the country or region. However, the point is that lung cancer has been reported from almost all parts of the world and recently there is a trend to increase of this malignancy

TABLE 22.2: The ten highest and lowest incidence rates of lung cancer per 100,000 population (trachea, bronchus, and lung) in both males and females[6]

Males Country		Females Country	
Highest Incidence		**Highest Incidence**	
New Zeland, Maori	119.1	NewZeland, Maori	62.2
USA, New Orleans: Black	115.9	Canada, NWT and Yukon	51.8
USA, S.Sanfrancisco Bay area Black	107.4	USA, Hawaiian	39.5
USA, Detroit, Black	107.2	USA, Alameda, White	37.9
USA, Alameda, Black	106.8	USA, Sanfrancisco Bay area White	36.9
UK, West Scotland	97.2	USA, Alameda, Black	36.5
USA, Hawaiian	96.1	USA, Hawaii, White	36.1
USA, LosAngeles, Black	93.1	USA, Detroit, Black	36.0
USA, New Orleans, White	92.0	USA, Seattle	36.0
Poland. Lower Silesia	88.4	USA, S.Sanfrancisco Bay area, Black	35.9
Lowest Incidence		**Lowest Incidence**	
India, Ahmedabad	13.5	Spain, Tarragona	3.0
Costa Rica	12.7	France, Martinique	3.0
Algeria, Setif	11.7	Mali, Bamako	2.6
France, Martinique	11.0	Spain, Murcia	2.5
India, Bangalore	10.1	Spain, Granada	2.5
Peru, Trujillo	9.5	India, Ahmedabad	2.1
India, Madras	8.5	India, Bangalore	1.9
Ecuador, Quito	8.3	Algeria. Setif	1.7
Mali, Bamako	4.8	India, Madras	1.4
The Gambia	1.0	The Gambia	—

in almost all countries. Part of this increase is due to improved diagnostic facilities available, but mostly there is a true increase.

International trends in lung cancer mortality as available from the WHO Data Bank,[8] gives a close approximation to that for the incidence of the disease. Mortality data from nine different countries revealed that both truncated and overall age-adjusted mortality rates increased rapidly in males since 1955 and started levelling off between mid 70s and 80s in some of these countries and even a decline in some. However, the mortality rate is showing a consistently rising trend in women.

Lung Cancer in the World

Recent Trends

Lung cancer is the most common cancer in terms of both incidence and mortality. 1.3 million new cases/year reported and of this there were 1.2 million deaths worldwide in 2002. It is the most common cancer killer close to 20 percent of all cancer deaths (WHO). Highest rates are reported from Europe and North America. The 5 year survival rate for lung cancer fluctuates between 8 percent and 12 percent and smoking is found in 90 percent of lung cancer cases. The age standardized

incidence rates in males and females are shown in the Figures 22.1A and 22.1B.

The estimated numbers of new cancer cases (Incidence) and deaths (Mortality) in 2002 in the world are shown in the Figures 22.2A and 22.2B (Parkin DM et al. CA Cancer J Clin 2005;55:74-108).

Age-standardized Incidence Rates for Lung Cancer data are shown in the Figure 22.3 per 100,000 by sex. (Parkin, DM et al. CA Cancer J Clin 2005;55:74-108).

In the USA more people die from lung cancer than from any other type of cancer. This is true for both males and females. In 2004, lung cancer accounted for more deaths than did breast, prostate, and colorectal cancers combined. Further 89,575 men and 68,431 women in the United States died of lung cancer. That same year, 108,355 men and 87,897 women were diagnosed with lung cancer. Trends in age-standardized lung cancer incidence and death rates by sex, in the United States, between 1975-2005 is shown in the Figures 22.4A and 22.4B. (Jemal A et al. J Natl Cancer Inst 2008;100:1672-1694; doi:10.1093/jnci/djn389)

The lung cancer mortality trends in the European Union for both sexes are shown in the Figures 22.5A and 22.5B.

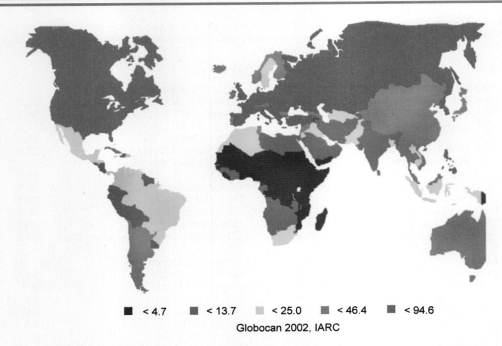

FIGURE 22.1A: Lung cancer in males: Age-standardized incidence rate per 100,000

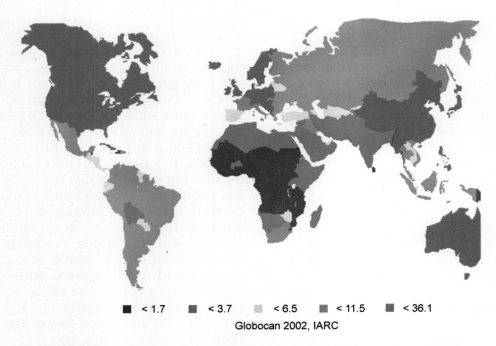

FIGURE 22.1B: Lung cancer in females: Age-standardized incidence rate per 100,000

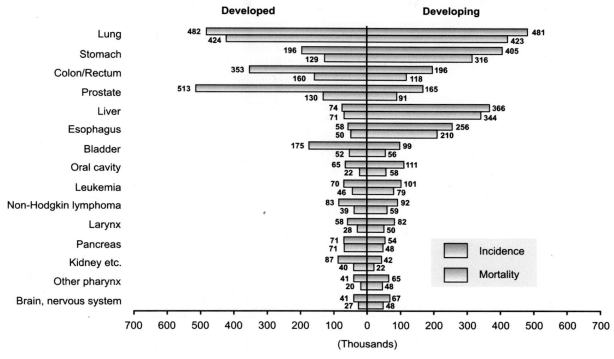

FIGURE 22.2A: New cancer cases (All types) and deaths in the world for 2002 in males

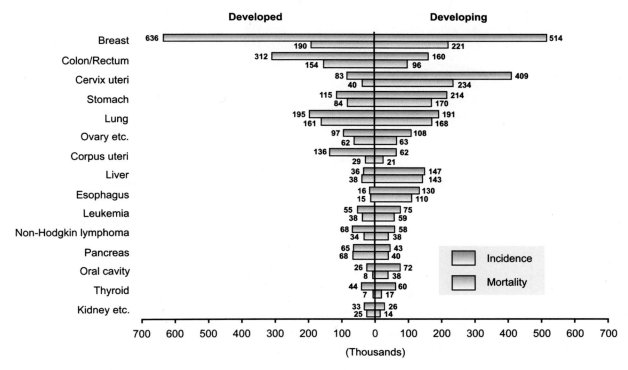

FIGURE 22.2B: New cancer cases (All types) and deaths in the world for 2002 in females

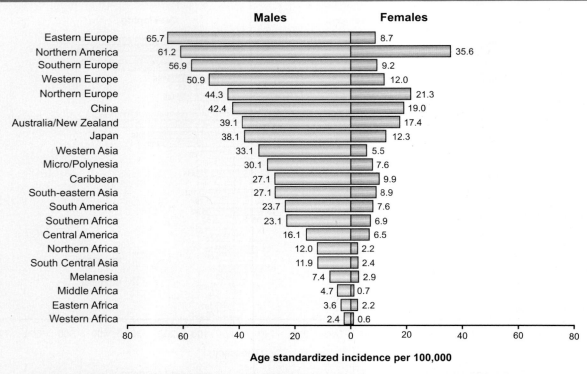

FIGURE 22.3: Age-standardized lung cancer incidence rates for both sexes in different countries of the world

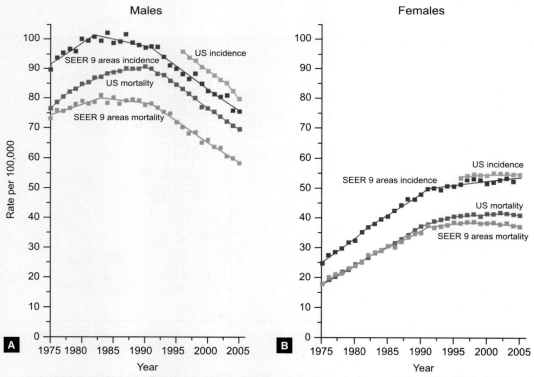

FIGURES 22.4A and B: Trends in age-standardized lung cancer incidence in the USA (1975-2005)

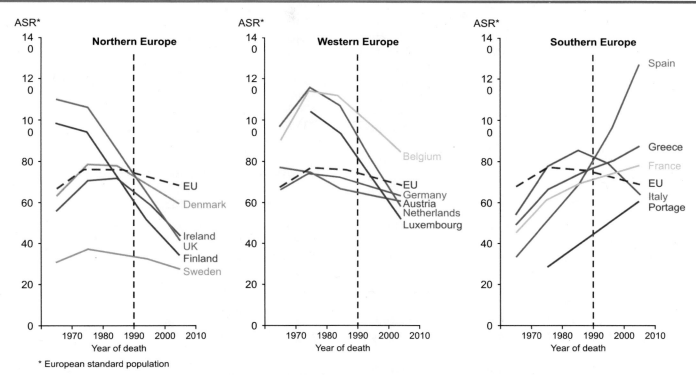

FIGURE 22.5A: Lung cancer mortality trends in the European Union in males

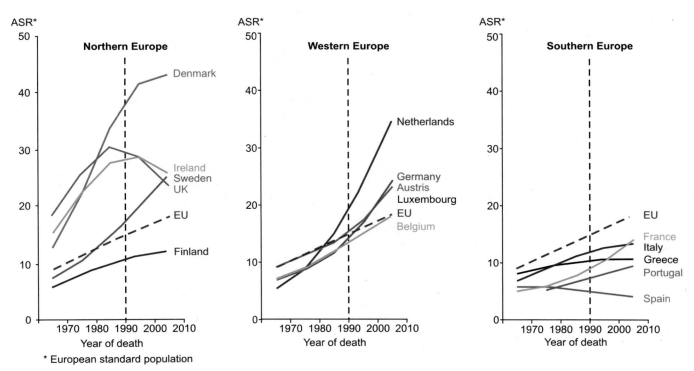

FIGURE 22.5B: Lung cancer mortality trends in the European Union in females

There are variations in the risk of different cancers by geographic area. Most of the international variation is due to exposure to known or suspected risk factors related to lifestyle or environment that provides a clear challenge to prevention. Lung cancer is the most common cancer in the world since 1985. A big change has occurred since 1980 as 69 percent were in developed countries, but now half (49.9%) of the cases occur in the developing countries. Worldwide, it is by far the most common cancer of men.

Lung Cancer in India

Primary lung cancer in India was reported to be rare or very infrequent in earlier published reports. An increase in the trend was recognized about a quarter of a century ago in the early 60s. Since then sporadic reports on clinical and pathological features of lung cancer have appeared from different parts of India.[9] Studies from India have emphasized the association of smoking habit and differences in relative risk rates in different communities based on the smoking habit. Significant epidemiological and cell type differences exist in this country compared to that is reported from the West.

The disease was rare in 1940s. However sporadic reports appeared in 1960s (Table 22.3). In the 1980s the ICMR established the cancer registry programme and subsequently the Cancer Atlas Programme covering the whole country. The data from this record is shown in the Table 22.4. Out of the 12 centers, lung cancer is the commonest in 6 in men and in the remaining 6 centers, it is either the second or third common malignancy. Further data revealed that the NE region is the *hotspot* having the highest incidence.

TABLE 22.3: Lung cancer in India in the 1960's

- Extremely infrequent *(Nath and Grewal 1935)*
- Most frequent finding in all Chest Diseases *(Wig et al 1961)*

Author	Incidence/prevalence	Comments
Banker 1953	14.4% of all cancers	Autopsy
Sirsat 1958	1% of all cancers	TMCH
Sinha 1961 (1955-59)	34/44,000 admissions	Calcutta
1957-62	342/10,313 (3.2%)	Citranjan Cancer Hosp
Viswanathan 1961		
1950	27.4/mil. hospital population	Data Hosp
1959	78.6/mil. hospital population	15 centres
Mishra 1966	4.2/10,000 hospital admn. 2.1% of all cancers survey	UP

TABLE 22.4: ICMR population based data from 12 centers

1st Common site	2nd Common site	3rd Common site
Bhopal	Chennai	Bangalore
Delhi	Thiruvananthapuram	Nagpur
Mumbai	Pune	
Ahmedabad		
Karungappally		
Kolkota		

Kolkota : CNCI – 13.8% of all cancers
Cancer Care and Welcome Home - 13.6% of all cancers.

International comparison of Age-Adjusted Rate (AAR) and Trunketed Rate (TR) – 35-64 Years – of lung cancer are shown in the Tables 22.5 and 22.6.

TABLE 22.5: International comparison of AAR,TR (35-64 Years) incidence rate per 100,000. Trachea, bronchus and lung in males

Year studied	Registry	AAR*	TR*
1979-82	UK (West Scotland)	100.4	120.7
1977-81	Finland	74.2	93.2
1979-82	UK (Oxford)	68.8	68.1
1978-82	USA (Bay area) White	64.3	81.1
	Black	89.8	140.1
1977-82	Columbia (Cali)	19.5	25.5
1977-86	China	22.8 (both males and females)	
1995	France	66.5	
	India		
	Bombay	14.6	24.7
	Bhopal	14.1	24.5
	Delhi	11.9	23.3
	Madras	11.1	23.2
	Bangalore	8.6	13.2
	Barshi	2.0	3.9

TABLE 22.6: International comparison of AAR, TR (35-64 Years) incidence rate per 100,000. Trachea, bronchus and lung females

Year studied	Registry	AAR*	TR*
1979-82	UK (West Scotland)	33.3	54.4
1977-81	Finland	28.6	46.3
1979-82	UK (Oxford)	25.3	41.5
1978-82	USA (Bay area) White	21.9	41.1
1978-82	USA (Connecticut) White	19.5	25.6
	Black	7.0	10.0
1977-82	Columbia (Cali)	5.4	9.5
1977-86	China	16.1 (both males and females)	
1995	France	8	
1996	Czech	22.7	
1989	India		
	Bombay	3.7	5.3
	Bhopal	3.2	6.3
	Delhi	2.2	4.5
	Madras	1.7	4.5
	Bangalore	1.6	4.1
	Barshi	0.0	0.0

TABLE 22.7: Lung cancer as reported from different parts of India

Authors	Total	M:F	Age (yrs)	Sm:NS	Squam.	Anapla.	Adeno.	Uncla.
1. Wig et al 1961	65	4.9	55.8	-	-	-	-	-
2. Sinha 1961	33	4.5	57.1	-	-	-	-	-
3. Viswanathan et al 1962	95	-	-	-	50.5	-	28.4	21.1
4. Karal et al 1967	100	24	52.1	-	41.0	-	20.0	39.0
5. Shankar 1967	20	All M	54.0	5.7	73.3	6.7	20.0	-
6. Nagrath et al 197	35	4.0	47.7	1.9	25.7	-	34.3	40.0
7. Reddy 1970	46	6.4	50	0.1	50	25	25	-
8. Guleria et al 1971	120	7.6	57.2	2.0	46.2	36.5	17.3	-
9. Basu et al 1971	24	7.0	48.3	5.0	62.5	8.3	25.0	4.2
10. Jha et al 1972	25	2.9	46.6	5.3	44.0	20.0	20.0	20.0
11. Nafar et al 1973	25	All M	51.0	7.3	56.0	20.0	12.0	12.0
12. Malik et al 1976	136	5.2	48.5	3.5	40.4	21.3	16.9	7.3
13. Narang et al 1977	58	8.7	51.3	4.8	37.9	51.8	10.4	-
14. Jindal et al 1979	150	5.5	51.7	2.4	32.5	19.3	15.8	21.9
15. Notani et al 1974	520	-	-	3.9	27.5	11.3	7.3	53.4
16. Garg et al 1973	82	-	-	-	46.3	28.0	20.7	-
17. Malhotra et al 1986	70	7.8	49.6	4.8	50.0	17.0	14.3	17.1
18. Jindal & Behera 1990	1009	4.5	54.3	2.7	34.3	27.6	25.9	12.2
19. Arora et al 1990	100	4.05	40-60	1.2	27	1	21	41
20. Rao	539	-	-	-	-	-	-	-
21. Rajasekaran etal 1993	232	7.9	53	2.7	72	4.3	3.9	15.1
22. Gupta et al 1998	279	7.41	56.7	4.5	42.3	32.2	19.9	5.6
23. Thippanna et al 1998	160	8.4	40-60	4	67.5	8.8	18.7	5.1
24. Arora 1998	200	-	-	-	-	-	-	-
25. Gupta D et al 2001	265	7.8	50-70	3.6	60	21.5	16.2	2.3
26. Kashyap et al 2001	638	6.17	54.6	2.4	58.3	-	10.81	-

TABLE 22.8: Clinical presentation of Indian lung cancer patients

Symptoms	Jindal and Behera 1990	Other Indian studies (range)
Anorexia	90	20.5-70
Weakness	90	4-60
Loss of weight	90	11.4-77
Cough with expectoration	88	40-94.3
Haemoptysis	69.2	8-60
Chest pain	52.2	16-66.67
Hoarseness of voice	29.9	9-33
Breathlessness	–	24-59
Dysphagia	20.8	2.9-6
Puffiness of the face	19.8	2.9-8.33
Fever	19.6	22-68.6
Nausea and vomiting	6	25.00
Other	30.5	25.00

The National Cancer Registry Program of the Indian Council of Medical Research, which collected data from six different parts of the country, both rural and urban areas, showed varying figures at different areas.[10] While cancer of the trachea, bronchus and lungs was the most common form of malignancy in males in 1989 from Bombay, Delhi, and Bhopal, it was the second most common in Madras, third in Bangalore, and was most unusual in Barshi, a rural area. The disease was most uncommon in females and only in Bombay it was the sixth common malignancy and in Bhopal it was the seventh in rank. Tables 22.5 and 22.6 shows the International comparison incidence rates of lung cancer vis a vis that is seen in India.[10]

Lung cancer has been reported from all parts of India and is shown in the Table 22.7.

Various clinical presentation of lung cancer in India is shown in the Table 22.8:

Hospital data from different parts of the country showed different patterns (see Table 22.7). In a large referral Northern Indian hospital (Postgraduate Institute of Medical Education and Research, Chandigarh), all cancers constituted about 4 percent of all hospital admissions, lung cancer was the fifth common malignancy. Males were affected more than females and about 19.46 percent of all cases of lung cancer were below the age of 40 years.[11] Jindal and Behera[12] has summarized the clinical features and cell type patterns of lung cancer which appeared in Indian literature in the past 30 years along with their own series of more than 1000 cases, which is perhaps the largest Indian series published. According to that report, the male female ratios have differed widely, although males were the predominant sufferers in most series. The average age as derived from the means of age group tables, has been quite similar in most of the studies, i.e. around 54 years, although some studies, the mean age was less than 50 years. This younger age of Indian patients is similar to the contemporary studies from Western countries of about 40 to 50 years ago.[13] The smoker: nonsmoker ratios have been lower compared to those in the West. The cell type pattern also differed in different series, although squamous cell carcinoma was the commonest. However, there was an increase in the incidence of small cell carcinoma and adenocarcinoma. The cell type pattern also varied with age.[14]

ETIOLOGY

(1) SMOKING

The single most major cause of lung cancer is smoking. All types of products including cigarette and *bidi* are responsible for this. The association has been well established both from epidemiological studies and experimental results.[15] The subject has been reviewed recently by Boyle and Maisonneuve.[16] Tobacco has been associated with cancer for at least 200 years[17] and the causal nature of the association with lung cancer has been reported for decades. Tobacco smoking is at present the most clearly defined and important cause of cancer in developed countries with lung cancer being the leading tobacco-related cancer site.[18] The association of tobacco smoking and lung cancer was suggested in the United Kingdom as early as in 1927.[19] Subsequently, the overwhelming role of tobacco smoking in the causation of lung cancer has been repeatedly demonstrated over the past 50 years.[20-27]

One of the earliest epidemiological studies on the relationship of amount of smoking and lung cancer is available from the report by Muller in 1940 which is quoted by Cornfield in 1951.[27] According to the study by Muller, smokers were classified as *moderate* (1-3 cigars/1-15 cigarettes/1-20 gm of tobacco per day); *heavy* (4-6 cigars/16-25 cigarettes/21-35 gm of tobacco per day); *very heavy* (7-9 cigars/26-35 cigarettes/26-50 gm tobacco per day); or *excessive smokers* (10-15 cigars/over 35 cigarettes/over 50 gm of tobacco per day). The risk of lung cancer among smokers was as follows: moderate smokers—3.07; heavy smokers—2.75; very heavy

smokers—16.80; and excessive smokers—29.16. Similar dose-response relationship was also reported by Schairer and Schoniger in 1943 (quoted in ref 16). Subsequently five major epidemiological studies (from VA Hospital Hines, Illinois; Buffalo; Detroit and Cincinnati, and Ohio; and St. Louis hospitals) contributed to the establishment of such relationship during 1950s although there may be some methodological deficiencies compared to present standards.[20,26,28-30] One more important information that came out from the study of Doll and Hill[20] was that duration of smoking was also an important contributor.

Subsequent epidemiological research on the association of smoking and lung cancer based on better quantification risk and identification of those smoking behavior and tobacco use which further modify the risk has established the fact which was reported 40 to 50 years ago.[16] More than 80 percent of the cases of lung cancer are due to smoking only. The risk increases in proportion to the fourth or fifth power of the duration of smoking and is thus strongly related to the age of onset of smoking. The rise in mortality is much more consistent with the effect of smoking, with the delayed peak in women explained by the fact that smoking became popular among women later than among men. No other known cause of lung cancer explains the recent trends of mortality as well as smoking does.

The three principal types of lung cancer—the squamous cell, small cell, and adenocarcinoma—are caused by smoking, although the relative risk is least extreme for adenocarcinoma. In various populations, particularly those of Chinese and Indian origin, the incidence of adenocarcinoma in nonsmokers appears to approach that of smokers.[31-33] However, adequate data are not available to quantify the phenomenon. Further studies are required to understand the etiology of such type of lung cancer better.

The Surgeon General USA, in his report in 1964 had summarized the causal relationship of cigarette smoking and lung cancer.[34] The association was strong in men and far outweighs all other factors. The data in women also pointed in the same direction. The risk of lung cancer increases with the duration of smoking and number smoked per day. Discontinuation of smoking reduces the risk of lung cancer. Compared to nonsmokers, average smokers have a 9 to 10 folds risk of lung cancer and in heavy smokers the risk is at least 20-fold. Risk for pipe and cigar smokers is less than cigarette smokers but far more than that in nonsmokers.[35] Filter cigarettes also have low risk than non-filter cigarettes. Various other studies also have confirmed these findings. While the risk of smokers smoking < 1/2 pack cigarettes per day is about 15 times compared to that in nonsmokers, the risk is more than 60 times in those smoking > 2 packs/day. Cigarette smoking also enhances the carcinogenic effect in certain occupations, like asbestos workers, and uranium miners, compared to that in nonsmokers with the same occupation. The risk is almost 14 times for the former and 5 times more in the later. Quieting smoking reduces the risk of lung cancer regardless of duration of smoking or the quantity smoked per day. It decreases slowly over 10 to 20 years, and after 20 years, the risk is the same to that in a nonsmoker. Besides, cigarettes, cigars, and pipes, *bidi*, and *hooka* smoking also increase the risk of lung cancer. In large parts of Asia including India, *bidi* smoking is an important cause of lung cancer. Studies from Bombay by Notani et al[36,37] revealed that the relative risk of all types of smokers to nonsmokers is 2.45, of *bidi* smokers 2.64 to 3.38, and of cigarette smokers 2.23 to 2.36. Studies from Chandigarh[12] has shown a smoker:nonsmoker ratio of 2.7:1. Thus, studies from India has shown that the risk of cigarette smokers is much lower in Indian population than the risk estimated for the Western population. Whether this is due to differences in the mode of inhalation or to differences in the age of starting the habit, or to some other environmental or genetic differences in the population is a matter of conjecture. The risk of *bidi* smoking is almost identical, or even more from these data. *Hooka* smoking is another risk factor as reported from Kashmir valley.[38]

Other aspects of smoking behavior apart from type of product smoked and risk of lung cancer, include daily dose of tobacco, duration of smoking, and the type of cigarette used. It is consistently found that, among otherwise similar cigarette smokers, there is a direct relationship between the daily dose and the increased risk of lung cancer in both men and women. The relationship is almost in a linear proportionate manner. As mentioned above, damage to the lungs accumulates with continuous smoking, and therefore duration of smoking is directly related to the development of lung cancer. In fact, to express this relationship a smoking index is described. Smoking index is expressed as the number of *bidis* or cigarettes smoked per day multiplied by the number of years smoked. It is graded as mild, when the smoking index is below 100; moderate when it is between 100 to 299; and severe when it is 300 or more. As the smoking index increases the risk of lung cancer is also increased. Those who start to smoke in adolescence and continue to smoke are at the greatest risk of developing lung cancer in adult life and importantly there is a delay of several decades between the widespread adoption of cigarette smoking by young adults

and the emergence of the full effects on national lung cancer rates. Even smokers of many years, who have not yet developed lung cancer, by ceasing to smoke, can avoid most of their subsequent life long risk.[23] Once the relationship of cigarette smoking and risk of lung cancer was established, efforts were made to change the design and smoke composition, including the introduction of filters, porous papers, and change in types of tobacco. These changes affected the tar yield of cigarette. Although it has not been possible to assess the direct impact of these changes on lung cancer, it has been shown that tar content have some effect.[39,40] Cigarettes delivering less than 17.6 mg tar were associated with a lower risk of lung cancer than those delivering more than 25.7 mg tar. Other case control studies have shown a fairly consistent tendency for lung cancer risks to be lower among users of filter than of nonfilter cigarettes and the reduction was to the tune of 40 to 50 percent.[41]

Various carcinogens (about 108 chemicals) identified in tobacco smoke include dimethyl-nitrosamine, diethyl-nitrosamine, methyl-ethyl-nitrosamine, N-nitrosopyrrolidine, and N-nitrosopiperidine in the gas phase; and benzo (a) pyrene, methyl-benzo (a) pyrenes, dibenz (a,h) acridine, dibenz (a,j) acridine, dibenz (c) carbazone, b-naphthylamine, benzanthracene, polonium-210, and arsenic, etc.[42-45] Of these the polynuclear aromatic hydrocarbons (PAH) are important. 2-naphthylamine and 4-α, minobiphenyl, are considered by the International Agency for Research on Cancer (IARC) to be human carcinogens. Benzo (a) pyrene, N-nitroso-dimethylamine, formaldehyde, and acetamide are suggested to be probable carcinogens, while 1,3-butadiene, nitrosonornicotine, N-nitrosopyrrolidine and indino [1,2,3-cd]pyrene are listed as possible carcinogens. Out of all these substances benzo(a)pyrene, is the most extensively studied. A number of studies have shown the concentrations of benzo(a)pyrene to be elevated in the urine of smokers. Smoking induces the enzyme aryl hydrocarbon hydroxylase (AHH), which metabolizes certain PAH to active carcinogens. There is perhaps a variation in the inducibility of the enzyme AHH, in different smokers, which may explain the differential susceptibility to development of tumors.

The relationship of smoking and lung cancer. [Peto, R., *et al.* (2000)] is shown below in Figure 22.6.

Passive Smoking

Nonsmoking women exposed to husband's smoke (passive smoking) or vice versa have a risk of 1.4 to 1.9 times than that of nonsmokers.[46-58] There is now strong evidence of the adverse health consequences of Environ-

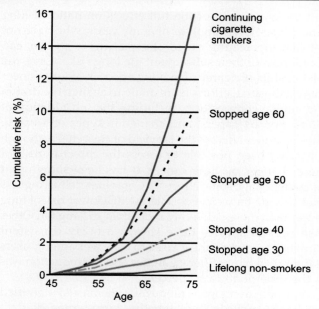

FIGURE 22.6: Relationship of smoking and lung cancer

mental Tobacco Smoke (ETS) or passive smoking. On the basis of available epidemiological data, the United States Environmental Protection Agency declared that ETS was a proven lung carcinogen in humans.[53] However, certain other reports have expressed some doubt about this association.

(2) OCCUPATIONAL RISKS

Major occupational respiratory carcinogens are shown in Table 22.9.[59-82] In terms of the number of cases produced, asbestos is by far the most important, and may account for as many as 5 percent of deaths from lung cancer in the USA. Apart from hematite mining the hazards are all more prevalent in industrial towns and cities than in the countries. Experimental and human studies suggest an association between exposure to crystalline silica and an excess of pulmonary malignancies. Although the data available are not sufficient to establish a clear cut causal relationship in humans, an association between the onset of pneumoconiosis and pulmonary malignancy is probable. Clinical and experimental evidences suggest a link between exposure to radiation and lung cancer. The agents responsible are radon and uranium. The combining effect of gamma radiation and smoking appears to be additive. Occupational exposures have been estimated to account for 5 to 36 percent of the lung cancers among men in different geographic areas in the Western countries.

(3) DIET

There is increasing evidence that some dietary factors may be protective for lung cancer, and some may increase the risk.[83-107] Although most consistent evidence

TABLE 22.9: Occupational risk of lung cancer		
Agent	Occupation	Comment
1. *Definitely known*		
Asbestos	Insulation worker	Some increase in risk after 10
	Shipyard workers	years. Substantial after 20 years
		Smoking increases risk 90 folds
Arsenic	Smelter workers	More in upper lobes. Dose related
	Vineyard workers	May have multiple primaries
Nickel Refinery workers	Squamous cell type common	
Radiation	Uranium mining	Majority oat cell type
	Haematite mining,	Due to radon exposure
	Hard rock mining	
Chromium	Chromium ore processing	Mostly squamous cell type
	Pigment manufacturers	
Chloromethyl	Workers in industries produc-	Oat cell common
ethers	ing these compounds.	
Mustard gas	Mustard gas producing workers	Squamous and undifferentiated
		cell carcinomas more common
Soots, tars,	Coke oven workers	
oils, coke	Gas house workers,	
	roofers, rubber workers	
2. *Suspected causes*		
Acrylonitrile		
Beryllium and beryllium compounds		
Dimethyl sulphate.		

relates to a protective effect of β-carotene, some more recent work suggests that other protective factors may be found in vegetables. Doll et al[104] have proposed that the risk for developing squamous cell carcinoma is significantly increased when smoking is combined with a deficiency of vitamin A. Case control studies from China have shown that vegetable intake is a protective factor for lung cancer.[105] In laboratory studies, preliminary experiments using both experimental animals and human bronchial epithelial cells show that a deficiency of retinoids in the culture media is accompanied by squamous cell transformation, simultaneous with increased B[a]P-DNA adduct formation. Both cellular and molecular changes can readily be reversed by the addition of retinoids.[105,106] On the otherhand, report by Heinonen et al[107] from a placebo controlled study performed on 29,133 male smokers who received alpha-tocoferol and beta-carotene supplement for 5 to 8 years showed no reduction in the incidence of lung cancer. The first cohort study in Norway, had showed that an index of vitamin A intake was negatively associated with lung cancer incidence. Other studies also showed similar observations. Recently, a large number of trials are on to utilize this information and beta carotene is used as chemoprophylactic agent for lung cancer. A recent case control study of diet and lung cancer in South India[103] has shown that green vegetables and bananas have a protective association with lung cancer. Pumpkins and onions have the most consistent protective effect. Animal protein foods and dairy products were found to have a predisposing effect on lung cancer in that study. Dietary cholesterol and animal fat increase the risk of lung cancer.

(4) AIR POLLUTION

The strongest evidence that air pollution causes carcinoma of the bronchus lies in the consistent urban-rural difference in incidence and mortality.[108-119] An excess mortality has been reported from many countries including UK, and USA. Urban air contains several known lung carcinogens including asbestos and arsenic, and polycyclic aromatic hydrocarbons from incomplete combustion of fuel. Some studies also show higher incidence of smoking in urban areas. Besides, occupational exposure to the above discussed carcinogens is more in urban areas. The lung cancer cases are more often reported in subjects residing in neighborhoods where the outdoor air is smoky.[117-119]

The possible role of indoor air pollutants to the human cancer burden has been a contentious issue in environmental risk assessment as the measurement of actual exposure to these substances over time is extremely difficult. The nature of these pollutants vary and fluctuate over time, and the concentration may be affected by a number of known and unknown factors like ventilation and human responses, etc. A symposium on this aspect has summarized the role of indoor air pollution in the causation of lung cancer.[120] Studies from China has stressed that coal burning at home is a significant risk factor for female lung cancer, particularly in nonsmoking females. Burning coal at home is responsible for elevated levels of SO_2, CO, TSP (total suspended particles), B[a]P, radon, and thoron. Exposure to cooking fumes is also a significant risk factor for lung cancer in nonsmoking females. However, incense burning used commonly in many homes as a part of worship did not significantly increase the risk.[121-123]

(5) CHRONIC LUNG DISEASES AND LUNG CANCER

Individuals with chronic nonneoplastic lung diseases have a documented high risk to develop lung cancer.[124,125] Tuberculosis, pneumonia, and emphysema were found to be associated with increased risk of lung cancer even after adjusting for smoking.[124,125] Lung cancers developing in association with old scars—"scar carcinoma", is commonly described with systemic sclerosis with lung involvement. In a retrospective cohort study of tuberculosis in Shanghai involving 30,373 cases of pulmonary tuberculosis revealed an elevated risk of lung cancer which was independent of smoking.[126] Treatment with isoniazid nor exposure to X-rays explained the higher risk. It is reported that lung cancer in association with chronic lung diseases result due to an impaired lung ventilation and concomitant increase in pulmonary carbon dioxide, which in turn causes pronounced hyperplasia of pulmonary neuroendocrine (PNE) cells.[127-129] This effect, perhaps, is mediated by a receptor with sensitivity for O_2/CO_2. These cells produce a number of autocrine growth factors which in turn may contribute to the increased burden of lung cancer in individuals with chronic lung diseases.

(6) OTHER HOST FACTORS AND LUNG CANCER

In a case control study (population based) from China it was observed that risk of lung cancer, particularly adenocarcinoma, was higher among women with shorter menstrual cycles with a strong dose-response relationship.[123] Further, among women aged 55 and above with natural menopause, the risk of adenocarcinoma increased with total number of lifetime menstrual cycles. Risk of lung cancer was positively associated with the age of menopause.[121] Although these data may be preliminary, they suggest that sex hormones, as well as levels and functions of oestrogen and progesterone receptors may be involved in controlling the growth of lung cells.

(7) FAMILIAL PREDISPOSITION TO LUNG CANCER

Since vast majority of heavy smokers do not develop lung cancer, it seems that an inherited predisposition or cofactors such as additional carcinogens might exist Although smoking is the major cause of lung cancer, only about 10 percent of heavy smokers die of this disease. The relative susceptibility of these 10 percent or the resistance of the remaining 90 percent to development of lung cancer is poorly understood and may be relative to some genetic events. There is some evidence that lung cancer develops in the family members of lung cancer patients. However, if it is truly hereditary or related to some common familial factors is not exactly known. The suspicion is strong enough to suggest that blood relatives of lung cancer patients are at increased risk of getting the disease. First degree relatives of lung cancer patients have a strong excess risk of 2.4 folds for the disease.

There appears to be a strong association between inheritance of the high metabolic phenotype for 4-debrisoquine hydroxylase and the development of lung cancer. Extensive metabolizers of debrisoquine have a 10 fold increase in the risk of developing lung cancer.

Earlier Studies comparing risk factors in subjects with lung cancer to individuals with other smoking related cancers have shown a lack of increased risk of developing lung cancer when only lung cancer in relatives was considered.[130] However, there was a significant excess of cancers in other sites in relatives of lung cancer patients. This indicates a heritable variation in the response to carcinogens. Development of lung cancer in subjects younger than 50 years showed a Mendelian codominant inheritance or a rare autosomal gene.[131] This gene was not involved for older subjects suggesting non-carriers having long-term exposure to tobacco.

(6) ONCOGENES AND LUNG CANCER

Recently, it has been identified that genes contribute to the process of malignant transformation. These are altered forms of normal genes normally present in eukaryotic cells. The gene families implicated in carcinogenesis include *proto-oncogenes* or *dominant oncogenes* and the *recessive* or *tumor suppressor genes*. While the *proto-oncogenes* (normal homologous of the oncogene) participate in critical cell functions, including signal transduction and transcription. Only a single mutant allele is required for malignant transformation. Primary modifications in these genes that confer the ability for transforming function include point mutations, amplifications, translocations, and rearrangements.

Tumor suppressor genes appear to require homozygous loss of function either by mutation, deletion, or a combination of the two. Cytogenetic studies have identified many chromosomal changes in lung cancer with numerical abnormalities, and structural aberrations including deletions and translocations.[132-135] These mutations include activation of the dominant cellular *proto-oncogenes* (which promote oncogenesis) of the *ras* and *myc* family and inactivation of the *recessive* or *tumor suppressor genes* (these genes help suppression of tumor development). Many of these changes are associated with true losses of DNA from the tumor cell. The most prominent of these changes is the deletion of the short arm of chromosome 3. These changes are seen in all types of lung cancer. More recently DNA losses have been noted on other chromosomes like 13, 17, 1, 7,9, 13-16, and 21. The DNA loss has been localized to the *rb* locus on chromosome 13.

Oncogenes of several different families also suffer genetic changes in lung cancer. These include point mutations in members of the *ras* family and changes in the *c-myc, N-myc, L-myc,* and *c-myb*. The changes in the *myc* family member expression have been associated with gene amplification, gene rearrangement and other alterations. Frequently involved genes in lung cancer are shown below:

Dominant oncogenes
c-myc, N-myc, L-myc	(Deregulated expression)
K-ras, H-ras, N-ras	(Activating mutation)
Her-2/neu	(Deregulated Expression)

Tumor Suppressor genes (Recessive oncogenes)
3p14
3p21,3
3p24-25
5q
9p
11p15
13q14
17p13 (p53 gene).

In small cell lung cancer amplified expression of the *c-myc, N-myc, L-myc* and *c-myb* oncogenes have been demonstrated and *c-myc,* amplification in extensive stage patients was associated with a history of prior chemotherapy and a poor prognosis.[136-138] *ras* gene point mutations have been found in non-small cell lung cancer, particularly adenocarcinoma, but not in small cell lung cancer.[139] The most frequent site of mutation was in the K-*ras* codon 12 and this site of mutation is associated with smoking.[140] This transformation is associated with poor survival.[141,142] Other oncogenes identified recently are the *bcl*-1 locus in 14 percent of squamous cell carcinomas[143] and the proto-oncogene *c-kit* in small cell lung carcinoma.[144]

Many chromosomal changes (see above) have also been identified in lung carcinoma cell lines. The most frequent change involves the deletion of the short arm of chromosome 3-3p.[137,145-147] Almost all small cell lung cancers and about 50 percent of the nonsmall cell lung cancers have an allele loss in this area[148] found by restricted fragment length polymorphism studies. On chromosome 11p there are two putative loci for tumor suppressor genes involved in nonsmall cell lung cancer and one of these is potentially related to the Wilms tumor gene.[149-151] The retinoblastoma gene (*rb*) on chromosome 13q is inactivated in virtually all small cell lung cancers and in about 10 to 20 percent of nonsmall lung cancer.[152,153] Chromosomal deletion in 17p have led to the identification of the p53 tumor suppressor gene. p53 is muted in all small cell lung cancers and about 50 percent of nonsmall cell lung cancers.[154-159]

HISTOLOGICAL CLASSIFICATION OF LUNG CANCER

There are mainly 5 different classifications for lung cancer described. But, the WHO classification is the one that is widely accepted and used. The first WHO classification was published in 1967. The purpose was to provide a light microscopic criteria for the various types so that these can be practised worldwide. That classification identified 14 categories of lung tumors/tumor like lesions. Over 90 percent of them fell into the 4 cell types (epidermoid, adeno-, small cell- and large cell carcinomas. The remaining types included combined epidermoid/adenocarcinoma. Carcinoid, bronchial gland tumors, papillary tumors of bronchial surface epithelium, mixed tumors including carcinosarcomas, unclassified tumors, mesotheliomas, melanomas, and tumorlike lesions. Although specific criteria was given for the major cell types, criteria for subtypes was minimal and sometimes misleading. In 1977, the classification was simplified to clarify the terminology and to recognize the impact of cytology as a diagnostic tool. This revised edition was published in 1981 and identified 7 categories.[160-162] Epithelial, Soft tissue, Mesothelial; Miscellaneous, Secondary, Unclassified, and Tumorlike lesions. The malignant epithelial tumors are shown in Table 22.10.

The above classification is based on light microscopic data. However impressive data have accumulated to invalidate the light microscopic interpretation of lung cancers. Electron microscopy have identified multiple

TABLE 22.10: WHO classification of lung tumors. Gr.C: malignant epithelial tumors,1981[160]

1. Squamous cell carcinoma (Epidermoid carcinoma)
   Variants: Spindle cell carcinoma
2. Small cell carcinoma
   (a) Oat cell carcinoma
   (b) Intermediate cell types
   (c) Combined oat cell carcinoma (squamous- or adeno-)
3. Adenocarcinoma
   (a) Acinar adenocarcinoma
   (b) Papillary adenocarcinoma
   (c) Brochiolo-alveolar cell carcinoma
4. Large cell carcinoma
   Variants:
   (a) Giant cell carcinoma
   (b) Clear Cell carcinoma
5. Adeno-squamous carcinoma
6. Carcinoid tumor
7. Bronchial gland carcinoma
   (a) Adenoid-cystic carcinoma
   (b) Mucoepidermoid carcinoma
   (c) Others
8. Others

differentiated ultrastructural characteristics within a tumor and, even within a single cell. Immunohistological and biochemical studies show distinct neuroendocrine products in classic nonsmall cell tumors (usually adenocarcinoma). Thus a multitude of new lung cancer classifications have been devised based on these data.[163-166] However, the clinical relevance of these classifications has not been proven to be superior to the already available classification based on light microscopy.

For practical purposes, the lung cancer is described as 5 main types:
(1) Squamous cell carcinoma (SQCC)
(2) Small cell carcinoma (SCLC)
(3) Adenocarcinoma (AC)
(4) Large cell anaplastic carcinoma (LCC)
(5) Undifferentiated cell carcinoma (UDCC).

SQCC and AC are further subdivided into well, moderate and poorly differentiated cancers (or Grades 1-4 or 1-3), depending upon how similar the histology of the tumor is to its cell of origin or how differentiated it appears.

The incidence of various histological types varies in different series. In general, earlier reports indicated that squamous cell carcinoma is the predominant cell type, occurring in more than 40 percent of cases. The incidence of various cell types is as follows: squamous cell carcinoma (40-60%); small cell carcinoma (7-25%); adenocarcinoma (10-25%); and large cell carcinoma (5-1%). However, recently there is a changing histopathology of lung cancer, although the above pattern is still maintained in other series.[12,167-173] There is an increase in the incidence of adenocarcinoma, and particularly bronchiolo-alveolar carcinoma, in USA, Japan and several other countries of the world. Traditionally, adenocarcinoma including the bronchiolo-alveolar carcinoma, has been the most frequent types of lung cancer to occur in nonsmokers, women, and young people, suggesting that major changes in the pathogenesis of lung tumors are in progress. Squamous and small cell carcinomas are more common in smokers and they are usually of central in origin. In a review of 1151 cases over a 20 years period (1970-1989) from Kyushu University in Japan, Ikeda et al[171] reported that the incidence of adenocarcinoma has increased from 26 to 45 percent in males and from 45 to 69 percent in females. In addition, the proportion of subtypes adenocarcinoma, classified in an electron microscopic study, underwent marked changes during the period 1982 to 1985; thus 71 percent of all adenocarcinomas were classified as being of the bronchiolo-alveolar type. The role of some etiologic factors other than smoking, like dietary or ecological, has been suggested.

Although the above classification based on light microscopy depending solely on hematoxylin and eosin histology, is of practical use in clinical practice, recent studies have brought out some of its shortcomings. Electron microscopic studies have shown that the presence of multiple lines of differentiation are common in lung cancer[174] supporting the common stem cell theory for the histogenesis of lung cancer. Large cell lung cancer can often be classified into at least one of either type of differentiated tumors, i.e. SQCC or AC. In addition, imprint smears of fresh surgical tumor specimens have shown similar observations. Further, recent reports indicate that lung tumors can be classified in a different ways, particularly the neuroendocrine tumors. Neuroendocrine cells and tumors are characterized morphologically by the presence of intracytoplasmic neurosecretory granules at the ultrastructural level and functionally by the production and secretion of neurohormonal factors (see biology of lung tumors below). Immunohistochemical markers can be directed against the content of these cells.[175] The original WHO classification has subdivided SCLC into oat cell and intermediate subtypes (Table 22.5). The distinction between these subtypes is not biologically significant, and the oat cell subtype is probably an artifact due to ischemia. Recently, morphological and biochemical studies have sufficient grounds to subclassify SCLC into "classic" and "variant" types.[176] Further, genetic studies and other tumor markers have added further light into various types of lung cancer.[172]

SQUAMOUS CELL CARCINOMA

These are mainly central in location and are associated with smoking. They typically arise from major bronchi, usually the lobar or the first segmental bronchus. The earliest form of the carcinoma is in the form of intraepithelial, noninfiltrating foci presenting grossly as localized, slightly red granular plaques or as gray white leukoplakia. Infiltrating malignancies present as bulky fungating gray white or yellow intraluminal bronchial masses, obstructing the bronchus easily and early in the course of the disease producing obstructive symptoms. About 10 percent of the growths show central necrosis, and cavitation (Fig. 22.7).

The adjacent bronchial mucosa shows evidence of squamous metaplasia, dysplasia, or intraepithelial neoplasia. Squamous metaplasia is not a necessary precursor. In its earliest recognizable form, "carcinoma in situ', the normally delicate translucent columnar epithelium of the bronchial mucosa is replaced by a thickened, stratified squamous epithelium composed of malignant squamous cells. Grossly the mucosa is granular, and opaque and gray, rugal folds are effaced, and pits of bronchial gland orifices are obscured. The cells exfoliate easily at this stage and can be identified in sputum specimens. As the carcinoma grows within the bronchial lumen and into and through the bronchial wall, the bronchus is obstructed with development of collapse (partial or complete depending on the size of lumen obstructed) and pneumonia. These carcinomas may grow to relatively large size locally before metastasizing. Even then, the metastasis is limited to regional lymph nodes for quite some time, enabling early stage squamous cell carcinoma to be amenable to surgery.

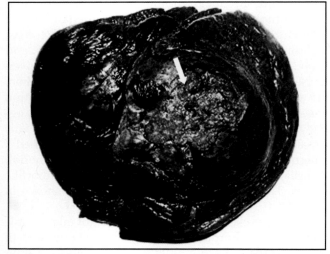

FIGURE 22.7: Pneumonectomy specimen from squamous cell carcinoma, infiltrating the pleural surface

The histological appearance of the tumor is composed of sheets of epithelial cells with abundant cytoplasm and hyperchromatic nuclei with coarse chromatin structure. They are classified into well-, moderately-, and poorly-differentiated cell types according to the frequency with which these histological features are found. In the well-differentiated types, there is abundant keratin formation. Cells grow in stratified or pseudoductal patterns and may form small whorls or nests. Squamous cells are connected by intercellular bridges which give the cell a prickle appearance. Individual cells may show intracellular keratinization or may coalesce to form epithelial pearls. Atypical mitotic features are present in plenty. Nuclei are enlarged, and have irregular membranes and dense chromatin patterns. Moderately differentiated neoplasms show less evidence of keratin formation, less cellular organization, and more marked nuclear atypia. Poorly differentiated types show stratification, intercellular bridge formation, and/or occasional foci of individual cell keratinization. The tumor cells are predominantly anaplastic with no attempt to show maturation. Nuclei are bizarre and enlarged with prominent nucleoli and inclusion bodies. The well- and moderately-differentiated tumors tend to grow slowly with local invasive properties, whereas the poorly differentiated cell types are more aggressive with more extrathoracic metastases (Fig. 22.8).

SMALL CELL CARCINOMA

These carcinomas usually arise centrally in major lobar or segmental bronchi and only rarely in the periphery. They probably originate endodermally from a common precursor cell that is capable of endocrine differentiation. This cell type is the most aggressive form of bronchogenic

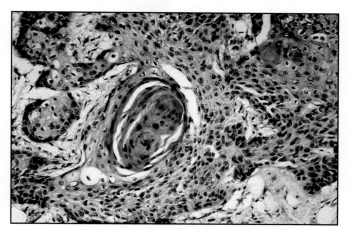

FIGURE 22.8: The cells have squamoid differentiation and show pleomorphism with round to oval nuclie and eosinophilic cytoplasm. The center of field shows a keratin pearl

carcinoma with many different biological characteristics than other cell types. They tend to metastasize early in the course of the disease. In fact, by the time the disease is diagnosed, it is often a systemic disease with metastasis to lymph nodes, liver, bone and brain in a majority of cases. They secret many hormones and biological markers distinct from other cell types and their response to therapy is equally dramatic.

The tumor provokes minimal bronchial changes with the mucosa being elevated very slightly. The tumor tend to spread in a centrifugal pattern to involve intrathoracic lymph nodes and other structures, particularly the superior vena cava quite early. Frequently the tumor produces red hemorrhagic masses and nodules. The bronchial lumen may be stenosed, but bulky intraluminal masses are not usual.

The oat cell subtype is composed of cells with small round to oval cells with a high nuclear/cytoplasmic ratio. The cells are almost twice the size of the lymphocytes. Nuclei are vesicular, with indistinct nucleoli and a fine salt-and-pepper chromatin distribution. Sometimes, the cells tend to have dense smudged hyperchromatic nuclei. The cells in intermediate subtypes are less regular in shape than the oat cells, and some of these tumors may also contain a mixture of small and large cells. When the large cells are more than 1 percent, the prognosis is worse because of resistance to chemotherapy. The combined oat cell carcinoma subgroup contain either small cell carcinoma with areas of squamous cell carcinoma or small cell carcinoma with areas of adenocarcinoma (Figs 22.9 to 22.12). Their behavior is same as small cell carcinoma and should be managed as such.

ADENOCARCINOMA

Most of the adenocarcinoma arise from the periphery and unrelated to the bronchi except by contiguous spread or lymphatic dissemination. A small percentage arise from the bronchial surface epithelium. Occasionally, the tumor is associated with scar tissues. The tumors tend to provoke a desmoplastic response and grossly they present as firm, circumscribed subpleural masses with gray-white mucoid surface on cut section. The overlying pleura tend to br thickened and puckered. The size is much smaller than the other cell types (Fig. 22.13). About 5 percent of the large tumors cavitate. In autopsy they may be missed as pleural scars. Pleural dissemination rarely occurs. The adenocarcinomas are divided histologically into categories based on growth pattern of the tumor. All begin as a solitary nodule. The acinar and papillary adenocarcinomas grow by destruction and invasion of tissue, much like adenocarcinoma of other organs. They form glandular patterns, and in some cases

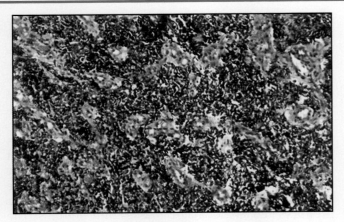

FIGURE 22.9: H&E stain, 50X, small cell carcinoma in transbronchial lung biopsy

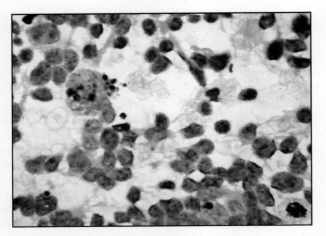

FIGURE 22.10: Small cell carcinoma - Pleomorphic poorly cohesive cells with little or no cytoplasm, nuclear moulding and smear artifact (H&E, 20X)

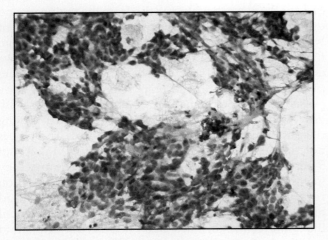

FIGURE 22.11: Small cell carcinoma - Pleomorphic poorly cohesive cells with little or no cytoplasm, nuclear moulding and smearing artifact (H&E, 20X)

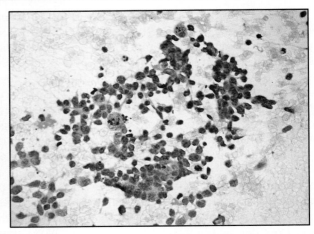

FIGURE 22.12: Small cell carcinoma - Pleomorphic poorly cohesive cells with absent cytoplasm, nuclear moulding, tear drop cells and inconspicuous nucleoli (H&E, 40X)

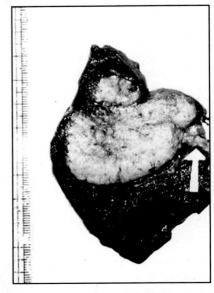

FIGURE 22.13: Gross specimen of adenocarcinoma of lung reaching upto pleural surface

may be difficult to distinguish from metastatic adeno-carcinoma to the lung. The acinar and papillary subtypes of adenocarcinoma tend to produce mucin. Because they are peripheral in location, they do not exfoliate cancer cells into the bronchus and are unlikely to be detected by sputum cytology unless they are large and invade major bronchial divisions. On the otherhand, because they are present within the aerated lung tissue, their detection by radiology is easier. Another variant is the solid growth pattern, but it behaves in similar pattern. All of these glandular carcinomas metastasize first to regional lymph nodes like squamous cell carcinoma, but are more likely metastasis occurs to distant sites earlier via blood stream. Carcinomas that are subpleural in origin can spread through the pleural lymphatics and more often produce pleural effusion containing cancer cells (Figs 22.14 to 22.17).

Bronchiolo-alveolar cell carcinomas may resemble subpleural nodules. Less often they present as multi-centric unilateral or bilateral nodules, being mistaken as lobar type of pneumonias. These tumors originate from Type II pneumocytes, ciliated, mucinous or Clara cells in the bronchiolar epithelium, and bronchiolar mucosal cells. The usual location is within or distal or to the terminal bronchioles (Figs 22.18 to 22.20).

They spread in lipidic fashion along the walls of alveoli and bronchioles, using these structures as a supporting stroma, with little destruction of pulmonary parenchyma. Tumor cells closely resemble the columnar or cuboidal, mucinous or nonmucinous bronchial

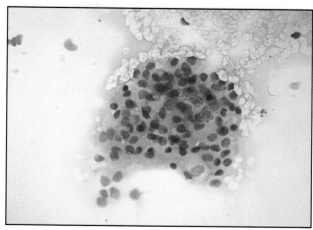

FIGURE 22.16: Adenocarcinoma - Loosely cohesive cluster of pleomophic tumor cells with coarse chromatin and conspicuous nucleoli (H&E, 40X)

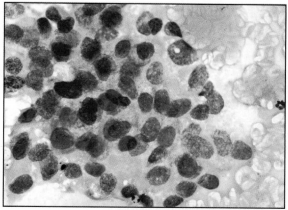

FIGURE 22.14: Adenocarcinoma - Loosely cohesive cluster of pleomorphic tumor cells with coarse chromatin with acinar formation (H&E 100X)

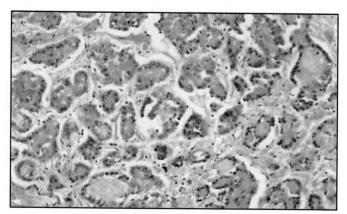

FIGURE 22.17: H&E stain, 50X, photomicrograph from adeno-carcinoma of lung

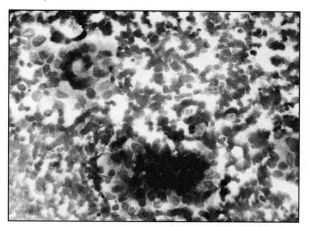

FIGURE 22.15: Adenocarcinoma - Loosely cohesive cluster of pleomorphic tumor cells in a hemorrhagic background (MGG, 40X)

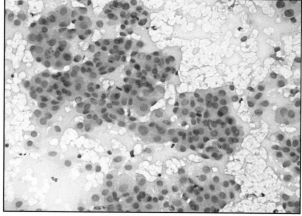

FIGURE 22.18: Flat monolayered sheets or cell clusters of regular small cell with moderate cytoplasm and fine chromatin-BAC (H&E, 40X)

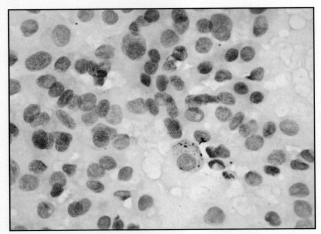

FIGURE 22.19: BAC - Flat monolayered sheets or cell clusters of regular small cell with moderate cytoplasm, fine chromatin and inconspicuous nucleoli (H&E, 100X)

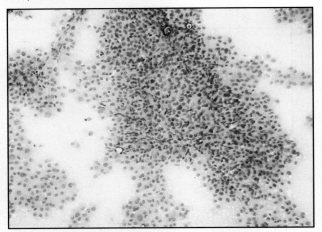

FIGURE 22.20: Bronchoalveolar cell carcinoma - Note flat monolayered sheets or cell clusters of regular small cell with moderate cytoplasm and fine chromation (H&E, 40X)

epithelium and spread throughout the lung by aerogenous dissemination. The gross appearance and radiologic presentation are those of a consolidation or pneumonic lung. Lymph node metastasis are common, but death is commonly due to respiratory failure.

LARGE CELL CARCINOMA

These tumors are epithelial tumors that show no obvious evidence of maturation to form squamous cells, acini or glands. Thus they constitute the left over tumors that do not show the features of any of the other cell types. Grossly, they are peripheral and subpleural in location and tend to present as large, bulky, and circumscribed masses. Cavitation may be present. Majority of the tumors are unrelated to bronchi except by contiguous growth.

On light microscopy, they are seen as large polygonal, spindle, or oval cells with abundant cytoplasm and large irregular pleomorphic nuclei with prominent nucleoli. Individual cells may have giant nuclei or may form syncytial multinucleated giant cells. Cells tend to be arranged in small nests, clusters, sheets, or in individual cell patterns (Fig. 22.21). The two variants of large cell carcinoma, the giant cell and clear cell carcinomas, are very rare. The giant cell type contains bizarre cells with giant nuclei and abundant cytoplasm. Clear cell types consist of large rounded cells with clear cytoplasm and with small central nuclei, simulating renal cortical carcinoma.

PATHOGENESIS AND BIOLOGY OF LUNG CANCER

In recent years it has become clear that considerable overlap exist between small cell lung cancer and non-small cell lung cancer. Histologic evaluation of specimens from lung cancer patients reveals more than one cell type in 10 percent or more of patients (e.g. mixed small cell/adenocarcinoma or squamous cell carcinoma). In autopsy studies of small cell lung cancer who died following systemic chemotherapy, mixed histologies were noted in 40 percent of patients which suggests either the emergence of a second tumor or that individual lung tumors can undergo differentiation to other cell types. It is now believed that all types of lung cancer arise from a common stem cell and this common stem cell theory for the histogenesis of lung cancer is now widely accepted. This has been depicted in Figure 22.22.

Searching for stem cells in the bronchial epithelium, it is reported that re-epithelialization of denuded tracheal grafts by basal cell clones give rise to goblet cells, ciliated cells, and secretory cells. In the bronchioles Clara cells

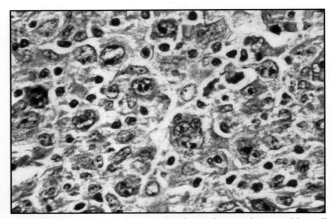

FIGURE 22.21: Photomicrograph shows large pleomorphic cells present in sheets. The cells have high NC ratio, large vsicular nuclei, prominent nucleoli and scanty cytoplasm

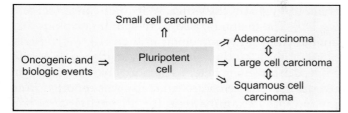

FIGURE 22.22: Common pathogenetic origin

give rise to ciliated cells and other Clara cells only. Such findings are significant in that they indicate that two different stem cell populations govern renewal of the epithelial lining: basal cells in the trachea and bronchi, and Clara cells in the bronchioles.[165]

The mechanisms of initiation of lung cancer by various carcinogens, be it in the smoke (Benzo(a)pyrene), or acquired from occupational exposures, the target of biologic actions have been the DNA. These actions have implicated DNA as a critical target molecule The metabolism of carcinogens are important in the generation of the chemically reactive form of the carcinogen which can bind to macromolecules. Similarly N-nitroso compounds require metabolism to form chemically reactive intermediates and those which transfer small alkyl groups to DNA show affinities for respiratory tissues.[177-181]

Understanding the origins and biology of lung cancer has been enhanced in recent years by the development of laboratory systems that permit the growth and characterization of tumor cells taken from patients. Most of these work has been done by establishing small cell lung cancer cell lines in tissue cultures.[178-180, 182,183] Ectopic production of polypeptides and steroid hormones and other factors has been well documented in patients with small cell lung cancer and in small cell lung cancer xenografts.[182] These have been summarized in Table 22.11.

TABLE 22.11: Factors synthesized by small cell lung cancer[183]

Adrenocorticotrophin	*Lipotropin*
Atrial natriuretic peptide	Neurotensin
Bombesin/gastrin releasing peptide	Neuromedin B
Calcitonin	Oestradiol
Calcitonin gene related peptide	Opioid peptides
Cholecystokinin	Oxytocin
Chorionic gonadotrophin	Parathyroid hormone
Endothelin	Physalaemin
Follicle stimulating hormone	Prolactin
Gastrin	Serotonin
Glucagon	Somatostatin
Granulocyte colony stimulating factor	Substance K
Growth hormone	Substance P
Growth hormone releasing factor	Transferrin
Insulin like growth factor binding proteins	Vasoactive intestinal peptide
Insulin like growth factor I	Vasopressin

The correlation of these hormone production and clinical extent and response is not clearly defined. Production of four other biological markers by small cell lung cancer cell lines have been reported recently. They are: neurone specific enolase (NSE), the BB isoenzyme of creatine kinase (CK-BB), the neuropeptide bombesin/gastrin-releasing peptide (GRP), and the key APUD enzyme L-dopa decarboxylase. A good correlation between serum concentrations and both disease extent and response to treatment has been demonstrated for both NSE and CK-BB. Lung cancer cells both produce and exhibit a mitogenic response to a variety of growth factors, indicating that these factors behave like "autocrine growth factors". In fact lung cancer cells can grow in media supplemented with only a few or no added growth factors. Autocrine peptides produced by lung cancer cells include GRP, and those with growth factor (TGF) and insulin-like-1 (IGF-1) activities. In some cases lung cancer cells can express multiple growth factors.[184,185] Nonsmall cell lung cancers (NSCLC) show varying degrees of differentiation and can express a range of growth factors. They include epidermal growth and transforming growth factor (TGF), both of which bind to the epidermal growth factor receptor.[186-189] Other factors that are found to be associated with NSCLC include p185[neu], the product of the HER2/neu oncogene (a transmembrane protein having homology with the epidermal growth factor receptor), platelet derived growth factor, bombesin/gastrin releasing peptide, neurone specific enolase, and chromogranin A.[190] The expression of growth factors and their receptors in some NSCLC appears to be related to aggressive clinical behavior and increased likelihood of response to chemotherapy.[191-193] Elevated circulating hormones in patients with lung cancer has been reported as follows: human chorionic gonadotrophin 12 to 14 percent; luteinizing hormone in 26.6; follicular stimulating hormone in 4.4 percent; prolactin in 37.8 percent; thyroid stimulating hormone in 3.2 percent; and cortisol in 30 percent of cases.[194,195] Altered levels of RNA and DNA in blood has also been noted in lung cancer patients.[196,197] Recently, more and more growth factors, antigens, and genetic abnormalities are being identified which have been useful to study the biology, therapy, and prognosis of both small cell and non-small lung cancer.[198-224]

Over the last decade, many cell surface molecules associated with lung tumors have been identified.[201] Monoclonal antibodies to most of these antigens for small cell lung cancer have been identified and can be grouped into 8 clusters.[223,225] Antibodies to cluster-1 antigen is known as neural cell adhesion molecule (NCAM) which functions as a hemophiliac adhesion molecule. This antigen is expressed in all small cell lung cancer cells. Polysialylated NCAM can be used as a useful tumor marker to distinguish SCLC from carcinoid tumors. Cluster-2 is a 40kDa surface protein with wide distribution on epithelial tissues. The antigen is most likely identical with a transmembrane protein cloned from adenocarcinoma cell line. Cluster-w4 antigen, a 40kDa phosphoinsitol-linked membrane glycoprotein expressed in all small cell lung cancer cells. Cluster-5 and cluster-5A antigens are sialoglycoproteins expressed on a large proportion of small cell lung cancer with little expression on normal epithelial tissues and no expression on nervous tissues or WBCs. Cluster-6 and cluster-8 antigens are blood group related carbohydrate structures and cluster-w7 antigen is a mucin related carbohydrate structure. Other well defined antigens like CD11b and CD57 have recently been described. It is reported that within a group of NSCLC patients, who were blood group A negative had a poor prognosis after surgery. Neuroendocrine markers in resected NSCLC are associated with worse prognosis.

Successful growth of colonies of lung cancer cells in agar and other selected media has been reported in specimens obtained from various cell lines. The overall success rate is 50 to 80 percent irrespective of histological type. The small cell lung cancer cell lines are of two kinds: the "classic" and the "variant" types based on morphology, growth properties, biochemistry, and radiosensitivity.[180,226-228] The characteristics of lung cancer cell lines are shown in Table 22.12.

SCREENING FOR LUNG CANCER

Studies in the USA (Mayo Lung Project) and other countries have been conducted in randomized controlled trials to evaluate the efficacy of lung cancer screening.[229-231] The methods used were sputum cytology and annual chest X-ray screening in high risk individuals. None of these studies showed any evidence of benefit from such screening in terms of mortality reduction from the disease. A case controlled study was reported from Japan, X-ray examinations for all participants and sputum cytology for high risk individuals were offered annually.[232] Although the result did not reach statistical significance, the study suggested that lung-cancer screening by miniature chest X-ray for all screens and sputum cytology for high-risk screenees can reduce mortality of the disease by 28 percent, at most in those who were screened within 12 months, as compared to those who did not undergo screening. However when the duration for comparison was extended to 60 months, the effect of screening on reduction of mortality decreased. Thus it seems that early screening for high risk subjects will not reduce the overall mortality from lung cancer. At best the disease can be diagnosed sometimes earlier. Moreover, such exercise involves a lot of expenditure. The efficacy of the lung cancer screening is still controversial because of the high costs of programs directed to this goal.[233-235] Low-dose spiral CT scanning fluorescent bronchoscopy and use of molecular markers have recently been utilized for lung cancer screening.

STAGING OF LUNG CANCER

Accurate subclassification of tumor cell types and determination of the extent of the disease at presentation are the most important steps that allow treatment decision and outcome of treatment. The one that is commonly used for the determination of anatomic extent is that developed by the American Joint Committee on Cancer.[236] The system uses the letters T, N, and M

TABLE 22.12: *In vitro* characteristics of lung cancer cell lines			
Property	SCLC(Classic)	SCLC(Variant)	NSCLC
Culture appearance	Tight aggregates	Loose aggregates	Adherent growth
Nucleoli	Inconspicuous	Prominent	Prominent
Nuclear/cytoplasmic ratio	High	Medium	Variable
Dense core granules	Present	Absent or rare	Absent
Doubling time	72 hrs	33 hrs	~ 50 hrs
Cloning efficiency	1-5%	10-30%	0.5-40%
L-dopa decarboxylase	Increased	Absent	Absent
Bombesine	Increased	Absent	Absent
NSE	Increased	Increased	Absent/Low
Creatine kinase	Increased	Increased	Absent/Low
Hormone production	Common	Seldom	Seldom
Radiation sensitivity	Sensitive	Resistant	Resistant
C-myc oncogene	Not amplified	Often amplified	Occasionally amplified

SCLC-Small cell lung cancer, NSCLC-Nonsmall cell lung cancer, NSE-Neurone specific enolase

representing the primary tumor, regional lymph nodes, and distant metastases. Another classification in use was that developed by the International Union Against Cancer.[237] As investigators throughout the world have put these staging systems to work, the need for refinements to meet their individual practices has resulted in variations in the use of the classification. Subsequently some modifications were made to these classifications based on retrospective investigations or reclassifications. Thus a new International Staging System for Lung Cancer has emerged and is shown in Table 22.13.[238]

For carcinoma of the bronchus the new classification differs from the old one with a new category of T4 for extensive extra-pulmonary extension of the disease, and a new N3 for cases with contralateral and/or supra-clavicular lymph node involvement. T1N1M0 was dropped from stage I to stage II; stage III was subdivided into IIIA and IIIB.

Because lung cancer is a dynamic process, the result of the disease stage may differ at various points of the course. Similarly, the extent may differ, as for example on clinical grounds, the metastasis to a distant organ may not be appa-

---

TABLE 22.13: International TNM definitions of lung cancer

Primary tumor (T)

Tx	Tumor proven by the presence of malignant cells in bronchopulmonary secretions, but not visualized on X-ray or by bronchoscopy, or any tumor that can not be assessed as in a re-treatment staging.
T0	No evidence of primary tumor.
TIS	Carcinoma *in situ*.
T1	A tumor that is 3.0 cm or less in greater dimension, sorrounded by lung or visceral pleura, and without evidence of invasion proximal to a lobar bronchus at bronchoscopy. (The uncommon superficial tumor of any size with its invasive component limited to the bronchial wall which may extend proximal to the main bronchus is also included in T1).
T2	A tumor more than 3.0 cm in greatest dimension, or a tumor of any size that either invades the visceral pleura or has associated atelectasis or obstructive pneumonitis extending to the hilar region. At bronchoscopy, the proximal extent of demonstrable tumor must be within a lobar bronchus or at least 2.0 cm distal to the carina. Any associated atelectasis or pneumonitis must involve less than an entire lung.
T3	A tumor of any size with direct extension into the chest wall (including superior sulcus tumors), diaphragm, or the mediastinal pleura or pericardium without involving the heart, great vessels, trachea, esophagus or vertebral body, or a tumor in the main bronchus within 2 cm of the carina without involving the carina.
T4	A tumor of any size with invasion of the mediastinum or involving the heart, great vessels, trachea, esophagus, vertebral body or carina or the presence of malignant pleural effusion. (Most pleural effusions associated with lung cancer are due to tumor. There are, however, some few patients in whom cytopathological examination of pleural fluid on more than one specimen, is negative for tumor, the fluid is nonbloody and is not an exudate. In such cases where these elements and clinical judgment dictate that the effusion is not related to the tumor, the patient should be staged T1, T2, or T3, excluding effusion as a staging element).

Nodal involvement (N)

N0	No demonstrable metastasis to regional lymph nodes.
N1	Metastasis to lymph nodes in the peribronchial or the ipsilateral hilar region, or both, including direct extension.
N2	Metastasis to ipsilateral mediastinal lymph nodes and subcarinal lymph nodes.
N3	Metastasis to contralateral mediastinal lymph nodes, contralateral hilar lymph nodes, ipsilateral or contralateral scalene or supraclavicular lymph nodes.

Distant metastasis (M)

M0	No (known) distant metastasis.
M1	Distant metastasis present-Specify site(s).

Stage grouping

Occult carcinoma	Tx	N0	M0
Stage 0	TIS	Carcinoma in situ	
Stage I	T1/T2	N0	M0
Stage II	T1/T2	N1	M0
Stage IIIA	T3	N0	M0
	T3	N1	M0
	T1-3	N2	M0
Stage IIIB	Any T	N3	M0
	T4	Any N	M0
Stage IV	Any T	Any N	M1

Other reports have validated this staging system subsequently.[239,240]

TABLE 22.13A: IASLC Proposed TNM Classification (2009)

T (Primary tumor)

TX   Primary tumor cannot be assessed, or tumor proven by the presence of malignant cells in sputum or bronchial washings but not visualized by imaging or bronchoscopy

T0   No evidence of primary tumor

Tis   Carcinoma *in situ*

T1   Tumor less than or equal to 3 cm in greatest dimension, surrounded by lung or visceral pleura, without bronchoscopic evidence of invasion more proximal than the lobar bronchus (i.e. not in the main bronchus)[a]

     T1a   Tumor less than or equal to 2 cm in greatest dimension

     T1b   Tumor > 2 cm but less than or equal to 3 cm in greatest dimension

T2   Tumor > 3 cm but less than or equal to 7 cm or tumor with any of the following features (T2 tumor with these features are classified T2a if less than or equal to 5 cm)
Involves main bronchus, greater than or equal to 2 cm distal to the carina
Invades visceral pleura
Associated with atelectasis or obstructive pneumonitis that extends to the hilar region but does not involve the entire lung

T2a   Tumor > 3 cm but less than or equal to 5 cm in greatest dimension

T2b   Tumor > 5 cm but less than or equal to 7 cm in greatest dimension

T3   Tumor > 7 cm or one that directly invades any of the following: chest wall (including superior sulcus tumors), diaphragm, phrenic nerve, mediastinal pleura, parietal pericardium; or tumor in the main bronchus (< 2 cm distal to the carina[a] but without involvement of the carina; or associated atelectasis or obstructive pneumonitis of the entire lung or separate tumor nodule(s) in the same lobe

T4   Tumor of any size that invades any of the following: mediastinum, heart, great vessels, trachea, recurrent laryngeal nerve, esophagus, vertebral body, carina, separate tumor nodule(s) in a different ipsilateral lobe

N (Regional lymph nodes)

NX   Regional lymph nodes cannot be assessed

N0   No regional lymph node metastases

N1   Metastasis in ipsilateral peribronchial and/or ipsilateral hilar lymph nodes and intrapulmonary nodes, including involvement by direct extension

N2   Metastasis in ipsilateral mediastinal and/or subcarinal lymph node(s)

N3   Metastasis in contralateral mediastinal, contralateral hilar, ipsilateral or contralateral scalene, or supraclavicular lymph node(s)

M (Distant metastasis)

MX   Distant metastasis cannot be assessed

M0   No distant metastasis

M1   Distant metastasis

M1a   Separate tumor nodule(s) in a contralateral lobe; tumor with pleural nodules or malignant pleural (or pericardial) effusion[b]

M1b   Distant metastasis

[a] The uncommon superficial spreading tumor of any size with its invasive component limited to the bronchial wall, which may extend proximally to the main bronchus, is also classified as T1a

[b] Most pleural (and pericardial) effusions with lung cancer are due to tumor. In a few patients, however, multiple cytopathologic examinations of pleural (pericardial) fluid are negative for tumor, and the fluid is nonbloody and is not an exudate. Where these elements and clinical judgment dictate that the effusion is not related to the tumor, the effusion should be excluded as a staging element and the patient should be classified as M0.

rent, but either on biopsy or surgery the true extent may be different. Thus, it is recommended that staging of the patient with lung cancer should be made at one or more of the following times during the course of the disease.

1. A clinical diagnostic stage after clinical examination and various laboratory procedures
2. A postsurgical treatment-pathologic stage, based on the above plus the pathologists report
3. A re-treatment staging, when there is recurrence of the disease or a new treatment is planned
4. An autopsy stage for those who die and an autopsy is performed.

Thus the new International staging of lung cancer has six levels with five stages of the disease, including a stage 0, that provide for the classification of six groups of patients who have similar prognostic expectations and therapeutic options. Stage I includes only patients with the best prognostic expectations (only T1 or T2 tumors without any metastasis). Stage II disease includes patients with T1, T2 primary tumors and metastasis confined to intrapulmonary lymph nodes including the hilar nodes. Stage IIIA disease with extra-pulmonary extension of the primary tumor and ipsilateral mediastinal lymph node metastasis, falls within the operable range. Stage IIIB includes more extensive extra-pulmonary extensions of the primary tumor than the potentially operable group. Stage IV includes patients with more distant metastasis.

International Association for the Study of Lung Cancer (IASLC) Prospective Lung Cancer Staging Project

In 1996, the International Association for the Study of Lung Cancer (IASLC) launched a worldwide TNM staging project to inform the next edition (seventh) of the TNM lung cancer staging system expected to be published in mid 2009. The committee recommended certain changes to the T, N, and M descriptors. Data on 100,869 patients were submitted to the international database, and data for 18,198 of these patients fulfilled the inclusion criteria for the T component analysis. Survival was calculated for clinical and pathologic T1, T2, T3, T4NOMO completely resected (R0), and for each T descriptor. A running log-rank test was used to assess cutpoints by tumor size. Results were internally and externally validated. On the basis of the optimal cutpoints, pT1NOR0 was divided into pT1a <= 2 cm (n = 1816) and pT1b > 2 to 3 cm (n = 1653) with 5 year survival rates of 77 and 71% (p < 0.0001). The pT2NOR0 cutpoints resulted in pT2a > 3 to 5 cm (n = 2822), pT2b > 5 to 7 cm (n = 825), and pT2c > 7 cm (n = 364). Their 5 year survival rates were 58, 49, and 35% (p < 0.0001). For clinically staged N0, 5 year survival was 53% for cT1a, 47% for cT1b, 43% for cT2a, 36% for cT2b, and 26% for cT2c. pT3NO (n = 711) and pT4 (any N) (n = 340) had 5 year survival rates of 38 and 22%. pT4 (additional nodule(s) in the same lobe) (n = 363) had a 5 year survival rate of 28%, similar to pT3 (p = 0.28) and better than other pT4 (p = 0.0029). For pM1 (ipsilateral pulmonary nodules) (n = 180), 5 year survival was 22%, similar to pT4. For cT4-malignant pleural effusion/nodules, 5 year survival was 2%. Recommended changes in the T classification are to subclassify T1 into T1a and T1b, and T2 into T2a and T2b; and to reclassify T2c and additional nodule(s) in the same lobe as T3, nodule(s) in the ipsilateral nonprimary lobe as T4, and malignant pleural or pericardial effusions as M1.

Further data were contributed from 46 sources in more than 19 countries. Adequate data were available on 67,725 cases of nonsmall cell lung cancer treated by all modalities of care between 1990 and 2000. The recommendations for changes to the T, N, and M descriptors were incorporated into TNM subsets. Candidate stage groupings were developed on a training subset and tested in a validation subset. The suggestions include additional cut-offs for tumor size, with tumors > 7 cm moving from T2 to T3; reassigning the category given to additional pulmonary nodules in some locations; and reclassifying pleural effusion as an M descriptor. In addition, it is suggested that T2b N0 M0 cases be moved from stage IB to stage IIA, T2a N1 M0 cases from stage IIB to stage IIA, and T4 N0-1 M0 cases from stage IIIB to stage IIIA.

Detailed suggested new IASLC staging system for lung cancer is shown in Table 22.8A.

For the T2 category, visceral pleural invasion is defined as invasion to the surface of the visceral pleura or invasion beyond the elastic layer. Based on a review of published literature, the IASLC Staging Committee recommends the elastic stains be used in cases where it is difficult to identify invasion of the elastic layer by hematoxylin and eosin (H&E) stains. A tumor that falls short of completely traversing the elastic layer is defined as PL0. A tumor that extends through the elastic layer is defined as PL1 and one that extends to the surface of the visceral pleural as PL2. Either PL1 or PL2 status allows classification of the primary tumor as T2. Extension of the tumor to the parietal pleura is defined as PL3 and categorizes the primary tumor as T3. Direct tumor invasion into an adjacent ipsilateral lobe (i.e. invasion across a fissure) is classified as T2a.

CLINICAL FEATURES

The disease is common in the 5th decade, although younger age groups can also be affected.[12,13, 241-244] the incidence increases rapidly from age 50 years, but the disease is uncommon among subjects in their 30s and 40s. The peak frequency of bronchogenic carcinoma occurs between the ages of 61 to 70 years, but in Indian patients the peak occurs a decade earlier, i.e. 51 to 60 years.[13,241] About 15 percent of the patients can be less than 40 years of age[13] and about 40 percent of patients are less than 50 years of age.[12] The prevalence of smoking is less pronounced in younger patients. The sex distribution depends upon the smoking habit in each country, although there is a male preponderance in most series, because of the higher prevalence of smoking in them. Lung cancer has already surpassed breast cancer as a cause of death among US women.[245] The overall male to female ratio in Indian series has been 4.5:1 although this differs in different age groups. The neoplasm occurs most frequently in smokers as discussed earlier[246] or in persons exposed to asbestos or other occupational agents.[247] Women are more likely to be nonsmokers.

Symptoms due to bronchogenic carcinoma may be due to (a) primary tumor as such, (b) due to extra-pulmonary extension, (c) due to metastasis, or (d) due to systemic nonmetastatic symptoms including para-neoplastic syndromes. Symptoms due to primary tumor include cough, expectoration, hemoptysis, dyspnea, chest pain, and fever. Symptoms of extra-pulmonary extension will be chest pain, (involvement of chest wall, soft tissue, bone, nerves, pleura, etc.), dyspnea, hoarseness of voice (vocal cord paralysis), superior vena caval obstruction, dysphagia, and cardiac symptoms. Bron-chorrhea as a symptom is reported to occur in about 10 percent of cases in bronchiolo-alveolar cell carcinoma. Metastasis to different organs will give rise to symptoms pertaining to that particular organ and may include lymph node masses, central nervous system symptoms, liver enlargement, bone pain and cutaneous lesions. Anorexia, weight loss, fever, and weakness are some of the prominent and important systemic symptoms.

A thorough clinical history including that of smoking and occupation should be taken. The onset of the symptoms is acute to subacute with the patient presenting within weeks to few months after the onset of symptoms. The progression is quite rapid with a downhill course. The initial cough may be mistaken as that of a smoker's cough. However a change in pattern, severity and associated systemic features should arouse the suspicion. The other disease that has similar symptoms is tuber-culosis. But the later is of more insidious in onset with a slowly progressive course.

Physical examination of the patient may give impor-tant clues. Emaciation, clubbing, hypertrophic pulmo-nary osteoarthropathy, metastatic lymph nodes parti-cularly in the supraclavicular and other cervical regions, and anemia, may be common findings. Evidence of superior vena caval obstruction may be present. Upper airways obstruction due to enlarged lymph nodes may be manifested as stridor and respiratory distress. Among the right sided node positive lung cancer patients, the highest incidence of nodal involvement occurs in the ipsilateral tracheobronchial group (77%), followed by the ipsilateral hilar nodes group (34.2%). Low mediastinal lymph nodes are involved in about a third of the contralateral tracheobronchial group, 27.3 percent of the anterior tracheal group and in half the subcarinal lymph node group. Among the left sided node positive lung cancer patients, the figures are 76.2 percent, 41.9 percent,

43.8 percent, 25.7 percent, and 44.8 percent respectively. Involvement of supraclavicular, contralateral hilar and upper mediastinal lymph nodes involvement is lower and varies from 0.6 to 19 percent in the right sided lesions and less than 9.5 percent in left sided tumors.[248]

Examination of the chest usually reveals evidence of collapse of a lobe, segment, or the whole lung. This may be either complete or partial according to the extent of occlusion of the bronchial lumen. Obstructive pneu-monitis (or lung abscess) with findings of both conso-lidation and collapse may be another frequent finding. Paradoxical diaphragmatic movement may be seen as a result of the involvement of phrenic nerves. Rarely, obvious chest wall swelling may be the clue to the diagnosis. Pleural effusion, often hemorrhagic, and usually moderate to massive may be present.

A thorough search should be made to find out any possible site of metastasis, including lymph nodes in other sites, bone, skin and scalp. All systems should be examined including the cardiovascular system, nervous system, gastrointestinal system, and the endocrine system. Pericardial effusion, hepatomegaly, ascites, gynecomastia, and various neurological abnormalities may be detected. Particular attention should be given to the presence of extrapulmonary paraneoplastic syn-dromes. Clinical examination may entirely be normal in 5 to 10 percent of cases.

Superior sulcus tumor or Pancoast's tumor is an uncommon form of bronchogenic carcinoma arising in the extreme apex of the lung. Originally described by Pancoast,[249] this is characterized by a distinct group of clinical symptoms and radiographic findings. The tumor is manifested by involvement of the cervical nerves and is characterized by pain along the lower part of the shoulder and inner aspect of the arm along C8, T1 and T2 nerve root distribution. The other features are wasting, and weakness of the small muscles of the hand and sensory loss in the same distribution of nerves. Horner's syndrome (ipsilateral partial ptosis, enophthalmos, meiosis, hypohidrosis, and absent spino-ciliary reflex) is another characteristic feature of this tumor. The incidence is between 2 to 5 percent in bronchogenic carcinoma, and most often it is associated with squamous cell carcinoma. Lung cancers are located predominantly on the right upper lobe regardless of histological characteristics. By definition it is a T3 lesion, and the N stage may be N0-2. Although by and large, the tumor was considered inoperable, and the treatment consisted of radiotherapy only, currently the best results are achieved with preoperative radiotherapy followed by extensive resection.[250]

Superior vena cava syndrome is usually associated with right upper lobe tumors of small cell histology. It is often common in men and include a feeling of fullness in the head or face, dyspnea with orthopnea, cough and swelling of face and upper extremities. Hoarseness of voice can occur due to laryngeal edema, which is worse in the morning and improves once the patient becomes ambulatory postural hoarseness). Syncope may occur and be precipitated by coughing. The initial physical findings are the presence of dilated veins over the anterior chest wall, with flow from above down wards. Subsequently jugular veins dilate and finally the facial and arm veins. Initially the distention of the neck veins may be limited to the right side if only the innominate vein is obstructed. Edema of the face and upper extremities may be accompanied by varying degrees of cyanosis. There may be epistaxis due to rupture of distended nose veins. The conjunctival veins may be dilated. Funduscopy will reveal dilated veins with papilledema in extreme cases. Drowsiness, and lethargy are terminal events because of cerebral edema—*the wet brain syndrome*. The cause of the obstruction is either due to direct extension of the tumor causing compression or intramural invasion or extrinsic compression by secondaries in lymph nodes, or thrombosis. Similar clinical picture is seen with other causes of superior vena caval obstruction. Such causes include lymphomas mainly non-Hodgkin's lymphoma, thymoma, primary sarcoma, extragonadal germinal cell tumor, and rarely granulomatous or fibrosing mediastinitis due to tuberculosis, histoplasmosis, syphilitic aneurysm, intrathoracic goiter, trauma, and idiopathic. Incipient superior vena caval obstruction can be made prominent by infusion of fluid in the upper limb veins, when the swelling becomes more prominent. However, for the confirmation of the diagnosis, venacavogram or contrast CT scan may have to be done. The obstruction may be described as pre-azygous or post-azygous type depending upon the site of obstruction, whether the obstruction occurs before or after the azygous vein joining the superior vena cava. In the later, veins in the abdomen and in the back will be more prominent and distended with an attempt to drain into the inferior vena cava.

A review of over 1000 patients from a large hospital from North India revealed that the male: female ratio was 4.5:1, with smoker: nonsmoker ratio being 2.68:1.[12] Occupation wise they were involved in farming (46.5%), white-collar jobs (24.1%), road working (7.6%), and industrial labor (11.6%). The other 10.1 percent were either unemployed or house-wives. The mean age was 54.6 years in males, and 52.8 years in females. The total

TABLE 22.14: Clinical features of bronchogenic carcinoma

Feature	Clinical (%)	Radiological (%)
Mass lesion with/ without collapse	68	70.7
Cavitary mass	2.3	6.0
Pleural effusion	19.9	25.1
Superior mediastinal obstruction	16	16.7
Clubbing	27.9	-
Hypertrophic pulmonary osteoarthropathy	2.8	-
Horner's syndrome	1.6	-
Rib erosion	-	4.8
Lymphangitis carcinomatosis	-	2.8
Phrenic nerve palsy	-	3.8
COPD	15	20.1
Tuberculosis	1.2	3.8
Normal	6.4	0.4

duration of symptoms at the time of presentation was less than three months in about a third of the patients, three to six months in 46 percent of the cases and more than six months in the remaining 21 percent of the patients. The major symptoms were weakness, anorexia, and weight loss (90%); cough and/or expectoration (88%); hemoptysis (69.2%); chest pain (52.2%); and hoarseness of voice (30%). Other symptoms were fever (20%); dysphagia (21%); facial swelling (20%); and others (31%). The clinical and radiological features are presented in Table 22.14.

Cough (92%), expectoration (79%), dyspnea (67%), and thoracic pain (58%) were the predominant symptoms in a large series reported from Mexico.[241] Another study from Austria[251] reported the common symptoms as dyspnea, hemoptysis, cough, and chest pain. In about 1/5th of the cases the initial diagnosis was something other than lung cancer. Although in most Western series the total duration of symptoms at the time of presentation was much earlier, the same in Indian studies was less than 3 months in about a third of cases, three to six months in 46.4 percent of cases, and about a fifth of the cases presents 6 months after the initial symptom.[12]

Most often, the disease is confused as tuberculosis in areas of high prevalence of the later, particularly in India. Therefore a delay in diagnosis occurs and it is not uncommon to see such patients are on antituberculosis drug therapy for varying lengths of time before a correct diagnosis is made. All the symptoms described above are common in tuberculosis. But certain clues can raise a suspicion for the diagnosis of lung cancer. The points are described in Table 22.15.

The paraneoplastic syndromes are very rare and are seen in less than 5 percent of cases . Various paraneo-

TABLE 22.15: Differentiating points between tuberculosis and lung cancer

Factors	Lung cancer	Pulmonary tuberculosis
Age	Usually elderly	Young and old
Duration of symptoms	Shorter	Longer
Smoking	Common	±
Clubbing	+	Rare
Chest pain	Common	Uncommon
SVC obstruction	Common cause	Very very rare
Hoarseness	Common	Rare (except laryngitis)
Collapse	Common	Unusual in adults
Mass lesion	Favors	Not a finding

TABLE 22.16: Paraneoplastic syndromes due to lung cancer

1. *Paraendocrinal syndromes*
   Cushing's syndrome (5%)
   Syndrome of inappropriate secretion of ADH (SIADH)
   Gynecomastia
   Severe skin darkening due to excess MSH
   Oncogenic osteomalacia
   Hypercalcemia (more common in squamous cell carcinoma)
2. *Nervous system*
   Myasthenia gravis-like syndrome (Eaton-Lambert Syndrome)
   Malignant cachexia
   Neuromyopathy
   Peripheral nerve involvement
   Primary or subacute sensory neuropathy
   Motor neuron disease
   Sensory motor neuropathy
   Limbic encephalitis
   Necrotizing myelopathy
   Central pontine myelinosis
   Cerebellar degeneration
   Retinopathy
3. *Hematological complications*
   Granulocytosis/granulocytopenia
   Thrombocytosis
   Lymphocytopenia
4. *Renal complications*
   Nephrotic syndrome
5. *Skeletal abnormalities*
   Hypertrophic pulmonary osteoarthropathy
6. *Cutaneous complications*
   Sign of Lesser-Trelat (appearance of sudden seborrheic keratosis)
   Acanthosis nigricans
   Erythema gyratum repens
   Polymyositis and dermatomyositis

plastic syndromes produced by lung cancer are shown in Table 22.16.

However, common ones like weakness, anorexia, and weight loss are very common. Other nonmetastatic complications occur in the following frequency:[12,252-255]

Clubbing	27.9%
Hypertrophic osteoarthropathy	2.8%
Gynecomastia	2.8%
Myopathy	0.7%
Neuropathies	0.9%
Cerebellar syndromes	0.4%
Thromboembolic	0.5%
Miscellaneous	1.7%

The mechanisms involved in the production of paraneoplasia include such possibility as the cancer's secretion of a profusion of biologically active products with hormone like specificity, directed at specific receptors within certain tissues, comparable to actions of cachectin. Autoimmune phenomena also play part in certain situations.

DIAGNOSIS

Various diagnostic methods for lung cancer include chest radiograph, CT scan, sputum cytology, bronchoscopy, cytologic and histologic examination of various specimens including that of the pleural fluid, bronchoscopic washings and brushings, bronchial biopsy specimens, and material obtained from metastatic tissues.

CHEST SKIAGRAM

This is the first line of investigation in any suspected case of bronchogenic carcinoma. Both posteroanterior, and lateral views are the minimal requirements. Tomography may be done in some selected cases to detect calcification or to detect pulmonary nodules not visible on standard skiagrams. The most common abnormality is a homogenous opacity with evidence of a mass, or collapse. Malignant lesions will have irregular margin with radiating strands. When lymphatics are blocked, one sees sun rays appearance radiating from the hilum. This is usually associated with lymph node enlargement in the hila or mediastinum. Unresolved pneumonias may be due to bronchogenic carcinoma causing proximal obstruction. About 10 percent of cases will cavitate. The characteristic cavitation, or breakdown, is usually eccentric, irregular in margin with nodularity. This is commonly seen in cases of squamous cell carcinoma. Pleural effusion, and distal pneumonitis are other findings. Mediastinal involvement in the form of lymph node enlargement is suggestive of metastasis to the node. However, absence of lymph node enlargement in chest skiagram does not rule out the possibility of secondaries. Diaphragm may be raised due to phrenic nerve paralysis or due to a volume shrinkage as a result of collapse. Rib erosion should be looked for very carefully, since the presence of this finding in association with a mass lesion, is almost pathognomonic of bronchogenic carcinoma, although there are other rare causes of rib erosion including tuberculosis, hydatid cyst, etc. Evaluation of a solitary pulmonary nodule is discussed earlier in the chapter on diagnostic methods.

Although chest skiagram is not diagnostic of lung cancer, it is the most common and the first line of investigation. Besides a strong suggestion of the disease, disease extension is more accurately assessed when they are present. As for example in a case of lung cancer, hilar/mediastinal lymphadenopathy suggests metastasis, rib erosion, or pleural effusion suggest the involvement of these structures. Although there is a great overlap in different cell types, each group has certain predominant features. Adenocarcinoma presents frequently as a small peripheral mass. Bronchiolo-alveolar cell carcinoma classically presents with multiple alveolar shadows, although nodular or solitary forms can be present.[256] Large cell carcinoma is peripheral in location, but is usually large. A hilar or perihilar mass with or without collapse and/or obstructive pneumonia is the most common finding in squamous cell carcinoma. A central lesion with a hilar or perihilar mass is also commonly seen in small cell carcinoma, although parenchymal masses are not uncommon (Figs 22.23 to 22.61).

Chest skiagram has been used as a screening test in the vulnerable subjects, particularly male smokers above the age of 45. Annual chest skiagram in these subjects may detect the malignancy in an earlier stage, when that can be operable.[229-235]

CT SCAN

Although CT scan has been used increasingly in recent years since its first introduction in the 1970s, its utility in the treatment of bronchogenic carcinoma is not clear,[257,258] although more and more clinicians and surgeons are using this investigation for various purposes. However, a number of potential benefits can be obtained through the use of CT scan. The potential benefits of CT scan include (i) distinguishing benign from malignant nodules; (ii) identifying endobronchial abnormalities; (iii) staging of mediastinal nodes; (iv) evaluation of involvement of contiguous structure; and (v) CT guided biopsy or fine needle aspiration cytology biopsy can be undertaken to obtain histological diagnosis. The main advantage of this investigation is that it is a noninvasive way of evaluating the mediastinal lymph nodes and extent of involvement of other intrathoracic structures. However both false positive and false negative results are possible, particularly for lymph nodes. Enlargement of a mediastinal lymph node may be either due to previous inflammation (i.e. tuberculosis) or hyperplasia, or due to metastasis. Therefore, detection

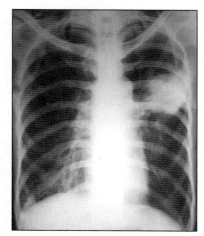

FIGURE 22.23: Dense irregular mass in the left midzone - squamous cell carcinoma

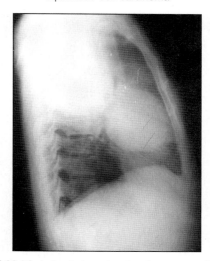

FIGURE 22.24: Lateral view showing the mass to be on the posterial and apical segment of the right upper lobe

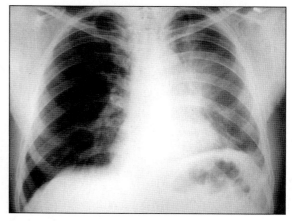

FIGURE 22.25: Carcinoma of lung. Note hilar mass with collapse of left lung with elevated left hemidiaphragm

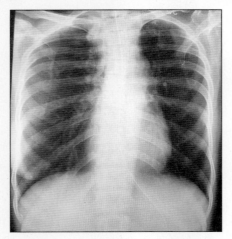

FIGURE 22.26: Carcinoma of the lung with left lung occlusion with local hyperlucency and mosaic perfusion

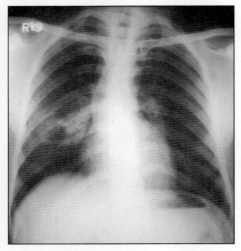

FIGURE 22.27: Cavitating lung cancer

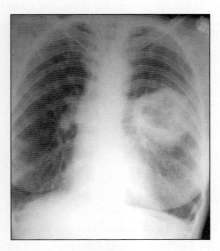

FIGURE 22.28: Cavitating squamous cell carcinoma

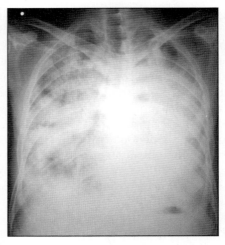

FIGURE 22.29: Bronchioloalveolar cell carcinoma

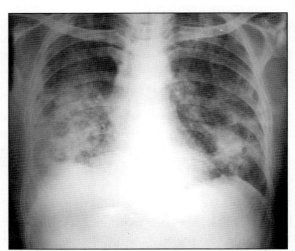

FIGURE 22.30: Bronchioloalveolar cell carcinoma

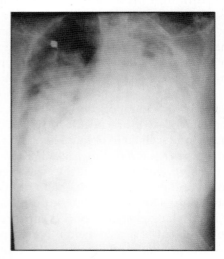

FIGURE 22.31: Bronchioloalveolar cell carcinoma

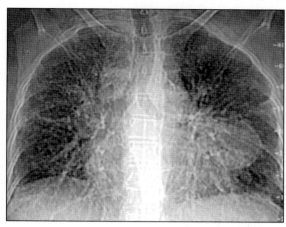

FIGURE 22.32: CXR - Mass lesion in left paracardiac region with thin rim of calcification

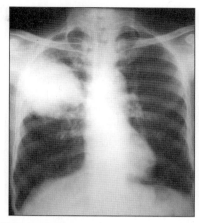

FIGURE 22.35: Dense homogenous opacity due to squomous cell carcinoma

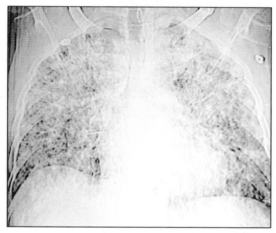

FIGURE 22.33: CXR - Reticular shadowing in both lungs - Lymphangitis carcinomatosis

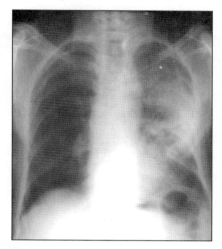

FIGURE 22.36: Adenocarcinoma of left lung. Note the opacity is peripheral

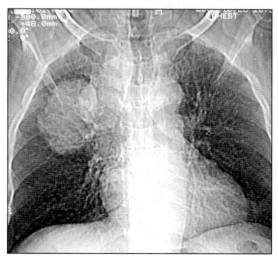

FIGURE 22.34: CXR - Right lung mass with right paratracheal lymphadenopathy

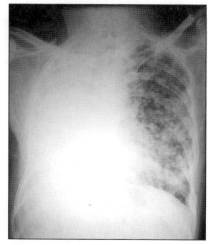

FIGURE 22.37: Right sided mass lesion with metastasis to the left lung

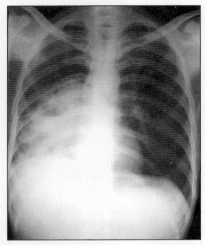

FIGURE 22.38: Eccentric cavitation in lung cancer (Squamous cell carcinoma)

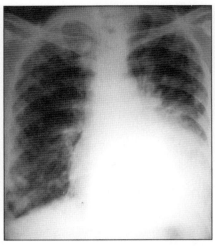

FIGURE 22.41: Left lower lobe mass with metastatic pericardial effusion and right lower lobe metastasis

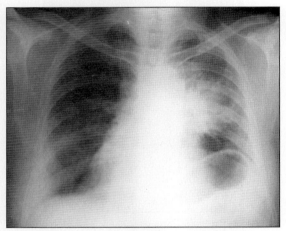

FIGURE 22.39: Left hilar mass with Sun-ray appearance. Note pleural effusion and diaphragmatic palsy

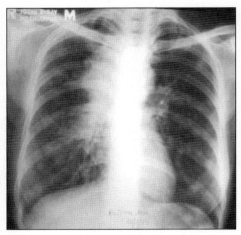

FIGURE 22.42: Left paratracheal mass with hilar involvement

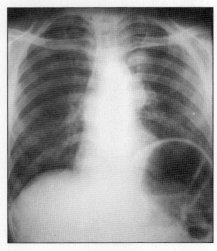

FIGURE 22.40: Left hilar prominence with diaphragmatic paralysis

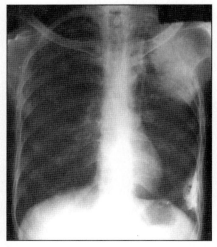

FIGURE 22.43: Left upper lobe mass with rib and chest wall involvement

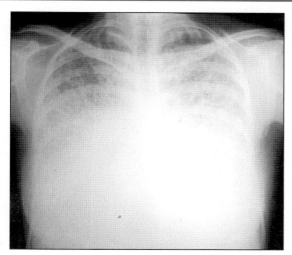

FIGURE 22.44: Lymphangitis carcinomatosis

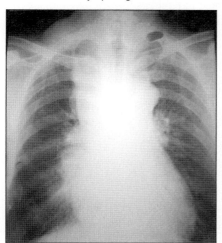

FIGURE 22.45: Mediastinal widening along with bilateral
hilar lymphadenopathy

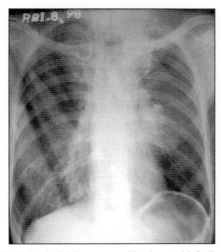

FIGURE 22.46: Left hilar mass with elevated left diaphragm

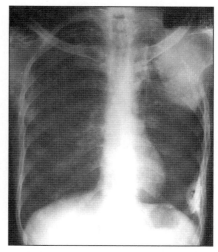

FIGURE 22.47: The mass lesion has eroded the rib
and thoracic cage

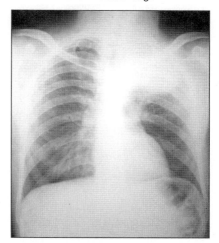

FIGURE 22.48: Primary lung cancer

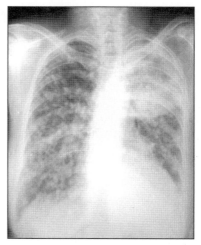

FIGURE 22.49: Primary lung cancer in the left upper lobe
with metastasis to the right lung

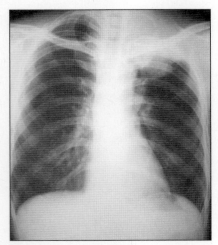

FIGURE 22.50: Rght upper lobe mass lesion with erosion of ribs (Pancoast's tumor)

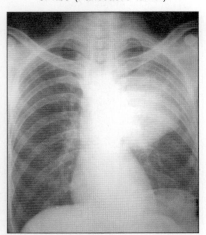

FIGURE 22.51: Right hilar mass with irregular but smooth margins suggestive of lung cancer

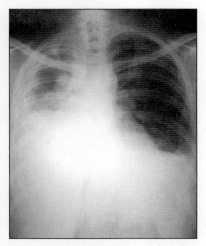

FIGURE 22.52: Right paracardiac mass with bilateral pleural effusion (metastatic)

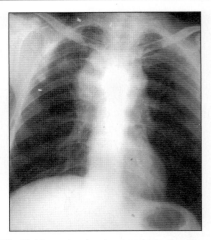

FIGURE 22.53: Right paratracheal mass. Note the hilum is pulled up due to lung collapse with obstructive hyperinflation of the right middle and lower lobe

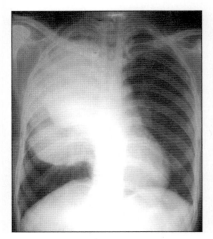

FIGURE 22.54: Right upper lobe mass lesion

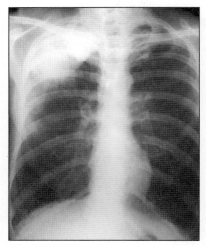

FIGURE 22.55: Right upper lobe mass with dense calcification (squamous cell carcinoma) with changes of COPD

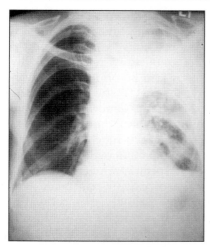

FIGURE 22.56: Right upper zone opacity with left lung collapse. Note hyperluscent right lung

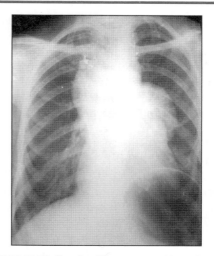

FIGURE 22.59: Small cell lung cancer. Note elevation of left diaphragm

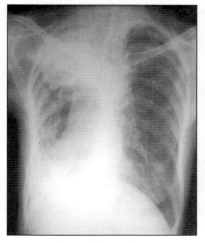

FIGURE 22.57: Scar carcinoma in a fibrosed lung

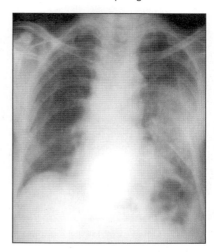

FIGURE 22.60: The lesion has eroded the rib. This is diagnostic of lung cancer

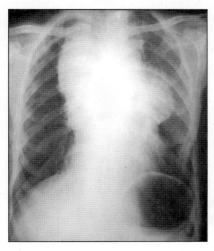

FIGURE 22.58: Small cell lung cancer

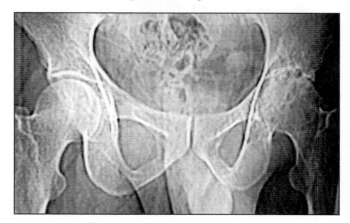

FIGURE 22.61: X-ray Pelvis - Reduced left hip joint space with erosion due to metastasis

of an enlarged lymph node does not necessarily represent metastasis. However, it is suggested that a lymph node size of more than 1.5 to 2 cm is almost due to metastasis. On the other hand, metastasis can be present in a normal sized gland. The other usefulness of the CT scan is the evaluation of involvement of the thoracic wall, pleura, ribs, or vertebrae by the tumor and the detection of calcification. Several studies have compared CT staging of the mediastinum with mediastinoscopy and postsurgical staging. Investigators using the first generation CT scanners with scanning times of 18 to 20 seconds found a low sensitivity in detecting mediastinal lymphadenopathy in 44 to 77 percent of cases. With the use of newer models with a scanning time of 2 to 3 seconds the

sensitivity has improved to 80 to 94 percent. Thus the use of CT scan in lung cancer can be summarized as follows. (i) The predictive value of a negative CT scan is in the order of 90 to 95 percent and in such cases mediastinoscopy can be omitted before thoracotomy. (ii) Similarly, when CT shows the mediastinum is normal, but the hilum is abnormal, mediastinal exploration can be omitted before thoracotomy. The predictive value of a positive scan is much more variable (50-100%) and therefore mediastinal exploration should possibly be undertaken. Specific appearances on CT scan for particular type of cancer has been described. For example, in bronchiolo-alveolar cell carcinoma three patterns has been described as: solitary; pneumonic; and the diffuse forms[259] (Figs 22.62 to 22.72).

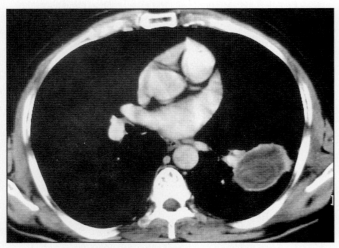

FIGURE 22.62: CT Chest - Left lower lobe mass with central low attenuating necrosis

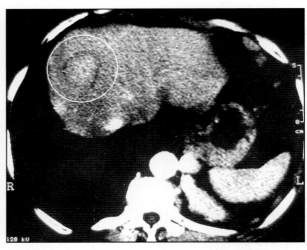

FIGURE 22.64: CT Abdomen - Isodense mass with peripehral halo - Liver metastasis

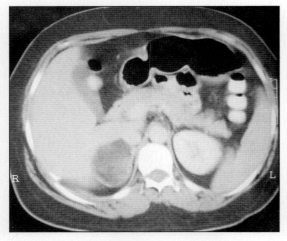

FIGURE 22.63: Abdominal CT. Rt suprarenal region mass lesion - Metastasis

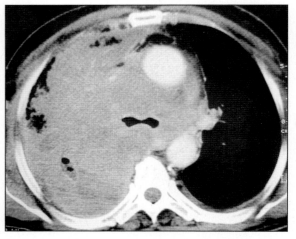

FIGURE 22.65: CT Chest - Carcinoma of right lung infiltrating mediastinum, SVC compression and AP window infiltration

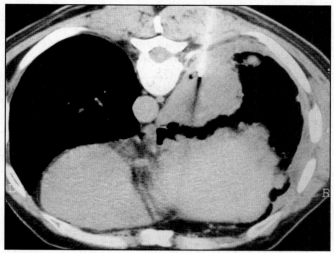

FIGURE 22.66: CT Chest - CT guided FNAC from right posterior lung mass

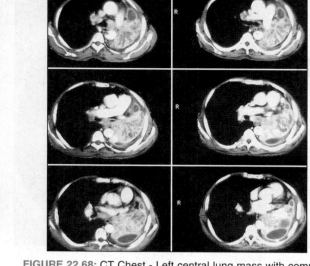

FIGURE 22.68: CT Chest - Left central lung mass with complete bronchial obstruction

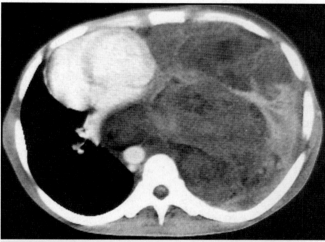

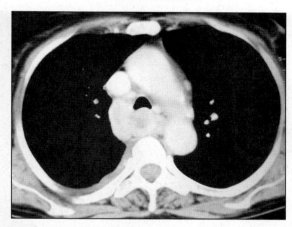

FIGURE 22.69: CT Chest - Mass in retrotracheal region with pressure over trachea

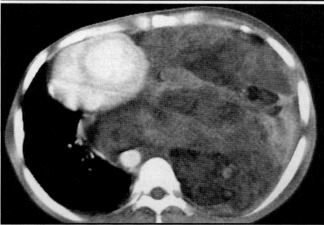

FIGURE 22.67: CT Chest - Huge necrotising mass in left hemithorax - Malignant

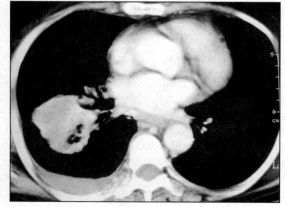

FIGURE 22.70: CT Chest - Mass lesion in right lower lobe with eccentric cavitation

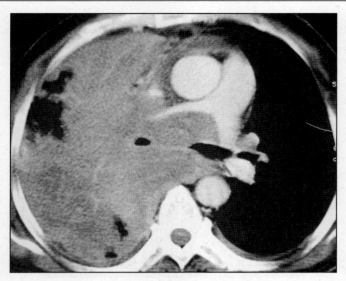

FIGURE 22.71: CT Chest - Right lung malignancy compressing SVC and right main pulmonary artery and sub-carinal invasion

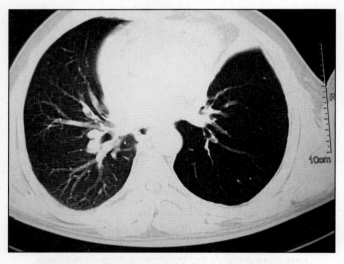

FIGURE 22.72: CT scan of the chest of the same patient with mosaic perfusion

MEDIASTINOSCOPY[260]

Metastasis to the mediastinal lymph nodes is a common problem in lung cancer. CT scan will indicate the presence of enlarged lymph nodes, but can not decide whether this is due to metastasis or not and there is possibility that normal sized glands may have micro-metastasis. Therefore anterior cervical mediastinoscopy has been used for many years to make a biopsy of these nodes to decide the diagnosis and stage of the disease. Recent results show that patients with a normal mediastinal appearance on chest X-ray will show positive findings at mediastinoscopy in about 25 percent of cases. Of those patients who did not undergo resection as a result of mediastinoscopy, 79 percent died within one year and in whom pulmonary resection was done on the basis of negative mediastinoscopy, there was a five year survival in 25 percent of cases. The procedure is carried out under general anesthesia and has a very low mortality rate of 0.09 percent. For most lesions mediastinal exploration is best undertaken by cervical mediastinoscopy, which allows assessment of both paratracheal chains and a limited examination of the main cranial nodes. For patients with left upper lobes tumors, many prefer to do a left anterior mediastinotomy, as the arch of the aorta makes examination of the nodes in the aortic window very difficult. The procedure, however is not entirely without risk and a 3 percent incidence of hemorrhage and minor complications of 2.6 percent has been reported.[261]

MAGNETIC RESONANCE IMAGING (MRI)

This procedure has recently been introduced into the diagnostic evaluation of lung cancer. Initial reports suggest that MRI evaluation of the mediastinum and hilum is approximately to that of the CT. The multiplanar capability of MRI is probably advantageous in assessment of the superior sulcus tumors and possibly evaluation of the aortic-pulmonary window region, an area difficult for CT. Also MR may have advantage over CT in assessment of chest wall invasion.

RADIONUCLIDE SCANS

Isotope scans of the brain, liver, and bones using technetium 99m, or radiolabelled albumin, gallium-67, and 57-Co-labelled bleomycin have been used to detect metastasis in these regions, particularly to evaluate symptoms suggesting the possibility of metastatic cancer to these organs. Some investigators have reported these techniques to be of value in detecting asymptomatic metastases from bronchogenic carcinoma especially searching for bone metastases. Gallium-67 shows an abnormal accumulation in 80 to 90 percent of all bronchogenic carcinoma. However, such accumulation also can occur in inflammatory lesions limiting the usefulness of the technique. Recently, immunoscintigraphy using iodine-131 anti-carcinoembryonic antigen and anti-carbohydrate 19 to 9 monoclonal antibodies has been used to detect mediastinal lymph node metastasis.[262] However, these tests have no extra advantage over CT scan and they are not cost-effective.

PET SCANS

Some investigators use PET scan to delineat hilar lymph node involvement as well as to evaluate lung nodules. It is discussed in detail in earlier section.

CYTOLOGY

With experienced personnel and using multiple, combined proper techniques, 70 to 90 percent of all lung cancers can be diagnosed by cytopathological examination. The various methods used to collect material for these examinations include sputum obtained from spontaneous cough or by induction; tracheobronchial secretions collected during bronchoscopy; percutaneous transthoracic needle aspiration; direct fine needle aspiration cytology of the metastatic sites like lymph nodes, subcutaneous nodules etc., and the pleural or pericardial fluids, transcarinal and transbronchial aspiration cytology.[263-277]

Sputum. Spontaneous cough is the most accessible and important pulmonary material for cytological examination. The method is simple, inexpensive, and without risk. However various factors including the method of collection, time of the day collected, number of samples examined, type of neoplasm, and location of the lesion, etc. decide the diagnostic yield. The most valuable specimen is the early morning sputum, which has the maximum yield. The cytological examination may be negative, even if, the tumor is large and central. When spontaneous sputum production is not enough, it can be aided by chest percussion or vibration of the chest wall. Sputum brought up during the first two hours and the next morning after bronchoscopy is frequently of great diagnostic value. For patients who can not produce sputum spontaneously, induction is a great help to them. Various methods are available including nebulization of tap water, and hyper- or hypotonic saline. Diagnostic yields of the sputum examination is reported to be 60 to 75 percent depending on the cell type and location of the tumor and provided the sampling is adequate and examination is done properly. Central lesions and squamous cell carcinoma are diagnosed most often easily by sputum examination. Examination of at least 5 specimen samples is recommended for better diagnostic yield. However, the examination is time consuming for the cytologists and in view of the other easily available cytological material including bronchoscopic washings and brushings, many centers do not take up this time consuming method of examination.

Sputum cytology has been used as a screening procedure in many early detection of lung cancer programs. Unfortunately, the yield of sputum cytology is very low. In the John Hopkins lung cancer screening project, among 5426 smokers, 233 had lung cancer on the basis of sputum cytology, over a period of 9 years.[278] Sputum cytology specimens obtained at initial screening showed cancer cells in only 11 subjects. Recently, a new, quantitative solid-state microscopy system has been developed at the British Columbia Cancer Research Center, which can produce a larger vision wherein details of the cell structure can be studied with automatic cell focus.[263] This will enhance the identification of atypical cells in the sputum in earlier stages of development of lung cancer.

Bronchial washings and brushings. Examination of bronchial brushings and washings obtained during bronchoscopy yields 70 to 90 percent cytologic detection in clinically suspected lesions. With the availability of fiberoptic bronchoscopes, samples from more peripheral lesions can be collected, and both central and peripheral malignancies can be diagnosed more easily. Cytological samples can be obtained also during bronchoscopy through transbronchial needle aspiration of carinal/ mediastinal lymph nodes and peripheral masses.

Transthoracic needle aspiration is used more frequently now a days in many centers.[278] The method is usually employed when other methods like sputum and bronchoscopy results are negative. Even some will prefer this as the first method provided the lesion is quite superficial and can easily be reached by the needle. The procedure can also be performed for deep seated lesions under fluoroscopic or CT guides. The diagnostic yield is to the tune of 80 to 90 percent. Failure of the method can usually be attributed to inadequate cellular samples, aspiration from the necrotic center of the tumor, or aspiration of the inflammatory area surrounding the neoplasm. When the pleura or pericardium are involved the cytological yield varies from 33 to 87 percent.

BRONCHOSCOPY

After the first discovery of bronchogenic carcinoma by Ikeda, the main indication of fiberoptic bronchoscopy has been suspected bronchogenic carcinoma all over the world and this is perhaps the most used method of diagnosis of lung cancer.[279-295] After the advent of fiberoptic bronchoscopes, rigid bronchoscopes are virtually not been used for this purpose. The advantages and the procedure has been described earlier. In bronchogenic carcinoma, the entire tracheobronchial tree can be examined. The lesions can be visualized under direct vision. The various abnormalities include growth, abnormal mucosa with areas of inflammation, easy bleeding, granularity, nodularity, and areas of bronchial stenosis. The Japan

Lung Cancer Society has identified 11 categories of findings: epithelial tumor, subepithelial tumor, heightened longitudinal relief, indistinct bronchial cartilage, mucosal irregularity, vascular engorgement, bleeding, redness, edema, accentuated irregular folds, and compression.[296] The correlation of broncoscopic findings with histological extent has also been reported.[281] The bronchoscopic findings in case of subepithelial invasion consisted of vascular engorgement, bleeding, subepithelial tumor, and emphasized longitudinal relief; irregularity of the mucosa is observed in cases of epithelial or muscular invasion; indistinct bronchial cartilage is observed in cases of invasion proximal to the extramural layer; accentuated irregular folds are observed in cases of invasion of the extramural or cartilage layers; and edema and redness are not specific for malignancy (Figs 22.73 to 22.75).

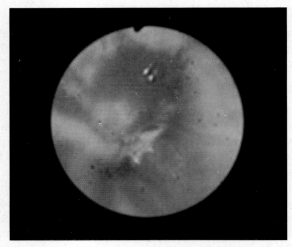

FIGURE 22.75: Bronchogenic carcinoma showing mucosal infiltration

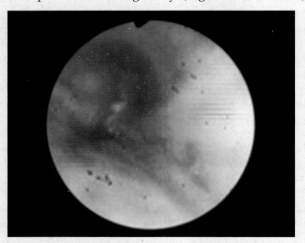

FIGURE 22.73: Endobronchial growth as seen in a case of carcinoma of lung. Note an ILBT catheter in position for brachytherapy

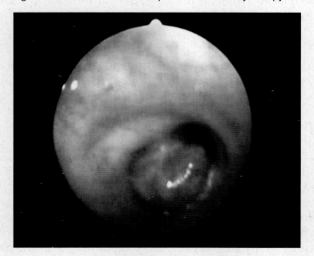

FIGURE 22.74: Endobronchial growth as seen through a FOB

Location of the tumor with extension to the carina or trachea is helpful for the staging of lung cancer. Recently hematoporphyrin derive (HPD) has been used to detect early abnormalities of the bronchial mucosa by detection of the fluorescence through the bronchoscope.[262] Biopsy, washings, brushings, transbronchial aspiration biopsy of the mediastinum and peripheral masses, transcarinal aspiration, and transendobronchial aspiration can be undertaken to obtain material for cytological and histological examination. The diagnostic yield of bronchial biopsy specimens varies from 70 to 90 percent depending upon the site of the tumor, type of the tumor, number of specimens examined, and experience of the pathologist and the endoscopist. Central lesions, with visible tumors and multiple samples give better diagnostic yield.

Wang has described a staging system based on the bronchoscopy and material obtained during the procedure.[295]

HEMATOLOGICAL AND BIOCHEMICAL INVESTIGATION

Routine blood tests are of little help in the evaluation of the patient with bronchogenic carcinoma. Anemia is common in these patients. However the presence of anemia, thrombocytopenia, and leukopenia in a patient with lung cancer may suggest the presence of bone marrow metastasis and a biopsy of the bone marrow is indicated. Routine blood biochemistry although nonspecific, may show hyponatremia due to syndrome of inappropriate antidiuretic hormone production, or hypercalcemia, or an abnormally elevated alkaline phosphatase due to metastasis in liver or bones.

TUMOR MARKERS/PRODUCTS

Malignant cells produce and release several substances which are classified as hormones, enzymes, and tissue antigens (see above). Of the lung cancer cell types, small cell cancer type produces most of these ectopic substances, although other cell types are also capable of producing some of these. Various hormones, and other substances that are reported to be produced by lung cancer cells are shown in Table 22.17.

Some of the other biological markers and oncofetal antigens that are produced in lung cancer include neurone specific enolase (NSE), the BB isoenzyme of creatine kinase (CK-BB), the neuropeptide bombesin/gastrin-releasing peptide (GRP), the key APUD enzyme L-dopa decarboxylase, carcinoembryonic antigens (CEA), beta$_2$-macroglobuline, and serum ferritin. However, their usefulness as diagnostic markers are not very clear, although some of them may be useful to follow the course and prognosis of the disease.

MANAGEMENT

Before deciding the treatment modality, histological diagnosis, performance status and staging of the disease is very essential. The assessment of the performance status of the patient is shown in Table 22.18. While the international staging system discussed earlier is suitable for nonsmall cell cancers, the same is not applicable for small cell lung cancers, because of the early spread of the later. Very rarely, however, one may see a small cell lung cancer in the early TNM stages.

Treatment of lung cancer is divided into:
(i) Surgery
(ii) Radiotherapy
(iii) Chemotherapy
(iv) A combination of the above
(v) Immunotherapy
(vi) General care of the patient.

The choice of a particular mode of therapy will depend upon the cell type and the stage of the disease. From management point of view, lung cancer is divided into small cell lung cancer (SCLC) and nonsmall cell lung cancer (NSCLC). The later includes entities like squamous cell carcinoma, adenocarcinoma and the large cell anaplastic carcinoma. SCLC differs from NSCLC in its cell of origin, rapidity of growth, propensy of rapid metastasis, production of ectopic hormones and amines and response to therapy While chemotherapy is the accepted mode of therapy for SCLC, surgery is rarely feasible in these cases because of widespread metastasis at the time of diagnosis. On the otherhand, NSCLC is relatively resistant to chemotherapy and surgery is the only definite form of therapy in the early stage of the disease. The problem of radiotherapy is that it is only a local mode of treatment and therefore, will not be able to control metastatic disease. However, all the three modalities of treatment have some role in each of the cell types.

TABLE 22.17: Ectopic production of hormones in lung cancer[194,195,297,298]

Hormones	Incidence (%)
ACTH (Adrenocorticotropic hormone)	24-30
HCG-β (Human chorionic gonadotropin)	6-13
MSH (Melanocyte-stimulating hormone)	19
Calcitonin	
ADH (Antidiuretic hormone)	65
Cortisol	33
Estrogen and progesteron	2-3
Prolactin	
Growth hormone	9
Other Peptide Hormones	
β-endorphin	45
Oxytocin	30
parathormone	27
Insulin	5
Gastrin	20
Glucagon	11

TABLE 22.18: The performance status of lung cancer patients[299]

A. *The Kornofsky Performance Scale*

Normal. No complaints. No evidence of disease	100%
Able to carry on normal activity, minor signs or symptoms of disease	90%
Normal activity with effort, some signs or symptoms of disease	80%
Cares for self' unable to carry on normal activity or to do active work	70%
Requires occasional assistance but is able to care for most of his needs	60%
Requires considerable assistance and frequent medical care	50%
Disabled; requires special care and assistance	40%
Severely disabled, hospitalization is indicated although death may not be imminent	30%
Very sick, hospitalization necessary, active supportive treatment necessary	20%
Moribund, fatal processes progressing rapidly	10%

B. *ECOG (ZUBROD) Scale*

Grade	Definition
0	Fully active, able to carry on all pre-disease activities without restriction (Kornofsky 90-100)
1	Restricted in physically strenuous activity but ambulatory and able to carryout work of a light or sedentary nature like office work and light house work (Kornofsky 70-80)
2	Ambulatory and capable of all self-care but unable to carryout any work activity, up and about more than 50 percent of waking hours (Kornofsky 50-60)
3	Capable of only limited self care, confined to bed or chair 50 percent or more of waking hours (Kornofsky 30-40)
4	Completely disabled, cannot carryout any self care, totally confined to bed or chair (Kornofsky 10-20).

ECOG-Eastern Cooperative Oncology Group.

APPROACH TO STAGING OF LUNG CANCER

The stage of disease is important for the type of treatment, an approach to correctly stage the disease is an essential component of management of lung cancer. (a) Nonsmall cell lung cancer (NSCLC): The International Association for Study of Lung Cancer (IASLC) has recommended the following pretreatment staging at the third IASLC workshop on therapy of NSCLC, in 1993.[300] The main objective of the recommendations of the expert group was that the (i) histological diagnosis must be proved before proceeding to the staging; (ii) the staging procedure must be simple and widely applicable without being limited to the lowest common denominator; (iii) the staging protocol must identify patients suitable for treatment with curative intent since there is no purpose to staging for palliative therapy; (iv) the staging protocol is applicable to good clinical practice with all forms of therapy. However, each institution can prefer additional investigations either for treatment or trial purposes. The protocol is TNM based (UICC or AJC equivalent). However, patient suitability is to be separately assessed.

The staging protocol involves 3 steps and is shown in Table 22.19.

(b) Small cell lung cancer: Two systems are Small cell lung cancer: Two systems are currently available for staging small cell carcinoma; the systems proposed by the VALG and the revised TNM system as above. The system of the VALG classified patients into two categories of "limited" and "extensive" small cell lung cancer, depending on whether all known tumors can be treated within a tolerable single radiotherapy port or not. This system is usually used in clinical practice, is sufficient for treatment decisions regarding local radiotherapy, and carries prognostic information independent of whether chemotherapy is used or not.[301] The IASLC study group has recommended the following classification and procedures required as shown in Table 22.20.[302,303]

It has been suggested that the staging should be based on clinical staging, pathological staging after surgery, and restaging can be undertaken after a particular therapy is administered.[304-306]

SMALL CELL LUNG CANCER

1. Chemotherapy

Small cell carcinoma at the time of diagnosis is considered to be a systemic disease because of early metastasis. Autopsy studies have shown that about 1/3rd of cases will have metastasis to brain, bone, and the liver each. Logically therefore, chemotherapy is considered to be the treatment of choice. The usual TNM system of classification is not well suited for SCLC as more than 95 percent of the patients will be classified as having stage IIIB or IV disease. Of all modalities of treatment available chemotherapy is the cornerstone of treatment for this type of lung cancer. Fortunately small cell lung cancer responds well to chemotherapy. Therefore world wide attention has been paid to treat the disease with more aggressive combination chemotherapy. In fact a large number of trials have established this fact.[307-351] Current trials in patients aged 70 years or less provide a response rate of 80 percent with complete response in 50 percent of cases and median survival of 14 to 16 months with a 2 years disease-free survival in 10 to 20 percent of cases in limited stage disease. For extensive stage disease the values are 8 to 11 months and 1 to 2 percent respectively. Some more recent analysis of data have shown that 24 percent of the patients with limited stage disease survived 2 years or more, and 7 percent survived 5 years or more. In the extensive disease population, 23 percent lived 1 year or more, 4 percent lived 2 years or more, and only 1 percent lived for 5 years. The other prognostic factors besides age, are performance status (higher the performance status, better is the prognosis), sex (females do better than males), presence or absence of pleural effusion and serum LDH levels.

The ideal therapeutic goal of chemotherapy in SCLC is to develop a treatment protocol which produces the highest percentage of long term disease free survival (cure) with the less possible morbidity due to the therapy itself. Many agents have shown antitumor activity against this cell type and they are shown in Table 22.21.[329]

However, it is established conclusively that a combination of drugs is superior to single agents. Many studies of combination chemotherapy have been carried out during the last decade. The most commonly used combinations are shown in Table 22.22. In the last few years there have been a tendency to include VP-16 in the treatment based on studies which show that combinations with this drug are superior to those without it.

The duration of treatment is uncertain. Most trials are maintaining chemotherapy for periods of 6 to 12 months, with a tendency to shorten the therapy during the last few years, provided that it was intensive. After about three to six months a restaging is done including a liver and bone marrow and bronchoscopy. If there is a complete remission, treatment can be stopped after six months. It is also true that even with complete remission after one year of therapy about 1/3rd of all patients will relapse.

In spite of advances in the chemotherapeutic regimens, the median survival for this cell types remains

TABLE 22.19: IASLC staging protocol for Nonsmall cell lung cancer

Investigation	Patient group	Confirmatory test
STEP I		
Clinical history (weight loss, performance status)	All	As appropriate
Clinical examination	All	As appropriate
Chest radiograph (PA, lateral)	All	Aspiration of effusion
Blood tests (Hb, Alkaline phosphatase transaminases, LDH)	All	As for high risk patients
If still thought suitable for curative therapy then proceed to step II.		
STEP II		
Bronchoscopy	All patients with central tumor or in whom central extension is suspected mediastinal exploration.	The features of proximal, extrinsic compression are unreliable and require further evaluation of mediastinum by CT and/or
Bone scan	High risk group (nonspecific symptoms)	Skeletal X-rays ± CT/MRI of bone if doubtful result
CT chest and upper abdomen (to lower pole of kidneys, with IV contrast study of mediastinal vessels)	Dubious finding confirmed All patients if available	
Liver ultrasound	High risk group, if CT not available	
Brain assessment by CT or MRI	High risk group	
If still thought suitable for curative therapy then proceed to step III.		
STEP III		
Bronchoscopy if not previously done	All patients	
Thoracoscopy or video-assisted	If pleural effusion is present, thoracoscopy. Cytology negative but clinically suspected	
Mediastinal exploration	To be done preoperatively by	
	• Transcarinal aspiration • Cervical mediastinoscopy	In whom CT suggests mediastinal invasion or if CT shows nodes > 1 cm
	• Additional evaluation of the subaortic fossa by left anterior mediastinotomy	The above group with tumors of the left upper lobe and left main bronchus
	• This must be performed intraoperatively and preoperatively • Palpation insufficient • Careful and extensive mediastinal dissection	All patients including those whose mediastinum has been assessed
	• Separate labeling as per ATS of excised nodes for subsequent histological examination (only N1 nodes on resected specimens) • Re-evaluation of T stage	

unchanged since the 1970s, but in the last decade several studies have suggested means to improve the results of chemotherapy. These are: (i) use of alternating noncross-resistant chemotherapy to delay or prevent the emergence of drug resistance during therapy; (ii) administration of drugs according to the cell cycle kinetics; (iii) incorporation of new drugs like JM-8, JM-9 and VM-26, having high antitumor activity; (iv) intensive high dose chemotherapy with or without bone marrow rescue; (v) simultaneous use of synergistic compounds; (vi) use of drugs according to the tumor cell culture and sensitivity; (vii) use of immunostimulants; and (viii) use of anti-

TABLE 22.20: Staging of small cell carcinoma	
Limited	- Disease confined to one hemithorax - With or without ipsilateral or contralateral mediastinal or supraclavicular lymph node metastasis - With or without ipsilateral pleural effusions independent of cytology
Extensive	- Any disease sites beyond the definition of limited disease

Staging procedures

General

History, physical examination, blood counts, serum biochemistry, histology/cytology

For local disease

Chest X-ray, Chest CT, fibreoptic bronchoscopy, mediastinoscopy, cytology of effusion and supraclavicular node

For distant disease

Bone scan and X-rays, ultrasound or CT abdomen, fine needle aspiration cytology, aspiration or biopsy of bone marrow, brain CT. *All these procedures are not required for routine management and may be necessary for clinical trials.*

TABLE 22.21: Active agents against small cell lung cancer[329]

Drugs	Approximate response rate (%)
Ifosfamide	50
Teniposide	50
Etoposide	40
Carboplatin	40
Cyclophosphamide	40
Vincristine	35
Methotrexate	35
Doxorubicin	30
Hexamethylmelamine	30
Vinblastine	30
Vindesine	30
Cisplatin	15
Lomustine	15
Newer drugs	
Taxanes	
Paclitaxel	34-41
Docitaxale	28
Camptothecins	
CPT-11	47-78
Topotecan	35-39
Gemcitabine	30

coagulants (warfarin). These methods are experimental at present and can not be recommended for routine use.

Associated complications like superior vena caval obstruction can be treated with chemotherapy alone with similar results to that of radiotherapy. If the effect is not observed within first few days, palliative radiotherapy may be tried for relief of obstruction.

Treatment of primary central nervous system metastasis is systemic chemotherapy with concomitant radiotherapy because of the poor penetration of many

TABLE 22.22: Selective chemotherapy regimens for small cell carcinoma of the lung		
Regimens		**Dose and schedule**
1.	Cyclophosphamide	1 gm/m^2 iv day 1 q 4 weeks
	CCNU	70 mg/m^2 PO day 1 q 4 weeks
	Vincristine	1.3 mg/m^2 iv (maximum 2 mg) day 1 q 4 weeks, except weekly for the first 4 weeks
	VP-16	70 mg/m^2 PO daily on days 2-5 q 4 week
2.	Cyclophosphamide	1.5 g/m^2 iv q 3 weeks
	Adriamycin	40 mg/m^2 q 3 weeks
	Vincristine	2 mg/m^2 q 3 weeks
3.	VP-16	50 mg/m^2 iv daily × 5 q 3 weeks
	Adriamycin	45 mg/m^2 iv × 1 q 3 weeks
	Cyclophosphamide	1 gm/m^2 iv q 3 weeks
4.	Ifosfamide	5 g/m^2 iv day 1 or 1.5 g/m^2 day 1-5
	VP-16	100-120 mg/m^2 iv day 1-3
5.	Carboplatin	300 mg/m^2 iv day 1
	VP-16	100 mg/m^2 iv days 1-3
6.	Ifosfamide	5 g/m^2 iv day 1
	Etoposide (VP-16)	100 mg/m^2 iv days 1-3
	Carboplatin	400 mg/m^2 iv day 1
7.	Irinotecan	100 mg/m^2 day 1
	Cisplatin	60 mg/m^2 day 1

The dose is calculated per sq. meter of body surface area. iv—intravenous; po—per oral.

antineoplastic drugs, although many recent studies have questioned the benefits of radiotherapy.

Results of treatment of relapse have been disappointing. Most patients usually relapse within 10 to 12 months. This may occur either locally or at sites of metastasis. A multifocal relapse will usually lead to a change in chemotherapy and the regimen has to include other active agents that were not used initially.

The palliation of symptoms such as syndrome of inappropriate ADH secretion will almost exclusively depend on the general response to systemic chemotherapy.

As administration of maximum chemotherapy is necessary, a considerable degree of complications is anticipated.[352-354] These include drug specific effects (e.g. nephrotoxicity with cisplatin and neuropathy with vincristine) and myelosuppression with serious infection problems during episodes of leucopenia. In general serious problems develop in less than 25 percent of cases and mortality occurs in less than 5 percent of cases due to this. Late side effects like acute myeloblastic leukaemia develop in long term survivors particular in those treated with regimens containing alkylating agents.

2. Radiotherapy

Small cell lung cancer is the most radiosensitive of all lung cancers.[355,356] Indications of radiotherapy in this type of cancer are: (i) Palliative therapy; (ii) Local irradiation as an adjuvant to systemic therapy; and (iii) prophylactic cranial irradiation. While there is no controversies about the use of radiotherapy in SCLC for palliative purposes, there is still considerable debate about its role as prophylactic cranial irradiation and as primary therapy. SCLC is highly sensitive to both radiotherapy and chemotherapy, but it is also regarded as disseminated from diagnosis; hence the ultimate ability to survive really depends on the efficacy of systemic agents used. For years radiotherapy has been used for the treatment because it was proved to be superior to surgery by prolonging survival. This was proved in the 1960s by the British Medical research Council. In the 1970s systemic chemotherapy was used as the cornerstone of treating SCLC. The problem of course was the local recurrence. It was therefore, important in controlling the local disease, at least to prevent/control recurrences which is more common in the primary site. Combined chemotherapy and radiotherapy has superiority over chemotherapy alone in all aspects except toxicity, both in terms of tumor response and median and long-term survival. The combined therapy has yielded twice fewer chest failures, longer long-term survival, and similar tumor responses and median survival, but also higher fatal toxicities.[357-363] A recent meta-analysis from the first 13 world wide randomized studies evaluating chemotherapy with or without chest irradiation[364] showed that the relative risk of death for the combined modality therapy compared with chemotherapy alone was 0.86 (p = 0.001).

The timing of radiotherapy is also not settled for localized SCLC. There are 5 conceptual combinations that have been explored: (i) sequential administration, when chemotherapy follows full course radiotherapy; (ii) simultaneous or concurrent administration; (iii) alternating radiotherapy between chemotherapy cycles (sandwich technique), radiotherapy either given early in divided fashion between chemotherapy cycles or given later, halfway through induction chemotherapy; (iv) sequential with radiotherapy following full induction chemotherapy (consolidation approach); and a (v) combination of concurrent and alternating. Three recent studies suggest that chest radiotherapy should be given concurrently with chemotherapy or in alternation with the radiotherapy starting not later than the third cycle of chemotherapy.[365-368] The total daily dose of radiotherapy is unresolved. However most studies use a total dose of 45 to 50 Gy in divided fractions.

The use of half-body irradiation, while promising, is still investigational. While the technique is valuable, it is limited by its systemic toxicity, which can be increased with adriamycin and perhaps with other drugs. Half body irradiation may very well be equivalent to an effective systemic cycle and in this fashion either consolidate or help treat disease. Other modes of therapy like total body irradiation, use of radiosensitizers, hypothermia and neutrons remain at experimental levels. With the use of computer dosimetry, including multiplane dosimetry with three dimensional display, a better definition of treatment volume can be achieved thereby minimizing radiation damage to normal lung tissue and adjacent tissues. There is no clear consensus regarding the optimal fraction size of radiotherapy. Large radiotherapy fractions have been associated with unacceptable and potentially lethal late toxicities.[369] Majority of trials have used standards fractions of 1.8 to 2.8 Gy/day, although fractions as high as 3.0 Gy has been used by some investigators. More recently, the concept of multiple daily fractionation (MDF) of radiotherapy is being investigated.[370]

Prophylactic cranial irradiation (PCI) or elective brain irradiation (EBI) has proved to substantially decrease the incidence of brain metastasis. However, there is no effect on survival, mainly because more effective systemic control of the disease is essential.[371-373] Some long-term adverse effects particularly on the central nervous system has been observed in long term survivors. In general the view is that it should be given to patients only who show complete response within the first two to three months after initial therapy. Most centers use 25 to 35 Gy in 8 to 14 fractions over two to two and a half weeks.

Other than for palliative purposes, there is no use for radiotherapy in extensive disease of SCLC. However, for patients with chest recurrences, consideration for chest radiotherapy and perhaps etoposide-platinum chemotherapy may be tried.

3. Surgery

The role of surgery in patients with SCLC is still uncertain and earlier, this form of therapy was abandoned. However, in recent years, the role of surgery has been re-examined.[374] Less than 5 percent of patients who present with T1 or T2 N0M0 disease may benefit from surgery followed by chemotherapy. A five year survival rate of 23 percent is achieved compared to less than 15 percent for patients treated with surgery alone. The 5 year survival correlates with stage of the disease: T1N0M0, 60 percent; T1N1M0 or T2N0M0 approximately 30 percent. Others have reported longer survival following surgery alone.[375-377] Comparable results however, have been obtained in this category of patients with chemotherapy alone.

More recently secondary surgery has been tried in patients who have obtained complete remission after combination chemotherapy given for two to four months.[377-381] However, the number of patients in these studies is too small to allow firm conclusion.

4. Immunotherapy and Others

Immunotherapy has been used in a limited extent in SCLC. The use of BCG, BCG-methanol extract, levamisole and interferon together with chemotherapy has shown disappointing results.

Various hematopoietic growth factors like erythropoietin, granulocyte colony stimulating factor (G-CSF), Granulocyte-macrophage colony stimulating factor (GM-CSF), and autologous bone marrow transplants have been used in conjunction with intensification of chemotherapy as a bone marrow rescue measure.[382]

NONSMALL CELL LUNG CANCER (NSCLC)

1. Surgery

The best treatment for these group of carcinoma, is perhaps surgery, if they are operable and is the only potentially curative treatment for non-small cell lung cancer.[383-389] Since both operability and survival of the depend upon the stage of the disease, it is very important that a proper staging is done before such a decision is taken. The recommendations for such procedures is discussed earlier. However a practical approach to such a staging is shown in Figure 22.76. The fitness of the patient for undergoing surgery is also important. Many

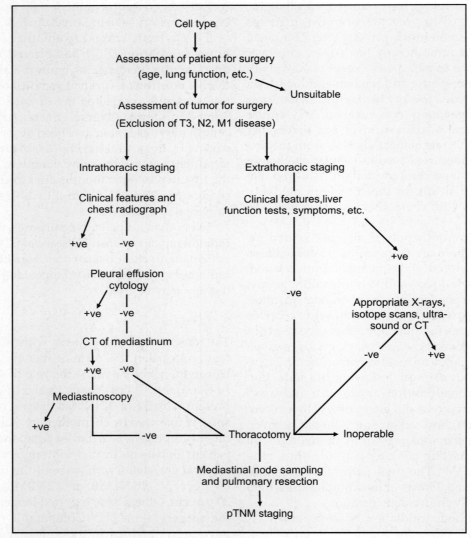

FIGURE 22.76: Diagnostic procedures for proper staging of NSCLC. pTNM-postsurgical pathological staging

TABLE 22.23: Preoperative evaluation

Very low risk	Very high risk	Moderate risk
Normal cardiac size and function, blood pressure, and ECG	Congestive cardiac failure ventricular arrhythmias, uncontrolled malignant hypertension, recent myocardial infarction	Coronary artery disease, arrhythmias, systemic hypertension, myocardial dysfunction
Normal arterial blood gases, and FEV_1 70% or more	$PaCO_2 > 45$ mm Hg, FEV_1 35% or less. Pulmonary hypertension	Hypoxia with normal $PaCO_2$, FEV_1 35-70%

patients with lung cancer have other diseases common to their particular age group, socioeconomic status, and smoking habits. These may include chronic bronchitis, emphysema, hypertension, coronary artery disease, diabetes mellitus, pulmonary infections and tuberculosis, etc. Therefore a detailed preoperative assessment of the patient is essential.[390-392] The preoperative evaluation of the patient is shown in Table 22.23.

In the earlier TNM staging system, stages I and II were considered operable. In the new International Staging system, lesions with IIIA stage can also be considered for surgery. 5 years survival after diagnosis is in the range of 50 percent in stage I and 35 percent in stage II. This survival decreases to less than 10 percent in more advanced cases. The survival data after surgery in different stages according to TNM type is shown in Table 22.24.[387,393] In general squamous cell carcinoma has a better survival followed by adenocarcinoma and large cell anaplastic carcinoma. Unfortunately, more than 80 percent (in series more than 90-95%) of the patients have advanced stage of the disease in stage IIIB or IV, so that they are inoperable. Recent reports have indicated that patients detected at stage I had a survival of 5 years in 705 of cases after surgery.[394]

The failure of surgery in more advanced cases is related to the metastasis which often exists, even if unrecognized clinically. The results are essentially the same since the early 60s, if one compares data from large institutions or from cooperative groups. If there has been any improvement in recent years, that is because of a more accurate preoperative staging using CT scans and mediastinoscopy with the overall resectability having declined. The reported cumulative 5 year survival for patients managed by resection increased from 23 to 40 percent between 1960 and 1985 can be attributable to better preoperative selection.[395]

Resection is the best treatment of localized, nonsmall cell lung cancer. It is desirable to have more accurate preoperative diagnosis and staging, only patients in whom a complete resection is anticipated (T1 to T4 stages, N0-1, and selected N2 cases, and an intraoperative staging to get the best results. The standard methods of surgery for primary lung cancer are pneumonectomy, and lobectomy. Lesser, or limited operations include wedge resection, segmental resection, nonanatomic limited resection, and sleeve lobectomy. The lesser resections are usually indicated in patients with poor cardiopulmonary reserve, and tumors in the T1 stage and are usually N0. Extended resections are usually undertaken in Stage III A disease, with T3 and T4 disease, N2, 3 disease, and in some selected cases of M1 disease, and superior sulcus tumor, but the overall prognosis is not good. Tumors that have locally invaded diaphragm, mediastinal pleura, and pericardium can be resected with results equivalent to other tumors of the same stage. Tumors less than 2 cm distal to carina can be resected with a sleeve lobectomy or pneumonectomy, although the operative mortality is high.

Adjuvant or neoadjuvant therapy like pre- and postoperative radio- and/or chemotherapy has not shown any advantage as regards the median survival,[396-404] although some studies some survival benefit. However, in uncontrolled trials, postoperative radiotherapy, particularly in superior sulcus tumors, have shown improved results. In a US lung Cancer Study Group trial, patients with stage II and III adenocarcinoma and large cell carcinomas showed significantly longer disease free

TABLE 22.24: Survival data in NSCLC after surgery

Stage	12 m %	24 m %	36 m %	48 m %	60 m %
I	85	72	64	59	55-85
T1N0M0					69
T2N0M0					59
II	72	49	36	31	29-55
T1N1M0					54
T2N1M0					40
III					
T3N0M0					44
T3N1M0					18
any T,N2M0					29

*Nonsquamous disease has worst prognosis.

survivals when they received chemotherapy after surgery than when they received immunotherapy with BCG. However the study did not show whether chemotherapy is better than no treatment.

A large number of randomized trials have used adjuvant immunotherapy after surgery.[405] This consisted of levamisole, intrapleural BCG, BCG cell wall skeleton, given intrapleurally or intradermally, mainly in patients with stage I and II squamous cell carcinoma after resection. However, the evidence is not convincing for their usefulness and these agents are no more used.

2. Radiotherapy

Radiotherapy in NSCLC can be used in the following circumstances: (i) As a palliation in inoperable cases; (ii) as a curative treatment in inoperable cases; (iii) as an adjuvant with surgery and/or chemotherapy and (iv) as preoperative therapy in patients with marginally resectable tumors. Postoperative radiotherapy can have an impact on survival only in patients without occult metastases at the time of initial treatment and in whom residual tumor has been left by the surgeon.[406-411] The role of preparative radiotherapy with or without adjuvant chemotherapy has not been defined clearly. It is however, generally agreed that radiotherapy is the standard treatment for unresectable tumors. There are two strategies for this. First, radiotherapy is intended to be palliative. If so the dose should be limited to 30 Gy. Second, radiotherapy is to be delivered with a curative intend, the dose should then be high and between 60 to 70 Gy.

Indications

Radiotherapy can be used under the following circumstances. (a) In operable cases of NSCLC, the superiority of radiotherapy over surgery is not appreciable, but in a group of selective patients this may be even curative. About 8 percent of subjects survive for 10 years or more. Patients who refuse surgery, or in old age, or in cases of contraindication of surgery because of medical reasons, radiotherapy is a good substitute and the overall survival rate is 16. The figure is higher (38%) if the tumor size is less than 2.0 cm.[412] (b) Radiotherapy can also be used preoperatively, either to reduce the tumor volume or to convert unresectable or marginally resectable tumors to resectable tumors. This can either be used as high dose radiotherapy or radical radiotherapy in doses of 40 to 60 Gy to sterilize the tumor and regional lymph nodes or in lower doses of 30 Gy, termed as 'adjuvant' radiotherapy followed by en bloc resection. (c). Post-operative radiotherapy may be used to take care of

residual tumor or hilar or mediastinal metastasis, with the hope of better survival. (d) Since patients of inoperable NSCLC has a poor prognosis, many uncontrolled studies have reported the value of radiotherapy. An 1 year survival rate has been reported to vary from 29 to 58 percent and a 5 year survival rate ranging from 4 to 10 percent.[413,414] (e) In combination with chemotherapy. Although there is no distinct advantage of combination chemo-radiotherapy, it seems logical that while chemotherapy will take care of the distant metastasis, radiotherapy will be able to control the local disease either by irradicating the tumor or by reducing the total tumor burden. The combined therapy can be administered either *sequentially*, i.e. one modality begins when the previous modality has concluded; *concurrently*, i.e. both modalities are given simultaneously, or in an *alternating fashion*, i.e. the modalities alternate. Available data indicate that patients with stage III NSCLC will benefit from combined treatment modality. The chemotherapy should be cisplatin based. But whether radiotherapy should be given before, during, or after chemotherapy is still unclear, and so also the precise role of combined therapy.

Treatment Schedules

Considerable technical advancement has occurred within the last few years in the administration of radical radiation therapy. Particularly, important is the computed guidance determination of the exact site, thereby minimizing radiation damage to normal tissue and giving higher dose to the tumor tissue. Radiotherapy can be given as continuous, 'split-course', hypo- and hyper-fractionation therapy.[415-418]

a. In **continuous radiotherapy** treatment, usually 1.5 to 2 Gy/day is given in 4 to 5 fractions/week through stationary A-P opposing fields. The target volume is the visible tumor with a safety margin of 1.5 to 2 cm. This is usually the conventional radiotherapy where a total of 60 Gy is delivered in 6 weeks. This schedule has a primary tumor control of up to 23 percent with a 1 and 2 year survival of the order of 35 percent and 12 percent respectively.

b. **Split-course therapy** is the periodic radiotherapy given to the same area but separated in time by a planned rest period when the normal cells can recover and there will be reduced morbidity. The primary tumor can shrink leading to better oxygenation and a smaller treatment volume. After the rest period the patient can be reassessed and those who have deteriorated can be excluded from further treatment. The problem with this form of treatment, however, is that viable tumor cells can also repopulate during the rest period.

c. **Hypofractionation** therapy is the delivery of radiotherapy in reduced treatment fractions. Usually 1 to 3 fractions are given per week, up to a total dose equal to a normal continuous treatment dose. This can be either given alone or in combination with radiosensitizers or hyperbaric oxygen.

d. Hyperfractionation is the delivery of multiple daily treatments separated by 4 to 8 hours

e. **CHART regimen** (continuous, hyperfractionated, accelerated radiotherapy) is a combination of all these features.

Other recent advances in radiotherapy are the use of Iodine 125 implants in primary tumor and Iridium 192 implants in mediastinum for better local control. Other irradiation techniques include higher LET (linear energy transfer) irradiation, use of hypoxic radiosensitizers, neutrons, and hyperthermia; but these are still investigational. Endobronchial irradiation through placement of catheters (Internal radiotherapy) is helpful in growths occluding the bronchial lumen or after external radiotherapy is given, so that residual tumor can be controlled with less doses of radiation.

The role of prophylactic cranial irradiation in NSCLC has not been clearly defined, although few reports claim benefit.

3. Chemotherapy

The role of chemotherapy in NSCLC in general is undefined. In spite of the fact that responses can be obtained in 20 to 40 percent of all patients, the survival benefits of chemotherapy has not been defined. A comparison of combination chemotherapy with those of the supportive care alone on the survival and quality of life in patients with advanced disease has produced not only conflicting but also very unimpressive results in studies from different countries.[419-424] However subsequent meta-analyses of individual studies have shown benefit of chemotherapy in NSCLC.[425-428] In a recent review of articles on chemotherapy trials in NSCLC published over the last 15 years in 6247 patients,[429] the objective and complete response rates for the overall population were 25 percent and 3 percent; for the patients with limited disease 34 percent and 5 percent; and for those with disseminated disease 22 percent and 3 percent, respectively. The response rate was significantly lower for single agent chemotherapy than for combination chemotherapy. When applying combination chemotherapy, the best results were obtained with regimens containing cisplatin, vindesine, vinblastine,

mitomycin C ifosfamide, doxorubicin, and etoposide. Many other drugs used earlier had response rates of less than 10 percent. A high dose of cisplatin (100 mg/m^2 or more) was also associated with better response rates than a lower dose. These differences were more marked in limited disease. Many more studies in hundreds are available in literature regarding the use of chemotherapy in NSCLC.[430-440]

Since NSCLC comprise of the major histological types of lung cancer, and more than 80 percent of the cases are unresectable by the time of presentation, there is a good reason for to try chemotherapy in these patients, although some do not agree with this assumption. Some firmly believe that all new patients with unresectable NSCLC should be offered chemotherapy. On the contrary, others do not favor this idea of using potentially toxic and costly drugs, with marginal or no benefits. In spite of these controversies, many centers treat these cases with chemotherapy and radiotherapy with some hope of benefit. A few selected regimens are shown in Table 22.25. The essence of all chemotherapy combination is that cisplatin is an essential component of these regimens.

At present no standardized chemotherapeutic regimen can be recommended a additional chemotherapy in resectable NSCLC (stages I-IIIA) is controversial. Combined modality treatment using radiotherapy and chemotherapy in advanced lung cancer has also been recommended by many, although the overall survival benefit is doubtful.[441-443] Although the use of chemotherapy has improved when compared with best supportive care (20-37 weeks vs 9-22 weeks) as is evident from large prospective studies[444,445] and there is improvement in symptomatic relief,[446] the question of quality of life,[447] cost factors[448,449] and toxicity should be taken into account before deciding therapy. In view of all these, patient selection is important. Various prognostic factors that indicate a good or poor outcome are shown in Table 22.226.[450-454]

TABLE 22.25: Selected chemotherapy regimens for NSCLC

1.	Cisplatin +	120 mg/m^2 day 1 and 29 then every 6 weeks
	Vinblastine	iv 6 mg/m^2
	or	weekly × 5 then q 3 weeks iv
	Vindesine	3 mg/m^2
2.	Cisplatin +	as above
	Vindesine +	as above
	Mitomycin-C	8 mg/m^2 on day 1, 29, and 71
3.	Mitomycin C	6 mg/m^2 day 1 i.v.
	Ifosfamide	3 g/m^2 i.v. infused over 3 hrs day 1
	Cisplatin	50 mg/m2 infused over 1 hr day 1.
The cycle is repeated every 3 weeks.		

TABLE 22.26: Prognostic factors in nonsmall cell lung cancer

- Performance status (Zubrod)
- Weight loss
- Serum albumin
- Staging (presence or absence of metastasis)
- Lymphocytes
- Lactic dehydrogenase
- Hoarseness
- Age and histological type were irrelevant sex and hoarseness only important when integrated within a multifactorial model

It is hoped that with newer advancements, human lung cancer can be studied in the laboratory with establishment of cell lines, heterotransplants of tumor tissues (xenografts in nude mice) and direct cloning of tumor cells using a soft agar assay which might help to select drugs for clinical use in future. Over the last decade, several new agents with significant activity have been identified and are being used in human trials with a hope to achieve better results.[455,456] These drugs include, *navelbine,* the *taxanes (taxol, and taxotere), gemcitabine, edatrexate,* and the *camptothecins (irinotecan and topotecan).*

Various other biological agents like retinoids, interferons, interleukins, LAK cells, and monoclonal antibodies have been explored as alternatives to traditional chemotherapies.[456-458]

SYMPTOMATIC TREATMENT OF LUNG CANCER

Management of associated complications is equally important for symptomatic relief as in any terminal illness. Besides, infections, nutrition, and psychological managements, pain and pleural effusion (when present are important which need attention. Local radiotherapy sometimes help in amelioration of pain. Most of the time stronger analgesics like dextromethorphan, morphine and its analogues, and mixtures of pain killer-cocktails like MCLA mixtures (morphine, cocaine, largactil, and alcohol) may be used judiciously, and may need to be administered as often as necessary. Management of pleural effusion is discussed in subsequent chapter on pleural diseases.

BRONCHOSCOPIC TREATMENT

Several bronchoscopic techniques have been used to treat patients with tracheobronchial pathology during the last decade. Palliation is the main aim, although according to some experts, in early stage tumor bronchoscopic treatment may have a curative potential.[459] Relief of dyspnea, hemoptysis, obstructive pneumonia, and improvement of gas exchange are possible after bronchoscopic treatment. The usefulness of this procedure consists of mechanical tumor removal, electrocautery, cryotherapy, endobronchial brachytherapy, photodynamic therapy, putting a stent in case of extrabronchial tumor, and the Nd-YAG laser resection.[460-462]

Laser (Light Amplification by Simulated Emission of Radiation) therapy has been in use for the treatment of many years in various disorders. This form of surgery refers to the transformation into heat of a unique form of light, which is being characterized by being monochromatic and coherent. Treatment of intrabronchial lesions is performed either through a rigid or fiberoptic bronchoscope under local or general anesthesia. The most frequently used instruments are the carbon dioxide laser, the argon laser, and the neodymium YAG (yttrium-aluminium-garnet, Nd-Yag) laser. The carbon dioxide laser has been used to treat tracheobronchial obstruction and can be repeated as required. Some prefer this for treating benign lesions only. The argon laser has been used mainly in conjunction with hematoporphyrin, a photosensitizing material. The Nd-YAG laser has greater depths of penetration and achieves better hemostasis.

The indications of laser therapy are to relieve hemoptysis and to improve lung function by removing airway obstruction and correcting lung collapse. Thus the goal of such therapy is just palliation of symptoms in non-curable patients, and may be useful in cases of recurrences after other forms of therapy are no longer useful. The complications of the procedure are hemorrhage, exsanguination, hypoxemia caused by obstruction by secretion or by debris, perforation, fire, pneumonia, and pneumothorax.

TREATMENT OF PANCOAST'S SYNDROME

The treatment strategy of superior sulcus tumor is a matter of controversy. While some consider radiotherapy alone is sufficient, others feel that radiotherapy followed by aggressive therapy is the best approach. Although initially it was thought that the tumor is resistant to radiotherapy, subsequent experience proved it to be the contrary. However, the controversy seems to be due to staging of the tumor. Survival is better in those without nodal involvement following surgery 3 weeks after radiotherapy (5 years survival in 44%), compared to those with hilar and mediastinal node involvement.

TREATMENT OF SUPERIOR VENA CAVA OBSTRUCTION

Treatment varies with the histology of the tumor as discussed earlier. In the past radiotherapy was considered as the first line of treatment. However, chemotherapy is equally effective in view of the fact that majority of cases are due to chemotherapy-sensitive small cell carcinoma. Radiotherapy is preferred for non-small cell lung cancers. A total dose of 50 Gy is recommended for better results. Prednisolone or hydrocortisone should be given prior to radiotherapy since this will increase edema and may worsen the obstruction during the first few days. Symptomatic relief of obstruction with steroids and diuretics are controversial. Perhaps diuretics have no role in obstructive edema. On the otherhand, by volume depletion, they may create more problems in sick patients. Another precaution to be taken in such cases is that intravenous fluid infusion should be avoided in upper limbs. The patient should sleep with the head-up position.

PREVENTION OF LUNG CANCER

Since smoking is the single most important causative factor for development of lung cancer, and lung cancer epidemic is in continuous expansion world wide, efforts to prevent smoking is the critical factor in prevention of lung cancer. In most countries, which has national programs for primary prevention of lung cancer, like Austria, China, Egypt, Japan, Sweden, and the United Kingdom, smoking control programs are given high priority.[463] The International association for Study of Lung Cancer (IASLC) have developed a 10 point policy recommendation in 1994 in the hope that their implementation would help eradicate tobacco induced diseases world wide including lung cancer on a global basis.[464] These recommendations are in line with those advocated by the WHO expert Committee on Smoking Control[465] and the report of the International union Against Cancer.[466] These include points on taxation to discourage smoking, regulation of tobacco advertising and promotion, education and counter-advertising, restrictions of children's access to tobacco, control of international tobacco trade, prevention of exposure to environmental tobacco smoke, reduced nicotine contents in smoking material, providing/alternative incentives to tobacco farmers, role of health personnel, and last but not the least, the early diagnosis and treatment of lung cancer.

Besides smoking other environmental factors, such as dietary deficiency of vitamins, and micronutrients may act as potential modifiers of lung cancer risk. The protective effect of vitamin A (retinol), vitamin E, beta-carotene, and selenium are known protectors. Therefore natural retinol and synthetic retinoids, beta-carotene, selenium, N-acetyl-cystine, and folate have shown chemopreventive properties.[467-470]

RECENT ADVANCES IN THE CHEMOTHERAPY AND NOVEL TARGETED THERAPY FOR LUNG CANCER

Nonsmall Cell Lung Cancer

As mentioned earlier, lung cancer is one of the most common malignancies in the world[471] and remains the leading cause of cancer-related deaths in Western countries.[472,473] The incidence is increasing especially among women, in whom lung cancer is now the leading cause of cancer death in the United States.[474] Patients with advanced disease who receive best supportive care survive for a few months, and approximately 90 percent do not survive 1 year.[471]

Chemotherapy for advanced nonsmall-cell lung cancer is often considered ineffective or excessively toxic. However, meta-analyses have demonstrated that, as compared with supportive care, chemotherapy results in a small improvement in survival in patients with advanced nonsmall-cell lung cancer.[475-477] In addition, randomized studies comparing chemotherapy with the best supportive care have shown that chemotherapy reduced symptoms and improves the quality of life.[478]

Over the past decade, a number of new agents have become available for the treatment of metastatic non-small-cell lung cancer, including the taxanes, gemcitabine, and vinorelbine. The combination of one or more of these agents with a platinum compound has resulted in high response rates and prolonged survival at one year in phase 2 studies.[479-483] However, there have been few comparisons of these newer chemotherapy regimens, which are now used frequently, with each other.

Chemotherapy affords only a marginal survival advantage in non-small-cell lung cancer (NSCLC). Results from different meta-analyses have shown that platinum-based combination chemotherapy regimens prolong survival in patients with chemotherapy regimens prolong survival in patients with advanced NSCLC when compared with best supportive care.[484,485] During the past few years, several drugs with novel mechanisms of action and significant activity against NSCLC have been identified, including paclitaxel, vinorelbine, gemcitabine, irinotecan, and tirapazamine.[486]

Gemcitabine as single-agent therapy has been studied extensively and has shown response rates of approximately 20 percent in patients with chemotherapy-native advanced NSCLC.[487-489] Gemcitabine has also shown preclinical and clinical evidence of synergism with cisplatin, with remission rates of 52 to 54 percent for the combination in phase II trials.[490,491]

Paclitaxel has produced overall response rates ranging from 20 to 42 percent in previously untreated patients with advanced NSCLC, with a 1-year survival rate of approximately 40 percent.[492-495] The combination of paclitaxel and cisplatin has produced good responses in both chemotherapy-native and previously treated patients with NSCLC, with neurotoxicity found to be the dose-limiting factor.[496,497]

Carboplatin, a cisplatin analog, has produced the best 1-year survival rate with the lowest toxicity as a single agent in a five-arm Eastern Cooperative Oncology Group (ECOG) study.[498] Carbolated is less nephrotoxic and less emetogenic than cisplatin and it lacks neurotoxicity, but has an overall efficacy that is comparable to cisplatin, with improved patient convenience because of the ease with which it can be administered.[499,500]

When paclitaxel and carboplatin are combined, response rates range from 27 to 62 percent, median survival time from 10 to 12 months, and 1-year survival time from 22 to 54 percent without major toxicity.[500-504] The combination of paclitaxel and gemcitabine is of particular interest among the nonplatinum combinations because of the agent' differing mechanisms of action, nonoverlapping toxicities, and activity. Paclitaxel possibly enhances the antitumor activity of gemcitabine and the combination has an additive effect.[505] Several phase I and II studies using a gemcitabine-paclitaxel combination in previously untreated patients with NSCLC have shown responses from 25 to 47 percent, with mild toxicity.[506-508]

Vinorelbine is a third generation vinca alkaloid, which has been in clinical development for 15 years. Recent exploration of its preclinical activity has revealed unexpected evidence of potential synergy with taxane compounds and early clinical results support the suggestion of enhanced efficacy particularly in breast cancer. The initial studies establishing the clinical activity of vinorelbine in breast cancer and non-small cell lung cancer have been extended to encompass a thorough evaluation of its contribution to combination chemotherapy for these disorders. In the treatment of breast cancer useful activity has been established for vinorelbine in combination with anthracyclines, anthracenediones, antimetabolites and the taxanes; additive toxicity is not a limiting factor. The activity of vinorelbine in the treatment of non-small cell lung cancer is significantly extended by incorporation into schedules utilizing cisplatin and other agents. Vinorelbine has also demonstrated useful activity in the treatment of a wide range of other malignancies including prostatic carcinoma, multiple myeloma, cancer of the ovary, cervix and head and neck and malignant lymphomas.

During the last decade, several new agents with single-agent activity in advanced nonsmall-cell lung cancer (NSCLC) have been identified.[509-512] When tested in the stage IV setting, usually in combination with cisplatin or carboplatin these agents have been shown to increase the median survival time compared with signle-agent cisplatin and chemotherapy regimens of the 1980s.[509-520] In addition, their use has led to improved quality of life.

For patient with locoregionally advanced unresectable disease (stage IIIB and some stage IIIa), the role of chemotherapy as a component of curative intent therapy has expanded in recent years.[509,521] Both sequentital and concomitant bimodality strategies have been investigated. The Cancer and Leukemia Group B (CALGB) and other have established that two cycles of induction chemotherapy with cisplatin and vinblastine followed by chest radiotherapy lead to an approximately 4 month increase in median survival time when compared with radiotherapy alone.[522-525] The effects of induction chemotherapy seem to be due primarily to a reduction of systemic failure rates without affecting local control.[525] Concomitant chemoradiotherapy has also been shown to lead to superior survival when compared with radiotherapy.[521,526,527] The combination of cisplatin and etoposide administered with concurrent radiotherapy has lead to encouraging data in the phase II setting when tested by the Southwest Oncology Group (SWOG), although a direct comparison with radiotherapy alone was not pursued.[528-530] The improved survival after concomitant chemoradiotherapy seems to be mediated primarily through increased local and regional control.[526] Thus, through complimentary mechanisms, both sequential and concomitant combined-modality therapy strategies lead to improved survival. In direct comparison, concomitant therapy is statistically superior to induction chemotherapy, although it is also associated with more severe acute toxicity.[531,532]

Significant advances in the treatment of advances NSCLC prompted a formal evaluation of the efficacy of gemcitabine-platinum combinations, in comparison with standard and emergent (novel) treatments. A literature review defined the primary focus to any randomized trial of gemcitabine plus cisplatin or carboplatin versus a platinum based regimen. Accordingly a meta-analysis of overall survival (OS) and time to progression (TTP) was performed.

A comprehensive search of published and unpublished sources was performed to identify all trials to December 2002. The hazard ratio (HR) was the summary statistic of choice, accounting for censoring and time-to-event. Where not reported or supplied by the investigator survival probabilities were estimated from Kaplan-Meier curves. The pooled HR was produced using a fixed effects meta-analysis. Statistical heterogeneity was addressed with a random effects model where appropriate. Estimation of absolute treatment benefit at one year was also performed.

In total, 13 of the 15 potentially eligible trials were included (one trial was excluded due to flawed randomization and one trial for data unavailability), resulting in pool of 4556 patients. A total of 17 comparators were analyzed: 12 against platinum-based doublets (11 novel agent-based doublets, VC -6), PC -2), PCb -2), DC -1) and one established agent doublet, EC), plus 5 against singlet/triplet agent regimens (MVC/MIC -4) and C -1)).

For OS a significant reduction in mortality in favor of the gemcitabine-based arms was observed, HR 0.90 (0.84 to 0.96, p < 0.001), using the fixed effects model, with an absolute survival improvement of 3.9 percent at 1 year. There was a significant reduction in TTP in favor of the gemcitabine regimens, HR 0.87 (0.82 to 0.93, p < 0.001), with the fixed effects model, with an absolute improvement of progression-free survival of 4.2 percent at 1 year. Overall the results demonstrate a slight but significant improvement in efficacy of gemcitabine plus a platinum agent when compared with platinum based comparators in survival and time to disease progression.

The Eastern Cooperative Oncology Group (ECOG) conduced a randomized clinical trial to compare the efficacy of three commonly used regimens with that of a reference regimen of cisplatin and paclitaxel.[533] The primary objective of this study was to compare overall survival in patients treated with cisplatin and gemcitabine, cisplatin and docetaxel, carboplatin and paclitaxel, or cisplatin and paclitaxel.

The response rate for all 1155 eligible patients was 19 percent, with a median survival of 7.9 months (95% confidence interval, 7.3 to 8.5), a 1- year survival rate of 33 percent (95% confidence interval, 30-36%), and a 2 year survival rate of 11 percent (95% confidence interval, 8-12%). The response rate and survival did not differ significantly between patients assigned to receive cisplatin and paclitaxel and those assigned to receive any of the three experimental regimens. Treatment with cisplatin and paclitaxel and those assigned to receive any of the three experimental regimens. Treatment with cisplating and gemcitabine was associated with a significantly longer time to the progression of disease than was treatment with cisplatin and paclitaxel but was more likely to cause grade 3, 4 of 5 renal toxicity (in 9% of patients, *vs* 3% of those treated with cisplatin plus

paclitaxel). Patients with a performance status of 2 had a significantly lower rate of survival than did those with a performance status of 0 or 1. None of four chemotherapy regimens offered a significant advantage over the others in the treatment of advanced non-small-cell lung cancer.

Platinum-based chemotherapy is an evidence-based standard of care for patients with advanced nonsmall-cell lung cancer (NSCLC) and good performance status. Drug discovery efforts in the 1980s led to the identification of several new chemotherapeutic drugs, including docetaxel, gemcitabine, irinotecan, paclitaxel, and vinorelbine, as discussed above with efficacy in the initial treatment of advanced NSCLC. When used as monotherapy and compared with best supportive care alone, these agents cause improved symptom palliation and longer survival than supportive care alone. Combination platinum-based chemotherapy further improves survival compared to single agents. Results of large randomized trials have demonstrated that docetaxel-platinum and docetaxel-non-platinum combinations have favorable activity as first-line treatment for patients with advanced NSCLC.

Docetaxel-platinum-based Doublets

Docetaxel has been evaluated in several randomized phase III trials in patients with chemotherapy-native advanced NSCLC. The Eastern Cooperative oncology group (ECOG) 1594 trial compared 3 different platinum-based combinations with a control arm of cisplatin and paclitaxel. One thousand two hundred and seven patients with advanced NSCLC were treated. The 3-investigatinal arms included carboplatin plus paclitaxel, cisplatin plus gemcitabine, and cisplatin plus docetaxel. The overall response rate in all evaluable patients was 19 percent with a median survival of 7.9 months. There were no significant differences in efficacy between the 4 treatment arms. The study initially included patients with an ECOG performance status (PS) of 2; however, after noting a high incidence of serious adverse events in the first 64 patients with a PS of 2, the protocol was amended to include only patients with a PS of 0 or 1.

The TAX 326 trial was a large randomized trial that compared docetaxel plus cisplatin or docetaxel plus carboplatin with vinorelbine plus cisplatin as first line treatment in 1,218 PS 0-2 patients with advanced NSCLC. The overall response rate was 31.6 percent for docetaxel/cisplatin versus 24.5 percent for vinorelbine/cisplatin (P =.029). Patients treated with docetaxel/cisplatin has an improved survival compared with those treated with vinorelbine/cisplatin.

The introduction of nay new chemotherapy agent for nonsmall cell lung cancer (NSCLC) ought to be considered carefully in light of both costs and measurable benefits. Decision-making is straight forward if a new treatment is relatively cheaper and more effective (i.e. introduce new therapy) or more expensive and less effective (i.e. reject new treatment) than standard therapies. However, if a treatment is more expensive ad also more effective, or less expensive but also less effective, decision making becomes more complicated. An economic evaluation of the cost-effectiveness of gemcitabine in advanced NSCLC was performed as a case study. A comprehensive literature search for published economic evaluations of gemcitabine was carried out. Economic studies examining treatment for advanced NSCLC were limited to cost-minimization analyses and cost-effectiveness analyses. The analyses included primary economic studies, e.g. trials that included an integral economic evaluation, and secondary research, e.g. analyses based on published trial data and modeling. Overall, gemcitabine regimens proved cost-effective against standard therapies in this analysis. Prospective economic and quality-of-life analyses should be incorporated into study designs to help identify treatments that will maximize societal health benefits.

Small Cell Lung Cancer

Although SCLC[534] in highly responsive to initial chemotherapy, the vast majority of patients experience tumor progression within 6 to 12 months after completion of first-line treatment.[535] Results of second-line chemotherapy are usually poor. The most active single agents yield response rates in the range of 10 to 30 percent,[536] and activity of combination chemotherapy regimens is usually < 40 percent.[534,537] In addition, duration of response to second line chemotherapy is short with a median survival that rarely exceeds 6 months.[538] There is no standard chemotherapy for second-line treatment of SCLC. However, for patients progressing after first line platinum-etoposide, cyclophosphamide adriamycin-vincristine-like regimens are widely used, whereas for patients relapsing after a nonplatinum based chemotherapy, such as cyclophosphamide-adriamycin-vincristine/adriamycin-cyclophosphamide-etoposide, a cisplatin based regimen, such as platinum-etoposide, is common practice.[539,540]

Small-cell lung cancer (SCLC) accounts for 15 to 20 percent of lung cancers diagnosed in the United States. The cornerstone of the treatment of SCLC is chemotherapy. SCLC is divided into limited disease (LD) and extensive disease (ED). Current treatment of LD-SCLC consists of concurrent chemotherapy and radiation therapy.[541] The 5 year survival rates with appropriate therapy are 15 to 25 percent. The use of hyperfractionated (twice-daily) radiation therapy with chemotherapy appears superior to that used with daily radiation therapy.[542] In the United States, the chemotherapy used with the radiation therapy is etoposide (VePesid, VP-16)/cisplatin (Platinol) (EP).

In ED-SCLC, the median survival following chemotherapy is 8 to 10 months. Etoposide/carboplatin (Paraplatin) is as effective as etoposide/cisplatin in treating patients with ED-SCLC.[543] More recently, irinotecan (CPT-11, Camptosar)/cisplatin was shown to be significantly superior to etoposide/cisplatin in patients with ED-SCLC.[544] For relapsed SCLC, chemotherapy is more effective in patients that have sensitive rather than refractory disease.[545]

Recommended Modes of Therapy

Schiller et al[546] conducted a randomized study to determine whether any of three chemotherapy regimens was superior to cisplatin and paclitaxel in patients with advanced non–small-cell lung cancer. A total of 1207 patients with advanced non–small-cell lung cancer were randomly assigned to a reference regimen of cisplatin and paclitaxel or to one of three experimental regimens: cisplatin and gemcitabine, cisplatin and docetaxel, or carboplatin and paclitaxel. Patients with non–small-cell lung cancer that was classified as stage IIIB (with malignant pleural or pericardial effusion), stage IV, or recurrent disease were randomly assigned to one of four treatment groups. The first group received the reference treatment: 135 mg of paclitaxel per square meter of body-surface area, administered over a 24 hour period on day 1, followed by 75 mg of cisplatin per square meter on day 2. The cycle was repeated every three weeks. In the second group, gemcitabine, at a dose of 1000 mg per square meter, was administered on days 1, 8, and 15, and cisplatin, at a dose of 100 mg per square meter, was administered on day 1 of a four-week cycle. Patients in the third group received 75 mg of docetaxel per square meter and 75 mg of cisplatin per square meter on day 1 of a three-week cycle. Those in the fourth group were treated with 225 mg of paclitaxel per square meter, given over a three-hour period on day 1, followed on the same day by carboplatin at a dose calculated to produce an area under the concentration–time curve of 6.0 mg per milliliter per minute, in a three-week cycle. The response rate for all 1155 eligible patients was 19 percent, with a median survival of 7.9 months (95 percent confidence interval, 7.3 to 8.5), a 1 year survival rate of 33 percent (95 percent confidence interval, 30 to 36 percent), and a 2 year survival rate of 11 percent (95 percent confidence interval, 8 to 12 percent). The response rate and survival did not differ significantly between patients assigned to receive cisplatin and paclitaxel and those assigned to receive any of the three experimental regimens. Treatment with cisplatin and gemcitabine was associated with a significantly longer time to the progression of disease than was treatment with cisplatin and paclitaxel but was more likely to cause grade 3, 4, or 5 renal toxicity (in 9 percent of patients, vs. 3 percent of those treated with cisplatin plus paclitaxel). Patients with a performance status of 2 had a significantly lower rate of survival than did those with a performance status of 0 or 1. Thus none of four chemotherapy regimens offered a significant advantage over the others in the treatment of advanced non–small-cell lung cancer. (See figure)

Kaplan–Meier Estimates of Overall Survival (Panel A) and the Time to Progression of Disease (Panel B) in the Study Patients, According to the Assigned Treatment.

Thus any one of the four described combination chemotherapy can be used in non-small cell lung cancer. Recently Pemetrexed has been recommended as the first-line treatment of non-small cell lung cancer. (Esteban E,

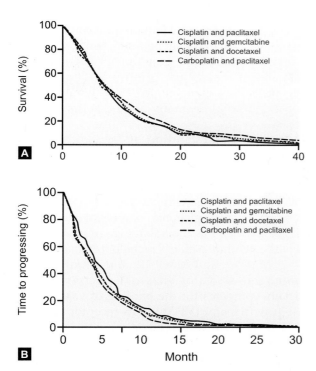

FIGURE 22.77: Comparison of 4 regimens on survival and times to progression in NSCLC (Ref No 546)

Casillas M, Cassinello A. Cancer Treatment Reviews, 2009;35:364-73).

NEWER STRATEGIES FOR LUNG CANCER TREATMENT (NOVEL THERAPEUTIC APPROACHES)

Lung cancer is a worldwide public health problem of immense proportions affecting both men and women. In the United States in 2002 more than 169,400 new cases of lung cancer are expected to be diagnosed.[547] Approximately 80 percent of these cases will have non-small-cell lung cancer (NSCLC) histology and > 70 percent of these patients will have advanced stage III and IV disease at diagnosis. With the best current treatments, only about 15 percent of these individuals will be alive 5 years later.[548] Therefore, there is a great need of development of newer agents those may help in the management of lung cancer.

Aside from a limited survival benefit, traditional chemotherapy has many limitations in NSCLC. It often causes unacceptable toxicity, which cannot be tolerated in patients already weakened by major surgery, old age, or who is compromised by prior chemotherapy and symptomatic late-stage disease. Newer, targeted approaches offer the potential for sparing healthy tissues and for a reduction in therapy-associated toxicity, by virtue of replacement of all or part of standard chemotherapeutic regimens. Arguably, the most promising therapies for NSCLC and other solid tumors include agents targeting cell-signaling pathways, such as the human epidermal growth factor receptor (HER) family. These include: small-molecule tyrosine-kinase inhibitors, such as epidermal growth factor receptor (HER1/EGFR)-specific cetuximab and HER2-specific trastuzumab (Herceptin; in clinical use for breast cancer); farnesyl transferase inhibitors; and agents targeting tumor angiogenesis, such as bevacizumab a MAb against vascular endothelial growth factor.

With the recent understanding of biology of cancer, it may be possible that cancer might be controlled and even cured by combining three potential therapeutic strategies aimed at (i) cancer-specific targets, (ii) universally-vital targets with selective protection of normal cells (the selective combinations) and (iii) tissue-specific targets. Although (i) targeting cancer-specific pathways (e.g. by imatinib and gefitinib) is probable, it alone will not be sufficient to control cancer. This strategy is limited to oncogene (kinase)-dependent cancers and is further limited by therapy-induced resistance and tumor progression. Thus, targeting cancer-specific pathways needs to be complemented by two divergent therapeutic strategies: (ii) selective combinations and (iii) tissue-selective therapy. With selective protection of normal cells (based on cell cycle and apoptosis manipulation), combinations of selective and chemotherapeutic drugs can be effective in most common cancers. Alternatively, tissue-selective therapy can suppress cancer cells in a tissue-selective manner, sparing other tissues. While alone, each therapeutic strategy may cause drug resistance and even tumor progression; these obstacles can be overcome and even exploited by using all three strategies in sequence. And finally, these strategies will benefit from molecular diagnostics and can be used for chemoprevention.[549]

The current understanding of the cellular and molecular events involved in the development of cancer identify six major alterations in cell physiology that collectively dictate malignant growth: self-sufficiency in growth signals, insensitivity to antigrowth signals, evasion of apoptosis, unlimited replicative potential, tissue invasion and sustained angiogenesis.[550] All of these processes are highly complex, but, in each case, several key regulatory mechanisms governing the development of malignancy have been identified, providing novel drug targets amenable for therapeutic intervention.[551] Among these events, the targeting of tumor-induced angiogenesis as a means of blocking tumor progression has generated a growing interest in recent years.[551] This interest stems from several observations that tumor cells cannot grow significantly in the absence of blood vessels[552] and that molecules interfering with angiogenesis have potent antitumor properties in animal models.[553] Moreover, since endothelial cells (Ecs) are genetically stable, inhibitors specific to these cells should not induce resistance in tumors in contrast to cytotoxic compounds (antimitotic, antimetabilites and alkylating agents) for which resistance is commonly observed.[554] Advanced in the understanding of tumor biology have enabled the identification of a number of new targets with potential to interfere with the mechanisms essential for tumor spread, growth, and survival. In order to fully explore the anticancer properties of these novel approaches, a broad pipeline of agents targeting a variety of key processes in tumor progression and metastasis are being developed.

Agents currently in preclinical development include Src kinase inhibitors. Src kinase is a signal transduction modulator that is highly regulated and active only at low levels in the majority of normal cells. In several human tumors, Src kinase activity is increased and may be associated with increasing the invasive potential of tumor cells. AZDO530 is an orally available Src kinase inhibitor with potential for activity in a wide range of tumors.

Extensive studies on the cellular and molecular processes underlying antiogenesis have identified key events associated with tumor-induced neovascularization: (i) stimulation of Ecs by tumor-derived angiogenic cytokines, such as the vascular endothelial growth factor (VEGF), resulting in increased EC proliferation and migration, (ii) secretion of matrix-degrading enzymes, such as matrix metalloproteinases and plasminogen activators, resulting in the digestion of surrounding extracellular matrix (ECM), and (iii) formation of three-dimensional capillary network in the vicinity of tumor cells, allowing their sustained growth by providing oxygen and essential nutrients. These cellular and molecular steps all represent attractive antiangiogenic targets, and have led to the identification and development of a variety of compounds targeting EC proliferation, migration or vessel formation.[555] At the present time, almost 300 angiogenesis inhibitors have been identified and developed, and more than 75 are under clinical evaluation, from which only three are under investigation in phase III clinical trials.

Angiogenesis plays in important role in vessel development and homeostasis during wound healing, female reproduction, and tissue regeneration. However, the upregulation of angiogenesis plays a central role in the development of several pathological conditions, such as age-related macular degeneration, psoriasis, rheumatoid arthritis, and tumor growth.[556,557] The growth and metastasis of malignant tumors is dependent on angiogenesis.[558] Blocking angiogenesis would appear to be a good strategy in many angiogenesis-dependent diseases.

Increased understanding of the complex factors involved in angiogenesis has led to the development of agents that can interfere with the specific components of the angiogenic process.[556,559] Among the angiogenesis inhibitors in late-stage clinical development is AE-941 (neovastar), an antiangiogenic component extracted from cartilage,[560] which has the advantage of being administered orally. It inhibits matrix metalloproteinases (MMPs) MMP-2, MMP-9, and MMP-12, and stimulates tissue plasminogen activator enzymatic activities.[561,562] It selectively competes for the binding of vascular endothelial growth factor (VEGF) to its receptor (VEGFR),[563] causing disruption to this signaling pathway. Finally, AE-941 induces apoptotic activities in endothelial cells.[564] Oral treatment with AE-941 induces a dose-dependent decrease in tumor growth in mice grafted with DA3 mouse mammary adenocarcinoma cells and reduces the number of lung metastases in mice grafted with M27 Lewis lung carcinoma cells.[565,566] Tumor necrosis has been observed following oral administration of AE-941 in human glioblastoma models in mice.[562]

A recently held international meeting on 'New Drugs in Cancer Therapy' at the National Tumor Institute of Naples, on 17 to 18 June 2004 reviewed the analogs of conventional anticancer drugs, such as taxanes, platinum compounds, anthracyclines and topoisomerase I inhibitors. The data of a phase II trial of BMS-247550, an epothilone B analog, in patients with renal cell carcinoma were reported. Data were also presented on BBR-3464, a trinucleate platinum analog that was developed on the grounds of greater potency, a more rapid rate of DNA binding and the ability to induce apoptosis regardless of the p53 status of the cell. Pegylated-coated liposomal formulation doxorubicin (Caelyx) has shown efficacy in metastatic breast cancer and in advanced ovarian cancer; sabarubicin is a third-generation anthracycline with equal or superior potency to doxorubicin or idarubicin in a variety of human tumor cell lines of different histotypes. The main mechanisms of resistance to topoisomerase I inhibitors were discussed; data on diflomotecan were reported, showing a narrow therapeutic index of the drug. The second session of the meeting focused on the ErbB family as a target for anticancer therapy. Recent evidence of a correlation between epidermal growth factor receptor (EGFR) mutations at exons 18 to 21 and clinical response of advanced nonsmall-cell lung cancer to gefitinib therapy was commented on. The issue of the association between ErbB2 expression and gefitinib activity was addressed, while clinical data of a phase II study of gefitinib in advanced breast cancer were presented. Monoclonal antibodies targeting EGFR represent another worthwhile way to interfere with EGFR-driven signal transduction. Cetuximab is reaching market registration in advanced colorectal cancer; in particular, due to the results of the BOND study. The recently presented results of the Bonner study strongly support the activity of this drug in head and neck cancer. A step forward in the research on anti-EGFR monoclonal antibodies may be represented by humanized monoclonal antibodies, such as EMD 72000 and ABX-EGF. Imatinib mesylate is probably the most outstanding example of an effective targeted therapy-its activity in gastrointestinal stromal tumors was so exciting that the drug reached the market without undergoing phase III evaluation. The third session of the meeting was on angiogenesis inhibitors. Drugs may interfere with the angiogenic process via different mechanisms and there is a sound rationale for combining antiangiogenic agents with chemotherapy or multiple antiangiogenic strategies. Clinical results obtained with direct antiangiogenic agents have been negative up to now, but some exciting results have been seen with bevacizumab, a monoclonal antibody targeting vascular endothelial growth factor (VEGF). A few VEGF-tyrosine kinase inhibiting small molecules, such as ZD6474, AZD2171 and PTK/ZK, are undergoing clinical trials. The fourth session of the meeting was on interference with intracellular signal transduction. Farnesyl transferase inhibitors exert their action by interfering with either pro-Ras or RhoB farnesylation. Several clinical studies of different phases with compounds belonging to this class have been carried out, either alone or in combination with chemotherapy; unfortunately, all of them have turned out to be negative. Cell cycle inhibitors, such as CYC-202 and BMS-387032, represent a class of interesting compounds which are in the early phase of development and whose clinical results are eagerly awaited. Another strategy to achieve cell cycle inhibition is to target heat shock protein 90, a molecular chaperone required for protein folding. Clinical data on depsipeptide, a histone deacetylase (HDAC) inhibitor with activity in T cell lymphoma, were presented. Suberoylanilide hydroxamic acid is another small molecular weight inhibitor of HDAC activity. Phase I/II clinical trials have shown low toxicity and evidence of antitumor activity; on the other hand, this compound has potential for synergism with radiotherapy, chemotherapy and biologicals.[567] In order to grow and metastasize, tumor cells must quickly develop a blood supply. Targeting the tumor vasculature is an approach that has received much research focus in recent years, resulting in the evolution of two distinct therapeutic strategies: antiangiogenic agents, which inhibit the antiogenic process and thereby prevent blood vessel formation: and vascular-targeting agents, which target and destroy existing tumor vasculature. Vascular endothelial growth factor (VEGF) is thought to be crucial for blood vessel formation and maintenance. ZD6474 is a novel inhibitor of VEGF receptor-2 (KDR) tyrosine kinase, with additional activity against epidermal growth factor receptor (EGFR) tyrosine kinase. Chronic once-daily oral administration of ZD6474 results in dose-dependent inhibition of tumor growth in a range of histologically distinct human xenograft models (breast, lung, prostate, colon, ovary and vulva), as well as including profound tumor regression in established PC-3 prostate xenografts. In Phase I clinical studies, cases of tumor regression have been observed in patients with nonsmall-cell lung cancer receiving ZD6474 therapy (currently in Phase II clinical development). In addition AZD2171, an extremely potent inhibitor of VEGFR tyrosine kinase activity of VEGF signaling, but without activity against EGFR tyrosine kinase, is in Phase I clinical development and has demonstrated preclinical antitumor activity in a broad spectrum of human xenograft models.

ZD6126 is a novel vascular-targeting agent that functions through the active species ZD6126 phenol to bind tubulin and thereby disrupt the microtublar network responsible for maintaining the shape of immature endothelial cells. In proliferating endothelial cells, such as those of the tumor neovasculature, this results in rapid morphological changes that lead to endothelial cell detachment and tumor vessel congestion. In normal mature endothelium, the presence of a supporting actin cytoskeleton means that endothelial cell conformation is maintained. ZD6126 treatment has been shown in induce selective disruption of tumor blood vessels, resulting in extensive central necrosis in a range of tumor xenograft models, leaving only a thin rim of viable tumor tissue at the periphery. Phase II clinical evaluation of ZD6126 is currently ongoing.

AZD3409 is a novel, oral prenyl transferase inhibitor (PTI). It is a novel antiproliferative agent that, in preclinical studies, achieves up to 90 percent inhibition of farnesyl transferase (Ftase) at well-tolerated doses, and has been shown to provide 24 hrs inhibition of Ftase following once-daily oral dosing. AZD3409 also inhibits other enzymes involved in protein prenylation and has potential for broad antitumor activity.

Agents in early preclinical development include a novel, oral, selective cyclin-dependent kinase inhibitor that is selective for tumor cells ad induces cell cycle arrest and tumor cell apoptosis. Also in early preclinical development are aurora kinase inhibitors that are anticipated to be selectively toxic to proliferating tumor cells and therefore have potential to be developed as novel anticancer agents.

Gefitinib is an orally active epidermal growth factor receptor tyrosine kinase inhibitor (EGFR-TKI) that blocks signal transduction pathways responsible for cellular proliferation. This agent has shown antitumor activity against a broad range of human tumors (both as monotherapy and in combination). Phase I clinical trials indicated that daily oral administration of IRESSA was associated with an acceptable tolerability profile and had promising clinical activity, particularly in patients with nonsmall-cell lung cancer (NSCLC). Further large phase II trials have confirmed that the drug has clinically meaningful antitumor activity and provides symptom relief in patients with locally advanced or metastatic NSCLC who are refractory to both platinum-containing

and docetaxel chemotherapy. In addition, the recommended dose (250 mg/day) has a favorable adverse-event profile, which is maintained on continued therapy.[568]

Oblimersen sodium is a first-in-class bcl-2 antisense oligonucleotide, which specifically targets bcl-2 mRNA, thus reducing the production of Bcl-2 protein. Oblimersen sodium has an 18-nucleotide sequence that is complementary to the first 6 codons of the bcl-2 mRNA. Oblimersen sodium binds to the bcl-2 mRNA, forming a heteroduplex, which enables the enzyme RNaseH to cleave the RNA sequence, degrading the bcl-2 message. This releases the olimersen sodium oligonucleotide to bind to additional targets.[569]

Preclinical studies in tumor cell lines and animal models of human cancer have demonstrated that oblimersen sodium is active against the production of Bcl-2 and acts in combination with a broad range of chemotherapy agents. Outcome measures in these studies included reduced Bcl-2 expression, increased apoptosis, inhibition of tumor growth, tumor reduction or elimination, and increased survival of the animal host.[569-574]

In a mouse xenograft model of human breast cancer, mice treated with oblimersen sodium in combination with docetaxel, paclitaxel, or cisplatin remained tumor-free for more than 5 months.[572]

Treatment with oblimersen sodium led to the survival of nude mice transplanted with imatinibresistant BCR-ABL-TF-1-R cells. These cells cause tumor transformation in nude mice.[573]

HER1/EGFR is pivotal in regulating several functions that determine cell proliferation and survival. Dysregulation of this receptor occurs frequently in NSCLC, and leads to poor prognosis and resistance to chemotherapy.[575-577] Agents such as erlotinib, which block HER1/EGFR activation and associated downstream signaling pathways, offer many opportunities to optimize NSCLC treatment. A kinder safety profile allows consideration for use in patients unsuitable for, and/or unresponsive to, aggressive chemotherapy.

REFERENCES

1. Parkin DM, Laara E, Muir CS. Estimates of the world wide frequency of sixteen major cancers in 1980. Int J Cancer 1988;41:184.
2. World Health Organization. Cancer in developed countries: Assessing the trends. WHO Chron 1985;39:109.
3. Parkin DM. Trends in lung cancer incidence worldwide. Chest 1989;96(Suppl):5S.
4. Hammond EC, Horn D. Smoking and death rates-Report on 44 months of follow up of 187,783 men. II. Death rates by cause. JAMA 1958:166:1294.

5. Parkin DM, Pisani P, Ferlay J. Estimates of the world-wide incidence of eighteen major cancers in 1985. Int J Cancer 1993;54:594-606.

6. Parkin DM, Muir CS, Whelan S, Gao YT, Ferlay J, Powell J (Eds): Cancer incidence in five continents Lyon. IARC 1992;6:120.

7. Negri E, La Vecchia C. Epidemiology of lung cancer: Recent trends in mortality with emphasis on Europe. Lung Cancer 1995;12(Suppl 1): S3-S11.

8. La Vecchia C, Lucchini F, Negri E, Boyle P, Maisonneuve P, Levi F. Trends in cancer mortality in Europe 1955-89. II. Respiratory tract, bone, connective and soft tissue sarcomas, and skin. Eur J Cancer 1992;28: 514-99.

9. Behera D. Lung cancer in India—A perspective. Indian J Chest Dis Allied Sci. 1992;34:91-101.

10. National Cancer Registry Programme. Biennial Report. An Epidemiological Study. Indian Council of Medical Research, New Delhi. Cancer Incidence 1988-1989; 2:3-42.

11. Behera D, Kashyap S. Pattern of malignancy in a North Indian hospital. J Ind Med Ass 1988;86:28-29.

12. Jindal SK, Behera D. Clinical spectrum of Primary lung cancer—Review of Chandigarh experience of 10 years. Lung India 1990;8:94-98.

13. Jindal SK, Malik SK, Dhand R, Gujral JS, Malik AK, Datta BN. Bronchogenic carcinoma in Northern India. Thorax 1982;37:343-47.

14. Jindal SK, Malik SK, Datta BN. Lung cancer in Northern India in relation to age, sex, and smoking habits. Eur J Respir Dis 1987;70:23-28.

15. IARC (International Agency for Research on Cancer). Tobacco smoking. Monographs on the evaluation of carcinogenic risk to humans. Lyon: IARC 1986;(38).

16. Boyle P, Maisonneuve P. Lung cancer and tobacco smoking. Lung Cancer 1995;12:167-81.

17. Redmond DE. Tobacco and cancer: The first clinical report. 1761. N Engl J Med 1970;282:18-23.

18. Doll R, Peto R. The causes of cancer: Quantitative estimates of avoidable risks of cancer in the United states today. J Natl Cancer Inst 1981;66:1191-1308.

19. Tylecote FE. Cancer of the lung. Lancet 1927;2:256-59.

20. Doll R, Hill AB. A study of the aetiology of carcinoma lung. Br Med J 1952:ii:1271-86.

21. Doll R, Hill AB. Smoking and carcinoma of lung. Br Med J 1950;ii:739-48.

22. Clemmesen J. Statistical studies in malignant neoplasms. I. Review and results. Copenhagen: Munksgaard 1965.

23. Doll R, Peto R, Wheatley K, Gray R, Sutherland I. Mortality in relation to smoking: 40 years observation on male British doctors. Br Med J 1994;309:901-11.

24. La Vecchia C, Boyle P, Franceschi S, et al. Smoking and cancer with emphasis on Europe. Eur J Cancer 1991;27: 94-104.

25. US Surgeon General: The health consequences of smoking: Cancer, Washington DC, US Department of Health and Human Services 1982;82-50179.

26. Wynder EL, Graham EA. Tobacco smoking as possible aetiological factor in bronchogenic carcinoma: A study of 684 proved cases. J Am Med Ass 1950;143:329-36.

27. Cornfield J. A method of estimating comparative rates from clinical data: Applications to cancer of the lung, breast, and cervix. J Natl Cancer Inst 1951;11:1269-75.

28. Schrek R, Baker LA, Ballard GP, Dolgoff S. Tobacco smoking as an aetiological factor in disease. I. Cancer. Cancer Res 1950;10:49-58.

29. Mills CA, Porter M. Tobacco smoking habits and cancer of the mouth and respiratory system. Cancer Res 1950;10:539-42.

30. Levin ML, Goldstein H, Gerhardt PR. Cancer and tobacco smoking. J Am Med Ass 1950;143:336-38.

31. Gao YT, Blot WJ, Zheng W. Lung cancer among chinese women. Int J Cancer 1987;40:604-09.

32. MacLennan R, de Costa J, Day NE, et al. Risk factors for lung cancer in Singapore Chinese: A population with high female incidence rates. Int J Cancer 1977;20: 854-60.

33. Behera D, Jindal SK, Malik SK. Primary adenocarcinoma of lung. Bull PGI (Chandigarh) 1984;18:176-79.

34. United States Public Health Service. Smoking and Health. PHS Publication Number 1103; Washington DC: United States Department of Health, Education and Welfare 1964.

35. Lubin JH, Li JY, Xuan XZ, et al. Risk of lung cancer among cigarette and pipe smokers in Southern China. Int J Cancer 1992;51:390-95.

36. Notani P, Sanghvi LD. A retrospective study of lung cancer in Bombay. Br J Cancer 1974;29:477-82.

37. Notani PN, Rao DN, Sirsat MV, Sanghvi LD. A study of lung cancer in relation to bidi smoking in different religious communities in Bombay. Ind J Cancer 1977;14:115-21.

38. Nafae A, Misra SP, Dhar SN, Shah SNA. Bronchogenic carcinoma in Kashmir valley. Ind J Chest Dis All Sc 1973;15:285-95.

39. Hammond EC, Garfinkel L, Seidman H, Lew EA. 'Tar' and nicotine content of cigarette smoke in relation to death rates. Environ Res 1976;12:262-74.

40. Kaufman DW, Palmer JR, Rosenberg L, et al. Tar content of cigarettes in relation to lung cancer. Am J Epidemiol 1989;129:703-11.

41. Lubin JH, Blot WJ, Berrino F, et al. Pattern of lung cancer risk according to type of cigarette smoked. Int J Cancer 1984;33:569-74.

42. Preston-Martin S. Evaluation of the evidence that tobacco-specific nitrosamines (TSNA) cause cancer in humans. Crit Rev Toxicol 1991;21:295-98.

43. Hoffman D, Djordjevic MV, Rivenson A, et al. A study of tobacco carcinogenesis. relative potencies of tobacco-specific nitrosamines as inducers of lung tumors in A/J mice. Cancer Lett 1993;71:25-30.

44. Hoffman D, Brunnemann KD, Prokopczyk B, Djordjevic MV. Tobacco-specific N-nitrosamines and area-

derived N-nitrosamines: Chemistry, biochemistry, carcinogenicity, and relevance to humans. J Toxicol Environ Health 1994;41:1-52.

45. IARC Monograph on the Evaluation of Carcinogenic Risks to Humans.1987;Suppl 7:17-74.

46. Hirayama T. Lung cancer in Japan. Effects of nutrition. and passive smoking. In Mizell M, Correa P (Eds): Lung cancer, causes and prevention. Verlag Chemi International, Deerfield Beach, 1984;175.

47. Hirayama T. Non-smoking wives of heavy smokers have a higher risk of lung cancer: A study from Japan. Br Med J 1981;282:183-85.

48. Trichopoulos D, Kalandidi A, Sparros L, MacMohan B. Lung cancer and passive smoking. Int J Cancer 1981;27:1-4.

49. Burns DM. Environmental tobacco smoke: The price of scientific certainty. J Natl Cancer Inst 1992;84:1387-88.

50. Stockwell HG, Goldman AL, Lyman GH, et al. Environmental tobacco smoke and lung cancer risk in nonsmoking women. J Natl Cancer Inst 1992;84:1417-22.

51. Reif JS, Dunn K, Ogilvie GK, Harris CK. Passive smoking and canine lung cancer risk. Am J Epidemiol 1992;135:234-39.

52. Katzenstein AW. Environmental tobacco smoke and lung cancer risk: Epidemiology in relation to confounding factors. Environ Int 1992;18:341-45.

53. United States Environmental Protection Agency. Respiratory health effects of passive smoking: Lung cancer and other disorders. Office of Health and Environmental assessment; office of Research and Development, US Environmental Protection Agency, EPA/600/6-90/006F, December 1992.

54. Wynder EL. The aetiology, epidemiology, and prevention of lung cancer. Semin Respir Med 1982;3:135.

55. Gross AJ, Van Leuwen FE. Presentation and dissent. The association of lung cancer in nonsmokers in the united states and its reported association with environmental tobacco smoke. J Clin Epidemiol 1995;48:587-606.

56. Brownson RC, Alavanja MCR, Hock ET, Loy TS. Passive smoking and lung cancer in nonsmoking women. Am J Public Health 1992;82:1525-30.

57. Darby SC, Pike MC. Lung cancer and passive smoking: Predicted effects from a mathematical model for cigarette smoking and lung cancer. Br J Cancer 1988;58:825-31.

58. Wells AJ. An estimate of adult mortality in the United States from passive smoking. Environ Int 1988;14: 249-65.

59. Coggon D, Achenson ED. Trends in lung cancer mortality. Thorax 1983;38:721.

60. Pairon JC, Brochard P, Jaurand MC, Bignon J. Silica and lung cancer: A controversial issue. Eur Respir J 1991;4:730-44.

61. Chia SE, Chia KS, Phoon WS, Lee HP. Silicosis and lung cancer among Chinese granite workers. Scand J Work Environ Health 1991;17:170-74.

62. Hnizdo E, Sluis-Cremer GK. Silica exposure, silicosis, and lung cancer: A mortality study of South African gold miners. Br J Ind Med 1991;48:53-60.

63. Amandus H, Costello J. Silicosis and lung cancer: In US miners. Arch Environ Health 1991;46:82-89.

64. Carta P, Cocco PL, Casula D. Mortality from lung cancer among Sardinian patients with silicosis. Br J Ind Med 1991;48:122-29.

65. Burns PB, Swanson GM. The occupational cancer incidence surveillance study (OCISS): Risk of lung cancer by usual occupation and industry in the Detroit metropolitan area. Am J Ind Med 1991;19:655-71.

66. Coultas DB, Samet JM. Occupational lung cancer. Clin Chest Med 1992;13:341-54.

67. Jockel KH, Ahrens W, Wichmann HE, et al. Occupational and environmental hazards associated with lung cancer. Int J Epidemiol 1992;21:202-13.

68. Finkelstein MM. Occupational associations with lung cancer in two Ontario cities. Am J Ind Med 1995;27:127-36.

69. McLaughlin JK, Jing-Qiong C, Dosemeci M, et al. A nested case-control study of lung cancer among silica exposed workers in china. Br J Ind Med 1992;49:167-71.

70. Miller AB. Environmental carcinogenesis. Radiation as a lung carcinogen. Chest 1986;89:312SS.

71. Wilkinson P, Hansell DM, Janssens J, et al. Is lung cancer associated with asbestos exposure when there are no small opacities on the chest radiograph? Lancet 1995;345:1074-78.

72. Highes JM, Weill H. Asbestosis as a precursor of asbestos related lung cancer: Results of a prospective mortality study. Br J Ind Med 1991;48:229-33.

73. Karjalainen A, Anttila S, Vanhala E, Vainio H. Asbestos exposure and the risk of lung cancer in a general urban population. Scand J work environ Health 1994;20:243-50.

74. Lubin JH, Boice JD Jr, Edling C, et al. Lung cancer in radon-exposed miners and estimation of risk from indoor exposure. J Natl cancer Inst 1995;87:817-27.

75. Chen R, Wei L, Huang H. Mortality from lung cancer among copper miners. Br J Ind Med 1993;50:505-09.

76. Vineis P, Thomas T, Hayers RB, et al. Proportion of lung cancers in males, due to occupation in different areas of the USA. Int J Cancer 1988;42:851-56.

77. Kusiak RA, Ritchie AC, Muller J, Springer J. Mortality from lung cancer in Ontario Uranium miners. Br J Ind med 1993;50:920-28.

78. Jarvholm B, Larsson S, Hagberg S, et al. Quantitative importance of asbestos as a cause of lung cancer in a Swedish industrial city: A case-referent study. Eur Respir J 1993;6:1271-75.

79. Wiernik PH, Sklarin NT, Dutcher JP, Sparano JA, Greenwald ES. Adjuvant radiotherapy for breast cancer as a risk factor for the development of lung cancer. Med Oncol 1994;11:1215.

80. Wang QS, Boffeta P, Parkin DM, Kogevinas M. Occupational risk factors for lung cancer in Tianjin, China. Am J Ind Med 1995;28:353-62.

81. Whitessell PL, Drage CW. Occupational lung cancer. Mayo Clin Proc 1993;68:183-88.

82. Becher H, Jedrychowski W, Wahrendorf J, et al. Effects of occupational air pollutants on various histological types of lung cancer: A population based case-control study. Br J Ind Med 1993;50:136-42.

83. Pastorino U. Lung cancer chemoprevention: Facts and hopes. Lung Cancer 1991;7:133-50.

84. Scali J, Astre C, Segala C, Gerber M. Relationship of serum cholesterol, dietary and plasma β-carotene with lung cancer in male smokers. Eur J Cancer Prev 1995;4:169-74.

85. Benner Se, Lippman SM, Hong WK. Current status of retinoid chemoprevention of lung cancer. Oncology 1995;9:205-10.

86. Hoffman D, Rivenson A, Abbi R, Wynder EL. A study of tobacco carcinogenesis: Effect of the fat content of the diet on the carcinogenic activity of 4-(methyl-nitrosamino)-1-(3-pyridyl)-1-butanone in F344 rats. Cancer Res 1993;53:2758-61.

87. Alavanja MCR, Brown CC, Swanson C, Brownson RC. Saturated fat intake and lung cancer risk among nonsmoking women in Missouri. J Natl Cancer Inst 1993;85:1906-16.

88. Lee JS, Lippman SM, Benner SE, et al. Randomized placebo-controlled trial of isoretinoin in chemo-prevention of bronchial squamous metaplasia. J Clin Oncol 1994;12:937-45.

89. Sidney S, Caan BJ, Friedman GD. Dietary intake of carotene in nonsmokers with and without passive smoking at home. Am J Epidemiol 1989;129:1305-09.

90. Omenn GS, Goodman G, Thornquist M, et al. The b carotene and retinol efficacy trial (CARET) for chemoprevention of lung cancer in high risk popu-lations: Smokers and asbestos-exposed workers. Cancer Res 1994;54(Suppl): 2038S-43S.

91. Lippman SM, Benner SE. Retinoid chemoprevention studies in upper aerodigestive and lung carcinogenesis. Cancer Res 1994;54(Suppl):2025S-28S.

92. Goodman MT, Kolonel LN, Yoshizawa CN, Hankin JH. The effect of dietary cholesterol and fat on the risk of lung cancer in Hawaii. Am J Epidemiol 1988;128:1241-55.

93. Heinonen OP, Huttunen JK, Albanes D, et al. The alpha-tocoferol, Beta-carotene Lung Cancer Prevention Study: Design, methods, participant characteristics, and compliance. Ann Epidemiol 1994;4:1-10.

94. Goodman MT, Hankin JH, Wilkens LR, Kolonel LN. High-fat foods and the risk of lung cancer. Epidemio-logy 1992;3:288-99.

95. Pastorino U, Pisani P, Berrino F, et al. Vitamin A and female lung cancer: A case control study on plasma and diet. Nutr Cancer 1987;10:171-79.

96. Shekelle RB, Tangney CC, Rossof AH, Stamler J. Serum cholesterol, beta-carotene, and risk of lung cancer. Epidemiology 1992;3:282-87.

97. Candelora EC, Stockwell HG, Armstrong AW, Pinkham PA. Dietary intake and risk of lung cancer in women who never smoked. Nutr Cancer 1992;17:263-70.

98. Swanson CA, Mao BL, Li JY, et al. Dietary determinants of lung cancer risk: Results from a case control study in Yunnan Province, China. Int J Cancer 1992;50:876-80.

99. Goodman Mt, Kolonel LN, Wilkens LR, et al. Dietary factors in lung cancer prognosis. Eur J Cancer 1992; 28:495-501.

100. Forman MR, Yao SX, Graubard BI, et al. The effect of dietary intake of fruits and vegetables on the odds ratio of lung cancer among Yunnan Tin miners. Int J Epidemiol 1992;21:437-41.

101. Wynder EL, Taioli E, Fujita Y. Ecologic study of lung cancer risk factors in the US and Japan with special reference to smoking and diet. Jpn J Cancer Res 1992;83:418-23.

102. Suzuki I, Hamnada GS, Zambonic MM, et al. Risk factors for lung cancer in Rio de Janeiro, Brazil: A case control study. Lung Cancer 1994;11:179-90.

103. Sankarnarayanan R, Varghese C, Dugffy SW, Padmakumary G, Day NE, Nair MK. A case control study of diet and lung cancer in Keral, South India. Int J Cancer 1994;58:644-49.

104. Doll R, et al. The strategy for detection of lung cancer hazards to men. Nature 1977;265:589-95.

105. Du Y, Cha Q, Chen X, et al. An epidemiological study of risk factors for lung cancer in Guangzhou, China. Lung Cancer 1996;14(Suppl 1);S9-S37.

106. Gupta MP, Khanduja KL, Koul IB, Sharma RR. Effect of cigarette smoke inhalation on benzo(a)pyrene induced lung carcinogenesis in Vitmin A deficiency in the rat. Cancer Letter 1990;55:83-93.

107. Heinonen O. The effect of vitamin E and beta carotene on the incidence of lung cancer and other cancers in male smokers. New Engl J Med 1994;330:1029-35.

108. Barbone F, Bovenzi M, Cavallieri F, Stanta G. Air pollution and lung cancer in Trieste, Italy. Am J Epidemiol 1995;141:1161-69.

109. Tao X, Hong CJ, Yu S, Zhu H. Risk of male lung cancer attributed to coal combustion indoors in Shanghai. Public Health Rev 1992;19:127-34.

110. Ger LP, Hsu WL, Chen KT, Chen CJ. Risk factors of lung cancer by histological category in Taiwan. Anticancer Res 1993;13:1491-1500.

111. Crawford WA. On air pollution, environmental tobacco smoke, radon, and lung cancer. J Air Pollut Control Assc 1988;38:1386-91.

112. Buffler PA, Cooper SP, Stinnett S, et al. Air pollution and lung cancer mortality in Harris County, Texas, 1979-1981. Am J Epidemiol 1988;128:683-99.

113. Freeman DJ, Cattell PCR. The risk of lung cancer from polycyclic aromatic hydrocarbons in Sydney air. Med J Aust 1988;149:612-15.

114. Xu YZ, Blot WJ, Xiao HP, et al. Smoking, air pollution, and the high rate of lung cancer in Shenyang, China. J Natl Cancer Inst 1989;81:1800-16.

115. Mumford JL, Chapman RS, Harris DB, et al. Indoor air exposure to coal and wood combustion emissions associated with a high lung cancer rate in Xuan Wei, China. Environ Int 1989;15:315-20.

116. Chapman RS, Mumford JL, He X, et al. Assessing indoor air pollution exposure and lung cancer risk in Xuan Wei, China. J Am Coll Toxicol 1989;8:941-48.

117. Xu ZY, Brown L, Pan GW, et al. Lifestyle, environmental pollution and lung cancer in cities of Lioning in northeastern China. Lung Cancer 1996;14(Suppl 1):S149-S160.

118. Brown lM, Pottern LM, Blot WJ. Lung cancer in relation to pollutants emitted from industrial sources. Environ Res 1984;34:250-61.

119. Pershengen G. Lung cancer mortality among men living near an arsenin-emitting smelter. Am J Epidemiol 1985;122:684-94.

120. Wu JM, Du YX. Summary of papers and research recommendations presented at the International Symposium on life style factors and human lung cancer, Guangzhou, China. Lung Cancer 1996;14(Suppl 1):S223-S234.

121. Wu-Williams AH, Dai XD, Blot WJ, et al. Lung cancer among women in North east China. Br J Cancer 1990;62:982-87.

122. Gao YT, Blot WJ, Zheng W, et al. Lung cancer among Chinese women. Int J Cancer 1987;40:604-09.

123. Gao YT. Risk factors for lung cancer among non-smokers with emphasis on lifestyle factors. Lung Cancer 1996;14(Suppl 1):S39-S45.

124. Wu AH, Fontham ETH, Reynolds P, et al. Previous lung disease and risk of lung cancer among life-time nonsmoking women in the United States. Am J Epidemiol 1995;141:1023-32.

125. Weiss W. COPD and lung cancer. In: Cherniak NS (Ed): Obstructive Pulmonary Disease, Philadelphia: WB Saunders 1991;344-47.

126. Gao YT, Zheng W, Jin F, et al. A case control study on the association of lung cancer with pulmonary tuberculosis. J Epidemiol (Jpn Epidemiol Assoc) 1992;2 (Suppl)S82-S88.

127. Johnson DE, Geogieff MK. Pulmonary perspective: Neuroendocrine cells in health and disease. Am Rev Respir Dis 1989;140:1807-12.

128. Youngson C, Nurse C, Yeger H, et al. Oxygen sensing in airway chemoreceptors. Nature 1993;365:153-55.

129. Schuller HM, Miller MS, Park PD, Orloff MS. Promoting mechanisms of CO_2 on neuroendocrine cell proliferation mediated by nicotine receptor stimulation. Significance for lung cancer risk in individuals with chronic lung disease. Chest 1996;109(Suppl):20S- 21S.

130. Ool WL, Elston RC, Chen VW, et al. Increased familial risk for lung cancer. J Natl Cancer Inst 1986;76:217-22.

131. Sellers TA, Bailey-Wilson JE, Elston RC, et al. Evidence for Mendelian inheritance on the pathogenesis of lung cancer. J Natl Cancer Inst 1990;82:1272-79.

132. Minna JD. Genetic events in the pathogenesis of lung cancer. Chest 1989;96:17S.

133. Sikora K, Ong G. Cancer genes. Thorax 1990;45:409.

134. Minna JD, Bader S, Bansel A, et al. Molecular genetics of lung cancer. Multiple genetic lesions are involved in the pathogenesis of lung cancer. In Lung Cancer. Frontiers in Science and Treatment. Ed: Motta G, Genoa, Italy, 1994:25-47.

135. Buchhagen DL. Molecular mechanisms in lung pathogenesis. Biochem Biophys Acta 1991;1972:159-76.

136. Brennan J, O'Connor T, Mackuch RW, et al. *myc* family DNA amplification in 107 tumors and tumor cell lines from patients with small cell lung cancer treated with different combination chemotherapy regimens. Cancer Res 1991;51:1708-12.

137. Whangpeng J, Kao SC, Lee EC, et al. Specific chromosome defect associated with human small cell lung cancer; deletion 3p(14-23). Science 1982;215:181-82.

138. Funa K, Steinholtz L, Nou E, et al. Increased expression of N-*myc* in human small cell lung cancer biopsies predict lack of response to chemotherapy and poor prognosis. Am J Clin Pathol 1987;88:216-20.

139. Rodenhuis S, Slebos R, Boot A, et al. Mutational activation of the K-*ras* oncogene: A possible pathogenetic factor in adenocarcinoma of the lung. N Engl J Med 1987;317:929-35.

140. Slebos RJ, Hruban RH, Dalesion O, et al. Relationship between K-*ras* oncogene activation and smoking in adenocarcinoma of lung. J Natl Cancer Inst 1991;83:1024-27.

141. Slebos RJ, Kibbelaar RE, Dalesio O, et al. K-ras oncogene activation as a prognostic marker in adenocarcinoma of lung. New Engl J Med 1990;323:561-65.

142. Mitsodomi T, Steinberg SM, Oie H, et al. Ras gene mutation in non-small lung cancers are associated with shortened survival irrespective of treatment. Cancer Res 1991;100:429-38.

143. Berenson JR, Koga H, Yang J, et al. Frequent amplification of the bcl-1 locus in poorly differentiated squamous cell carcinoma of the lung. Oncogene 1990;5:1343-48.

144. Sekido Y, Obata Y, Ueda R, et al. Preferential expression of c-kit proto-oncogene transcripts in small cell lung cancer. Cancer Res 1991;51:2416-19.

145. Whang-Peng J, Bumm PJ, Kao SC, et al. A non-random chromosomal abnormality, deletion 3-p(14-23), in human small cell lung cancer (SCLC). Cancer Genet Cytogenet 1982;6:119-34.

146. Harris CC, Reddel R, Pfeifer A, et al. Role of oncogenes and tumor suppressor genes in human lung carcinogenesis. In O'Neil IKO, Chen J, Bartch (Eds): Relevance

to human cancer of nitroso compound, tobacco smoke, and mycotoxins. Lyon, International Agency for Research on Cancer 1991;294-303.

147. Carney DN. Oncogenes and genetic abnormalities in lung cancer. Chest 1989;96:27S.

148. Rabbitts P, Douglas J, Daly M, et al. Frequency and extent of allelic loss in the short arm of chromosome 3 in non-small cell lung cancer. Genes Chrom Cancer 1989;1:95-195.

149. Ludwig CU, Raefle G, Dalquen P, et al. Allelic loss on the short arm of chromosome 11 in non-small lung cancer. Int J Cancer 1991;49:661-65.

150. Skinner MA, Vollmer R, Huper G, et al. Loss of heterozygosity for genes on 11p and the clinical course of patients with lung carcinoma. Cancer Res 1990;50: 2303-06.

151. Weston A, Willey JC, Modali R, et al. Differential DNA sequence deletion from chromosomes 3,11,13, and 17 in squamous cell carcinoma, large cell carcinoma, and adenocarcinoma of the human lung. Proc Natl Acad Sc USA 1989;86:3968-73.

152. Hensel CH, Hsieh CL, Gazdar AF, et al. Altered structure and expression of the human retinoblastoma susceptibility gene in small cell lung cancer. Cancer Res 1990;50:3067-72.

153. Horowitz JM, Park SH, Bogenmann E, et al. Frequent inactivation of the retinoblastoma anti-oncogene is restricted to a subset of human tumor cells, Proc Natl Acad Sci USA 1990;87:2775-79.

154. Chiba I, Takahashi T, Nau MM, et al. Mutations in the p53 gene are frequent in primary, resected non-small cell lung cancer. Oncogene 1990;5:1603-10.

155. Takahashi T, Nau Mm, Chiba I, et al. p53: A frequent target for genetic abnormalities in lung cancer. Science 1989;246:491-94.

156. Lung ML, Wong MP, Skaanild CL, et al. p53 mutation in non-small cell lung carcinomas in Hong Kong. Chest 1996;109:718-26.

157. Naylor SL, Marshall A, Johnson AB, et al. Chromosome 3p in small cell lung cancer. Lung Cancer 1988;4:117-20.

158. Kadowaki MH, Ferguson MK. The role of chromosome 3 deletions in lung cancer. Lung Cancer 1990;6:165-70.

159. Hosoe S, Shigedo Y, Ueno K, et al. Detailed deletion mapping of the short arm of chromosome 3 in small cell and non-small cell carcinoma of the lung. Lung Cancer 1994;10:297-306.

160. WHO International histological classification of tumors, No 1. In Histological typing of lung tumors (2nd edn),WHO: Geneva 1981.

161. The WHO histological typing of lung tumors. Am J Clin Pathol 1982;77:123-36.

162. Mathews MJ. World Health Organization lung cancer classification. Chest 1986;89:315S.

163. Lamb D. Histological classification of lung cancer. Thorax 1984;39:161.

164. Yesner R. Update in pathology. Chest 1986;89:307S.

165. Report on the 3rd IASLC Lung Tumor Biology Workshop, 6-9 August, 1990. Lung Cancer 1991;7:171-78.

166. Carr DT, Holoye PY. Bronchogenic carcinoma. In Murray JF, Nadel JA (Eds): Textbook of Respiratory Medicine. WB Saunders Company: Philadelphia 1988;50:1174.

167. Vincent RG, Pickren JW, Lane WW, et al. The changing histopathology of lung cancer Cancer 1977;39:1647.

168. Beard CM, Jedd MB, Woolner LB, et al. Fifty-year trend in incidence rate of bronchogenic carcinoma by cell type in Olmsted county, Minnesota. J Natl Cancer Inst 1988;80:1404-07.

169. Tanaka I, Matsubara O, Kasuga T, et al. Increasing incidence and changing histopathology of primary lung cancer in Japan. Cancer 1988;62:1035-39.

170. Waggenar SSC, Tazelaar HD, Grimbrere CHF, et al. Second primary lung cancer. An update and International comparison. In G Motta (Ed): Lung Cancer. Frontier in Sciences and Treatment: G Motta Public, Genoa, Italy 1994;527-34.

171. Ikeda T, Kurita Y, Inusuka S, et al. The changing pattern of lung cancer by histological type: A review of 1151 cases from a university hospital in Japan, 1970-1989. Lung Cancer 1991;7:157-64.

172. Wagenaar SSC, Tazelaar HD. Ten years after the WHO classification for lung cancer: Where are we? Lung Cancer 1994;11(Suppl 3):S39-S43.

173. Choi JH, Chung HC, Yoo NC, et al. Changing trends in histological types of lung cancer during the last decade (1981-1990) in Korea: A hospital-based study. Lung Cancer 1994;10:287-96.

174. Mooi WF, Dingemans KP, Wagenaar SS, et al. Ultrastructural heterogeneity of lung carcinomas: Representatives of samples for electron microscopy in tumor classification. Hum Pathol 1990;21:1227-34.

175. Gazdar AF, Helman LJ, Israel MA, et al. Expression of neuroendocrine cell markers L-dopa decarboxylase, chromogranin A, and dense core granules in human tumors of endocrine and nonendocrine origin. Cancer Res 1988;48:4078-82.

176. Garney DN, Gazdar AF, Bepler G, et al. Establishment and identification of small cell lung cancer cell lines having classic and variant features. Cancer Res 1985;45:2913-23.

177. Carney DN. Recent advances in the biology of small cell lung cancer. Chest 1986;89(Suppl):253S.

178. Fergusson RJ, Smyth JF. Studying lung cancer in the laboratory: 1-development of model systems. Thorax 1987;42:753-58.

179. Fergusson RJ, Smyth JF. Studying lung cancer in the laboratory: 2-chemosensitivity testing. Thorax 1987;42: 833-37.

180. Fergusson RJ, Smyth JF. Studying lung cancer in the laboratory: Use of cell lines to investigate the biology of lung cancer. Thorax 1987;42:922-25.

181. Connor PJ. Molecular mechanisms in chemically induced cancer. Chest 1989;96;24S.

182. Sheppard MN. Neuroendocrine differentiation in lung tumors. Thorax 1991;46:843-50.

183. Woll PJ. Growth factors and lung cancer. Thorax 1991;46:924-29.

184. Stahel RA. Monoclonal antibodies in lung cancer. Chest 1989;96:27S.

185. Yamaguchi K, Imanishi K, Maruno K, et al. Lung cancer and autocrine growth factors. Chest 1989;96:31S.

186. Haeder M, Rotsch M, Bepler G, et al. Epidermal growth factor expression in human lung cancer cell lines. Cancer Res 1988;48:1132-36.

187. Soderdahl G, Betsholtz C, Johansson A, Nilsson K, Bergh J. Differential expression of platelet-derived growth factor and transforming growth factor genes in small- and non-small cell human lung carcinoma lines. Int J Cancer 1988;41:636-41.

188. Veale D, Kerr N, Gibson GH, Harris AL. Characterization of epidermal growth factor receptor in primary human non-small cell lung cancer. Cancer Res 1989;49:1313-17.

189. Tateishi M, Ishida T, Mitsudomi T, Kaneko S, Sugimachi K. Immunohistochemical evidence of autocrine growth factors in adenocarcinoma of the human lung. Cancer Res 1990;50:7077-80.

190. Kern JA, Schwartz DA, Nordberg JE, et al. p185^{neu} expression in human lung adenocarcinomas predicts shortened survival. Cancer Res 1990;50:5184-91.

191. Mooi WJ, Dewar A, Springall D, Polak JM, Addis BJ. Non-small cell lung carcinomas with neuroendocrine features. A light microscopic, immunohistochemical, and ultrastructural study of 11 cases. Histopathology 1988;13:329-37.

192. Graziano SL, Mazid R, Newman N, et al. The use of neuroendocrine immunoperoxidase markers to predict chemotherapy response in patients with non-small cell lung cancer. J Clin Oncol 1989;7:1398-1406.

193. Hamid QA, Corrin B, Dewar A, Hoefler H, Sheppard MN. Expression of gastrin-releasing peptide (human bombesin) gene in large cell undifferentiated carcinoma of the lung. J Pathol 1990;161;145-51.

194. Behera D, Malik SK, Sharma BR, Dash RJ. Circulating hormones in lung cancer. Ind J Med Res 1984;79: 636-40.

195. Behera D, Dash S, Malik SK, Dash RJ. Serum hCG in bronchogenic carcinoma. Ind J Chest Dis All Sc 1984;26:238-41.

196. Behera D, Malik SK, Dani HM, Gumbhir K. Circulating blood RNA in lung cancer. J Assc Phys Ind 1986;34: 579-80.

197. Behera D, Gumbhir K, Malik SK, Dani HM. Lung cancer and circulating DNA. Ind J Chest Dis All Sc 1986;28: 54-55.

198. Lau-Wong MM, Kwan SYL, Yew WW, et al. Application of squamous cell carcinoma associated antigen mono-clonal radioimmunoassay in the diagnosis of broncho-genic carcinoma. Lung Cancer 1991;7:151-56.

199. Thomas F, Brambrilla E, Friedman A. Transcription of siomatostatin receptor subtype 1 and 2 genes in lung cancer. Lung Cancer 1994;11:111-14.

200. Kiriakogiani-Psaropoulou P, Malamou-Mitsi V, Martino-poulou U, et al. The value of neuroendocrine markers in non-small lung cancer: A comparative immunohisto-pathologic study. Lung Cancer 1994;11:353-64.

201. Stahel RA. Biology of lung cancer. Lung Cancer 1994;10(Suppl 1):S59-S66.

202. Szturmowicz M, Roginska E, Roszkowski K, et al. Prognostic value of neuron-specific enolase in small cell lung cancer patients. Lung Cancer 1993;8:259-64

203. O'Byrne KJ, Carney DN. Somatostatin and the lung. Lung Cancer 1993;10:151-72.

204. Muller LC, Gasser R, Huber H, Klingler A, Salzer GM. Neuron-specific enolase in small cell lung cancer: Longitudinal tumor marker evaluation. Lung Cancer 1992;8:29-36.

205. Nakamura H, Sayami P, Hayata Y. Analysis of G-CSF producing lung cancer cell lines and non-growth stimulatory effects of rhG-CSF on lung cancer cells *in vitro* and *in vivo*. Lung Cancer 1992;8:141-52.

206. Kayser K, Gabius HJ, Kohler A, Runtsch T. Binding of neuroendocrine markers and biotinylated sex hor-mones and the survival in human lung cancer. Lung Cancer 1990;6:171-83.

207. Hirsch FR, Holst JJ, Spang-Thomsen M, Larson MT. Immunocytochemical demonstration of bombesin in immunoreactivity in small cell carcinoma of the lung. Lung Cancer 1990;6:1-8.

208. Schneider PM, Hung MC, Ames RS, et al. A novel alteration in the epidermal growth factor receptor gene is frequently detected in human non-small cell lung cancer. Lung Cancer 1990;6:65-72.

209. International Conference on Hormones, Growth Factors, and Oncogenes in Pulmonary Carcinoma. Lung Cancer 1988;4, Special Issue.

210. Buccheri G, Ferrigno D, Vola F. Carcinoembryonic antigen (CEA), tissue polypeptide antigen (TPA) and other prognostic indicators in squamous cell lung cancer. Lung Cancer 1993;10:21-33.

211. Saito S, Tanio Y, Tachibana I, et al. Complimentary DNA sequence encoding the major neural cell adhesion molecule isoform in a human small cell lung cancer cell line. Lung Cancer 1994;10:307-18.

212. Buccheri G, Ferrigno D. Monitoring lung cancer with tissue polypeptide antigen: An ancilliary, profitable serum test to evaluate treatment response and posttreatment disease status. Lung Cancer 1995;13: 155-68.

213. Moro D, Villemain D, Vuillez JP, Delord CA, Brambilla C. CEA, CYFRA21-1, and SCC in non-small cell lung cancer. Lung Cancer 1995;13:169-76.

214. Splinter TAW. Serum tumor markers and management of non-small cell lung cancer. Lung Cancer 1995;13: 177-79.

215. Mitshuhashi N, Takahashi T, Sakurai H, et al. Establishment and characterization of a new human lung poorly differentiated adenocarcinoma cell line, GLL-1, producing carcinoembryonic antigen (CEA) and CA19-9. Lung Cancer 1995;12:13-24.

216. Scagliotti GV, Masiero P, Pozzi E. Biological prognostic factors in non-small cell lung cancer. Lung Cancer 1995;12(Suppl 1):S13-S25.

217. Johnson BE, Kelly MJ. Biology of small cell lung cancer. Lung Cancer 1995;12(Suppl3):S5-S16.

218. Roth JA. Molecular events in lung cancer. Lung Cancer 1995;12(Suppl 2):S3-S15.

219. Kwa HB, Michalides RJAM, Dijkman JH, Mooi WJ. The prognostic value of NCAM, p53, and cyclin D1 in resected non-small cell lung cancer. Lung Cancer 1996;14:207-18.

220. Norgaard P, Damstrup L, Rygaard K, Spang-Thompsen M, Poulsen HS. Acquired TGF beta-1 sensitivity and TGF beta-2 expression in cell lines established from a single small cell lung cancer patient during clinical progression. Lung Cancer 1996;14:63-74.

221. Timoshenko AV, Kayser K, Kaltner H, Andre S, Gabius HJ. Binding capacity of two immunomodulatory lectins, carrier-immobilized glycoligands and steroid hormones in lung cancer and the concentration of nitrite/nitrate in pleural effusions. Lung Cancer 1996;14:75-84.

222. 4th IASLC lung tumor biology workshop. Brief Report. Lung Cancer 1994;10:339-46.

223. Minna JD. The molecular biology of lung cancer pathogenesis. Chest 1993;103:449S-456S.

224. Beverly PCL, Bobrow LG, Souhami RS. Second International workshop on Small Cell Lung Cancer Antigens. Br J Cancer 1991;63:Suppl XIV.

225. Souhami RS, Beverly PCL, Bobrow LG, Ledermann JA. Antigens of lung cancer: Results of the Second International Workshop on Lung Cancer antigens. J Natl Cancer Inst 1991;83:609-12.

226. Koros AMC, Atchison RW, Mitchell DL. Small cell lung cancer antigen expression differs on 'classic' and 'variant' SCLC and carcinoid cells. Lung Cancer 1991;7:225-34.

227 Souhami RL. The antigens of lung cancer. Thorax 1992;47:53-56.

228. Weynants P, Humblet Y, Canon JL, Symann M. Biology of small cell lung cancer: An overview. Eur Respir J 1990;3:699-14.

229. Sanderson DR. Lung cancer screening. The Mayo study. Chest 1986;89:324S.

230. Woolner LB, Farrow GM. Mayo Lung Project: Pathological findings in occult bronchogenic carcinoma detected through lung cancer screening. Clin Oncol 1982;1:513-26.

231. Gabrielli M, Cattelani L, Rusca M, et al. The efficacy of sputum occult blood screening (SOBS) for the cytological diagnosis of lung atypias: Preliminary results of a lung Cancer (LC) screening in a little county community near Parma. In: Lung Cancer = Frontiers in science and treatment. Motta G (Ed): Italy 1993; 209-16.

232. Sobue T, Suzuki T, Naruke T, The Japanese Lung-Cancer-Screening Research Group. A case control study for evaluating lung cancer screening in Japan. Int J Cancer 1992;50:230.

233. Fontana R, Sanderson DR, Woolner LB, et al. Screening for lung cancer. A critique of the Mayo Lung Project. Cancer 1991;67:1155-64.

234. Strauss GM, Gleason RE, Sugarbaker DJ. Screening for lung cancer re-examined. A reinterpretation of the Mayo Lung Project. Randomized trials on lung cancer screening. Chest 1993;103:337S-341S.

235. Melamed MR, Flehinger BJ, Zaman MB. Impact of early detection on the clinical course of lung cancer. Surg Clin North Am 1987;67:909-35.

236. American Joint Committee on Cancer, Task force on Lung: Staging of Lung Cancer. Chicago: American Joint Committee on Cancer 1979.

237. Harmer EM. TNM classification of malignant tumors, Geneva, Union Internationale Contre le Cancer 1978; 41-45.

238. Mountain CF. A new International staging system for lung cancer. Chest 1986;89(Suppl):225S-233S.

239. Spiro SG, Goldstraw P. The staging of lung cancer. Thorax 1984;39:401.

240. Bulzebruck H, Drings P, Kayser K, et al. Classification of lung cancer: First experience with the new TNM classification (4th edn). Eur Respir J 1991;4:1197.

241. Medina FM, Barrera RR, Morales JF, et al. Primary lung cancer in Mexico city: A report of 1019 cases. Lung Cancer 1996;14:185-93.

242. Lam WK, So SY, Yu DYC. Clinical features of bronchogenic carcinoma in Hong Kong. Review of 480 patients. Cancer 1983;52:369-76.

243. Gupta RC, Behera D, Malik SK. Bronchogenic carcinoma in the young adults below the age of 35 years. Ind J Chest Dis 1984;26:3-5.

244. Green LS, Fortoul TI, Ponciano G, Robles C, Rivero O. Bronchogenic cancer in patients under 40 years old. The experience of a Latin American County. Chest 1993; 104:1477-81.

245. Samet JM, Wiggins CL, Humble CG, Pathak DR. Cigarette smoking and lung cancer in New Mexico. Am Rev Respir Dis 1988;1327:1110-13.

246. Capewell S, Sankaran K, Lamb D, Mc Intyre M, Sudlow MF. Lung cancer in life long non- smokers. Thorax 1991;46:565-65.

247. Coultas DHB, Samet JM. Occupational lung cancer. Clin Chest Med 1992;13:341-54.

248. Kiricuta IC, Mueller G, Stiess J, Bohndorf W. The lymphatic pathways of non-small cell lung cancer and their implication in curative irradiation treatment. Lung Cancer 1994;11:71-82.

249. Pancoast HK. Importance of careful roentgen-ray investigations of apical chest tumors. JAMA 1924;83: 1407-11.

250. Sartori F, Rea F, Breda C, et al. Resection for superior sulcus tumor. In Motta G (Ed): Lung Cancer. Frontiers in Science and Treatment. Genoa 1993;469-72.

251. Vituc C, Kunze M. From anmnesis to diagnosis in male lung cancer patients. International Congress Series No. 558. Lung Cancer. Etiology, Epidemiology, Prevention, Early diagnosis, Treatment. Proceedings of the 1st European Symposim on Lung Cancer, Chalkidiki, 1980;94-99.

252. Gabaza EC, Taguchi O, Yamakami T, et al. Evaluating prethrombotic state in lung cancer using molecular marker. Chest 1993;103:196-200.

253. Behera D, Kalra S, Nalini K, Malik SK, Jindal SK, Dash RJ. Galactorrhoea with gynecomastia in a male with lung cancer. Indian J Chest Dis Allied Sci 1987;29: 112-14.

254. Thirkill CE. Lung cancer-induced blindness. Lung Cancer 1996;14:253-64.

255. Matsubara S, Yamaji Y, Fijita T, et al. Cancer-associated retinopathy syndrome: A case of small cell lung cancer expressing recover in immunoreactivity. Lung Cancer 1996;14:265-71.

256. Donovan WD, Yankelevitz DF, Henschke CI, Altorki N, Nash TA. Endobronchial spread of bronchiolo-alveolar carcinoma. Chest 1993;104:951-53.

257. Elliot JA. Preoperative mediastinal evaluation in primary bronchial carcinoma: A review of staging investigations. Postgrad Med J 1984;60:83-91.

258. Colice GL. Chest CT for known or suspected lung cancer. Chest 1994;106:1538-50.

259. Akata S, Fukushima A, Kakizaki D, Abe K, Amino S. CT scanning of bronchiolo-alveolar cell carcinoma: Specific appearances. Lung Cancer 1995;12:221-30.

260. Larsson S. Mediastinoscopy in bronchogenic carcinoma. Scand J Thorac Cardiovasc Surg 1976;19(suppl).

261. Boilleau G, Pujol JL, Ychou M, et al. Detection of lymph node metastasis in lung cancer: Comparison of 131I-Anti-CEA-Anti-CA 19-9 immunoscintigraphy versus computed tomography. Lung Cancer 1994;11:209-19.

262. Lam S, MacAulay C, Palcic B. Detection and early localization of early lung cancer by imaging techniques. Chest 1993;103(Suppl):12S-14S.

263. Avasthi PS, Chakrabarty SN, Gupta SP. Needle biopsy of the lung. J Ind Med Ass 1962;39:289-91.

264. Chaubey VS, Dubey GK. Observations on percutaneous lung biopsy. Ind J Chest Dis All Sc 1972;14:151-57.

265. Chaudhury R, Ajmani NK, Mishra RC, Chuttani HK. Percutaneous needle biopsy of the lung. Ind J Chest Dis 1976;18:245-50.

266. Gupta SK, Dhand R, Kaul K, Jindal SK, Malik SK. Aspiration cytology of lung lesions. Ind J Chest Dis All Sc 1979;21:108-15.

267. Sharma SK, Verma V, Pande JN, Guleria JS. Fine needle aspiration biopsy cytology for diagnosis of intrathoracic lesions. Ind J Chest Dis All Sc 1983;25:41-45.

268. Gera ML, Parmar MS, Raj B, Mehrotra MC. Role of percutaneous needle lung biopsy in the diagnosis of pulmonary lesions. Ind J Chest Dis 1983;25:109-12.

269. Singh NM, Gupta RKJ, Das DK, Pant CS. Ultrasonically guided fine needle aspiration biopsy (FNAB) of intrathoracic lesions. Ind J Chest Dis All Sc 1987;29: 81-89.

270. Rajwanshi A, Jayaram N, Behera D, Gupta SK, Malik SK. Fine needle aspiration cytology of intrathoracic lesions: a reappraisal. Ind J Pathol Microbiol 1989;32: 306-09.

271. Verma K. Cytological diagnosis in lung diseases. Ind J Chest Dis All Sc 1983;26:89-90.

272. Erozan YS, Frost JK. Cytopathologic diagnosis of lung cancer. In Straus MJ (Ed): Lung Cancer: Clinical diagnosis and treatment. Grune and Straton: New York 1977;7:95.

273. Dhand R, Jindal SK, Malik SK. Diagnostic methods in lung cancer. Ind J Cancer 1982;19:77-80.

274. Guber A, Cohen R, Ronah R, et al. Flow cytometric analysis and cytokeratin typing of human lung tumors. Chest 1994;105:138-43.

275. Utz JP, Patel AM, Edell EC. The role of transcarinal aspiration in the staging of bronchogenic carcinoma. Chest 1993;104:1012-16.

276. Jones DF, Chin R Jr, Cappellari JO, Haponik EF. Endobronchial needle aspiration in the diagnosis of small cell carcinoma. Chest 1994;105:1151-54.

277. Frost JK, Ball WC Jr, Levin ML, et al. Sputum cyto-pathology: Use and potential in monitoring the work place environment by screening for biological effects of exposure. J Occup Med 1986;28:692-703.

278. Gulati M, Kumar S, Suman K, Kumar S, Suri S, Behera D, Jindal SK. Ultrasound guided aspiration biopsy of peripheral pulmonary lesions. Indian J Chest Dis Allied Sci 1996;38:19-23.

279. Zavala DC. Diagnostic fibreoptic bronchoscopy. Techniques and results of biopsy in 600 patients. Chest 1975;68:12-19.

280. Kvale PA, Bode FR, Kini S. Diagnostic accuracy in lung cancer. Comparisons of techniques used in association with flexible fibreoptic bronchoscopy. Chest 1976;69: 752-56.

281. Gemma A, Takenaka K, Andou M, et al. Bronchoscopic findings of extramural lung cancer invading the subepithelium or submucosa. Lung Cancer 1995;12: 35-44.

282. Kvale PA. Collection and preparations of bronchoscopic specimens. Chest 1978;73(Suppl):707-12.

283. Chuang MT, Marchevsky A, Teirstein A, et al. Diagnosis of lung cancer by fibreoptic bronchoscopy: Problems in the histological classification of non-small cell lung cancer. Thorax 1984;39:175.

284. Saltzstein SL, Harrell JH, Cameron T. Brushings, washings, or biopsy? Obtaining maximum value from flexible fibreoptic bronchoscopy in the diagnosis of cancer. Chest 1977;71:630-32.

285. Richardson RH, Zavala DC, Mukerjee PK, Bedell GN. The use of fibreoptic bronchoscopy and brush biopsy in the diagnosis of suspected pulmonary malignancy. Am Rev Respir Dis 1974;109:63-69.

286. Mitchell DM, Emerson CJ, Collyer J, Collins JV. Fibreoptic bronchoscopy: Ten years on. Br Med J 1980;2:360-63.

287. Lam WK, So SY, Hsu C, Yu DYC. Fibreoptic bronchoscopy in the diagnosis of lung cancer: Comparison of washings, brushings and biopsies in central and peripheral tumors. Clin Oncol 1983;9:35-42.

288. Jindal SK, Behera D, Dhand R, Kashyap S, Malik SK. Flexible fibreoptic bronchoscopy in clinical practice: A review of 1000 procedures. Ind J Chest Dis All Sc 1985;27:153-58.

289. Pande JN, Sharma SK, Tondon M, Verma K, Guleria JS. Fibreoptic bronchoscopy in the diagnosis of malignant lesions of lung: A 3 years experience. Ind J Chest Dis All Sc 1982;24:244-50.

290. Kulpati DDS, Kumar V, Hira HS, Chauhan MR. Flexible fibreoptic bronchoscopy in endoscopically visible bronchogenic carcinoma. Ind J Chest Dis All Sc 1985;27:207-10.

291. Kapoor SC. Comparative study of fibreoptic bronchoscopy and rigid bronchoscopy. Lung India 1982;1:25-28.

292. Minami H, Ando Y, Nomura F, et al. Interbronchoscopist variability in the diagnosis of lung cancer by flexible bronchoscopy. Chest 1994;105:1658-62.

293. Poe RH, Levy PC, Israel RH, et al. Use of fibreoptic bronchoscopy in the diagnosis bronchogenic carcinoma. A study in patients with idiopathic pleural effusions. Chest 1994;105:1663-67.

294. Keicho N, Oka T, Takeuchi K, et al. Detection of lymphomatous involvement of the lung by broncho-alveolar lavage. Application of immunophenotypic and gene rearrangement analysis. Chest 1994;105:458-62.

295. Wang KP. Staging of bronchogenic carcinoma by bronchoscopy. Chest 1994;106:588-93.

296. The Japan Lung Cancer Society. General rule for clinical and pathological record of lung cancer (3rd edn), Tokyo; Kanehara Shuppan Ltd. 1987;59-68.

297. Recchione C, Galante E, Secreto G, Cavalleri A, Dati V. Abnormal serum hormone levels in lung cancer. Tumori 1983;69:293-98.

298. Calciano A, Khaw KT, Barrett-Conner E, Garland C. Sex hormones, sex hormone binding globulin, and lung cancer: A 12 year prospective study in a cohort of men aged 50-79. Br Med J 1988;4:569-70.

299. Monfardine S, et al. UICC Technical Report Series (3rd edn). Geneva 1981;56:21.

300. Goldstraw P, Rocmans P, Ball D, et al. Pre-treatment minimal staging for non-small cell lung cancer: An updated consensus report. Lung Cancer 1994;11(Suppl 3):S1-S4.

301. Zelen M. Key note address on biostatistics and data retrieval. Cancer Chemother Rep 1973;4:31-42.

302. Stahel RA, Ginsberg R, Havemann K, et al. Staging and prognostic factors in small cell lung cancer: A consensus report. Lung Cancer 1989;5:119-26.

303. Jensen LI, Hirsch FR, Peters K, Jensen F, Thomsen C. Diagnosis of abdominal metastases in small cell carcinoma of the lung: A prospective study of computer tomography and ultrasonography. Lung Cancer 1992;8:37-45.

304. Mitchel F, Soler M, Imhof E, Perruchoud AP. Initial staging of non-small cell lung cancer: Value of routine isotope bone scanning. Thorax 1991;46:469.

305. Glazer GM. Radiologic staging of lung cancer using CT and MRI. Chest 1989;96:44S.

306. Sagel MSS. Computed tomography in the evaluation of lung cancer. Chest 1986;89:318S.

307. Hansen HH. Chemotherapy of small cell carcinoma: A review. Q J Med 1987;63:275-82.

308. Hansen HH, Kristjansen PEG. Changing concepts in the management of patients with lung cancer. Med J Australia 1988;149:77.

309. Debevec M, Orel J. Treatment of small cell lung cancer by surgery, chemotherapy, and irradiation. Lung Cancer 1991;7:339.

310. Albain KS, Crowley JJ, Livingston RB. Long-term survival and toxicity in small cell lung cancer. Expanded Southwest Oncology Group experience. Chest 1991;99:1425.

311. Behera D. Therapy of lung cancer-recent progress. Lung India 1990;8:53.

312. Behera D. Recent advances in the management of lung cancer. J Asso Phys India 1991;39:337.

313. Behera D, Malik SK. Chemotherapy of inoperable bronchogenic carcinoma. Ind J Chest Dis All Sci 1985;27:175.

314. Kristjansen PEG, Hansen HH. Brain metastases from small cell lung cancer treated with combination chemotherapy. Eur J Cancer Clin Oncol 1988;24:345-9.

315. Iredale JP, Hooi LM, Kerr KM, Sudlow MF, Wathen CJ. Vindesine and etoposide chemotherapy in the management of patients with small cell lung cancer and poor prognosis. Respiration 1991;58:77.

316. Pastan I, Gottesman MM. Multidrug resistance. Annu Rev Med 1991;42:277-312.

317. Behera D. Lung cancer to treat or not to treat. Bull Postgrad Inst Med Edu Res 1995;29:7-14.

318. Behera D, Jindal SK, Sharma SC. Etoposide (VP-16) containing combination chemotherapy for treatment of patients with small cell lung cancer. Ind J Chest Dis All Sc 1995;37:15-19.

319. Johnson D. Treatment of limited-stage small cell lung cancer: Recent progress and future directions. Lung Cancer 1993;9(Suppl 1):S1-S19.

320. Comis RL. Extensive small cell lung cancer. Lung Cancer 1993;9(Suppl 1):S27-S39.

321. Loeherer PJ Sr, Ansari R, Einorn LH. Extensive small cell lung cancer: Trials of Indiana University and the Hoosier Oncology Group. Lung Cancer 1993;9(Suppl 1):S41-S49.

322. Thatcher N. Ifosfamide/carboplatin/etoposide (ICE) regimen in small cell lung cancer. Lung Cancer 1993;9 (Suppl 1):S51-S67.

323. Bishop JF. The role of colony-stimulating factors in small cell lung cancer. Lung Cancer 1993;9(Suppl 1):S75-S83.

324. Greco FA. Treatment options for patients with relapsed small cell lung cancer. Lung Cancer 1993;9(Suppl 1):S85-S89.

325. Keane M, Carney DN. Treatment of elderly patients with small cell lung cancer. Lung Cancer 1993;9(Suppl 1):S91-S98.

326. Aisner J. Strategies for new drug identification in small cell lung cancer. Lung Cancer 1993;9(Suppl 1):S99-S107.

327. Turrisi AT III. Current perspectives in the treatment of small cell lung cancer. Lung Cancer 1993;9(Suppl 1):S109-S117.

328. Turrisi AT III. Combined platinum etoposide with radiation therapy in limited stage small cell lung cancer: An effective treatment strategy. Lung Cancer 1995;12 (Suppl 3):S41-S51.

329. Ettinger DS. New drugs for treating small cell lung cancer. Lung Cancer 1995;12(Suppl 3):S53-S61.

330. Postmus PE, Smit EF. Oral therapy for small cell lung cancer. Lung Cancer 1994;12(Suppl 3):S63-S70.

331. Johnson DH. Future directions in the management of small cell lung cancer. Lung Cancer 1995;12(Suppl 3):S71-S75.

332. Carney DN. Carboplatin/etoposide combination chemotherapy in the treatment of poor prognosis patients with small cell lung cancer. Lung Cancer 1995;12 (Suppl 3):S77-S83.

333. Greco FA, Hainsworth JD. Etoposide phosphate or etoposide with cisplatin in the treatment of small cell lung cancer: Randomized phase II trial. Lung Cancer 1995;12(Suppl 3):S85-S95.

334. Souhami RL, Ruiz de Elvira MC. Chemotherapy dose intensity in small cell lung cancer. Lung Cancer 1994;10(Suppl 4):S175-S185.

335. Stephens RJ, Girling DJ, Machin D. Treatment related deaths in small cell lung cancer trials: Can patients at risk be identified? Lung Cancer 1994;11:259-74.

336. Morere JF, Duran A, Tcherakian F, et al. Cisplatin-5-fluorouracil in small cell lung cancer. A phase II study in 109 patients. Lung Cancer 1994;11:275-81.

337. Jassem J, Karnicka-Mlodkowska H, Jassem E, et al. Combination chemotherapy with cyclophopsphamide, epirubicin and etoposide in small cell lung cancer. Lung Cancer 1994;11:283-91.

338. Talbot DC, Smith IE. New drugs in lung cancer. Thorax 1992;47:188-94.

339. Sandler AB, Buzaid AC. Lung cancer: A review of current therapeutic modalities. Lung 1992;170:249-65.

340. O'Dwyer PJ, Leyland-Jones B, Alonso MT, Marsoni S, Wittes RE. Etoposide (VP-16-213). New Eng J Med 1985;312:692-700.

341. Smyth JF, Hansen HH. Current status of research into small cell carcinoma of the lung: Summary of the second workshop of the International Association of the Study of Lung Cancer (IASLC). Eur J Cancer Clin Oncol 1985;21:1295-98.

342. Hirsch FR, Hansen HH, Hansen M, et al. The superiority of chemotherapy including etoposide based *in vivo* cell cycle analysis in the treatment of extensive small cell lung cancer: A randomized trial of 288 consecutive patients. J Clin Oncol 1987;5:585-91.

343. Roed H, Vindelov LL, Christensen IBJ, Spang-Thomsen M, Hansen HH. The cytotoxic activity of cisplatin, carboplatin, and tenoposide alone and combined determined on four small cell lung cancer cell lines by the clonogenic assay. Eur J Cancer Clin Oncol 1988;24:247-53.

344. Livingston RB. Small cell carcinoma of the lung. Blood 1980;56:575-84.

345. Ihde DC, Makuch RW, Carney DN, et al. Prognostic implications of stage of disease and sites of metastases in patients with small cell carcinoma of the lung treated with intensive combination chemotherapy. Am Rev Respir Dis 1981;123:500-07.

346. Sibille Y, Steyaer J, Francis C, Bosly A, Prignot J. Three drug chemotherapy combined with radiation therapy in small cell carcinoma of the lung. Eur J Respir Dis 1983;64:113-20.

347. Chahinian AP, Mandel EL, Holland JF, Jaffrey IS, Terstlin AS. MACC (methotrexate, adriamycin, cyclophosphamide and CCNU) in advanced lung cancer. Cancer 1979;43:1590-97.

348. Morstyn G, Ihde DC, Lichter AS, et al. Small cell lung cancer 1973-1983: Early progress and recent obstacles. J Radiat Oncol Biol Phys 1984;10:515-39.

349. Broder LE, Selawry OS, Charyulu KN, Ng A, Bagwell S. A controlled clinical trial testing two potentially non-cross-resistant chemotherapeutic regimens in small cell carcinoma of the lung. Chest 1981;79:327-35.

350. Behera D. Chemotherapy of lung cancer: Experience from PGI, Chandigarh. Ind J Med Paed Oncol 1995;16:121-26.

351. Oldham RK, Greco FA. Small cell lung cancer. A curable disease. Cancer Chemother Pharmacol 1980;4:173-77.

352. Anonymous. Cancer, Cancer therapy, and hair. Lancet 1983;19:1177-78.

353. Kris MG, Gralla RJ, Clark RA, et al. Incidence, course, and severity of delayed nausea and vomiting following the administration of high dose cisplatin. J Clin Oncol 1985;3:1379-84.

354. Kris MG, Gralla RJ, Tyson LB, et al. Improved control of cisplatin-induced emesis with high dose metoclo-

pramide and with combination of metoclopramide, dexamethasone, and diphenhydramine. Cancer 1985;55: 527-34.

355. Bunn PA Jr, Kelly K. The role of routine chest radiotherapy in small cell lung cancer. An issue of timing and stage. Chest 1993;104:661-62.

356. Ohnosi T, Ueoka H, Kiura K, et al. Delayed chest irradiation for patients with limited small cell lung cancer. Lung Cancer 1994;10(Suppl 1):S338.

357. Feld R, Pringle JF, Evans WK, et al. Combined modality treatment of small cell carcinoma of the lung. Arch Intern Med 1981;141:469-73.

358. Ihde DC. Current status of therapy for small cell carcinoma of the lung. Cancer 1984;54:2722-28.

359. Osterlind K, Hansen HH, Hansen HS, et al. Chemotherapy versus chemotherapy plus irradiation in limited small cell lung cancer. Results of a controlled trial with 5 years follow-up. Br J Cancer 1986;54:7-17.

360. Turrisi A III. Innovations in multimodality therapy for lung cancer; combined modality management of limited small-cell lung cancer. Chest 1993;103:56S-59S.

361. Johnson BE. Current approaches to combined chemotherapy and chest radiotherapy for the treatment of patients with limited stage small cell lung cancer. Lung Cancer 1994;10(Suppl 1):S281-S288.

362. Arriagada R, Le Chevalier T, Ruffie P, et al. Alternative radiotherapy and chemotherapy in limited small cell lung cancer: The IGR protocol. Lung Cancer 1994; 10(Suppl 1):S289-S298.

363. Gregor A. Factors influencing use of alternating chemotherapy and radiation schedules in mall cell lung cancer. Lung Cancer 1994;10(Suppl 1):S299-S306.

364. Pignon JP, Arriagada R, Ihde DC, et al. Effects of thoracic radiotherapy on mortality in limited small cell lung cancer: A meta-analysis of 13 randomized trials among 2140 patients. New Engl J Med 1992;327:1618-24.

365. Perry MC, Eaton WL, Propert KJ, et al. Chemotherapy with or without radiotherapy in limited small cell carcinoma of the lung. N Engl J Med 1987;316:912-18.

366. Joss R, Alberto P, Bleher E, Kapanei Y, Cavalli F. Combined modality treatment of small cell lung cancer (SCLC): Randomized comparison of three induction chemotherapies followed by maintenance chemotherapy with or without radiotherapy to the chest. Proceedings of the fourth World Conference on lung Cancer, Toronto 1985;141.

367. Murray N, Coy P, Peter I, et al. The importance of timing for thoracic irradiation (TF) in the combined modality treatment of limited stage small cell lung cancer. (SCLC). Proc Am Soc Clin Oncol 1991;10:243.

368. Labeau B, Chastang C, Brechot JM, Capron F. A randomized trial of delayed thoracic radiotherapy in complete responder patients with small cell lung cancer. Chest 1993;104:726-33.

369. Payne DG, Arriagada R, Dombernowsky P, et al. The role of thoracic radiation therapy in small cell lung cancer: A consensus report. Lung Cancer 1989;5:135-38.

370. Turrisi A, Wagner H, Glover D, et al. Limited small cell lung cancer: Concurrent BID thoracic radiotherapy with platinum-etoposide ; an ECOG study. Proc Am Soc Clin Oncol 1990;230.

371. Kristjansen PEG. Should current management of small cell lung cancer include prophylactic cranial irradiation? Lung Cancer 1994;10(Suppl 1):S319-S330.

372. Ihde DC. Prophylactic cranial irradiation: Current controversies. Lung Cancer 1993;9(Suppl 1):S69-S74.

373. Kristjansen PEG, Hansen HH. Prophylactic cranial irradiation in small cell lung cancer an update. Lung Cancer 1995;12(Suppl 3):S23-S40.

374. Shields TW, Higgins GA, Mathews MJ, Heehn RJ. Surgical resection in the management of small cell carcinoma of lung. J Thorac Cardiovasc Surg 1982;84:481-88.

375. Johnson DH, Greco FA. Small cell carcinoma of the lung. CRC Crit Rev Oncol Hematol 1986;4:303-06.

376. Seifter EJ, Ihde DC. Therapy of small cell lung cancer: A perspective on two decades of clinical research. Semin Oncol 1988;15:278-99.

377. Shepherd FA, Ginsberg RJ, Feld R, Evans WK, Johansen E. Surgical treatment of limited small cell lung cancer. The University of Toranto Lung Oncology experience. J Thorac Cardiovasc Surg 1991;101:385-93.

378. Johnson DH, Einhorn LH, Mandelbaum I, Williams SD, Greco FA. Postchemotherapy resection of residual tumor in limited stage small cell lung cancer. Chest 1987;92:241-46.

379. Williams CJ, McMillan I, Lea R, et al. Surgery after initial chemotherapy for localized small cell carcinoma of the lung. J Clin Oncol 1987;5:1579-88.

380. Prager RL, Foster JM, Hainsworth JD, et al. The feasibility of adjuvant surgery in limited-stage small cell carcinoma: A prospective evaluation. Ann Thorac Surg 1984;38:622-26.

381. Meyer JA, Comis RL, Ginsberg SJ. Phase II trial of extended indications for resection in small cell carcinoma of the lung. J Thorac Cardiovasc Surg 1982;83:12-19.

382. Thatcher N. Haematopoietic growth factors and lung cancer treatment. Thorax 1992;47:119-26.

383. Eschapasse H, Gaillard J, Dahan M. Sleeve lobectomy for carcinoma of lung. Chest 1986;89:336S.

384. Crabbe MM, Pattrissi GA, Fontenelle LJ. Minimal resection for bronchogenic carcinoma: An update. Chest 1991;99:1421.

385. Ginsberg RJ. Limited resection in the treatment of stage I non-small cell lung cancer. Chest 1989;96:50S.

386. Pearson FG. Current status of surgical resection for lung cancer. Chest 1994;106:337S-339S.

387. Roth JA. Surgical approach to locally advanced potentially resectable non-small cell lung cancer. Lung Cancer 1994;11(Suppl 3):S25-S30.

388. Ginsberg RJ. Multimodality therapy for non-small cell lung cancer: The role of surgery. Lung Cancer 1993;9 (Suppl 2): S25-S30.

389. Feld R. Current perspectives in the treatment of non-small cell lung cancer. Lung Cancer 1993;9(Suppl 2):S1-S4.

390. Drings P. Preoperative assessment of lung cancer. Chest 1989;96:42S.

391. Ali MK, Ewer MS. Preoperative cardiopulmonary evaluation of patients undergoing surgery for lung cancer. Cancer Bull 1980;32:100.

392. Busch E, Verazin G, Antkowiak JG, et al. Pulmonary complications in patients undergoing thoracotomy for lung carcinoma. Chest 1994;105:760-66.

393. Klastersky J. Therapy of non-small cell lung cancer. Lung Cancer 1995;12(Suppl 1):S133-S145.

394. Ihde DC. Chemotherapy of lung cancer. N Engl J Med 1992;327:1434-1441.

395. Pearson FG. Lung cancer: The past twenty five years. Chest 1986;89:200S-205S.

396. Faber LP. Current status of neoadjuvant therapy for non-small cell lung cancer. Chest 1994;106:355S-358S.

397. Pujol JL, Hayot M, Rouanet P, et al. Long-term results of neoadjuvant ifosfamide, cisplatin, and etoposide combination in locally advanced non-small cell lung cancer. Chest 1994;106:1451-55.

398. Burkes RL, Ginsberg RJ, Shepherd FA, et al. Induction chemotherapy with mitomycin, vindesine, and cisplatin for stage III unresectable: Results of the Toranto phase II trial. J Clin Oncol 1992;10:580-86.

399. Johnson DH, Strupp J, Greco FA, et al. Neoadjuvant cisplatin plus vendesine chemotherapy in locally advanced non-small cell lung cancer. Cancer 1991;68:1216-20.

400. Rossel R, Gomez-Codina J, Camps C, et al. A randomized trial comparing preoperative chemotherapy plus surgery with surgery alone in patients with non-small cell lung cancer. New Engl J Med 1994;330:153-58.

401. Roth JA, Fossela F, Komaki R, et al. A randomized trial perioperative chemotherapy and surgery alone in resectable stage IIIA non-small cell lung cancer. J Natl Cancer Inst 1994;86:673-80.

402. Holms EC. Postoperative chemotherapy for non-small cell lung cancer. Chest 1993;103:30S-34S.

403. Wagner H. Rational integration of radiation and chemotherapy in patients with unresectable stage IIIA or IIIB NSCLC. Chest 1993;103:35S-42S.

404. Albain KS. Induction therapy followed by definitive local control for stage III non-small cell lung cancer. Chest 1993;103:43S-50S.

405. Thatcher N, Honeybourne D, Wagstaff J, et al. Moderate to high dose cyclophosphamide and intercalated Corynebacterium parvum in patients with metastatic lung cancer. Br J Dis Chest 1984;78:89-97.

406. Damstrup L, Poulsen HS. Review of the curative role of radiotherapy in the treatment of non-small cell lung cancer. Lung Cancer 1994;11:153-78.

407. Schaake-Koning C. Radiotherapy in non-small cell lung cancer: Optimal doses and schedules. Lung Cancer 1995;12(Suppl 1):S119-S124.

408. Withers HR. Biological basis of radiation therapy for cancer. Lancet 1992;339:156.

409. Tobias JS. Clinical practice of radiotherapy. Lancet 1992;339:159.

410. Cox JD, Byhardt RW, Perez K, et al. Altered fractions for non-small cell carcinoma of the lung. Chest 1989;96:68S.

411. Brach B, Buhler C, Hayman MH, Joyner LR, Liprie SF. Percutaneous computed tomography guided fine needle brachytherapy of pulmonary malignancies. Chest 1994;106:268-74.

412. Noordijk EM, Clement EP, Hermans J, Wevar AMJ, Leer JWH. Radiotherapy is an alternative to surgery in elderly patients with resectable lung cancer. Radiother Oncol 1988;13:83-89.

413. Coy P, Kennelly GM. The role of curative radiotherapy in the treatment of lung cancer. Cancer 1980;45:698-702.

414. Choi NCH, Doucette JA. Improved survival of patients with unresectable non-small cell bronchogenic carcinoma by an innovated high-dose en-bloc radiotherapeutic approach. Cancer 1981;48:101-09.

415. Herrmann T, Voigtman L, Knorr A, Lorenz J, Johanssen U. The time-dose relationship for radiation induced lung damage in pigs. Radiat Oncol 1986;5:127-35.

416. Steel GG, Deacon JM, Duchesne GM, et al. The dose-rate effect in human tumor cells. Radiat Oncol 1987;9:299-310.

417. Bentzen SM, Thames HD. Is there an influence of overall treatment time in the response of lung to fractionated radiotherapy? Radiat Oncol 1989;14:171-73.

418 Saunders MI. Fractionation and dose in thoracic radiotherapy. Lung Cancer 1994;10(Suppl 1):S245-S252.

419. Cormier Y, Bergeron D, La Forge J, et al. Benefits of polychemotherapy in advanced non-small cell bronchogenic carcinoma. Cancer 1982;50:845-49.

420. Rapp E, Pater JL, Willan A, et al. Chemotherapy can prolong survival in patients with advanced non-small cell lung cancer; reports of a Canadian multicenter randomized trial. J Clin Oncol 1988;633-34.

421. Ganz PA, Figlin RA, Haskel CM, La Soto N, Siau J. The UCLA Solid Tumor Study Group. Supportive care versus supportive care and combination chemotherapy in metastatic non-small cell lung cancer: Does chemotherapy make a difference? Cancer 1989;63:1271-78.

422. Woods RL, Williams CJ, Levi J, et al. A randomized trial of cisplatin and vindesine versus supportive care only in advanced non-small cell lung cancer. Br J Cancer 1990;61:608-11.

423. Cellerino R, Tummarello D, Guidi F, et al. A randomized trial of alternating chemotherapy versus best supportive care in advanced non-small cell lung cancer. J Clin Oncol 1991;9:1453-61.

424. Kassa S, Lund E, Thorud E, Hatlevoll R, Host H. Symptomatic treatment versus combination chemotherapy for patients with extensive non-small cell lung cancer. Cancer 1991;67:2443-47.

425. Vokes EE, Bitran JD. Non-small cell lung cancer. Towards the next plateau. Chest 1994;106:659-60.

426. Grilli R, Oxman AD, Julian JM. Chemotherapy for advanced non-small cell lung cancer: How much benefit is enough? J Clin Oncol 1993;11:1866-72.

427. Souquet PJ, Chauvin H, Boissel JP, et al. Polychemotherapy in advanced non-small cell lung cancer: A meta-analysis. Lancet 1993;342:19-21.

428. Marino P, Pampallona S, Preatoni A, Cantoni A, Invernizzi F. Chemotherapy vs supportive care in advanced non-small cell lung cancer. Results of a meta-analysis of the literature. Chest 1994;106:861-65.

429. Donnadieu N, Paesmans M, Sculier JP. Chemotherapy of non-small cell lung cancer according to disease extent: A meta analysis of the literature. Lung Cancer 1991;7: 243-52.

430. Buccheri G. Chemotherapy and survival in non-small cell lung cancer. Three years later. Chest 1994;106:990-92.

431. Mugia FM, Blum RH, Foreman JD. Role of chemotherapy in the treatment of lung cancer: Evolving strategies for non-small cell histologies. Int J Radiation Oncol Bio Phys 1984;10:137-45.

432. O'Connell JP, Kris MG, Gralla RJ, et al. Frequency and prognostic importance of pretreatment clinical characteristics in patients with advanced non-small cell lung cancer treated with combined chemotherapy. J Clin Oncol 1986;4:1604-14.

433. Kris MG, Gralla R, Wertheim MS, et al. Trial of the combination of mitomycin, vindesine, and cisplatin in patients with advanced non-small cell cancer. Cancer Treat Rep 1986;(7):1091-96.

434. Vokes EE, Bitran JD, Vogelzang NJ. Chemotherapy for non-small cell lung cancer. The continuing challenge. Chest 1991;99:26.

435. Kris MG, Gralla R, Kalman L, et al. Randomized trial comparing vindesine plus cisplatin with vinblastin plus cisplatin in patients with non-small cell lung cancer, with an analysis of methods of response assessment. Cancer Treat Rep 1985;69:387-95.

436. Kris MG, Gralla R, Kelsen D, et al. Trial of vindesine plus mitomycin in stage-3 non-small cell lung cancer. An active regimen for outpatient treatment. Chest 1985;87:368-72.

437. Buccheri G. Chemotherapy and survival in non-small cell lung cancer. The old vexata questio. Chest 1991;99:1328.

438. Haskell CM. Chemotherapy and survival of patients with non-small cell lung cancer. A contrary view. Chest 1991;99:1325.

439. Backowski MT, Creach JC. Chemotherapy of non-small cell cancer: A reappraisal and a look to the future. Cancer Treat Rev 1983;10:159-73.

440. Cullen MH. The MIC regimen in non-small cell lung cancer. Lung Cancer 1993;9(Suppl 2):S81-S89.

441. Johnson DH. Combined modality treatment for locally advanced non-small cell lung cancer-which control arm? Lung Cancer 1994;10(Suppl 1):S231-S238.

442. Le Chevalier T, Arriagada R, Quoix E, et al. Radiotherapy alone *vs* combined chemotherapy and radiotherapy in unresectable non-small cell lung carcinoma. Lung Cancer 1994;10(Suppl 1):S239-S244.

443. Schaake-Koning C, van den Bogaert W, Dalesio O, et al. Radiosensitization by cytotoxic drugs. The EORTC experience by the Radiotherapy and Lung Cancer Cooperative Groups. Lung Cancer 1994;10(suppl 1): S263-S270.

444. Cellerino R, Tummarello D, Piga A. Chemotherapy or not in advanced non-small cell lung cancer. Lung Cancer 1990;6:99-109.

445. Marino P, Preatoni A, Cantoni A, Buccheri G. Single agent chemotherapy versus combination chemotherapy in advanced non-small cell lung cancer: A quality and meta-analysis study. Lung Cancer 1995;13:1-12.

446. Klastersky J. Therapy of non-small cell lung cancer. Lung Cancer 1995;12(suppl 1):S133-S145.

447. Bergman B. Psychosocial issues in the treatment of patients with lung cancer. Lung Cancer 1992;8:1-20.

448. Boyer M. The economics of lung cancer. Lung Cancer 1996;14:13-17.

449. Evans WK, Will BP, Berthelot JM, Wolfson MC. The economics of lung cancer management in Canada. Lung Cancer 1996;14:19-29.

450. Jeremic B, Shibamoto Y. Pre-treatment prognostic factors in patients with stage III non-small cell lung cancer. Treated with hyperfractionated radiation therapy with or without concurrent chemotherapy. Lung Cancer 1995;13:21-30.

451. Moro D, Villemain D, Vuillez JP, Delord CA, Brambilla C. CEA, CYFRA 21-1 and SCC in non-small cell lung cancer. Lung Cancer 1995;13:169-76.

452. Feld R, Borges M, Giner V, et al. Prognostic factors in non-small cell lung cancer. Lung Cancer 1994;11(suppl 3):S19-S23.

453. Hespanhol V, Queiroga H, Magalhães A, Santos AR, Coelho M, Marques A. Survival predictors in advanced non-small cell lung cancer. Lung Cancer 1995;13:253-67.

454. Scagliotti GV, Masiero P, Pozzi E. Biological prognostic factors in non-small cell lung cancer. Lung Cancer 1995;12(Suppl 1):S13-S25.

455. Sorensen JB. Treatment of non-small cell lung cancer: New cytotoxic agents. Lung Cancer 1993;10:173-87.

456. Comis RL, Friedland DM. New chemotherapy agents in the treatment of advanced non-small cell lung cancer: An update including data from the Seventh World Conference on Lung cancer. Lung Cancer 1995;12(suppl 2):S63-S99.

457. Kimura H, Yamaguchi Y. Adjuvant immunotherapy with interleukin 2 and lymphokine-activated killer cells after non-curative resection of primary lung cancer. Lung Cancer 1995;13:31-44.

458. Stein R, Goldenberg M. Prospects for the management of non-small cell carcinoma of the lung with monoclonal antibodies. Chest 1991;99:1466.

459. Hayata Y. Photoradiation. Chest 1986;89:332S.

460. Arabian AA. Experience with Nd: YAG laser for lung cancer. Chest 1986;89:332S.

461. Use of CO_2 laser bronchoscope for palliation of tracheo-bronchial malignancy (airway obstruction): Advantages and disadvantages. Chest 1986;89:333S.

462. Macha HN, Becker KO, Kemmer HP. Pattern of failure and survival in endobronchial laser resection. A matched pair study. Chest 1994;105:1668-72.

463. A WHO meeting. Reappraisal of the present situation in prevention and control of lung cancer. Bull WHO 1982;60:809-19.

464. Tobacco policy recommendations of the International Association for study of Lung cancer (IASLC): A ten point program. Lung Cancer 1994;11:405-07.

465. WHO Technical report Series, No 636, 1979 (Controlling the smoking epidemic: Report of a WHO Expert Committee.

466. International Union against Cancer. In Gray N, Daube M (Eds): Guidelines for smoking control (2nd edn), UICC Technical Report Series: Geneva 1980;52.

467. Saito M, Kato H, Tsuchida T, Konaka C. Chemo-prevention effects on bronchial squamous metaplasia by folate and vitamin B_{12} in heavy smokers. Chest 1994;106:496.

468. Pastorino U. Lung cancer chemoprevention: Facts and hopes. Lung Cancer 1991;7:133-50.

469. Lippman SM, Benner SE, Hong WK. Chemoprevention strategies in lung carcinogenesis. Chest 1993;103:15S-19S.

470. Pastorino U. Lung cancer chemoprevention. In Motta G Grafica LP (Eds): Lung Cancer. Frontiers in Science and Treatment: Genoa, 1994;535-47.

471. Ginsberg RJ, Vokes EE, Rosenzweig K. Non small cell lung cancer. In De Vita Jr, Hellman S, Roseberg SR (Eds): Cancer: Principles and Practice of Oncology (6th edn). Philadelphia, PA: Lippincott-Raven, 2001;925-83.

472. Landits SM, Murray T, Bolden S, et al. Cancer statistics, 1998. CA Cancer J Clin 1998;48:6-29.

473. Lubin JM. Lung and larynx. In Bethesda, MD (Ed): Cancer Rates and Risks (4th edn). National Institutes of Health, National Cancer Institute, 1996;158-61.

474. Greenlee RT, Hill-Harmon MB, Murray T, et al. Cancer statistics 2001. CA Cancer J Clin 2001;51:15-36.

475. Marino P, Pampallona S, Preatoni A, Cantoni A, Invernizzi F. Chemotherapy vs supportive care in advanced non-small-cell lung cancer: results of a meta-analysis of the literature. Chest 1994;106:861-65.

476. Chemotherapy in non-small-cell lung cancer: A meta-analysis using up dated data on individual patients from 52 randomised clinical trails. Br Med J 1995;311:899-909.

477. Grilli R, Oxman AD, Julian JS. Chemotherapy for advanced non-small-cell lung cancer: How much benefit is enough? J Clin Oncol 1993;11:1866-72.

478. Cullen M, Billingham J, Woodraffe C, et al. Mitomycin, ifosfamide, and cisplatin in unresectable non-small-cell lung cancer: Effect on survival and quality of life. J Clin Oncol 1999;17:3188-94.

479. Sandler AB, Ansari R, McClean J, Fisher W, Dorr A, Einhorn LH. A Hoosier Oncology Group phase II study of gemcitabine plus cisplatin in non-small-cell lung cancer (NSCLC). Prog Proc Am Soc Clin Oncol 1995;14:357.

480. Abratt RP, Bezwoda WR, Goedhals L, Hacking DJ. A phase 2 study of gemcitabine with cisplatin in patients with non-small-cell lung cancer. Prog Proc Am Soc Clin Oncol 1995;14:375.

481. Crino L, Scagliotti G, Marangolog M, et al. Cisplatin-gemcitabine combination in non-small-cell lung cancer (NSCLC): A phase II study. Prog Proc Am Soc Clin Oncol 1995;14:352.

482. Langer CJ, Leighton JC, Comis RL, et al. Paclitaxel and carboplatin in combination in the treatment of advanced non-small-cell lung cancer: A phase II toxicity, response, and survival analysis. J Clin Oncol 1995;13: 1860-70.

483. Le Chevalier T, Belli L, Monnier A, et al. Phase II study of docetaxel (Toxotere) and cisplatin in advanced non-small-cell lung cancer (NSCLC): an interim analysis. Prog Proc Am Soc Clin Oncol 1995;14:350.

484. Chemotherapy in non-small cell lung cancer: A meta-analysis using updated data on individual patients from 52 randomized clinical trials. Non-small Cell Lung Cancer Collaborative Group. Br Med J 1995;311:899-909.

485. Cullen MH, Billingham LJ, Woodroffe CM, et al. Mitomycin, ifosfamide and cisplatin in unresectable non-small-cell lung cancer: Effects on survival and quality of life. J Clin Oncol 1999;17:3188-94.

486. Lilenbaum RC, Green MR. Novel chemotherapeutic agents in the treatment of non-small-cell lung cancer. J Clin Oncol 1993;11:1391-1402.

487. Barton-Burke M, Gemcitabine. A pharmacologic and clinical overview. Cancer Nurs 1999;22:176-83.

488. Shepherd FA. Phase II trials of single-agent activity of gemcitabine in patients who advanced non-small cell lung cancer: An over. Anticancer Drugs 1995;6:19-25.

489. Gatzemeier U, Shepherd FA, Le Chevalier T, et al. Activity of gemcitabine in patients with non-small cell lung cancer: A multicentre, extended phase II study. Eur J Cancer 1996;32A:243-48.

490. Crino L, Scagliotti G, Marangolo M, et al. Cisplatin-gemcitabine combination in advanced non-small-cell lung cancer: A phase II study. J Clin Oncol 1997;15:297-303.

491. Abratt RP, Bezwoda WR, Goedhals L, et al. Weekly gemcitabine and monthly cisplatin: Effective chemo-therapy for advanced non-small-cell lung cancer. J Clin Oncol 1997;15:744-49.

492. Rowingsky EK, Donehower RC. Taxol: Twenty years later, the story unfolds. J Natl Cancer Inst 1991;83: 1778-81.

493. Murphy WK, Fosella FV, Winn RJ, et al. A phase II study of taxol in patients with untreated advanced non-small-cell lung cancer. J Natl Cancer Inst 1993;85: 384-88.

494. Gatzemeier U, Heckmayer M, Neuhauss R, et al. Chemotherapy of advanced inoperable non-small-cell lung cancer with paclitaxel: A phase II trial. Semin Oncol 1995;22:24-28 (6 suppl 15).

495. Hainsworth JD, Thompson DS, Greco FA. Paclitaxel by 1-hour infusion: An active drug in metastatic non-small-cell lung cancer. J Clin Oncol 1995;13:1609-14.

496. Rowinsky EK, Gilbert MR, McGuire WP, et al. Sequences of taxol and cisplatin: A phase I and pharmacologic study. J Clin Oncol 1991;9:1692-1703.

497. Rowinsky EK, Chandbry V, Forastiere AA, et al. Phase I and pharmacologic study of paclitaxel and cisplatin with granulocyte colony-stimulating factor: Neuromuscular toxicity is dose-limiting. J Clin Oncol 1993; 11:2010-20.

498. Bonomi PD, Finkelstein DM, Ruckdeschel JC, et al. Combination chemotherapy versus single agents followed by combination chemotherapy in stage IV non-small-cell lung cancer. A study of the Eastern Cooperative Oncology Group. J Clin Oncol 1989;7:1602-1613.

499. Calvert AH, Newell DR, Gumbrell LA, et al. Carboplatin dosage: Prospective evaluation of a simple formula based on renal function. J Clin Oncol 1989;7: 1748-56.

500. Kosmidis PA, Mylonakis N, Fountizilas G, et al. Paclitaxel and carboplatin in inoperable non-small cell lung cancer: A phase II study. Ann Oncol 1997;8:697-99.

501. Langer CJ, Leighton JC, Comis RL, et al. Paclitaxel and carboplatin in combination in the treatment of advanced non-small-cell lung cancer: A phase II toxicity, response, and survival analysis. J Clin Oncol 1995;13: 1860-70.

502. Johnson DH, Paul DM, Hande KR, et al. Paclitaxel plus carboplatin in advanced non-small-cell lung cancer: A phase II trial. J Clin Oncol 1996;14:2054-2060.

503. Kelly K, Pan Z, Murphy J, et al. A phase I trial of paclitaxel plus carboplatin in untreated patients with advanced non-small-cell lung cancer. Clin Cancer Res 1997;3:1117-23.

504. Kosmidis P, Mylonakis N, Skarlos D, et al. Paclitaxel (175 mg/m²) plus carboplatin (6AUC) versus paclitaxel (225 mg/m²) plus carboplatin (6 AUC) in advanced non-small-cell lung cancer (NSCLC): A multicenter randomized trial-Hellenic Cooperative Oncology Group (HeCOG). Ann Oncol 2000;11:799-805.

505. Kroep JR, Giaccone G, Voon DA, et al. Gemcitabine and paclitaxel: Pharmacokinetic and pharmacodynamic interactions in patients with non-small-cell lung cancer. J Clin Oncol 1999;17:2190-97.

506. Giaccone G, Smith EF, van Meerbeeck JP, et al. A phase I-II study of gemcitabine and paclitaxel in advanced non-small-cell lung cancer patients. Ann Oncol 2000;11:109-12.

507. Monnier A, Douillard JY, Lerouge D, et al. Results of a phase II study with Taxol (paclitaxel) and Gemzar (gemcitabine) in metastatic non-small cell lung cancer (NSCLC). Proc Am Soc Clin Oncol 2000;19:516a.

508. Auerback M, Chaudhry M, Richards P, et al. Phase II study of gemcitabine and paclitaxel in metastatic non-small cell lung cancer. Proc Am Soc Clin Oncol 2000; 10:522a.

509. Ginsberg R, Vokes EE, Rosenzweig K. Non-small-cell lung cancer. In DeVita JV, Hellman S, Rosenberg SA (Eds): Cancer-Principles and Practice of Oncology (6th edn). Philadelphia, PA: JB Lippinoctt Co, 2001;925-82.

510. Bunn PA Jr, Kelly K. New chemothrapeutic agents prolong survival and improve quality of life in non-small-cell lung cancer: A review of the literature and future directios. Clin Cancer Res 1998;4:1087-1100.

511. Hoffman PC, Mauer AM, Vokes EE. Lung Cancer. Lancet 2000;355;479-485, (published erratum appears in Lancet 355: 1280, 2000).

512. Johnson DH. Treatment strategies for metastatic non-small-cell lung cancer. Clin Lung Cancer 1999;1:34-41.

513. Schiller JH, Harrington D, Belani CP, et al. Comparison of four chemotherapy regimens for advanced non-small-cell lung cancer. N Engl J Med 2002;346;92-98.

514. Bonomi P, Kim K, Fairclough D, et al. Comparison of survival and quality of life in advanced non-small-cell lung cancer patients treated with two dose levels of paclitaxel combined with cisplatin versus etoposide with cisplatin: Results of an Eastern cooperative Oncology group Trial. J Clin Oncol 2000;18:623-31.

515. Giaccone G, Splinter TA, Debruyne C, et al. Randomized study of paclitaxel-cisplatin versus cisplatin-teniposide in patients with advanced non-small-cell lung cancer: The European Organization for Research and Treatment of Cancer, Lung Cancer Cooperative Group J Clin Oncol 1998;16:2133-41.

516. Le Chevalier T, Brisgand D, Douillard JY, et al. Randomized study of vinorelbine and cisplatin versus vindesine and cisplatin versus vinorelbine alone in advanced non-small-cell lung cancer: Results of a European multicenter trial including 612 patients. J Clin Oncol 1994;12:360-67.

517. Wozniak AJ, Crowlet JJ, Balcerzak SP, et al. Randomized trial comparing cisplatin with cisplatin plus vinorelbine in the treatment of advanced non-small-cell lung cancer: A Southwest Oncology Group Study. J Clin Oncol 1998;16:2459-65.

518. Sandler AB, Nemunaitis J, Denham C, et al. Phase III trial of gemcitabine plus cisplatin versus cisplatin alone in patients with locally advanced or metastatic non-small-cell lung cancer. J Clin Oncol 2000;18:122-30.

519. Vokes EE, Bitran JD. Non-small-cell lung cancer: Toward the next plateau. Chest 1994;106:659-61.

520. Shepherd FA. Chemotherapy for non-small cell lung cancer: Have we reached a new plateau? Semin Oncol 1999;26:3-11.

521. Gordon FS, Vokes EE. Chemoradiation for locally advanced, unresectable NSCLC: New standard of care, emerging strategies. Oncology (Huntingt) 13:1075-1088; discussion, 1999;1091-94.

522. Dillman RO, Herndon J, Seagren SL, et al. Improved survival in stage III non-small-cell lung cancer: Seven-year follow-up of cancer and leukemia group

B (CALGB) 8433 tiral. J Natl Cancer Inst 1996;88: 1210-15.

523. Vokes EE, Green MR. Clinical studies in non-small-cell lung cancer. The CALGB experience. Cancer Invest 1998;16:72-79.

524. Sause W, Kolesar P, Taylor SI, et al. Final results of phase III trial in regionally advanced unresectable non-small-cell lung cancer: Radiation Therapy Oncology Group, Eastern Cooperative Oncology Group, and Southwest Oncology Group. Chest 2000;117:358-64.

525. Le Chevalier T, Arriagada R, Quoix E, et al. Radiotherapy alone versus combined chemotherapy and radiotherapy in nonresectable non-small-cell lung cancer: First ananlysis of a randomized trial in 353 patients. J Natl Cancer Inst 1991;83:417-23.

526. Schaake-Koning C, van den Bogaert W, Dalesio O, et al. Effects of concomitant cisplatin and radiotherapy on inoperable non-small-cell lung cancer. N Engl J Med 1992;326:524-30.

527. Jeremic B, Shibamoto Y, Actimovic L, et al. Randomized trial of hyperfactionated radiation therapy with or without concurrent chemotherapy for stage III non-small-cell lung cancer. J Clin Oncol 1995;13:452-58.

528. Albain KS, Rusch VW, Crowlet JJ, et al. Concurrent cisplatin/etoposide plus chest radiotherapy followed by surgery for stage III A (N₂) and IIIB non-small-cell cancer: Mature results of Southwest Oncology Group phase II study 8805. J Clin Oncol 1995;13:1880-92.

529. Albain K, Crowlet JJ, Turrist AT, et al. Concurrent cisplatin/etoposide plus radiotherapy (PE+RT) for pathologic stage (path TN) IIIB non-small-cell lung cancer (NSCLC): A Southwest Oncology Group (SWOG) phase II study (S9019). Proc Am Soc Clin Oncol 1997;16:128a (abstr 450).

530. Gaspar L, Gandara D, Chansky K, et al. Consolidation docetaxel following concurrent chemoradiotherapy in pathologic stage IIIb non-small-cell lung cancer (NSCLC) (SWOG 9504): Patterns of failure and updated survival. Proc Am Soc Clin Oncol 20:315a, 2001 (abstr 1255).

531. Furuse K, Fukuoka M, Kawahara M, et al. Phase III study of concurrent versus sequential thoracic radiotherapy in combination with mitomycin, vindersine, and cisplatin in unresectable stage III non-small-cell lung cancer. J Clin Oncol 1999;17:2692-99.

532. Curran W, Scott C, Langer C. Phase III comparison of sequential versus concurrent chemoradiation for patients with unresected stage III non-small cell lung cancer: Report of Radiation Therapy Oncology Group 9410, 9th World Conference on Lung Cancer. Lung Cancer 2000;29:93.

533. Schiller JH, Harrington D, Belani CP, Langer C, Sandler A, Krook J, Zhu J, Johnson DH. Eastern Cooperative Oncology Group. Comparison of four chemotherapy regimens for advanced non-small-cell lung cancer. N Engl J Med 2002;346:92-98.

534. Postmus PE, Smit EF. Treatment of relapsed small cell lung cancer. Semin Oncol 2001;28:48-52.

535. Simon G, Ginsberg RJ, Ruckdeschel JC. Small cell lung cancer. Chest Surg Clin N Am 2001;11:165-88.

536. Grant SC, Gralla RJ, Kriss MG, Orazem J, Kitsis EA. Single agent chemotherapy trials in small cell lung cancer, 1970-1990: The case for studies in previously treated patients. J Clin Oncol 1992;10:484-98.

537. Figoli F, Veronesi A, Ardizzoni A, Canobbio L, Bruschi G, Mazza F, Zagonel V, Lo Re G, Rosso R, Monfardini S. Cisplatin and etoposide as second line chemotherapy in patients with small cell lung cancer. Cancer Investig 1988;6:1-5.

538. Albain KS, Crowley JJ, Hutchins L, Gandara D, O'Bryan RM, Von Hoff DD, Griffin B, Livngston RB. Predictors of survival following relapse or progression of small cell lung cancer. Cancer (Phila) 1993;72:1184-91.

539. Roth BJ, Johnson DH, Einhorn LH, Schacter LP, Cherng NC, Cohen HJ, Crawford J, Randolph JA, Goodlow JL, Broun GO, et al. Randomized study of cyclophosphamide, doxorubicin and vincristine versus etoposide versus alteration of these regimens in small cell lung cancer: Phase III trial of Southeastern Cancer Study Group. J Clin Oncol 1992;10:282-91.

540. Fukuoka M, Furuse K, Saijo N, Nishiwaki Y, Ikegami H, Tamura T, Shimoyama M, Suemasu K. Randomized trial of cyclophosphamide, doxorubecin and vincristine versus cisplatin and etoposide versus alteration of these regimens in small cell lung cancer. J Natl Cancer Inst (Bethesda), 1991;83:855-61.

541. Takadda M, Fukuoka M, Kawahara M, et al. Phase III study of concurrent versus sequential thoracic radiotherapy in combination with cisplatin and etoposide for limited-stage small-cell lung cancer: Results of the Japan Clinical Oncology Group Study 9104. J Clin Oncol 2002;20:3054-60.

542. Turrisi AT 3rd, Kim K, Blum R, et al. Twice-daily compared with once-daily thoracic radiotherapy in limited small-cell lung cancer treated concurrently with cisplatin and etoposide. N Engl J Med 1999;340:265-71.

543. Kosmidis PA, Smantas E, Fountizilas G, et al. Cisplatin/etoposide versus carboplatin/etoposide chemotherapy and irradiation in small cell lung cancer: A randomized phase III study. Hellenic Cooperative Oncology Group for Lung Cancer Trials. Semin Oncol 1994;21(3 Suppl 6):23-30.

544. Noda K, Nishiwaki Y, Kawahara M, et al. Irinotecan plus cisplatin compared with etoposide plus cisplatin for extensive small-cell lung cancer. N Engl J Med 2002; 346:85-91.

545. Ardizzoni A, Hansen H, Dombernowsky P, et al. Topotecan, a new active drug in the second-line treatment of small cell lung cancer: A phase II study in patients with refractory and senstitive disease. The European Organization for Research and Treatment of Cancer Early Clinical Stidies Group and New Drug Development Office, and the Lung Cancer Cooperative Group. J Clin Oncol 1997;15:2090-96.

546. Schiller JH, Harrington D, Belani CP, Langer C, Sandler A, Krook J, Zhu J, Johnson DH; Eastern Cooperative

Oncology Group. Comparison of four chemotherapy regimens for advanced non-small-cell lung cancer. N Engl J Med 2002;346:92-98.

547. Cancer Facts and Figures 2002. Atlanta, GA: American Cancer Society 2002.

548. American Society of Clinical Oncology. Clinical practice guidelines for the treatment of unresected non-small-cell lung cancer. J Clin Oncol 1997;15:2996-3016.

549. Blagosklonny MV. How Cancer Could Be Cured by 2015. Cell Cycle 2005 Feb 21;4 [Epub ahead of print].

550. Hanahan D, Weinberg RA. The hallmarks of cancer. Cell 2000;100:57-70.

551. Hanahan D, Folkman J. Patterns and emerging mechanisms of the angiogenic switch during tumorigenesis. Cell 1996;86:353-64.

552. Foldman J. Tumor angiogenesis inhibitors and their therapeutic implications. N Engl J Med 1971;285:1182-86.

553. Cao Y. Endogenous angiogenesis inhibitors and their therapeutic implications. Int J Biochem Cell Bio 2001;33:357-69.

554. Kerbel RS. Inhibition of tumor angiogenesis as a strategy to circumvent acquired resistance to anti-cancer therapeutic agents. Bio Essays 1991;13:31-36.

555. Scappaticci FA. Mechanisms and future directions for angiogenesis-based cancer therapies. J Clin Oncol 2002; 20:3906-27.

556. Folkman J. Angiogenesis in cancer, vascular, rheumatoid and other disease. Nat Med 1995;1:27-31.

557. Folkman J. Tumor angiogenesis: Therapeutic implications. New Engl J Med 1971;285:1182-86.

558. Folkman J, Shing Y. Angiogenesis. J Biol Chem 1992;267:10931-84.

559. Ribatti D, Vacca A, Bertossi M, et al. Anti-angiogenesis: A multipurpose therapeutic tool? Int J Clin Lab Res 1993;23:177-20.

560. Dupont E, Brazeau P, Junear C. Extracts of shark cartilage having an antiangiogenic activity and an effect on tumor progression: Process of making thereof. US Patent 1997;5618-25.

561. Gingras D, Renaud A, Mousseau N, et al. Matrix proteinase inhibition by Neovastat, a multifunctional antiangiogenic compound. Anticancer Res 2001;21: 145-55.

562. Berger F, Jourdes P, Benabid AL. AE-941 (Neovastat) shows a beneficial effect in experimental glioma and is associated with high angiostain level in treated tumors. Proc Am Assoc Cancer Res 2001;42:724.

563. Beliveau R, Gingras D, Kruger, et al. The antiangiogenic agent Neovastar (AE-941) inhibits VEGF-mediated biological effect. Clin Cancer Res 2002;8:1242-50.

564. Boivin D, Gendron S, Beaulieu E, et al. The antiangiogenic agent Neovastat (AE-941) induces endothelial cell apoptosis. Molecular Cancer Ther 2002;1:795-802.

565. Castronovo V, Dimitriadou V, Savard P, et al. Cartilage as a source of natural inhibitors of angiogenesis. In

566. Teicher BA (Ed): Antiangiogenic Agent in Cancer Therapy. Totowa, NJ: Human Press 1999;175-82. Dupont E, Moussa SA, Dimitriadou V, et al. Antiangiogenic and antimetastatic properties of AE-941, an orally active extract derived from cartilage. Clin Exp Metastasis 2002;19:145-53.

567. Caponigro F, Basile M, Rosa VD, Normanno N. New Drugs in Cancer Therapy, National Tumor Institute, Naples, 17-18 June 2004. Anticancer Drugs 2005;16: 211-21.

568. Razis E, Skarlos D, Briasoulis E, Dimopoulos M, Fountzilas G, Lambropoulos S, Rigatos S, Kopterides P, Efstathiou H, Tzamakou E, Bakoyannis C, Pectasides D, Makatsoris T, Varthalitis G, Papadopoulos S, Kosmidis P. Treatment of non-small cell lung cancer with gefitinib ('Iressa', ZD1839): the Greek experience with a compassionate-use program. Anticancer Drugs 2005;16:191-8.

569. Klasa RJ, Gillum AM, Klem RE, Frankel SR. Oblimersen Bcl-2 antisense: facilitating apoptosis in anticancer treatment. Antisense Nucleic Acid Drug Dev 2002; 12:193-13.

570. Morris MJ, Tong W, Osman l, et al. A phase I/IIA dose-escalating trial of bcl-2 antisense (G3139) treatment by 14-day continuous intravenous infusion (CI) for patients with androgen-indepndent prostate cancer or other advanced solid tumor malignancies. Presented at the 35th Annual Meeting of the American Society of Clinical Oncology; May 15-18, 1999;Atlanta, GA. Abstract 1243.

571. Jansen B Wacheck V, Heere-Ress E, et al. Chemosensitisation of malignant melanoma by Bcl2 antisense therapy. Lancet 2000;356:1728-33.

572. Yang D, Ling Y, Almazan M, et al. Tumor regression of human breast carcinomas by combination therapy of anti-Bcl-2 antisense oligonucleotide and chemotherapeutic drugs. Proc Amer Assoc Cancer Res 1999;Abstract 4814.

573. Tauchi T, Nakajima A, Sumi M, Shimamoto T, Sashida G, Ohyashiki K. G3139 (Bcl-2 antisense oligonucleotide) is active aginast imatinib-resistant BCR-ABL-positive cells. Presented at the 93rd Annual Meeting of the American Association for Cancer Research; April 6-10, 2002; San Francisco, CA. Abstract 4702.

574. Lacy J, Loomis R. Bcl-2 antisense (G3139, Genasense™) enhances the *in vitro* and *in vivo* response of EBV-associated lymphoproliferative disease to rituximab. Presented at the 93rd Annual Meeting of the American Association for Cancer Research; April 6-10, 2002; San Francisco, CA. Abstract 2853.

575. Ryan PD, Chabner BA, On receptor inhibitors and chemotherapy. Clin Cancer Res 2000;6:4607-09.

576. Carbone DP. The biology of lung cancer. Semin Oncol 1997;24:388-401.

577. Carbone D. Molecular modalities in the treatment of lung cancer. Oncology (Huntingt) 1999;13:142-47.

Chapter 23

Pulmonary Neoplasms other than Bronchogenic Carcinoma

There are different types of tumors of the lung and the tracheobronchial tree although the incidence is much less than bronchogenic carcinoma. There are many different classifications of these tumors, without any accepted uniformity. Table 23.1 outlines some of these according to their cell of origin.[1-4]

EPITHELIAL TUMORS

These tumors are rare and comprise of about 1 to 2 percent of all pulmonary neoplasms.[1-4] True bronchial adenoma must be distinguished from the more commonly occurring epithelial tumors; carcinoids, cylindromas, and mucoepidermoid tumors. The **bronchial adenoma** is a benign tumor that arises from the bronchial glands and present as small polypoid tumors projecting into the bronchial lumen. They may cause obstructive pneumonitis or hemoptysis. They are most often confused with other endobronchial tumors. Histology will distinguish this form from other tumors. Conservative resection is the proper treatment and the prognosis is very good.

CARCINOID TUMOR

These tumors are the next most common form of bronchogenic neoplasms second to bronchogenic carcinoma. They constitute about 2 to 4 percent of all bronchial tumors. The tumors originate in the neuroendocrine cells (Kulchitsky's cells) or APUD cells of the bronchial mucosa. These tumors are potentially malignant.

TABLE 23.1: Pulmonary tumors (other than bronchogenic carcinoma)

Epithelial tumors	*Mesothelial tumors*
Papilloma	Benign mesothelioma
Adenoma	Malignant mesothelioma
Carcinoid	*Miscellaneous tumors*
Adenoid cystic carcinoma (cylindroma)	Hodgkin's lymphoma
Mucoepidermoid carcinoma	Non-Hodgkin's lymphoma
Melanoma	Leukemia
Clear cell tumor	Histiocytic tumors
Sclerosing pneumocytoma	Lymphoproliferative disorders
Soft tissue tumors	Teratoma
Lipoma/liposarcoma	Hamartoma
Fibroma/fibrosarcoma	Carcinosarcoma
Chondroma/chondrosarcoma	Tuberous sclerosis
Neurofibroma/neurofibrosarcoma	Angiosarcoma
Lymphangioma	Arteriovenous malformations
Hemangioma/hemangiosarcoma	Lymphangiectasis
Leiomyoma/leiomyosarcoma	Secondary tumors
Myeloblastoma	Blastoma
Chemodectoma	Eosinophilic granuloma
Lymphangioleiomyomatoma	Tumorlet
Rhabdomyosarcoma	Inflammatory pseudotumors
Hemangiopericytoma	
Plasmacytoma	
Myxoma	
Neurilemmoma	

No definite etiological agent, smoke, occupation, or other carcinogen, has particularly been implicated for the causation of this tumor. The tumor usually arises from a main or segmental bronchus and is often visible bronchoscopically.

Pathologically bronchial carcinoid tumors are classified as neuroendocrine carcinomas, and are divided into typical and atypical forms, with variable grade of malignancy.[5] The typical form consists of sheets or aggregates of small cells with dark central nuclei and pale cytoplasm in a vascular stroma. The small, polyhedral cells are grouped in nests, ribbons, or broad sheets. The arrangement of the cells in the stroma is orderly. The atypical carcinoid shows increases mitotic activity, irregular nuclei, and prominent nucleoli. These cells have a greater potential for secondaries and they are difficult to distinguish from oat cell carcinoma.[6,7]

The disease can occur at any age including the young and the old. The patients are usually younger than that in bronchogenic carcinoma. Peripheral tumors may be asymptomatic and are detected only on a routine chest X-ray. Clinical symptoms and signs vary according to the location of tumor. They are slow growing tumors presenting with hemoptysis or symptoms/signs of bronchial obstruction, including repeated infections. Both men and women are affected equally. Other symptoms may be wheezing, or cough. Central neoplasms are symptomatic due to bronchial obstruction (i.e. pneumonia, atelectasis, bronchiectasis, emphysema and/or lung abscess); if airway obstruction is partial, then cough, wheezing and recurrent pulmonary infections occur. Peripheral tumors are generally asymptomatic and they are discovered occasionally, when chest X-ray is made for other reasons. Occasionally "carcinoid syndrome", characterized by episodic flushing, bronchospasm, hypotension, tachycardia, and diarrhea. These symptoms are seen in about 1 percent of carcinoids of the bronchus. Other features may include abdominal cramps, edema of the face, pellagra like symptoms, and involvement of tricuspid, pulmonary or mitral valves. The syndrome is related to the tryptophane metabolism by the carcinoid cells with production of serotonin. The diagnosis of the syndrome is made by measuring 5-hydroxyindoleacetic acid.[8,9]

Most patients have an abnormal chest X-ray, although in few cases the changes may not be apparent. The radiological findings may demonstrate a mass in the pulmonary parenchyma of varying sizes, obstructive emphysema, obstructive collapse or obstructive pneumonia. Occasionally metastasis to mediastinal nodes may be common. Radiographic features are similar in typical and atypical bronchial carcinoid tumors. In central tumors a rounded well-circumscribed hilar mass is noted, with lobulated or bumpy margins. Central cavitation is not referred to. Peripheral bronchial carcinoid tumors appear as a solitary nodule, inferior then 3 cm in size, marginated, surrounded by normal pulmonary tissue. Signs and symptoms of BCT are evasive and vague. No current clinical or laboratory procedures are useful in confirming the diagnosis; particularly, no imaging modalities are able to differentiate between bronchial carcinoid tumors and other pulmonary tumors. For this reason, a clinical radiologic endoscopic and histopathologic approach is necessary. CT is more sensitive than conventional radiography, especially in detecting small lesions, calcification and enlarged lymph nodes. MRI may be useful in those patients, who cannot tolerate IV contrast media. Scintigraphy may be employed in discovering relapses and long standing metastases (Figs 23.1 to 23.4).

Bronchoscopic biopsy is the definite way of establishing the diagnosis. However, biopsy of this lesion is associated with high incidence of complications, since the tumors are vascular and liable to bleed. The bronchoscopic appearance of a carcinoid tumor is described as smooth, glistening, and well circumscribed. Very rarely, carcinoids present as diffuse multicentric endobronchial lesions or as multiple peripheral tumors. Bronchography, shows a smooth narrowing or cutoff in the bronchial tree (Figs 23.5 to 23.12).

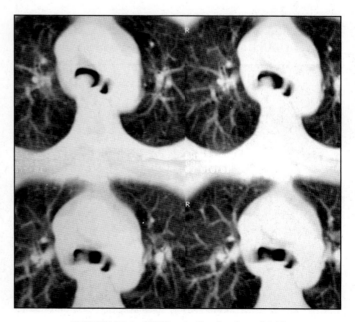

FIGURE 23.1: CT Chest - Tracheal carcinoid

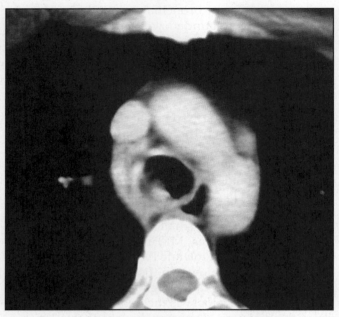

FIGURE 23.2: Magnified view of CT Chest - Showing mass lesion in trachea - Inflammatory pseudotumor

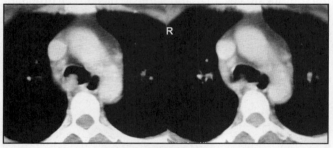

FIGURE 23.3: CT Scan Chest - Tracheal mass

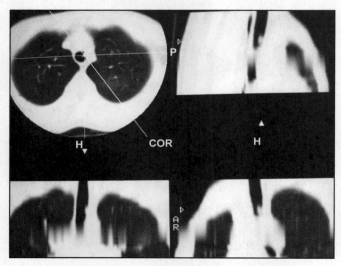

FIGURE 23.4: CT Reconstruction showing tracheal mass

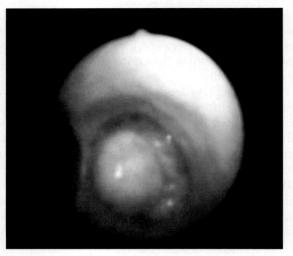

FIGURE 23.5

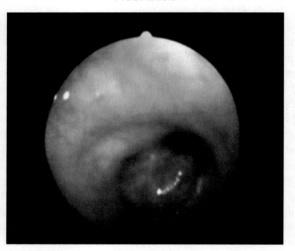

FIGURE 23.6

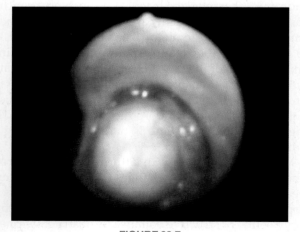

FIGURE 23.7

FIGURES 23.5 TO 23.7: Carcinoid as seen through a FOB

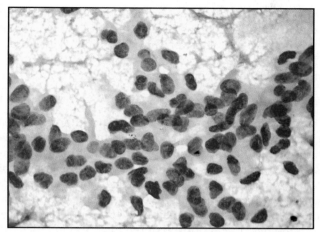

FIGURE 23.8: Neuroendocrine tumor-Loose aggregate of small tumor cells, little pleomorphism, stippled chromatin, prominent acinar, rosette – like structure (MGG, 40X)

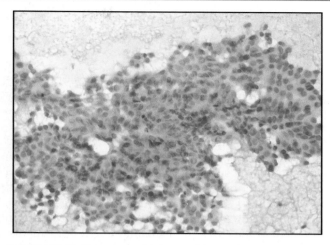

FIGURE 23.11: Neuroendocrine tumor of lung - Loose aggregate of regular round to oval tumor cells in a clean background (H&E, 20X)

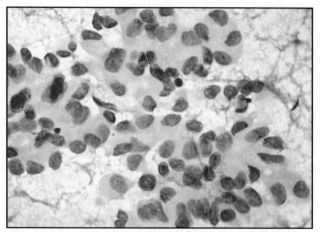

FIGURE 23.9: Neuroendocrine tumor of lung - A highly cellular smear showing tumor cells adhering to the capillaries and dispersed regular tumor cells (MGG, 10X)

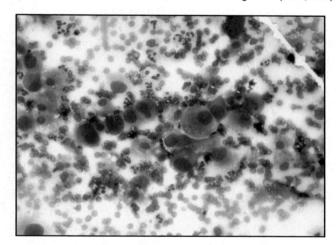

FIGURE 23.12: Neuroendocrine tumor of lung

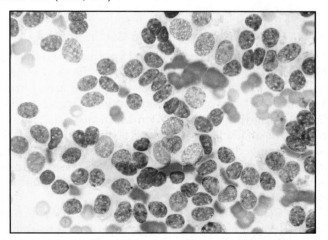

FIGURE 23.10: Neuroendocrine tumor of lung - A highly cellular tumor

All carcinoids are potentially capable of metastasis, and the incidence is about less than 10 percent. The usual sites of such metastasis are lymph nodes, liver, and bone. The bony lesions are typically osteoblastic. The over all prognosis is good in spite of the presence of metastasis.

The usual method of treatment is surgical removal. Five-year survival rates have been reported in over 90 percent of the cases after surgery. Atypical variety has a 5 year survival in about 70 percent of cases. The nature of surgery depends upon the extent of the tumor and may vary from wedge tracheobronchotomy, a lobectomy with sleeve resection of the contiguous bronchus, a pneumonectomy, or a simple wedge or segmental resection of the involved pulmonary parenchyma.

Recurrent or metastatic recurrence of the disease has been treated with chemotherapy (streptozotocin and 5-

fluorouracil/chlorambucil) and radiotherapy with varying success.[6-10]

LYMPHOMAS

The lungs and pleura are the common sites of involvement by lymphomas. Rarely the lung may be the primary site of origin of either Hodgkin's or non-Hodgkin's lymphoma.[11-15]

Hodgkin's lymphoma primarily affects adults and commonly involves the hilar and mediastinal lymph nodes. In a large series of cases, 52 percent were found to have intrathoracic involvement; lungs being affected in 43 percent of cases; hilar nodes in 34 percent cases; mediastinum in 23 percent of the cases; and pleura in 11 percent of the cases. Apart from these involvements, other radiological features include: infiltration of the peribronchial tissue, direct extension from the involved nodes, patchy infiltrates, diffuse pneumonic consolidation, and nodular lesions. All histological types can involve lungs, although the lymphocyte predominance type does so less frequently than the others. *Primary Hodgkin s disease of the lung* is rare.[15] The diagnostic criteria of such diagnosis include histologic proof of disease; restriction of the disease to the lung without hilar lymph node involvement; and exclusion of the presence of the disease at other sites. Primary Hodgkin's disease of the lung is common in women having a bimodal age distribution with a tendency toward an older age group. Diagnosis of both intrathoracic disease and primary disease is made by appropriate histological examination on specimens obtained from fine needle aspiration, bronchoscopy, mediastinoscopy, mediastinotomy or thoracotomy. Treatment of lymphoma will depend upon the stage of the disease.

Non-Hodgkin's lymphoma is characteristically a disease of the older age group with a peak incidence in the 60s and 70s. The disease is present commonly at extra-nodal sites in most of the cases. Thoracic involvement is in the form of enlarged hilar or mediastinal nodes, diffuse consolidation, peribronchial infiltration, nodular lesions, and pleural effusion. Intrathoracic involvement occurs in 20 to 25 percent of cases. Enlarged nodes may occur with all pathological types, but lung infiltration is commonly seen with the low-grade lymphocytic type whereas nodular lesions occur in the high-grade lymphoblastic type of non-Hodgkin's lymphoma. Primary lung involvement in this form of lymphoma is very rare. The symptoms are usually nonspecific. The chest X-ray usually shows a single area of diffuse infiltration, which may be nodular. The whole lung may be involved. Pathologically primary non-Hodgkin's lymphomas are often low-grade lymphoplasmacytoid type or immunocytomas. The diagnosis can be made in the same way as that for the Hodgkin's lymphoma. Treatment depends upon the stage of the disease. The prognosis is less favorable than Hodgkin's lymphoma.

PULMONARY BLASTOMA

These malignant cells are rare pulmonary tumors derived from both the epithelial and connective tissue.[16-18] The glandular tubules usually lie in a malignant mesenchymal stroma. These tumors resemble lung tissues of fetal type and are believed to arise from pulmonary blastoma. It occurs both in children and adults and more common in males than females. The tumor usually arises from the peripheral portion of the lung and invades the bronchial tissue. The clinical features and metastatic characteristics are those that of the bronchogenic carcinoma. Surgery is the treatment of choice if possible. In inoperable cases, radiotherapy and chemotherapy have benefited some patients.

CARCINOSARCOMA

This is a rare pulmonary tumor (0.2%) and histologically is a mixture of carcinoma of the nonsmall cell type, and sarcoma, usually of the spindle cell type.[19] The tumor is more common in men past middle age. The presentation is similar to that any other bronchogenic carcinoma. Radiologically it is seen as a peripheral mass with obstructive pneumonitis. The diagnosis is confirmed by examination of the sputum or examination of the bronchoscopic specimens. Metastases are common. Surgical resection is the treatment of choice if there is no demonstrable metastasis at the time of presentation. In other cases, chemotherapy containing adriamycin regimens is beneficial.

CYLINDROMA (Adenoid Cystic Carcinoma)

This tumor represents only about 15 percent of epithelial, tumors of the bronchus. However it is the commonest malignant tumor of the trachea. The tumor arises from the mucous glands of the airways and may infiltrate into the surrounding tissues. Microscopically, the tumor consists of small pleomorphic and stellate cells with dark nuclei arranged in trabecular, cylinders, or tubes, as the tumor's name suggests. The cells show increased mitosis and the surrounding stroma may show myxomatous changes (Figs 23.13 to 23.17).

The symptoms are like those of any endobronchial lesion like hemoptysis, cough, sputum wheezing, dyspnea, and obstructive pneumonia. Radiology may

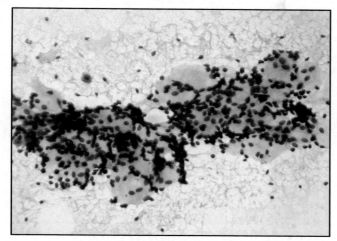

FIGURE 23.13: Adenoid cystic carcinoma - Small uniform cells with hyperchromatic nuclei embedded in hyaline stroma globules (H&E, 20X)

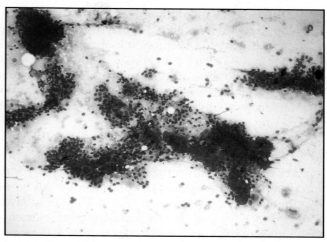

FIGURE 23.16: Adenoid cystic carcinoma - Small uniform cells with hyperchromatic nuclei embedded in hyaline stromal globules (MGG, 10X)

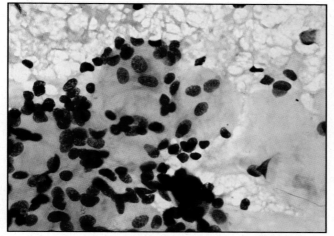

FIGURE 23.14: Adenoid cystic carcinoma - Small uniform cells with hyperchromatic nuclei embedded in hyaline stromal globules (H&E, 40X)

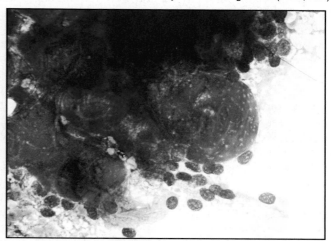

FIGURE 23.17: Adenoid cystic carcinoma - Small uniform cells with hyperchromatic nuclei embedded in hyaline stromal globules (MGG, 40X)

show a hilar tumor or collapse or consolidation, or even may be normal in some cases. Bronchoscopy usually reveals a polypoidal or infiltrating mass that bleeds easily. Biopsy is usually diagnostic.

Ideal treatment is surgery if feasible. Because of central location of the tumor, this may not be possible in some cases. Tracheal reconstruction procedures have been tried in some of these cases. Radiotherapy may be beneficial. Laser therapy may be of help in relieving the obstruction in cases where surgery is not possible. The overall prognosis is worse than carcinoids.

MUCOEPIDERMOID TUMOR

These rare tumors arise in the mucous glands of the trachea and bronchi. They are composed of mixed well-differentiated mucous cells and sheets of squamous cells with keratinization and intercellular bridging. Patholo-

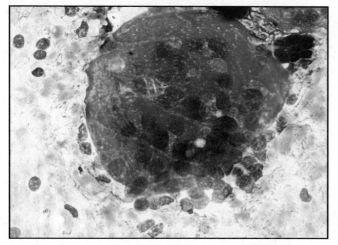

FIGURE 23.15: Adenoid cystic carcinoma - Small uniform cells with hyperchromatic nuclei embedded in hyaline stromal globules (MGG, 100X)

gically they may be of high-grade or low-grade tumors. The symptoms are usually due to that of any obstructive lesion. Chest X-ray, CT scan, and tomograms will reveal the tumor in the airway. Bronchoscopically the tumor is seen as a polypoid or a sessile mass. Biopsy confirms the diagnosis. Surgical resection of the tumor with various reconstructive procedures is the treatment of choice.

SARCOMAS

Primary sarcomas of the lungs of all types are very rare tumors and account for less than 1 percent of all types of pulmonary neoplasms (Fig. 23.18). They may arise from the bronchial wall, or from almost all tissue elements of the lung (nerves, connective tissue, vascular tissue, fibrous tissue, etc.). Uncommonly, they may arise from the pulmonary parenchyma and may remain silent for a long period of time till they produce pressure symptoms on the surrounding structures. The tumor may be undifferentiated or may reveal differentiation into a subtype of the above elements like angiosarcoma, chondrosarcoma, fibrosarcoma, leiomyosarcoma, neurofibrosarcoma, osteosarcoma, rhabdomyosarcoma and liposarcoma, etc. (Figs 23.19 to 23.22). Besides producing symptoms depending upon the location (bronchogenic, obstructive, pneumonitis), hypertrophic pulmonary osteoarthropathy and hypoglycemia, though rare, are two characteristic presentations of pulmonary sarcomas. The diagnosis is based on the biopsy. A primary sarcoma from extrathoracic sites should be excluded, since secondaries from these sites may mimic primary

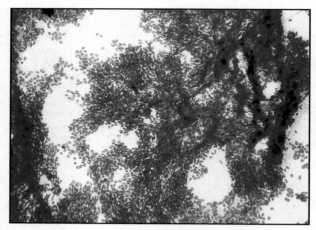

FIGURE 23.19: Sarcoma—Fascicles of spindle cells - Ovoid to spindle uniform nuclei having tapering ends with minimal nuclear atypia (MGG, 20X)

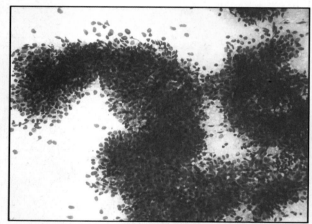

FIGURE 23.20: Sarcoma - Highly cellular smear with small fascicle of round to oval tumor cells with blunt ends with moderate nuclear atypia (MGG, 20X)

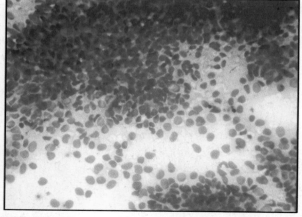

FIGURE 23.21: Sarcoma—Highly cellular smear with small fascicle of round to oval tumor cells with blunt ends with moderate nuclear atypia (MGG, 40X)

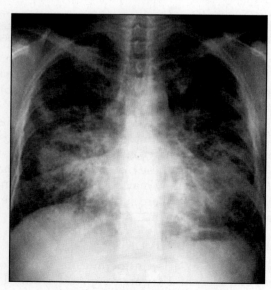

FIGURE 23.18: Kaposi sarcoma

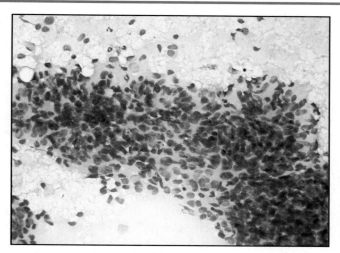

FIGURE 23.22: Fibrosarcoma—Fascicles of spindle cells - Ovoid to spindle cells; ovoid to spindle uniform nuclei having tapering ends with minimal nuclear atypia (MGG, 20X)

sarcomas of the lung. Surgical resection should be taken up whenever possible. The 5 year survival rate varies from 5 to 25 percent. More differentiated types have a better prognosis than the undifferentiated type. Unresectable tumors may be treated with radiotherapy and chemotherapy.

EOSINOPHILIC GRANULOMA

This is one of the three conditions together known as histiocytosis-X.[20-24] Hystiocytosis X was originally thought to be a lipid storage disease, but is now classified as a condition of abnormal histiocyte proliferation. The three conditions included under this term are: eosinophilic granuloma, Hand-Schuller-Christian disease, and Letterer-Siwe disease. Hand-Schuller-Christian disease occurs in children and young adults, is slowly progressive, and manifested by exophthalmos, diabetes insipidus, and multiple osteolytic lesions. Letterer-Siwe disease is a generalized fulminating disease of the infants and children with involvement of the skin, viscera and bone that is rapidly fatal. Eosinophilic granuloma is a disseminated disease of the adults and mainly affects the lungs and bones. Although the interrelationship of these three is not exactly known, they are grouped together because of a similar histopathological picture. There is a granulomatous infiltration with proliferation of histiocytes with vesicular and lobulated nuclei, basophilic nucleoli and eosinophilic cytoplasm. The histiocytes contain characteristic X-bodies or tennis requite bodies on electron microscopy. Deposits of lipids may be seen in the cytoplasm of the histiocytes.

Eosinophilic granuloma, now often called pulmonary Langerhans' cell histiocytosis, is a nodular infiltration of the interstitium of the lung by histiocytes, plasma cells, lymphocytes, and eosinophils and produces a symmetric cystic interstitial lung disease that affects the upper zones and spares the bases.[25-28] Eosinophilic granuloma is highly associated with smoking and may occur at any age. In adults, the disease affects men and women in similar numbers.[26,29] Isolated pulmonary disease is a frequent finding at presentation, as are bone lesions and diabetes insipidus. Eosinophilic granuloma may be asymptomatic at presentation, but commonly reported symptoms include cough, dyspnea, fever, anorexia, and weight loss;[26] chest pain and hemoptysis are less common. Other manifestations of disseminated disease (such as bone pain, polydipsia, polyuria, rash, lymphadenopathy, and hepatosplenomegaly) occur in only 15 percent of affected adults. Most patients have no abnormal results on routine laboratory tests, with the exception of an elevated erythrocyte sedimentation rate.[30] Patients with late-stage disease associated with peribronchiolar cysts often have airway obstruction and increased lung volumes.[25-28,31,32] While radiologic findings of nodules and small cystic spaces of the upper lung zones are present, surgical biopsy is required for diagnosis.[23] Though rare in eosinophilic granuloma, a slow progression to fibrosis and honeycombing has been described.[33] The transformation of nodules into cysts is a well-recognized radiologic pattern.[32,34] In addition, the combination of symptomatic disease and continued smoking placed this patient at high risk for progression of the disease.[35,36] Cancer, including lymphoma, leukemia, and pulmonary adenocarcinoma, may develop in patients with eosinophilic granuloma.[33]

Histopathologically, the predominant finding is stellate scars, 1 to 2 mm in diameter, composed of central fibrosis with dense collagen. At the edge of the scars there is extension of lymphocytes and fibrosis in a configuration resembling that of an octopus. Cysts are present, with fibrous walls containing smooth muscle and lined by reparative cuboidal pneumocytes. Although only scattered Langerhans' cells are identified on staining for S-100 and CD1a antigens, the size and shape of the scars and cysts are characteristic of eosinophilic granuloma in a late, burned-out phase.[35-43] The cysts resulted from bronchiolar destruction by the proliferating Langerhans' cells in an earlier phase of the disease, with mechanical weakening of the lung architecture, air trapping, or both. In the lungs, in contrast to most organs, healing often results in smooth-muscle proliferation, which is seen in the walls of these cysts. They are analogous to the cysts seen in honeycomb lung, except that they originate in the bronchioles rather than the alveoli.

The conventional treatment strategy includes cessation of smoking and the administration of corticosteroids for progressive disease, possibly followed by the use of cytotoxic agents such as vinblastine or cyclophosphamide. Finally, lung transplantation is considered for progressive disease that is refractory to these treatments. Interleukin-2 has an inhibitory effect on Langerhans' cells. Studies have shown that tobacco glycoprotein, a potent immunostimulator isolated from tobacco smoke, causes weak production of interleukin-2 from lymphocytes in patients with eosinophilic granuloma.[44] This deficit of interleukin-2 is thought to lead to enhanced local survival and proliferation of Langerhans' cells. Therefore, replacing interleukin-2 might theoretically prevent the progression of eosinophilic granuloma. There are case reports that intravenous interleukin-2 leads to a clinical remission[44] but the general usefulness of such therapy remains to be seen.

The patients usually survive a median of 12.5 years after the diagnosis. However, the course of illness varies, and at least some patients live longer (for 23 years) after the diagnosis is made. Approximately half the deaths are associated with respiratory failure, and airway obstruction on lung-function testing and decreased diffusing capacity indicated a poor prognosis. Examination of transbronchial biopsy specimens is often nondiagnostic, and the typical CT findings in the upper lung zones are frequently absent. A link with hematologic cancers or lung cancers is suggested but not confirmed.

LYMPHANGIOLEIOMYOMATOSIS (LAM)

This is a rare disease that almost exclusively affects women of childbearing age, and is of unknown etiology and was described about 60 years ago.[45-49] It is due to a benign diffuse nodular proliferation of the smooth muscle cells around the lymphatic vessels, blood vessels, and airway and other tissues of the abdomen and thorax. The atypical hyperplastic muscles involve the bronchioles, venules, arterioles and small air spaces. In later stages, the smooth muscle cells form nodular aggregates. Although the cause is not known, because of tits occurrence in women of childbearing age, it is thought that the disorder is related to endocrine dysfunction and partly driven by hormonal stimuli. This is further supported by the fact that LAM has an onset predominantly in the premenopausal women, exacerbations during pregnancy, and the therapeutics benefits of hormonal therapy. Even there is no *in vitro* or *in vivo* data to support the hypothesis that the proliferation of LAM cells is dependant on hormonal stimuli, there are considerable indirect evidence that steroid hormones influence smooth muscle cell growth in pulmonary LAM. This evidence includes, in addition to the above, the presence of ER and PR in pulmonary LAM cells, exacerbation of LAM during estrogen therapy, and the apparent therapeutic response in the form of clinical improvement or stabilization to exogenous hormonal agents in some patients. Immunohistochemical studies of LAM specimens for estrogen and progesterone receptors (ER and PR) immunoreactivity however, have been variable.

The median age of onset is usually 33 years and the disease is clinically characterized by shortness of breath, hemoptysis, cough, chest pain, recurrent pneumothorax, and chylous pleural effusion.[50,51] Chest X-ray typically reveals reveals hyperinflated lungs with fine linear and nodular opacities more in the lower lung fields (diffuse interstitial infiltrates). Pulmonary function abnormalities include an increased total lung capacity, and residual volume, airflow obstruction, ventilation-perfusion mismatch, and decreased diffusing capacity. The small airway function is grossly abnormal. There is both a hypoxia and hypocarbia. The disease is usually progressive with a slowly declining clinical course[51] with death due to respiratory failure in few years. Although most LAM is pulmonary, retroperitoneal and pelvic lymph node involvement can also occur.[52] LAM can occur as an isolated disorder, which is referred to as sporadic LAM, or it may occur in association with tuberous sclerosis (TSC). LAM affects about 2.3 percent of individuals (or 4.6% of women) with TSC.[53] Renal angiolipomas occur in 70 percent of TSC patients and in 33 to 63 percent of women with sporadic LAM.[49,54-56] This association may reflect a common underlying genetic basis for both diseases.[57] Estrogen and progesterone receptor immunoreactivity in renal angiolipomas has been reported from women with pulmonary LAM.[58]

The disease was thought to be invariably fatal. But treatment with high-dose progesterone, bilateral oophorectomy, or tamoxifen may benefit some patients by reducing the amount of abnormal intrapulmonary muscles. Lung transplantation is the only effective therapy for end-stage disease.

METASTATIC TUMORS IN THE LUNG

Any tumor including bronchogenic carcinomas may metastasize into the lungs.[59-62] There are various patterns of metastasis, which may be helpful in the differential diagnosis of the primary sites. These are shown in Table 23.2 (Figs 23.23 to 23.28).

TABLE 23.2: Metastasis to lungs from primaries

Pattern of metastasis	Primary sites
Solitary metastasis	Large bowel, breast, cervix, kidney, sarcomas
Multiple cannonball tumors	Hypernephroma, seminoma, sarcomas, colon, choriocarcinoma, breast
Diffuse, nodular infiltration	Breast, stomach, thyroid, colon
Lymphangitis carcinomatosis	Breast, stomach, pancreas, prostate, bronchogenic carcinoma
Endobronchial metastasis	Breast, kidney, colon, cervix, hypernephroma
Carcinomatous embolization	Prostate, breast, stomach, colon, pancreas, liver, cervix, choriocarcinoma
Bilateral hilar node metastasis	Lymphomas, oat cell carcinoma, Kidney, head and neck, testis, breast, malignant melanoma

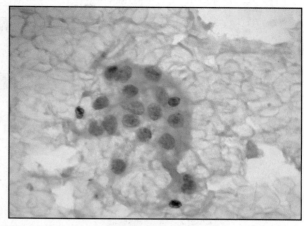

FIGURE 23.25: Loosely cohesive cluster of tumor cells, low NC ratio, abundant cytoplasm 2nd conspicious nucleoli in a case of metastatic renal cell carcinoma (H&E, 100X)

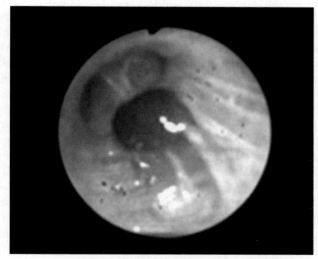

FIGURE 23.23: Endobronchial melanoma as seen through a FOB

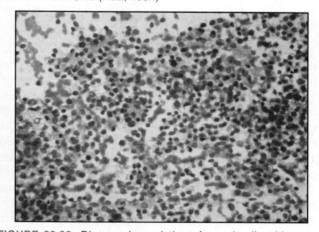

FIGURE 23.26: Dispersed population of round cells with coarse chromatin and occasional rosette formation in a case of metastatic round cell tumor (MGG, 20X)

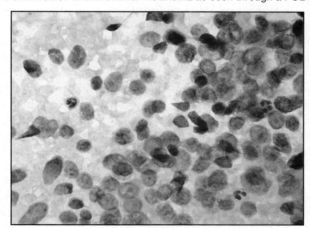

FIGURE 23.24: Dispersed population of round cells with coarse chromatin and conspicuous nucleoli in a case of metastatic round cell tumor (H&E, 100X)

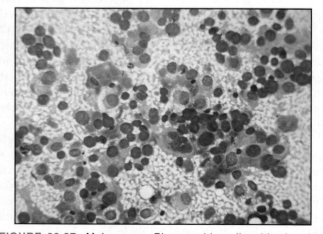

FIGURE 23.27: Melanoma - Pleomorphic cells with abundant eosinophilic cytoplasm, eccentric dark nuclei, prominent nucleoli occasional cells showing intracytoplasmic pigment

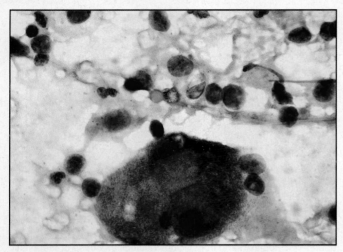

FIGURE 23.28: Melanoma - Dispersed population of pleomorphic cells with multinucleation and presence of abundant intracytoplasmic melanin pigment (H&E, 100X)

PSEUDOTUMORS

Inflammatory pseudotumors of the lung are uncommon. These masses resemble carcinoma of the lung radiographically and are discovered only at time of the histologic review of the resected specimen.[63] A large number of pulmonary lesions may present as pseudotumors. The importance lies in the fact that they are most often confused with neoplasms, especially on chest X-rays. The lesions are frequently asymptomatic. The groups of diseases included in this category are: pseudolymphomas, plasma cell granulomas, xanthomatous pseudotumors, paraffinomas, endometriosis of the lung, intrapulmonary hematomas, amyloidosis, localized Wegener's granulomatosis, and round atelectasis. A localized collection of pleural fluid in the horizontal fissure may simulate a tumor on chest X-ray and this has been called a "phantom tumor" or "vanishing tumor" because it may disappear on lateral decubitus X-ray films, and after control of congestive cardiac failure, with which it is associated. Other diagnostic clues for this type of localized effusion are that in right lateral films, the shadow is not spherical and small triangular opacities extend anteriorly and posteriorly into the fissure.

Inflammatory pseudotumor (also called plasma cell granuloma, histiocytoma and xanthofibroma) is a benign, slow growing lesion which may present with cough, dyspnea, hemoptysis and unresolving pneumonia or can be discovered radiographically as a localized lesion. It has been reported in individuals up to 70 years old, but approximately two-thirds have developed in individuals under 30 years of age. The sex incidence is approximately equal. Inflammatory pseudotumors of the

lung are usually peripheral lesions but may occasionally be endobronchial.[64] The presenting features can also be nonspecific like chest pain and cough.[65] The disease can occur rarely in children and in association with extrapulmonary pseudotumors.[66] Bronchial mucus has tomodensitometric features and MR signal intensity similar to that of water. However, chronic entrapped mucus collections, due to water reabsorption and higher protein content, can have CT attenuation values higher than 20 and reaching even 130 HU. Higher protein concentration also causes a sensible reduction in T1 relaxation time. The demonstration of mucus within a mediastinal, bronchial or pulmonary lesion is an important diagnostic clue permitting remarkable shortening of the list of differential diagnoses.[67]

They may be confused with pulmonary "mass" suspected as malignant tumor. They may be originally diagnosed as malignant lung tumor although in reality they are inflammatory pseudotumor in about 30 percent of cases. Pulmonary inflammatory pseudotumors, may be a pitfall diagnosing a lung mass and implicate legal problems. Surgical resection leads to the final diagnosis in doubtful cases. A wide resection has a diagnostic aim and may preserve healthy parenchyma. Clinicians, pathologists and surgeons should accurately inform patients with doubtful diagnosis of pulmonary malignancy. Any decision should be kept altogether either choosing the simple observation or the timely surgical diagnostic and therapeutical approach.[68]

Pulmonary inflammatory pseudotumors of the fibrous histiocytoma type shares several clinical attributes with inflammatory sarcomatoid carcinoma and shows closely similar histological features, except that the inflammatory pseudotumors lacks mitoses and invasiveness, and contained xanthoma cells or multinucleated elements in some cases. Immunohistochemical analyses shows consistent dissimilarities between inflammatory sarcomatoid carcinoma and inflammatory pseudotumors; keratin and epithelial membrane antigen were present in inflammatory sarcomatoid carcinoma but not inflammatory pseudotumors, whereas actin was observed only in the proliferating spindle cells of inflammatory pseudotumors. In summary, the potential clinicopathologic overlap between inflammatory sarcomatoid carcinoma and inflammatory pseudotumors suggests that caution should be exercised in the separation of these two lesions. In particular, it is unwise to attempt to make this distinction in an intraoperative frozen section setting.[69]

Between February 1946 and September 1993, 56,400 general thoracic surgical procedures were performed at the Mayo Clinic. Twenty-three patients (0.04%) had resection of an inflammatory pseudotumor of the lung.[70] There were 12 women and 11 men. Median age was 47 years (range, 5 to 77 years). Six patients (26%) were less than 18 years old. All pathologic specimens were re-reviewed, and the diagnosis of inflammatory pseudotumor was confirmed. Eighteen patients (78%) were symptomatic which included cough in 12, weight-loss in 4, fever in 4, and fatigue in 4. Four patients had prior incomplete resections performed elsewhere and underwent re-resection because of growth of residual pseudo-tumor. Wedge excision was performed in 7 patients, lobectomy in 6, pneumonectomy in 6, chest wall resection in 2, segmentectomy in 1, and bilobectomy in 1. Complete resection was accomplished in 18 patients (78%). Median tumor size was 4.0 cm (range, 1 to 15 cm). There were no operative deaths. Follow-up was complete in all patients and ranged from 3 to 27 years (median, 9 years). Overall 5-year survival was 91 percent. Nineteen patients are currently alive. Cause of death in the remaining 4 patients was unrelated to pseudotumor. The pseudotumor recurred in 3 of the 5 patients who had incomplete resection; 2 have had subsequent complete excision with no evidence of recurrence 8 and 9 years later. The authors concluded that inflammatory pseudotumors of the lung are rare. They often occur in children, can grow to a large size, and are often locally invasive, requiring significant pulmonary resection. Complete resection, when possible, is safe and leads to excellent survival. Pseudotumors, which recur, should be re-resected.[70]

REFERENCES

1. Carr DT, Holoye PY. Neoplasms of the lungs. General principles and diagnostic approach. In Murray JF, Nadel JA (Eds): Textbook of Respiratory Medicine. WB Saunders Company: Philadelphia 1988;49-52:1169.
2. Frazer RG, Pare JAP. Neoplastic diseases of the lungs. In diagnosis of diseases of the chest. WB Saunders Company: Philadelphia 1978;2:981.
3. Whimster WF. Tumors of the trachea, bronchus, lung and pleura. Pitman Books: London 1983.
4. Seaton A, Seaton D, Leitch AG. Other pulmonary neoplasms and related conditions. In Crofton and Douglas's respiratory diseases (4th edn). Blackwell Scientific Publications: London 1989;36,975.
5. Squerzanti A, Basteri V, Antinolfi G, D'agostino F, Scutellari PN, Ravenna F, Ghirardi R, Cavallesco G. Bronchial carcinoid tumors: Clinical and radiological correlation. Radiol Med (Torino) 2002;104:273-84.
6. Hurt R, Bates M. Carcinoid tumors of the bronchus: A 33 years of experience. Thorax 1984;39:617-23.
7. Okike N, Bernatz P, Woolner LB. Carcinoid tumors of the lung. Ann Thorac Surg 1976;22:270-77.
8. Blondal T, Grimelius L, Nou E, et al. Argyrophil carcinoid tumors of the lung: Incidence, clinical study, and follow-up of 46 patients. Chest 1980;78:840-44.
9. Mc Caughan BC, Martini N, Bains MS. Bronchial carcinoids: Review of 124 cases. J Thorac Cardiovasc Surg 1985;89:8-17.
10. Betelsen S, Aasred A, Lund C, Jacobsen M, Skov Jensen B, Ludwigsen E, Paulsen P, Paulsen SM, Bodsberg E, Christoffer-Sen I, et al. Bronchial carcinoid tumors: A clinicopathological study of 82 cases. Scand J Thorac Cardiovasc Surg 1985;19:105-11.
11. Ellman P, Bowdler AJ. Pulmonary manifestations of Hodgkin's disease. Br J Dis Chest 1960;54:59-71.
12. Macdonald JB. Lung involvement in Hodgkin's disease. Thorax 1977;32:664-67.
13. Manoharan A, Pitney WR, Schonell ME, Bader LV. Intrathoracic manifestations in Non-Hodgkin's lymphoma. Thorax 1979;34:29-32.
14. Jenkins PF, Ward MJ, Davies P, Fletcher J. Non-Hodgkin's lymphoma, chronic lymphocytic leukaemia and the lung. Br J Dis Chest 1981;75:22-30.
15. Yousem SA, Weiss LM, Colby TV. Primary pulmonary Hodgkin's disease. Cancer 1986;57:1217-24.
16. Parker JC Jr, Payene WS, Woolner LB. Pulmonary blastoma (embryoma). J Thorac Cardiovasc Surg 1966;51:694-99.
17. Peacock MJ, Whitewell F. Pulmonary blastoma. Thorax 1976;31:197-204.
18. Jacobsen M, Francis D. Pulmonary blastoma. Acta Pathol Microbiol Immunol Scand 1980;88:151-60.
19. Cabarcos A, Dorronsoro MG, Beristain JLL. Pulmonary carcinosarcoma: A case study and review of literature. Br J Dis Chest 1985;79:83-94.
20. Davidson AR. Eosinophilic granuloma of the lung. Br J Dis Chest 1976;70:125-28.
21. Zinkham WH. Multifocal eosinophilic granuloma: Natural history, aetiology and management. Am J Med 1976;60:457-63.
22. Friedman PJ, Liebow AA, Sokoloff J. Eosinophilic granuloma of lung: Clinical aspects of primary pulmonary histiocytosis in adults. Medicine 1981;60:385-96.
23. Wheeler RB, Sofka CM, Amorosa JK, Raska K, Nosher JL. Radiology-pathology conference: Robert Wood Johnson Medical School. Eosinophilic granuloma of the lung. N J Med 1995;92:526-28.
24. Rajagopol J, Mark EJ. Case records of the Massachusetts General Hospital. Weekly clinicopathological exercises. Case 32-2002. A 58-year-old man with interstitial pulmonary disease. N Engl J Med 2002;347:1262-68.
25. Basset F, Corrin B, Spencer H, et al. Pulmonary histiocytosis X. Am Rev Respir Dis 1978;118:811-20.

26. Vassallo R, Ryu JH, Schroeder DR, et al. Clinical outcomes of pulmonary Langerhans'-cell histiocytosis in adults. N Engl J Med 2002;346:484-90.

27. Friedman PJ, Liebow AA, Sokoloff J. Eosinophilic granuloma of the lung: Clinical aspects of primary histiocytosis in the adult. Medicine (Baltimore) 1981; 60:385-96.

28. Schonfeld N, Frank W, Wenig S, et al. Clinical and radiologic features, lung function and therapeutic results in pulmonary histiocytosis X. Respiration 1993;60:38-44.

29. Malpas JS. Langerhans cell histiocytosis in adults. Hematol Oncol Clin North Am 1998;12:259-68.

30. Nezelof C, Basset F. Langerhans cell histiocytosis cell research: Past, present, and future. Hematol Oncol Clin North Am 1998;12:385-406.

31. Schwarz MI, King TE Jr. Interstitial lung disease (3rd edn). Hamilton, Ont: BC Decker 1998.

32. Lacronique J, Roth C, Battesti JP, Basset F, Chretien J. Chest radiological features of pulmonary histiocytosis X: A report based on 50 adult cases. Thorax 1982;37: 104-09.

33. Dail DH, Hammar SP (Eds). Pulmonary pathology (2nd edn). New York: Springer-Verlag, 1994.

34. Brauner MW, Grenier P, Tijani K, Battesti JP, Valeyre D. Pulmonary Langerhans cell histiocytosis: Evolution of lesions on CT scans. Radiology 1997;204:497-502.

35. Von Essen S, West W, Sitorius M, Rennard SL. Complete resolution of roentgenographic changes in a patient with pulmonary histiocytosis X. Chest 1990;98:765-67.

36. Mogulkoc N, Veral A, Bishop PW, Bayindir U, Pickering CA, Egan JJ. Pulmonary Langerhans' cell histiocytosis: Radiologic resolution following smoking cessation. Chest 1999;115:1452-55.

37. Tazi A, Montcelly L, Bergeron A, Valeyre D, Battesti JP, Hance AJ. Relapsing nodular lesions in the course of adult pulmonary Langerhans cell histiocytosis. Am J Respir Crit Care Med 1998;157:2007-10.

38. Powers MA, Askin FB, Cresson DH. Pulmonary eosinophilic granuloma: A 25-year follow-up. Am Rev Respir Dis 1984;129:503-07.

39. Hoffman L, Cohn JE, Gaensler EA. Respiratory abnormalities in eosinophilic granuloma of the lung: Long-term study of five cases. N Engl J Med 1962; 267:577-89.

40. Case Records of the Massachusetts General Hospital (Case 5-1978). N Engl J Med 1978;298:327-32.

41. Corrin B, Basset F. A review of histiocytosis X with particular reference to eosinophilic granuloma of the lung. Invest Cell Pathol 1979;2:137-46.

42. Housini I, Tomashefski JF Jr, Cohen A, Crass J, Kleinerman J. Transbronchial biopsy in patients with pulmonary eosinophilic granuloma: Comparison with findings on open lung biopsy. Arch Pathol Lab Med 1994;118:523-30.

43. Kohalmi F, Strausz J, Egervary M, Szekeres G, Timar J. Differential expression of markers in extensive and restricted Langerhans cell histiocytosis (LCH). Pathol Oncol Res 1996;2:184-87.

44. Hirose M, Saito S, Yoshimoto T, Kuroda Y. Interleukin-2 therapy of Langerhans cell histiocytosis. Acta Paediatr 1995;84:1204-06.

45. Van Stossel E. Uber muskulare cirrhose dur lunge. Beitr Klin Tuberk 1937;90:432-42.

46. Kalassian KG, Doyel R, Kao P, et al. Lymphangioleiomyomatosis: New insights. Am J Respir Crit Care Med 1997;155:1183-86.

47. Sullivan EG. Lymphangioleiomyomatosis: A review. Chest 1998;114:1689-1703.

48. Workshop NHLBI. Report of Workshop on Lymphangioleimyomatosis. Am J Respir Crit Care Med 1999; 159:679-83.

49. Chu SC, Horiba K, Usuki J, et al. Comprehensive evaluation of 35 patients with lymphangioleiomyomatosis. Chest 1999;115:1041-52.

50. Taylor JR, Ryu J, Colby TV, et al. Lymphangioleiomyomatosis: Clinical course in 32 patients. N Engl J Med 1990;323:1254-60.

51. Johnson SE, Davey DD, Cibull ML, et al. Lymphangioleiomyomatosis. Am Surg 1993;59:395-99.

52. Torres VE, Bjornsson J, King BF et al. Extrapulmonary lymphangioleiomyomatosis and lymphangiomatous cysts in the tuberous sclerosis complex. Mayo Clin Proc 1995;70:641-48.

53. Castro M, Shepherd CW, Gomez MR, et al. Pulmonary tuberous sclerosis. Chest 1995;107:189-95.

54. Bernstein SM, Newell JD, Adamczyk D, et al. How common are renal angiomyolipomas in patients with pulmonary lymphangioleiomyomatosis? Am J Respir Crit Care Med 1995;152:2138-43.

55. Kerr LA, Blute ML, Ryu JH, et al. Renal angiolipomas in association with pulmonary lymphangioleiomyomatosis: Forme froste of tuberous sclerosis. Urology 1993;41:440-44.

56. Maziak DE, Kesten S, Rappaport DC, et al. Extrathoracic angiomyolipomas in lymphangioleiomyomatosis. Eur Respir J 1996;9:402-05.

57. Smolarek TA, Wessner LL, McCormack FX, et al. Evidence that lymphangioleiomyomatosis is caused by TSC2 mutations: Chromosome 16p13 loss of heterozygosity in angiomyolipomatosis. Am J Hum Genet 1998;62:810-15.

58. Logginidou HL, Ao X, Russo I, Henske EP. Frequent estrogen and progesterone receptor immunoreactivity in renal angiomyolipomas from women with pulmonary lymphangioleiomyomatosis. Chest 2000;117:25-30.

59. Baumgartener WA, Mark JB. Metastatic malignancies from distant sites to the tracheobronchial tree. J Thorac Cardiovasc Surg 1980,79:499-503.

60. Shepherd MP. Endobronchial metastatic disease. Thorax 1982;37:362-70.

61. Behera D, Malik SK, Jindal SK. Solitary endobronchial metastasis. Ind J Chest Dis All Sci 1983;25:155.

62. Crow J, Slavin G, Kreel L. Pulmonary metastasis. A pathologic and radiologic study. Cancer 1981;47:2595.

63. Tuncozgur B, Ustunsoy H, Bakir K, Ucak R, Elbeyli L. Inflammatory pseudotumor of the lung. Thorac Cardiovasc Surg. 2000;48:112-13.

64. Hajjar WA, Ashour MH, Al-Rikabi AC. Endobronchial inflammatory pseudotumor of the lung. Saudi Med J 2001;22:366-68.

65. Omasa M, Kobayashi T, Takahashi Y, Tamada J. Surgically treated pulmonary inflammatory pseudotumor. Jpn J Thorac Cardiovasc Surg 2002;50:305-98.

66. Janik JS, Janik JP, Lovell MA, Hendrickson RJ, Bensard DD, Greffe BS. Recurrent inflammatory pseudotumors in children. J Pediatr Surg 2003;38:1491-95.

67. Gaeta M, Vinci S, Minutoli F, Mazziotti S, Ascenti G, Salamone I, Lamberto S, Blandino A. CT and MRI findings of mucin-containing tumors and pseudotumors of the thorax: Pictorial review. Eur Radiol 2002;12:181-89.

68. Rizzo S, Marchesi R, Ronchi V, Scicchitano D, Luinetti O, Pandolfi U. Inflammatory pseudotumor of the lung. Diagnostic-therapeutic effectiveness of its radical resection. Minerva Chir 2000;55:807-14.

69. Wick MR, Ritter JH, Nappi O. Inflammatory sarcomatoid carcinoma of the lung: Report of three cases and clinicopathologic comparison with inflammatory pseudotumors in adult patients. Hum Pathol 1995;26: 1014-21.

70. Cerfolio RJ, Allen MS, Nascimento AG, Deschamps C, Trastek VF, Miller DL, Pairolero PC. Inflammatory pseudotumors of the lung. Ann Thorac Surg 1999; 67:933-36.

Sarcoidosis

INTRODUCTION

Sarcoidosis is a systemic granulomatous disease that primarily affects the lung and lymphatic systems of the body. A diagnosis of the disorder usually requires the demonstration of typical lesions in more than one organ system and exclusion of other disorders known to cause granulomatous disease. Since sarcoidosis was first described in 1877, it has continued to fascinate both clinicians and scientists. Much progress has been made in terms of understanding the protean clinical and unique immunological and pathological features of the disorder. Less is known about the epidemiology and genetic factors that contribute to the development and expression of the disease. The appropriate therapy for the disorder also has not been well defined for all patients. Most importantly, sarcoidosis is a disease of unknown etiology.

DEFINITION

The Joint Committee of the American Thoracic Society (ATS), the European Respiratory Society (ERS), and the World Association of Sarcoidosis and Other Granulomatous disorders (WASOG) recommended the following definition in 1999:[1] "Sarcoidosis is a multisystem disorder of unknown cause(s).[2] It commonly affects young and middle-aged adults and frequently presents with bilateral hilar lymphadenopathy, pulmonary infiltration, and ocular and skin lesions. The liver, spleen, lymph nodes, salivary glands, heart, nervous system, muscles, bones, and other organs may also be involved. The diagnosis is established when clinicoradiological findings are supported by histological evidence of noncaseating epithelioid cell granulomas. Granulomas of known causes and local sarcoid reactions must be excluded. Frequently observed immunological features are depression of cutaneous delayed-type hypersensitivity and a heightened helper T cell type 1 (Th1) immune response at sites of disease. Circulating immune complexes, along with signs of B cell hyperactivity, may also be found".

Although, the etiology of this disease is unknown, most clinicians and investigators around the world agrees on the descriptive definition[3-8] which suggested the fact that: it is a multisystem disorder of unknown cause(s), most commonly affecting young adults, and frequently presenting with hilar lymphadenopathy, pulmonary infiltrations, ocular and skin lesions. The diagnosis is established most securely when well-recognized clinicoradiographic findings are supported by histological evidence of widespread epithelioid granulomas in more than one system. Multisystem sarcoidosis must be differentiated from local sarcoid-tissue reactions. There is imbalance of CDT4: T8 subsets, an influx of Th1 helper cells to sites of activity, hyperreactivity of B cells, and circulation of immune complexes. Markers of activity include raised levels of serum angiotensin converting enzyme (SACE), abnormal calcium metabolism, a positive Kveim-Siltzbach skin test, intrathoracic uptake of radioactive gallium, and abnormal fluorescence angiography. The course and prognosis correlate with the mode of onset. An acute onset usually heralds self-limited course of spontaneous resolution, whereas an insidious onset may be followed by relentless progressive fibrosis. Corticosteroids relieve symptoms, suppress the formation of granulomas including the Kveim-Siltzbach granulomas, and normalize both levels of SACE and the uptake of gallium. A synthesis of clinical features, radiology, histology, biochemical changes, and immunological abnormalities helps to distinguish it from nonspecific local sarcoid-tissue reactions.

The course and prognosis may correlate with the mode of the onset and the extent of the disease. An acute onset with erythema nodosum or asymptomatic bilateral hilar lymphadenopathy usually heralds a self-limiting course, whereas an insidious onset, especially with multiple extrapulmonary lesions, may be followed by relentless, progressive fibrosis of the lungs and other organs.

History

1877-1898: The initial description of sarcoidosis was given by an English physician, Jonathon Hutchinson, who, in 1877, described a patient whose hands and feet had multiple, raised, purplish cutaneous patches that which had developed over 2 year.[9] Hutchinson attributed these lesions to a manifestation of gout. In a subsequent publication,[10] he described additional cases and suggested this phenomenon represented a "form of skin disease which has . . . hitherto escaped special recognition." The subsequent reports of the salient histopathological and clinical features of sarcoidosis described primarily dermatological manifestations or limited site involvement (e.g. ocular, parotid glands, bones) and the systemic nature of the disorder was not appreciated.

Some of the important landmarks on the description of sarcoidosis are as follows:

1899: Carl Boeck, a Norwegian dermatologist, provided drawings of skin lesions on the hand of a Norwegian sailor; his illustrations were seen by Hutchinson but never published.[11] His nephew, Caesar Boeck, described a case of cutaneous lesions in 1899 resembling Hutchinson's report, and he termed it "multiple benign sarcoid of the skin"; epithelioid cells and giant cells were noted on histologic examination.[12] He used the term *sarkoid* (sarcoid → sarcoidosis) because he felt that the lesions resembled sarcoma, but were benign. The term *sarcoidosis* stemmed from this report. Caesar Boeck subsequently published 24 cases of "miliary lipoids," with involvement of lung, bone, lymph nodes, spleen, nasal mucosa, or conjunctivae, underscoring the systemic nature of the disease.[8]

1889-1892: Besnier, of France, first described lupus pernio in 1889.[13] The histological features of lupus pernio were delineated 3 year later.[14]

1904-1920: In 1904, Kreibich, a professor of dermatology in Prague, described sarcoid bone cysts in a patient with lupus pernio.[15] Sarcoid bone lesions were often attributed to tuberculosis or other specific diseases.[16]

1909: In 1909, the Danish ophthalmologist, Heerfordt, described uveoparotid fever in three patients (characterized by a chronic, febrile course, enlarged parotid glands, and uveitis; two had unilateral facial nerve palsy).[17] At the time, the syndrome was ascribed to mumps.

1915: The involvement of internal organs was appreciated by Kuznitsky and Bittorf, who described a 27 years old soldier with multiple skin and subcutaneous nodules, histological confirmation of Boeck's sarcoid, enlarged hilar nodes, and pulmonary infiltrates on chest radiographs.[18]

1916-17: Jorgen Schaumann, a Swedish dermatologist, decribed patients with involvement of multiple organs including lung, bone, tonsils, gums, spleen, and liver.[19]

1919-34: In an article submitted in 1919 (ultimately published in 1934), Schaumann suggested that features previously attributed to separate diseases likely represented a systemic disorder, which he termed "lymphogranulomatose benigne".[20] He and many other investigators believed that sarcoidosis likely represented a variant of tuberculosis.[11]

1939: An association between sarcoidosis and hypercalcemia or hypercalciuria was first observed in 1939.[21]

1935-1963: This is the period during which important developments in the diagnosis and description of clinical features of sarcoidosis were described. In 1941, Ansgar Kveim, a Norwegian dermatologist, observed that intradermal inoculation of sarcoid lymph node tissue elicited a papular eruption in 12 of 13 patients with sarcoidosis.[22] He concluded that an unknown agent distinct from tuberculosis caused the papules. A similar reaction had been noted earlier by investigators in the United States, but was largely ignored.[23] Louis Siltzbach developed a revised test using splenic suspension, affirmed its specificity, and organized an international study.[24] The test was termed the Kveim-Siltzbach test, recognizing the contributions of these investigators. Sven Löfgren contributed significant new insights to the clinical features of sarcoidosis and delineated a syndrome that often occurs at the onset of sarcoidosis in Caucasians, characterized by erythema nodosum, bilateral hilar lymphadenopathy, fever, and polyarthritis.[25] This constellation of features has since been termed Löfgren's syndrome. Necropsy studies[26] and a large clinical series.[27] further defined the clinical spectrum and natural history of sarcoidosis.

In 1951, corticosteroids were first used to treat sarcoidosis, with anecdotal successes.[28,29] Numerous uncontrolled studies affirmed favorable responses in a subset of patients.[29-31] Interpretation of efficacy was obscured by the high rate of spontaneous remissions noted, particularly, in patients with early disease, Löfgren's syndrome, or bilateral hilar lymphadenopathy on chest radiographs.[27,30,31] In 1958, Wurm and colleagues proposed a radiographic staging system,[32] which was adopted by clinical investigators as a prognostic guide[30,31,33,34] and still remains in widespread clinical use. Using this radiographic schema to stratify patients, several prospective, randomized trials were carried out over the next three decades to evaluate the role of corticosteroids in the treatment of pulmonary sarcoidosis.[35] While these diverse studies failed to define the role and impact of corticosteroids in modifying the course of sarcoidosis, they did affirm the heterogeneous clinical course and expression of the disorder. By the mid-1970s, the availability of the fiberoptic bronchoscope enabled the diagnosis of sarcoidosis to be confirmed with minimal morbidity and high sensitivity.[36] In addition, retrieval of immune effector cells via bronchoalveolar lavage (BAL) at the time of bronchoscopy contributed enormously to the understanding of the pathogenesis of sarcoidosis and other inflammatory lung disorders.[37]

Until the late 1960s, research efforts and the international scope of sarcoidosis investigations were limited. The first International Meeting on Sarcoidosis was convened by Geraint James in London in 1958.[8] In 1963, the International Committee on Sarcoidosis was formed to develop a wider base for research and epidemiological studies.[11] Research investigations and publications escalated dramatically. At the Seventh International Conference in New York in 1975, immunological aberrations associated with sarcoidosis were defined[38] and serum angiotensin-converting enzyme (ACE) was first recognized as a possible biochemical marker of active sarcoidosis.[39] By the late 1970s and early 1980s, a plethora of studies dissected the immunological, biochemical, and pathogenetic mechanisms operative in sarcoidosis.[40,41] Compartmentalization of the immune response and involvement of helper T lymphocytes and activated immune effector cells at sites of disease activity were appreciated.[37,40-42] Ancillary studies to "stage" disease activity were developed (e.g. gallium-67 citrate scanning,[40,43] and bronchoalveolar lavage;[37,42] however, the clinical value of these procedures remains controversial. In the past three decades, hundreds of scientific studies have evaluated immunologic, pathogenic, or epidemiologic aspects of sarcoidosis. A MEDLINE search of the English language literature cited more than 6,500 publications since 1965 relevant to sarcoidosis. The number of scientific forums devoted to sarcoidosis has also increased. In 1984, the journal *Sarcoidosis* was started in Milan, by Gianfranco Rizzato.[8] In 1987, at the Milan World Congress on Sarcoidosis, the World Association of Sarcoidosis and Other Granulomatous Disorders

(WASOG) were formed, replacing the old International Committee.[8] These developments provided an infrastructure for fostering collaborative studies of this disease.

Sarcoidosis in India

The disease was considered rare in this country. Till about 1990 only few case reports and series were described and still many respiratory physicians looked upon this diagnosis with suspicion. However, by this time it is now well recognized and accepted as a distinct clinical entity and cases are being reported from all parts of the country with study of different aspects of the disease.[44-104]

Epidemiology

Sarcoidosis occurs throughout the world, affecting both sexes and all races and ages. The epidemiology of sarcoidosis remains problematic for several reasons, including lack of a precise, consistent case definition, variable methods of case ascertainment, variability in disease presentation, lack of sensitive and specific diagnostic tests, resulting in underrecognition and misdiagnosis of the disease particularly in areas of high prevalence of tuberculosis, and the paucity of systematic epidemiologic investigations of cause.[105]

Age and Sex

Sarcoidosis is most common in the age group of 20 to 40 years, although young children and aged may have the disease. In Indian patients, the age distribution is slightly higher than that reported from the western countries. Most large series report a greater frequency of sarcoidosis in women than men, although there is some discrepancy in the data. The disease shows a consistent predilection for adults less than 40 year of age, peaking in those 20 to 29 year old.[106] In Scandinavian countries and Japan, there is a second peak incidence in women more than 50 year of age.[107] Most studies suggest a slightly higher disease rate for women. The disease is most common in northern Europe, Great Britain and USA. The highest prevalence rates of the disease have been reported from Sweden (64/100,000 population) followed by Denmark and Germany. In the developing nations, the exact incidence of the disease is difficult to establish because of the common occurrence of diseases like tuberculosis, which is easily confused with sarcoidosis. However, in recent years the existence of the entity is being recognized increasingly, either because of increasing awareness of the existence of the disease with improvements in diagnostic techniques or because of a true increase in the incidence. For example, while in India, the disease was hardly described few years ago, since the mid 80s there are reports of over 1000 cases of Sarcoidosis . In United States, blacks are 10 to 17 times more likely to develop Sarcoidosis than whites. Black females in USA are affected nearly twice as frequently as black males, but prevalence in males and females is approximately the same in all other groups. In the only population-based incidence study of sarcoidosis in the United States, rates were 5.9 per 100,000 person-years for men and 6.3 per 100,000 person-years for women[108-110] on the basis of cumulative incidence estimates, the lifetime risk of sarcoidosis is 0.85 percent for US whites and 2.4 percent for US blacks.[111] Estimates of the prevalence of sarcoidosis range from fewer than 1 case to 40 cases per 100,000, with an age-adjusted annual incidence rate in the United States of 35.5 per 100,000 for blacks and 10.9 per 100,000 for whites.[110,112] Swedes, Danes, and US blacks appear to have the highest prevalence rates in the world.[113] Sarcoidosis is rarely reported in Spain, Portugal, India, Saudi Arabia, or South America,[113,114] partly because of the absence of mass screening programs and also because of the presence of other, more commonly recognized granulomatous diseases (tuberculosis, leprosy, fungal infection) that obscure sarcoidosis recognition.

Significant heterogeneity in disease presentation and severity occurs among different ethnic and racial groups. Several studies suggest that sarcoidosis in blacks is more severe, while whites are more likely to present with asymptomatic disease.[22,25,111,115-118] Extrathoracic manifestations are more common in certain populations, such as chronic uveitis in US blacks, lupus pernio in Puerto Ricans, and erythema nodosum (EN) in Europeans. Sarcoid-related EN is uncommon in blacks and Japanese.[119] Cardiac and ocular sarcoidosis appear to be more common in Japan, where the most frequent cause of death for sarcoid patients is from myocardial involvement.[108,120,121] Elsewhere, mortality is due most commonly to respiratory failure.[115,122] Overall mortality from sarcoidosis is 1 to 5 percent. Intriguing spatial clusters of illness have suggested person-to-person transmission or shared exposure to an environmental agent. A 1987 case-control study of residents of the Isle of Man observed that 40 percent of sarcoidosis cases reported prior contact with a person known to have the disease, compared with 1 to 2 percent of the controls.[123,124] Of these contacts, 14 pairs occurred in the same household, only 9 of who were blood relatives. Nine pairs came in contact with one another at work, 2 were

neighbors, and 14 were noncohabiting friends. Other case reports of husband-wife sarcoidosis fuel speculation of shared environmental or infectious exposure. Some studies have observed a seasonal clustering of sarcoidosis cases in winter and early spring.[125,126] Geographic and spatial clusters of disease have also been described, although problems with disease misclassification and study design hamper interpretation. Early observations of increased disease prevalence in the rural southeastern and middle Atlantic United States led to studies that examined potential etiologic factors in meteorology and soil, plants, pine, pollen, proximity to forests, water supply, use of firewood, proximity to lumbering and wood milling, and exposure to farm animals and pets, among others.[127] Neither animal experiments nor human studies have yet proven these hypotheses.

Etiology

Sarcoidosis is a systemic granulomatous disease of unknown etiology that primarily affects the lungs. The etiology remains unclear; however, environmental, genetic, ethnic, and familial factors probably modify expression of the disease. As an example, African Americans are at greater risk of mortality and morbidity than are white Americans, and more often have a family history of sarcoidosis. Although the cause(s) of sarcoidosis remain unknown, there are three different lines of evidence supporting the idea that sarcoidosis results from exposure of genetically susceptible hosts to specific environmental agents: (a) the aforementioned epidemiological studies (b) the inflammatory response in sarcoidosis, which is characterized by large numbers of activated macrophages and T lymphocytes bearing the CD4 helper phenotype, with a pattern of cytokine production in the lungs that is most consistent with a Th1-type immune response triggered by an antigen; and (c) the implications of studies concerning the T cell receptor (TCR) in patients with sarcoidosis.

Role of Genetic Factors

Familial sarcoidosis Over 200 cases of familial sarcoidosis have been described in literature. However, no clear Mendelian pattern of inheritance has emerged. Brother-sister and mother-child associations are common in these cases, but father-child association is rare. The severity and clinical presentations are not different from that in the nonfamilial cases. There is a preponderance of monozygotic over dizygotic twins. Although there is no conclusive proof, possible role of genetic and environmental factors shared by these families have been postulated. There are numerous reports of familial clustering of sarcoidosis. In the United States, familial clusters occur more commonly among blacks (with a rate of at least 19% in affected black families) than whites (with a rate of 5%).[128] In the Republic of Ireland, there is a high national prevalence of sarcoidosis, and a high prevalence (2.4%) also occurs among siblings.[129] An increased prevalence of sarcoidosis has been described in the Furano district of northern Japan, with some evidence of familial clustering.[130] HLA analyses of affected families suggest that the mode of inheritance of risk for sarcoidosis is likely polygenic, with the most common genotype frequencies being class I HLA-A1 and -B8 and class II HLA-DR3.[131] It is likely that genetically predisposed hosts are exposed to antigens that trigger an exaggerated cellular immune response leading to granuloma formation. The frequency of HLA typings in patients with sarcoidosis has not shown any preponderance of any particular type over the others. However, it is reported that individuals with sarcoidosis and HLA-B7 are more likely to be symptomatic. Other reports suggest that white sarcoid patients with HLA-B8 are more likely to have arthritic symptoms with or without erythema nodosum. Other reports suggest that frequency of sarcoidosis is 5.5 times greater in black patients with HLA-Bwl5 than in those lacking the antigen. Patients with B8 HLA types have greater chances of clearance of pulmonary fibrosis.

The recognition of race as an important risk factor clearly suggests a genetic predisposition to develop sarcoidosis.[132] Race as mentioned previously the disease is 10 to 17 times more common in blacks than whites, and more common in Europeans than that in the South-East Asians. The most compelling argument for a genetic mechanism of acquiring this predisposition is that there is occasional familial clustering of cases.[133] In general, genetic differences in candidate genes that could predispose an individual to sarcoidosis may reside in loci that influence T cell function, the regulation of antigen recognition and processing, or the regulation of matrix deposition that favors granuloma formation and progressive fibrosis.[134] But it is also likely that genetic factors may be important in defining the pattern of disease presentation and progression as well as its overall prognosis. This is illustrated by an investigation of the relationship between sarcoidosis and HLA phenotypes in two different countries in Europe, the Czech Republic and Italy.[135] A common observation for both countries was the association of certain manifestations of sarcoidosis with HLA-A1, -B8, and -DR3; whereas a negative association was observed for the

phenotypes HLA-B12 and -DR4. Findings that were restricted to only one of the countries were the association of disseminated systemic disease and HLA-B22, among the Italians, and the association of some specific clinical features and HLA-B13, among the non-Italians. In a study using genomic typing of a homogeneous Scandinavian population, a favorable prognosis was related to the DR17[134] haplotype, whereas DR15[136] and DR16[135] indicated a more protracted disease course.[137] DR17,[134] which was overrepresented among Scandinavian patients with sarcoidosis, has also been shown by others to be related to a good outcome.[135,138] In a totally different ethnic population from Japan, restriction fragment length polymorphism showed several restriction fragments of the DRβ gene only in DRw52-positive patients,[139] and these patients were likely to have limited-stage disease without ophthalmic involvement. In contrast, DR5J-positive Japanese patients often get a poorly resolving disease.[140] Analyses of the HLA specificity allow ethnic comparisons, and enable studies of the relationship between the HLA phenotype and the clinical outcome.

The Role of Environmental Agents

As the cause of sarcoidosis has remained unknown, the list of possible causative agents has continuously expanded since pine tree pollen was suggested. Some of the proposed agents are listed in Table 24.1.

TABLE 24.1: Possible etiological factors[1,8,141]

Infectious agents	Organic substances
• Viruses (herpes, Epstein-Barr, retrovirus, coxsackie B virus, cytomegalovirus, rubella, measles, retrovirus)	• Pine tree pollen • Clay • Peanut dust • Immune complexes
• Borrelia burgdorferi	
• Propionibacterium acnes	
• Mycobacterium tuberculosis and other mycobacteria	
• Phage transformed mycobacteria	
• Cell wall deficient mycobacteria	
• Streptococcal cell wall	
• Mycoplasma	
• Nocardia	
• Histoplasma	
• Corynebacterium species	
Inorganic substances	
Occupation	
• Aluminum	
• Zirconium	
• Talc	
• Beryllium	
• Oxalosis	
Miscellaneous	

Already in 1969, Mitchell and Rees[142] suggested a transmissible agent in the etiology of sarcoidosis. Ever since, there have been reports supporting such a notion, including the findings of sarcoidosis in recipients of transplants from patients with sarcoidosis.[143] Several infectious organisms have been implicated as potential causes of sarcoidosis, e.g. viruses, *Borrelia burgdorferi,* and *Propionibacterium acnes* (*see* Table 24.1). Also, non-infectious environmental agents can elicit a granulo-matous response with many features that are similar to sarcoidosis, e.g. beryllium, aluminum, and zirco-nium.[144-146] Therefore, the accurate diagnosis of sarcoidosis depends on a stringent inquiry concerning potential exposures to both organic and inorganic antigens. Finally, the host itself has been considered a potential source of granuloma-inducing antigens. However, the possibility that sarcoidosis is an auto-immune disorder is now considered less likely.

Because granulomatous inflammation is the histo-logic hallmark of sarcoidosis, investigators continue to improve and apply modern diagnostic tools in the search for infectious agents such as mycobacteria, which are known to induce a host granulomatous response.[141,147] Although the techniques are now more sophisticated, this principle has been applied for decades. Using various techniques, different groups have been able to detect antibodies to mycobacteria in patient sera in 50 to 80 percent of cases,[148,149] whereas fewer of the controls were positive. In the absence of specific patterns, it is difficult to interpret this type of data because patients with sarcoidosis may exhibit a generalized polyclonal synthesis of immunoglobulins resulting in higher titers than normal against a variety of common antigens. Failure to detect anti-mycobacterial antibodies or to culture mycobacteria does not exclude them in the pathogenesis of the disease, but it highlights the importance of seeking the antigen within the affected tissue. The demonstration of tuberculostearic acid[150] and muramyl dipeptide,[151] both components of the myco-bacterial cell wall, in sarcoid nodules has been used as indirect evidence for the presence of mycobacteria, and acid-fast L (mycobacteria cell wall-deficient) forms have been grown from the blood of patients with sarcoidosis.[152] To date, there is no evidence that sarcoidosis is caused by an infectious agent.

The evidence for an infective etiology, particularly mycobacterial, is becoming more appealing. Unfortu-nately, even with the advent of molecular tools, such as the highly sensitive polymerase chain reaction, the debate has not been resolved. The advantages and pitfalls of these techniques were elegantly reviewed by Mangiapan and Hance.[147] Their overview elucidates the need for caution in interpreting positive as well as negative findings. Failure to demonstrate mycobacteria may depend on insensitive methods, whereas positive findings may be due to contamination. The latter obser-vation demonstrates the need for sufficient control samples to appreciate the frequency with which false-positive results are occurring. Recent findings of mycobacterial DNA or ribosomal RNA in tissue speci-mens or BAL cells from patients with sarcoidosis must be interpreted in this context.[153,154] Altogether, these data suggest that if mycobacterial DNA is present in most sarcoid tissue, the amount must be relatively small. Alternatively, some of the patients diagnosed as having sarcoidosis may have a disorder initiated by myco-bacterial infection,[147] while other antigens trigger the disease in other patients.

A number of agents are postulated to be the respon-sible agents (*see* Table 24.1). These include exposure to pine pollen or beryllium, and infective agents like myco-bacteria, viruses, and fungi besides occupations, genetic and familial factors.[155-182] However, all these suggestions are discarded because of lack of any substantial evi-dence. Recent animal inoculation studies have suggested the possibility an unidentified transmissible agent, which needs further confirmation. Several studies have explored occupational risk factors for sarcoidosis. In the 1940s, cases of "sarcoidosis" in women in the fluores-cent light industry in Salem, Massachusetts led to the recognition of beryllium exposure as the cause of "Salem sarcoid." Exposure to other metal dusts, fumes, and organic antigens can cause granulomatous lung diseases that are difficult to distinguish clinically from sarcoidosis, emphasizing the importance of a careful occupational and environmental exposure history.[183] The Isle of Man study[184] observed that 18.8 percent of sarcoidosis cases were health care workers (mainly nurses), compared with 4.2 percent of the controls, an observation that has been made in several other studies.[185,186] This finding may reflect a more frequent use of chest radiographs in this population. A report of three sarcoidosis cases clustered among 57 firefighters who apprenticed together suggests a shared environmental exposure.[187] A significant association was identified between increased risk for sarcoidosis and ever having served on US Navy aircraft carriers, perhaps, again, only reflecting increased detection rates arising from more frequent use of routine chest radiographs in this setting.[188] Sarcoidosis appears to occur more commonly in nonsmokers than in smokers.[189] The extent to which environmental and occupational exposures confer increased risk for sarcoidosis awaits further investigation.

There is an elevated risk of sarcoidosis for workers with industrial organic dust exposures, especially in Caucasian workers. Workers for suppliers of building materials, hardware, and gardening materials were at an increased risk of sarcoidosis as were educators. Work providing childcare was negatively associated with sarcoidosis risk. Jobs with metal dust or metal fume exposures were negatively associated with sarcoidosis risk, especially in Caucasian workers.[180]

Sarcoidosis has occurred in conjunction with HIV infection, although this is rare.[190-192]

IMMUNOLOGY AND PATHOGENESIS OF SARCOIDOSIS

Sarcoidosis is characterized by granulomas consisting of a circumscribed collection of phagocytic cells in various states of activation and differentiation, including monocytes, macrophages, and multinucleated giant cells.[193-207] The most characteristic is the epithelioid cell. Although the granulomas occur in the peribronchial, subpleural, and perivascular areas of the lung, most concentration occurs in the pulmonary interstitium. Mononuclear cell infiltration into the interstitium is an important initiating factor in granuloma formation. These cells consist of a large number of T lymphocytes. Antigenic invasion is met by a granulomatous inflammatory response, which depends on close interaction between activated macrophages bearing increased expression of MHC class II molecules and CD 4 TH lymphocytes. The dual signal of the MHC-antigen complex and interleukin 1, secreted by macrophages, activates the T cells and a cascade of other cytokines to be released, which further enhance or suppress macrophage function. The T cells and macrophages are found in plenty at the site of sarcoid inflammation, but they are less evident at distant sites as evidenced by circulatory lymphopenia with an absolute decrease in T helper cells. Bronchoalveolar lavage has shown lymphocytic alveolitis with accumulation of macrophages and T cells within the alveolar structure. Monoclonal antibody studies have shown that macrophages with double phenotype RFD1+ D7+ may have an important immunomodulatory role in sarcoid inflammation, with the help of interferon, which is a potent activator of HLA-DR molecular expression on the surface of macrophages.

Various immunological abnormalities include both T cells and B cells. The T cell abnormalities are characterized by complete or partial anergy to skin tests (delayed hypersensitivity); depressed proliferative responses to antigens, mitogens, and mixed lymphocyte culture; and lymphocytopenia in the form of decreased number of circulating T cells and normal or decreased helper T suppressor T cells. The humoral or B cell abnormalities in sarcoidosis include polyclonal elevation of serum immunoglobulins; exaggerated humoral response to certain antigens; high serum antibodies to Mycoplasma, viruses (Epstein-Barr, rubella, parainfluenza, herpes simplex); autoantibodies to rheumatoid factor, antinuclear antibody and T cells; circulating immune complexes, Platelet aggregation, Raji cell and rheumatoid factor, Raji cell and Clq binding; and decreased number of B cells. The early sarcoid reaction is characterized by the accumulation of activated T cells and macrophages at sites of ongoing inflammation, notably in the lung.[201,202] Studies of sarcoid T lymphocytes in involved areas have shown that, in most patients, cells bear the helper CD4 phenotype; in rare cases the accumulating cells are predominantly CD8+ lymphocytes.[203] These cells spontaneously release interferon γ(IFN-γ) and interleukin 2 (IL-2) and other cytokines.[204,205] Further, sarcoid alveolar macrophages (AMs) behave as versatile secretory cells that release a great variety of cytokines, including tumor necrosis factor α (TNF-α), IL-12, IL-15, and growth factors.[206,207]

Various immunological abnormalities as observed in sarcoidosis are as follows:

- Intraalveolar and interstitial accumulation of CD4+ cells with helper-inducer activity and release of IL-2.
- Expansion of T cells bearing a restricted TCR repertoire in involved tissues. This pattern is consistent with a TCR oligoclonality. Expansion of the lung γ/β TCR cell pool in a subset of patients.
- Increased *in situ* production of Th1 cell-derived cytokines (IL-2 and IFN-γ) during granuloma formation.
- Increased expression of members of TNF-ligand and TNF-receptor superfamilies by sarcoid T cells.
- B cell hyperactivity and spontaneous *in situ* production of immunoglobulins.
- Increased spontaneous rate of proliferation of lung immunocompetent cells.
- Increased spontaneous rate of proliferation of lung immunocompetent cells.
- Accumulation of monocyte-macrophages with antigen-presenting cell capacity and expressing increased levels of activation markers (HLA-DR, HLA-DQ, CD71) and adhesion molecules (CD49a, CD54, CD102).

- Increased release of macrophage-derived cytokines (IL-1, IL-6, IL-8, IL-15, TNF-α, IFN-γ, GM-CSF) and chemokines (RANTES, MIP-1α, IL-16). Most of these cytokines favor granuloma formation and lung damage.
- Increased production of macrophage-derived fibrogenic cytokines (TGF-β and related cytokines, PDGF, and IGF-I), favoring evolution toward fibrosis.

(GM-CSF = granulocyte-macrophage colony-stimulating factor; IFN-γ = interferon γ; IGF-I = insulin-like growth factor I; IL-2 = interleukin 2; MIP-1α = macrophage inflammatory protein 1α; PDGF = platelet-derived growth factor; RANTES = regulation on activation, normal T cell expression and secretion; TCR = T cell receptor; TGF-β = transforming growth factor β; Th1 = helper T cell type 1; TNF = tumor necrosis factor).

The accumulation of immunocompetent cells likely represents the earliest step in the series of events that leads to granuloma formation, with activated CD45RO+ Th1-type T lymphocytes as the central cell in this phenomenon. From a pathogenic point of view, two mechanisms account for the increased number of cells in tissues involved by the sarcoid inflammatory process: a cellular redistribution from the peripheral blood to the lung and an *in situ* proliferation.[208] In the first mechanism, chemoattractant cytokines (including IL-8, IL-15, IL-16, and RANTES [regulation on activation, normal T cell expression and secretion]) cooperate to expand the intraalveolar pool of CD4+ memory cells within the inflamed area.[209,210] The second mechanism responsible for the accumulation of CD4+ helper T cells at sites of granuloma formation is *in situ* IL-2-mediated proliferation. A large number of BAL lymphocytes from patients with sarcoidosis are CD4+/HLA-DR+ T cells spontaneously releasing IL-2 and expressing a functional IL-2 receptor system.[209,211,212] Various studies indicate that IL-2 acts as a local growth factor for T lymphocytes infiltrating the lung parenchyma and other involved sarcoid tissues.[213,214] T cells isolated from patients with active sarcoidosis also show elevated mRNA and protein levels of IFN-γ, proliferation of activated T cells and are involved in the differentiation of Th0 cells into Th1 cells.[215] Thus, a Th1-type T cell response (secreting IL-2, IL-12, IFN-γ, and TNF-β) is likely to favor the granulomatous response at sites of disease activity.

No studies have shown why lung disease persists in some patients but not other patients. In addition, no studies have shown how persistent disease results in lung injury and fibrosis. However, the immunological pattern of cells in the sarcoid infiltrate suggests that (*a*) sarcoid granulomas are formed in response to a persistent and likely poorly degradable antigenic stimulus that induces a local Th1-type T cell-mediated immune response with an oligoclonal pattern; in fact, these cells are biased[216] in expression of genes for the α- and β-chain variable region of the T cell receptor (TCR); and (*b*) as a consequence of their chronic stimulation, macrophages release mediators of inflammation, locally, leading to accumulation of Th1 cells at sites of ongoing inflammation and contributing to the development of the granuloma structure. Experimental data from the *Schistosoma mansoni* model suggest one mechanism by which fibrosis may develop with persistent disease, i.e. there is a shift in the cytokine pattern from a Th1 to a Th2 phenotype with secretion of IL-4, IL-5, IL-6, IL-9, and IL-10. In the model, this results in a fibroproliferative response with substantial extracellular matrix deposition, and subsequent evolution toward pulmonary fibrosis.[217] Alternatively, in sarcoidosis, a persistent Th1 response may be associated with fibrosis. Studies of the Th1/Th2 secretory pattern in humans during the various phases of the sarcoid inflammatory process are needed to elucidate the regulatory immune mechanisms that govern matrix modifications in this disease.

In addition to understanding the pathogenesis of sarcoidosis, another goal of the immunological studies includes the identification of discrete markers (surface antigens, cytokine production, etc.) that may aid in the management of patients, not only in terms of prognosis, but also to define the different phases of the disease.

The T Cell Receptor

The majority of T lymphocytes use the α/β TCR to recognize antigenic peptides in the context of MHC molecules, and the variable regions of the TCR are constructed through rearrangement of noncontiguous germline gene segments. It has been proposed that analyses of the TCR may reveal the existence of T cells with a restricted TCR usage, suggesting a specific antigen triggering the development of sarcoidosis.[216,218] In addition, it has been shown in animal models that T cells with highly restricted TCR V (variable segment) gene usage can mediate an experimental model of autoimmune disease, and that modulation of these cells can affect the disease.

One potential problem with this strategy for identifying an antigen in sarcoidosis is that the duration of the disease may have an influence on the TCR usage, resulting in a more heterogeneous T cell response later on in the disease process. Further, because the onset of disease in sarcoidosis is relatively insidious, it may be difficult to estimate any possible influence of disease duration on the heterogeneity of the T cell response. In addition, the variations in TCR V gene usage that have been reported from different groups may be affected by differences in the ethnic origin of the populations that have been studied. Although many of the findings in this field of research are intriguing, it is still unclear how helpful they will be in eliciting the etiology of sarcoidosis.

Pathology

Histologically, sarcoidosis is characterized by noncaseating miliary granulomas involving many organs, including the lungs, lymph nodes, liver, spleen, skin, eyes, salivary glands, respiratory tract, joints, nervous system, and testes. The most commonly involved organs are the lungs followed by the lymph nodes. Fine miliary patterns affecting mainly the upper lobes and a relative sparing of the lower lobes, are common gross findings on autopsy. Fibrotic changes with honeycombing and thin walled emphysematous changes are common in the end stage disease.[219]

The characteristic lesion of sarcoidosis is a discrete, compact, noncaseating epithelioid cell granuloma. The epithelioid cell granulomas consist of highly differentiated mononuclear phagocytes (epithelioid cells and giant cells) and lymphocytes. Giant cells may contain cytoplasmic inclusions such as asteroid bodies and Schaumann bodies.[220,221] The central portion of the granuloma consists of predominantly CD4+ lymphocytes, whereas CD8+ lymphocytes are present in the peripheral zone.[222,223] Sarcoid granulomas may develop fibrotic changes that usually begin at the periphery and travel centrally, ending with complete fibrosis and/or hyalinization. Granulomas may occasionally exhibit focal coagulative necrosis.[222] It has been suggested that necrotizing sarcoid granulomatosis (NSG) may be a variant of sarcoidosis.[223,224] On electron microscopy, well-developed epithelioid cells show numerous cytoplasmic projections with frequent interdigitations. The morphology suggests a secretory function.[222,225]

The early lesions of sarcoidosis are composed of confluent, well-circumscribed epithelioid granulomas, which have a predilection for peribronchial, perivascular, subpleural, and interseptal septa. Such granulomas are also seen in the submucosa of the bronchus and bronchial gland and in the peribronchial connective tissue. Sarcoid granulomas tend to undergo perigranulomatous fibrotic changes and are sometimes replaced by hyalinous changes in the chronic stage. Alveolar septa away from the granulomas are essentially normal, except for perigranulomatous alveolar septa, which may show interstitial infiltration mainly of lymphocytes.

Although pleural involvement occurs up to 35 percent of the cases microscopically, clinical manifestation is uncommon. Sarcoid granulomas are common in the veins and arteries, specially the perivascular connective tissue. *True necrosis is not a feature of sarcoid granuloma,* although a small number of sarcoid granulomas may undergo a mild degree of coagulative necrosis in the central portion of granulomas During the development of sarcoid granuloma cytoplasmic structures including vacuoles, asteroid bodies, Schaumann bodies, and birefringent crystals, may be seen within the giant cells. Although these findings are not specific for sarcoidosis, they are uncommon in granulomas due to tuberculosis. The cytoplasmic vacuoles or *centrospheres sire* multiple and foamy in character and may be centrally or peripherally located. *Asteroid bodies* are stellate-shaped structures in the cytoplasm with deeply eosinophilic spokes radiating from a central core. *Schaumann bodies* are concentrically laminated hematoxylin staining bodies and are often seen in sarcoidosis. They are composed of calcium and iron salts. They are also seen in other granulomatous diseases like beryllium pneumonitis, in which case they are larger and called as conchoid bodies. Extracellular Schaumann bodies are seen in areas of fibrosis due to sarcoidosis also, and perhaps represent the residual structures in areas of previous active granuloma (Figs 24.1 to 24.3).

Lymph nodes (especially intrathoracic), lungs, liver, spleen, and skin are common sites of sarcoid granulomas, which are of a similar nature when found in any organ[220,222,226,227] In the lung, about 75 percent of the granulomas are located close to or within the connective tissue sheath of bronchioles and subpleural or perilobular spaces (a lymphangitic distribution).[221,223,228]

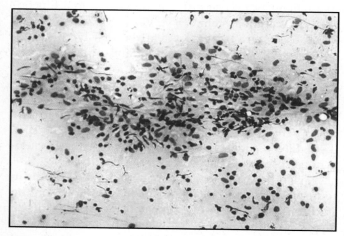

FIGURE 24.1: Giemsa stain, 50X, FNA of supraclavicular lymphnode showing non-necrotizing epithelioid cell granuloma

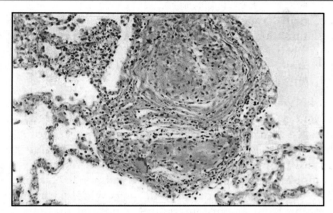

FIGURE 24.2: H&E stain, 50X, non-necrotizing epithelioid cell granuloma of sarcoidosis

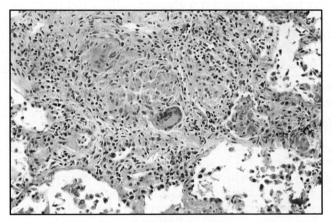

FIGURE 24.3: H&E stain, 200X, non-necrotizing epithelioid cell granuloma in transbronchial lung biopsy

Vascular involvement is observed in more than half of the patients with open lung biopsy or autopsy studies.[221-223,229]

Because of the lack of knowledge about the etiology of sarcoidosis, diagnosis is established when clinico-radiologic findings are supported by histologic evidence of granulomas. Because important differential diagnoses are infectious diseases, the need for microbiologic studies and cultures continues, especially when the patient has fever or when there are necrotic lesions in the biopsy specimens. Special stains for acid-fast bacilli and fungi are justified for the diagnosis, especially when there are atypical features for sarcoidosis such as necrosis or an airspace predominance of granulomas.[221]

The morphologic diagnosis of pulmonary sarcoidosis relies on three main findings: the presence of tight, well-formed granulomas and a rim of lymphocytes and fibroblasts in the outer margin of granulomas; peri-lymphatic interstitial distribution of granulomas (which allows transbronchial biopsies to be used as sensitive

diagnostic tools); and exclusion of an alternative cause.[221,230,231]

The differential diagnosis of sarcoid granulomas varies according to the sites of biopsy, such as lymph node, skin, liver, bone marrow, and spleen.[232]

Tumor-related Sarcoid Reactions

Regional lymph nodes of carcinomas show noncaseating epithelioid cell granulomas (sarcoid reactions) with an average frequency of 4.4 percent.[233,234] Biopsy specimens of liver and spleen obtained at laparotomy for the staging of Hodgkin's disease and non-Hodgkin's lymphomas show epithelioid cell granulomas with an average frequency of 13.8 and 7.3 percent, respectively[233,234] Three to 7 percent of patients with carcinoma may show granulomas in the primary tumors,[233] as in seminoma and dysgerminoma.[235,236]

Granulomatous Lesions of Unknown Significance (The GLUS Syndrome)

Fifteen to twenty percent of biopsy samples with granulomatous lesions have an undetermined etiology. These patients have a disease process that has been named the GLUS (granulomatous lesions of unknown significance) syndrome.[237] Immunohistologically, GLUS syndrome granulomas are B cell positive, as are tumor-related sarcoid reactions and toxoplasmosis. However, granulomas in sarcoidosis and mycobacterial infection are B cell negative.[238]

Sarcoid granulomas may completely resolve with only residual scars. Progressive and chronic disease is represented by extensive pulmonary fibrosis and honey-combing. The differentiating features in this late stage of the disease from diffuse fibrosing interstitial pneumonitis are that, in the latter the process is more diffuse rather than patchy as in sarcoidosis, and the cyst walls of sarcoidosis are thinner.[222,223] Pulmonary artery hypertrophy and thickening may be seen in the late stage of the disease. Various factors responsible for progression/inhibition from granuloma to fibrosis are as follows:[5]

Promoting factors	Inhibitors
Th2 cytokines	Th1 cytokines
Il-1	Interferon gamma
IL-4	IL-12
RANTES	Corticosteroids
Type I procollagen	Prostaglandin E
Type 1 collagen	Perfenidone
Fibronectin	Pentoxyphylline

Contd...

Contd...

Promoting factors	Inhibitors
Tumor necrosis factor	Thalidomide
Platelet derived growth factor	Bosentan
Endothelin-1	Halofuginone
	Transforming growth factor antibody
	Tumor necrosis factor antibody
	Infiximab
	Entanercept

Summary of Immunopathological March in Sarcoidosis

Formation of granulomas occur in a step-wise manner following a series of events.[239] It starts when T helper cells recognize protein peptides presented to them by antigen presenting cells earing HLA class II molecules. This immunological reactivity or inflammation attracts monocytes, macrophages that coalesce to form multi-nucleated giant cells and then epithelioid cells. Granuloma formation is further aided by a series of chemotactic factors. These include; Th1 cells induce IL-2, interferon gamma and tumor necrosis factor with the help of IL-12 and co-stimulator B7. This leads to formation of exuberant granulomas which further is associated with active cell mediated hypersensitivity and tissue destruction. These series of events are further remodeled by cytokines, adhesion molecules, matrix receptors of the integrin family, co-stimulator B7 and CD28, IL-12, and RANTES (regulated on activation normal T cells as secreted). These changes are reflected in the bronchoalveolar fluid. Angiotensin converting enzyme is generated within active granulomas. Monocyte chemoattract protein-1 is detected in macrophages peripheral to the granulomas but not within it. Both reflect early sarcoid activity.

Anergy is a form of immune apathy due to cytokine dysregulation and signal transduction. With CD28 co-stimulator there is active T cell proliferation, without it there is ignorance, apathy and anergy. CD28 and B7 are transmembrane glycoprotein signals on helper T cells and antigen presenting cells respectively. The signals induce the T cells to produce Il-2, which in turn activates the T cells to proliferate and interact with B cells and cytotoxic T cells. In due course this costimulation must end and the activated helper T cells are brought under control. This is done by cytotoxic T lymphocytes antigen 4 gene (CTLA-4), a regulatory molecule on the surface of activated T helper cells.

Apoptosis is another mechanism to switch off granulomatous inflammation. This is achieved via Fas antigen (Fas) and Fas ligand (FasL). Apoptosis may be an useful mechanism in resolving granulomatous inflammation and preventing postinflammatory scarring and fibrosis.

CLINICAL FEATURES

Although the clinical features of sarcoidosis may be absent or confined to a single organ, it is a generalized disease that may involve almost every organ of the body.[240-266] The individual with sarcoidosis may be asymptomatic or may present with constitutional symptoms and pulmonary or extra pulmonary features. The clinical course of sarcoidosis is widely variable, ranging from asymptomatic but abnormal findings in chest radiography to progressive multiorgan disease, which leads to fibrosis with organ failure and functional impairment. The common age of affection is between 20 to 40 years.

Nonspecific Constitutional Manifestations

Constitutional symptoms like fever, fatigue, malaise, anorexia, and weight loss are mild and may not be present. Sarcoidosis is a multiorgan disorder. Because of diverse manifestations, patients with sarcoidosis may present to clinicians with different specialties. The clinical picture of the disease depends on ethnicity, duration of the illness, site and extent of organ involvement, and activity of the granulomatous process.[267,268] Nonspecific constitutional symptoms such as fever, fatigue, malaise, and weight loss may occur in about one-third of patients with sarcoidosis. Fever is generally low grade but temperature elevations of 39 to 40°C may be seen. Weight loss is usually limited to 2 to 6 kg during the 10 to 12 weeks before presentation. Fatigue, when present, can be quite disabling. Occasionally, night sweats may occur. The constitutional symptoms are more frequent in African-Americans and Asian Indians than in white individuals and in Asian patients. Sarcoidosis is an important and frequently overlooked cause of fever of unknown origin (FUO).[269] The GLUS syndrome (Granulomatous lesions of unknown significance) has some of the features of sarcoidosis, including fever and hepatosplenomegaly.[270]

Intrathoracic Sarcoidosis

Respiratory symptoms or abnormal chest radiographs are the most common manifestation of sarcoidosis. The lungs are affected in more than 90 percent of patients with sarcoidosis. Dyspnea, dry cough, and chest pain occur in one-third to one-half of all patients. Although retrosternal in location, chest pain is usually no more than a vague tightness of the thorax, but can occasionally be severe and indistinguishable from cardiac pain.[271] Hemoptysis is rare. Clubbing rarely occurs and lung crackles are present in fewer than 20 percent of patients. Cough, dyspnea, chest pain, and nasal complaints may herald the onset of the disease and these symptoms are noted in 30 to 50 percent of most studies. Although the precise pathogenesis is not clear, clinical evidence suggests that lung is the first site of involvement. Then the process extends into the hilar and mediastinal nodes by lymphatics. Dyspnea is the most common respiratory symptom and is present in about one-third of the newly detected cases. In contrast, some patients may be completely asymptomatic in spite of marked radiological changes. Intrathoracic disease may be classified into several stages as follows:

Stage*	Finding
0	Normal chest radiograph
I	Bilateral hilar lymphadenopathy (BHL)
II	BHL plus pulmonary infiltrations
III	Pulmonary infiltrations (without BHL)
IV	Pulmonary fibrosis

*Classification is based on the posteroanterior chest radiogram only. Sometimes a CT scan or ⁶⁷Ga lung scan gives information suggesting a different stage. The staging of these patients is presently an open question, but at the moment it is not necessary to change the staging criteria because a CT or ⁶⁷Ga scan is indicated in a limited number of patients.

Stage 0 In this stage the chest radiograph is normal and only extrapulmonary disease is apparent, although histologically the lungs and the mediastinum may be involved. About 5 to 10 percent of patients with sarcoidosis will have a normal chest X-ray at the time of initial presentation.

Stage I Sarcoidosis is characterized by bilateral symmetrical hilar lymphadenopathy with or without enlargement of the paratracheal glands. This is the earliest clinically detectable form of the disease and the most common mode of presentation of sarcoidosis (40-60%). Although the parenchyma of the lung appears to be clear radiologically, there may be histological changes. The inferior group of right paratracheal nodes is commonly affected. Patients in this stage have minimal or no symptoms unless there is associated erythema nodosum. Mild cough and minimal substernal discomfort are the usual respiratory symptoms. The extrathoracic organs are involved in about 10 percent of cases with this stage. Noncaseating granuloma of the liver, or scalene lymph nodes is present in about 75 percent of the patients. Majority of the patients with this stage show clearance of their disease spontaneously within about 1 to 2 years. About 10 to 15 percent progress to stage II.

Stage II In this stage pulmonary opacity is associated with hilar lymphadenopathy and is present in about 25 to 35 percent of the patients. The opacities may be localized or unilateral, but more often diffuse and symmetrical. Fine or coarse reticular shadows are recognized. Miliary lesions are also commonly seen. The nodulations may be coarse and well defined, or fluffy, ill-defined cotton-wool patches known as alveolar sarcoidosis may develop. A combination of all these changes are also noted clinical features in this stages may be nil or low-grade fever, cough, malaise, weight loss, or tachypnea, particularly with miliary infiltrations. When there is extensive pulmonary involvement with fibrosis, dyspnea is a prominent symptom. Radiological resolution occurs. In about one-half to two-thirds of the patients. Irreversible pulmonary fibrosis may be present in some of the patients (15-20%). Hilar and mediastinal lymph nodes may undergo egg shell calcification.

Clearing of intrathoracic lymph nodes with persistent or progression of the parenchymal infiltrations characterizes stage III Sarcoidosis. The absence of lymph nodes on chest X-ray may however be detected on CT scan, and other imaging techniques in bout 5 to 15 percent of the patients in this stage. The changes are usually bilateral and more prominent in the mid-lung fields. Dense fibrosis, loss of lung volume, honeycombing, and bulla formation, pulmonary hypertension, right ventricular enlargement and fungal balls in the cavities may be the other changes. Pneumothorax is another complication in this group of patients. Some designate patients with diffuse fibrosis, as stage IV or IIIB disease.

Clinical features in this late stage of the disease are mainly dominated by dyspnea accompanied by dry cough. Extrathoracic manifestations like skin and ocular features accompany stage III disease more often than other stages.

Stage IV consists of advanced fibrosis with evidence of honeycombing, hilar retraction, bullae, cysts, and emphysema. Transition from stage I to III is usual, but a reversal from stage III to stage II and I is usual. If hilar lymphadenopathy is seen in a case of stage III sarcoidosis, another etiology for the lymph node enlargement should be sought.

The extrathoracic manifestations of sarcoidosis are summarized in the Table below.

System	Manifestations
Upper respiratory tract involvement	Nasal mucosal changes, epistaxis, bleeding, ulceration, perforation, stuffiness, crusting. Laryngeal involvement less than 1 percent. Commonly associated with lupus pernio.
Endobronchial involvement	Pathologic evidence of involvement not infrequent. Frequency of such involvement in 30 to 100 percent of cases. Although parenchymal lung disease is more common, the airways (larynx, trachea, and bronchi) may also be involved, leading to airway obstruction and bronchiectasis. Airway hyperactivity has been reported in up to 20 percent of patients.[272]
Pleura	Unusual. Histological changes in a few. Other uncommon manifestations include pleural effusion, chylothorax, pneumothorax, pleural thickening and calcification, lymph node calcification, and cavity formation.[273]
Skin	Transient or chronic. Erythema nodosum (EN) commonest and more frequent in Europeans; and in women; mostly in stage I disease. Plaques and nodules (lupus pernio). Subcutaneous nodules. Infiltration of old scars. Psoriasiform cutaneous sarcoidosis.
Ocular	Occur in about 25 percent of patients. Common in blacks and if slit lamp examination is done routinely. Uveal tract is most commonly affected, although any part may be involved. May appear first. Bilateral subacute or chronic anterior uveitis with iridocyditis commonest followed by conjunctival involvement. May be associated with *Heerfordt s syndrome* or uveoparotid fever; with parotid gland enlargement, with cranial nerve palsy, and systemic symptoms). "Mutton fat" keratitic precipitates seen in anterior chamber. Others include choroidoretinitis, phlyctenular conjunctivitis, follicles and nodules in conjunctiva, keratoconjunctivitis sicca, periphlebitis retinae with retinal hemorrhage, and retinitis proliferans, painless enlargement of lacrimal glands.
Bones and joints	Incidence 1-13 percent. Osteoporosis, cortical thinning, cysts, common in phalanges, metacarpals and metatarsals. Arthralgia or arthritis with EN. Larger joints are affected. Migratory polyarthralgia/polyarthritis may be seen.
Skeletal muscles	Rare. Nodules and tenderness, chronic myopathy, wasting and weakness may be seen.

Contd...

Contd...

System	Manifestations
Central nervous system	Incidence 1 to 5 percent. Both central and peripheral system affected. Encephalopathy, meningitis, space-occupying lesions, seizures, arid involvement of any part of brain, cranial nerve palsies (facial nerve commonest, II, IX, X, VIII, XI, XII, in order of frequency); Mono- or polyneuropathy.
Heart	Clinically 5 percent, autopsy 20 percent. Cor pulmonale, granulomas in left ventricle, ventricular septum, right ventricle, papillary muscles, and atria. Common in older people. Arrhythmias (ventricular), ST and T wave changes. A-V blocks, complete bundle branch block, sudden death, congestive heart failure, angina pectoris, papillary muscle dysfunction, ventricular aneurysm, pericardia! effusion, and cardiomegaly.
Lymph nodes	Peripheral lymphadenopathy common. Cervical nodes followed by epitrochlear, axillary, and retroperitoneal nodes are also involved.
Hepatic	Clinically may not be apparent. More common in stage II and III disease, and less often in fibrotic stage of the disease. Liver enlargement in less than 20 percent. Biochemically normal except alkaline phosphatase which may be raised. The clinical spectrum may include normal liver, portal fibrosis, obliteration of hepatic venous bed, portal fibrosis, and cholestasis with or without biliary cirrhosis.
Spleen	Splenomegaly is observed in 5 to 20 percent. Pathological involvement in more than 50 percent of cases.
Genitourinary system	Granulomas rare. Most common is nephrocalcinosis due to hypercalcemia (2%) and hypercalciuria. Involvement very rare.
Lymphoid system.	About one-third of patients with sarcoidosis have palpable peripheral lymph glands. The most frequently involved glands are cervical, axillary, epitrochlear, and inguinal. In the neck, the posterior triangle nodes are more commonly affected than the nodes in the anterior triangle. Enlarged glands are discrete, movable, and nontender. They do not ulcerate and do not form draining sinuses. Splenic enlargement is usually minimal and silent, but it may cause pressure symptoms, anemia, leukopenia, and thrombocytopenia.[274]

Heart. Clinical evidence of myocardial involvement is present in about 5 percent of patients with sarcoidosis.[275] However, the autopsy incidence may be higher. The course of the disease is variable and ranges from benign arrhythmias or high-degree heart block to sudden death. An electrocardiogram (ECG) may be negative, while 24 hr. Holter monitoring reveals ventricular tachycardia, heart block, or ventricular ectopic beats. A Doppler echocardiogram can detect diastolic dysfunction but thallium-201 imaging is superior for showing segmental contraction abnormalities.[275] Myocardial imaging with thallium-201 may also reveal segmental defects that correspond either to a granulomatous disease or a fibrous scar. The clinical significance of abnormal thallium scans in patients with asymptomatic sarcoidosis is not known. Long-term studies suggest that the risk of cardiac dysfunction or sudden death in these patients is low.[276] Coronary angiography is needed to exclude the possibility of coronary artery disease if the thallium-201 imaging suggests cardiac involvement. Endomyocardial biopsy showing granulomas does confirm the diagnosis of cardiac sarcoidosis, but the diagnostic yield from the procedure is low because of the inhomogeneous distribution of the granulomatous process. Thus, sarcoid patients with cardiac dysfunction, ECG abnormalities, or thallium-201 imaging defects should be presumed to have cardiac sarcoidosis even when endomyocardial biopsy specimens show no granuloma.

Liver. Although granulomas are found in as many as 50 to 80 percent of liver biopsy specimens, the liver is palpable in less than 20 percent of patients.[277,278] Hepatic involvement rarely causes portal hypertension, hepatic failure, or increased mortality related to liver dysfunction. Abnormalities of liver function tests are common.[279,280] Asymptomatic patients with only hepatic sarcoidosis and mild liver function abnormalities do not require treatment. Corticosteroids may improve severe liver dysfunction.[278,281,282]

Skin. Cutaneous involvement occurs in about 25 percent of all patients.[283] Two clinically important and easily recognizable skin lesions are erythema nodosum and lupus pernio. Erythema nodosum, the hallmark of acute sarcoidosis, is commonly seen in European, Puerto Rican, and Mexican patients, particularly in women of childbearing age. It is rare in Japanese and African-American patients. The lesion consists of raised, red, tender bumps or nodules on the anterior aspects of the legs. Granulomas are not characteristic of these biopsy specimens. Adjacent joints are usually swollen and painful. Erythema nodosum usually remits within 6 to 8 wk. Recurrent episodes of erythema nodosum are rare.[284] Löfgren's syndrome consists of fever, bilateral hilar adenopathy, erythema nodosum, and arthralgia.[285] Lupus pernio represents chronic sarcoidosis and consists of

indurated plaques associated with discoloration of the nose, cheeks, lips, and ears. The lesion is more common in African-American women. The nasal mucosa is frequently involved. Lupus pernio is often associated with bone cysts and pulmonary fibrosis. The course of the disease with lupus pernio is prolonged; spontaneous remissions are rare. Other skin lesions in chronic sarcoidosis include plaques, maculopapular eruptions, subcutaneous nodules, changes in old scars, alopecia, and hypo- and hyperpigmented areas. As a rule, chronic sarcoidosis skin lesions do not cause pain or itch, nor do they ulcerate (Figs 24.4 and 24.5).

Ocular lesions. Ocular involvement may occur in 11 to 83 percent of patients with sarcoidosis.[279] Any part of the eye or orbit may be affected; uveitis is the most common

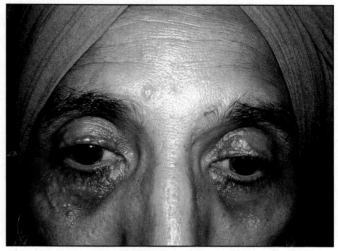

FIGURE 24.4

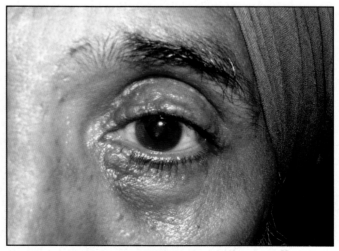

FIGURE 24.5

FIGURES 24.4 AND 24.5: Sarcoidosis of skin

of all sarcoid eye lesions. Acute anterior uveitis clears spontaneously or after local therapy with corticosteroids (eye drops); chronic uveitis may lead to adhesions between the iris and the lens, causing glaucoma, cataract, and blindness. Fluorescence angiography is a sensitive test of microvascular involvement and should be considered if posterior uveitis is suspected.[286] Other eye lesions include conjunctival follicles, lacrimal gland enlargement, keratoconjunctivitis sicca, dacryocystitis, and retinal vasculitis.

Neurosarcoidosis. Clinically recognizable involvement of the nervous system occurs in less than 10 percent of patients with sarcoidosis.[287,288] The disease has a predilection for the base of the brain. Cranial nerve involvement, particularly facial palsies and hypothalamic and pituitary lesions, are common. These lesions tend to occur early and respond favorably to treatment.[289] Space-occupying masses, peripheral neuropathy, and neuromuscular involvement occur later and portend a chronic course. Serum angiotensin-converting enzyme levels are of limited value. Both computed tomography (CT) and magnetic resonance imaging (MRI) have been used to support the diagnosis of neurosarcoidosis. Gadolinium-enhanced MRI is the preferred test for evaluating brain parenchyma, meninges, and spinal cord. MRI manifestations are, however, nonspecific.[290] Whenever possible, an effort should be made to secure histological confirmation. Cerebrospinal fluid (CSF) reveals lymphocytosis and elevated proteins in about 80 percent of the patients. Other CSF features of neurosarcoidosis include elevated ACE (about half of patients), lysozyme, and β_2-macroglobulins, and an increased CD4/CD8 ratio.[279] CSF analysis is also important in excluding tuberculosis and fungal infections.

Musculoskeletal system. While joint pains occur in 25 to 39 percent of patients with sarcoidosis, deforming arthritis is rare.[273] The joints most commonly affected are knees, ankles, elbows, wrists, and small joints of the hands and feet. The articular involvement may be acute and transient or chronic and persistent. Symptomatic muscle involvement is rare. Chronic myopathy occurs more commonly in women and may be the sole presentation of the disease. Corticosteroid-induced myopathy should be excluded. Proximal muscle weakness, a common clinical manifestation, must be distinguished from corticosteroid-induced myopathy. Appropriate synovial or muscle biopsy specimens may reveal non-caseating granulomas.[291] Bone cysts occur only in association with chronic skin lesions.[283]

Gastrointestinal tract. The incidence of gastrointestinal (GI) tract involvement is less than 1.0 percent. The stomach is the most commonly involved part of the GI tract. Esophagus, appendix, rectum, and pancreas are involved less frequently. Sarcoidosis may mimic Crohn's disease, tuberculosis, fungal infection, or pancreatic neoplasm.[292,293]

Hematological abnormalities. Hematologic abnormalities, particularly those involving the red and white cell lines, are frequent but not diagnostic. Anemia (hemoglobin of less than 11 g/dL) occurs in 4 to 20 percent of patients with sarcoidosis. Hemolytic anemia is rare. Leukopenia occurs in as many as 40 percent of patients but is rarely severe.[280] In the absence of splenomegaly, leukopenia may reflect bone marrow involvement, however, the most common mechanism is a redistribution of blood T cells to sites of disease.[277,294] Leukemoid reaction, eosinophilia, and thrombocytopenia are rare.

Parotid glands. The combination of fever, parotid enlargement, facial palsy, and anterior uveitis is called Heerfordt's syndrome. Unilateral or bilateral parotitis with swollen, painful enlargement of the gland occurs in less than 6 percent of patients. In about 40 percent of the patients, parotid enlargement is self-limiting.

Endocrine manifestation. Hypercalcemia occurs in about 2 to 10 percent of patients with sarcoidosis; hypercalciuria is about three times more frequent.[295,296] These abnormalities are due to dysregulated production of 1,25-(OH)$_2$-D$_3$ (calcitriol) by activated macrophages and granulomas.[295,296] Undetected, persistent hypercalcemia and hypercalciuria can cause nephrocalcinosis, renal stones, and renal failure.[297] Diabetes insipidus may occur owing to pituitary or hypothalamic involvement. Hypothyroidism, hyperthyroidism, hypothermia, adrenal suppression, and anterior pituitary involvement are rare.[298]

Reproductive organs. Asymptomatic granulomas may occur in any part of the female reproductive system, including the breast. The uterus is the organ most commonly affected. The male reproductive tract is rarely affected. However, because of concerns about possible testicular malignancy, one-third of male patients with this type of involvement may receive unnecessary orchiectomies.[299]

The kidneys. Rarely, the granulomatous process may produce interstitial nephritis by directly involving the kidneys. More commonly, renal failure is related to hypercalcemia and nephrocalcinosis. Renal sarcoidosis may mimic a tumor.[300,301]

Special Situations

Sarcoidosis in children. Kendig reviewed 104 cases in which the patients were 15 yr of age or younger and found that the distribution of organs involved in children was similar to that in adults.[302] The diagnosis of sarcoidosis should be considered in a child of any age who experiences a skin rash, uveitis, lymphadenopathy, and pulmonary involvement. The prognosis for children is more favorable than for adults.[303]

Sarcoidosis in pregnancy. Sarcoidosis does not affect pregnancy adversely, but the disease may worsen after parturition; therefore, a chest roentgenogram should be obtained within 6 months of delivery. The incidence of spontaneous abortion, miscarriage, and congenital fetal abnormalities for patients with sarcoidosis is no different from that found in mothers without sarcoidosis.[304,305]

Sarcoidosis in the elderly. Although many patients with sarcoidosis live with the disease through their later years, only a few patients develop it after the age of 65 years. In managing the disease in the aged, it is important to appreciate that a malignant disease of the lung, stomach, intestine, and even uterus may give rise to a granulomatous reaction in the draining lymph nodes. This local sarcoid reaction must be distinguished from multisystem sarcoidosis.[306,307]

COURSE AND PROGNOSIS

The disease can be arbitrarily divided into a subacute and a chronic phase, when the duration is less than and more than two years respectively. Subacute sarcoidosis develops in patients below 30 years of age and they are often asymptomatic with the disease being detected accidentally by chest radiography. Erythema nodosum may be the initiating feature with uveitis, peripheral lymphadenopathy or parotid enlargement. Kveim test is usually positive with noncaseating granulomas being present in many organ systems. The prognosis is usually good with spontaneous resolution.

Chronic sarcoidosis has an insidious onset with the patient being usually over 30. Parenchymal lesions are often present. In contrast to the subacute phase, skin lesions, and chronic ocular findings are more common. Manifestations pertaining to other systems may rarely be present. The Kveim test is usually negative at this stage except when mediastinal lymphadenopathy is present. Spontaneous remission is unlikely and the prognosis is unfavorable because of progressive fibrosis with striking functional derangements in the affected organs. The subacute phase might not have been noticed.

INVESTIGATIONS

The joint statement of the American Thoracic Society (ATS), the European Respiratory Society (ERS) and the World Association of Sarcoidosis and Other Granulomatous Disorders (WASOG) recommends the following investigations.[1]

1. History (occupational and environmental exposure, symptoms)
2. Physical examination
3. Posteroanterior chest radiography
4. Pulmonary function tests: spirometry and DL_{CO}
5. Peripheral blood counts: White blood cells, red blood cells, platelets
6. Serum chemistries: calcium, liver enzymes (alanine aminotransferase, aspartate aminotransferase, alkaline phosphatase), creatinine, blood urea nitrogen
7. Urine analysis
8. ECG
9. Routine ophthalmologic examination
10. Tuberculin skin test.

Radiology

Radiological changes and stages of pulmonary sarcoidosis have been discussed earlier. The most common mediastinal glands involved are hilar (97%), nodes in the aortopulmonary window (76%), right paratracheal (71%), anterior mediastinal nodes (16%), and posterior mediastinal glands in 2 percent of cases. Various parenchymal lesions including fibrosis have also been described in clinical manifestations.[308-312]

Other Chest Imaging Techniques

In the evaluation of sarcoidosis, CT provides a detailed pictorial display of the lymph nodes including those not routinely detected by chest X-rays. However, in the routine management of a patient, CT is not necessary. The investigations may be of help in guiding a fine needle aspiration biopsy, to detect bronchiectasis or bullae with air fluid levels suggesting infections, and the evaluation of obstruction of vital structures like superior vena cava.[313,314]

MRI may be of help in outlining the mediastinal structures including the soft tissues and blood vessels. However, like CT, this investigation is not required for routine management of patients.[315]

Pulmonary Function Tests

Reduction of lung volumes can be detected in 20 percent of the patients with stage I disease, and in about

70 percent of cases with stage II or III disease. A restrictive ventilatory type of defect with reduced forced vital capacity and total lung capacity to a greater extent than residual volume and functional residual capacity is characteristically seen in sarcoidosis as with other interstitial fibrosis. The reduced lung volumes are due to a decrease in static lung compliance. The diffusing capacity for carbon monoxide ($D_L CO$) is common, which may precede lung volume changes. In stage I disease, the reduction is related to a decreased D_M (membrane conductance), whereas in more advanced cases the reduction is due to a decreased Q_c (capillary blood volume).

Obstructive ventilatory defects have recently been recognized in sarcoidosis. In earlier stages, (stage I), there is an increased bronchial hyperreactivity. This may be due to inflammatory granulomatous bronchial involvement. These changes are recognized on bronchoscopy as "cobblestone appearance" and lymphocytosis on bronchoalveolar lavage much more commonly obstructive defects are observed in patients with more advanced stage III disease. The causes of such defects at this stage probably include bronchial distortion due to fibrosis, and endobronchial inflammation resulting in peribronchial or peribronchial fibrosis. In extreme cases, bronchial compression due to lymph nodes may produce obstruction in earlier stages. Laryngeal involvement may cause upper airway obstruction.[316-319]

DIAGNOSIS

Since clinical features and pathological changes in sarcoidosis are similar to many other diseases, it is important to have a reasonably confirmed diagnosis. This is particularly important to exclude other serious causes. A careful clinical history and examination and laboratory studies should be performed. These include radiographic and pulmonary physiologic studies, as well as a review of the previous chest X-ray if available. Since it is a multisystemic disease, it is important to search for sites of involvement in the extrapulmonary organs. Thus routine studies of blood biochemistry, urine, and electrocardiogram should be done. Examination of the eyes with slit-lamp should be done routinely in all suspected cases of sarcoidosis.

The diagnosis of sarcoidosis needs a compatible clinical picture, histologic demonstration of noncaseating granulomas, and exclusion of other diseases capable of producing a similar histologic or clinical picture. The presence of noncaseating granulomas in a single organ such as skin does not establish a diagnosis of sarcoidosis. The diagnostic work-up for patients with sarcoidosis

should attempt to accomplish four goals: (*a*) provide histologic confirmation of the disease, (*b*) assess the extent and severity of organ involvement, (*c*) assess whether the disease is stable or is likely to progress, and (*d*) determine if therapy will benefit the patient.

Biopsy

In the presence of a compatible clinical picture, the first step is to choose the site for a proper biopsy. Transbronchial lung biopsy (TLB) is the recommended procedure in most cases. Its diagnostic yield depends largely on the experience of the operator, ranging from 40 percent to more than 90 percent when four to five lung biopsies are carried out.[320] The risk of the procedure in experienced hands is low.

A careful examination of the patient may disclose other possible sites for biopsy, such as skin, lip, or superficial lymph nodes. A granulomatous scar (a fresh granulomatous reaction on the site of an old scar) may be a very useful site for biopsy. It is not useful to biopsy erythema nodosum lesions because they will not show granulomas. Liver biopsy is rarely indicated, even if there is biochemical or clinical evidence of liver involvement. The use of scalene biopsy also is no longer recommended. In some instances, ^{67}Ga scans may indicate a site for biopsy.[321-323]

When bronchial or transbronchial biopsies are nondiagnostic, and no other accessible sites for biopsy are identified, surgical lung biopsy may be indicated, if there are readily identified abnormalities on the chest roentgenogram or lung CT scan. The finding of mediastinal adenopathy on the conventional CT scan should prompt biopsy by mediastinoscopy before video-assisted thoracoscopic lung biopsy (VTLB) or open lung biopsy.[324,325] The diagnostic yield of all of these procedures is reported to be more than 90 percent. The complication rate and hospital stay of patients undergoing mediastinoscopy are significantly lower than for patients undergoing surgical lung biopsy. VTLB has the advantage of permitting biopsy of both lung and lymph nodes.

The Patient without Histology

Some patients refuse biopsy and in others the pulmonary impairment is too severe for a lung biopsy. Clinical and/or radiological features alone may be diagnostic for patients with stage I (reliability of 98%) or Stage II (89%) disease, but are less accurate for patients with Stage III (52%) or Stage 0 (23%) disease.[326] A patient who presents with a classic Löfgren's syndrome of fever, erythema nodosum, arthralgias, and bilateral hilar lymphadenopathy may not require biopsy proof if resolution of disease is rapid and spontaneous. In some instances, bronchoalveolar lavage (BAL) and studies on lymphocyte subpopulations are helpful. According to Costabel, a CD4/CD8 ratio greater than 3.5 has a sensitivity of 53 percent, a specificity of 94 percent, a positive predictive value of 76 percent, and a negative predictive value of 85 percent.[327,328] In other words, a CD4/CD8 ratio > 3.5 provides a diagnosis of sarcoidosis with a specificity of 94 percent even if the TLB has not been diagnostic. Bronchial muscosal biopsy may be performed during the same procedure; it is positive for noncaseating granulomata in 41 to 57 percent of patients with sarcoidosis.[329] The appearance of a Panda pattern combined with a Lambda pattern on a total body ^{67}Ga scan may support the diagnosis of sarcoidosis and obviate the need for invasive diagnostic procedures.[330] However, these findings are present in only a small number of patients.[321] In selected centers, the Kveim-Siltzbach test may be available and helpful for diagnosis.[331] It may still be indicated when the chest X-ray and CT scan are normal in cases of uveitis of unknown origin, hypercalciuria, hepatic granulomatous disease, suspected neurosarcoidosis, or recurrent erythema nodosum.[332] Transmission of infective agents is possible by this procedure, if the antigen is poorly prepared or controlled. A mildly elevated angiotensin-converting enzyme is never diagnostic because elevations may be seen in many diseases.[333] Elevations greater than two times the upper limits of normal are much less common in other diseases but, unfortunately, can occasionally be seen in other granulomatous diseases, such as tuberculosis, Gaucher's disease, and hyperthyroidism.

Findings of Further Investigations

Once history and clinical and radiological features establish the diagnosis, an additional work-up is recommended for all patients. Pulmonary function tests are important to measure initial lung impairment and to provide a baseline to assess improvement or deterioration of the lung disease. Therefore, like the history, physical examination, and chest roentgenograph, they are indicated for all patients. Aberrations in lung function tests are found in only 20 percent of patients with stage I disease, compared with 40 to 70 percent of patients with stage II, III, or IV disease. The most common parameters indicating functional impairment are the diffusion capacity and the vital capacity.[334] Both restrictive and obstructive pulmonary function abnormalities may be found. Other tests that should be routinely performed on all patients are indicated above.

For some patients, lung CT scans are indicated. The usual indications for lung CT scans are as follows: (i) atypical clinical and/or chest radiograph findings, (ii) detection of complications of the lung disease, such as bronchiectasis, aspergilloma, pulmonary fibrosis, traction emphysema, or a superimposed infection or malignancy, and (iii) a normal chest radiograph but a clinical suspicion of the disease. In most patients, the classic findings of the disease on lung CT scans are as follows:[335] (i) widespread small nodules with a bronchovascular and subpleural distribution, (*ii*) thickened interlobular septae, (iii) architectural distortion, and (iv) conglomerate masses. Less common findings are: (a) honeycombing, (b) cyst formation and bronchiectasis, and (c) alveolar consolidation.

Extrapulmonary sarcoidosis should be studied with appropriate tests like Holter monitoring, echocardiography and thallium scans to detect myocardial involvement, and MRI or head CT scans to detect CNS involvement.

Clinical activity is assessed on the basis of onset, worsening, or persistence of symptoms or signs directly related to sarcoidosis. A long list of markers of activity has been suggested as potential diagnostic aids or indices of "activation".[336,337] Some of these markers are consistent with the ability of the disease to progress in one organ, but they often do not detect progression in other organs. Some commonly used markers of activity are shown in Table 24.2.

An attempt should be made in all cases to obtain a histological diagnosis to look for noncaseating granulomas. The number of sites of biopsy will depend upon the clinical situation. More is the number of sites of biopsies, better and greater are the chances of certainty of the diagnosis. A single positive biopsy, however, is enough for most clinical purposes. Any enlarged lymph node, old scar tissues, conjunctival tissue, liver, or biopsy from a skin lesion are usually sufficient for histological diagnosis. Transbronchial lung biopsy through the bronchoscope is positive in most cases with involvement of lung parenchyma. Although in countries with less frequent tuberculosis, a chest X-ray with bilateral hilar lymphadenopathy may be characteristic of sarcoidosis, and a histological proof may not be necessary, in countries with high prevalence of tuberculosis, this "no biopsy approach" may not be appropriate and acceptable.

Since the histological changes are nonspecific in sarcoidosis and such findings are also possible with many other conditions including tuberculosis, fungal infection, hypersensitivity pneumonitis, granulomatous

	TABLE 24.2: Markers of activity[364]	
Clinical	Biochemical or instrumental	Imaging
Fever	Serum ACE	Progressive changes on chest radiographs or lung, CT scans
Uveitis	Hypercalcemia	Ground-glass attenuation on HRCT scan
Erythema nodosum	Positive ^{67}Ga uptake	
Lupus pernio	Worsening lung function	Fluorescein angiography of the eyes
Changing scar	BAL fluid: lymphocyte alveolitis and high CD4/CD8 ratio	Brain MRI or CT scan
Polyarthralgia	Bone cysts	
Splenomegaly		
Lymphadenopathy	Abnormal ECG, echocardiogram, or thallium scan	
Salivary and lacrimal gland enlargement	Abnormal liver function tests	
Myocardial disease Facial palsy or other neurological symptoms or signs		
Progressive respiratory symptoms (dyspnea or cough)		

Definition of abbreviations: ACE = angiotensin-converting enzyme; CT = computed tomography; HRCT = high-resolution CT; MRI = magnetic resonance imaging

vasculitides, lymphomatoid granulomatosis, and berylliosis, these should be excluded with appropriate skin and serologic tests, cultures, and special stains.

Fiberoptic Bronchoscopy

In most of the cases fiberoptic bronchoscopy and transbronchial biopsy are the preferred procedures to obtain tissue for histological examination. In stage I disease, the accuracy may be increased by transbronchial or transtracheal needle aspiration of the lymph nodes. In addition the bronchial biopsy itself may be helpful since the mucosa may show granulomas frequently. The positivity is more if the biopsy is taken from an abnormal-looking area. Bronchoalveolar lavage can be done simultaneously to assess the activity of the disease (see below[338-352]):

Other Biopsy Procedures

Mediastinoscopy and open lung biopsy are rarely necessary to diagnose pulmonary sarcoidosis: Blind biopsy of other sites are now rarely required after the availability of fiberoptic bronchoscope and trans-bronchial biopsy.

Kveim-Siltzbach Test

Although a variety of test materials are used for the purpose by various investigators, the most potent test materials are those prepared from sarcoidal spleen or lymph nodes. Although used over the past 50 years, its role, as, a diagnostic test remains controversial. While some reports show the test to be sensitive and specific, others demonstrate that it is nonspecific and insensitive. Most often the poor results are attributed to the use of unreliable test material, unfortunately one such reliable preparation is not available widely. The drawbacks of the test are the 4 to 6 weeks necessary for maturation of the nodule, the need for a biopsy, insufficient number of test materials, and the problems in the histological inter-pretation of the test. Another drawback is the need to defer steroid therapy till the test is complete.[353-363]

The effective principle in the test material is parti-culate and is located intracellularly. The reaction is difficult to classify into none of the conventional types I to IV immunological reactions. There is little correlation between the intensity of granulomatous involvement of the tissue extracted and its granuloma inducing potency. The frequency of positive Kveim test is highest in patients with erythema nodosum, cutaneous sarcoidosis, and stage I disease. Apart from this, the test does not give any particular prognostic information. With the advent of transbronchial biopsies, one gets a quick and better result than that from the Kveim test.

Mantoux Test

This test is negative in most patients of sarcoidosis with a high predictive value.

Assessment of Activity of Sarcoidosis

Assessment of activity of sarcoidosis is important to distinguish active inflammation from inactive fibrosis or hyalinization to help in deciding the institution of steroid therapy. Moreover, the intensity of inflammation is an important determinant for progression of the disease to the stage of fibrosis. Several different approaches have been tried to assess this activity, and they include bronchoalveolar lavage, gallium scanning, and measurement of angiotensin converting enzyme activity.[1]

Presence of lymphocytosis in bronchoalveolar lavage and a count of more than 28 percent of T lymphocytes were considered to be the predictors for responsiveness to therapy and deterioration in the lung function respectively, although all investigators do not confirm these observations.

Gallium-67, a radionuclide is detected very little in the normal lung after intravenous injection. However, in diseased lungs, as in sarcoidosis, gallium accumulates in areas of active granulomatous inflammation due to their uptake by activated macrophages. Thus, after 48 hours after intravenous injection of gallium, the radionuclide is frequently detected over the lungs, mediastinal lymph nodes, lacrimal and parotid glands. The intensity of uptake in the lungs is then graded on a scale of 0 to 4. Prognostic 'value of the scan in pulmonary sarcoidosis, has shown that normal scans (grade 0) are associated with stability of lung function. However, the correlation is poor with stage II disease and I. Another disadvantage of the test is that the uptake is nonspecific. Such abnormal scans are also possible with any other inflammation in the lungs.

Angiotensin-converting enzyme is a halide-activated exopeptidase that catalyzes the conversion of angiotensin I to angiotensin II. Normally, the highest levels are found in the pulmonary vascular endothelium. Epithelioid cells in sarcoid granuloma secrete this enzyme and the elevation in the serum concentrations of angiotensin-converting enzyme occurs in about 70 percent of the patients. However, elevations also occur in other disease states like miliary tuberculosis, atypical mycobacterial disease, silicosis, asbestosis, histoplasmosis, and other conditions simulating sarcoidosis. Many believe that the magnitude of elevation of the enzyme reflect the granuloma load in sarcoidosis. The levels show decline with either a spontaneous remission or with steroid therapy. Thus, it may be a useful marker for monitoring the effect of therapy.

Various markers of activity are shown in Table 24.2.

TREATMENT

Although vast majority of patients with newly diagnosed sarcoidosis remit spontaneously, and prediction of progression to fibrosis is difficult, it is clear that the administration of corticosteroids usually produce at least short-term improvement in symptoms, chest X-ray, lung functions and dyspnea. The indications of corticosteroid therapy are:[365-380]

1. Vital impairment in liver, heart, kidneys, central nervous system, and eyes.
2. Radiographic stage II or III disease with dyspnea severe enough to incapacitate the patient or alter the life-style of the patient.
3. Active disease (see earlier discussion).

Those with radiographic stage I disease without dyspnea need no steroid therapy. The most controversial group are those in stage II and III radiographic disease but without dyspnea. Some believe that presence of radiographic abnormalities is enough indication for such therapy even in the absence of symptoms. Others recommend watching these patients and treating only when there is worsening and development of symptoms, progression of radiological findings, or deterioration of lung function test results.

A suggested protocol for prednisolone therapy is to begin therapy with 40 mg daily. After 2 weeks, the daily dose is to be reduced by 5 mg at 2 week intervals. If no objective improvement occurs after 6 to 8 weeks, therapy should be discontinued. If improvement has occurred, prednisolone therapy is continued for 6 to 8 months in a dose of 15 mg daily. Then the drug is to be tapered by 2.5 mg decrements each month. If relapse occurs, the dosage is to be increased to the previously documented satisfactory level. High dose pulse therapy with methyl prednisolone of 30 mg/kg intravenously once a week has not been shown to be more beneficial than the standard oral therapy. Alternate-day treatment may be equally effective although initial responses tend to occur more slowly.

Oral (OCS) or inhaled steroids (ICS) are widely used in its treatment, but there is no consensus about when and in whom therapy should be initiated, what dose should be given and for how long. Corticosteroids given for several months have deleterious side effects so it is important to know whether they have any maintained benefit in pulmonary sarcoidosis. A recent Cochrane review using *MEDLINE, EMBASE* and *CENTRAL* searched. Twelve randomized control trials of variable quality involving 1051 participants who met the inclusion criteria of the review. The oral steroid dose was equivalent to prednisolone 4 to 40 mg/day. With oral corticosteroid there was an improvement in chest X-ray over 3 to 24 months (Relative Risk (RR): 1.46 [1.01 to 2.09], 3 studies), but the authors concluded that this finding requires cautious interpretation. No other significant differences were identified on secondary outcomes. For the role of inhaled corticosteroids data were inadequate to perform meaningful analysis of data on chest X-ray. Two studies showed no improvement in lung function, In one study there was an improvement in diffusing capacity in the treated group. There were no data on side effects. In one study, symptoms improved at the end of six months of treatment. The authors concluded that oral steroids improved the chest X-ray and a global score of chest X-ray, symptoms and spirometry over 3 to 24 months. However, there is little evidence of an improvement in lung function. There are limited data beyond two years to indicate whether oral steroids have any modifying effect on long-term disease progression. Oral steroids may be of benefit for patients with Stage 2 and 3 diseases with moderate to severe or progressive symptoms or chest X-ray changes.[381]

Alternatives to corticosteroids for immunosuppression in sarcoidosis have been tried with chlorambucil, chloroquine, and methotrexate.[5,382-384] But there is no evidence that these agents, alone or in combination with prednisolone, are more effective than corticosteroids alone. Some of these commonly used alternative drugs are as follows:

Drugs	Dosages
Methotrexate	10-25 mg/week
Azathioprine	50-200 mg/d
Cyclophosphamide	50-150 mg/d orally
	or 500-2,000 mg
	or 500-2,000 mg
	every 2 weeks intravenously
Hydroxychloroquine	200-400 mg/d
Experimental/novel drugs[5]	

Drugs	Mechanism of action
Chlorambucil	Helpful in chronic fibrotic skin and lung lesions
Calcium chelating agents Effervescent phosphate Sodium cellulose phosphate	
Potassium	Softens fibrotic skin lesion
p-aminobenzoate, thalidomide, pentoxyphylline	Inhibitors of tumor necrosis factor
Cyclosporin	Prevents T cells producing cytokines (IL-2)
Tacrolimus, Sirolimus	Blocks intercellular signal transduction by IL-2 receptor
Mycophenolate	
Monoclonal antibodies OK3	T cell receptor blockade
Cytotoxic T lymphocyte	Block costimulatory signal CD28
Antigen-4-gene (CTLA-4)	Prevents graft vs host disease
Infliximab	Human mouse chimeric antitumor necrosis factor (TNF) antibody
Etanercept	Human protein of recombinant p 75 TNF receptors fused with Fc portion of human IgG1

Lung Transplantation

After COPD, sarcoidosis is the second most common condition for which lung transplantation may be a treatment option.[385] However, since most patients run a benign course and only about 10 to 20 percent sustain permanent sequelae, sarcoidosis patients constitute only 2.5 percent of all lung transplant recipients. Sarcoidosis is the fifth most common indication for lung transplantation but is likely to become the fourth leading indication as the need for transplantation in IPAH patients continues to decrease with the increase in effective medical therapies. In the guideline statement from 1998,[386-388] sarcoidosis was not among the diseases for which there were specific recommendations.

Since there is the chance in earlier stages of disease for spontaneous reversal, only those patients with stage IV sarcoidosis should be considered for transplantation. This stage is characterized by advanced fibrotic changes, honeycombing, hilar retraction, bullae, cysts, and emphysema. Needless to say, there is little chance for spontaneous remission at this stage.

There are many different factors that need to be accounted for when deciding to evaluate and list patients for lung transplantation. These decisions are best made by transplant pulmonologists who have a more intimate knowledge of local waiting times. When there is doubt about the severity of a patient's disease, it is prudent to err on the side of early referral. Even when patients are reticent about transplantation, it is always best to encourage them to be seen at a local transplant center where the necessary education can be provided, thus enabling a fully informed decision on the part of the patient.[389]

REFERENCES

1. American Thoracic Society. The European Respiratory Society. The World Association of Sarcoidosis and Other Granulomatous Disorders. Statement on sarcoidosis: Joint statement of the American Thoracic Society (ATS), the European Respiratory Society (ERS) and the World Association of Sarcoidosis and Other Granulomatous Disorders (WASOG) adopted by the ATS Board of Directors and by the ERS Executive Committee, February 1999. Am J Respir Crit Care Med 1999; 160,736-55.
2. Yamamoto M, Sharma OP, Hosoda Y. Special report: The 1991 descriptive definition of sarcoidosis. Sarcoidosis 1992;9:33-34.
3. Scadding JG, Mitchell DN. Definition. Sarcoidosis. Chapman and Hall. London, UK: 1985,36-42.
4. Mitchel DN, Scadding JG. Sarcoidosis. Am Rev Respir Dis 1974;110;774-802.
5. James DG. Sarcoidosis. Postgrad Med J 2001; 77:177-180.
6. Martin WJ 2nd, Iannuzzi MC, Gail DB, Peavy HH. Future directions in sarcoidosis research: Summary of an NHLBI working group. Am J Respir Crit Care Med 2004;170:567-71.
7. Sarcoidosis and other granulomatous diseases of the lung. In Fanburg BLP (Ed): Lung Biology in Health and Disease. Marcel Dekker: New York 1983;3.
8. James DG. Descriptive definition and historic aspects of sarcoidosis. Clin Chest Med 1997;18:663-79.
9. Hutchinson J. Case of livid papillary psoriasis. In illustrations of clinical surgery, J & A Churchill: London 1877;1:42-43.
10. Hutchinson J. On eruptions which occur in connection with gout: Case of Mortimer's malady. Arch Surg 1898;9:307-14.
11. Hosoda Y, Odaka M. History of sarcoidosis. Semin Respir Med 1992;13:359-67.
12. Boeck C. Multiple benign sarcoid of the skin. J Cutan Genitourinary Dis 1899;17:543-50.
13. Besnier M. Lupus pernio de la face: Synovitis funguses (scrofulo-tuberculoses) symetriques des extremities superieures. Ann Dermatol: Syphiligr 1899;10:33-36.
14. Tenneson M. Lupus pernio (Lupus pernio). Bull Soc Fr Dermatol Syphiligr 1892;3: 417-19.
15. Kreibich K. Ueber lupus pernio. Arch Derm Syph (Wien) 1904;71:13-16.
16. Jüngling O. Osteitis tuberculosa multiplex cystica. Fortschr Geb Roentgenstr 1920;27:375-83.
17. Heerfordt C. Ubereine Febris uveo-parotidea subchronica. Von Graefe's Arch Opthalmol 1909;70:254-73.
18. Kuznitsky E, Bittorf A. Sarcoid mit Beteiligung innerer Organe. Münch. Med Wochenschr 1915;1349-53.
19. Schaumann J. Etude sur le lupus pernio et ses rapports avec les sarcoides et la tuberculoses. Ann Dermatol Syphiligr 1916-1917;357-63.
20. Schaumann J. Etude anatomo pathologique et histologique sur les localizations viscerales de la lymphogranulomatoses benigne. Bull Soc Fr Dermatol Syphiligr 1934;1167-22.
21. Harrell G, Fisher S. Blood chemical changes in Boeck's sarcoid with particular reference to protein, calcium, and phosphatase values. J Clin Invest 1939;18:687-93.
22. Kveim A. En ny og spesifikk kutan-reaksjon ved Boecks sarcoid. Nord Med 1941;9:69-172.
23. Williams R, Nickerson D. Skin reactions in sarcoid. Proc Soc Exp Biol Med 1935;33:403-05.
24. Siltzbach L. The Kveim test in sarcoidosis: A study of 750 patients. JAMA 1961;178: 476-82.
25. Löfgren S. Erythema nodosum: Studies on etiology and pathogenesis in 185 adult cases. Acta Med Scand 1946;124:1-197.
26. Longscope W, Frieman D. A study of sarcoidosis based on a combined investigation of 160 cases including 30 autopies from the Johns Hopkins Hospital and Massachusetts General Hospital. Medicine 1952;31:1-142.
27. Maycock RI, Bertrand P, Morrison CE, Scott JH. Manifestations of sarcoidosis: analysis of 145 patients with review of nine series selected from the literature. Am J Med 1963;35:67-89.
28. Sones M, Israel HL, Dratman MB, Frank JH. Effect of cortisone in sarcoidosis. N Engl J Med 1951;244:209-13.
29. Siltzbach LE. Effects of cortisone in sarcoidosis: A study of 13 patients. Am J Med 1952;12:139-60.
30. Scadding J. Prognosis of intrathoracic sarcoidosis in England: A review of 136 cases after 5 years' observations. Br Med J 1961;2:1165-72.
31. Siltzbach LE, James DG, Neville E, Turiaf J, Battesti JP, Sharma OP, Hosoda Y, Mikami R, Odaka M. Course and prognosis of sarcoidosis around the world. Am J Med 1974;57: 847-52.
32. Wurm K, Reindell H, Heilmeyer L. Der Lungenboeck in Röntgenbild. Thieme, Stuttgart, Germany 1958.
33. Neville E, Walker AN, James DG. Prognostic factors predicting the outcome of sarcoidosis: an analysis of 818 patients. Q J Med 1983;52:525-33.
34. Romer FK. Presentation of sarcoidosis and outcome of pulmonary changes. Dan Bull Med 1982;29:27-32.

35. Eule H, Weinecke A, Roth I, Wuthe H. The possible influence of corticosteroid therapy on the natural course of pulmonary sarcoidosis: Late results of a continuing clinical study. Ann NY Acad Sci 1986;465: 695-701.

36. Koerner SK, Sakowitz AJ, Appelman RI, Becker NH, Schoenbaum SW. Transbronchial lung biopsy for the diagnosis of sarcoidosis. N Engl J Med 1975;293:268-70.

37. Hunninghake GW, Crystal RG. Pulmonary sarcoidosis: A disorder mediated by excess helper T-lymphocyte activity at sites of disease activity. N Engl J Med 1981;305:429-34.

38. James DG, Neville E, Walker A. Immunology of sarcoidosis. Am J Med 1975;59:388-94.

39. Lieberman J. Elevation of serum angiotensin-converting-enzyme (ACE) level in sarcoidosis. Am J Med 1975;59:365-72.

40. Crystal RG, Roberts RC, Hunninghake GW, Gadek JE, Fulmer JD, Line BR. Pulmonary sarcoidosis: A disease characterized and perpetuated by activated lung T-lymphocytes. Ann Intern Med 1981;94:73-94.

41. Daniele RP, Dauber JH, Rossman MD. Immunologic abnormalities in sarcoidosis. Ann Intern Med 1980; 92:406-16.

42. Thomas PD, Hunninghake GW. Current concepts of the pathogenesis of sarcoidosis. Am Rev Respir Dis 1987;135:747-60.

43. Line BR, Hunninghake GW, Keogh BA, Jones AE, Johnston GS, Crystal RG. Gallium-67 scanning to stage the alveolitis of sarcoidosis: Correlation with clinical studies, pulmonary function studies, and bronchoalveolar lavage. Am Rev Respir Dis 1981;123: 440-6.

44. Gupta SK. A survey of sarcoidosis. J Indian Med Assoc 1961;37:116-20.

45. Gupta SK. Erythema nodosum and its aetiology. With special reference to sarcoidosis. J Indian Med Assoc 1963;40:202-06.

46. Gupta SK. Sarcoidosis: A study in Eastern India. J Indian Med Assoc 1977;68:245-47.

47. Gupta SK. Clinical profile of sarcoidosis in Eastern India. Indian J Chest Dis Allied Sci 1981;23:173-78.

48. Gupta SK. Sarcoidosis in India: Long-term follow-up report of a series. J Assoc Physicians India 1982;30:304-08.

49. Behera D, Malik SK, Sehgal S. Pulmonary sarcoidosis. Review of 9 cases. Ind J Chest Dis 1984;26:77-80.

50. Gupta SK, Mitra K, Roy M, Dutta SK. Sarcoidosis in India. Indian J Chest Dis Allied Sci 1985;27:55-63.

51. Bambery P, Behera D, Kaur U, Gupta A, Jindal SK, Malik SK, Deodhar SD. Profile of sarcoidosis in North India. Sarcoidosis 1987;4:155-58.

52. Bambery P, Bharati B, Bushnurmath SR, Behera D, Jindal SK, Kaur U, Deodhar SD, Sakhuja V, Chugh KS. Non-tubercular pulmonary vasculitis with granulomas in North India: Clinicopathological study of 39 patients (Abstract). Sarcoidosis 1989; 6 (Suppl.1):103.

53. Bambery P, Gupta A, Saini JS, Behera D, Jindal SK, Malik SK, Jain IS. Ocular sarcoidosis in North India: Prospective study of 25 patients (Abstract). Sarcoidosis 1989;6 (Suppl. 1):106.

54. Behera D, Varma S, Bambery P, Chakrabarti S. High-dose methyl prednisolone for autoimmune thrombocytopenia in sarcoidosis. Sarco Vascu and Diffuse Lung Dis 1997;14:188-92.

55. Bambery P, Behera D, Gupta A, Kaur U, Jindal SK, Sehgal S, Malik SK and Deodhar SD. In Grassi C, Rizzato G, Pozzi E (Eds): Sarcoidosis in North India An emerging clinical spectrum in sarcoidosis and other granulomatous disorders." Elsevier Science Publishers BV (Biomedical Division),1998;311-12.

56. Jindal SK, Gupta D, Aggarwal AN. Sarcoidosis in India: Practical issues and difficulties in diagnosis and management. Sarcoidosis Vasc Diffuse Lung Dis 2002;19:176-84.

57. Jindal SK, Gupta D, Aggarwal AN. Sarcoidosis in developing countries. Curr Opin Pulm Med 2000;6:448-54.

58. Jindal SK, Gupta D. Incidence and recognition of interstitial pulmonary fibrosis in developing countries. Curr Opin Pulm Med 1997;3:378-83.

59. Mohan A, Sood R, Shariff N, Gulati MS, Gupta SD, Dutta AK. Sarcoidosis manifesting as massive splenomegaly: A rare occurrence. Am J Med Sci 2004;328:170-72.

60. Gupta SK. Clinical profile of sarcoidosis in Himachal Pradesh. Assoc Physicians India 1998;46:243.

61. Gupta SK. Sarcoidosis: A journey through 50 years. Indian J Chest Dis Allied Sci 2002;44:247-53.

62. Gupta SK, Mitra K, Chatterjee S, Chakravarty SC. Sarcoidosis in India. Br J Dis Chest 1985;79:275-83.

63. Gupta SK. Pediatric sarcoidosis in India. Indian J Pediatr 2001;68:931-35.

64. Gupta SK, Mitra K. Paediatric sarcoidosis. J Assoc Physicians India 1988;36:150-53.

65. Gupta SK, Mitra K. Sarcoidosis in children. Indian Pediatr 1988;25:88-92.

66. Gupta SK, Gupta S. Sarcoidosis in India: A review of 125 biopsy-proven cases from eastern India. Sarcoidosis 1990;7:43-49.

67. Gupta SK. The first published case of sarcoidosis in India. J Assoc Physicians India. 1988;36:676-77.

68. Gupta SK. Sarcoidosis. J Assoc Physicians India. 1988;36:573-74.

69. Sharma SK, Mohan A. Uncommon manifestations of sarcoidosis. J Assoc Physicians India 2004;52:210-14.

70. Sharma SK, Mohan A. Sarcoidosis: global scenario & Indian perspective. Indian J Med Res 2002;116:221-47.

71. Sharma SK, Balamurugan A, Pandey RM, Saha PK, Mehra NK. Human leukocyte antigen-DR alleles influence the clinical course of pulmonary sarcoidosis in Asian Indians. Am J Respir Cell Mol Biol 2003;29: 225-31.

72. Sharma SK, Pande JN, Mukhopadhay AK, Goulatia RK, Wali JP, Guleria JS. Bilateral recurrent spontaneous pneumothoraces in sarcoidosis. Jpn J Med 1987;26:69-71.

73. Sharma SK, Pande JN, Guleria JS. Diffuse interstitial pulmonary fibrosis. Indian J Chest Dis Allied Sci 1984;26:214-19.

74. Sharma SK, Mohan A, Guleria JS. Clinical characteristics, pulmonary function abnormalities and outcome of prednisolone treatment in 106 patients with sarcoidosis. J Assoc Physicians India 2001;49:697-704.

75. Sharma SK, Mohan A, Guleria R, Padhy AK. Diagnostic dilemma: Tuberculosis? or, sarcoidosis? Indian J Chest Dis Allied Sci 1997;39:119-23.

76. Gupta S. Autologous mixed lymphocyte reaction in health and disease states in man. Vox Sang 1983;44:265-88.

77. Behera D, D' Souza G, Rajwanshi A, Jindal SK. Broncho-alveolar lavage-cellular characteristics in patients with idiopathic pulmonary fibrosis and sarcoidosis. Ind J Chest Dis All Sci 1990;32:107-10.

78. Pande JN, Sharma SK, Verma K. Value of enumerating cellular constituents of bronchoalveolar lavage fluid in differentiating sarcoidosis and cryptogenic fibrosing alveolitis. Sarcoidosis 1990;7:96-100.

79. Sharma SK, Pande JN, Verma K, Guleria JS. Broncho-alveolar lavage fluid (BALF) analysis in interstitial lung diseases—A 7-year experience. Indian J Chest Dis Allied Sci 1989;31:187-96.

80. Sharma SK, Pande JN, Verma K, Guleria JS. Inter-relationship between bronchoalveolar lavage cellular constituents and pulmonary functions in sarcoidosis. Indian J Chest Dis Allied Sci 1989;31:77-84.

81. Sharma SK, Verma U, Pande JN, Murugesan K, Verma K, Guleria JS. Glucocorticoid receptors in broncho-alveolar lavage fluid in sarcoidosis. A preliminary report. Chest 1988;93:577-79.

82. Gupta SK, Mitra K, Chatterjee S, Banerjee D, Roy M. Multiple biopsies in the diagnosis of sarcoidosis. Indian J Chest Dis Allied Sci 1984;26:65-73.

83. Gupta D, Mahendran C, Aggarwal AN, Joshi K, Jindal SK. Endobronchial vis a vis transbronchial involvement on fiber-optic bronchoscopy in sarcoidosis. Sarcoidosis Vasc Diffuse Lung Dis 2001;18:91-92.

84. Behera D, Arvinndan AN, Bambery P, Majumdar S. Surfactant levels in bronchoalveolar lavage in sarco-idosis. Chest 2002;122/4 (Suppl):152S.

85. Gupta D, Jorapur V, Bambery P, Joshi K, Jindal SK. Pulmonary sarcoidosis: Spirometric correlation with transbronchial biopsy. Sarcoidosis Vasc Diffuse Lung Dis 1997;14:77-80.

86. Bala M, Gupta S, Pasha MA. Angiotensin-converting enzyme assay optimization: Influence of various buffers and their concentrations. Clin Biochem 2000;33:687-89.

87. Gupta SK. Mantoux test site granuloma: An appraisal of the diagnostic value in sarcoidosis. Indian J Chest Dis Allied Sci 1997;39:13-18.

88. Gupta SK, Dutta SK. Comparative merits of different tissue biopsies in the diagnosis of sarcoidosis: Indian perspective. J Assoc Physicians India 1996;44:609-11.

89. Gupta SK. Markers of activity in sarcoidosis with a special reference to serum angiotensin converting enzyme (SACE). Indian J Chest Dis Allied Sci 1993;35:117-27.

90. Gupta SK, Chakraborty M, Mitra K. Serum angiotensin converting enzyme in respiratory diseases. Indian J Chest Dis Allied Sci. 1992;34:19-24.

91. Gupta SK. Treatment of sarcoidosis patients by steroid aerosol: A ten-year prospective study from Eastern India. Sarcoidosis. 1989;6:51-54.

92. Dutta SK, Gupta SK, Mitra K. Cell mediated immunity in sarcoidosis. J Indian Med Assoc 1988;86:259-61.

93. Gupta SK, Mitra K. Appraisal or SACE. J Assoc Physicians India 1988;36:525.

94. Gupta SK, Mitra K, Dutta SK. Dinitrochlorobenzene test in sarcoidosis. J Assoc Physicians India 1986;34:786-87.

95. Gupta SK. Diagnostic value of SACE. J Assoc Physicians India 1986;34:827.

96. Gupta SK, Mitra K, Chakraborty M. Serum angiotensin converting enzyme in respiratory diseases. J Assoc Physicians India 1985;33:651-52.

97. Das A, Chatterjee S, Bagchi SC, Gupta SK. Ocular involvement in sarcoidosis. Indian J Ophthalmol 1984;32:195-99.

98. Roy M, Gupta SK. Interpretation of Kveim test in sarcoidosis. Indian J Pathol Microbiol 1983;26:27-30.

99. Gupta SK, Chatterjee S. Systemic and neuro-sarcoidosis in a child. Indian Pediatr 1983;20:380-82.

100. Gupta SK, Chatterjee S. The roentgenographic staging of sarcoidosis. Historic and contemporary perspectives. Chest 1984;85:141.

101. Kashyap S, Kumar M, Thami GP, Saini V. Umbilicated papular sarcoidosis. Clin Exp Dermatol 1996;21:395-96.

102. Kashyap S, Kumar M, Thakur S. Sarcoidosis presenting as polycythemia. A case report. J Assoc Physicians India 1995;43:795-96.

103. Sharma SK, Khanna M, Sharma S, Srivastava LM, Verma K, Khilnani GC, Pande JN. Effect of corticosteroid treatment on various serological and bronchoalveolar lavage abnormalities in patients with sarcoidosis. Indian J Med Res 1995;101:207-12.

104. Sharma SK, Rao DN, Pande JN, Guleria JS. Serum angiotensin-converting enzyme activity in sarcoidosis. Indian J Med Res 1987;85:638-44.

105. Hennessy TW, Ballard DJ, DeRemee RA, Chu CP, Melton LJ. The influence of diagnostic access bias on the epidemiology of sarcoidosis: A population-based study in Rochester, Minnesota, 1935-1984. J Clin Epidemiol 1988;41:565-70.

106. Gordis L. Sarcoidosis: Epidemiology of Chronic Lung Diseases in Children. The John Hopkins University Press: Baltimore 1973;53-78.

107. Alsbirk PH. Epidemiologic studies on sarcoidosis in Denmark based on a nationwide central register: A preliminary report. Acta Med Scand 1964;176:106-9.

108. Iwai K, Sekiguti M, Hosoda Y, DeRemee RA, Tazelaar HD, Sharma OP, Maheshwari A, Noguchi TI. Racial difference in cardiac sarcoidosis incidence observed at autopsy. Sarcoidosis 1994;11:26-31.

109. Milman N, Selroos O. Pulmonary sarcoidosis in the Nordic countries 1950-1982: Epidemiology and clinical picture. Sarcoidosis 1990;7:50-57.

110. Henke CE, Henke G, Elveback LR, Beard CM, Ballard DJ, Kurland LT. The epidemiology of sarcoidosis in Rochester, Minnesota: A population-based study of incidence and survival. Am J Epidemiol 1986;123: 840-45.

111. Rybicki BA, Major M, Popovich J Jr, Maliarik MJ, Iannuzzi MC. Racial differences in sarcoidosis incidence: A 5-year study in a health maintenance organization. Am J Epidemiol 1997;145: 234-41.

112. Bresnitz EA, Strom BL. Epidemiology of sarcoidosis. Epidemiol Rev 1983;5:124-56.

113. James GD. Sarcoidosis and other granulomatous disorders. Marcel Dekker: New York 1994.

114. Mana J, Badrinas F, Morera J, Fite E, Manresa F, Fernandez-Nogues F. Sarcoidosis in Spain. Sarcoidosis 1992;9:118-22.

115. Keller AZ. Hospital, age, racial, occupational, geographical, clinical and survivorship characteristics in the epidemiology of sarcoidosis. Am J Epidemiol 1971;94: 222-30.

116. Mitchell DN, Scadding JG. Sarcoidosis. Am Rev Respir Dis 1974;110:774-802.

117. McNicol MW, Luce PJ. Sarcoidosis in a racially mixed community. JR Coll Physicians Lond 1985;19:179-83.

118. Edmondstone WM, Wilson AG. Sarcoidosis in Caucasians, Blacks and Asians in London. Br J Dis Chest 1985;79:27-36.

119. Pietinalho A, Ohmichi M, Hiraga Y, Lofroos AB, Selroos O. The mode of presentation of sarcoidosis in Finland and Hokkaido, Japan: A comparative analysis of 571 Finnish and 686 Japanese patients. Sarcoidosis Vasc. Diffuse Lung Dis 1996;13:159-66.

120. Iwai K, Tachibana T, Takemura T, Matsui Y, Kitaichi M, Kawabata Y. Pathological studies on sarcoidosis autopsy: I. Epidemiological features of 320 cases in Japan. Acta Pathol Jpn 1993;43:372-6.

121. Iwai K, Takemura T, Kitaichi M, Kawabata Y, Matsui Y. Pathological studies on sarcoidosis autopsy: II. Early change, mode of progression and death pattern. Acta Pathol Jpn 1993;43:377-85.

122. Gideonc NM, Mannino DM. Sarcoidosis mortality in the United States 1979-1991: An analysis of multiple-cause mortality data. Am J Med 1996;100: 423-27.

123. Parkes SA, Baker SB, Bourdillon RE, Murray CR, Rakshit M. Epidemiology of sarcoidosis in the Isle of Man: 1. A case controlled study. Thorax 1987;42:420-26.

124. Hills SE, Parkes SA, Baker SB. Epidemiology of sarcoidosis in the Isle of Man: 2. Evidence for space-time clustering. Thorax 1987;42:427-30.

125. Bardinas F, Morera J, Fite E, Plasencia A. Seasonal clustering of sarcoidosis. Lancet 1989;2:455-56.

126. Glennas A, Kvien TK, Melby K, Refvem OK, Andrup O, Karstensen B, Thoen JE. Acute sarcoid arthritis: Occurrence, seasonal onset, clinical features and outcome. Br J Rheumatol 1995;34:45-50.

127. Gentry JT, Nitowsky HM, Michael M. Studies on the epidemiology of sarcoidosis in the United States: The relationship to soil areas and to urban-rural residence. J Clin Invest 1955;34:1839-56.

128. Harrington DW, Major M, Rybicki B, Popovich J, Maliarik M, Iannuzzi MC. Familial sarcoidosis: Analysis of 91 families. Sarcoidosis 1994;11:240-43.

129. Brennan NJ, Crean P, Long JP, Fitzgerald MX. High prevalence of familial sarcoidosis in an Irish population. Thorax 1984;39:14-18.

130. Hiraga Y, Hosoda Y, Zenda I. A local outbreak of sarcoidosis in northern Japan Z Erkr. Atmungsorgane 1977;149:38-43.

131. Pasturenzi L, Martinetti M, Cuccia M, Cipriani A, Semenzato G, Luisetti M. HLA class I, II, and III polymorphism in Italian patients with sarcoidosis: The Pavia-Padova Sarcoidosis Study Group. Chest 1993;104:1170-75.

132. Rybicki BA, Major M, J Popovich Jr, MJ Maliarik, MC Iannuzzi. Racial differences in sarcoidosis incidence: A 5-year study in a health maintenance organization. Am J Epidemiol 1997;145:234-41.

133. Buck AA. Epidemiologic investigations of sarcoidosis: IV. Discussion and summary. Am J Hyg 1961;74:189-202.

134. Perez RL, Roman J, Staton Jr GW, Hunter RL. Extravascular coagulation and fibrinolysis in murine lung inflammation induced by the mycobacterial cord factor trehalose-6,6'-dimycolate. Am J Respir Crit Care Med 1994;149:510-18.

135. Martinetti M, Tinelli C, Kolek V, MCuccia, Salvaneschi L, Pasturenzi L, Semenzato G, Cipriani A, Bartova A, Luisetti M. "The sarcoidosis map": A joint survey of clinical and immunogenetic findings in two European countries. Am J Respir Crit Care Med 1995;152:557-64.

136. Moller DR, Konishi K, Kirby M, Balbi B, Crystal RG. Bias toward use of a specific T cell receptor beta-chain variable region in a subgroup of individuals with sarcoidosis. J Clin Invest 1988;82:1183-91.

137. Berlin M, Fogdell-Hahn A, Olerup O, Eklund A, Grunewald J. HLA-DR predicts the prognosis in Scandinavian patients with pulmonary sarcoidosis. Am J Respir Crit Care Med 1997;156:1601-05.

138. Gardner J, Kennedy HG, Hamblin A, Jones E. HLA associations in sarcoidosis: a study of two ethnic groups. Thorax 1984;39:19-22.

139. Kunikane H, Abe S, Yamaguchi E, Aparicio JM, Wakisaka A, Yoshiki T, Kawakami Y. Analysis of restriction fragment length polymorphism for the HLA-DR gene in Japanese patients with sarcoidosis. Thorax 1994;49:573-76.

140. Abe S, Yamaguchi E, Makimura S, Okazaki N, Kunikane H, Kawakami Y. Association of HLA-DR with sarcoidosis: Correlation with clinical course. Chest 1987;92:488-90.

141. Kon OM,du Bois RM. Mycobacteria and sarcoidosis. Thorax 1997;52(Suppl 3):S47-S51.

142. Mitchell DN, Rees RJ. A transmissible agent from sarcoid tissue. Lancet 1969;2:81-84.

143. Heyll A, Meckenstock G, Aul C, Sohngen D, Borchard F, Hadding U, Modder U, Leschke M, Schneider W. Possible transmission of sarcoidosis via allogeneic bone marrow transplantation. Bone Marrow Transplant 1994;14:161-64.

144. De Vuyst P, Dumortier P, Schandene L, Estenne M, Verhest A, Yernault JC. Sarcoidlike lung granulomatosis induced by aluminum dusts. Am Rev Respir Dis 1987;135:493-97.

145. Skelton HGD, Smith KJ, Johnson FB, Cooper CR, Tyler WF, Lupton GP. Zirconium granuloma resulting from an aluminum zirconium complex: A previously unrecognized agent in the development of hypersensitivity granulomas. J Am Acad Dermatol 1993;28: 874-76.

146. Newman LS. Beryllium disease and sarcoidosis: Clinical and laboratory links. Sarcoidosis 1995;12:7-19.

147. Mangiapan G, AJ Hance. Mycobacteria and sarcoidosis: An overview and summary of recent molecular biological data. Sarcoidosis 1995;12:20-37.

148. Milman N, Andersen AB. Detection of antibodies in serum against *M. tuberculosis* using Western blot technique: Comparison between sarcoidosis patients and healthy subjects. Sarcoidosis 1993;10:29-31.

149. Chapman JS, Speight M. Further studies of mycobacterial antibodies in the sera of sarcoidosis patients. Acta Med Scand Suppl 1964;425:61-67.

150. Hanngren A, Odham G, Eklund A, Hoffner S, Stjernberg N, Westerdahl G. Tuberculostearic acid in lymph nodes from patients with sarcoidosis. Sarcoidosis 1987;4:101-04.

151. Eishi Y, Ando N, Takemura T, Matui Y. Pathogenesis of granuloma formation in lymph nodes with sarcoidosis. Sarcoidosis 1992;9:669.

152. Almenoff PL, Johnson A, Lesser M, Mattman LH. Growth of acid fast L forms from the blood of patients with sarcoidosis. Thorax 1996;51:530-33.

153. Saboor SA, Johnson NM, McFadden J. Detection of mycobacterial DNA in sarcoidosis and tuberculosis with polymerase chain reaction. Lancet 1992;339:1012-15.

154. Mitchell IC, Turk JL, Mitchell DN. Detection of mycobacterial rRNA in sarcoidosis with liquid-phase hybridisation. Lancet 1992;339:1015-17.

155. British Thoracic and Tuberculosis Association. Familial association in sarcoidosis. Tubercle 1973;54:87.

156. Reich JM. What is sarcoidosis? Chest 2003;124,367-71.

157. DeRemee RA. The sarcoid polemic. Chest 1969;55, 445-46.

158. David M, Skillrud DM. Sarcoidosis Cycle. Chest 2004;125:1171-72.

159. Berlin M, Fogdell-Hahn A, Olerup O, et al. HLA-DR predicts the prognosis in Scandinavian patients with pulmonary sarcoidosis. Am J Respir Crit Care Med 1997;156,1601-05.

160. McGrath DS, Goh N, Foley PJ, et al. Sarcoidosis: Genes and microbes—soil or seed? Sarcoidosis Vasc Diffuse Lung Dis 2001;18,149-64.

161. M Schurmann R, Valentonyte J, Hampe J, Muller-Quernheim, E Schwinger, S Schreiber. CARD15 gene mutations in sarcoidosis. Eur Respir J 2003;22:748-54.

162. Anthony W, O'Regan, Jeffrey S, Berman JS. The Gene for Acute Sarcoidosis? Am J Respir Crit Care Med 2003; 168:1142-43.

163. GM Verleden, RM du Bois D, Bouros M, Drent A, Millar, J Muller-Quernheim, G Semenzato, S Johnson, G Sourvinos, D Olivieri, A Pietinalho, A Xaubet. Genetic predisposition and pathogenetic mechanisms of interstitial lung diseases of unknown origin. Eur Respir J 2001;18(32-suppl):17S-29S.

164. Janssen R, Sato H, Grutters JC, Ruven HJT, Bois RM du, Matsuura R, Yamazaki M, Kunimaru S, Izumi T, Welsh KI, Nagai S, van den Bosch JMM. The Clara Cell 10 Adenine 38 Guanine Polymorphism and Sarcoidosis Susceptibility in Dutch and Japanese Subjects. Am J Respir Crit Care Med 2004;170:1185-87.

165. Thomeer MJ, Costabel U, Rizzato G, Poletti V, Demedts M. Comparison of registries of interstitial lung diseases in three European countries. Eur Respir J 2001;18(32-suppl): 114S-18S.

166. Grunewald J, Eklund A. Human leukocyte antigen genes may outweigh racial background when generating a specific immune response in sarcoidosis. Eur Respir J 2001;17:1046-48.

167. Iannuzzi MC, Rybicki BA. Genetics of sarcoidosis: Candidate genes and genome scans. Proc Am Thorac Soc 2007;4:108-16.

168. Schwarz J, Vanek J. Demonstration of acid fast rods in sarcoidosis. Am Rev Respir Dis 1970;101,395-400.

169. Baum GL, Schwarz J, Barlow PB. Sarcoidosis and specific etiologic agents: A continuing enigma. Chest 1973;63, 488-94.

170. Judson M. The etiologic agent of sarcoidosis: What if there isn't one? Chest 2003;124,6-8.

171. Wheat LJ, French ML, Wass JL. Sarcoidlike manifestations of histoplasmosis. Arch Intern Med 1989; 149,2421-26.

172. Reich JM. Deciphering histoplasmosis, systemic noncaseating granuloma, and sarcoidosis in the literature. Chest 1998;113,1143.

173. Scadding JG. Mycobacterium tuberculosis in the aetiology of sarcoidosis. BMJ 1960;2,1617-23.

174. Thomas PD, Hunninghake GW. State of the art: Current concepts of the pathogenesis of sarcoidosis. Am Rev Respir Dis 1987;135,747-60.

175. Reich JM, Mullooly JP, Johnson RE. Linkage analysis of malignancy-associated sarcoidosis. Chest 1995;107, 605-13.

176. Meyer KC. Beryllium and lung disease. Chest 1994; 106,942-46.

177. Drent M, Bomans PHH, Van Suylen RJ, et al. Association of man-made mineral fiber exposure and sarcoidlike granulomas. Respir Med 2000;94,815-20.

178. Hughes JM, Jones RN, Glindemeyer HW, et al. Follow up study of workers exposed to man made mineral fibres. Br J Ind Med 1993;50,658-67.

179. Newman LS, Rose CS, Bresnitz EA, Rossman MD, Barnard J, Frederick M, et al. The ACCESS Research Group. A Case Control Etiologic Study of Sarcoidosis: Environmental and Occupational Risk Factors. Am J Respir Crit Care Med 2004;170:1324-30.

180. Barnard J, Rose C, Newman L, Canner M, Martyny J, McCammon C, et al. ACCESS Research Group. Job and industry classifications associated with sarcoidosis in A Case-Control Etiologic Study of Sarcoidosis (ACCESS). J Occup Environ Med 2005;47:226-34.

181. Rabin DL, Thompson B, Brown KM, Judson MA, Huang X, Lackland DT, Knatterud GL, Yeager H Jr, Rose C, Steimel J. And on behalf of the ACCESS Research Group. Sarcoidosis: Social predictors of severity at presentation. Eur Respir J 2004;24:601-08.

182. Planck A, Eklund J, Grunewald S Vene. No serological evidence of Rickettsia helvetica infection in Scandinavian sarcoidosis patients. Eur Respir J 2004;24:811-13.

183. Redline S, Barna BP, Tomashefski JF Jr, Abraham JL. Granulomatous disease associated with pulmonary deposition of titanium. Br J Indian Med 1986;43:652-56.

184. Parkes SA, Baker SB, Bourdillon RE, Murray CR, Rakshit M, Sarkies JW, Travers JP, Williams E. Incidence of sarcoidosis in the Isle of Man. Thorax 1985;40: 284-87.

185. Bresnitz EA, Stolley PD, Israel HL, Soper K. Possible risk factors for sarcoidosis: a case-control study. Ann NY Acad Sci 1986;465:632-42.

186. Edmondstone WM. Sarcoidosis in nurses: Is there an association? Thorax 1988;43:342-43.

187. Kern DG, Neill MA, Wrenn DS, Varone JC. Investigation of a unique time-space cluster of sarcoidosis in firefighters. Am Rev Respir Dis 1993;148:974-80.

188. Sarcoidosis among US. Navy enlisted men, 1965-1993. MMWR 1997;46:539-43.

189. Douglas JG, Middleton WG, Gaddie J, Petrie GR, Choo-Kang YF, Prescott RJ, Crompton GK. Sarcoidosis: A disorder commoner in non-smokers? Thorax 1986; 41:787-91.

190. Trevenzoli M, Cattelan AM, Marino F, Marchioro U, Cadrobbi P. Sarcoidosis and HIV infection: A case report and a review of the literature. Postgrad Med J 2003;79: 535-38.

191. Fasano MB, Sullivan KE, Sarpong SB, et al. Sarcoidosis and common variable immunodeficiency: Report of 8 cases and review of the literature. Medicine 1996;75, 251-61.

192. Gomez V, Smith PR, Burack J, et al. Sarcoidosis after antiretroviral therapy in a patient with acquired immunodeficiency syndrome. Clin Infect Dis 2000;31, 1278-80.

193. Daniele RP. Immunology of sarcoidosis. Semin Respir Med 1991;12:204.

194. Balbi B, Moller DR, Kirby M, Holroyd K, Crystal RG. Increased numbers of T lymphocytes with p6 T antigen receptors in a subgroup of individuals with pulmonary sarcoidosis. Clin Invest 1990;85;1353.

195. Fehrenbach H, Zissel G, Goldmann T, Tschernig T, Vollmer E, Pabst R, Muller-Quernheim J. Alveolar macrophages are the main source for tumour necrosis factor-(alpha) in patients with sarcoidosis. Eur Respir J 2003;21: 421-28.

196. Kobayashi S, Kaneko Y, Seino KI, Yamada Y, Moto-hashi S, Koike J, Sugaya K, Kuriyama T, Asano S, Tsuda T, Wakao H, Harada M, Kojo S, Nakayama T, Taniguchi M. Impaired IFN-{gamma} production of V{alpha}24 NKT cells in non-remitting sarcoidosis. Int Immunol. 2004;16:215-22.

197. Psathakis K, Papatheodorou G, Plataki M, Panagou P, Loukides S, Siafakas NM, Bouros D. 8-Isoprostane, a marker of oxidative stress, is increased in the expired breath condensate of patients with pulmonary sarcoidosis. Chest 2004;125:1005-11.

198. Sawyer RT, Parsons CE, Fontenot AP, Maier LA, Gillespie MM, Gottschall EB, Silveira L, Newman LS. Beryllium-induced Tumor Necrosis Factor-{alpha} Production by CD4+ T Cells Is Mediated by HLA-DP. Am J Respir Cell Mol Biol 2004;31:122-30.

199. Pujols L, Xaubet A, Ramirez J, Mullol J, Roca-Ferrer J, Torrego A, Cidlowski JA, Picado C. Expression of glucocorticoid receptors {alpha} and {beta} in steroid sensitive and steroid insensitive interstitial lung diseases. Thorax 2004;59: 687-93.

200. Ziora D, Kaluska K, Kozielski J. An increase in exhaled nitric oxide is not associated with activity in pulmonary sarcoidosis. Eur Respir J 2004;24:609-14.

201. Hunninghake GW, Crystal RG. Pulmonary sarcoidosis: A disorder mediated by excess helper T-lymphocyte activity at sites of disease activity. N Engl J Med 1981;305:429-34.

202. Semenzato G, Pezzutto A, Chilosi M, Pizzolo G. Redistribution of T lymphocytes in the lymph nodes of patients with sarcoidosis. N Engl J Med 1982;306: 48-49.

Sarcoidosis **1411**

203. Agostini C, Trentin L, Zambello R, Bulian P, Siviero F, Masciarelli M, Festi G, Cipriani A, Semenzato G. CD8 alveolitis in sarcoidosis: Incidence, phenotypic characteristics, and clinical features. Am J Med 1993;95: 466-72.

204. Konishi K, Moller DR, Saltini C, Kirby M, Crystal RG. Spontaneous expression of the interleukin 2 receptor gene and presence of functional interleukin 2 receptors on T lymphocytes in the blood of individuals with active pulmonary sarcoidosis. J Clin Invest 1988;82: 775-81.

205. Robinson RBW, McLemore TL, Crystal RG. Gamma interferon is spontaneously released by alveolary macrophages and lung T lymphocytes in patients with pulmonary sarcoidosis. J Clin Invest 1988;75:1488-1505.

206. Baughman RP, Strohofer SA, Buchsbaum J, Lower EE. Release of tumor necrosis factor by alveolar macrophages of patients with sarcoidosis. J Lab Clin Med 1990;115: 36-42.

207. Kreipe H, Radzun HJ, Heidorn K, Barth J, Kiemle-Kallee J, Petermann W, Gerdes J, Parwaresch MR. Proliferation, macrophage colony-stimulating factor, and macrophage colony-stimulating factor-receptor expression of alveolar macrophages in active sarcoidosis. Lab Invest 1990;62:697-703.

208. Crystal RG, Bitterman PB, Rennard SI, Hance AJ, Keogh BA. Interstitial lung diseases of unknown cause: Disorders characterized by chronic inflammation of the lower respiratory tract. N Engl J Med 1984;310:235-44.

209. Agostini CL, Trentin M, Facco R Sancetta, Cerutti A, Tassinari C, Cimarosto L, Adami F, Cipriani A, Zambello, Semenzato G. Role of IL-15, IL-2, and their receptors in the development of T cell alveolitis in pulmonary sarcoidosis. J Immunol 1996;157:910-18.

210. Agostini C, Zambello R, Sancetta R, Cerutti A, Milani A, Tassinari C, Facco M, Cipriani A, Trentin L, Semenzato G. Expression of tumor necrosis factor-receptor superfamily members by lung T lymphocytes in interstitial lung disease. Am J Respir Crit Care Med 1996;153:1359-67.

211. Saltini C, Spurzem JR, Lee JJ, Pinkston P, Crystal RG. Spontaneous release of interleukin 2 by lung T lymphocytes in active pulmonary sarcoidosis is primarily from the Leu3+DR+T cell subset. J Clin Invest 1986;77:1962-70.

212. Semenzato G, Agostini C, Trentin L, Zambello R, Chilosi M, Cipriani A, Ossi E, Angi MR, Morittu L, Pizzolo G. Evidence of cells bearing interleukin-2 receptor at sites of disease activity in sarcoid patients. Clin Exp Immunol 1984;57:331-37.

213. Pinkston P, Bitterman PB, Crystal RG. Spontaneous release of interleukin-2 by lung T lymphocytes in active pulmonary sarcoidosis. N Engl J Med 1983;308:793-800.

214. Hunninghake GW, Bedell GN, Zavala DC, Monick M, Brady M. Role of interleukin-2 release by lung T-cells in active pulmonary sarcoidosis. Am Rev Respir Dis 1983;128:634-38.

215. Moller DR, Forman JD , Liu MC, Noble PW, Greenlee BM, Vyas P, Holden DA, Forrester JM, Lazarus A, Wysocka M, Trinchieri G, Karp C. Enhanced expression of IL-12 associated with Th1 cytokine profiles in active pulmonary sarcoidosis. J Immunol 1996;156: 4952-60.

216. Grunewald J, Olerup O, Persson U, Ohrn MB, Wigzell H, Eklund A. T-cell receptor variable region gene usage by CD4+ and CD8+ T cells in bronchoalveolar lavage fluid and peripheral blood of sarcoidosis patients. Proc Natl Acad Sci USA. 1994;91: 4965-69.

217. Kunkel SL, Lukacs NW, Strieter RM, Chensue SW. Th1 and Th2 responses regulate experimental lung granuloma development. Sarcoidosis Vasc Diffuse Lung Dis 1996;13:120-28.

218. Heyll A, Meckenstock G, Aul C, Sohngen D, Borchard F, Hadding U, Modder U, Leschke M, Schneider W. Possible transmission of sarcoidosis via allogeneic bone marrow transplantation. Bone Marrow Transplant 1994;14:161-64.

219. Mitchell DN, Scadding JG, Heard BE, et al. Sarcoidosis: Histopathological definition and clinical diagnosis. J Clin Pathol 1977;30,395-408.

220. Longscope W, Frieman D. A study of sarcoidosis based on a combined investigation of 160 cases including 30 autopies from the Johns Hopkins Hospital and Massachusetts General Hospital. Medicine 1952;31:1-42.

221. Kitaichi M. Pathology of pulmonary sarcoidosis. Clin Dermatol 1986;4:108-15.

222. Rosen Y. Sarcoidosis. In Dail DH, Hammer SP (Eds): Pulmonary Pathology (2nd edn). Springer-Verlag, New York 1994;13-645.

223. Colby TV. Interstitial lung diseases. In Thurlbeck W, Churg A (Eds): Pathology of the Lung (2nd edn). Thieme Medical Publishers: New York. 1995;589-737.

224. Churg A, Carrington CB, Gupta R. Necrotizing sarcoid granulomatosis. Chest 1979;76:406-13.

225. Sheffield EA, Williams WJ. Pathology. In DG James (Eds): Sarcoidosis and Other Granulomatous Disorders. Marcel Dekker, New York. 1994;45-67.

226. Iwai K, Tachibana T, Takemura T, Matsui Y, Kitaichi M, Kawabata Y. Pathological studies on sarcoidosis autopsy: I. Epidemiological features of 320 cases in Japan. Acta Pathol Jpn 1993;43:372-76.

227. Perry A, Vuitch F. Causes of death in patients with sarcoidosis: A morphologic study of 38 autopsies with clinicopathologic correlations. Arch Pathol Lab Med 1995;119:167-72.

228. Lacronique J, Bernaudin J, Loler P, Lange F, Kawanami O, Saumon G, Geroges R, Basset F. Alveolitis and granulomas: Sequential course in pulmonary sarcoidosis. In Chretien J, Marsac J, Saltiel J (Eds): Sarcoidosis and other granulomatous Disorders. Pergamon Press: Paris 1983;36-42.

229. Takemura T, Matsui Y, Saiki S, Mikami R. Pulmonary vascular involvement in sarcoidosis: A report of 40 autopsy cases. Hum Pathol 1992;23:1216-23.

230. Tuder RM. A pathologist's approach to interstitial lung disease. Curr Opin Pulm Med 1996;2:357-63.

231. Freiman DG, Hardy HL. Beryllium disease: The relation of pulmonary pathology to clinical course and prognosis based on a study of 130 cases from the US beryllium case registry. Hum Pathol 1970;1:25-44.

232. Woodard BH, Rosenberg SI, Farnham R, Adams DO. Incidence and nature of primary granulomatous inflammation in surgically removed material. Am J Surg Pathol 1982;6:119-29.

233. Brincker H. Sarcoid reactions in malignant tumors. Cancer Treat Rev 1986;13:147-56.

234. Romer F. Sarcoidosis and Cancer. In J James (Eds): Sarcoidosis and Other Granulomatous Disorders. Marcel Dekker, New York 1994;401-15.

235. Pickard WR, Clark AH, Abel BJ. Florid granulomatous reaction in a seminoma. Postgrad Med J 1983;59: 334-35.

236. Dietl J, Horny HP, Ruck P, Kaiserling E. Dysgerminoma of the ovary: An immunohistochemical study of tumor-infiltrating lymphoreticular cells and tumor cells. Cancer 1993;71: 2562-68.

237. Brincker H. Granulomatous lesions of unknown significance: The GLUS syndrome. In James D (Ed): Sarcoidosis and other granulomatous disorders. Marcel Dekker: New York 1994;69-86.

238. Brincker H, Pedersen NT. Immunohistologic separation of B-cell-positive granulomas from B-cell-negative granulomas in paraffin-embedded tissues with special reference to tumor-related sarcoid reactions. Apmis 1991;99:282-90.

239. James DG. What makes granulomas tick ? Thorax 1991;46:734.

240. Porzezinska M, Slominski JM. Sarcoidosis—Clinical features, diagnosis and treatment. Przegl Lek 2004;61: 972-77.

241. Sharma OP. Airway obstruction in sarcoidosis. A study of 123 nonsmoking black American patients with sarcoidosis. Chest 1988;94:343.

242. Baculard, Blanc N, Boule M, Fauroux B, Chadelat K, Boccon-Gibod L, Tournier G, Clement A. Pulmonary sarcoidosis in children: A follow-up study. Eur Respir J 2001;17:628-35.

243. Demedts M, Wells AU, Anto JM, Costabel U, Hubbard R, Cullinan P, Slabbynck H, Rizzato G, Poletti V, Verbeken EK, Thomeer MJ, Kokkarinen J, Dalphin JC, Newman Taylor A. Interstitial lung diseases: An epidemiological overview. Eur Respir J 1,2001; 18(32_suppl): 2S-16S.

244. Ryu JH, Myers JL, Swensen SJ. Bronchiolar Disorders. Am J Respir Crit Care Med 2003;168:1277-92.

245. Chambellan P, Turbie H, Nunes M, Brauner JP, Battesti D. Valeyre. Endoluminal Stenosis of Proximal Bronchi in Sarcoidosis: Bronchoscopy, function, and evolution. Chest 2005;127: 472-81.

246. Awasthi A, Nada R, Malhotra P, Goel R, Joshi K. Fatal renal failure as the first manifestation of sarcoidosis diagnosed on necropsy in a young man: A case report. J Clin Pathol 2004;57:1101-03.

247. Presas FM, Colomer PR, Sanchon BR. Bronchial hyper-reactivity in fresh stage I Sarcoidosis. Ann NY Acad Sci 1986;465;523.

248. Lewis MI, Horak DA. Airflow obstruction in Sarcoi-dosis. Chest 1987;92;582.

249. Elgart ML. Cutaneous Sarcoidosis: Definition and types of lesions. Clin Dermatol 1986;4;35.

250. James DJ. Ocular Sarcoidosis. Ann Ny Acad Sci 1986;465;551.

251. Roberts WC, McAllister HA, Ferrance VJ. Sarcoidosis of the heart. A clinicopathological study of 35 necropsy patents (Group I) and review of 78 previously described necropsy patients. (Group II). Am J Med 1977;63;86.

252. Thrasher DR, Briggs DD. Pulmonary Sarcoidosis. Clin Chest Med 1982;3;537.

253. Hypercalcemia in a patient with common variable immunodeficiency and renal granulomas. Am J Kidney Dis 2005;45:e90-e93.

254. Kaiboriboon K, Olsen TJ, Hayat GR. Cauda equina and conus medullaris syndrome in sarcoidosis. Case report and literature review. Neurologist 2005;11:179-83.

255. Karmaniolas K, Liatis S, Dalamaga M, Mourouti G, Digeni A, Migdalis I. A case of ovarian sarcoidosis mimicking malignancy. Eur J Gynaecol Oncol 2005;26: 231-32.

256. Campbell SE, Reed CM, Bui-Mansfield LT, Fillman E. Vertebral and spinal cord sarcoidosis. AJR Am J Roentgenol 2005;184:1686-87.

257. Behbehani R, Sergott RC, Frohman L, Behbehani R, Sergott RC, Frohman L. Foggy vision. Surv Ophthal-mol 2005;50:285-89.

258. Heinz C, Steuhl KP, Heiligenhaus A. Uveitis in child-hood sarcoidosis. Klin Monatsbl Augenheilkd 2005; 222:348-52.

259. Keitzer R, Pleyer U. Uveitis in childhood sarcoidosis. Klin Monatsbl Augenheilkd 2005;222:346-47.

260. Matsuo T, Fujiwara N, Nakata Y. First presenting signs or symptoms of sarcoidosis in a Japanese population. Jpn J Ophthalmol 2005;49:149-52.

261. Ashraf O, Zubairi AB, Aslam F, Ashraf K, Muzaffar S. A case of non-resolving cough and weight loss. J Pak Med Assoc 2005;55:127-30.

262. Purroy Garcia F, Comabella M, Raguer N, Majo J, Montalban. Lambert-Eaton Myasthenic syndrome associated with sarcoidosis. J Neurol 2005;252(9):1127-28.

263. Lindstedt EW, Baarsma GS, Kuijpers RW, van Hagen PM. Anti-TNF-{alpha} therapy for sight threatening uveitis. Br J Ophthalmol 2005;89:533-36.

264. Johns CJ, Scott PP, Schonfield SA. Sarcoidosis. Annu Rev Med 1989;40;353.

265. Kizer JR, Zisman DA, Blumenthal NP, Kotloff RM, Kimmel SE, Strieter RM, Arcasoy SM, Ferrari VA,

Hansen-Flaschen J. Association Between Pulmonary Fibrosis and Coronary Artery Disease. Archives of Internal Medicine 2004;164:551-56.

266. Gibbons WJ, Levy RD, Nava S, et al. Subclinical cardiac dysfunction in sarcoidosis. Chest 1991;100:44.

267. Iwai K, Sekiguti M, Hosoda Y, DeRemee RA, Tazelaar HD, Sharma OP, Maheshwari A, Noguchi TI. Racial difference in cardiac sarcoidosis incidence observed at autopsy. Sarcoidosis 1994;11:26-31.

268. Teirstein AS, Padilla ML, De Palo LR, Schilero GJ. Sarcoidosis mythology. Mt Sinai J Med 1996;63:335-41.

269. Telenti A, Hermans PE. Idiopathic granulomatosis manifesting as fever of unknown origin. Mayo Clin Proc 1989;64:44-50.

270. Brincker H. Granulomatous lesions of unknown significance: The GLUS syndrome. In James D (Ed): Sarcoidosis and Other Granulomatous Disorders. Marcel Dekker: New York 1994;69-86.

271. Hendrick DJ, Blackwood RA, Black JM. Chest pain in the presentation of sarcoidosis. Br J Dis Chest 1976;70:206-10.

272. Bechtel JJ, Starr TD, Dantzker DR, Bower JS. Airway hyperreactivity in patients with sarcoidosis. Am Rev Respir Dis 1981;124:759-61.

273. Lynch JP III, Kazerooni EA, Gay SE. Pulmonary sarcoidosis. Clin Chest Med 1997;18:755-85.

274. Salazar A, Mana J, Corbella X, Albareda JM, Pujol R. Splenomegaly in sarcoidosis: A report of 16 cases. Sarcoidosis 1995;12:131-34.

275. Fahy GJ, Marwick T, McCreery CJ, Quigley PJ, Maurer BJ. Doppler echocardiographic detection of left ventricular diastolic dysfunction in patients with pulmonary sarcoidosis. Chest 1996;109:62-66.

276. Kinney EL, Caldwell JW. Do thallium myocardial perfusion scan abnormalities predict survival in sarcoid patients without cardiac symptoms? Angiology 1990;41:573-76.

277. Maycock RI, Bertrand P, Morrison CE, Scott JH. Manifestations of sarcoidosis: Analysis of 145 patients with review of nine series selected from the literature. Am J Med 1963;35:67-89.

278. Maddrey WC, Johns CJ, Boitnott JK, Iber FL. Sarcoidosis and chronic hepatic disease: A clinical and pathologic study of 20 patients. Medicine 1970;49:375-95.

279. Lynch JP III, Sharma OP, Baughman RP. Extrapulmonary sarcoidosis. In Process Citation. Semin Respir Infect 1998;13:229-54.

280. Lower EE, Smith JT, Martelo OJ, Baughman RP. The anemia of sarcoidosis. Sarcoidosis 1988;5:51-55.

281. Valla D, Pessegueiro-Miranda H, Degott C, Lebrec D, Rueff B, Benhamou JP. Hepatic sarcoidosis with portal hypertension: A report of seven cases with a review of the literature. Q J Med 1987;63:531-44.

282. Vatti R, Sharma OP. Course of asymptomatic liver involvement in sarcoidosis: Role of therapy in selected cases. Sarcoidosis Vasc Diffuse Lung Dis 1997;14:73-76.

283. Sharma OP. Cutaneous sarcoidosis: Clinical features and management. Chest 1972;61:320-25.

284. James D. Sarcoidosis of the skin. Semin Respir Med 1992;13:422-41.

285. Löfgren S. Erythema nodosum: Studies on etiology and pathogenesis in 185 adult cases. Acta Med Scand 1946;124:1-197.

286. Karma A. Ophthalmic changes in sarcoidosis. Acta Ophthalmol Suppl 1979;141:1-94.

287. Oksanen VE. Neurosarcoidosis. In DG James (Ed): Sarcoidosis and Other Granulomatous Disorders, Marcel Dekker: New York. 1994;73:285-309.

288. Chapelon C, Ziza JM, Piette JC, Levy Y, Raguin G, Wechsler B, Bitker MO, Bletry O, Laplane D, Bousser MG, et al. Neurosarcoidosis: Signs, course and treatment in 35 confirmed cases. Medicine 1990;69:261-76.

289. Sharma OP. Neurosarcoidosis: A personal perspective based on the study of 37 patients. Chest 1997;112:220-28.

290. Williams DWD, Elster AD, Kramer SI. Neurosarcoidosis: Gadolinium-enhanced MR imaging. J Comput Assist Tomogr 1990;14:704-07.

291. Gran JT, Bohmer E. Acute sarcoid arthritis: A favourable outcome? A retrospective survey of 49 patients with review of the literature. Scand J Rheumatol 1996;25:70-73.

292. Garcia C, Kumar V, Sharma OP. Pancreatic sarcoidosis. Sarcoidosis Vasc Diffuse Lung Dis 1996;13:28-32.

293. Sharma O, Kadakia J. Gastronintestinal sarcoidosis. Semin Respir Med 1992;13:442-49.

294. Browne PM, Sharma OP, Salkin D. Bone marrow sarcoidosis. JAMA 1978; 240: 2654-55.

295. Goldstein RA, Israel HL, Becker KL, Moore CF. The infrequency of hypercalcemia in sarcoidosis. Am J Med 1971;51:21-30.

296. Sharma OP. Vitamin D, calcium, and sarcoidosis. Chest 1996;109: 535-39.

297. Rizzato G, Colombo P. Nephrolithiasis as a presenting feature of chronic sarcoidosis: A prospective study. Sarcoidosis Vasc Diffuse Lung Dis 1996;13:167-72.

298. Papadopoulos KI, Hornblad Y, Liljebladh H, Hallengren B. High frequency of endocrine autoimmunity in patients with sarcoidosis. Eur J Endocrinol 1996;134:331-36.

299. Carmody JP, Sharma OP. Intrascrotal sarcoidosis: Case reports and review. Sarcoidosis Vasc Diffuse Lung Dis 1996;13:129-34.

300. Sato A. Renal dysfunction in patients with sarcoidosis. Intern Med 1996;35:523-24.

301. Cruzado JM, Poveda R, Mana J, Carreras L, Carrera M, Grinyo JM, Alsina J. Interstitial nephritis in sarcoidosis: Simultaneous multiorgan involvement. Am J Kidney Dis 1995;26:947-51.

302. Kendig EL Jr. The clinical picture of sarcoidosis in children. Pediatrics 1974;54:289-92.

303. James DG, Kendig EL Jr. Childhood sarcoidosis. Sarcoidosis 1988;5:57-59.
304. Siltzbach LE. Sarcoidosis. In Rovinsky JJ, Guttmacker FC (Eds): Medical, Surgical and Gynecologic Complications of Pregnancy. William and Wilkins, Baltimore. 1965;150.
305. Given FR, DiBendetto RL. Sarcoidosis and pregnancy. Obstet Gynecol 1963;22:355.
306. Stadnyk AN, Rubinstein I, Grossman RF, Baum GL, Hiss Y, Solomon A, Rosenthal T. Clinical features of sarcoidosis in elderly patients. Sarcoidosis 1988;5: 121-23.
307. Conant EF, Glickstein MF, Mahar P, Miller WT. Pulmonary sarcoidosis in the older patient: Conventional radiographic features. Radiology 1988;169:315-19.
308. De Remee RA. The radiographic staging of sarcoidosis History and contemporary perspectives. Chest 1983; 83;128.
309. Berkmen YM. Radiologic aspects of intrathoracic sarcoidosis. Semin Roentgenol 1985;20:356.
309A. Marten K, Rummeny EJ, Engelke C. The CT halo: A new sign in active pulmonary sarcoidosis. Br J Radiol 2004;77:1042-45.
310. Pipavath S, Godwin JD. Imaging of interstitial lung disease. Radiol Clin North Am 2005;43:589-99.
311. Warshauer DM, Lee JK T. Imaging manifestations of abdominal sarcoidosis. Am J Roentgenol 2004;182: 15-28.
312. Koyama T, Ueda H, Togashi K, Umeoka S, Kataoka M, Nagai S. Radiologic manifestations of sarcoidosis in various organs. Radio Graphics 2004;24:87-104.
313. Austin JHM. Pulmonary Sarcoidosis. What are we learning from CT? Radiology 1989;171;603.
314. Bergeron JP, Laissy P, Loiseau E, Schouman-Claeys, Hance AJ, Tazi A. Computed tomography of pulmonary sarcoid-like granulomas induced by complete Freund's adjuvant in rats. Eur Respir J 2001;18:357-61.
315. Gamsu G, Sostman D. Magnetic resonance imaging of the thorax. Am Rev Respir Dis 1989;139;254.
316. Thunnel M. Pulmonary function in patients with sarcoidosis: A three year follow-up. Sarcoidosis 1987;4;129.
317. Coates EO, Comroe JK. Pulmonary function studies in Sarcoidosis. Clin Invest 1951;30;848
318. Lamberto C, Nunes H, Le Toumelin P, Duperron F, Valeyre D, Clerici C. Membrane and Capillary Blood Components of Diffusion Capacity of the Lung for Carbon Monoxide in Pulmonary Sarcoidosis: Relation to Exercise Gas Exchange. Chest 2004;125:2061-68.
319. Leuchte HH, Neurohr C, Baumgartner R, Holzapfel M, Giehrl WM, Vogeser J Behr. Brain natriuretic peptide and exercise capacity in lung fibrosis and pulmonary hypertension. Am J Respir Crit Care Med 2004;170:360-65.
320. Gilman MJ, Wang KP. Transbronchial lung biopsy in sarcoidosis: An approach to determine the optimal number of biopsies. Am Rev Respir Dis 1980;122:721-24.
321. Israel HL, Albertine KH, Park CH, Patrick H. Wholebody gallium 67 scans: Role in diagosis of sarcoidosis. Am Rev Respir Dis 11991;44:1182-86.
322. Rizzato G, Blasi A. A European survey on the usefulness of ^{67}Ga lung scans in assessing sarcoidosis: Experience in 14 research centers in seven different countries. Ann NY Acad Sci 1986;465:463-78.
323. Thomeer MJ, Dehaes B, Mortelmans L, Demedts M. Pertechnegas lung clearance in different forms of interstitial lung disease. Eur Respir J 2002;19:31-36.
324. Raghu G. Interstitial lung disease: A diagnostic approach. Are CT scan and lung biopsy indicated in every patient? Am J Respir Crit Care Med 1995;151:909-14.
325. Gossot DL, Toledo S, Fritsch M Celerier. Mediastinoscopy vs thoracoscopy for mediastinal biopsy: Results of a prospective nonrandomized study. Chest 1996;110:1328-31.
326. Hiraga Y, Hosoda Y. Acceptability of epidemiological diagnostic criteria for sarcoidosis without histological confirmation. In Mikami R, Hosoda Y (Eds): Sarcoidosis. University of Tokyo Press: Tokyo 1981;373-77.
327. Costabel U. Sensitivity and specificity of BAL findings in sarcoidosis. Sarcoidosis 1992;9(Suppl. 1):211-14.
328. Winterbauer RH, Lammert J, Selland M, Wu R, Corley D, Springmeyer SC. Bronchoalveolar lavage cell populations in the diagnosis of sarcoidosis. Chest 1993;104:352-61.
329. Bjermer L, Thunell M, Rosenhall L, Stjernberg N. Endobronchial biopsy positive sarcoidosis: Relation to bronchoalveolar lavage and course of disease. Respir Med 1991;85:229-24.
330. Sulavik SB, Spencer RP, Weed DA, Shapiro HR, Shiue ST, Castriotta RJ. Recognition of distinctive patterns of gallium-67 distribution in sarcoidosis. J Nucl Med 1990;31:1909-14.
331. Siltzbach L, Ehrlich J. The Nickerson-Kveim reaction in sarcoidosis. Am J Med 1954;16:790-803.
332. James DG.Sarcoidosis today. Sarcoidosis 1991;8:163-65.
333. Allen RK. A review of angiotensin converting enzyme in health and disease. Sarcoidosis 1991;8:95-100.
334. Keogh BA, Hunninghake GW, Line BR, Crystal RG. The alveolitis of pulmonary sarcoidosis: Evaluation of natural history and alveolitis-dependent changes in lung function. Am Rev Respir Dis 1983;128: 256-65.
335. Wells A. High resolution computed tomography in sarcoidosis: A clinical perspective. Sarcoidosis Vasc Diffuse Lung Dis 1998;15:140-46.
336. Costabel U, Bois RD, Eklund A. Consensus conference: Activity of sarcoidosis. Sarcoidosis 1994;11:27-33.
337. Semenzato G. Assessment of disease activity in sarcoidosis: Deeds and misdeeds. Sarcoidosis 1993;10: 100-03.
338. Mitchell DN, Scadding JG, Heard BE, et al. Sarcoidosis: Histopathological definition and clinical diagnosis. J Clin Pathol 1977;30,395-408.

339. Sharma OP. Sarcoidosis. A clinical approach. Spring field, IL Charles C Thomas 1974.
340. Mitchell DM, Mitchell DN, Collins JV, Emersion CJ. Transbronchial lung biopsy through fibreoptic bronchoscope in diagnosis of sarcoidosis. Br Med J 1980;280:679.
341. Check IJ, Gowitt GT, Staton GW. Bronchoalveolar lavage cell differential in the diagnosis of sarcoid interstitial lung disease. Likelihood ratios based on computerized data base. Am J Clin Pathol 1985;84;744.
342. Hollinger WM, Staton GW, Fazman WA, et al. Prediction of therapeutic response in steroid treated pulmonary sarcoidosis. Evaluation of clinical parameters, bronchoalveolar lavage, gallium-67 scanning, and serum angiotensin-converting enzyme levels. Am Rev Respir Dis 1985;132;65.
343. Trisolini R, Agli LL, Cancellieri A, Poletti V, Tinelli C, Baruzzi G, Patelli M. The value of flexible transbronchial needle aspiration in the diagnosis of stage I sarcoidosis. Chest 2003;124:2126-30.
344. Stjernberg N, Bjornstad-Pettersen H, Truedsson H. Flexible fiberoptic bronchoscopy in sarcoidosis. Acta Med Scand 1980;208:397-99.
345. Armstrong JR, Radke JR, Kvale PA, Eichenhorn MS, Popovich J Jr. Endoscopic findings in sarcoidosis: Characteristics and correlations with radiographic staging and bronchial mucosal biopsy yield. Ann Otol Rhinol Laryngol 1981;90:339-43.
346. Costabel U, Bross KJ, Guzman J, Nilles A, Ruhle KH, Matthys H. Predictive value of bronchoalveolar T cell subsets for the course of pulmonary sarcoidosis. Ann NY Acad Sci 1986;465:418-26.
347. Takahashi T, Azuma A, Abe S, Kawanami O, Ohara K, Kudoh S. Significance of lymphocytosis in bronchoalveolar lavage in suspected ocular sarcoidosis. Eur Respir J 2001;18:515-21.
348. Jouveshomme S, Fardeau C, Finet JF, Akakpo JP, Beigelman C, Hoang PL, Derenne JP. Alveolar lymphocytosis in patients with chronic uveitis: Relationship to sarcoidosis. Lung 2001;179:305-17.
349. Ward K, O'Connor C, Odlum C, et al. Prognostic value of bronchoalveolar lavage in sarcoidosis: The critical influence of disease presentation. Thorax 1989;44,6-12.
350. Valeyre D, Saumon G, Georges R, et al. The relationship between disease duration and noninvasive pulmonary explorations in sarcoidosis with erythema nodosum. Am Rev Respir Dis 1984;129,938-43.
351. Foley NM, Coral AP, Tung K, et al. Bronchoalveolar lavage cell counts as a predictor of short term outcome in pulmonary sarcoidosis. Thorax 1989;44,732-8.
352. Haslam PL. Clinical evaluation of different markers of inflammation in relation to disease activity and long-term outcome in pulmonary sarcoidosis. Sarcoidosis 1992;(Suppl 1),37-42.
353. James DG, Thompson DG. The Kveim test in sarcoidosis. Q J Med 1995;24,49-60.
354. Munro CS, Mitchell DN. The Kveim response: Still useful, still a puzzle. Thorax 1987;42;321.
355. Douglas SD, Siltzbach LE. Electron microscopy of Kveim biopsies in sarcoidosis. In Iwai K, Hosoda K (Eds): Sixth International Conference on Sarcoidosis, University Press. Tokyo: Japan 1974,54-56.
356. Mishra BB, Poulter LW, Janossy G, et al. The distribution of lymphoid and macrophage like cell subsets of sarcoid and Kveim granulomata: Possible mechanism of negative PPD reaction in sarcoidosis. Clin Exp Immunol 1983;54,705-15.
357. Hart DP, Mitchell DN, Sutherland I. Associations between Kveim test results, previous BCG vaccination, and tuberculin sensitivity in healthy young adults. Br Med J 1964;5386,795-804.
358. Munro CS, Mitchell DN, Poulter LW, et al. Early cellular responses to intradermal injection of Kveim suspension in normal subjects and those with sarcoidosis. J Clin Pathol 1986;39,176-82.
359. Martin AG, Kleinherz ME, Elmets CA. Immunohistologic identification of antigen-presenting cells in cutaneous sarcoidosis. J Invest Dermatol 1986;86,625-28.
360. Munro CS, Campbell DA, du Bois, RM, et al. Dendritic cells in cutaneous, pulmonary and lymph node lesions of sarcoidosis. Scand J Immunol 1987;25,461-67.
361. Munro CS. The Kveim response: Still useful, still a puzzle. Thorax 1987;42,321-31.
362. Munro CS, Mitchell DN, Poulter LW, et al. Immunological processes active in developing Kveim responses differ in normal and sarcoidosis subjects [abstract]. Am Rev Respir Dis 1986;132(Suppl),A244.
363. Hillerdal G, Nou E, Osterman K, et al. Sarcoidosis: Epidemiology and prognosis: A 15-year European study. Am Rev Respir Dis 1984;130,29-32.
364. Janssen R, Sato H, Grutters JC, Bernard A, van Velzen-Blad H, du Bois RM, van den Bosch JMM. Study of Clara Cell 16, KL-6, and Surfactant Protein-D in Serum as Disease Markers in Pulmonary Sarcoidosis. Chest 2003;124:2119-25.
365. Brown JK. Pulmonary sarcoidosis. Clinical evaluation and management. Semin Respir Med 1991;12;215.
366. Bascom R, Johns CJ. The natural history and management of sarcoidosis. Adv M Med 1986;31:213.
367. Hunninghake GW, Gilbert S, Pueringer R, Dayton C, Floerchinger C, Helmers R, Merchant R, Wilson J, Galvin J, Schwartz D. Outcome of the treatment for sarcoidosis. Am J Respir Crit Care Med 1994;149:893-98.
368. Turner-Warwick M. Treatment of pulmonary sarcoidosis. State of the art. Excerpta Medico 1988;621-30.
369. Israel HL, Fouts DW, Beggs RA. A controlled trial of prednisone treatment of sarcoidosis. Am Rev Respir Dis 1973;107;609.
370. Johns CJ, Macgregor MI, Zachary JB, Ball WC. Extended experience in the long-term corticosteroid treatment of

pulmonary sarcoidosis. Ann Ny Acad Med Sci 1976;278;722.

371. Alenezi B, Lamoureux E, Alpert L, Szilagyi A. Alenezi B, Lamoureux E, Alpert L, Szilagyi A. Effect of ursodeoxycholic acid on granulomatous liver disease due to sarcoidosis. Dig Dis Sci 2005;50:196-200.

372. DeRemee RA. The present status of treatment of pulmonary sarcoidosis: A house divided. Chest 1977;71,388-93.

373. Milburn HJ, Poulter LW, Dilmec A, et al. Corticosteroids restore the balance between locally produced Th1 and Th2 cytokines and immunoglobulin isotypes to normal in sarcoid lung. Clin Exp Immunol 1997;108,105-13.

374. Reich JM. Mortality of intrathoracic sarcoidosis in referral vs population-based settings: Influence of stage, ethnicity, and corticosteroid therapy. Chest 2002;121, 32-39.

375. Young RL, Harkleroad LE, Lordon RE, et al. Pulmonary sarcoidosis: A prospective evaluation of glucocorticoid therapy. Ann Intern Med 1970;73,207-12.

376. Harkleroad LE, Young RL, Savage PJ, et al. Pulmonary sarcoidosis: Long-term follow-up of the effects of steroid therapy. Chest 1982;82,84-87.

377. Israel HL, Fouts DW, Beggs RA. A controlled trial of prednisone treatment of sarcoidosis. Am Rev Respir Dis 1973;107,609-14.

378. Eule H, Weinecke A, Roth I. The possible influence of corticosteroid therapy on the natural course of sarcoidosis. Ann N Y Acad Sci 1986;465,695-701.

379. Selroos O, Niemistö M, Riska N. A follow-up study of treated and untreated early sarcoidosis. In Iwai K, Hosoda Y (Eds): Proceedings of the VI International Conference on Sarcoidosis, Tokyo, University of Tokyo Press. Tokyo: Japan 1972-1974,525-28.

380. Viskum K, Vestbo J. Vital prognosis in intrathoracic sarcoidosis with special reference to pulmonary function and radiographic stage. Eur Respir J 1993;6,349-53.

381. Paramothayan N, Lasserson T, Jones P. Corticosteroids for pulmonary sarcoidosis. Cochrane Database Syst Rev 2005;18:CD001114.

382. O Gluck, G Colice. Recognizing and treating glucocorticoid-induced osteoporosis in patients with pulmonary diseases. Chest 2004;125:1859-76.

383. Kataria YP. Chlorambucil in sarcoidosis. Chest 1980; 78:36.

384. Siltzbach Le, Teirstein AS. Chloroquine therapy in 43 patients with intrathoracic and cutaneous sarcoidosis. Ada Med Scand 1964;176(suppl 425);302.

385. Lacher M. Spontaneous remission or response of sarcoidosis with methotrexate. Ann Int Med 1968; 69:1247.

386. Nathan SD. Lung transplantation: Disease-specific considerations for referral. Chest 2005;127:1006-16.

387. F Shorr, Davies DB, Nathan SD. Predicting mortality in patients with sarcoidosis awaiting lung transplantation. Chest 2003; 124:922-28.

388. American Society for Transplant Physicians. American Thoracic Society. European Respiratory Society. International Society for Heart and Lung Transplantation. International guidelines for the selection of lung transplant candidates: The American Society for Transplant Physicians (ASTP)/American Thoracic Society (ATS)/European Respiratory Society (ERS)/ International Society for Heart and Lung Transplantation (ISHLT). Am J Respir Crit Care Med 1998; 158,335-39.

389. Cox CE, Donohue JF, Brown CD, Kataria YP, Judson MA. Health-related quality of life of persons with sarcoidosis Chest 2004;125:997-1004.

Pulmonary Vasculitides

Vasculitis is a morphological phenomenon observed in several clinically different conditions that have a tendency to involve blood vessels in an inflammatory process, either due to an immunological mechanism or by direct involvement. The vasculitides are a heterogeneous group of syndromes characterized by blood vessel inflammation. Since Zeek's initial proposal of five separate types of vasculitis in 1952, many schemes have been developed to classify vasculitis according to the size of blood vessel involvement (that is, small arteries compared with medium-sized or large arteries),[1,2] scope of involvement (limited compared with systemic),[3] or whether the vasculitis occurs secondary to other conditions.[4] These include a range of diseases with variable clinical and pathological features. The involvement of vessels leads on to ischemia of the distal circulation causing a variety of structural and functional derangements. Vasculitis may occasionally be a minor component of a systemic illness. Some form of the Vasculitides is indolent, self-limiting, and clinically mild; whereas others may be rapidly fatal. However, a vast majority lies in between these two spectra.

The epidemiology of systemic vasculitis is becoming increasingly well understood.[5-7] Giant cell arteritis is the commonest type of vasculitis with an incidence that is highest in populations of Scandinavian descent, where the annual incidence reaches 15 to 35/100,000 aged > 50 years. The ANCA-associated vasculitides have an overall incidence of 20/million with a peak age of onset at 65 to 74 years. Wegener's granulomatosis appears to be more common in northern Europe compared with microscopic polyangiitis, which seems to be more common in southern Europe. Henoch-Schönlein purpura is the commonest form of childhood vasculitis in the West with an incidence of 20/100,000 aged < 17 years, but it is much rarer in adults (13/million). Kawasaki disease is commonest in the childhood population of southeast Asia; in Japan the incidence is 500/million

aged 5 years, 50 percent of cases occur in those aged < 2 years. Behçet's disease occurs along the Silk Road and in the Mediterranean littoral with prevalence in Turkey of 380/100,000. The various types of vasculitis have very different geographical and ethnic distributions, which provide clues to the pathogenesis.[5-7] The systemic vasculitides are very rare in childhood and peak in the 65 to 70 year old age group. Wegener's granulomatosis appears to be more common in the North of Europe compared with the South. All are more common in whites compared with other populations. Genetic and environmental factors, including infection, drugs, and silica, are important in etiology. Giant cell arteritis is predominantly a disease of whites over the age of 50. It appears more common in individuals with Nordic descent. Incidence may be increasing over time and cyclical variation in disease may reflect an infectious etiology. Takayasu arteritis is a disease of the aorta and its branches, however pulmonary and cardiac arteries may be involved. Patients are usually under 40 years of age at presentation and there are no apparent differences in incidence or clinical characteristics/aortic involvement across the globe. Takayasu's arteritis has a relatively uniform global incidence of one to two/million. Kawasaki disease (KD) and Henoch-Schönlein purpura are diseases of children and rarely affect adults. Both have been reported to be more common in Asians than whites. The incidence of KD is higher in Japan and China compared with other regions. No definite trigger factors have been found, but KD has been linked to infection, house dust mite and chemicals, and Henöch-Schonlein purpura to a pesticide and drugs.[7] Results of a population-based vasculitis register over 5 years for the incidence of primary systemic vasculitis (PSV) among 2.78 million habitants in northern Germany revealed a stable incidence for all PSV. Compared with other European studies coming from small regions or referral centers, the incidence rates for ANCA-associated PSV were the same as in Norway, lower than those in United Kingdom, but higher than those in Spain.[7]

Till recently, Wegener's granulomatosis (WG) was considered a rare disease in India. However, Wegener's granulomatosis is being recognized with increasing frequency in India. Few case series from tertiary care centers have been reported.[8-14b] Histologically confirmed patients have a clinical profile similar to that described from developed countries. Delayed diagnosis leads to the death of most patients, usually within days of hospital admission, due to extensive vasculitis and renal failure. Tuberculosis is the most frequently considered diagnosis and most patients have been treated for it in spite of progressive clinical deterioration. Those who could be adequately treated with low dose daily cyclophosphamide and corticosteroids do well. Majority of patients who could be diagnosed and treated have better prognosis and they can be well 1 to 8 years later. The Indian authors believe that if prompt lung biopsy and ANCA determination are resorted to in patients with the so called "resistant tuberculosis", it will greatly expedite case detection, diagnosis and optimum treatment of this remediable disease.

Different workers classify these disorders differently. While earlier investigators divided vasculitides according to the vessel size involved, more recent classifications use pathogenic as well as histologic features. All remain controversial because of differences of opinion and terminology, incomplete knowledge of the pathogenesis, occurrence of overlap syndromes, and some cases that do not fit well into any particular group. A simplified classification of these disorders is presented in Table 25.1.[15-24]

TABLE 25.1: Pulmonary vasculitides

I. Distinct clinicopathological syndromes with invariable lung involvement
   1. Wegener's granulomatosis
   2. Churg-Strauss syndrome
   3. Lymphomatoid granulomatosis
   4. Necrotizing sarcoid granulomatosis
   5. Bronchocentricgranulomatosis
   6. Polyarteritis nodosa (PAN)

II. Nonspecific arteritis with variable lung involvement
   1. Takayasu's aortoarteritis
   2. Sarcoidosis
   3. Goodpasture's syndrome
   4. Collagen vascular disorders
   5. Henoch-Schonlein purpura
   6. Behcet's disease, mixed cryoglobulinemia, giant cell arteritis
   7. Pulmonary vasculitis due to infections (tuberculosis, fungal infections, syphilis, parasitic, bacterial infections, and septicemias)

The entities listed under group I mostly affect the small and medium sized vessels, and this group is conventionally known as the *vasculitides disorders*. Vasculitides have also been classified on the basis of pathologic and serologic criteria into three general categories: those mediated by (i) anti-basement membrane antibody (Goodpasture's syndrome); (ii) those mediated by immunecomplex [collagen vascular disorders, poly arteritis nodosal (PAN), leukocytoblastic angiitis, Henoch-Schonlein purpura, mixed cryoglobulinemia]; and (iii) those without any immune deposits and ANCA associated (Wegener's granulomatosis, pulmonary capillarities, PAN, leukocytoblastic angiitis).

To facilitate communication among researchers, the American College of Rheumatology (ACR) proposed classification criteria in 1990 for seven vasculitides, including Wegener granulomatosis, giant-cell arteritis, polyarteritis nodosa, and hypersensitivity vasculitis.[25] The ACR vasculitis criteria were developed and validated on the basis of multicenter data.[26,27] Rheumatologists from 48 centers in the United States, Canada, and Mexico participated in this effort by contributing data from 1020 consecutive patients with a new diagnosis of vasculitis (established < 2 years before study entry) to a central database between 1982 and 1987.[26] The rheumatologists provided each patient's diagnosis and information on symptoms; physical findings; and any relevant results of laboratory, biopsy, or angiographic studies that influenced the diagnosis of vasculitis.[26] Neither biopsy nor angiography was required for inclusion in the data set, although most patients had biopsy.[26,28] In fact, to increase the representativeness of the sample, the data set included some patients with vasculitis who had not had biopsy or had a negative biopsy result.[26,28] Thus, the referring rheumatologist's diagnosis served as the gold standard in developing the ACR classification criteria.[26,27] These criteria have been associated with sensitivities ranging from 71 to 94 percent and specificities ranging from 87 to 92 percent for each specific diagnosis compared with other forms of vasculitis.

In general, the ACR criteria for rheumatologic syndromes,[29-33] including the ACR vasculitis criteria sets,[25] were developed as classification criteria for research. In particular, the ACR vasculitis criteria were established to distinguish a specific type of vasculitis among patients with various vasculitides, not to differentiate patients who have vasculitis from those who do not have vasculitis for diagnostic purposes.[25] However, clinicians, particularly nonrheumatologists, often apply

ACR classification criteria as diagnostic criteria for various rheumatologic syndromes in individual patients, particularly those with positive results on serologic tests.[34] This phenomenon is entirely understandable given the reported high sensitivity and specificity of ACR criteria sets for classification of patients.

Usually, classifications of vasculitic syndromes are based on clinical and histopathologic findings because pathogenetic mechanisms are poorly understood. As mentioned above, a subcommittee of the Diagnostic and Therapeutic Criteria Committee of the American College of Rheumatology (ACR) developed classification criteria for seven major vasculitic disorders through the analysis of prospectively collected patient data from 48 centers. Using two classification methods, the subcommittee derived criteria for polyareritis nodosa, Churg-Strauss syndrome, Wegner's granulomatosis, hypersensitivity vasculitis, Henoch-Schönlein purpura, giant cell (temporal) arteritis, and Takayasu's arteritis. Although such criteria may identify typical patients with a distinct form of vasculitis, they are not intended to establish a diagnosis in an individual patient; rather, they should aid comparability of different patient groups in various research endeavors.[35] However, the 1990 ACR classification criteria function poorly in the diagnosis of specific vasculitides.[36]

The clinical and pathological features of some of these necrotizing vasculitides are shown in Table 25.2.[37]

WEGENER'S GRANULOMATOSIS (WG)

Friedrich Wegener first described the symptoms of the granulomatosis in 1936 and 1939. Wegener's granulomatosis is an uncommon disease characterized by vasocentric necrotizing granulomatous lesions of the upper and lower respiratory tract, glomerulonephritis, and small vessel vasculitis (systemic necrotizing arteritis). This *classic* triad may not be present in all patients and a *limited* form with minor renal disease has also been described. The presentations of the disease are sinusitis (67%), nasal discharge (22%) that may be blood stained, and multiple cavitating pulmonary nodules (71%). In about half of the cases, it may be asymptomatic. Hemoptysis is the most

TABLE 25.2: Pathological and clinical features of some vasculitides

Features	Churg-Strauss syndrome	PAN	Microscopic PAN	Wegener's granulomatosis
Age	15-69	6-80	14-73	14-75
Asthma(%)	100	15	0	0
Hemoptysis	—	3	32	18
Organs affected (%)				
Lung	40	33	40	95
Sinuses	–	3	9	91
Cardiovascular system	40	23	9	12
Skin	70	49	60	45
Eyes	–	6	24	58
Central nervous system	62	14	18	11
Peripheral nervous system	65	61	27	11
Gastrointestinal system	51	27	50	0
Kidneys	28	46	100	85
Joints	23	49	71	67
Histology				
Vessel size	Medium	Medium small	Small small	Small
Granulomas	+	±	–	+
Kidneys				
Arteries	+	+	Rare	Rare
Infarcts	–	+	–	–
Interstitial nephritis	+	+	+	–
Glomerulonephritis	Mild focal	–	Focal to necrotizing	Focal to necrotizing
Granulomas	+	–	+	Rare
Eosinophilic infiltrates	+	–	–	–

PAN-polyarteritis nodosa

common respiratory symptom and massive alveolar hemorrhage can occur. Middle ear disease secondary to sinusitis and eye disease with proptosis has been described. Hypertension is uncommon despite renal involvement, and renal involvement in the form of abnormal histology occurs in over 70 percent of cases. WG and MPA (Microscopic polyangitis) are often grouped together as the antineutrophil cytoplasmic antibody (ANCA)-associated small vessel vasculitides. However, up to 10 percent of these cases will be ANCA negative.[38] They can affect many organ systems, and clinically are differentiated by their predilection for the pulmonary system. No single test is capable of diagnosing or distinguishing between these conditions. Therefore, a combination of clinical, serological and histopathological factors must be considered to provide a final diagnosis. WG is a granulomatous vasculitis that, in contrast to Churge-Strauss syndrome, does not cause asthma, although the two may coexist because of the prevalence of asthma in the population. Nasal, oropharyngeal, or pulmonary involvement is essentially universal at diagnosis. Ear, nose and throat disease includes epistaxis, nasal and oral ulceration and necrosis, sinus pain and hearing loss. Pulmonary involvement includes hemorrhage, pleural effusions and large airway inflammation and stenosis. Pulmonary hemorrhage may be extensive before hemoptysis or other overt clinical signs become apparent. Renal involvement ranges from a subclinical glomerulonephritis (blood and protein on the urine bedside test) to rapidly progressive glomerulonephritis, and it is nearly universal.[39] A respiratory limited form of the diseases has been touted, but over 80 percent of these cases go on to develop renal disease, and so the distinction is of little use.[40] The presence of renal disease is arbitrarily used to define generalized. MPA is a nongranulomatous vasculitis that has less of a predilection for the lungs, although pulmonary involvement is still seen in up to 40 percent of cases.[41] Renal involvement is again common. Cardiac involvement can occur in both, manifesting as myocarditis, coronary arteritis, valvulitis, endocarditis, conduction disturbances and pericarditis. Acute pericardial inflammation may lead to life threatening tamponade.[42] The musculoskeletal, neurological and cutaneous systems are also frequently affected, in WG more than in MPA.

The disease can rarely involve any of the other organs of the body, although rarely.[43-76]

Pathogenesis

Wegener's granulomatosis (WG) is a complex autoimmune syndrome that is characterized by upper/lower respiratory necrotizing granulomatosis, glomerulonephritis and small-vessel vasculitis. Since Wegener's 1936 description, considerable advances in recognition and treatment have changed this disease from a rapidly and uniformly fatal illness to a chronic disease characterized by remissions and relapses. The serendipitous discovery of antineutrophil cytoplasmic antibodies (ANCAs) as a marker associated with WG focused attention on the potential pathogenic role of these antibodies and has recently led to the development of novel animal models that might facilitate our understanding of the disease pathogenesis. Future animal models of this disease will have to account for the role of both ANCA-mediated pathology and granulomatous inflammation to enable us to understand the chronic and persistent features of WG in humans.[77]

In Wegener's granulomatosis (WG), antiproteinase 3 (PR3) autoantibodies (PR3-ANCA) are crucial in the development of generalized vasculitis. Within WG these ANCAs are usually (80-90%) directed against the azurophilic enzyme proteinase 3, the so-called PR3-ANCA. Wegener's pathognomonic lesion, a granulomatous inflammation of the upper and lower respiratory tract, contains abundant lymphocytes and macrophages. Lymphocyte clusters in germinal center-like formation within the granulomatous lesion are frequently observed, which suggests antigen-driven B cell maturation. Wegener's autoantigen PR3, the target for autoreactive B and T cells, is expressed in granulomatous lesions. Disease progression in WG is accompanied by a profound generalized alteration of T cell differentiation with an increase of effector memory T cells [CD4(+) CD28(-)]. The cytokine profile suggests an aberrant Th1-type response either to an environmental trigger and/or the autoantigen PR3 itself. *Staphylococcus aureus*, a risk factor for disease exacerbation, is widely present in the upper airways in WG. The Ig gene repertoire from WG lesions indicates a predominance of VH3+ B cells with affinity to PR3 as well as to the *S. aureus* B cell superantigen SPA. Hence, within the WG lesion, *S. aureus* might support the maturation of PR3-affinity B cells that enter a germinal center reaction in contact with PR3 and T cells and expand, leading to PR3-ANCA production. Thus, granulomatous lesions could represent a potential lymphoid tissue-maintaining autoantibody production rather than a simple, random leukocyte accumulation in WG.[78]

A pathophysiological role for these autoantibodies, supported by numerous *in vitro* and *in vivo* studies, is specifically based on their capacity to bind and activate neutrophils and potentially may damage vessels. In this review, the pathogenic potential of different developmental stages of the neutrophil in the pathogenesis of

WG is discussed. After release from the bone marrow into the circulation, neutrophils can be primed by TNF-alpha and become attached to locally activated endothelium. Once attached to the endothelium, ANCAs can fully activate these primed neutrophils. In this activation process, the degree of activation after stimulation with PR3-ANCAs associates with the level of PR3 expression on the membrane of the neutrophil. Following activation, infiltrated neutrophils become apoptotic with further membrane expression of PR3. In WG patients, clearance of apoptotic neutrophils can be disturbed due to the opsonization of PR3-expressing apoptotic neutrophils with PR3-ANCAs, thereby perpetuating inflammation by the release of proinflammory cytokines during clearance; or it may favor autoimmunity by PR3 presentation in an inflammatory environment. Furthermore, the presence of ANCAs and the release of the vessel-related pentraxin PTX3 may lead to the persistence of late apoptotic neutrophils in tissues, thereby inducing leukocytoclastic lesions that are characteristic in patients with WG. All together, alive neutrophils as well as apoptotic neutrophils play a key role in different inflammatory phenomena seen in patients suffering from WG.[79]

Thus, it may be summarized pulmonary vasculitis are strongly associated with antineutrophil cytoplasmic autoantibodies (ANCA) directed against enzymes contained in the primary granules of neutrophils and peroxidase-positive lysosomes of monocytes. There is strong evidence for a pathogenic role of ANCA. *In vitro,* ANCAs can activate cytokine-primed neutrophils and monocytes resulting in oxygen radical formation and release of lysosomal enzymes. *In vivo,* antimyeloperoxidase ANCA has been shown to induce crescentic glomerulonephritis and systemic vasculitis. Overall, the available data suggest that ANCA are indeed a pathogenic factor in the development of small-vessel vasculitis. Antiglomerular basement membrane (anti-GBM) disease also causes pulmonary vasculitis through immune attack on alveolar capillaries and glomerulonephritis through antibody mediated injury to glomerular capillaries. Thus, there is evidence that antibodies are important pathogenic factors in both ANCA disease and anti-GBM disease, however, there are also indications that T cells may play important pathogenic roles in both categories of disease as well.[80] Cytoplasmic ANCA specifically prime CD14-dependent monocytes and neutrophils for activation. The resulting enhanced responsiveness to bacterial pathogens may contribute to the development and maintenance of inflammatory lesions during active WG.[80,81]

Antineutrophil Cytoplasmic Antibodies (ANCA)

In 1985, van der Woude et al first reported that IgG autoantibodies against cytoplasmic components of neutrophils, granulocytes, and monocytes have a immunodiagnostic potential for WG. The titers of antineutrophil cytoplasmic antibodies (ANCA) too, often correlated well with the activity of the disease. The methods used in the demonstration of ANCA are indirect immunofluorescence (IIF) test or enzyme-linked immunosorbent assays (ELISAs), either using a purified neutrophil cytoplasmic extract called as 'a granules (G)' or using purified neutrophil cytoplasmic granules like myeloperoxidase (MPO) or Proteinase3 (PR3). Immunofluorescence is still the method of choice for ANCA detection, and is the most commonly used technique where perinuclear ANCA (P-ANCA), cytoplasmic ANCA (C-ANCA), and atypical ANCA (X-ANCA) patterns could be well distinguished. Cytoplasmic ANCA pattern is mostly associated with WG and is less often seen in other conditions, and its major target antigen is PR3. Particularly important in both the diagnosis and pathogenesis of the small vessel vasculitides is the ANCA. Indirect immunofluorescence identifies two clinically important patterns of staining: cytoplasmic ANCA (cANCA) and perinuclear ANCA (pANCA). In WG and MPA, these are directed against specific constituents of neutrophil granules, namely the antigens proteinase (PR)-3 and myleoperoxidase (MPO), respectively. In practice this is demonstrated by an enzyme-linked immunosorbent assay. Binding of ANCAs to these molecules on activated neutrophils is felt to be an important mechanism of tissue injury in vasculitis.

There is some crossover of cANCAs and pANCAs between WG and MPA. pANCAs directed against MPO are found in up to 24 percent of WG cases, whereas up to 27 percent of MPA cases will be cANCA positive.[33] Pragmatically, because distinguishing WG from MPA does not change therapy in the ICU, it is only necessary to identify the presence of a small vessel vasculitis and not to classify it. By using testing with both indirect immunofluorescence and enzyme-linked immunosorbent assay for the combination of cANCA and PR-3 or pANCA and MPO, the sensitivity for diagnosing the presence of either WG or MPA can be increased to approximately 73 percent, while the specificity remains at approximately 99 percent.[82] However, the presence or absence of ANCAs cannot be used in isolation to diagnose or exclude WG or MPA. Other conditions may also produce a positive ANCA (up to 50% of CSS patients will give a positive result for PR-3 or MPO,[33] and other antigens can produce a similar staining pattern (especially the pANCA). Furthermore, the PPV and negative predictive value (NPV) of any diagnostic test depend on the prevalence of the disease in the population being investigated. ANCA has the highest PPV and the lowest NPV in patients, who have the most classical clinical presentation, but neither value ever reaches 100 percent; a negative result, while decreasing the likelihood of the diagnosis, never excludes it. For example, when attempting to diagnosis renal vasculitis in the context of significant renal impairment and other clinical features consistent with WG or MPA, the presence or absence of pANCA–MPO or cANCA–PR-3 combinations have a PPV of 92 to 98 percent and a NPV of 80-93 percent.[83] Therefore, a negative ANCA still leaves a likelihood of up to a 20 percent that such a patient has a small vessel vasculitis.

A meta-analysis has shown that the sensitivities of cANCA testing for overall Wegener granulomatosis ranged from 34 to 92 percent, and the specificities ranged from 88 to 100 percent. The pooled sensitivity was 66 percent (95% CI, 57-74%), and the pooled specificity was 98 percent (CI, 96% to 99.5%). Four articles provided data on disease activity. For active disease, the pooled sensitivity was 91 percent (CI, 87-95%), and the pooled specificity was 99 percent (CI, 97-99.9%). For inactive disease, the pooled sensitivity and specificity were 63 percent and 99.5 percent, respectively. Although cANCA test results may serve clinicians as adjunct evidence for the diagnosis of Wegener granulomatosis, these results must be viewed in the context of the patient's clinical picture and disease activity and the prevalence of Wegener granulomatosis in the clinical setting in which the patient is seen.[84-109]

An increase in cANCA titer often precedes relapse of WG while a decrease in cANCA is seen with remission. Treatment, based on changes in serum cANCA titers, prevents disease relapses.[110] Monitoring of cANCA, in most cases, would therefore be of great value in distinguishing between changes due to WG and symptoms caused by other diseases. The present study was undertaken to identify the specificities and strength of ANCA and its subtypes in classical and limited WG cases by IIF and ELISA, and to correlate them with systemic or organ involvement and with other laboratory parameters.[111,112] No genetic marker has been identified yet for its diagnosis.[113,114]

Imaging

Radiological techniques can be used to help confirm the involvement of multiple organs in the disease process, but there are few features that are specific to WG or MPA

alone. Granulomata, pulmonary infiltrates, or hemorrhage can be identified on chest radiography or, with more sensitivity, on high-resolution computed tomography. However, there are many other conditions (e.g. tuberculosis, sarcoidosis and malignancy) that can mimic these changes. Their presence adds to the overall picture but should not be interpreted in isolation. A computed tomography scan of the sinuses may be more helpful, especially in WG, in which a mucosal thickening, bony destruction and infiltration to the orbits can all suggest WG[115,116] (Figs 25.1 to 25.3).

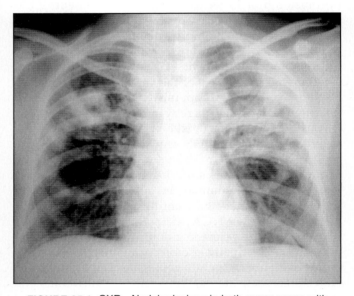

FIGURE 25.1: CXR - Nodular lesions in both upper zones with cavitation - A case of Wegener's granulomatosis

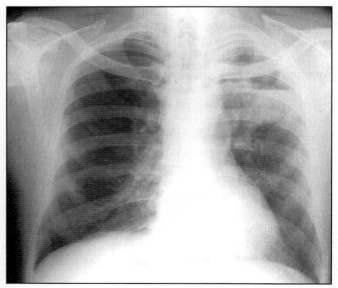

FIGURE 25.2: Wegener's lung. Note the nodular and cavitary lesions on the left upper zone and cavity on the right lower zone

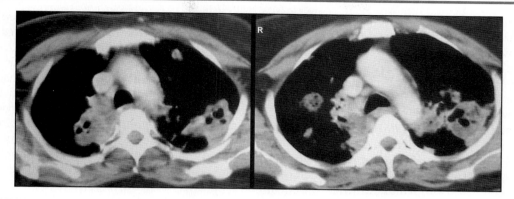

FIGURE 25.3: CT Chest - Nodular lesions with cavitation in both upper lobe – A case of Wegner's granulomatosis

Multiple pulmonary nodules on chest skiagram have been described in limited WG.[117] Five years after disease onset a quarter of the WG patients reported pulmonary symptoms, had severe abnormalities on HRCT, and abnormal PFT. The correlation between these abnormalities was poor, but the number of pulmonary involvements was a risk factor for reduced gas diffusion, obstructive lung disease, parenchymal bands, and pleural thickening. Treatment variables had no discernible negative pulmonary effects.[118]

Histology

Where possible, biopsy of an affected organ is desirable. Skin biopsy shows a leukocytoclastic vasculitis, which confirms the presence of a vasculitic process, but it is also seen in many conditions other than MPA and WG. Nasopharyngeal biopsy is useful if lesions are present and may provide diagnostic information for WG if granulomatous disease is identified. However, relatively small amounts of tissue are often obtained and only one-third of biopsies show features distinguishable as active vasculitis.

When no easily accessible lesions are present, then a decision on the next most appropriate site for biopsy must be made based on the clinical picture. Renal biopsy shows a segmental necrotizing crescentic glomerulonephritis, with no immunoglobulin deposition (so called 'pauci-immune'). This contrasts with other causes of cresentic glomerulonephritis, such as bacterial endocarditis or the collagen vascular diseases, which have immunoglobulin deposited in the glomerulus. Although diagnostic of a primary small vessel vasculitis, this histological picture rarely distinguishes WG from MPA because granulomas are seen infrequently. The histological changes may vary from mild focal and segmental glomerulonephritis with little impairment of renal function to a severe necrotizing glomerulonephritis with

crescent formation (rapidly progressive glomerulonephritis, RPGN) leading on to renal failure. Granulomas and arteritis are rarely seen in biopsy specimens. Anemia, leukocytosis, and raised erythrocyte sedimentation rate (ESR) are usual at presentation, and mild eosinophilia can also be present. Lung biopsy reveals a granulomatous inflammation and vasculitis. Open or thoroscopic biopsy has a far higher diagnostic yield (up to 90% if specific lesions can be identified) than transbronchial biopsy, which provides diagnostic material in only 10 percent of cases.[119] Pathological features are distinct in each type of vasculitis. As mentioned, there are three major vasculitis syndromes that affect the lung: Wegener's granulomatosis (WG), Churg-Strauss syndrome (CSS), and microscopic polyangiitis (MPA). The pathology of pulmonary vasculitis is complicated because it requires correlation with clinical, laboratory, and radiological features; there is overlap in some histological features among the vasculitis syndromes; biopsies early in the course of disease or after therapy may show atypical or incomplete histological features; the differential diagnosis is complex and includes infection that should not be treated with corticosteroids or immunosuppressive agents; and few pathologists have much experience with these cases. Major histological features of necrosis, granulomatous inflammation, and vasculitis characterize WG. The inflammatory consolidation consists of a mixture of neutrophils, lymphocytes, plasma cells, macrophages, giant cells, and eosinophils. Necrosis may take the form of neutrophil microabscesses or geographic necrosis. Granulomas may take several forms, including scattered or loose clusters of giant cells, palisading histiocytes or giant cells lining the border of geographic necrosis or microabscesses, and palisading microgranulomas. Sarcoidal granulomas are very rare. CSS may show eosinophilic pneumonia, allergic granulomas, and eosinophilic vasculitis.

Asthmatic bronchitis may also be present. Biopsies from CSS patients are rare because this syndrome is usually diagnosed clinically. Microscopic polyangiitis demonstrates neutrophilic capillarities and diffuse alveolar hemorrhage.[120-123]

Criteria for the classification of Wegener's granulomatosis (WG) were developed by the ACR comparing 85 patients who had this disease with 722 control patients with other forms of vasculitis. For the traditional format classification, 4 criteria were selected: abnormal urinary sediment (red cell casts or greater than 5 red blood cells per high power field), abnormal findings on chest radiograph (nodules, cavities, or fixed infiltrates), oral ulcers or nasal discharge, and granulomatous inflammation on biopsy. The presence of 2 or more of these 4 criteria was associated with a sensitivity of 88.2 percent and a specificity of 92.0 percent. A classification tree was also constructed with 5 criteria being selected. These criteria were the same as for the traditional format, but included hemoptysis. The classification tree was associated with a sensitivity of 87.1 percent and a specificity of 93.6 percent. We describe criteria, which distinguish patients with WG from patients with other forms of vasculitis with a high level of sensitivity and specificity. This distinction is important because WG requires cyclophosphamide therapy, whereas many other forms of vasculitis can be treated with corticosteroids alone.[124] Two of the following four criteria are required to meet ACR classification criteria for Wegener granulomatosis: 1) nasal or oral inflammation; 2) nodules, fixed infiltrates, or cavities on a chest radiograph; 3) microscopic hematuria or more than 5 erythrocytes per high-power field; and 4) granulomatous inflammation on biopsy. These criteria have a reported sensitivity of 88.2 percent and a reported specificity of 92 percent for the classification of Wegener granulomatosis compared with other vasculitides.[124]

Treatment

Immunosuppressive drugs are important in the management of autoimmune pulmonary diseases.[125] Sequential immunosuppression combining remission induction with cyclophosphamide with less toxic maintenance therapy such as azathioprine, methotrexate, or mycophenolate mofetil is useful in Wegener's granulomatosis, systemic vasculitis, and lupus. Less aggressive forms of diseases that have been routinely treated with cyclophosphamide have been treated with alternate regimens (e.g. methotrexate treatment of limited Wegener's granulomatosis, and mycophenolate mofetil for lupus). Finally, strategies to minimize severe side effects of immunosup-

pression include genetic testing for predisposition to drug toxicity and proposed techniques for fertility preservation during cyclophosphamide treatment.[125]

Treatment strategies are evolving. Cyclophosphamide (CYC) plus corticosteroids (CS) is the mainstay of therapy for generalized, multisystemic WG. Historically, the combination of CYC plus CS was used for a minimum of 12 months, but concern about late toxicities associated with CYC has led to novel treatment approaches. Currently, short-course (3-6 months) induction treatment with CYC plus CS, followed by maintenance therapy with less toxic agents (e.g. methotrexate, azathioprine) is recommended. Further, recent studies suggest that methotrexate combined with CS may be adequate for limited, nonlife threatening WG. The role of other immunomodulatory agents (including trimethoprim-sulfamethoxazole) is also being explored.[126] Methotrexate may be useful in some cases.[127]

Some authors have used induction therapy with pulses and oral administration of methylprednisolone (MP) with oral administration of cyclophosphamide (CP) and plasma exchange in patients with alveolar hemorrhage and serum creatinine (SCr) levels >/ = 6 mg/dL. CP was then converted to azathioprine (AZA) or mycophenolate mofetil (MMF) after 3 to 6 months of therapy. Low doses of MP with or without AZA or MMF were administered until the end of follow-up. Therapy institution resulted in remission of disease in all patients. They concluded that induction therapy with MP and CP seems to be the regimen of choice in patients with ANCA-associated glomerulonephritis. Early diagnosis and therapy institution as well as long-term treatment lead to acceptable renal survival.[128] Damage from both active disease and its treatment remain important problems for patients with WG. Despite the dramatic improvements in patient survival achieved over the last several decades, only a few patients with WG emerge from a period of active disease without sustaining some damage from the disease itself, its treatment, or both. An important measure of future therapeutic approaches will be their ability to reduce the damage accrued over time.[129] High-dose azathioprine pulse (HAP) therapy has also been used in the induction of remission in patients with active Wegener's granulomatosis (WG) refractory to or intolerant of cyclophosphamide. HAP (1200-1800 mg) applied monthly as continuous intravenous infusions at 50 mg/h. Patients received a total of 50 courses of intravenous azathioprine (AZA) therapy. HAP therapy represents a well-tolerated regimen in patients with active WG intolerant of or refractory to cyclophosphamide. A partial or complete remission is observed in about 68 percent of patients.[130]

Rituximab (RIT) is a monoclonal anti-CD20 antibody, which depletes B-lymphocytes but not plasma cells. RIT is used for treatment of B-cell lymphomas, but has also shown beneficial effects in autoimmune diseases. Patients particularly resistant to conventional therapy or who relapse repeatedly after cessation of cyclophosphamide, show promise with rituximab therapy.[131-134]

A number of newer novel methods of treating Wegener's granulomatosis have been reported recently that include Extracorporeal membrane oxygenation with lepirudin anticoagulation in heparin induced thrombocytopenia, autologous peripheral blood stem cell transplantation, Etanercept, 15-deoxyspergualin, and methyl prednisolone,[135-144] Plasmapheresis is also used to manage severe pulmonary hemorrhage or rapidly progressive renal failure. Recently, it is reported that antibiotics, particularly cotrimoxazole is helpful in the successful treatment of Wegener's granulomatosis. It is speculated that the disease is precipitated by infection in a susceptible host. Plasma exchange can be considered for first-line therapy in patients with acute renal failure and/or pulmonary hemorrhage. Refractory disease is rare and is usually due to inadequate treatment. The vasculitides provide a particular challenge for the critical care team. Particular aspects of major organ support related to these conditions are essential.

Effective treatment has revolutionized the prognosis of these conditions (vasculitis). However, mortality is still approximately 50 percent for those requiring admission to intensive care unit. Furthermore, there is a high morbidity associated with both the diseases themselves and the treatment.

CHURG-STRAUSS SYNDROME (CSS) OR ALLERGIC GRANULOMATOSIS AND ANGIITIS

The classic presentation of Churg-Strauss syndrome is with asthma and subsequently with evidence of vasculitis, at which time asthma usually abates. The development of vasculitis is accompanied by fever; weight loss, anemia, leucocytosis, and eosinophilia in most of the patients (81%) with an absolute eosinophil count over $1.5 \times 10^9/L$, and a raised ESR. The hematological findings are good indicators of disease activity. The chest X-ray usually shows patchy pneumonic or nodular infiltrates in 30 to 80 percent of cases. Cardiovascular system is involved in a large number of cases with death being due to cardiac failure in about a third. Pericardial and myocardial involvement are the common manifestations. Neurological disease is also common and the peripheral nervous system is usually affected causing mononeuritis multiplex.[145] Abdominal pain may be

present, although serious gastrointestinal problems are seen in about a fourth of the patients. Minor renal abnormalities occur, but progressive renal failure is rare.[146]

Clinical Features

Characteristically, the asthma precedes the vasculitic phase of the illness by up to 2 to 3 decades, although the two can appear simultaneously. Often this is problematic enough to warrant long-term steroids, which can have the effect of masking the development of future systemic features. As well as asthma, allergic rhinitis and skin lesions (tender subcutaneous nodules on the extensor surfaces, palpable purpura, hemorrhagic lesions or a maculopapular rash) are exceedingly common. Renal disease is more common than originally appreciated, with up to 84 percent of patients in one series of 19 patients exhibiting some degree of renal involvement, ranging from subclinical proteinuria to renal failure.[146] However, renal failure requiring replacement therapy is still relatively rare (around 10% of cases).

Other Investigations

There is no diagnostic laboratory test. A marked peripheral eosinophilia is the most common finding, but it is not specific. Furthermore, this can fluctuate rapidly, particularly in response to treatment, and can therefore easily be missed if steroids are started for the asthma before investigations are performed. IgE levels are also typically elevated, and there are circulating immune complexes. pANCA is positive against MPO, as in MPA, in around 50 percent of cases.[147] Churg-Strauss syndrome (CSS) is classified among the so-called antineutrophil cytoplasmic antibody-associated systemic vasculitides (AASVs) because of its clinicopathologic features that overlap with the other AASVs. However, while antineutrophil cytoplasmic antibodies (ANCAs) are consistently found in 75 to 95 percent of patients with Wegener's granulomatosis or microscopic polyangiitis, their prevalence in CSS varies widely and their clinical significance remains uncertain. ANCAs are present in approximately 40 percent of patients with CSS. A pANCA pattern with specificity for MPO is found in most ANCA-positive patients. ANCA positivity is mainly associated with glomerular and alveolar capillaritis.[148]

Imaging

Chest radiographic features can be very diverse, ranging from transient patchy opacities to the widespread shadowing of pulmonary hemorrhage. High-resolution computed tomography is more useful, and the findings of enlargement of the peripheral pulmonary arteries and alterations in their configuration may help to support the diagnosis (Figs 25.4 to 25.6).

Histology

Open or thoracoscopic lung biopsy is again more useful than transbronchial biopsy. Alternatively, sural nerve biopsy, in patients with evidence of a polyneuritis, may be helpful. Renal biopsy typically shows the nondiagnostic features of a focal segmental glomerulonephritis, and extravascular eosinophilic granulomas are rarely seen.[146] As such, renal biopsy adds little to the diagnosis that could not have been predicted from urine microscopy and analysis. Only a few glomeruli may show changes of focal or diffuse changes of glomerulonephritis in kidney biopsy. Eosinophilic infiltrates, granulomas, and

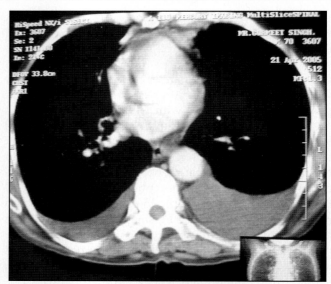

FIGURE 25.6: CT scan in a case of Churg-Strauss syndrome with pleural effusion

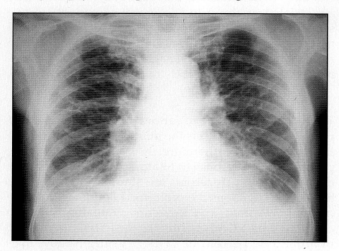

FIGURE 25.4: A case of Churg-Strauss syndrome with pleural effusion

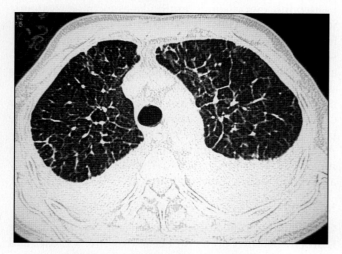

FIGURE 25.5: CT scan of the chest in a case of Churg-Strauss syndrome

necrotic vasculitis are the other features. CSS may show eosinophilic pneumonia, allergic granulomas, and eosinophilic vasculitis. Asthmatic bronchitis may also be present. Biopsies from CSS patients are rare because this syndrome is usually diagnosed clinically.

Diagnosis

The American Rheumatology Society has recommended the diagnostic criteria for CSS.[149] Criteria for the classification of Churg-Strauss Syndrome (CSS) were developed by comparing 20 patients who had this diagnosis with 787 control patients with other forms of vasculitis. For the traditional format classification, 6 criteria were selected:
- Asthma
- Eosinophilia greater than 10 percent on differential white blood cell count
- Mononeuropathy (including multiplex) or polyneuropathy
- Nonfixed pulmonary infiltrates on roentgenography
- Paranasal sinus abnormality
- Biopsy containing a blood vessel with extravascular eosinophils.

The presence of 4 or more of these 6 criteria yielded a sensitivity of 85 percent and a specificity of 99.7 percent. A classification tree was also constructed with 3 selected criteria: asthma, eosinophilia greater than 10 percent on differential white blood cell count, and history of documented allergy other than asthma or drug sensitivity. If a subject has eosinophilia and a documented history of either asthma or allergy, then that subject is classified as having CSS. For the tree classification, the sensitivity was 95 percent and the specificity was 99.2 percent,[145] although there are certain limitations of this classification.[36,149] The hallmarks of CSS are asthma (95%), allergic rhinitis (55-70%), a peripheral blood eosinophilia (> 1.5 × 10^9/l or > 10% of total white cell count) and evidence of a systemic vasculitis affecting two or more extrapulmonary organs. Particularly, important is cardiac involvement (acute pericarditis, constrictive pericarditis, heart failure and myocardial infarction), which accounts for up to 50 percent of deaths attributable to CSS.[146,150]

Treatment

Treatment regimens consist of an initial remission phase with aggressive immunosuppression, followed by a more prolonged maintenance phase using less toxic agents and doses. This review focuses on the initial treatment of fulminant vasculitis, the mainstay of which remains immunosuppression with steroids and cyclophosphamide.[142] Newer forms of therapy like Interferon-alpha has been found useful.[151-153]

POLYARTERITIS NODOSA

Polyarteritis nodosa (PAN), the prototype of systemic vasculitis, is a rare condition characterized by necrotizing inflammation of medium-sized or small arteries without glomerulonephritis or vasculitis in arterioles, capillaries, or venules. Signs and symptoms of this disease are primarily attributable to diffuse vascular inflammation and ischemia of affected organs. Virtually any organ with the exception of the lungs may be affected, with peripheral neuropathy and symptoms from osteoarticular, renal artery, and gastrointestinal tract involvement being the most frequent clinical manifestations, although less common clinical presentation may involve other organs.[154-172] A clear distinction between limited versus systemic disease and idiopathic versus hepatitis B related PAN should be done because there are differences in the implicated pathogenetic mechanisms, their treatment, and prognosis. Classical polyarteritis nodosa is a necrotizing vasculitis affecting medium sized muscular arteries. The common site of involvement is at the points of bifurcation, leading on to the formation of aneurysms. These may rupture or thrombose resulting in tissue necrosis. The aneurysms are common in the renal, mesenteric or hepatic vessels demonstrated by angiography or computed tomography.

PAN is a necrotizing vasculitis of the medium and small muscular vessels, which may affect any organ system. Historically it has often been considered part of

a spectrum of disease involving MPA and CSS. However, it is now clear that these are discrete conditions. In a subgroup of patients with PAN the disease process seems related to active hepatitis B infection. Clinically, this is indistinguishable from idiopathic PAN; however, the treatment strategies are quite different.[173] For this reason, testing for hepatitis B should be conducted early in the disease course.

Clinical Features

The characteristic features of PAN can be appreciated from the consequences of infarction and ischemia in critical organs because of the involvement of small and medium sized arteries. This commonly presents as a syndrome of multiorgan failure/compromise, on the background of constitutional upset (e.g. fever, malaise, weight loss). Hypertension is a common finding, particularly in relation to healed arteritis. The lung and spleen are characteristically spared. Areas of infarction and ischemia with fibrinoid necrosis of the large vessels are the major renal abnormalities. These patients present with systemic symptoms like fever, weight loss, and hypertension. The organs most commonly affected are skin, joints, and nervous system. Asthma may be present in 10 to 25 percent of the cases, in which eosinophilia is often noted. Although pulmonary shadowing occurs in some of these cases, hemoptysis is uncommon. This may involve the nervous system, skin, kidneys and gastrointestinal tract, although any organ can be affected. Pulmonary involvement is documented, but this is far less common than in the other vasculitides. Cardiac involvement occurs in only about 10 to 30 percent of cases.[174] but can produce significant compromise. Nerve involvement typically takes the form of mononeuritis multiplex, with both sensory and motor components. This can be present in up to 65 percent of cases and, in the absence of diabetes, is highly suggestive of PAN. Central nervous system involvement is increasingly recognized. Most commonly, this takes the form of stroke (either ischemic or hemorrhagic) or cranial nerve palsies, due to necrosis and narrowing of medium sized intracranial vessels. Renal involvement is clinically significant in up to 50 percent of cases,[174] but it is even more commonly found at autopsy. Narrowing of renal vessels leads to multiple areas of renal infarction, glomerular ischemia and hypertension. A true glomerulonephritis is not typically found, and so the urine is frequently normal (unlike in WG, MPA and CSS). Gastrointestinal tract involvement is heralded by abdominal pain, which may worsen after meals (abdominal angina). The spectrum then continues to include hemorrhage, infarction and perforation.

Imaging

In most vasculitides imaging techniques are of little value in diagnosis, but this is not the case for PAN. Angiography of either the gastrointestinal tract or kidneys characteristically shows multiple aneurysms and irregular constriction of the large vessels and occlusion of the penetrating vessels. This is often considered diagnostic in the correct clinical setting, making it possible to avoid the need to obtain a tissue diagnosis from a potentially very sick patient.

Histology

A tissue biopsy is still the 'gold standard' diagnostic test, and affected areas will show the classical necrotic inflammation of the medium sized arteries, which is diagnostic of PAN.

A subgroup of cases of polyarteritis nodosa is described affecting small vessels and characterized by a necrotizing glomerulitis with crescent formation and interstitial nephritis, and often without aneurysm formation. This group has been known as microscopic polyarteritis nodosa. The clinical presentation of these patients includes constitutional symptoms with fever, minor upper respiratory tract symptoms with sinusitis. About a third present with hemoptysis with radiographic and lung function evidence of intrapulmonary hemorrhage, and may be life-threatening. Pleuritis and pleural effusion may occur in few cases and usually uncommon. Abdominal hemorrhage is common, but nervous and cardiovascular system involvement is rare. All patients show evidence of anemia, raised ESR, microscopic hematuria, and raised serum creatinine, and are usually negative for hepatitis B surface antigen, distinct from those with classical polyarteritis nodosa Lymphomatoid granulomatosis.

Hepatitis B virus-associated polyarteritis nodosa (HBV-PAN) is a typical form of classic PAN whose pathogenesis has been attributed to immunecomplex deposition with antigen excess.[154] Thus, HBV-PAN, a typical form of classic PAN, can be characterized as follows: when renal involvement is present, so is renal vasculitis; glomerulonephritis due to vasculitis is never found; antineutrophil cytoplasmic antibodies (ANCA) are not detected; relapses are rare, and never occur once viral replication has stopped and seroconversion has been obtained. Combining an antiviral drug with PE facilitates seroconversion and prevents the development

of long-term hepatic complications of HBV infection. The major cause of death is gastrointestinal tract involvement. Importantly, the frequency of HBV-PAN has decreased in relation to improved blood safety and vaccination campaigns.

Three of the following 10 criteria are required to meet ACR classification criteria for polyarteritis nodosa: (1) Weight loss of at least 4 kg, (2) livedo reticularis, (3) testicular pain or tenderness, (4) myalgias, weakness, or tenderness, (5) mononeuropathy or polyneuropathy, (6) diastolic blood pressure greater than 90 mm Hg, (7) elevated blood urea nitrogen or creatinine level, (8) hepatitis B virus infection, (9) arteriographic abnormality, (10) biopsy specimen of small or medium-sized artery containing polymorphonuclear leukocytes.[175]

These criteria have a reported sensitivity of 82.2 percent and a reported specificity of 86.6 percent for the classification of polyarteritis nodosa compared with other vasculitides.[175]

Very rarely, polyarteritis nodosa has been reported after interferon treatment for chronic hepatitis C.[176]

Currently, corticosteroids plus cyclophosphamide is the standard of care for idiopathic PAN, in particular for patients with adverse prognostic factors (more severe disease), in whom this combination prolonged survival. In contrast for hepatitis B related PAN treatment consists of schemes that include plasmapheresis and antiviral agents. Although combining corticosteroids and cyclophosphamide has greatly improved the prognoses of severe necrotizing vasculitides, some patients continue to have fulminating disease and die within the first year of diagnosis.[177-180]

Recently, the French Vasculitis Study Group conducted a study to 1) analyze the frequency of HBV infection in patients with PAN, in light of the classification systems described since 1990; 2) describe the clinical characteristics of HBV-PAN; 3) compare the evolution according to conventional or antiviral treatment; and 4) evaluate long-term outcome. One hundred fifteen patients were included in therapeutic trials organized by the French Vasculitis Study Group and/or referred to our department for HBV-PAN between 1972 and 2002. To determine the frequency of HBV-PAN during the 30 year period, we analyzed a control group of patients with PAN without HBV infection, followed during the same period and diagnosed on the same bases. Depending on the year of diagnosis, different treatments were prescribed. Before the antiviral strategy was established, some patients were given corticosteroids (CS) with or without cyclophosphamide (CY). Since 1983, treatment for patients with HBV markers has combined 2 weeks of CS followed by an antiviral agent (successively, vidarabine, interferon-alpha, and lamivudine) combined with plasma exchanges (PE). Ninety-three (80.9%) patients entered remission during this period and 9 (9.7%) of them relapsed; 41 (35.7%) patients died. For the 80 patients given the antiviral strategy as intention-to-treat, 4 (5%) relapsed and 24 (30%) died vs 5 (14.3%) relapses (not significant [NS]) and 17 (48.6%) deaths (NS) among the 35 patients treated with CS alone or with CY or PE. HBe-anti-HBe seroconversion rates for the 2 groups, respectively, were: 49.3 percent vs 14.7 percent (p < 0.001). Patients who seroconverted obtained complete remission and did not relapse. They concluded that, HBV-PAN, a typical form of classic PAN, can be characterized as follows: when renal involvement is present, so is renal vasculitis; glomerulonephritis due to vasculitis is never found; antineutrophil cytoplasmic antibodies (ANCA) are not detected; relapses are rare, and never occur once viral replication has stopped and seroconversion has been obtained. Combining an antiviral drug with PE facilitates seroconversion and prevents the development of long-term hepatic complications of HBV infection. The major cause of death is gastrointestinal tract involvement. Importantly, the frequency of HBV-PAN has decreased in relation to improved blood safety and vaccination campaigns.[154] There are remarkable differences among pediatric patients with PAN, with different clinical manifestations and overall better survival and lower relapse rates when compared.[181]

Lymphomatoid Granulomatosis

This is a distinct clinical entity different from lymphomas, to which it bears histological similarities, and from limited Wegener's granulomatosis, to which it bears both clinical and histological similarities. The disease is characterized by lymphoreticular infiltrates, which are angiocentric and angio destructive. There is a male preponderance, and it affects all ages. Pulmonary symptoms are present in at least half of the cases and include cough, dyspnea, and chest pain. Constitutional symptoms like fever, weight loss, and malaise are common. Central nervous system and skin involvement occurs in about a third of the patients. Cranial and peripheral nerve involvement, and nasopharyngeal lesions may be present. Erythematous, macular or papular skin lesions may be the only presentations with abnormal chest X-rays. Chest radiograph may show bilateral nodular infiltrates, mistaken for metastatic tumors (Figs 25.7 and 25.8). Cavitations are less common. Since the disease may involve arteries adjacent to bronchi, involvement of the adjacent bronchus in the

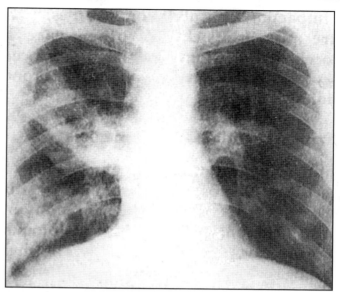

FIGURE 25.7: Chest skiagram of a patient with lymphomatoid granulomatosis. Note the areas of consolidation, nodules and cavities

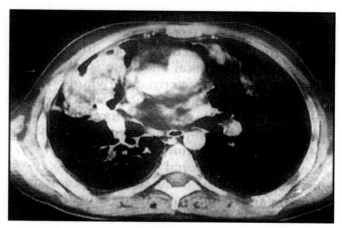

FIGURE 25.8: Corresponding CT scan of the same patient

form of bronchiolitis obliterans is common and obstructive pneumonia is seen occasionally.

Bronchocentric Granulomatosis

Bronchocentric granulomatosis is a necrotizing granulomatous disease of the lungs and is centered mainly around bronchi and bronchioles. It is often included as an eosinophilic lung disease.[182] Although the etiology has not been fully elucidated, the current pathogenetic mechanism is considered to be an immunologic reaction against endobronchial antigens, since most patients exhibit signs of bronchial asthma, eosinophilia and allergic bronchopulmonary aspergillosis.[183-190] However, nonasthmatic patients may develop bronchocentric granulomatosis without signs for endobronchial fungal infections, but probably as a consequence of other pulmonary infections. A possible association with an influenza-A virus infection has been suggested.[191] Rarely, it may be associated with bronchogenic carcinoma[192] or rheumatoid arthritis.[193]

Patients usually present with fever, cough, chest pain, and malaise. About half of the patients will have history of asthma with a few having history of allergies. Peripheral eosinophilia is present in only half of the cases and there is no correlation with the presence of asthma. Some patients have positive skin test for and serum precipitin to Aspergillus. Extrapulmonary involvement is not seen. The clinical and morphologic features are reported in 15 patients with bronchocentric granulomatosis. Patients were divided into two groups on the basis of the morphologic findings. Group I consisted of five patients with necrotizing granulomas containing abundant eosinophils in the areas of necrosis. Three of these patients were asthmatic, two had elevated blood eosinophil counts, and in one there were fungal hyphae within necrotizing granulomas. In another case a sputum culture was positive for Aspergillus. The findings in these cases support the contention that some bronchocentric granulomas associated with tissue eosinophilia may represent a hypersensitivity reaction to inhaled Aspergillus. Group II included 10 patients with bronchocentric granulomas showing many polymorphonuclear cells but few eosinophils. One of these 10 had asthma, and blood eosinophilia was found in only one patient. The etiology and pathogenesis of these bronchocentric granulomas is unclear. The differences in morphology and clinical symptomatology between the two groups suggest that these lesions may arise from more than one etiologic agent and pathogenetic mechanism. Follow-up information was available for 11 individuals. Corticosteroids were given to four patients and lesions were resected from five patients. Neither recurrence of bronchocentric granulomas nor death due to them was reported.[194]

The macroscopic pathological appearance includes consolidation and mass lesion. Microscopically, the typical histology of airway-centered necrotizing granulomata is present in all cases. Aspergillus hyphae may be identified in these cases. Nocardia specie can be cultured from the biopsy specimen in some cases.

Radiological features are variable. The roentgenographic manifestations of bronchocentric granulomatosis include mass lesions, alveolar infiltrates and reticulonodular infiltrates. Correlation of these radiographic patterns with the pathologic findings helps explain the varied morphologic appearance of this disease on the chest radiographs. Upper lobe involvement and uni-

lateral disease are usually predominant. Most patients present with solitary mass lesions. Pleural reaction is occasionally noted. Hilar adenopathy and cavitation are infrequent. There is little correlation between radiographic pattern and clinical presentation.[195] Most commonly, one lobe is involved although bilateral and multiple lobe involvement are also possible. Mucus impaction, consolidation, nodules, and cavitation are possible. Unlike other vasculitides, bronchocentric granulomatosis is not angiocentric or angiodestructive, and mainly affects the bronchi and bronchioles.

Treatment consists of immunosuppressive drugs (prednisone and cyclophosphamide), which led to complete clinical and radiological remission.

Necrotizing Sarcoidal Granulomatosis

This entity is characterized by granuloma, necrosis, and vasculitis. The etiology is obscure but an immune disturbance is suspected. Necrosis is a prominent feature and distinguishes this disorder from conventional sarcoidosis. In most of the cases, fever and systemic symptoms related to lung and extrapulmonary organs are present. Scleritis may be a feature.[196-198] The patients may be asymptomatic and are discovered only on chest X-rays. The changes in chest radiographs are usually bilateral and without hilar lymph node or extrapulmonary involvement. The course is usually benign. The disease is possibly steroid responsive.

Microscopic Polyangiitis[199-209]

Wegener's granulomatosis and microscopic polyangiitis are often grouped together as the antineutrophil cytoplasmic antibody (ANCA)-associated small vessel vasculitides. The following diagnostic criteria are proposed for microscopic polyangiitis: (i) Biopsy verified necrotizing vasculitis in small vessels and/or glomerulonephritis with few or no immune deposits and (ii) Involvement of more than one organ system as indicated by biopsy verified vasculitis in small to medium sized vessels or surrogate parameter for glomerulonephritis and (iii) Lack of biopsy and surrogate parameter for granulomatous inflammation in the respiratory system.[199]

TREATMENT

Untreated, the vasculitides are invariably fatal, with a 5 year survival of less than 15 percent. The use of corticosteroids has increased this survival rate to 60 percent in Churg-Strauss syndrome. Patients with polyarteritis nodosa also respond to treatment with corticosteroids, so also other vasculitic disorders. However, the treatment of choice for Wegener's granulomatosis and microscopic polyarteritis nodosa is a combination of cyclophosphamide with high dose prednisolone or intravenous methyl prednisolone for induction, which is reduced to maintenance doses. This has produced remission in over 90 percent of the cases.

REFERENCES

1. Lie JT. The classification and diagnosis of vasculitis in large and medium-sized blood vessels. Pathol Annu 1987;22:125-62.
2. Jennette JC, Falk RJ, Andrassy K, Bacon PA, Churg J, Gross WL, et al. Nomenclature of systemic vasculitides. Proposal of an international consensus conference. Arthritis Rheum 1994;37:187-92.
3. Alarcon-Segovia D. The necrotizing vasculitides. A new pathogenetic classification. Med Clin North Am 1980;61:241-60.
4. Lie JT. Nomenclature and classification of vasculitis: Plus ca change, plus c'est la meme chose. Arthritis Rheum 1994;37:181-86.
5. Watts RA, Scott DG. Epidemiology of the vasculitides. Semin Respir Crit Care Med 2004;25:455-64.
6. Lane SE, Watts R, Scott DG. Epidemiology of systemic vasculitis. Curr Rheumatol Rep 2005;7:270-75.
7. Reinhold-Keller E, Herlyn K, Wagner-Bastmeyer R, Gross WL. Stable incidence of primary systemic vasculitides over five years: Results from the German vasculitis register. Arthritis Rheum 2005;53:93-99.
8. Bambery P, Sakhuja V, Gupta A, Behera D, Kaur U, Bhusnurmath SR, Jindal SK, Malik SK, Deodhar SD, Chugh KS. Wegener's granulomatosis in north India. An analysis of eleven patients. Rheumatol Int 1987;7:243-47.
9. Malik SK, Deodhar SD, Chugh KS. Wegener's granulomatosis in north India. An analysis of eleven patients. Rheumatol Int 1987;7:243-47.
10. Bambery P, Gupta A, Sakhuja V, Kaur U, Gangwar DN, Jain IS, Deodhar SD. Ocular manifestations of Wegener's granulomatosis in north India. Sarcoidosis 1988;5:132-35.
11. Bambery P, Katariya S, Sakhuja V, Kaur U, Behera D, Malik SK, Deodhar SD. Wegener's granulomatosis in north India. Radiologic manifestations in eleven patients. Acta Radiol 1988;29:11-13.
12. Malaviya AN, Kumar A, Singh YN, Singh RR, Dash SC, Khare SD, Wali JP, Sharma SK, Handa R, Saluja S. Wegener's granulomatosis in India: Not so rare. Br J Rheumatol 1990;29:499-500.
13. Bambery P, Sakhuja V, Bhusnurmath SR, Jindal SK, Deodhar SD, Chugh KS. Wegener's granulomatosis: Clinical experience with eighteen patients. J Assoc Physicians India 1992;40:597-600.
14. Singh YN, Malaviya AN, Sharma SK, Kumar A, Wali JP, Dash SC, Bhuyan UN. Wegener's granulomatosis in northern India. J Assoc Physicians India. 1992;40:594-96.
14a. Kumar A, Pandhi A, Menon A, Sharma SK, Pande JN, Malaviya AN. Wegener's granulomatosis in India: Clinical features, treatment and outcome of twenty five patients. The Indian Journal of Chest Diseases and Allied Sciences 2001;43:1-7.
14b. Kaushal R, Dash SC, Kapur S, Bhuyan UN. Wegener's granulomatosis with rapidly progressive glomerulonephritis. J Assoc Physicians India 1987; 35:382-84.
15. Alarcon-Segovia D. The necrotizing vasculitides. A new pathogenic classification. Clin North Am1977;61:241-60.
16. Fauci AS, Haynes BF, Katz P. The spectrum of vasculitis: Clinical, pathologic, immunologic, and therapeutic considerations. Ann Intern Med 1978;89:660.
17. Cupps TR, Fauci AS. The vasculitic syndromes. Adv Intern Med 1982;27:315-44.
18. Leavitt RY, Fauci AS. Pulmonary vasculitis. Am Rev Respir Med 1986;134:149-66.
19. Leibow AA. Pulmonary angiitis and granulomatosis. Am Rev Respir Dis 1973;108:1-18.
20. DeRemee RA, Weiland MH, McDonald TJ. Respiratory vasculitis. Mayo Clin Proc 1980;55:492-98.
21. Edwards CW. Vaculitis and granulomatosis of the respiratory tract. Thorax 1982;37:81.
22. Chandler DB, Fulmer JD. Pulmonary vasculitis. Lung 1985;1985;163:257-73.
23. Cole SR, Johnson KJ, Ward PA. Pathology of sarcoidosis, granulomatous vasculitis, and other idiopathic granulomatous diseases of the lung. In sarcoidosis and other granulomatous diseases of the lung. In Lung Biology in Health and Disease: Fanburg BLP (Ed). Marcel Dekker, New York 1983;149.
24. Sawicka EH. The necrotizing vasculitides. Thorax 1987;42:913-17.
25. Hunder GG, Arend WP, Bloch DA, Calabrese LH, Fauci AS, Fries JF, et al. The American College of Rheumatology 1990 criteria for the classification of vasculitis. Introduction. Arthritis Rheum 1990;33:1065-67.
26. Bloch DA, Michel BA, Hunder GG, McShane DJ, Arend WP, Calabrese LH, et al. The American College of Rheumatology 1990 criteria for the classification of vasculitis. Patients and methods. Arthritis Rheum 1990;33:1068-72.
27. Bloch DA, Moses LE, Michel BA. Statistical approaches to classification. Methods for developing classification and other criteria rules. Arthritis Rheum 1990;33:1137-44.
28. Fries JF, Hunder GG, Bloch DA, Michel BA, Arend WP, Calabrese LH, et al. The American College of Rheumatology 1990 criteria for the classification of vasculitis. Summary. Arthritis Rheum 1990;33:1135-36.
29. Arnett FC, Edworthy SM, Bloch DA, McShane DJ, Fries JF, Cooper NS, et al. The American Rheumatism Association 1987 revised criteria for the classification of rheumatoid arthritis. Arthritis Rheum 1988;31:315-24.
30. Altman R, Asch E, Bloch D, Bole G, Borenstein D, Brandt K, et al. Development of criteria for the classification

and reporting of osteoarthritis. Classification of osteoarthritis of the knee. Diagnostic and Therapeutic Criteria Committee of the American Rheumatism Association. Arthritis Rheum 1986;29:1039-49.

31. Altman R, Alarcon G, Appelrouth D, Bloch D, Borenstein D, Brandt K, et al. The American College of Rheumatology criteria for the classification and reporting of osteoarthritis of the hand. Arthritis Rheum 1990;33:1601-10.

32. Altman R, Alarcon G, Appelrouth D, Bloch D, Borenstein D, Brandt K, et al. The American College of Rheumatology criteria for the classification and reporting of osteoarthritis of the hip. Arthritis Rheum 1991;34:505-14.

33. Tan EM, Cohen AS, Fries JF, Masi AT, McShane DJ, Rothfield NF, et al. The 1982 revised criteria for the classification of systemic lupus erythematosus. Arthritis Rheum 1982;25:1271-77.

34. Panush RS, Schur PH. Is it lupus? Bull Rheum Dis 1997;46:3-8.

35. Michel BA. Classification of vasculitis. Curr Opin Rheumatol 1992;4:3-8.

36. Rao JK, Allen NB, Pincus T. Limitations of the 1990 American College of Rheumatology Classification Criteria in the diagnosis of vasculitis. Am J Med 1998;129:345-52.

37. Bambery P, Bhushnurmath B, Jindal SK, Datta BN. Pulmonary vasculitis: An Indian perspective. Semin Respir Med 1991;12:115.

38. Savige J, Davies D, Falk RJ, Jennette JC, Wiik A. Antineutrophil cytoplasmic antibodies and associated diseases: A review of the clinical and laboratory features. A kidney Int 2000;57:846-62.

39. Hoffman GS, Kerr GS, Leavitt RY, Hallahan CW, Lebovics RS, Travis WD, Rottem M, Fauci AS. Wegener granulomatosis: An analysis of 158 patients. Ann Intern Med 1992;116:488-98.

40. Aasarod K, Iversen BM, Hammerstrom J, Bostad L, Vatten L, Jorstad S. Wegener's granulomatosis: Clinical course in 108 patients with renal involvement. Nephrol Dial Transplant 2000;15:611-18.

41. Nachman PH, Hogan SL, Jennette JC, Falk RJ. Treatment response and relapse in antineutrophil cytoplasmic autoanti-body-associated microscopic polyangiitis and glomerulonephritis. J Am Soc Nephrol 1996;7:33-39.

42. Soding PF, Lockwood CM, Park GR. The intensive care of patients with fulminant vasculitis. Anaesth Intensive Care 1994, 22:81-89.

43. Jones GL, Lukaris AD, Prabhu HV, Brown MJ, Bondeson J. Wegener's granulomatosis mimicking a parotid abscess. J Laryngol Otol 2005;119:746-49.

44. de Leeuw K, Kallenberg C, Bijl M. Accelerated atherosclerosis in patients with systemic autoimmune diseases. Ann NY Acad Sci 2005;1051:362-71.

45. Ponniah I, Shaheen A, Shankar KA, Kumaran MG. Wegener's granulomatosis: The current understanding. Oral Surg Oral Med Oral Pathol Oral Radiol Endod 2005;100:265-70.

46. Shah SP, Larkin G. Wegener's granulomatosis and mucous membrane pemphigoid: A diagnostic challenge of coexisting autoimmune disease. Eye 2006;20(7):856-58.

47. Shoda H, Kanda H, Tanaka R, Komagata Y, Misaki Y, Yamamoto K. Wegener's granulomatosis with eosinophilia. Intern Med 2005;44:750-53.

48. Jansen TL, van Houte D, de Vries T, Wolthuis A. ANCA seropositivity in HIV: A serological pitfall. Neth J Med 2005;63:270-74.

49. Short J, McKinney AM, Lucato LT, Teksam M, Truwit CL. Transalar encephalocele associated with Wegener's granulomatosis and meningeal enhancement: Case report. AJNR Am J Neuroradiol 2005;26:1873-75.

50. Peachell MB, Muller NL. Pulmonary vasculitis. Semin Respir Crit Care Med 2004;25:483-89.

51. Arista S, Sailler L, Astudillo L. Relapsing esophageal and gastric ulcers revealing Wegener's granulomatosis. Am J Med 2005;118:923-4.

52. Wang CR, Chang JM, Shen WL, Lin WJ, Lee JY, Liu MF. An unusual presentation of Wegener's granulomatosis mimicking thymoma. Ann Rheum Dis 2005;64:1238-40.

53. Gaber KA, Ryley NG, Macdermott JP, Goldman JM. Wegener's granulomatosis involving prostate. Urology 2005;66:195.

54. Langford CA. Vasculitis in the geriatric population. Clin Geriatr Med 2005;21(3):631-47.

55. Ahmed Hel S, Linthicum FH Jr. Wegener's granuloma. Otol Neurotol 2005;26(3):548-49.

56. Naz SM, Fairburn K. Pseudotumor of the breast: An unusual presentation of Wegener's granulomatosis. Breast J 2005;11:295-96.

57. Maramattom BV, Giannini C, Manno EM, Wijdicks EF. Wegener's granulomatosis and vertebro-basilar thrombosis. Cerebrovasc Dis 2005;20:65-68.

58. Feldmann H. A historic case of Wegener's granulomatosis: The physicist who discovered the electromagnetic waves: Heinrich Hertz. Laryngorhinootologie 2005;84:426-31.

59. Tumiati B, Zuccoli G, Pavone L, Buzio C. ENT Wegener's granulomatosis can hide severe central nervous system involvement. Clin Rheumatol 2005;24:290-93.

60. Onal IK, Ozcakar L, Temirel K, Aran R, Kurt M. Fatal endocarditis in Wegener's granulomatosis: Mitral valve involvement and an intracardiac mass. Joint Bone Spine 2005;72(6):585-87.

61. Düzgün N, Morris Y, Güllü S, Gürsoy A, Ensari A, Kumbasar OO, Duman M. Diabetes insipidus presentation before renal and pulmonary features in a patient with Wegener's granulomatosis. Rheumatol Int 2005; 26(1):80-82.

62. Rosmarakis ES, Kapaskelis AM, Rafailidis PI, Falagas ME. Association between Wegener's granulomatosis and increased antithyroid antibodies: Report of two cases and review of the literature. Int J Clin Pract. 2005;59:373-75.

63. [No authors listed] Summaries for patients. Venous thrombosis in Wegener granulomatosis. Ann Intern Med. 2005;142:154.

64. Krambeck AE, Miller DV, Blute ML. Wegener's granulomatosis presenting as renal mass: A case for nephron-sparing surgery. Urology 2005;65:798.

65. Said G, Lacroix C. Primary and secondary vasculitic neuropathy. J Neurol. 2005;252:633-41.

66. Bertelmann E, Liekfeld A, Pleyer U, Hartmann C. Cytomegalovirus retinitis in Wegener's granulomatosis: Case report and review of the literature. Acta Ophthalmol Scand 2005;83:258-61.

67. Ulinski T, Martin H, Mac Gregor B, Dardelin R, Cochat P. Fatal neurologic involvement in pediatric Wegener's granulomatosis. Pediatr Neurol. 2005;32:278-81.

68. Deurenberg RH, Nieuwenhuis RF, Driessen C, London N, Stassen FR, van Tiel FH, Stobberingh EE, Vink C. The prevalence of the *Staphylococcus aureus* tst gene among community- and hospital-acquired strains and isolates from Wegener's Granulomatosis patients. FEMS Microbiol Lett 2005;245:185-89.

69. Rosmarakis ES, Kapaskelis AM, Kasiakou SK, Falagas ME. Case report: Wegener's granulomatosis presents as pulmonary infection. Am Fam Physician 2005; 71:1062, 1064. Erratum in: Am Fam Physician 2005; 72:574.

70. Strivens RL, Bateman A, Arden NK, Edwards CJ. Intestinal perforation and jejunal haemorrhage due to Wegener's granulomatosis. Clin Exp Rheumatol 2005;23:124.

71. Talar-Williams C, Sneller MC, Langford CA, Smith JA, Cox TA, Robinson MR. Orbital socket contracture: A complication of inflammatory orbital disease in patients with Wegener's granulomatosis. Br J Ophthalmol 2005;89:493-97.

72. Costello F, Gilberg S, Karsh J, Burns B, Leonard B. Bilateral simultaneous central retinal artery occlusions in wegener granulomatosis. J Neuroophthalmol 2005;25:29-32.

73. Monteiro ML, Borges WI, do Val Ferreira Ramos C, Lucato LT, Leite CC. Bilateral optic neuritis in wegener granulomatosis. J Neuroophthalmol 2005;25:25-28.

74. Keni SP, Wiley EL, Dutra JC, Mellott AL, Barr WG, Altman KW. Skull base Wegener's granulomatosis resulting in multiple cranial neuropathies. Am J Otolaryngol 2005;26:146-49.

75. Dimeo DE, Ferguson PJ, Bishop WP. An unusual intestinal presentation of C-ANCA/PR-3 positive vasculitis in a child. J Pediatr Gastroenterol Nutr 2005;40:368-70.

76. Tsironi E, Eftaxias B, Karabatsas CH, Ioachim E, Kalogeropoulos C, Psilas K. An unusually longstanding, strictly ocular, limited form of Wegener's granulomatosis. Acta Ophthalmol Scand 2005;83:123-25.

77. Sarraf P, Sneller MC. Pathogenesis of Wegener's granulomatosis: Current concepts. Expert Rev Mol Med 2005;7:1-19.

78. Voswinkel J, Muller A, Lamprecht P. Is PR3-ANCA Formation Initiated in Wegener's Granulomatosis Lesions? Granulomas as Potential Lymphoid Tissue Maintaining autoantibody Production. Ann NY Acad Sci 2005;1051:12-19.

79. van Rossum AP, Limburg PC, Kallenberg CG. Activation, apoptosis, and clearance of neutrophils in Wegener's granulomatosis. Ann NY Acad Sci 2005; 1051:1-11.

80. Heeringa P, Schreiber A, Falk RJ, Jennette JC. Pathogenesis of pulmonary vasculitis. Semin Respir Crit Care Med 2004;25:465-74.

81. Hattar K, van Burck S, Bickenbach A, Grandel U, Maus U, Lohmeyer J, Csernok E, Hartung T, Seeger W, Grimminger F, Sibelius U. Anti-proteinase 3 antibodies (c-ANCA) prime CD14-dependent leukocyte activation. J Leukoc Biol 2005;78(4):992-1000.

82. Hagen EC, Daha MR, Hermans J, Andrassy K, Csernok E, Gaskin G, Lesavre P, Ludemann J, Rasmussen N, Sinico RA, et al. Diagnostic value of standardized assays for anti-neutrophil cytoplasmic antibodies in idiopathic systemic vasculitis. EC/BCR project for ANCA assay standardization. Kidney Int 1998;53:743-53.

83. Jennette JC, Wilkman AS, Falk RJ. Diagnostic predictive value of ANCA serology. Kidney Int 1998, 53:796-98.

84. Fauci AS, Haynes BF, Katz P, Wolff SM. Wegener's Granulomatosis: Prospective clinical and therapeutic experience with 85 patients over 21 years. Ann Intern Med 1983;98:76-85.

85. van der Woude FJ, Rasmussen N, Lobatto S, Wiik A, Permin H, van Es LA, et al. Autoantibodies against neutrophils and monocytes: A new tool for diagnosis and marker of disease activity in Wegener's granulomatosis. Lancet 1985;1:425-29.

86. Csernok E, Muller A, Gross WL. Immunopathology of ANCA-associated vasculitis. Intern Med 1999;38:759-65.

87. Hagen EC, Andrassy K, Csernok E, Daha MR, Gaskin G, Gross W, et al. The value of indirect immunofluorescence and solid phase techniques for ANCA detection: A report on the first phase of an international cooperative study on the standardization of ANCA assays. EEC/BCR Group for ANCA Assay Standardization. J Immunol Methods 1993;159:1-16.

88. Badakere SS, Pradhan VD. ANCA: Anti-neutrophil cytoplasmic antibodies and their role in vasculitis associated kidney disorders. Indian J Med Sci 2002;56: 335-39.

89. Jenne DE, Tschopp J, Ludemann J, Utecht B, Gross WL. Wegener's autoantigen decoded. Nature 1990;346:520.

90. Rao JK, Weinberger M, Oddone EZ, Allen NB, Landsman P, Feussner JR. The role of antineutrophil cytoplasmic antibody (c-ANCA) testing in the diagnosis of Wegener granulomatosis. A literature review and meta-analysis. Ann Intern Med 1995;123:925-32.

91. Sinico RA, Radice A, Corace C, Ditoma L, Sabadini E. Value of a New Automated Fluorescence Immunoassay

(EliA) for PR3 and MPO-ANCA in Monitoring Disease Activity in ANCA-Associated Systemic Vasculitis. Ann NY Acad Sci 2005;1050:185-92.

92. Teixeira L, Mahr A, Jaureguy F, Noel LH, Nunes H, Lefort A, Barry S, Deny P, Guillevin L. Low seroprevalence and poor specificity of antineutrophil cytoplasmic antibodies in tuberculosis. Rheumatology 2005;44:247-50.

93. Neumann IS, Mirzaei R, Birck K, Osinger R, Waldherr HD, Kohn, FT Meisl. Expression of somatostatin receptors in inflammatory lesions and diagnostic value of somatostatin receptor scintigraphy in patients with ANCA-associated small vessel vasculitis. Rheumatology 2004;43:195-201.

94. Blundell G, Roe S. Wegener's granulomatosis presenting as a pleural effusion. Br Med J 2003;327:95-96.

95. Campbell SM, Wernick R. Update in rheumatology. Ann Intern Med 1999;130:135-42.

96. Merkel PA, Polisson RP, Chang Y, Skates SJ, Niles JL. Prevalence of antineutrophil cytoplasmic antibodies in a Large Inception Cohort of Patients with Connective Tissue Disease. Ann Intern Med 1997;126:866-73.

97. Malnick SDH, Evron E, Sthoeger ZM. Testing with antineutrophil cytoplasmic antibody to diagnose. Wegener Granulomatosis. Ann Intern Med 1996; 125:622.

98. Hoffman GS. Testing with antineutrophil cytoplasmic antibody to diagnose wegener granulomatosis. Ann Intern Med 1996;125:622.

99. Mandl LA, Solomon DH, Smith EL, Lew RA, Katz JN, Shmerling RH. Using antineutrophil cytoplasmic antibody testing to diagnose vasculitis: Can test-ordering guidelines improve diagnostic accuracy? Archives of Internal Medicine 2002;162:1509-14.

100. Schönermarck U, Lamprecht P, Csernok E, Gross WL. Prevalence and spectrum of rheumatic diseases associated with proteinase 3-antineutrophil cytoplasmic antibodies (ANCA) and myeloperoxidase-ANCA. Rheumatology 2001;40:178-84.

101. Gross WL, Trabandt A, Reinhold-Keller E. Diagnosis and evaluation of vasculitis. Rheumatology 2000;39:245-52.

102. Potter MB, Fincher RK, Finger DR. Eosinophilia in Wegener's Granulomatosis. Chest 1999;116:1480-83.

103. Vassilopoulos D, Hoffman G. Clinical utility of testing for antineutrophil cytoplasmic antibodies. Clin Diagn Lab Immunol 1999;6:645-51.

104. Langford CA, Hoffman GS. Rare diseases bullet 3: Wegener's granulomatosis. Thorax 1999;54:629-37.

105. Wong SN, Shah V, Dillon MJ. Antineutrophil cytoplasmic antibodies in Wegener's granulomatosis. Arch Dis Child1998;79:246-250.

106. Pradhan VD, Badakere SS, Ghosh K, Almeida A. ANCA: Serology in Wegener's granulomatosis. Indian J Med Sci 2005;59:292-300.

107. Sinico RA, Radice A, Corace C, DI Toma L, Sabadini E. Value of a new automated fluorescence immuno-assay (EliA) for PR3 and MPO-ANCA in monitoring disease activity in ANCA-associated systemic vasculitis. Ann N Y Acad Sci 2005;1050:185-92.

108. Van Rossum AP, van der Geld YM, Limburg PC, Kallenberg CG. Human anti-neutrophil cytoplasm autoantibodies to proteinase 3 (PR3-ANCA) bind to neutrophils. Kidney Int 2005;68:537-41.

109. Damoiseaux JG, Slot MC, Vaessen M, Stegeman CA, Van Paassen P, Cohen Tervaert JW. Evaluation of a new fluorescent-enzyme immuno-assay for diagnosis and follow-up of ANCA-associated vasculitis. J Clin Immunol 2005;25:202-08.

110. Schultz DR, Diego JM. Antineutrophil cytoplasmic antibodies (ANCA) and systemic vasculitis: Update of assays, immunopathogenesis, controversies and report of a novel De novo ANCA associated vasculitis after kidney transplantation. Semin in Arthritis Rheum 2000;29:267-85.

111. Boomsma MM, Stegeman CA, van der Leij MJ, Oost W, Hermans J, Kallenberg CG, et al. Prediction of relapses in Wegener's granulomatosis by measurement of anti-neutrophil cytoplasmic antibody test levels: A prospective study. Arthritis Rheum 2000;49:2025-33.

112. Han WK, Choi HK, Roth RM, McCluskey RT, Niles JL. Serial ANCA titers: Useful tool for prevention of relapses in ANCA- associated vasculitis. Kidney Int 2003; 63:1079-85.

113. Cooley P, Taylor KH, Czika W, Seifer C, Taylor JF. Analysis of a biomarker for Wegener's granulomatosis. Int J Immunogenet 2005;32:237-43.

114. Chanseaud Y, Tamby MC, Guilpain P, Reinbolt J, Kambouchner M, Boyer N, Noel LH, Guillevin L, Boissier MC, Mouthon L. Analysis of autoantibody repertoires in small- and medium-sized vessels vasculitides. Evidence for specific perturbations in polyarteritis nodosa, microscopic polyangiitis, Churg-Strauss syndrome and Wegener's granulomatosis. J Autoimmun 2005;24:169-79.

115. Lloyd G, Lund VJ, Beale T, Howard D. Rhinologic changes in Wegener's granulomatosis. J Laryngol Otol 2002;116:565-69.

116. Lohrmann C, Uhl M, Kotter E, Burger D, Ghanem N, Langer M. Pulmonary manifestations of wegener granulomatosis: CT findings in 57 patients and a review of the literature. Eur J Radiol 2005;53:471-77.

117. Kaushik ML, Sinha PK, Pandey D, Pal LS, Kashyap S. Limited Wegener's granulomatosis presenting as multiple lung nodules. Indian J Chest Dis Allied Sci. 2004;46:39-42.

118. Koldingsnes W, Jacobsen EA, Sildnes T, Hjalmarsen A, Nossent HC. Pulmonary function and high-resolution CT findings five years after disease onset in patients

with Wegener's granulomatosis. Scand J Rheumatol 2005;34:220-28.

119. Semple D, Keogh J, Forni L, Venn R. Clinical review: Vasculitis on the intensive care unit—part 1: Diagnosis. Critical Care 2005,9:92-97.

120. Travis WD. Pathology of pulmonary vasculitis. Semin Respir Crit Care Med 2004;25:475-82.

121. Ferrario F, Rastaldi MP. Histopathological atlas of renal diseases: ANCA-associated vasculitis (first part). J Nephrol 2005;18:113-16.

122. Ferrario F, Rastaldi MP. Histopathological atlas of renal diseases: ANCA-associated vasculitis (Second part). J Nephrol 2005;18:217-20.

123. Lesavre P, Noel LH. ANCA-negative pauci-immune renal vasculitis: Histology and outcome. Nephrol Dial Transplant 2005;20:1392-99.

124. Leavitt RY, Fauci AS, Bloch DA, Michel BA, Hunder GG, Arend WP, Calabrese LH, Fries JF, Lie JT, Lightfoot RW Jr, et al. The American College of Rheumatology 1990 criteria for the classification of Wegener's granulomatosis. Arthritis Rheum 1990;33:1101-07.

125. Marder W, McCune WJ. Advances in immunosuppressive drug therapy for use in autoimmune disease and systemic vasculitis. Semin Respir Crit Care Med 2004;25:581-94.

126. Lynch JP, White E, Tazelaar H, Langford CA. Wegener's granulomatosis: Evolving concepts in treatment. Semin Respir Crit Care Med 2004;25:491-521.

127. Specks U. Methotrexate for Wegener's granulomatosis: What is the evidence? Arthritis Rheum 2005;52:2237-42.

128. Kokolina E, Alexopoulos E, Dimitriadis C, Vainas A, Giamalis P, Papagianni A, Ekonomidou D, Memmos D. Immunosuppressive therapy and clinical evolution in forty-nine patients with antineutrophil cytoplasmic antibody-associated glomerulonephritis. Ann N Y Acad Sci 2005;1051:597-605.

129. Seo P, Min YI, Holbrook JT, Hoffman GS, Merkel PA, Spiera R, Davis JC, Ytterberg SR, St Clair EW, McCune WJ, Specks U, Allen NB, Luqmani RA, Stone JH. WGET Research Group. Damage caused by Wegener's granulomatosis and its treatment: Prospective data from the Wegener's Granulomatosis Etanercept Trial (WGET). Arthritis Rheum 2005;52:2168-78.

130. Benenson E, Fries JW, Heilig B, Pollok M, Rubbert A. High-dose azathioprine pulse therapy as a new treatment option in patients with active Wegener's granulomatosis and lupus nephritis refractory or intolerant to cyclophosphamide. Clin Rheumatol 2005;24:251-57.

131. Omdal R, Wildhagen K, Hansen T, Gunnarsson R, Kristoffersen G. Anti-CD20 therapy of treatment-resistant Wegener's granulomatosis: Favourable but temporary response. Scand J Rheumatol 2005;34:229-32.

132. Eriksson P. Nine patients with anti-neutrophil cytoplasmic antibody-positive vasculitis successfully treated with rituximab. J Intern Med 2005;257:540-48.

133. Bachmeyer C, Cadranel JF, Demontis R. Rituximab is an alternative in a case of contraindication of cyclophosphamide in Wegener's granulomatosis. Nephrol Dial Transplant 2005;20:1274.

134. Ferraro AJ, Day CJ, Drayson MT, Savage CO. Effective therapeutic use of rituximab in refractory Wegener's granulomatosis. Nephrol Dial Transplant 2005;20:622-25.

135. Balasubramanian SK, Tiruvoipati R, Chatterjee S, Sosnowski A, Firmin RK. Extracorporeal membrane oxygenation with lepirudin anticoagulation for Wegener's granulomatosis with heparin-induced thrombocytopenia. ASAIO J 2005;51:477-79.

136. Tsukamoto H, Nagafuji K, Horiuchi T, Miyamoto T, Aoki K, Takase K, Henzan H, Himeji D, Koyama T, Miyake K, Inoue Y, Nakashima H, Otsuka T, Tanaka Y, Nagasawa K, Harada M. A Phase I-II Trial of autologous peripheral blood stem cell transplantation in the treatment of refractory autoimmune disease. Ann Rheum Dis 2006;65(4):508-14.

137. Goek ON, Stone JH. Randomized controlled trials in vasculitis associated with anti-neutrophil cytoplasmic antibodies. Curr Opin Rheumatol 2005;17:257-64.

138. Merkel PA, Lo GH, Holbrook JT, Tibbs AK, Allen NB, Davis JC Jr, Hoffman GS, McCune WJ, St Clair EW, Specks U, Spiera R, Petri M, Stone JH. Wegener's Granulomatosis Etanercept Trial Research Group. Brief communication: High incidence of venous thrombotic events among patients with Wegener granulomatosis: The Wegener's clinical occurrence of thrombosis (WeCLOT) study. Ann Intern Med 2005;142:620-6. Summary for patients in: Ann Intern Med 2005;142:I54.

139. Schmitt WH, Birck R, Heinzel PA, Gobel U, Choi M, Warnatz K, Peter HH, van der Woude FJ. Prolonged treatment of refractory Wegener's granulomatosis with 15-deoxyspergualin: An open study in seven patients. Nephrol Dial Transplant 2005;20:1083-92.

140. Torheim EA, Yndestad A, Bjerkeli V, Halvorsen B, Aukrust P, Froland SS. Increased expression of chemokines in patients with Wegener's granulomatosis-modulating effects of methylprednisolone in vitro. Clin Exp Immunol 2005;140:376-83.

141. Bellisai F, Morozzi G, Marcolongo R, Galeazzi M. Pregnancy in Wegener's granulomatosis: Successful treatment with intravenous immunoglobulin. Clin Rheumatol. 2004;23:533-35.

142. Semple D, Keogh J, Forni L, Venn R. Clinical review: Vasculitis on the intensive care unit—part 2: Treatment and prognosis. Crit Care 2005;9:193-97.

143. Daikeler T, Erley C, Mohren M, Amberger C, Einsele H, Kanz L, Kotter I. Fever and increasing cANCA titre after kidney and autologous stem cell transplantation for Wegener's granulomatosis. Ann Rheum Dis 2005;64:646-47.

144. Stone JH, Rajapakse VN, Hoffman GS, Specks U, Merkel PA, Spiera RF, Davis JC, St Clair EW, McCune J, Ross S, Hitt BA, Veenstra TD, Conrads TP, Liotta LA, Petricoin EF 3rd. Wegener's Granulomatosis Etanercept Trial Research Group. A serum proteomic approach to gauging the state of remission in Wegener's granulomatosis. Arthritis Rheum 2005;52: 902-10.

145. Kawakami T, Soma Y, Kawasaki K, Kawase A, Mizoguchi M. Initial cutaneous manifestations consistent with mononeuropathy multiplex in Churg-Strauss Syndrome. Arch Dermatol 2005;141:873-78.

146. Clutterbuck EJ, Evans DJ, Pusey CD. Renal involvement in Churg–Strauss syndrome. Nephrol Dial Transplant 1990;5:161-67.

147. Conron M, Beynon HL. Churg-Strauss syndrome. Thorax 2000, 55:870-77.

148. Sinico RA, Di Toma L, Maggiore U, Bottero P, Radice A, Tosoni C, Grasselli C, Pavone L, Gregorini G, Monti S, Frassi M, Vecchio F, Corace C, Venegoni E, Buzio C. Prevalence and clinical significance of antineutrophil cytoplasmic antibodies in Churg-Strauss syndrome. Arthritis Rheum 2005;52:2926-35.

149. Masi AT, Hunder GG, Lie JT, Michel BA, Bloch DA, Arend WP, Calabrese LH, Edworthy SM, Fauci AS, Leavitt RY, et al. The American College of Rheumatology 1990 criteria for the classification of Churg-Strauss syndrome (allergic granulomatosis and angiitis). Arthritis Rheum 1990;33:1094-100.

150. Heller I, Isakov A, Topilsky M. American College of Rheumatology criteria for the diagnosis of vasculitis. Ann Intern Med 1999;130:861.

151. Hasley PB, Follansbee WP, Coulehan JL. Cardiac manifestations of Churg-Strauss syndrome: Report of a case and review of the literature. Am Heart J 1990;120:996-99.

152. Watts RA, Scott DGI, Pusey CD, Lockwood CM. Vasculitis—Aims of therapy. An overview. Rheumatology 2000;39:229-32.

153. Tatsis E, Schnabel A, Gross WL. Interferon-alpha treatment of four patients with the Churg-Strauss syndrome. Annals 1998;129:370-74.

154. Guillevin L, Mahr A, Callard P, Godmer P, Pagnoux C, Leray E, Cohen P. French Vasculitis Study Group. Hepatitis B virus-associated polyarteritis nodosa: Clinical characteristics, outcome, and impact of treatment in 115 patients. Medicine (Baltimore) 2005;84:313-22.

155. Fathalla BM, Miller L, Brady S, Schaller JG. Cutaneous polyarteritis nodosa in children. J Am Acad Dermatol 2005;53:724-28.

156. Colmegna I, Maldonado-Cocco JA. Polyarteritis nodosa revisited. Curr Rheumatol Rep 2005;7:288-96.

157. Bourgarit A, Le Toumelin P, Pagnoux C, Cohen P, Mahr A, Le Guern V, Mouthon L, Guillevin L. French Vasculitis Study Group. Deaths occurring during the first year after treatment onset for polyarteritis nodosa, microscopic polyangiitis, and Churg-Strauss syndrome: A retrospective analysis of causes and factors predictive of mortality based on 595 patients. Medicine (Baltimore). 2005;84:323-30.

158. Kraemer M, Linden D, Berlit P. The spectrum of differential diagnosis in neurological patients with livedo reticularis and livedo racemosa A literature review. J Neurol 2005;252(10):1155-66.

159. Kato T, Fujii K, Ishii E, Wada R, Hidaka Y. A case of polyarteritis nodosa with lesions of the superior mesenteric artery illustrating the diagnostic usefulness of three-dimensional computed tomographic angiography. Clin Rheumatol 2005;24(6):628-31.

160. MacLaren K, Gillespie J, Shrestha S, Neary D, Ballardie FW. Primary angiitis of the central nervous system: Emerging variants. QJM 2005;98:643-54.

161. Ozen S. Problems in classifying vasculitis in children. Pediatr Nephrol 2005;20:1214-18.

162. Reddy SM, Pui JC, Gold LI, Mitnick HJ. Postirradiation morphea and subcutaneous polyarteritis nodosa: Case report and literature review. Semin Arthritis Rheum 2005;34:728-34.

163. Chanseaud Y, Tamby MC, Guilpain P, Reinbolt J, Kambouchner M, Boyer N, Noel LH, Guillevin L, Boissier MC, Mouthon L. Analysis of autoantibody repertoires in small and medium-sized vessels vasculitides. Evidence for specific perturbations in polyarteritis nodosa, microscopic polyangiitis, Churg-Strauss syndrome and Wegener's granulomatosis. J Autoimmun 2005;24:169-79.

164. Topaloglu R, Kazik M, Saatci I, Kalyoncu M, Cil BE, Akalan N. An unusual presentation of classic polyarteritis nodosa in a child. Pediatr Nephrol 2005;20: 1011-15.

165. Stephens RS, Brown C, Wiener CM. Persistent lower abdominal and groin pain: What is the diagnosis? Am J Med 2005;118:364-67.

166. Misdraji J, Graeme-Cook FM. Miscellaneous conditions of the appendix. Semin Diagn Pathol 2004;21:151-63.

167. Said G, Lacroix C. Primary and secondary vasculitic neuropathy. J Neurol 2005;252:633-41.

168. Fourcade G, Lequellec A, Blard JM, Pages M. Cerebral angiitis caused by periarteritis nodosa. Rev Neurol (Paris). 2005;161:323-25.

169. Lederlin M, Cales V, Parent Y, Strainchamps P. What is your diagnosis? J Radiol 2005;86(2 Pt 1):177-80.

170. Fernandes SR, Samara AM, Magalhaes EP, Sachetto Z, Metze K. Acute cholecystitis at initial presentation of polyarteritis nodosa. Clin Rheumatol 2005;24(6):625-27.

171. Mason A, Theal J, Bain V, Adams E, Perrillo R. Hepatitis B virus replication in damaged endothelial tissues of patients with extrahepatic disease. Am J Gastroenterol 2005;100:972-76.

172. Semple D, Keogh J, Forni L, Venn R. Clinical review: Vasculitis on the intensive care unit—part 2: Treatment and prognosis. Crit Care 2005;9:193-97.

173. Guillevin L, Lhote F, Jarrousse B, Bironne P, Barrier J, Deny P, Trepo C, Kahn MF, Godeau P. Polyarteritis nodosa related to hepatitis B virus. A retrospective study of 66 patients. Ann Med Interne (Paris) 1992; (Suppl 1):63-74.

174. Guillevin L, Le Thi Huong D, Godeau P, Jais P, Wechsler B. Clinical findings and prognosis of polyarteritis nodosa and Churg-Strauss angiitis: A study in 165 patients. Br J Rheumetol. 1988;27(4):258-64.

175. Lightfoot RW, Michel BA, Bloch DA, Hunder GG, Zvaifler NJ, McShane DJ, et al. The American College of Rheumatology 1990 criteria for the classification of polyarteritis nodosa. Arthritis Rheum 1990;33:1088-93.

176. de Dios Garcia-Diaz J, Garcia-Sanchez M, Busteros JI, Arcos P. Polyarteritis nodosa after interferon treatment for chronic hepatitis C. J Clin Virol 2005;32:181-82.

177. Levy Y, Uziel Y, Zandman G, Rotman P, Amital H, Sherer Y, Langevitz P, Goldman B, Shoenfeld Y. Response of vasculitic peripheral neuropathy to intravenous immunoglobulin. Ann NY Acad Sci 2005;1051:779-86.

178. Dauphine C, Kovar J, de Virgilio C. Successful non-operative management of acute intraperitoneal hemorrhage due to undiagnosed polyarteritis nodosa. Ann Vasc Surg 2005;19:724-27.

179. Al-Bishri J, le Riche N, Pope JE. Refractory polyarteritis nodosa successfully treated with infliximab. J Rheumatol 2005;32:1371-73.

180. Guillevin L. Virus-induced systemic vasculitides: New therapeutic approaches. Clin Dev Immunol 2004;11:227-31.

181. Ozen S, Anton J, Arisoy N, Bakkaloglu A, Besbas N, Brogan P, et al. Juvenile polyarteritis: Results of a multicenter survey of 110 children. J Pediatr 2004; 145:517-22.

182. Alberts WM. Eosinophilic interstitial lung disease. Curr Opin Pulm Med 2004;10:419-24.

183. Alves dos Santos JW, Torres A, Michel GT, de Figueiredo CW, Mileto JN, Foletto VG Jr, de Nobrega Cavalcanti MA. Non-infectious and unusual infectious mimics of community-acquired pneumonia. Respir Med 2004;98:488-94.

184. Paterson DL. New clinical presentations of invasive aspergillosis in non-conventional hosts. Clin Microbiol Infect 2004;10 (Suppl 1):24-30.

185. Moltyaner Y, Geerts WH, Chamberlain DW, Heyworth PG, Noack D, Rae J, Doyle JJ, Downey GP. Underlying chronic granulomatous disease in a patient with bronchocentric granulomatosis. Thorax 2003;58:1096-98.

186. Kim DH, Lee JH, Kim BH, Choi EK, Park JS, Kim KY, Choi YH, Myong NH, Lee KY. Chronic necrotizing bronchopulmonary aspergillosis with elements of bronchocentric granulomatosis. Korean J Intern Med 2002;17:138-42.

187. Yano S, Shishido S, Kobayashi K, Nakano H, Kawasaki Y. Bronchocentric granulomatosis due to Aspergillus terreus in an immunocompetent and non-asthmatic woman. Respir Med 1999;93:672-74.

188. Yano S, Kobayashi K, Shishido S, Nakano H. Intra-bronchial aspergillus nidulans infection in an immuno-competent man. Intern Med 1999;38:372-75.

189. Giroir BP, Squires J. Bronchocentric granulomatosis in a nonasthmatic adolescent. Pediatr Infect Dis J 1989; 8:181-83.

190. Sulavik SB. Bronchocentric granulomatosis and allergic bronchopulmonary aspergillosis. Clin Chest Med 1988;9:609-21.

191. van der Klooster JM, Nurmohamed LA, van Kaam NA. Bronchocentric granulomatosis associated with influenza-A virus infection. Respiration 2004;71:412-16.

192. Houser SL, Mark EJ. Bronchocentric granulomatosis with mucus impaction due to bronchogenic carcinoma. An association with clinical relevance. Arch Pathol Lab Med 2000;124:1168-71.

193. Bonafede RP, Benatar SR. Bronchocentric granulomatosis and rheumatoid arthritis. Br J Dis Chest 1987;81:197-201.

194. Koss MN, Robinson RG, Hochholzer L. Bronchocentric granulomatosis. Hum Pathol 1981;12:632-38.

195. Robinson RG, Wehunt WD, Tsou E, Koss MN, Hochholzer L. Bronchocentric granulomatosis: Roentgenographic manifestations. Am Rev Respir Dis 1982;125:751-56.

196. Stephen JG, Braimbridge MV, Corrin B, Wilkinson SP, Day D, Whimster WF. Necrotizing 'sarcoidal' angiitis and granulomatosis of the lung. Thorax 1976;31:356-60.

197. Li LY, Zhu YJ, He ZG. Pulmonary angitis and granulomatosis. Zhonghua Nei Ke Za Zhi 1992;31:424-7,445.

198. Riono WP, Hidayat AA, Rao NA. Scleritis: A clinicopathologic study of 55 cases. Ophthalmology 1999;106: 1328-33.

199. Sørensen SF, Slot O, Tvede N, Petersen J. A prospective study of vasculitis patients collected in a five year period: Evaluation of the Chapel Hill nomenclature. Ann Rheum 2000;59:478-82.

200. Altaie R, Ditizio F, Fahy GT. Microscopic polyangitis presenting with subacute reversible optic neuropathy. Eye 2005;19:363-65.

201. Yamagata K, Hirayama K, Mase K, Yamaguchi N, Kobayashi M, Takahashi H, Koyama A. Apheresis for MPO-ANCA-associated RPGN-indications and efficacy: Lessons learned from Japan nationwide survey of RPGN. J Clin Apher 2005;20(4):244-51.

202. Nagata H, Teramoto K, Suwa A, Abe T, Kimura T, Shibata R. A 73-year-old man with confusion, fever, and positive MPO-ANCA.Keio J Med. 2004;53:103-14.

203. Gupta RK. Pauci-immune crescentic glomerulonephritis. Indian J Pathol Microbiol 2003;46:357-66.

204. Funauchi M, Nozaki Y, Hashimoto K, Suk Yoo B, Ohno M, Kinoshita K, Kanamaru A. Microscopic polyangitis as a possible cause of diabetes insipidus. Clin Rheumatol 2002;21:540.

205. Metaxaris G, Prokopakis EP, Karatzanis AD, Sakelaris G, Heras P, Velegrakis GA, Helidonis ES. Otolaryngo-logic manifestations of small vessel vasculitis. Auris Nasus Larynx 2002;29:353-56.

206. Bakkaloglu A, Ozen S, Baskin E, Besbas N, Gur-Guven A, Kasapcopur O, Tinaztepe K. The significance of anti-neutrophil cytoplasmic antibody in microscopic polyangitis and classic polyarteritis nodosa. Arch Dis Child 2001;85:427-30.

207. Stratta P, Messuerotti A, Canavese C, Coen M, Luccoli L, Bussolati B, Giorda L, Malavenda P, Cacciabue M, Bugiani M, Bo M, Ventura M, Camussi G, Fubini B. The role of metals in autoimmune vasculitis: Epidemiological and pathogenic study. Sci Total Environ 2001;270: 179-90.

208. Rott T, Vizjak A, Koselj M. ANCA-associated vasculitis—an autopsy study. Wien Klin Wochenschr. 2000;112: 671-75.

209. Ara J, Mirapeix E, Rodriguez R, Saurina A, Darnell A. Relationship between ANCA and disease activity in small vessel vasculitis patients with anti-MPO ANCA. Nephrol Dial Transplant 1999;141667-72.

Chapter
26

Lungs in Systemic Diseases

The connective tissue disorders (also called collagen vascular diseases) represent an heterogeneous group of immunologically-mediated inflammatory disorders with a large variety of affected organs besides the lungs. They are a group of systemic disorders characterized by inflammation of vessels, connective tissues, and serosal surfaces. The respiratory system may be involved in all its components: airways, vessels, parenchyma, pleura, respiratory muscles, etc. The frequency, clinical presentation, prognosis and response to therapy vary, depending on the pattern of involvement as well as on the underlying connective tissue disorders.[1] In this section the most frequent types of lung disorders observed in patients with connective tissue disease (CTD) will be discussed. Each of these disorders may be associated with lung involvement including interstitial lung disease. The pulmonary manifestations in each of these disorders will be discussed in brief.

RHEUMATOID ARTHRITIS

Rheumatoid arthritis (RA) is the most common CTD. Pulmonary involvement is quite common in rheumatoid arthritis, even preceding the development of the disease.[2-4] Clinical and radiological detection of lung involvement may be late; with the availability of high resolution CT (HRCT) scans the abnormalities can be picked up quite early.[5,6] The HRCT may be abnormal in about two-thirds of patients. The most frequent abnormalities are reticulonodular patterns, which are found in 63 percent, ground-glass attenuation (20%), and bronchiectasis (17%). Pulmonary function results are normal in 37 percent. Titers of rheumatoid factor and erythrocyte sedimentation rate are significantly higher in those who have abnormal HRCT findings. Higher Larsen's score, advanced age, and severe disease are significant risk factors for lung involvement and are statistically significant predictors of lung involvement in RA.

The pleuropulmonary manifestations of RA are varied, pleural abnormalities and interstitial lung disease being the more common. Although RA affects women preferentially, men are more affected by pleuropulmonary manifestations of the disease. Novel serologic markers, more specific than rheumatoid factor, may help the diagnosis of RA: keratins antibodies (AKA) and cyclic citrullinated peptide antibodies (anti-CCP). Sensitivity is highest for IgM rheumatoid factor (75%), followed by anti-CCP antibodies (68%) and AKA (46%). Specificity is highest for anti-CCP antibodies (96%), followed by AKA (94%) and IgM rheumatoid factor (74%).

The pulmonary manifestations of rheumatoid arthritis are:
1. Pleural involvement
   - Pleural effusion
   - Pneumothorax
   - Empyema
   - Bronchopleural fistula.
2. Parenchymal involvement
   - Interstitial lung disease
   - Fibrobullous disease
   - Caplan's syndrome
   - Rheumatoid nodules.
3. Airways involvement
   - Lung function changes
   - Bronchiolitis
   - Bronchiectasis
   - Crycoaretynoid arthritis.
4. Vascular involvement
   - Pulmonary arteritis
   - Pulmonary artery hypertension
   - Alveolar hemorrhage.
5. Malignancy
   - Bronchogenic carcinoma.
6. Infection.
7. Drug induced lung diseases.

Pleural Involvement

Pleural involvement with or without effusion is the most common manifestation of rheumatoid lung disease. The pleural as well as pericardial disease is frequently asymptomatic and may only be detected only on routine X-rays for other reasons. About a third of cases with pleural disease, will have associated intrapulmonary lung disease. Pleural involvement may be in the form of pleuritis and pleural effusions, pneumothorax, pyopneumothorax, and pleural empyema. Histologic pleural disease is observed in 40 to 70 percent of RA patients at autopsy.[7] Pathologic findings vary. Pleural nodules, with a palisaded histiocytic reaction surrounding central areas of fibrinoid necrosis similar to that seen in rheumatoid nodules, affect preferentially the visceral pleura, so that they are rarely picked up by closed pleural biopsy. Acute inflammatory changes, pleural fibrosis or lymphoid hyperplasia are also seen.

Pleural involvement may be clinically silent. Symptomatic pleural involvement manifests with pain and/or dyspnea. Pleural chest pain occurs in 25 percent of RA patients; 5 percent of RA patients develop pleural effusions, usually small to moderate in volume, unilateral more often than bilateral. Effusions are usually spontaneously resolving within weeks, however chronic effusions are possible.

Examination of the pleural fluid is mandatory to ascertain its nature and determine its cause. Particularly, exclusion of cancer or infection is needed in patients who will receive immunosuppressants as a therapy. The pleural fluid is an exudates and sterile with high concentrations of protein and lactate dehydrogenase. The most characteristic feature of pleural fluid is a low glucose concentration in spite of a normal blood glucose level. The fluid may look chylous because of high cholesterol content (pseudochylous effusion). There may be evidence of complement activation and a decreased complement activity. Cytology will show large number of both mononuclear and polynuclear leukocytes that are present in the fluid. Rheumatoid factor is positive in the pleural fluid in higher concentrations than in the blood. Pleural biopsy may show nonspecific inflammatory changes and in some cases, there may be granulomatous reactions identical to that found in rheumatoid nodules. Typically, glucose concentration in pleural fluid is lower than 0.50 g/l, and lower than 0.1 g/l in 40 percent of patients. Low glucose level is thought to be due to a poor transport of glucose from blood to the pleura by an unknown mechanism. Low pleural fluid pH, elevated adenosine deaminase activity, elevated rheumatoid factor, increased neuron-specific enolase and soluble interleukin-2 receptor have all been associated with rheumatoid effusion, but none is specific.[8,9]

Pleural effusions associated with RA usually do not require a specific treatment. Although the effusion may resolve spontaneously, they may persist for longer periods of time. Effusion due to rheumatoid arthritis needs no treatment, except when they are symptomatic. Fluid can be removed and if it recurs, a course of corticosteroids or pleurodesis may be needed. Large pleural effusions causing dyspnea are treated with chest tube drainage and pleural sclerosis in refractory cases.

Pneumothorax, pyopneumothorax, pleural empyema. Rupture of a necrotic rheumatoid nodule in the pleura may induce a pneumothorax, or a pyopneumothorax if infected. The same mechanism probably explains the frequency of pleural empyema in RA. The treatment of these manifestations is based on chest tube drainage, with antibiotics if infection is present.

Interstitial Lung Disease

Interstitial lung disease is the predominant pulmonary manifestation of RA. Interstitial changes are observed in 80 percent of lung biopsies, in up to 50 percent of lung CT and < 5 percent of chest radiographs.[10,11] A decrease of the diffusing capacity of carbon monoxide is observed in up to 40 percent of RA patients. Bronchoalveolar lavage abnormalities are detected in 50 percent of asymptomatic RA patients with normal chest radiography, essentially a lymphocytic alveolitis. A neutrophil alveolitis is observed in patients with clinically evident interstitial lung disease. Symptomatic interstitial lung disease is less frequent than radiographical prevalence but the limitation of activity due to articular involvement may mask dyspnea on exercise. The interstitial lung disease associated with rheumatoid arthritis is similar to that of idiopathic pulmonary fibrosis. The pathogenesis of idiopathic pulmonary fibrosis as well as that of several other interstitial lung diseases is poorly understood. The role of autoimmunity in interstitial lung diseases associated with connective tissue disorders such as systemic sclerosis, systemic lupus erythematosus, and rheumatoid arthritis as well as the vasculitides is well established. There is at least some evidence in the literature that supports the role of autoimmunity as one of the mechanisms of alveolar injury responsible for idiopathic pulmonary fibrosis. This review is an attempt to summarize the studies on this subject. Repeated extraneous insults and exposures are considered to be responsible for recurrent alveolar injury, inflammation, dysregulated tissue repair, and fibroproliferation resulting in pulmonary fibrosis. The presence of autoantibodies in the sera of patients with idiopathic pulmonary fibrosis has been demonstrated in a few studies. Several autoantibodies, including anti-Sm antibodies, antibodies to U1 ribonucleoproteins, and antibodies to U3 ribonucleoproteins, have been demonstrated in connective tissue disorders, many of which are associated with interstitial lung involvement. Autoimmunity has been also suggested as a possible mechanism of rejection caused by bronchiolitis obliterans after lung transplantation.[12]

Histopathological findings in RA-associated interstitial lung disease disclose very different patterns, sometimes associated: usual interstitial pneumonia (UIP), NSIP, desquamative interstitial pneumonia (DIP), LIP, organizing pneumonia, eosinophilic infiltration.[13] Many cases are difficult to classify into one pattern. Follicular bronchiolitis consisting of lymphoid hyperplasia and reactive germinal centers along small airways is also detected, frequently associated with an LIP pattern. The NSIP pattern is the most prevalent although in one study, UIP was the most frequent pattern.

HRCT pattern vary according to the histopathological pattern with a good concordance.[14] The most common CT features of RA-related lung disease were ground glass opacity and reticulation.[14] The features that suggest the diagnosis of rheumatoid interstitial lung disease are a coexistent systemic disease, pleural effusion, and/or necrobiotic nodules. The natural history of the disease is not known. In general, the disease is less severe than that due to idiopathic variety (Fig. 26.1).

The prognosis of RA-associated interstitial lung disease is usually good as the deterioration of lung function is slow. However, one study reported a median survival of 3.5 years and a 5 year survival rate of 39 percent in 49 patients with RA hospitalized for interstitial pulmonary fibrosis, survival very similar to what is observed in patients with idiopathic pulmonary fibrosis.[15]

Treatment of RA-associated interstitial lung disease is not well defined. Ideally, it should be tailored according to the pattern of lung pathologic involvement. However, lung biopsy is rarely performed in these patients and therapy is essentially empirical. Treatment with corticosteroids is indicated if there is a progressive disease. Early intervention is essential before extensive fibrotic changes occur. For patients who do not respond to corticosteroid therapy or who have unacceptable side effects, cyclophosphamide or methotrexate may be used. Corticosteroids are first-line therapy (prednisone, 0.5 to 1 mg/kg);[16] responders are estimated to be 40 percent. Patients with acute lung disease, with more cellular lung infiltration, with an organizing pneumonia pattern, or with eosinophilic or lymphocytic alveolitis, are more susceptible to treatment. Cyclophosphamide, azathioprine, methotrexate, cyclosporine, have been used, isolated or in association with corticosteroids for maintenance treatment or for corticosteroid resistant forms. At this time, the best treatment regimen is not defined. Treatment should be adapted to clinical, radiographic and functional tests.

Secondary amyloidosis involving the lung with an interstitial pattern is a rare but possible complication of long lasting RA.[16] Apical fibrobullous disease, similar to what is observed in patients with ankylosing spondylarthritis, is observed in RA patients.[17]

Rheumatoid Nodules/Necrobiotic Nodules

These nodules in the lungs are similar to the subcutaneous nodules in the skin due to rheumatoid arthritis. They may be single, or multiple and are either intraparenchymal or may be present on the pleural surface. The size varies from few millimeters to few centimeters. They are usually associated with other manifestations of rheumatoid lung disease. The size may be decreased or increased with the activity of the disease. The nodules may cavitate, with secondary infection and may be associated with pleural effusion or bronchopleural fistula. The nodules do not compromise lung function, and need no treatment unless there is infection or bronchopleural fistula. The nodules are often associated with bronchogenic carcinoma.

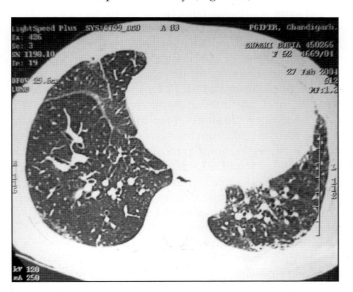

FIGURE 26.1: CT scan of chest showing ILD in a case of rheumatoid arthritis

Rheumatoid nodules are the only specific lesions observed in the lung of RA patients. Rheumatoid nodules are histologically similar to that observed in the subcutaneous tissue. Occasionally, giant cells and well-formed granulomas may be observed in the peripheral region of the nodule.[16] Very frequent at microscopic examination of the lung (30%), or on HRCT lung slices (20%), nodules are seldom seen on standard chest X-ray (< 1%). Nodules usually predominate in the upper and mid-lung regions, in the peripheral subpleural zone, although endobronchial nodules do exist. The nodules are more prevalent in males, and in patients with extra-articular manifestations or with subcutaneous nodules. Multiple widespread nodules have been described as *rheumatoid nodulosis*.[18] Detection of one or more lung nodules in a patient with RA poses the problem of their nature. A systematic diagnostic workup is needed in order not to miss an infectious or tumoral lesion.

Caplan's Syndrome

A syndrome of bilateral lung nodules in silica-exposed RA patients has been described as the Caplan's syndrome, also observed in other dust exposed RA patients.[19] The histopathological image of the nodules is similar to the rheumatoid nodule except for the presence of an additional peripheral pigmented dust surrounding the lesion.[10] Most patients have a preexisting mild pneumoconiosis. Caplan's syndrome is the presence of simple pneumoconiosis in a patient with rheumatoid arthritis. Although occurs most commonly in coal miners, it has also been associated with other occupations that result in exposure to silica. They include boiler scaling, roof tile manufacturing, asbestos mining, and aluminium production. The syndrome is characterized by the presence of single or multiple well-defined nodules measuring about 0.5 to 5.0 cm in diameter, and situated in the periphery of the lung. The nodules appear rapidly at the onset of rheumatoid arthritis, but usually appear in crops. Appearance of new nodules often is associated with an exacerbation of rheumatoid arthritis. The nodules themselves do not require specific therapy. If there is infection or bronchopleural fistula, these complications are to be treated routinely.

Pulmonary Arteritis and Pulmonary Hypertension

Lung vascular involvement is a rare finding in patients with RA. Although the most common cause of pulmonary hypertension in rheumatoid arthritis is interstitial fibrosis, in some cases the disease is primarily in the vasculature. The primary arteritis is manifested similar to that of the idiopathic pulmonary hypertension.[19] Alveolar hemorrhage related to pulmonary vasculitis has been reported,[20] sometimes with antineutrophil cytoplasmic antibodies.[21] No therapy has any effect on the natural history of the disease.

Upper Lobe Fibrobullous Disease

Recently, there are increasingly more reports of fibrobullous or cavitary disease of the upper lobe in patients of rheumatoid arthritis. The radiological features resemble that of ankylosing spondylitis with patchy upper lobe fibrosis and cystic spaces.[17]

Bronchiolitis and Bronchiectasis

The association of bronchiolitis with rheumatoid arthritis has been described in a number of patients. Initially, treatment with penicillamine was considered to be the contributory factor, although subsequently it was reported that such changes occur even without penicillamine treatment.[22] Histologically, an intense inflammatory infiltrate of lymphocytes and plasma cells are seen around the bronchiolar walls and in some cases complete fibrous obliteration of the airway lumen. These are described as bronchiolitis obliterans, and follicular bronchiolitis. Chest X-ray only shows hyperinflation. These patients present clinically with worsening dyspnea of RA patients present with bronchiectasis (associated with interstitial changes in one of evolution of RA is possible. Bronchiectasis is more common in women than in men (2.8 women/1 man), as is the case for RA.[23] In some studies, RA appears at a younger age in patients with bronchiectasis (46 *vs* 51 years). The coexistence of RA and bronchiectasis is associated with an alteration of lung function tests and a poor 5-year survival.[23] In a case-study, patients with RA and bronchiectasis were 7.3 times more likely to die than the general population, 5.0 times more likely than patients with RA and 2.4 times more likely than patients with bronchiectasis without RA.[23] An increased risk of death within the RA and bronchiectasis group was associated with a history of smoking, more severe RA and steroid usage;[24] in that study, 60 percent of the mortality was due to infections and acute respiratory failure. Bronchiectasis probably favors lung infections, a major cause of death in RA.[25] Bronchiectasis also increases the postoperative morbidity in RA patients.[26]

The reasons for an increased prevalence of bronchiectasis in RA are not very clear. Patients with RA have an increased susceptibility to airway infections perhaps due to a defect in humoral immunity.[27] The *yellow nail syndrome*, which associates recurrent bronchial and rhinosinusal infections, pleural effusions, lymphedema and typical changes of the nail has been described in RA.[28] Bronchiectasis in RA patients has been associated with some DR1 haplotypes and with DQB1*0601, *0301, *0501.[29] An excess of heterozygous mutations in the cystic fibrosis transmembrane regulator (CFTR) gene has been described in some.[30] Sjögren's syndrome (SS) does not seem to be overrepresented in patients with RA and bronchiectasis.

Pulmonary Function Changes (Airway Obstruction)

Pulmonary function studies in RA patients demonstrate an increased prevalence of chronic airway obstruction (16-38% of RA patients)[31,32] and an increased bronchial reactivity to metacholine (55% of RA patients in one study).[33] Patients may benefit of a treatment with inhaled corticosteroids and bronchodilators. Pathology studies demonstrate different patterns of airways involvement: follicular bronchiolitis, constrictive bronchiolitis, diffuse panbronchiolitis.[34] Despite the high prevalence of lung function abnormalities, severe airways obstruction in nonsmoking RA patients is a rare finding, which is clearly more frequent in patients treated with D-penicillamine even in non-RA patients,[35] although it may be observed in RA without D-penicillamine treatment.[36] The associated histology pattern is constrictive bronchiolitis (previously bronchiolitis obliterans). The prognosis is poor with 50 percent mortality within a few months.

Cricoarytenoid Arthritis

Cricoarytenoid arthritis is a frequent and may be present in 26 percent of cases of RA.[37] It is frequently an over-looked manifestation of RA that may present with poorly defined symptoms: sensation of foreign body in the throat, sore throat, hoarseness, fullness in the throat, dyspnea, difficulty with inspiration, pain radiating to the ears, stridor, dysphagia, odynophagia, and pain with speech. The diagnosis is clinically evident with direct or indirect laryngoscopy showing inflammatory changes of the arytenoids (erythema, swelling, thickening of mucosa) with reduced motility. CT scan confirms the diagnosis.[38] In some cases, ankylosis of the crico-arytenoid joint may induce an upper airway obstruction with a characteristic pattern on the flow-volume curve. Cricoarytenoid arthritis is treated with anti-inflammatory medications. In patients with dyspnea, surgery may be needed. Cricoarytenoid arthritis may favor obstructive sleep apnea, which is more frequent in RA patients.

Lung Cancer

Bronchogenic carcinoma is one of the recently recognized complications of rheumatoid arthritis. There is no specific cell type, which is predominant. Rheumatoid arthritis is an independent risk factor. This increased incidence of carcinoma is not entirely clear but is probably secondary to epithelial metaplasia and hyperplasia present in diffuse fibrotic lungs.[16]

Other Pulmonary Problems

The incidence of pulmonary infections occurs relatively more frequently in these patients. Bronchiectasis and cystic fibrosis patients have positive rheumatoid factor and polyarthritis. It is not clear whether the association is causal or by chance. Other complications described include eosinophilic pneumonia, progressive loss of lung volume, secondary diffuse amyloidosis, and bronchocentric granulomatosis.[2,3,16]

Lung Disease due to Drugs used for RA

Several drugs used for the treatment of RA have been associated with drug-induced lung disease. Undesirable respiratory side effects of methotrexate, gold salts, D-penicillamine, and nonsteroidal anti-inflammatory drugs are possible. However, new compounds (such as anti-TNF, sirolimus, leflunomide), and new clinicoradio-logical patterns are continuously described.[39-41]

Radiological Findings of RA

Rheumatoid arthritis is associated with four CT patterns: usual interstitial pneumonia, nonspecific interstitial pneumonia, bronchiolitis, and organizing pneumonia. The most common CT features of rheumatoid arthritis–related lung disease were ground-glass opacity and reticulation. Various CT findings are described in Table 26.1.[42]

REFERENCES

1. Crestani B. The respiratory system in connective tissue disorders. Allergy 2005;60:715-34.
2. Helmers R, Galvin J, Hunninghake GW. Pulmonary manifestations associated with rheumatoid arthritis. Chest 1991;100:235.
3. Hunninghake GW, Fauci AS. Pulmonary involvement in the collagen vascular diseases. Am Rev Respir Dis 1979;119:471.
4. Brannan MH, Good CA, Divertie MB, Baggenstoss AH. Pulmonary disease associated with rheumatoid arthritis. JAMA 1984;189;914.
5. Bilgici A, Ulusoy H, Kuru O, Celenk C, Unsal M, Danaci M. Pulmonary involvement in rheumatoid arthritis. Rheumatol Int 2005;25:429-35.

TABLE 26.1: CT findings of lung involvement in RA

Usual Interstitial pneumonia	Irregular linear opacities and honeycombing that predominantly involve basal and subpleural lung regions; may show traction bronchiectasis, architectural distortion, and ground glass opacities, CGO* (inconspicuous finding)
Nonspecific interstitial pneumonia	GGO*, usually bilateral with some predominance of subpleural and basal regions; may show fine reticulation or traction bronchiectasis within GGO*, airspace consolidation, and minor honeycombing
Organizng pneumonia	Patchy and multiple airspace consolidation usually with subpleural or peribronchial distribution associated with GGO*; may show centrilobular nodules or masses
Diffuse alveolar damage	Patchy or diffuse GGO* sometimes with panlobular distribution associated with airspace consolidation; may show intralobular reticulation or traction bronchiectasis and dependent area predominance
Lymphoid interstitial pneumonia	Poorly defined centrilobular nodules and GGO* that accompany thickening of interlobular septa and/or bronchovascular bundle; may show cystic airspaces and lymph node enlargement
Bronchiolitis obliterans	Mosaic perfusion with bronchial dilatation on inspiratory CT scans and air trapping on expiratory CT scans; may show centrilobular nodules and branching linear structures
Follicular bronchiolitis	Centrilobular and/or peribronchial nodules and branching linear structures, may show bronchial dilatation and braonchial wall thickening

*GGO—Ground glass opacity

6. Ayhan-Ardic FF, Oken O, Yorgancioglu ZR, Ustun N, Gokharman FD. Pulmonary involvement in lifelong non-smoking patients with rheumatoid arthritis and ankylosing spondylitis without respiratory symptoms. Clin Rheumatol 2006;25(2):213-18.
7. Murin S, Wiedemann HP, Matthay RA. Pulmonary manifestations of systemic lupus erythematosus. Clin Chest Med 1998;19:641-65.
8. Pettersson T, Soderblom T, Nyberg P, Riska H, Linko L, Klockars M. Pleural fluid soluble interleukin 2 receptor in rheumatoid arthritis and systemic lupus erythematosus. J Rheumatol 1994;21:1820-24.
9. Nyberg P, Soderblom T, Pettersson T, Riska H, Klockars M, Linko L. Neurone-specific enolase levels in pleural effusions in patients with rheumatoid arthritis. Thorax 1996;51:92-94.
10. Lamblin C, Bergoin C, Saelens T, Wallaert B. Interstitial lung diseases in collagen vascular diseases. Eur Respir J 2001;32:69s-80s.
11. Dawson JK, Fewins HE, Desmond J, Lynch MP, Graham DR. Fibrosing alveolitis in patients with rheumatoid arthritis as assessed by high resolution computed tomography, chest radiography, and pulmonary function tests. Thorax 2001;56:622-27.
12. Jindal SK, Agarwal R. Autoimmunity and interstitial lung disease. Curr Opin Pulm Med 2005;11:438-46.
13. Colby TV. Pulmonary pathology in patients with systemic autoimmune diseases. Clin Chest Med 1998;19:587-612.
14. Tanaka N, Kim JS, Newell JD, Brown KK, Cool CD, Meehan R, et al. Rheumatoid arthritis-related lung diseases: CT findings. Radiology 2004;232:81-91.
15. Hakala M. Poor prognosis in patients with rheumatoid arthritis hospitalized for interstitial lung fibrosis. Chest 1988;93:114-18.
16. Tanoue LT. Pulmonary manifestations of rheumatoid arthritis. Clin Chest Med 1998;19:667-85.
17. Yue CH, Park CH, Kushner I. Apical fibrocavitary lesions of the lung in rheumatoid arthritis. Am J Med 1986;81:741-46.
18. Wisnieski JJ, Askari AD. Rheumatoid nodulosis. A relatively benign rheumatoid variant. Arch Intern Med 1981;141:615-19.
19. Dawson JK, Goodson NG, Graham DR, Lynch MP. Raised pulmonary artery pressures measured with Doppler echocardiography in rheumatoid arthritis patients. Rheumatology 2000;39:1320-25.
20. Naschitz JE, Yeshurun D, Scharf Y, Sajrawi I, Lazarov NB, Boss JH. Recurrent massive alveolar hemorrhage, crescentic glomerulonephritis, and necrotizing vasculitis in a patient with rheumatoid arthritis. Arch Intern Med 1989;149:406-08.
21. Torralbo A, Herrero JA, Portoles J, Barrientos A. Alveolar hemorrhage associated with antineutrophil cytoplasmic antibodies in rheumatoid arthritis. Chest 1994;105:1590-92.
22. Cortet B, Flipo RM, Remy-Jardin M, Coquerelle P, Duquesnoy B, Remy J, et al. Use of high resolution computed tomography of the lungs in patients with rheumatoid arthritis. Ann Rheum Dis 1995;54:815-9.
23. McMahon MJ, Swinson DR, Shettar S, Wolstenholme R, Chattopadhyay C, Smith P, et al. Bronchiectasis and rheumatoid arthritis: A clinical study. Ann Rheum Dis 1993;52:776-79.

24. Swinson DR, Symmons D, Suresh U, Jones M, Booth J. Decreased survival in patients with co-existent rheumatoid arthritis and bronchiectasis. Br J Rheumatol 1997;36:689-91.

25. Suzuki A, Ohosone Y, Obana M, Mita S, Matsuoka Y, Irimajiri S, et al. Cause of death in 81 autopsied patients with rheumatoid arthritis. J Rheumatol 1994;21:33-36.

26. Grennan DM, Gray J, Loudon J, Fear S. Methotrexate and early postoperative complications in patients with rheumatoid arthritis undergoing elective orthopaedic surgery. Ann Rheum Dis 2001;60:214-17.

27. Snowden N, Moran A, Booth J, Haeney MR, Swinson DR. Defective antibody production in patients with rheumatoid arthritis and bronchiectasis. Clin Rheumatol 1999;18:132-35.

28. David-Vaudey E, Jamard B, Hermant C, Cantagrel A. Yellow nail syndrome in rheumatoid arthritis: A drug-induced disease? Clin Rheumatol 2004;23:376-78.

29. Hillarby MC, McMahon MJ, Grennan DM, Cooper RG, Clarkson RW, Davies EJ, et al. HLA associations in subjects with rheumatoid arthritis and bronchiectasis but not with other pulmonary complications of rheumatoid disease. Br J Rheumatol 1993;32:794-97.

30. Puechal X, Fajac I, Bienvenu T, Desmazes-Dufeu N, Hubert D, Kaplan JC, et al. Increased frequency of cystic fibrosis deltaF508 mutation in bronchiectasis associated with rheumatoid arthritis. Eur Respir J 1999;13:1281-87.

31. Geddes DM, Webley M, Emerson PA. Airways obstruction in rheumatoid arthritis. Ann Rheum Dis 1979;38:222-25.

32. Vergnenegre A, Pugnere N, Antonini MT, Arnaud M, Melloni B, Treves R, et al. Airway obstruction and rheumatoid arthritis. Eur Respir J 1997;10:1072-78.

33. Hassan WU, Keaney NP, Holland CD, Kelly CA. Bronchial reactivity and airflow obstruction in rheumatoid arthritis. Ann Rheum Dis 1994;53:511-14.

34. Homma S, Kawabata M, Kishi K, Tsuboi E, Narui K, Nakatani T, et al. Diffuse panbronchiolitis in rheumatoid arthritis. Eur Respir J 1998;12:444-52.

35. Epler GR, Snider GL, Gaensler EA, Cathcart ES, FitzGerald MX, Carrington CB. Bronchiolitis and bronchitis in connective tissue disease. A possible relationship to the use of penicillamine. JAMA 1979;242:528-32.

36. Pegg SJ, Lang BA, Mikhail EL, Hughes DM. Fatal bronchiolitis obliterans in a patient with juvenile rheumatoid arthritis receiving chrysotherapy. J Rheumatol 1994;21:549-51.

37. Lofgren RH, Montgomery WW. Incidence of laryngeal involvement in rheumatoid arthritis. N Engl J Med 1962;267:193-95.

38. Bayar N, Kara SA, Keles I, Koc C, Altinok D, Orkun S. Cricoarytenoiditis in rheumatoid arthritis: Radiologic and clinical study. J Otolaryngol 2003;32:373-78.

39. Libby D, White DA. Pulmonary toxicity of drugs used to treat systemic autoimmune diseases. Clin Chest Med 1998;19:809-21.

40. Camus P, Foucher P, Bonniaud P, Ask K. Drug-induced infiltrative lung disease. Eur Respir J 2001;18:93s-100s.

41. Foucher P, Camus P. Pneumotox on the web. http://www.pneumotox.com. [Accessed June 2009]

42. Tanaka N, Kim JS, Newell JD, Brown KK, Cool CD, Meehan R, Emoto T, Matsumoto T, Lynch DA. Rheumatoid arthritis-related lung diseases: CT findings. Radiology 2004;232:81-91.

SYSTEMIC LUPUS ERYTHEMATOSUS (SLE)

Systemic lupus erythematosus (SLE) is an autoimmune disorder that primarily affects women. SLE may affect virtually any organ and as such, the disease frequently involves the respiratory system. The majority of patients with SLE develop pleural or pulmonary disease in the course of their illness. Respiratory involvement is more common in men than in women. The American College of Rheumatology classification criteria for SLE were updated in 1997.[1] The criterion 'positive LE cell preparation' was deleted, and the item 'false-positive test for syphilis' was expanded to 'positive finding of antiphospholipid antibodies', including IgG or IgM anticardiolipin antibodies and lupus anticoagulant. Although lung involvement is not a criterion for SLE diagnosis, lung involvement has been associated with increased mortality.[2,3] The prognosis of SLE greatly improved in the past years and two prospective cohorts of 1000 European[2] and 644 Canadian[4] patients with lupus found 95 and 93 percent 5 year survival rates, respectively. Therefore, the respiratory physician is likely to see more and more of these complications.

The pulmonary manifestations of SLE may include:[5-14]
1. Pleural involvement
2. Lupus pneumonitis
3. Pulmonary hemorrhage
4. Interstitial fibrosis
5. Diaphragmatic dysfunction
6. Linear atelectasis
7. Infection, pulmonary embolism, pulmonary hypertension.

Pleural Involvement

Pleurisy and pleural effusion are the most frequently occurring clinical features of SLE and may be unilateral or bilateral. Pleural involvement may be asymptomatic although pleuritic pain is very common, affecting 45 to 60 percent of patients, and may occur without radiographically detectable chest effusion. Lupus pleuritis is typically associated with chest pain, dyspnea, cough and fever. Clinically apparent effusions have been reported in up to 50 percent of patients and pathological involvement at autopsy in up to 93 percent of patients. Pleural involvement may be the first manifestation of SLE. Pleuritis is commonly associated with pericarditis.[15] The involvement may be radiologically silent with findings of friction rub and chest pain or small effusions. On the other hand, the fluid may be sufficient enough to cause dyspnea. The pleural effusion is uni- or bilateral, small to moderate in size (but may be massive). Thoracocentesis is always needed in an SLE patient with pleural effusion as patients with SLE may have effusions for many different reasons, sometimes associated (infection, pulmonary embolism, renal failure, cardiac failure, etc.). The typical effusion is a serous or serosanguineous sterile exudate. The leukocyte differential count may show a predominance of neutrophils or mononuclear cells. Spontaneous hemothorax has been described. Biochemistry is nonspecific with increased lactate dehydrogenase and normal glucose levels. The pleural fluid antinuclear antibody assay is increased in SLE effusions. Typical lupus erythematosus cells (LE cells) are seen in pleural fluid but their search is not necessary. If performed, pleural biopsy will show lymphocytes and plasmocytes pleural infiltration with some degree of pleural thickening and fibrosis. Vasculitis involving the pleural vessels is a rare finding. Pleural biopsy is indicated to exclude other etiologies, such as tuberculosis or cancer.

Characteristically, the fluid is an exudate with a normal glucose level, and a high count of mononuclear, or at times polymorphonuclear leucocytes. Immune complexes, reduced levels of C_3 and C_4, LE cells, and ANF (antinuclear factor) may be present in the fluid. Pleural biopsy shows nonspecific changes. The effusion is usually self-limiting and if necessary, may need aspiration. In severe and persistent cases, steroid therapy helps in rapid resolution. The effusion should be differentiated from secondary infection and pulmonary infarction and other causes outlined above, which are the other complications of SLE. While the former can be excluded by culture and Gram stain, the latter should be suspected if the patient has lupus anticoagulant.

Spontaneous resolution of SLE effusions may occur. Lupus pleuritis is very sensitive to small doses of systemic corticosteroids, usually providing a rapid relief of symptoms within days. Resolution of effusions may be longer. Intrapleural corticosteroids have not been adequately studied and the available experience suggests that they have a limited efficacy. Chest drainage is rarely needed, as effusions are typically small. Exceptionally, pleurodesis or pleurectomy are needed for chronic effusions not controlled by medical therapy.

Lupus Pneumonitis

Acute pneumonia like presentation of SLE patients can be seen in up to 12% of cases in some series. It often reveals a previously unknown SLE 50% of the patients or may occur in the course of the disease. This is often a serious and life-threatening complication of SLE.

The clinical presentation is nonspecific, simulating an acute infectious pneumonitis, with cough, dyspnea and fever. Hemoptysis is occasionally seen. Ill look of the patient and findings of crepitations are the clinical findings. Severe hypoxemia is often present. Arterial blood gases analysis reveal hypoxemia with hypocapnia. Radiologically, the infiltrates are seen on both lungs, and predominantly on the bases. The infiltrations may also be diffusely distributed and patchy. Pleural effusion may be present.

The diagnostic dilemma is always between lupus pneumonitis and pneumonia due to secondary infection, which is very common in these patients. Sometimes such distinction is extremely difficult and only response to steroid therapy confirms the presence of lupus pneumonitis. However, this becomes dangerous, if the problem is secondary to infection. Careful microbiological assessment should be carried out, and if necessary (possibly safe) both antibiotic and steroids should be used. Chest radiography and CT scan show uni- or bilateral alveolar infiltrates which usually predominate in the lower lobes. Small pleural effusions are commonly associated. Occasionally, acute respiratory failure, requiring mechanical ventilation will occur. Apart from the rare occurrence of LE cells or the detection of hematoxylin-eosin bodies, histological features obtained are nonspecific and include alveolar wall damage and necrosis, alveolar edema, hyaline membranes, inflammatory cell infiltration and alveolar hemorrhage; capillary inflammation and thrombosis are also detected; deposits of immunoglobulins and complement are variably present.[16,17]

A syndrome of acute reversible hypoxemia with normal chest X-ray films, a normal CT scan and a rapid response to corticosteroids has been described in patients with SLE.[18,19] The syndrome was attributed to leukoaggregation in the lung capillaries. Available histology data are very limited but demonstrate an infraradiologic inflammation in the aleolar space.[19] This suggests that this syndrome is a form of less severe severity of acute lupus pneumonitis rather than a distinct entity.[19]

The clinicoradiographic presentation of lupus pneumonitis is absolutely nonspecific and may simulate lung infection, pulmonary embolism, or other acute pulmonary diseases. An invasive diagnostic workup must be set up and time is crucial as acute respiratory failure and death may develop. Bronchoalveolar lavage with a search for bacterial, viral, fungal and parasitic agents is required, but empirical antibiotherapy must not be delayed as lung infections remain the first cause of pulmonary infiltrates in SLE patients. CT scan will appropriately characterize the lesions and exclude the potential diagnosis of pulmonary embolism. Some have advocated lung biopsy to exclude some other diagnostic possibilities, however this procedure bears its own morbidity and mortality and lung histologic analysis is usually not diagnostic. Pathologically, the lungs show nonspecific inflammatory changes with both lymphocytic and polymorphonuclear alveolitis with alveolar wall edema, and small vessel arteritis. Immunoglobulin deposition and positive antinuclear antibodies can be detected in the alveolar walls and vessels.

The treatment of acute lupus pneumonitis is based upon high doses intravenous corticosteroids (prednisone, 1 kg/day).[20,21] Most patients will improve with this treatment despite 50 percent mortality has been reported in older series.[20] Pulse day for several days) have been used in patients with a severe initial presentation. Immunosuppressive or cytotoxic agents such as cyclophosphamide are used in patients with a poor response to corticosteroids. The place of new immunomodulatory agents such as anti-TNF[22] has not been evaluated. Once the diagnosis of lupus pneumonitis is made, it should be treated aggressively with high dose of prednisolone, in the above-mentioned dosage. If there is no response within 2 to 3 days, and there is renal involvement also, cyclophosphamide may be added. The dose is then to be reduced and maintained at the lowest level where the patient is free of recurrences.

Pulmonary Hemorrhage

Acute diffuse pulmonary hemorrhage can occur in SLE. Diffuse alveolar hemorrhage (DAH) is a rare but severe manifestation of SLE most series reporting 50 to 90 percent mortality[20,23,24] although a more favorable outcome has been reported.[25]

Immune complex-mediated injury, vasculitis with alveolar capillaritis, alveolar damage related to infection, probably plays a role in the pathogenesis of the condition. The histologic findings in DAH are similar to those of acute lupus pneumonitis. Acute inflammation and necrosis involving capillaries, arterioles, and small muscular arteries has been described.[26] The involvement of capillaries is manifested by an infiltrate of necrotic neutrophils within alveolar septa often associated with

destruction of the alveolar wall. This capillaritis is almost a universal finding,[26] while involvement of arterioles and small arteries is seen in about 3/4th of cases. Immunofluorescence and electron microscopy will demonstrate immune complexes. Capillaritis has also been described in alveolar hemorrhage associated with the antiphospholipid synpurpura, cryoglobulinemia, and Behçet's syndrome, and Wegener disease; and is not specific of SLE. It may also be seen in antibasement membrane antibody disease.

DAH reveals SLE in 11 to 20 percent of cases.[23] Patients with lupus nephritis are at increased risk of developing DAH, and renal involvement is observed in 60 percent of the patients at diagnosis of DAH. Microvascular renal and lung involvement appear to be pathogenetically similar.[27] The presentation ranges from asymptomatic to fulminant. Affected patients are young (mean age: 27 years) and present acutely ill with dyspnea, cough, fever and anemia. Symptoms are usually abrupt in onset, being present for less than 3 days in two-thirds of patients. Hemoptysis is initially present in less than half of patients. Bilateral lung infiltrates, ranging from limited ground glass opacities to dense consolidations are present. Arterial hypoxemia is common and more than 50 percent of the patients will need mechanical ventilation.

The diagnosis of DAH is usually easily obtained with bronchoalveolar lavage, which allows for a search for infectious agents. Concomitant lung infection, bacterial, fungal or viral, is observed in about one-third of patients, and bears a poor prognosis.[23] Lung biopsy, either transbronchial or surgical, is not useful once the diagnosis of SLE is ascertained with the presence of antinuclear antibodies, and may be dangerous in critically ill patients. Echocardiography is mandatory to evaluate the presence of valvular or myocardial dysfunction.

The treatment of SLE-associated DAH is not well defined. High-dose corticosteroid alone does not appear to be very effective. In a recent series, DAH developed in patients already treated with high dose corticosteroids for lupus nephritis.[24] Plasmapheresis has been anecdotally successful.[28] A combination of corticosteroids, cyclophosphamide and plasmapheresis has been used with promising results.[29] At this time, plasmapheresis should be reserved for patients with severe DAH refractory to corticosteroids and cyclophosphamide.[30] Survivors are exposed to the risk of developing pulmonary fibrosis.[31] The patient typically presents with cough, malaise, dyspnea, hemoptysis, and anemia. The chest X-ray will reveal bilateral diffuse fluffy shadows and the diagnostic clue comes from a low hemoglobin. Clinically, it is difficult to distinguish from Goodpasture's syndrome except for the absence of anti-basement membrane antibody. Extensive alveolar hemorrhage and non-specific alveolitis with neutrophilic inflammatory cell infiltration of small arteries, arterioles, and capillaries are characteristic pathologic findings. Uremia and thrombocytopenia can cause such hemorrhages secondarily, although inflammatory changes will be absent on histological sections.

The condition may be fatal despite therapy. Treatment consists of oxygenation, blood transfusion, and high dose corticosteroid and cyclophosphamide. Usefulness of plasmapheresis in SLE hemorrhage is not proven.

Interstitial Fibrosis

Although some evidence of alveolitis is possible, in autopsy cases of SLE, clinically evident interstitial fibrosis is relatively rare. This occasional occurrence of interstitial fibrosis is associated with immunecomplex deposition in the alveolar walls. Extensive lung fibrosis is rarely observed (~3% of the patients). However systematic CT evaluation of nonselected patients with SLE demonstrated the high prevalence of interstitial abnormalities, observed in 30 percent of the patients.[32] Pulmonary function tests were abnormal in about 40 to 50 percent of the patients with abnormal HRCT, but HRCT changes did not correlate with pulmonary function abnormalities.[32,33] A larger series[34] described 18 patients, identified over a 1 year period, with radiographic evidence of pulmonary fibrosis, representing less than 3 percent of the patients followed at that institution. All the patients had a restrictive functional pattern but only seven were symptomatic. The disease develops insidiously, sometimes with mild flares of lung involvement.[35] In some patients, lung fibrosis could be the sequela of acute pneumonitis. Lung involvement does not correlate with any biological characteristic, although in one series an association between anti-SS-A antibodies and chronic interstitial pneumonia was observed.[36] but this observation was not confirmed in later studies, which described an association between low DLCO and anti-U1 RNP antibodies.[37] Histologic reports describe nonspecific abnormalities with interstitial lymphocytic infiltrates, interstitial fibrosis, and honeycomb changes.[34,35] The place of nonspecific interstitial pneumonia (NSIP) in SLE is not well defined.[38] Lymphocytic interstitial pneumonia (LIP) has been described in a few patients with SLE, usually associated with Sjögren syndrome. The development of lung cysts should suggest the diagnosis of LIP. The clinicoradiologic syndrome of organizing pneumonia (formerly known as BOOP) characterized by patchy alveolar infiltrates and an histologic pattern of organizing pneumonia has been described in patients with SLE with a good response to corticosteroids.

Response to steroid and other immunosuppressive drugs is unsatisfactory.and treatment is poorly evaluated. Response is variable.[35] Improvement with oral methotrexate has been reported.[39]

Airway Involvement

Unlike in RA, upper airway involvement is uncommon in SLE. Laryngeal involvement is reported to occur in 0.3 to 13 percent of patients.[40] The glottis and cricoarytenoid joints seem to be the most commonly involved sites, although the epiglottis and subglottis have also been reported to be involved. Laryngeal symptoms rarely present as isolated findings. Hoarseness, throat pain, and/or dyspnea all may be presenting symptoms depending on the site of involvement. SLE-related vasculitis may directly involve the larynx causing a subglottic stenosis.[41] Lower airways obstruction is not a common finding in SLE patients as evidenced by the systematic evaluation of pulmonary function tests[42] although a few cases of significant airflow obstruction have been reported.

PULMONARY VASCULAR DISEASE

Pulmonary Hypertension

Some degree of pulmonary hypertension (PHT) complicates the course of SLE in 5 to 14 percent of the patients.[43-45] PHT prevalence and mean pulmonary pressure tend to increase with time.[46] In one study, PHT was associated with an overall 2 year mortality 50 percent.[47] There are only a few case reports in the literature of patients with SLE and severe PHT resulting in right heart failure. Autopsy findings from these patients have demonstrated pathologic changes of medial hypertrophy, intimal fibrosis, and plexiform lesions, which are virtually identical to the alterations seen in patients with idiopathic PHT.[48] Pulmonary veno-occlusive disease, a rare form of PHT with distinct histopathology, has also been reported.[49] Identification of pulmonary veno-occlusive disease is important as vasodilators are poorly tolerated in that form of disease.[50] The pathophysiology of PHT is poorly understood; antiphospholipid antibodies, antiendothelial cells antibodies,[51] vasculitis, vasospasm, and inflammation all contribute to the development of the typical proliferative lesions observed in the disease. Raynaud's phenomenon (75%) and antiphospholipid antibodies (60%) are more common in SLE patients with PHT. Interstitial lung disease may also be more frequent (60% compared with 19% without PHT). The diagnosis of PHT is suspected on echocardiography and must be confirmed by cardiac catheterization. Exclusion of chronic thromboembolic PHT with ventilation-perfusion scintigraphy is mandatory. Treatment is based on oral anticoagulants and vasodilators. Intravenous epoprostenol has given good results.[48,52] Newer vasodilators, such as sildenafil[53] may be useful in some patients. When possible, a trial of corticosteroids and cyclophosphamide should be performed before initiating vasodilators since anecdotal responses have been reported.[54]

Pulmonary Embolism

Pulmonary embolism is a particular risk in those patients having lupus anticoagulant. It interferes with the transformation of prothrombin to thrombin causing a prolonged partial thromboplastin time. Paradoxically, it causes thrombosis probably due to its inhibition of release of arachidonic acid metabolites from cell membrane and resulting in a loss of their inhibitory effects on platelet aggregation. Pulmonary hypertension is another complication possibly related to the presence of the lupus anticoagulants.

A prothrombic effect of SLE separate of the antiphospholipid syndrome has been suggested but not definitely proved.[55] The antiphospholipid syndrome is very common in SLE. Anticardiopin antibodies of the IgG or the IgM isotype are found in 24 and 13 percent of the patients with SLE, and are associated with an increased prevalence of thrombosis (30% with IgG, 31% with IgM, vs 9% without).[56] This point is controversial as in some studies, anticardiolipin antibodies are not associated with thrombosis, but prolonged activated partial thromboplastin is.[55] The antiphospholipid syndrome may develop in 50 to 70 percent of patients with both SLE and antiphospholipid antibodies after 20 years of follow-up.

Catastrophic Antiphospholipid Syndrome

The catastrophic antiphospholipid syndrome is a rare and excessively severe manifestation of the antiphospholipid syndrome, which is observed both in primary and secondary antiphospholipid syndrome.[55] The syndrome is characterized by multiple simultaneous vascular occlusions throughout the body. The lung is involved in 66 percent of the cases, with ARDS, pulmonary embolism, pulmonary artery thrombosis, pulmonary microthrombi, or alveolar hemorrhage, sometimes associated.[57]

Pulmonary Infections in SLE

Patients of SLE are prone to infections possibly because of an altered immune functions either because of the disease per se or because of the frequent use of immunosuppressants for treatment. There is some evidence of depressed macrophage function in these patients. Common organisms involved include *Pneumocystis carinii (jerovicii)*, Candida, *Toxoplasma gondii*, Aspergillus, Mycobacteria, and Staphylococci. About a third of the cases die of infection. Infection is a major cause of morbidity and mortality in patients with SLE, contributing for more than 50 percent deaths in some series. Lung infection is the most important cause of respiratory manifestations in SLE and is secondary to the immunosuppression associated with SLE itself and induced by corticosteroids and immunosuppressants. Patients with SLE are susceptible to usual pathogens and opportunistic pathogens. Mycobacterial and nocardial infections seem to be particularly important. The frequent occurrence of infection mandates an aggressive approach to the SLE patient with pulmonary infiltrates. Infection should be presumed and treated empirically until an alternative diagnosis is given. Bronchoscopic lung sampling should be the rule, especially if the patient is receiving immunosuppressants.

The Vanishing Lung Syndrome or the Shrinking Lung Syndrome

The term 'shrinking lung syndrome' has been applied to SLE patients presenting with progressive dyspnea, the characteristic chest radiographic findings of small lung volumes, elevated hemidiaphragms and bibasilar atelectasis, with a restrictive ventilatory defect and a preserved carbon monoxide transfer coefficient. This syndrome was attributed to diaphragmatic dysfunction on the basis of the demonstration of decreased inspiratory muscle strength in 11 SLE patients.[58] Conversely, others[59] using bilateral electrostimulation with the shrinking lung syndrome, failed to demonstrate diaphragm weakness. In a well-documented case, Hardy et al. described a patient with the syndrome and bilateral phrenic nerve paralysis.[60] With corticosteroids, the phrenic nerve function recovered whereas the restrictive functional pattern persisted, suggesting that reduced diaphragm muscle contractility per se does not explain the small volume lungs and respiratory symptoms in patients with the syndrome. Hawkins reached similar conclusions in a different patient.[61] Some improvement of dyspnea and restriction has been observed with corticosteroids.[20] Many patients seem to stabilize and have no worsening of lung function with time.

Respiratory Muscle Weakness

Diaphragmatic muscle weakness or elevation has been observed in about a third of the patients in addition to a possible respiratory muscle myositis.[13] These patients present with increasing exertional dyspnea and they are not able to take a full inspiration. Restrictive lung function abnormalities are common. Diaphragmatic excursion is limited on screening and transdiaphragmatic pressure is reduced. This is otherwise known as *"vanishing lung syndrome"*. Treatment with steroid often improves diaphragmatic function.

Other Pulmonary Abnormalities

Linear atelectasis is quite a common radiological finding in SLE, and may be due to infection, pleurisy, or elevated diaphragm.

The simultaneous occurrence of sarcoidosis and SLE has been reported in a few cases.[20] Nodular amyloidosis, excavating nodules, have also been observed.

REFERENCES

1. Hochberg MC. Updating the American College of Rheumatology revised criteria for the classification of systemic lupus erythematosus. Arthritis Rheum 1997;40:1725.
2. Abu-Shakra M, Urowitz MB, Gladman DD, Gough J. Mortality studies in systemic lupus erythematosus. Results 1.from a single center. II. Predictor variables for mortality. J Rheumatol 1995;22:1265-70.
3. Stoll T, Seifert B, Isenberg DA. SLICC/ACR Damage Index is valid, and renal and pulmonary organ scores are predictors of severe outcome in patients with systemic lupus erythematosus. Br J Rheumatol 1996;35:248-54.
4. Cervera R, Khamashta MA, Font J, Sebastiani GD, Gil A, Lavilla P, et al. Morbidity and mortality in systemic lupus erythematosus during a 5-year period. A multicenter prospective study of 1,000 patients. European Working Party on Systemic Lupus Erythematosus. Medicine (Baltimore) 1999;78:167-75.
5. Segal AM, Calabrese LH, Ahamad M, et al. The pulmonary manifestations of systemic lupus erythematosus. Semin Arthritis Rheum 1985;14:202-24.
6. Pines A, Kapilnsky N, Olchovsky D, Rozenman J, Franki O. Pleuropulmonary manifestations of systemic lupus erythematosus: Clinical features of its subgroups. Prognostic and therapeutic implications. Chest 1985;88:129-35.
7. Brasington RO, Firth DE. Pulmonary disease in systemic lupus erythematosus. Clin Exp Rheumatol 1985;3:269.
8. Miller RL, Greenberg SD, McLarty JW. Lupus lung. Chest 1985;88:265.
9. Matthay RA, Schwartz MI, Petty TL, et al. Pulmonary manifestations of systemic lupus erythematosus: Review of 12 cases of acute lupus pneumonitis. Medicine 1975;54:397.
10. Haupt HM, Moore GW, Hutchins GM. The lung in systemic lupus erythematosus. Analysis of the pathologic changes in 120 patients. Am J Med 1981;71:791-98.
11. Pertschuk LP, Moccia LF, Rosen Y, et al. Acute pulmonary complications in systemic lupus erythematosus: Immunofluorescence and light microscopic study. Am J Clin Pathal 1977;68:553-57.
12. Holgate ST, Glass DN, Haslam P, Maini RN, Turner Warwick M, et al. Respiratory involvement in systemic lupus erythematosus: A clinical and immunological study. Clin Exp Immunol 1976; 24:385-95.
13. Martens J, Demedts M, Vanmeenen MT, Dequeker J. Respiratory muscle dysfunction in systemic lupus-erythematosus. Chest 1984;84:170-76.
14. Hellman DB, Petri M, Whiting OKQ. Fatal infections in systemic lupus erythematosus: The role of opportunistic organisms. Medicine 1987;66:341.
15. Crestani B. The respiratory system in connective tissue disorders. Allergy 2005;60:715-34.
16. Haupt HM, Moore GW, Hutchins GM. The lung in systemic lupus erythematosus. Analysis of the pathologic changes in 120 patients. Am J Med 1981;71:791-98.
17. Colby TV. Pulmonary pathology in patients with systemic autoimmune diseases. Clin Chest Med 1998;19:587-612.
18. Abramson SB, Dobro J, Eberle MA, Benton M, Reibman J, Epstein H, et al. Acute reversible hypoxemia in systemic lupus erythematosus. Ann Intern Med 1991;114:941-47.
19. Susanto I, Peters JI. Acute lupus pneumonitis with normal chest radiograph. Chest 1997;111:1781-83.
20. Murin S, Wiedemann HP, Matthay RA. Pulmonary manifestations of systemic lupus erythematosus. Clin Chest Med 1998;19:641-65.
21. Raj R, Murin S, Matthay RA, Wiedemann HP. Systemic lupus erythematosus in the intensive care unit. Crit Care Clin 2002;18:781-803.
22. Aringer M, Smolen JS. Tumour necrosis factor and other proinflammatory cytokines in systemic lupus erythematosus: A rationale for therapeutic intervention. Lupus 2004;13:344-47.
23. Zamora MR, Warner ML, Tuder R, Schwarz MI. Diffuse alveolar hemorrhage and systemic lupus erythematosus. Clinical presentation, histology, survival, and outcome. Medicine (Baltimore) 1997;76:192-202.
24. Liu MF, Lee JH, Weng TH, Lee YY. Clinical experience of 13 cases with severe pulmonary hemorrhage in systemic lupus erythematosus with active nephritis. Scand J Rheumatol 1998;27:291-95.
25. Schwab EP, Schumacher HR Jr, Freundlich B, Callegari PE. Pulmonary alveolar hemorrhage in systemic lupus erythematosus. Semin Arthritis Rheum 1993;23:8-15.

26. Myers JL, Katzenstein AA. Microangiitis in lupus-induced pulmonary hemorrhage. Am J Clin Pathol 1986;85:552-56.

27. Hughson MD, He Z, Henegar J, McMurray R. Alveolar hemorrhage and renal microangiopathy in systemic lupus erythematosus. Arch Pathol Lab Med 2001;125: 475-83.

28. Erickson RW, Franklin WA, Emlen W. Treatment of hemorrhagic lupus pneumonitis with plasmapheresis. Semin Arthritis Rheum 1994;24:114-23.

29. Euler HH, Schroeder JO, Harten P, Zeuner RA, Gutschmidt HJ. Treatment-free remission in severe systemic lupus erythematosus following synchronization of plasmapheresis with subsequent pulse cyclophosphamide. Arthritis Rheum 1994;37:1784-94.

30. Keane MP, Lynch JP III. Pleuropulmonary manifestations of systemic lupus erythematosus. Thorax 2000;55:159-66.

31. Specks U. Diffuse alveolar hemorrhage syndromes. Curr Opin Rheumatol 2001;13:12-17.

32. Fenlon HM, Doran M, Sant SM, Breatnach E. High-resolution chest CT in systemic lupus erythematosus. AJR Am J Roentgenol 1996;166:301-07.

33. Sant SM, Doran M, Fenelon HM, Breatnach ES. Pleuropulmonary abnormalities in patients with systemic lupus erythematosus: Assessment with high resolution computed tomography, chest radiography and pulmonary function tests. Clin Exp Rheumatol 1997;15:507-13.

34. Eisenberg H, Dubois EL, Sherwin RP, Balchum OJ. Diffuse interstitial lung disease in systemic lupus erythematosus. Ann Intern Med 1973;79:37-45.

35. Weinrib L, Sharma OP, Quismorio FP Jr. A long-term study of interstitial lung disease in systemic lupus erythematosus. Semin Arthritis Rheum 1990;20:48-56.

36. Boulware DW, Hedgpeth MT. Lupus pneumonitis and anti-SSA(Ro) antibodies. J Rheumatol 1989;16:479-81.

37. Groen H, ter Borg EJ, Postma DS, Wouda AA, van der Mark TW, Kallenberg CG. Pulmonary function in systemic lupus erythematosus is related to distinct clinical, serologic, and nailfold capillary patterns. Am J Med 1992;93:619-27.

38. Tansey D, Wells AU, Colby TV, Ip S, Nikolakoupolou A, du Bois RM, et al. Variations in histological patterns of interstitial pneumonia between connective tissue disorders and their relationship to prognosis. Histopathology 2004;44:585-96.

39. Fink SD, Kremer JM. Successful treatment of interstitial lung disease in systemic lupus erythematosus with methotrexate. J Rheumatol 1995;22:967-69.

40. Loehrl TA, Smith TL. Inflammatory and granulomatous lesions of the larynx and pharynx. Am J Med 2001; 111:113-17.

41. Karim A, Ahmed S, Siddiqui R, Marder GS, Mattana J. Severe upper airway obstruction from cricoarytenoiditis as the sole presenting manifestation of a systemic lupus erythematosus flare. Chest 2002;121:990-93.

42. Andonopoulos AP, Constantopoulos SH, Galanopoulou V, Drosos AA, Acritidis NC, Moutsopoulos HM. Pulmonary function of nonsmoking patients with systemic lupus erythematosus. Chest 1988;94: 312-15.

43. Perez HD, Kramer N. Pulmonary hypertension in systemic lupus erythematosus: Report of four cases and review of the literature. Semin Arthritis Rheum 1981;11:177-81.

44. Badui E, Garcia-Rubi D, Robles E, Jimenez J, Juan L, Deleze M, et al. Cardiovascular manifestations in systemic lupus erythematosus. Prospective study of 100 patients. Angiology 1985;36:431-41.

45. Simonson JS, Schiller NB, Petri M, Hellmann DB. Pulmonary hypertension in systemic lupus erythematosus. J Rheumatol 1989;16:918-25.

46. Winslow TM, Ossipov MA, Fazio GP, Simonson JS, Redberg RF, Schiller NB. Five-year follow-up study of the prevalence and progression of pulmonary hypertension in systemic lupus erythematosus. Am Heart J 1995;129:510-15.

47. Orens JB, Martinez FJ, Lynch JP.III. Pleuropulmonary manifestations of systemic lupus erythematosus. Rheum Dis Clin North Am 1994;20:159-93.

48. Robbins IM, Gaine SP, Schilz R, Tapson VF, Rubin LJ, Loyd JE. Epoprostenol for treatment of pulmonary hypertension in patients with systemic lupus erythematosus. Chest 2000;117:14-18.

49. Kishida Y, Kanai Y, Kuramochi S, Hosoda Y. Pulmonary venoocclusive disease in a patient with systemic lupus erythematosus. J Rheumatol 1993;20:2161-62.

50. Resten A, Maitre S, Humbert M, Sitbon O, Capron F, Simoneau G, et al. Pulmonary arterial hypertension: Thin-section CT predictors of epoprostenol therapy failure. Radiology 2002;222:782-88.

51. Yoshio T, Masuyama J, Sumiya M, Minota S, Kano S. Antiendothelial cell antibodies and their relation to pulmonary hypertension in systemic lupus erythematosus. J Rheumatol 1994;21:2058-63.

52. Humbert M, Sanchez O, Fartoukh M, Jagot JL, Sitbon O, Simonneau G. Treatment of severe pulmonary hypertension secondary to connective tissue diseases with continuous IV epoprostenol (prostacyclin). Chest 1998;114:80S-82S.

53. Molina J, Lucero E, Luluaga S, Bellomio V, Spindler A, Berman A. Systemic lupus erythematosus-associated pulmonary hypertension: Good outcome following sildenafil therapy. Lupus 2003;12:321-23.

54. Goupille P, Fauchier L, Babuty D, Fauchier JP, Valat JP. Precapillary pulmonary hypertension dramatically improved with high doses of corticosteroids during systemic lupus erythematosus. J Rheumatol 1994;21: 1976-77.

55. Levine JS, Branch DW, Rauch J. The antiphospholipid syndrome. N Engl J Med 2002;346:752-63.

56. Cervera R, Khamashta MA, Font J, Sebastiani GD, Gil A, Lavilla P, et al. Systemic lupus erythematosus: Clinical and immunologic patterns of disease expression

in a cohort of 1,000 patients. The European Working Party on Systemic Lupus Erythematosus. Medicine (Baltimore) 1993;72:113-24.

57. Asherson RA, Cervera R, Piette JC, Font J, Lie JT, Burcoglu A, et al. Catastrophic antiphospholipid syndrome. Clinical and laboratory features of 50 patients. Medicine (Baltimore) 1998;77:195-207.
58. Wilcox P, Stein H, Clarke S, Pare P, Pardy R. Phrenic nerve function in patients with diaphragmatic weakness and systemic lupus erythematosus. Chest 1988;93: 352-58.
59. Laroche CM, Mulvey DA, Hawkins PN, Walport MJ, Strickland B, Moxham J, et al. Diaphragm strength in the shrinking lung syndrome of systemic lupus erythematosus. Q J Med 1989;71:429-39.
60. Hardy K, Herry I, Attali V, Cadranel J, Similowski T. Bilateral phrenic paralysis in a patient with systemic lupus erythematosus. Chest 2001;119:1274-77.
61. Hawkins P, Davison AG, Dasgupta B, Moxham J. Diaphragm strength in acute systemic lupus erythematosus in a patient with paradoxical abdominal motion and reduced lung volumes. Thorax 2001;56:329-30.

PROGRESSIVE SYSTEMIC SCLEROSIS (PSS)/SYSTEMIC SCLEROSIS (SSc)

Progressive systemic sclerosis (PSS) or Systemic Sclerosis (SSc) is a multisystem disease characterized by fibrosis of the epidermis and dermis (scleroderma) and fibrosis of other organs including kidneys, lungs, heart, gastrointestinal tract, and skeletal muscles. The most common characteristic of the disease is the involvement of smaller blood vessels and the damage to the endothelium, which allows toxic substances to enter into the perivascular tissue. Recent studies suggest that the presence of the anti-Scl 70 antibody is a strong predictor of lung disease in PSS.[1,2] Pulmonary involvement in systemic sclerosis is very common, both clinically and at autopsy, and bears a poor prognosis. Pulmonary complications are now the first cause of death in PSS.[3] Interstitial lung disease with progressive fibrosis is the most common pulmonary disease, affecting 75 percent patients at autopsy, followed by PHT, affecting up to 50 percent of SSc patients.[4] Systemic involvement usually appears within 5 years of diagnosis (essentially within 2 years), but later appearance is also possible and thus justifies a close follow-up of these patients.

Two forms of PSS have been individualized with characteristic clinical presentation, autoimmune signature and evolution. **Limited PSS** (70% of all PSS patients) is characterized by distal cutaneous sclerosis (below the knees, the elbows, and not affecting the thorax), a long history of Raynaud's phenomenon before the diagnosis and the presence of circulating anticentromere anti-

bodies (positive in 70% patients). Its typical form consists in the CREST syndrome with subcutaneous calcinosis, Raynaud's phenomenon, esophageal dysmotility, sclerodactily, and telangiectasias predominating on the face and the thorax. PHT typically occurs in patients with limited SSc. Survival has been estimated at 98 percent at 1 year, 80 percent at 6 years and 50 percent at 12 years after diagnosis.[5] **Diffuse PSS** (30%) is characterized by the proximal involvement of the skin, extending to the thorax. Cutaneous involvement occurs simultaneously to the appearance of the Raynaud's phenomenon. Antitopoisomerase antibodies are present in 30 percent of the patients, whereas anticentromere antibodies are usually absent (detected in 3% of the patients with diffuse SSc). Pulmonary fibrosis typically affects patients with diffuse SSc. Survival was poor: 80 percent at 1 year, 30 percent at 6 years, 15 percent at 12 years[5] but recent data suggest an improvement of the prognosis.[6] The pathophysiology of SSc is poorly understood, particularly the link between autoimmunity and fibroproliferation does not appear clearly. It may be the consequence of endothelial lesions.

The lung manifestations are:[1]
1. Interstitial fibrosis
2. Pulmonary hypertension
3. Aspiration pneumonias
4. Restriction of ventilation due to tight chest
5. Increased incidence of lung cancer.

Interstitial Lung Disease

Most patients with PSS and the CREST (calcinosis of the finger tips, Raynaud's phenomenon, esophageal dysfunction, sclerodactyly, and telangiectasia of the skin) syndrome ultimately develop pulmonary fibrosis. The clinical features, radiological changes, and pulmonary functional abnormalities are similar to those seen in other causes of interstitial fibrosis. The presence of clinical interstitial fibrosis and reduced lung function in a patient with PSS implies a reduced life expectancy, with about 60 percent of the patients surviving for 5 years. However, the disease is not rapidly progressive. Steroids have no effect on the course of the disease. However, penicillamine may improve lung function, particularly the diffusing capacity.

Interstitial lung disease may occur in limited or diffuse SSc. The onset of pulmonary involvement is usually progressive and rarely precedes scleroderma although a syndrome called SSc sine scleroderma has been described in men exposed to inhaled mineral particles.[7] About 25 percent of SSc patients will develop clinically significant interstitial lung disease and 13 percent a severe restrictive lung disease.[8]

For many years, idiopathic pulmonary fibrosis and pulmonary fibrosis associated with SSc were viewed as histologically similar, contrasting with the very different prognosis of the two diseases.[9] It is now clearly evident that NSIP is the main histological pattern in interstitial lung disease associated with SSc,[10-12] UIP being the pattern associated with idiopathic pulmonary fibrosis.[13] Deterioration of pulmonary function tests (a restrictive ventilatory defect and reduced DLCO) is arguments for a poor prognosis. Evolution of DLCO over the first year after diagnosis has a strong prognostic value.[12]

HRCT of the lung is the best tool to identify pulmonary fibrosis in SSc.[14] Abnormalities predominate in the basal and subpleural regions of the lungs, and combine reticular and ground glass opacities with honeycombing. Ground glass opacities are usually the predominant abnormality; they consist more of fine intralobular fibrosis than true alveolitis.[15,16] Disease extent on HRCT has a strong prognostic value.

Bronchoalveolar lavage has been extensively evaluated in patients with SSc. BAL lymphocytosis in SSc is associated with secondary SS and has a relatively better prognosis. BAL neutrophilia has been consistently associated with progressive disease as assessed by deterioration of lung function.[17-19] However, whether BAL neutrophilia is an independent factor for predicting progression of interstitial lung disease in SSc when other prognostic factors (such as pulmonary function tests and the extent of fibrosis on HRCT) are taken into account is debated.[14] BAL eosinophilia bears a poor prognosis in one study.[12]

The treatment of lung involvement in SSc is poorly defined. Indeed, controlled studies are lacking. Current data suggest that cyclophosphamide, either oral[19] or intravenous,[20-22] with low dose corticosteroids, stabilizes or improves lung function tests and HRCT, with subsequent decline in most patients after stopping cyclophosphamide. Unresolved issues concern the dose of corticosteroids to be administered with cyclophosphamide, the optimal dose and duration of cyclophosphamide, the optimal immunosuppressive treatment after initial cyclophosphamide treatment. A combination of low dose prednisone and azathioprine is often given after 12 months of cyclophosphamide. Hypofertility is possible after cyclophosphamide treatment and patients should be given the possibility to store ovules or sperm in view of future procreation. The decision when to begin treatment is difficult. The best criteria is probably the evidence of progression on successive evaluation.[14]

There is limited evidence for an antifibrotic activity of cyclosporine[23] or D-penicillamine in the lung.[24] Other treatments are being prospectively evaluated, such as bosentan (antagonist of ETA and ETB endothelin receptors) or autologous stem cell transplantation.[25] Lung transplantation has been successfully performed in patients with SSc. Esophageal dysmotility induces specific postoperative complications.

Pulmonary Hypertension

PHT is defined by mean pulmonary artery pressure > 25 mm Hg at rest, or > 30 mm Hg at exercise. PHT affects 5 to 33 percent of SSc patients, depending on the diagnostic criteria used. Clinically severe PHT affects 9 percent of CREST patients.[26] Severe PHT usually occurs in patients with the limited cutaneous form of the disease, although it may also be observed in patients with diffuse SSc in association with pulmonary fibrosis. In the later situation, PHT is rarely severe (mPAP < 35 mmHg). PHT is a late complication of SSc, occurring 7 to 9 years after diagnosis. Pathology shows fibrosis of the intima, hypertrophy of the media, and plexogenic arteriopathy as observed in idiopathic PHT.[27] A mononuclear inflammatory infiltrate may be seen.[28]

Invasive hemodynamic study is the gold standard diagnostic test. It has been suggested to perform an invasive hemodynamic study in patients with suspected raised pulmonary artery systolic pressures of > 35 mm Hg, carbon monoxide transfer factor (TLCO) < 50 percent predicted, or a precipitous fall in TLCO > 20 percent over a 1 year period with no pulmonary fibrosis, and patients with SSc with breathlessness with no pulmonary fibrosis.[29] Doppler-echocardiography has a good positive predictive value but it cannot be used safely to exclude PHT in patients with an high prediagnostic probability as is the case in patients with SSc.[29,30] Echocardiography must be performed annually in patients with SSc.

The natural history of PHT is almost always progressive deterioration with death. In a recent series, survival was 81, 63, and 56 percent at 1, 2, and 3 years from the diagnosis.[29] Hemodynamic indices of right ventricular failure: raised mRAP (hazard ratio: 21), raised mPAP (hazard ratio: 20), and low CI (hazard ratio: 11) predicted an adverse outcome. There was no significant difference in survival between patients with SSc PHT with and without pulmonary fibrosis.

Treatment of PHT in SSc is linked to the evidence obtained in idiopathic PHT. Physical effort and pregnancy must be avoided because of the risk for acute right ventricule failure and death. Warfarin is recommended. Supplemental oxygen is given in patients with hypoxemia (PaO$_2$ < 60 mm Hg). Diuretics may be used in patients with edema. Vasodilators may be useful in patients with a significant vasodilatory response with inhaled nitric oxide testing: nifedipine and diltiazem are the most useful drugs.[31] High doses are needed: nifedipine 90 to 180 mg/day and diltiazem 360 to 720 mg/day. The use of lower doses is not effective. Angiotensin-converting enzyme inhibitors are not useful in this context. Continuous infusion of prostacyclin (epoprostenol) or its analog isoproterenol improves hemodynamic parameters and the effort capacity although the effect on survival is uncertain.[32] In the experience of the Antoine Béclère center (Clamart, France), survival in patients with CREST syndrome-associated PHT appeared to be lower than in patients with the idiopathic form of the disease.[33] Acute pulmonary edema may occur at the initiation of vasodilators in patients with veno-occlusive disease or capillary hemangiomatosis[34] both abnormalities may be observed in patients with SSc. Oral, inhaled or subcutaneously administered analogs of prostacyclin have been developed and demonstrate beneficial effects in PHT, either idiopathic or associated with CTD.[32] The effect is always limited in the latter compared with the former. Bosentan, an oral ETA and ETB endothelin receptors antagonist, prevented deterioration in the walking distance among patients with scleroderma-associated PHT.[35] Successful treatment of SSc digital ulcers and pulmonary arterial hypertension with bosentan has been reported.[36] Therapeutic trials using sildenafil are underway.[37] Anecdotal case reports indicate that immunosuppressants improve PHT associated with CTD, SLE and MCTD rather than scleroderma. A trial of corticosteroids and cyclophosphamide should be performed in patients with PHT under a strict clinical and hemodynamic control. Lung transplantation is possible in case of epoprostenol failure.[38]

Lung Cancer

Lung cancer incidence is increased four- to sixteen-fold in patients with SSc compared with the general population and may affect up to 4 percent of SSc patients.[39,40] This is similar to the increased risk observed in patients with idiopathic pulmonary fibrosis. Lung cancer occurs essentially in patients with pulmonary fibrosis and is not related to tobacco smoke. Adenocarcinomas of the bronchoalveolar type are overrepresented but all cell types are observed. The mechanisms of this association are not perfectly understood.

Miscellaneous Syndromes

Organizing pneumonia, alveolar hemorrhage, sarcoidosis, cystic lung disease, pneumothorax, and respiratory muscle dysfunction have been observed repeatedly in patients with SSc.[4] Aspiration pneumonia is especially frequent in patients with severe esophageal dysfunction. Dysphagia and gastroesophageal reflux due to motility disorder of the esophagus may be responsible for recurrent aspiration pneumonias.

The rigid skin and the associated involvement of the thoracic muscles of respiration may ultimately cause ventilatory failure with a restrictive pattern of pulmonary function abnormality.

A very rare syndrome, called *relapsing organizing pneumonitis* is described in association with PSS and is characterized by increasing breathlessness and confluent areas of consolidation. The entity is steroid responsive.

REFERENCES

1. Owens GR, Follansbee WP. Cardiopulmonary manifestations of systemic sclerosis. Chest 1987;91:118-27.
2. Manoussakis MN, Constantopoulous SH, Gharavi AE, Moutsopoulos HM. Pulmonary involvement in systemic sclerosis: A Association with anti-Scl 70 antibody and digital pitting. Chest 1987;92:509-13.
3. Altman RD, Medsger TA Jr, Bloch DA, Michel BA. Predictors of survival in systemic sclerosis (scleroderma). Arthritis Rheum 1991;34:403-13.
4. Minai OA, Dweik RA, Arroliga AC. Manifestations of scleroderma pulmonary disease. Clin Chest Med 1998;19:713-31.
5. LeRoy EC, Black C, Fleischmajer R, Jablonska S, Krieg T, Medsger TA Jr, et al. Scleroderma (systemic sclerosis): Classification, subsets and pathogenesis. J Rheumatol 1988;15:202-05.
6. Ferri C, Valentini G, Cozzi F, Sebastiani M, Michelassi C, La Montagna G, et al. Systemic sclerosis: Demographic, clinical, and serologic features and survival in 1,012 Italian patients. Medicine (Baltimore) 2002;81:139-53.
7. Lomeo RM, Cornella RJ, Schabel SI, Silver RM. Progressive systemic sclerosis sine scleroderma presenting as pulmonary interstitial fibrosis. Am J Med 1989;87:525-27.
8. Steen VD, Conte C, Owens GR, Medsger TA Jr. Severe restrictive lung disease in systemic sclerosis. Arthritis Rheum 1994;37:1283-89.
9. Wells AU, Cullinan P, Hansell DM, Rubens MB, Black CM, Newman-Taylor AJ, et al. Fibrosing alveolitis associated with systemic sclerosis has a better prognosis than lone cryptogenic fibrosing alveolitis. Am J Respir Crit Care Med 1994;149:1583-90.
10. Fujita J, Yoshinouchi T, Ohtsuki Y, Tokuda M, Yang Y, Yamadori I, et al. Non-specific interstitial pneumonia as pulmonary involvement of systemic sclerosis. Ann Rheum Dis 2001;60:281-83.

11. Kim DS, Yoo B, Lee JS, Kim EK, Lim CM, Lee SD, et al. The major histopathologic pattern of pulmonary fibrosis in scleroderma is nonspecific interstitial pneumonia. Sarcoidosis Vasc Diffuse Lung Dis 2002;19: 121-27.

12. Bouros D, Wells AU, Nicholson AG, Colby TV, Polychronopoulos V, Pantelidis P, et al. Histopathologic subsets of fibrosing alveolitis in patients with systemic sclerosis and their relationship to outcome. Am J Respir Crit Care Med 2002;165:1581-86.

13. American Thoracic Society. Idiopathic pulmonary fibrosis: Diagnosis and treatment. International consensus statement. Am J Respir Crit Care Med 2000;161:646-64.

14. Latsi PI, Wells AU. Evaluation and management of alveolitis and interstitial lung disease in scleroderma. Curr Opin Rheumatol 2003;15:748-55.

15. Wells AU, Hansell DM, Corrin B, Harrison NK, Goldstraw P, Black CM, et al. High resolution computed tomography as a predictor of lung histology in systemic sclerosis. Thorax 1992;47:738-42.

16. MacDonald SLS, Rubens MB, Hansell DM, Copley SJ, Desai SR, du Bois RM, et al. Nonspecific interstitial pneumonia and usual interstitial pneumonia: Comparative appearances at and diagnostic accuracy of thin-section CT. Radiology 2001;221:600-05.

17. Silver RM, Miller KS, Kinsella M, Smith EA, Schabel SI. Evaluation and management of scleroderma lung disease using bronchoalveolar lavage. Am J Med 1990;88:470-76.

18. Behr J, Vogelmeier C, Beinert T, Meurer M, Krombach F, Konig G, et al. Bronchoalveolar lavage for evaluation and management of scleroderma disease of the lung. Am J Respir Crit Care Med 1996;154:400-06.

19. White B, Moore WC, Wigley FM, Xiao HQ, Wise RA. Cyclophosphamide is associated with pulmonary function and survival benefit in patients with scleroderma and alveolitis. Ann Intern Med 2000;132:947-54.

20. Pakas I, Ioannidis JP, Malagari K, Skopouli FN, Moutsopoulos HM, Vlachoyiannopoulos PG. Cyclophosphamide with low or high dose prednisolone for systemic sclerosis lung disease. J Rheumatol 2002;29: 298-304.

21. Giacomelli R, Valentini G, Salsano F, Cipriani P, Sambo P, Conforti ML, et al. Cyclophosphamide pulse regimen in the treatment of alveolitis in systemic sclerosis. J Rheumatol 2002;29:7316.

22. Griffiths B, Miles S, Moss H, Robertson R, Veale D, Emery P. Systemic sclerosis and interstitial lung disease: A pilot study using pulse intravenous methylprednisolone and cyclophosphamide to assess the effect on high resolution computed tomography scan and lung function. J Rheumatol 2002;29:2371-78.

23. Clements PJ, Lachenbruch PA, Sterz M, Danovitch G, Hawkins R, Ippoliti A, et al. Cyclosporine in systemic sclerosis. Results of a forty-eight-week open safety study in ten patients. Arthritis Rheum 1993;36:75-83.

24. Clements PJ, Furst DE, Wong WK, Mayes M, White B, Wigley F, et al. High-dose versus low-dose D-penicillamine in early diffuse systemic sclerosis: Analysis of a two-year, double-blind, randomized, controlled clinical trial. Arthritis Rheum 1999;42:1194-1203.

25. Farge D, Passweg J, van Laar JM, Marjanovic Z, Besenthal C, Finke J, et al. Autologous stem cell transplantation in the treatment of systemic sclerosis: Report from the EBMT/EULAR Registry. Ann Rheum Dis 2004;63:974-81.

26. Stupi AM, Steen VD, Owens GR, Barnes EL, Rodnan GP, Medsger TA Jr. Pulmonary hypertension in the CREST syndrome variant of systemic sclerosis. Arthritis Rheum 1986;29:515-24.

27. Cool CD, Kennedy D, Voelkel NF, Tuder RM. Pathogenesis and evolution of plexiform lesions in pulmonary hypertension associated with scleroderma and human immunodeficiency virus infection. Hum Pathol 1997;28: 434-42.

28. Dorfmüller P, Perros F, Balabanian K, Humbert M. Inflammation in pulmonary hypertension. Eur Respir J 2003;22:358-63.

29. Mukerjee D, St George D, Coleiro B, Knight C, Denton CP, Davar J, et al. Prevalence and outcome in systemic sclerosis associated pulmonary arterial hypertension: Application of a registry approach. Ann Rheum Dis 2003;62:1088-93.

30. Mukerjee D, St George D, Knight C, Davar J, Wells AU, Du Bois RM, et al. Echocardiography and pulmonary function as screening tests for pulmonary arterial hypertension in systemic sclerosis. Rheumatology 2004;43: 461-66.

31. Alpert MA, Pressly TA, Mukerji V, Lambert CR, Mukerji B, Panayiotou H, et al. Acute and long-term effects of nifedipine on pulmonary and systemic hemodynamics in patients with pulmonary hypertension associated with diffuse systemic sclerosis, the CREST syndrome and mixed connective tissue disease. Am J Cardiol 1991;68:1687-91.

32. Gugnani MK, Pierson C, Vanderheide R, Girgis RE. Pulmonary edema complicating prostacyclin therapy in pulmonary hypertension associated with scleroderma: A case of pulmonary capillary hemangiomatosis. Arthritis Rheum 2000;43:699-703.

33. Badesch DB, McLaughlin VV, Delcroix M, Vizza CD, Olschewski H, Sitbon O, et al. Prostanoid therapy for pulmonary arterial hypertension. J Am Coll Cardiol 2004;43:56S-61S.

34. Sanchez O, Humbert M, Sitbon O, Nunes H, Garcia G, Simonneau G. Pulmonary hypertension associated with connective tissue diseases. Rev Med Interne 2002;23: 41-54.

35. Rubin LJ, Badesch DB, Barst RJ, Galie N, Black CM, Keogh A et al. Bosentan therapy for pulmonary arterial hypertension. N Engl J Med 2002;346:896-903.

36. Humbert M, Cabane J. Successful treatment of systemic sclerosis digital ulcers and pulmonary arterial hypertension with endothelin receptor antagonist bosentan. Rheumatology 2003;42:191-93.

37. Rosenkranz S, Diet F, Karasch T, Weihrauch J, Wassermann K, Erdmann E. Sildenafil improved pulmonary hypertension and peripheral blood flow in a patient with scleroderma-associated lung fibrosis and the raynaud phenomenon. Ann Intern Med 2003;139: 871-73.

38. Rosas V, Conte JV, Yang SC, Gaine SP, Borja M, Wigley FM, et al. Lung transplantation and systemic sclerosis. Ann Transplant 2000;5:38-43.

39. Abu-shakra M, Guillemin F, Lee P. Cancer in systemic sclerosis. Arthritis Rheum 1993;36:460-64.

40. Hill CL, Nguyen AM, Roder D, Roberts-Thomson P. Risk of cancer in patients with scleroderma: A population based cohort study. Ann Rheum Dis 2003;62:728-31.

ANKYLOSING SPONDYLITIS

In this condition, progressive inflammation of the spinal joints leads to ankylosis. It occurs mainly in young adults. A strong genetic predisposition for this disease is proved with the occurrence of the disorder in subjects carrying the HLA-B27 antigen.

The lungs are only involved in long-standing cases of ankylosing spondylitis.[1,2] Severe involvement of the thoracic cage leads to a restrictive pattern of lung function, which may be sufficient to cause dyspnea.

About 1 percent of patients with long standing disease may develop upper lobe fibrosis. There is no correlation with the severity of the disease. Bronchiectasis develops secondary to this fibrosis, and may contain fungal balls causing hemoptysis. Colonization with atypical mycobacteria can occur. In that situation, it becomes difficult to know whether mycobacteria or ankylosing spondylitis is the cause of upper lobe disease.

REFERENCES

1. Gacad G, Hamosh P. The lung in ankylosing spondylitis. Am Rev Respir Dis 1973;107;286-89.

2. Rosenow SC, Strimlan CV, Muhn JR, Ferguson P. Pleuropulmonary manifestations of ankylosing spondylitis. Mayo Clin Proc 1977,52:641.

SJÖGREN'S SYNDROME (SS)

This autoimmune disease is characterized by the infiltration of different organs by CD4-positive T lymphocytes, the lacrymal and salivary glands being the most often involved. The classic triad associates xerostomia (dry mouth), xerophtalmia (dry eyes) and arthritis. Multiple diagnosis criteria have been proposed, and have been recently updated.

Criteria now require the presence of either an anti-SSa or anti-SSb autoantibody, or a typical lesion on the accessory gland biopsy (Chisholm grade 3 or 4). SS may be isolated (primary SS) or associated with a definite CTD (secondary SS, primarily with RA). Lung involvement is less common and less severe in primary SS than in secondary SS. The involvement of lungs in this condition has been reported to occur in 9 to 75 percent of patients. However, the prevalence of pulmonary disease in SS varies widely according to the diagnostic modalities used to identify the abnormalities. HRCT detects abnormalities in 34 to 65 percent of SS patients evaluated.[2,3] A comprehensive evaluation including lung function tests detected abnormalities in 75 percent of SS patients.[4] However, if one considers only clinically significant pulmonary disease, it is estimated to affect less than 10 percent of SS patients.[5,6] Airways involvement and interstitial lung disease are the most frequent manifestations of lung involvement in SS. The manifestations may be: (i) dry cough with dry tracheobronchial mucosa (xerotrachea); (ii) airway narrowing; (iii) interstitial fibrosis; (iv) Diffuse lymphocytic infiltrates; (v) malignant lymphoma or reticulum cell sarcoma; and (vi) respiratory tract infections and pneumonia due to lack of respiratory secretions.[4,5]

Airways Involvement

Lymphocytic infiltration involves the entire respiratory tract from nares to bronchioles and alveoli.[7,8] Symptoms are thought to be secondary to the desiccation of the respiratory tract, to abnormalities of the mucociliary clearance and to the chronic inflammatory state of the airways, although some patients have no symptoms despite lymphocytic infiltration of the bronchial mucosa. Upper respiratory tract involvement manifests as dryness, crusting, recurrent infections, nasal septal perforation, and recurrent otitis media. Lower airways involvement will produce a dry irritating cough, observed in up to 50 percent of the patients,[9] and recurrent bronchial and pulmonary infections in about 20 percent of the patients.[9]

Many studies have evaluated obstructive airway disease in SS patients. Although one study found no evidence of obstructive airway disease when compared with control populations,[10] most of the studies using sensitive tests observed abnormal expiratory flows in patients with SS.[11] The clinical importance of these abnormalities remains unproven. Bronchial hypereactivity is detected in 40 to 60 percent of SS patients;[12] its mechanism is probably different from asthma-associated hyperreactivity as it is not controlled by inhaled corticosteroids.[13] HRCT studies confirm the prevalence of bronchial changes in SS with quite different prevalence values in different studies: bronchial mucosa thickening (8-68%), bronchiolar nodules (6-29%), bronchiectasis (5-42%), air trapping (32%).[3,14-17]

Interstitial Lung Disease

Interstitial lung disease is common in patients with SS and may reveal the disease. It affects 8 to 38 percent of patients with primary SS. The histopathology of interstitial lung disease in SS is not specific. Different histological patterns may be observed, sometimes associated in a given individual: NSIP, UIP, LIP, follicular bronchiolitis, organizing pneumonia, end-stage lung. NSIP is the more common pattern.[12] Well-formed granulomas may be seen in up to 10 percent of samples. Accordingly, the HRCT pattern in SS is not specific. However, cystic lesions are reported in about 30 percent of the patients with SS, often associated with LIP.[18] Cysts form as a consequence of bronchiolar obstruction due to follicular bronchiolitis, and sometimes bullous destruction of the lung occurs.[18]

Bronchoalveolar lavage has demonstrated the high prevalence of subclinical lymphocytic and neutrophilic alveolitis, affecting 50 percent of SS patients.[19] Alveolitis is more frequent in patients with extrapulmonary involvement. An expansion of CD8+ T-lymphocytes has been associated with more frequent alteration of lung function tests.[20] Neutrophilic alveolitis was associated with alterations of lung function tests.[21]

Information concerning the evolution and the treatment of interstitial lung disease in SS are limited. Available data suggest that interstitial lung disease in primary SS has a good prognosis without evidence of clinically significant deterioration over time, although progression of lung disease is more likely to occur in patients with BAL fluid neutrophilia[21] or with an abnormal HRCT of the lung.[22]

Hydroxycholoroquine has been shown to reduce sicca symptoms in a retrospective study[23] but its effect on pulmonary involvement was not evaluated. Organizing pneumonia in the context of SS respond quite well to corticosteroids. The response of LIP to corticosteroids and immunosuppressive therapies is not well described in the literature. The evolution of other forms of interstitial lung disease is poorly documented. Deheinzelin reported the evolution of 11 patients treated with azathioprine alone or combined with prednisone.[2] The condition of seven patients improved (symptomatic relief and increase of FVC) and one patient deteriorated. Among five untreated patients, only one improved. The respective position of these treatments is not clear but a trial of prednisone and azathioprine should be performed in symptomatic patients.

Pulmonary Lymphoma

Patients with SS have an increased risk of developing a lymphoma (relative risk). The risk is maximal for primary SS (*2). Sjögren's associated lymphoma is usually a B-cell non-Hodgkin's lymphoma which arise primarily in the salivary glands, but also in mucosal sites including stomach and the lung. Pulmonary lymphoma will affect 1 to 2 percent of all patients with SS.[24] Pulmonary involvement occurs in 20 percent of the patients with Sjögren's associated lymphoma.[25,26] Radiographical presentation may vary: chronic alveolar opacities, reticular or reticulonodular opacities, diffuse nodular lesions, or pleural effusion with or without mediastinal disease.[24] Pulmonary lymphoma may be indolent and surgically removed,[27] may be controlled with cytotoxic drugs such as chloraminophene or cyclophosphamide, and may evolve to an aggressive disease requiring a systemic polychemotherapy with monoclonal B cell antibodies.[28] The nature and existence of pseudo-lymphoma, a tumor-like aggregate of lymphoid cells that does not meet the criteria for malignancy, is debated.

Others

Pleural thickening and pleural effusions are uncommon in SS and should be investigated to determine their specific cause (lymphoma, tuberculosis, etc.). Pulmonary hypertension, pulmonary amyloidosis, the association of sarcoidosis with SS, diaphragmatic dysfunction, have been described.

REFERENCES

1. Vitali C, Bombardieri S, Jonsson R, Moutsopoulos HM, Alexander EL, Carsons SE, et al. Classification criteria for Sjögren's Syndrome: A revised version of the European criteria proposed by the American-European consensus group. Ann Rheum Dis 2002;61:554-58.
2. Deheinzelin D, Capelozzi VL, Kairalla RA, Barbas Filho JV, Nascimento Saldiva PH, Ribeiro de Carvalho CR. Interstitial lung disease in primary Sjögren's syndrome: Clinical pathological evaluation and response to treatment. Am J Respir Crit Care Med 1996;154:794-99.
3. Franquet T, Giménez A, Monill JM, Diaz C, Geli C. Primary Sjögren's Syndrome and associated lung disease: CT findings in 50 patients. AJR 1997;169:655-58.

4. Constantopoulos SH, Papadimitriou CS, Moutsopoulos MH. Respiratory manifestations in primary Sjögren's Syndrome: A clinical, functional, and histologic study. Chest 1985;88:226-29.

5. Strimlan CV, Rosenow EC, Divertie MB, Harrison EG. Pulmonary manifestations of Sjögren's syndrome. Chest 1976;70:354-61.

6. Davidson BKS, Kelly CA, Griffiths ID. Ten year of follow up of pulmonary function in patients with primary Sjögren's Syndrome. Ann Rheum Dis 2000;59: 709-12.

7. Ryu JH, Myers JL, Swensen SJ. Bronchiolar disorders. Am J Respir Crit Care Med 2003;168:1277-92.

8. Papiris SA, Saetta M, Turato G, La Corte R, Trevisani L, Mapp CE et al. CD4-positive T-lymphocytes infiltrate the bronchial mucosa of patients with Sjögren's Syndrome. Am J Respir Crit Care Med 1997;156:637-41.

9. Mialon P, Barthélémy L, Sebert P, Le Hénaff C, Sarni D, Pennec YL, et al. A longitudinal study of lung impairment in patients with primary Sjögren's Syndrome. Clin Exp Rheumatol 1997;15:349-54.

10. Papathanasiou MP, Constantopoulos SH, Tsampoulas C, Drosos AA, Moutsopoulos HM. Reappraisal of respiratory abnormalities in primary and secondary Sjögren's Syndrome. Chest 1986;90:370-74.

11. Gudbjörnsson B, Hedenström H, Stalenheim G, Hällgren R. Bronchial hyperresponsiveness to methacholine in patients with primary Sjögren's syndrome. Ann Rheum Dis 1991;50:36-40.

12. Yamadori I, Fujita J, Bandoh S, Tokuda M, Tanimoto Y, Kataoka M, et al. Nonspecific interstitial pneumonia as pulmonary involvement of primary Sjögren's syndrome. Rheumatol Int 2002;22:89-92.

13. Stalenheim G, Gudbjörnsson B. Anti-inflammatory drugs do not alleviate bronchial hyperreactivity in Sjögren's syndrome. Allergy 1997;52:423-27.

14. Papiris A, Maniati M, Constantopoulos SH, Roussos C, Moustopoulos HM, Skopouli FN. Lung involvement in primary Sjögren's Syndrome is mainly related to the small airway disease. Ann Rheum Dis 1999;58:61-64.

15. Uffman M, Kiener HP, Bankier AA, Baldt MM, Zontsich T, Herold CJ. Lung manifestation in asymptomatic patients with primary Sjögren's Syndrome: assessment with high resolution CT and pulmonary function tests. J Thorac Imaging 2001;16:282-89.

16. Koyama M, Johkoh T, Honda O, Mihara N, Kozuka T, Tomiyama N, et al. Pulmonary involvement in primary Sjögren's syndrome: spectrum of pulmonary abnormalities and computed tomography findings in 60 patients. J Thorac Imaging 2001;16:290-96.

17. Taouli B, Brauner M, Mourey I, Lemouchi D, Grenier P. Thin-section chest CT findings of primary Sjögren's syndrome: Correlation with pulmonary function. Eur Radiol 2002;1:1504-11.

18. Johkoh T, Ichikado K, Akira M, Honda O, Tomiyama N, Mihara N et al. Lymphocytic interstitial pneumonia: Follow-up CT findings in 14 patients. J Thorac Imaging 2000;15:162-67.

19. Hatron PY, Wallaert B, Gosset D, Tonnel AB, Gosselin B, Voisin C, et al. Subclinical lung inflammation in primary Sjögren's syndrome. Relationship between bronchoalveolar lavage cellular analysis findings and characteristics of the disease. Arthritis Rheum 1987;30: 1226-31.

20. Wallaert B, Prin L, Hatron PY, Ramon P, Tonnel AB, Voisin C. Lymphocyte subpopulations in bronchoalveolar lavage in Sjögren's syndrome. Evidence for an expansion of cytotoxic/suppressor subset in patients with alveolar neutrophilia. Chest 1987;92:1025-31.

21. Wallaert B, Hatron PY, Grosbois JM, Tonnel AB, Devulder B, Voisin C. Subclinical pulmonary involvement in collagen-vascular diseases assessed by bronchoalveolar lavage. Am Rev Respir Dis 1986;133: 574-80.

22. Salaffi F, Manganelli P, Carotti M, Baldelli S, Blasetti P, Subiaco S, et al. A longitudinal study of pulmonary involvement in primary Sjögren's syndrome: Relationship between alveolitis and subsequent lung changes on high-resolution computed tomography. Br J Rheumatol 1998;37:263-69.

23. Fox RI. Sjögren's syndrome: Evolving therapies. Expert Opin Investig Drugs 2003;12:247-54.

24. Cain HC, Noble PW, Matthay RA. Pulmonary manifestations of Sjögren's syndrome. Clin Chest Med 1998;19:687-99.

25. Hansen LA, Prakash UB, Colby TV. Pulmonary lymphoma in Sjogren's syndrome. Mayo Clin Proc 1989;64:920-31.

26. Royer B, Cazals-Hatem D, Sibilia J, Agbalika F, Cayuela JM, Soussi T, et al. Lymphomas in patients with Sjögren's syndrome are marginal zone B-cell neoplasms, arise in diverse extranodal and nodal sites, and are not associated with viruses. Blood 1997;90:766-75.

27. Cordier JF, Chailleux E, Lauque D, Reynaud-Gaubert M, Dietemann-Molard A, Dalphin JC, et al. Primary pulmonary lymphomas. A clinical study of 70 cases in nonimmunocompromised patients. Chest 1993;103: 201-08.

28. Isaacson PG, Du MQ. MALT lymphoma: From morphology to molecules. Nat Rev Cancer 2004;4:644-53.

MIXED CONNECTIVE TISSUE DISEASE

Patients with mixed connective tissue disease (MCTD) exhibit clinical features of SLE, progressive SSc, and Polymyositis-dermatomyositis.[1,2] A prerequisite for the diagnosis of MCTD is the presence of high titers of antibodies against uridine-rich RNA-small nuclear ribonucleoprotein (anti-RNP). Although they were not reported in the original publication on MCTD, pleuropulmonary manifestations are common in MCTD and the incidence varies from 20 to 85 percent.[2] Respiratory and nonrespiratory features of the disease follow those seen in SLE, scleroderma, or polymyositis-dermatomyositis. Major respiratory manifestations include interstitial lung disease and pulmonary fibrosis (20-65%), pleural effusion (50%), and pulmonary hypertension (10-45%). Other pulmonary features consist of pulmonary vasculitis, pulmonary thromboembolism, pulmonary infections (secondary to aspiration pneumonia due to esophageal motility alterations and immunosuppression), alveolar hemorrhage, pulmonary nodules, pulmonary cysts, mediastinal lymphadenopathy, and respiratory muscles dysfunction. PHT is a major cause of mortality and morbidity. Principles for diagnosis and treatment are similar to those described for SLE, scleroderma, and polymyositis-dermatomyositis.

REFERENCES

1. Prakash UB, Luthra HS, Divertie MB. Intrathoracic manifestations in mixed connective tissue disease. Mayo Clin Proc 1985;60:813-21.
2. Prakash UB. Respiratory complications in mixed connective tissue disease. Clin Chest Med 1998;19: 733-46.

POLYMYOSITIS-DERMATOMYOSITIS (PM-DM)

These are a group of inflammatory myopathies and are often included in the connected tissue diseases. PM and dermatomyositis (DM) are those which are particularly associated with pulmonary involvement. Pulmonary involvement may precede by many years, or occur simultaneously or follow the muscular manifestations of PM-DM.[1,2] The *antisynthetase syndrome* includes PM or DM (63-100%), interstitial lung disease (40-100%), Raynaud's phenomenon (25-100%), thick cracked skin over the tips and sides of the fingers (mechanics hands), and the presence of one of the seven identified antisynthetase antibodies. Severe constitutional symptoms are common, with fever in 80 percent of the patients, asthenia and weight loss. This syndrome must be recognized because of the high prevalence of pulmonary disorders.[3] Interstitial lung disease with CD8+ lymphocytic alveolitis without muscle involvement may be observed.[4] Five to eight percent of cases in the antisynthetase syndrome manifest as overlap syndromes with other CTD including RA, lupus, scleroderma, and SS.[3] The antisynthetase syndrome carries a poor prognosis that seems related to the severity and frequent steroid resistance of interstitial lung disease.

Different elements of the respiratory system may be involved in patents with PM/DM: respiratory muscles dysfunction,[5] interstitial lung disease, lung cancer, aspiration pneumonia in patients with pharyngolaryngeal muscles involvement, pulmonary hypertension.[6] Cardiac involvement is common and may induce dyspnea and chest X-ray abnormalities. Pulmonary involvement is a predominant cause of death, due to aspiration pneumonia (particularly in elderly patients),[7] to the evolution of pulmonary fibrosis or to lung cancer.[8] About 15 percent of patients with PM-DM have a diagnosis of cancer in their medical history.[9] Lung cancer is one of the most frequent. Both PM and DM increase the risk of having a lung cancer and the risk is maximal for DM [standardized index ratio for DM: 5.9 (3.7-9.2), for PM: 2.8 (1.8-4.4)].[9] Most of the cases (70%) occur after the diagnosis of PM/DM. The risk is maximal in the first year of diagnosis but persists for 5 years in PM, and even more for DM.

REFERENCES

1. Bohan A, Peter JB, Bowman RL, Pearson CM. An computed assisted analysis of 153 patients with polymyositis and dermatomyositis. Medicine 1977;56:255-86.
2. Yang Y, Fujita J, Tokuda M, Bandoh S, Ishida T. Chronological evaluation of the onset of histologically confirmed interstitial pneumonia associated with polymyositis/dermatomyositis. Intern Med 2002;41:1135-41.
3. Imbert-Masseau A, Hamidou M, Agard C, Grolleau JY, Cherin P. Antisynthetase syndrome. Joint Bone Spine 2003;70:161-68.
4. Sauty A, Rochat T, Schoch OD, Hamacher J, Kurt AM, Dayer JM, et al. Pulmonary fibrosis with predominant CD8 lymphocytic alveolitis and anti-Jo-1 antibodies. Eur Respir J 1997;10:2907-12.
5. Dauriat G, Stern JB, Similowski T, Herson S, Belmatoug N, Marceau A, et al. Acute respiratory failure due to diaphragmatic weakness revealing a polymyositis. Eur J Intern Med 2002;13:203-05.
6. Grateau G, Roux ME, Franck N, Bachmeyer C, Taulera O, Forest M, et al. Pulmonary hypertension in a case of dermatomyositis. J Rheumatol 1993;20:1452-53.
7. Marie I, Hatron PY, Levesque H, Hachulla E, Hellot MF, Michon-Pasturel U, et al. Influence of age on characteristics of polymyositis and dermatomyositis in adults. Medicine (Baltimore) 1999;78:139-47.
8. Marie I, Hachulla E, Hatron PY, Hellot MF, Levesque H, Devulder B, et al. Polymyositis and dermatomyositis: Short-term and long-term outcome, and predictive factors of prognosis. J Rheumatol 2001;28:2230-37.
9. Hill CL, Zhang Y, Sigurgeirsson B, Pukkala E, Mellemkjaer L, Airio A, et al. Frequency of specific cancer types in dermatomyositis and polymyositis: A population-based study. Lancet 2001;357:96-100.

BEHÇET'S SYNDROME

This occasionally involves the lungs producing arteritic lesions.[1] The lesions are multiple recurrent infarcts with hemoptysis, which may be fatal. High dose prednisolone with cyclophosphamide is the treatment of choice. Fibrinolytic agents like stanozolol or phenformin may be helpful in resolving thrombosis and are useful in persistent hemoptysis.

REFERENCE

1. Efthimiou J, Johnston C, Spiro SG, Turner-Warwick T. Pulmonary disease in Behcet's syndrome. Q J Med 1986,58:259-80.

OTHER DISEASES

Pulmonary involvement can occur in a number of other systemic diseases, although very rarely.[1-10]

REFERENCES

1. Wood JR, Bellamy D, Child AH, Citron KM. Pulmonary disease in patients with Marfan's syndrome. Thorax 1984;39:780-84.

2. Streeten EA, Murphy EA, Pyeritz RE. Pulmonary function in Marfan's syndrome. Chest 1987;91:408-12.

3. Riccardi VM. Von Recklinghausen neurofibromatosis. New Engl J Med 1981;305:1617-27.

4. Massaro D, Katz S, Mathews MJ, Higgins G. Von Recklinghausen's neurofibromatosis associated with cystic lung disease. Am J Med 1975;38:233.

5. Liberman BA, Chamberlain DW, Goldstein RS. Tuberous sclerosis with pulmonary involvement. J Can Med Assoc 1984;130:287-89.

6. Wood JR, Bellamy D, Child AH, Citron KM. Pulmonary disease in Marfan syndrome. Thorax 1984;39:780-84.

7. Ayres JG, Pope FM, Reidy JF, Clark TJH. Abnormalities of the lung and thoracic cage in Ehlers-Danlos syndrome. Thorax 1985;40:300-05.

8. White DA, Smith GJW, Cooper JAD, et al. Hermansky-Pudlak syndrome and interstitial lung disease: Report of a case with lavage findings. Am Rev Respir Dis 1984;130:138-41.

9. Young RC, Castro O, Baxter RP, Dunn R, Armstrong EM, Cook FJ, Sampson CC, et al. The lung in sickle disease: A clinical overview of common vascular, infectious, and other problems. J Nat Med Assoc 1981;73: 19-26.

10. Davis SC, Luce PJ, Win AA, et al. Acute chest syndrome in sickle-cell disease. Lancet 1984;1:36-38.

Occupational and Environmental Lung Diseases

Occupational lung diseases comprise a group of disorders caused by the inhalation of a wide variety of harmful materials, dust, microorganisms, smoke, allergens, vapors, fumes, etc. Although these substances are present in general environment, most of them occur in work-related environments in greater concentrations resulting in a variety of lung reactions including the lung parenchyma, and airways.[1]

Dusts are solid particles of mineral or organic origin dispersed in air or other gaseous media and as such, are different from fumes, vapors, and smoke. Dusts are produced due to mechanical disintegration of rocks, minerals, and other materials by impulsive forces such as drilling, blasting, crushing, grinding, sawing, and polishing, etc. They are also produced due to agitation or breaking down of organic substances like cotton fibers, pollens, and fungal spores. Thus, the size of dust particles varies widely. For example, while sand grains are about 200 to 2000 μm in diameter, virus particles are 28 nm to 0.2 μm in size.

Fumes are oxides of metals formed by heating of metals to their melting points. The particle size ranges from 0.1 to 1 μm. These particles aggregate easily, when they are referred to as *vapors.*

Mists are liquid droplets formed due to condensation of vapors or the atomization of liquids around appropriate liquids. Many particles are less than 0.1 μm in diameter and therapeutic mists are usually less than 10 μm.

Aerosols are airborne particles, which include all of the above categories and thus, consist of both dispersed particles and droplets.

Occupational lung diseases include a wide variety of disorders including cancer, hypersensitivity pneumonitis, COPD, bronchial asthma, bronchial hyperreactivity including altered pulmonary function changes.[2-14] Hypersensitivity pneumonitis (HP) develops after inhalation of many different environmental antigens, causing variable clinical symptoms that often make diagnosis uncertain. The prevalence of HP is higher than recognized, especially its chronic form. Mechanisms of disease are still incompletely known. Strategies to improve detection and diagnosis are needed, and treatment options, principally avoidance, are limited. Population-based studies are needed to more accurately document the incidence and prevalence of HP; better classification of disease stages, including natural history; evaluation of diagnostic tests and biomarkers used to detect disease; better correlation of computerized tomography lung imaging and pathologic changes; more study of inflammatory and immune mechanisms; and improvement of animal models that are more relevant for human disease.

It is generally agreed that many lung diseases such as asthma and chronic obstructive pulmonary disease (COPD) have polygenic inheritance, and that the association of a specific genotype or genotypes with the disease is likely to vary between populations. Furthermore, it is recognized that the etiology of many lung diseases involves a complex interplay between genetic background and exposure to multiple environmental stimuli, and understanding the mechanisms through which genes and environment interact represents a major challenge. Experimental approaches and challenges must be overcome to identify disease genes for asthma, COPD and chronic bronchitis, and occupational lung diseases.[14,15] In particular, common polymorphisms in CD14, glutathione S-transferase, and tumor necrosis factor alpha have been found to be important in gene-environment interaction and asthma pathogenesis. An understanding of gene-environment interactions in complex lung diseases is essential to the development of new strategies for lung disease prevention and treatment.[16]

Fate of Inhaled Particles

The subject has been discussed in the chapter on lung defence mechanisms. Briefly, inhaled aerosols closely follow the movement of air in the respiratory tract. The depth to which they can penetrate depends upon the physical characteristics (size, shape, density and aerodynamic properties), and the volume of each respiration. The aerodynamic property (aerodynamic diameter = actual diameter multiplied by p, where p is the density) is one of the most important determinants of such deposition. Maximum deposition occurs with 2 to 5 µm diameter range. Majority of the inhaled particles less than 1 µm diameter are expelled in the exhaled air, their concentration in the inhaled air must be high to enable some of them to be retained and deposited in the lung.

There are various ways in which solid particles are deposited—sedimentation, inertial impaction, interception, Brownian movement, and diffusion. Anatomy and physiological protective mechanisms, both immunological and nonimmunological, help to get rid of these noxious, unwanted substances. The role of the mucociliary escalator, macrophages, and various immunoglobulins has been discussed previously.

Studies on health effects of airborne particulate matter (PM) have traditionally focused on particles < 10 µm in diameter (PM_{10}) or particles < 2.5 µm in diameter ($PM_{2.5}$). The coarse fraction of PM_{10}, particles > 2.5 µm, has only been studied recently. These particles have different sources and composition compared with $PM_{2.5}$.

Time series studies relating ambient PM to mortality have in some places provided evidence of an independent effect of coarse PM on daily mortality, but in most urban areas, the evidence is stronger for fine particles. The few long-term studies of effects of coarse PM on survival do not provide any evidence of association.[17]

In studies of chronic obstructive pulmonary disease, asthma and respiratory admissions, coarse PM has a stronger or as strong short-term effect as fine PM, suggesting that coarse PM may lead to adverse responses in the lungs triggering processes leading to hospital admissions. There is also support for an association between coarse PM and cardiovascular admissions. Therefore, special consideration should be given to studying and regulating coarse particles separately from fine particles.

Airborne particles come in all sorts of sizes, shapes and compositions. The smallest, "ultrafine" particles are generated by nucleation and condensation, largely from combustion emissions. Their numbers are large (easily > 10,000 per cc), their mass is small (mass concentration

usually reaches only a few µg·m^{-3}). Ultrafine particles are inherently unstable, and grow through coagulation and condensation to larger "accumulation" particles, which are mostly 0.1 to 1 µm in diameter. These particles usually make up more than half of the particle mass in ambient air. Sulphates, nitrates, and elemental and organic carbon often dominate their composition. Because combustion processes ultimately generate all of these, such particles are usually coined "combustion" particles. Particles > 1 to 2 µm usually have a quite different origin and composition. Primarily mechanical processes, such as wind or abrasion, generate them. Often, crustal material, such as silicates, is a large fraction of coarse particles but this depends on the specific sources: metals may be important when large metallurgic industries are a main source. Such coarse particles may vary in size all the way up to 100 µm, larger particles become too heavy to remain airborne for any length of time.

In the last 15 years, airborne particles have been characterized in many areas by measurement of particulate matter (PM) < 10 µm in diameter (PM_{10}), because particles of this size can penetrate into the thoracic part of the airways where they may have adverse effects. The more inclusive measure of total suspended particulates (TSP) did incorporate larger particles, but was considered to be too unspecific to be used as a basis for air quality standards aimed at protecting human health. Effectively, introduction of PM_{10} has removed the larger particles, which may still deposit in the upper airways (nose, throat) from consideration when studying and regulating health effects of particles. Because PM_{10} is often mostly consisting of particles smaller than a few micrometers, it cannot be easily distinguished in studies from fine particles (FP), often measured as particles < 2.5 µm or $PM_{2.5}$. That is not to say that the concentrations are the same; the issue is that temporal and spatial variation of $PM_{2.5}$ and PM_{10} are often similar, despite the difference in sources and composition between fine and coarse particles (CP), simply because $PM_{2.5}$ is such a large fraction of PM_{10}.

Only in recent years has the difference between coarse and fine particles come to be more explicitly appreciated. Investigators have included separate measurements of fine and coarse particles in their studies rather than measurements of $PM_{2.5}$ and PM_{10}. This has shown that, in contrast to the high correlation between PM_{10} and $PM_{2.5}$, there is often much less correlation between $PM_{2.5}$ and coarse particles, usually defined and measured as particles > 2.5 and < 10 µm. Of note is that sometimes this quantity is arrived at by subtracting a direct measurement of $PM_{2.5}$ from a direct measurement of PM_{10};

the disadvantage of this is that coarse particle measurement is then affected by two measurement errors rather than one. Other sampling configurations separate fine and coarse particles before they are collected on filters to be weighed, or are detected by other means. These recent studies have made it possible to investigate the role of fine and coarse particles without running into the complication that any statement about PM_{10} is likely to be also valid for (or even dominated by) $PM_{2.5}$, simply because $PM_{2.5}$ is such a large fraction of PM_{10}. The observation that the correlation between fine and coarse particles if often low has made it relatively easy to separate their effects in field studies. Separate collection of fine and coarse particles on appropriate media has also facilitated toxicology studies, allowing conclusions as to whether, on a mass basis, the two fractions have equal or different toxicities, qualitatively as well as quantitatively.

A detailed description of the occurrence, measurement and correlations of coarse and fine particles has been described by Wilson and Su.[18] These authors concluded "fine and coarse particles are separate classes of pollutants and should be measured separately in research and epidemiologic studies. $PM_{2.5}$ and $PM_{(10-2.5)}$ are indicators or surrogates, but not measurements, of fine particles." To illustrate the last point, it has been shown that in certain areas windblown dust significantly contributes to $PM_{2.5}$.[19] An early example of a study that addressed fine and coarse PM separately is a study from the USA[20,21] which found that daily mortality in six cities was associated with fine particles but not with coarse particles. Since then, a small body of evidence has emerged that allows further analysis of the relative importance of fine and coarse particles.

Lung Reactions to Inhaled Particles

The character and severity of lung reactions are determined by three important basic factors:
- The nature and properties of the dust.
- The amount of dust retained in the lungs and the duration of exposure to it (dose × time) and
- Individual idiosyncrasy and immunological reactivity of the individual.
- The possible lung responses are summarized in Table 27.1.

PNEUMOCONIOSIS

Pneumoconiosis or dust related lung disease is the permanent alteration of lung structure due to inhalation of mineral dust and the tissue reactions of the lungs to

TABLE 27.1: Lung reactions to work-related substances

Type of disease/reaction	Occupational exposure
Bronchial asthma	Isocyanates, and a large number of other substances.
Bronchitis	Dust, fumes
Emphysema	Coal
Fibrosis	
diffuse	Asbestos, Beryllium
nodular	Silica, Coal
Hypersensitivity pneumonitis	Fungi in hay, Drugs, etc.
ARDS	Toxic gases
Lung cancer	Asbestos, Radon
Mesothelioma	Asbestos

its presence excluding bronchitis and emphysema. Thus, *pneumoconiosis can be defined as the nonneoplastic reaction of the lungs to inhaled minerals or organic dust and the resultant alteration in their structure excluding asthma, bronchitis, and emphysema.*

The chest radiograph has been an important tool in the diagnosis of occupational lung diseases. The International Labor Organization has recommended a classification to be used and this is strictly for studying pneumoconiosis.[22,23] The shadows are categorized as *small* or *large* opacities. The small opacities are subclassified on the basis of their predominant size. *Rounded* shadows are denoted as *p* (up to 1.5 mm diameter); *q* (1.5-3.0 mm in diameter); and *r* (3-10 mm diameter). *Irregular* opacities are denoted as s (up to 1.5 mm diameter); *t* (1.5-3.0 mm diameter); and *u* (3-10 mm diameter). Profusion of the lesions is assessed by comparison with standard films on a 0 to 3 scale. The broad categories are subdivided on the basis of whether the film is thought to be, say category 1 but category 0 is also considered seriously, (1/0) or category 1 but category 2 was considered (1/2). The abnormalities are divided into a 12-point classification. They are expressed as follows:

Category 0	0/-, 0/0, 0/1
Category 1	1/0, 1/1, 1/2
Category 2	2/1, 2/2, 2/3
Category 3	3/2, 3/3, 3/+

The classification also requires description of the lung zones affected, and recording of any other abnormalities like pleural plaques, diffuse thickening, and calcification. Symbols are provided for recording other features like tuberculosis, emphysema, and bulla, etc. Film quality needs to be commented upon. Thus, a complete classification should include the film quality, presence, site and category of small shadows, predominant types of small shadows, presence of pleural changes, or any other feature. If massive fibrosis is present, it should be staged as follows:

Stage A   Greater than 1 cm and up to 5 cm in maximum diameter

Stage B   Above 5 cm but less than the volume of the equivalent of the right upper zone

Stage C   Greater than B.

If multiple lesions greater than 1 cm are present, their maximum diameters are summed and categorized.

SILICOSIS

Silicosis (Latin, *silex*, flint) is perhaps the oldest occupational disease, probably existing in the paleolithic period. Hippocrates and Pliny refer to the disorder. Some of the most tragic and wanton examples of occupational disease were due to silicosis, for example, how table blade grinding in Sheffield (1886) robbed workers of 25 years of life, or the Gauley Bridge disaster in West Virginia (1931). Although some would suggest that simple silicosis is no longer a problem as it is "not associated with impairment or disability and even without effect on longevity in many although not all". However, in a carefully designed pooled analysis a clear exposure-response relation for silicosis and mortality is shown.[24] Increased mortality is also seen at exposure levels below the current US Occupational Health and Safety Administration's permissible exposure limit (PEL) of 0.10 mg/m³ for respirable crystalline silica. This conclusion is the culmination of considerable new knowledge concerning dose-response relations and methodological developments in the past few decades. New knowledge has accumulated concerning associations between silica exposure and pneumoconiosis, *Mycobacterium tuberculosis*, and chronic obstructive pulmonary disease. A key development has been the classification of silica as a human carcinogen (class 1) in 1996 by the International Agency for Research on Cancer (IARC).[25] One of the silicosis related disappointments at the close of the past century were the failure to develop new treatments for pulmonary fibrosis based on the once promising tetrandrine and polyvinylpridine-N-oxide research.

Silicosis, the chronic fibrosing disease of the lungs due to prolonged and heavy exposure to free crystalline silica; have been recognized as an occupational hazard for centuries. Silicosis is a preventable occupational lung disease caused by inhaling dust containing crystalline silica;[26] no effective treatment for silicosis is available. Deaths from inhalation of silica-containing dust can occur after a few months' exposure.[26] However, many developed countries have reduced the mortality with better control measures. Analysis of data from the USA indicates a decline in silicosis mortality during 1968-2002 and suggested that progress has been made in reducing the incidence of silicosis in the United States. However, silicosis deaths and new cases still occur, even in young workers. Because no effective treatment for silicosis is available, effective control of exposure to crystalline silica in the workplace is crucial.[27] Two main factors are likely responsible for this trend. First, many of the deaths in the early part of the study period occurred among persons whose main exposure to crystalline silica dust probably occurred before introduction of national compliance standards for silica dust exposure use permissible exposure limits [PELs] based on the American Conference of Governmental Industrial Hygienists threshold limit value). These limits began to be applied in the early 1970s and included indirect control through regulation of mixed mine dust in underground coalmines by using the MSHA (the Mine Safety and Health Administration) formula.[28] These regulatory limits, coupled with other recommendations such as that by NIOSH in 1974 (i.e. recommended exposure limit [REL] to respirable crystalline silica shall not exceed 0.05 mg/m³),[29] likely has led to reduced silica dust exposures since the 1970s. Ancillary preventive measures (e.g. respiratory protection, posting warning signs, and record keeping or reporting occupational illnesses) might also have reduced personal exposures. The second major factor relates to declining employment in heavy industries (e.g. mining industry from 989,400 employees in 1980 to 512,200 in 2002), where silica exposures were prevalent. However, silicosis deaths and new cases are still occurring, even in young workers in the United States. Because no effective treatment for silicosis is available, primary prevention (i.e. engineering or other control of exposure) should be maintained or improved to reduce worker morbidity and mortality.

The greatest death toll from silicosis in the United States occurred with excavation of Hawk's Nest Tunnel, critical to the construction of a hydroelectric plant in West Virginia during 1930-1931. Approximately 5,000 workers bored through Gauley Mountain to create the tunnel; an estimated 2,500 worked inside. A subsequent study determined that silicosis claimed the lives of at least 764 workers at Hawk's Nest Tunnel[30] By the end of 1937, a total of 46 states had passed laws relevant to workers with silicosis.

Most of the earth's crust consists of compounds of silicon and oxygen. The compound that is responsible for silicosis is silicon dioxide, which occurs in nature in three different crystalline forms. They are; quartz, crystobalite, and tridymite. Quartz is a hard, colorless substance and is the most common of all minerals and is a constituent of many rocks including granite and sandstone. The uncombined forms of silicon dioxide are called "free silica", which are different from silicates, which contain cations. The ubiquitous presence of silicon dioxide in the earth's crust is mainly responsible for the frequent contact of workers of various occupations. Crystalline silica exposure and silicosis have been associated with work in mining, quarrying, tunneling, sandblasting, masonry, foundry work, glass manufacture, ceramic and pottery production, cement and concrete production, and work with certain materials in dental laboratories. The following is the list of main occupational sources of free silica:

1. Mining, quarrying, and tunneling. Mining of gold, tin, copper, and mica produces dust with high concentrations of free silica. Sandstone is also a good source of free silica.
2. Stone cutting, dressing, polishing, and cleaning monumental masonry.
3. Abrasives and abrasive blasting.
4. Glass manufacturing.
5. Foundry work.
6. Pottery, porcelain, and brick lining.
7. Boiler scaling.
8. Vitreous enameling.

The 10 topmost type of industry and occupations that are more prone for development for silicosis in USA are as follows (the same may be different in other countries):

INDUSTRY

- Metal mining
- Miscellaneous nonmetallic mineral and stone products
- Pottery and related products
- Nonmetallic mining and quarrying, except fuel
- Iron and steel foundries
- Structural clay products
- Coal mining
- Miscellaneous fabricated metal products
- Miscellaneous retail stores
- Blast furnaces, steel works, rolling, and finishing mills.

OCCUPATION

1. Miscellaneous metal and plastic-processing machine operators
2. Hand molders and shapers, except jewelers
3. Hand molding, casting, and forming occupations
4. Crushing and grinding machine operators

5. Molding and casting machine operators
6. Mining engineers
7. Mining machine operators
8. Mining occupations, (other than above)
9. Supervisors, extractive occupations
10. Construction trades, (not mentioned otherwise).

These occupations and industries may be different in different countries. For example, in countries like India, stone cutting and mining may be more important occupations for the development of silicosis. Many other occupations associated with silicosis has been reported from all over the world.[31-33]

SILICOSIS IN INDIA

Studies to assess the exposure to free silica and the possible concurrent exposure to other hazards by respirable dust analysis for crystalline silica and heavy metals; chromium, copper, iron and nickel have shown the mean percentage of crystalline silica in the respirable dust is 23.9. The calculations for severity of exposure to crystalline silica shows that 61 percent of the samples analyzed for crystalline silica resulted in integrated RSPM levels in excess of the Permissible Exposure Limit (PEL); 46 percent exceeded PEL in the first unit, 80 percent in the second and 54 percent in third unit. The average concentration of the measured metals in samples of respirable dust are found to be chromium 0.389 $\mu g/m$ to the power 3 (microgram per cubic meter), copper 1.95 $\mu g/m$ to the power 3, iron 17.73 $\mu g/m$ to the power 3 and nickel 5.55 $\mu g/m$ to the power 3. The maximum concentrations are; chromium 2.3 $\mu g/m$ to the power 3, copper 3.9 $\mu g/m$ to the power 3, iron 47.5 $\mu g/m$ to the power 3 and nickel 11.9 $\mu g/m$ to the power 3. The average as well as the maximum concentrations of the metals are well below the Threshold Limit Values (TLV) of 500 $\mu g/m$ to the power 3, 1000 $\mu g/m$ to the power 3, 5000 $\mu g/m$ to the power 3 and 1000 $\mu g/m$ to the power 3 for chromium, copper, iron and nickel respectively. Crystalline silica is responsible for silicosis in foundry workers. The presence of metals is linked to increased risk for developing lung cancer in the foundry workers. The foundry atmosphere, however, presents a multiple exposure environment. There are many important confounders as smoking. The best can be said is, that the various agents act together synergistically and potentiate the cancer risk in foundry workers. However, one thing is very clear that silica exposure remains a common and important exposure and engineering controls have not been implemented to achieve the capture of particulate to attain compliance.[34] Similarly, in order to find out the associated risk of coal workers' pneumoconiosis in coal mines. The drilling, blasting and loading are the major dusty operations. Exposures of driller and loader were varied between, 0.81 to 9.48 mg/m^3 and 0.05 to 9.84 mg/m3 respectively in B & P mining, whereas exposures of DOSCO loader, Shearer operator and Power Support Face Worker were varied between 2.65 to 9.11 mg/m^3, 0.22 to 10.00 mg/m^3 and 0.12 to 9.32 mg/m^3 respectively in LW mining. In open cast mining, compressor and driller operators are the major exposed groups. The percentage silica in respirable dusts found below 5 percent in all most all the workers except among query loaders and drillers of open cast mines.[35] In another study copper levels were not different in those suffering from silicosis or those who are exposed, but having no disease.[36]

A number of occupations are associated with silicosis and the prevalence varied according to the occupation. Silicosis has been reported in emery polishing workers in cycle factory.[37] In another survey of 300 workers it was observed that 32 (10.66%) workers were suffering from silicosis of which 20 (62.5%) workers were working in small-scale sector and 12 (37.5%) in large-scale industry. Workers with duration of more than 10 years comprised 62.5 percent of silicotics and 37.5 percent had worked for less than 10 years. The prevalence of silicosis was 22.47 percent (20 out of 89) in workers engaged for more than 10 years and 5.68 percent (12 out of 211) who were working for less than 10 years. Shortness of breath was the most frequent symptom (43.34%) followed by dry cough (29.65%) and expectoration (6.68%). Mean FEV$_1$ in silicotics was 2.25 plus minus 0.59 L/s (p less than 0.01) and mean FVC was 2.52 plus minus 0.64 L (p less than 0.05). Radiology, most of silicotics had grade III and IV disease (31.25% and 59.37% respectively). 8 out of 32 (25%) silicotics were suffering from tuberculosis. The authors concluded that prevalence of Silicosis in emery polishers is more in small-scale industry as compared to large-scale industry and it increased with longer duration of exposure.[38] Lung function has been found to be reduced in workers exposed to silica.[39] Other occupations known to cause silicosis include flour-mill workers,[40] stone quarrying, and mining. Stone quaring and other stone related work is an important occupational hazard for the development of silicosis. The workers employed in stone quarries, which is an unorganized sector of industry, are exposed to variable silica dust concentration at their work place. A very large extent of respiratory morbidity and lung function impairment is observed in this group of employees. Four hundred sixteen sand stone quarry workers of Jodhpur district were screened for prevalence of silicosis and pulmonary tuberculosis to estimate magnitude of the problem in this region. Their chest radiographs were taken at 300 mA and were read according to international classification of radiographs of pneumoconioses, 1980. Concentration of total and respirable dust in quarries was measured. Chronic symptoms persistent for six or more months were cough (49.5%), expectoration (42.1%), dyspnea (41.1%) and pain chest (24.8%). Radiological opacities suggestive of silicosis were seen in 9.9 percent radiographs, and radiological signs of pulmonary tuberculosis were seen in 15.6 percent radiographs. Prevalence of both conditions increased with duration of work. Examination of sputum smear of subjects with symptoms of tuberculosis revealed 3.6 percent prevalence of bacteriologically confirmed cases of tuberculosis. Minimum concentration of respirable quartz was 8893 micron/m to the power of 3 in air samples collected from breathing zone of quarry workers, while WHO suggests a safe upper limit of 40 microns/m to the power of 3. The study indicates a considerable prevalence of silicosis in desert but of lesser magnitude and severity as compared to other parts of India.[41] A case control study of deceased quarry workers and controls comparing their age at the time of death showed that the mean age at death was 49.3 +/- 12.1 years in quarry workers and 60.0 +/- 14.4 years in nonworker controls. In another prospective study, a sample of 314 quarry workers and 40 ex-workers was followed up for a period of 17.4 +/- 7.2 months to study their mortality rate. This study demonstrated that there was excess mortality in quarry works (stanardised mortality ratio (SMR) = 1.84,95 percent confidence interval 0.79-2.90). Mortality was higher in those with opacities suggestive of silicosis in chest skiagrams (age adjusted death rate 66.3 per thousand per year and SMR = 6.95), than in nonsilicotics (age adjusted death rate 19.97 per 1000 per year and SMR = 1.63). Workers with pulmonary tuberculosis had significantly higher mortality than other quarry workers. Even in the absence of tuberculosis, mortality was more in silicotics (age adjusted death rate 24.9 per thousand per year, SMR 2.8).[42] Another cross-sectional study was carried out to study the respiratory morbidity and lung function involvement in this group. This study has found 32.5 percent prevalence of respiratory morbidity in stone quarry workers, on the basis of radiological appearance. However, no case of silicosis was detected. The impairment of lung function was significantly associated with increasing age, duration of dust exposure, smoking status and presence of chronic obstructive airways disease on radiological appearance. However, the measured dust concentration levels were found to be in permissible range. Thus, it can be concluded from this study that even low dust level exposure for longer duration can result in lung and lung function involvement. Hence, stone quarry workers, because of their occupational exposure to silica dust, are at increased risk of lung and lung function involvement.[43] In another survey the prevalence of silicosis was reported to be 38.2 percent among workers of small scale agate industry situated in and around Khambhat, Gujarat State. Follow-up survey carried out after a period of 6 years among 91 workers from the main study to assess the progress of silicosis revealed higher prevalence of respiratory morbidity in these workers. Predominance of restrictive pattern was observed on ventilatory function evaluation among these workers.[44]

Silicosis is a pervasive disease because of the ubiquitous presence of silica. It is one of the most important occupational diseases because of its high prevalence, irreversibility occurrence and its close relationship with tuberculosis. The precise data on industry-wise incidence of silicosis are not available at present. However, there are strong reasons, from some of the survey work, to believe that there is a very high incidence of disease in many industries, particularly the small scale and cottage industries in the country. There is a need for formulating countrywide strategy for the prevention and control of silicosis in industrial populations.[45] Another study from Orissa was carried out in three factories at Barang (glass, refractory and ceramic). These factories employ around 1,500 workers who attend the local ESI dispensary when sick. During December, 1989 to December, 1990, a total of 531 patients attended the dispensary with chest symptoms. Of these, 63 cases (diagnosed as pulmonary tuberculosis 54, pneumonia 2, lung abscess 4, bronchiectasis 2 and bronchial asthma 1) were referred to Department of TB and Chest Diseases, SCB Medical College, where their final diagnosis was: pulmonary tuberculosis 28, silicosis 17, occupational asthma 11, silicotuberculosis 6 and pulmonary eosinophilia 1.[46] The prevalence of airway obstruction as judged by FEV_1 percentage value in different categories of silicosis in state pencil industry, Mandasaur was determined and related to smoking habits and respiratory symptoms. The overall prevalence of airway obstruction was seen in 18.8 percent workers and a linear relationship with category of silicosis noted. In all categories of silicosis, smokers demonstrated significantly higher obstruction than nonsmokers. Obstruction was worse in category two and three with symptoms. This prevalence of airway obstruction is attributable to the very high concentration of total and respirable dust containing high percentage of free silica to which the workers are exposed.[47] Other Indian authors have reported rare presentations of silicosis in other occupations[48-52] and the status of occupational lung disease in India is being highlighted to be an important respiratory problem.[53]

Pathogenesis

The sequence of events in the development of silicosis include (i) inhalation of silica particles, of less than 10 µm in size, their penetration and retention; (ii) ingestion of the particles by the macrophages; (iii) death of macrophages; (iv) release of the contents of the dead cells including silica particles; accumulation of other inflammatory cells; (vi) collagen production; (vii) hyalinization and (viii) possible complications.

The prevalence and severity of development of disease is determined by the intensity and duration of exposure. Sandstone predisposes to a greater intensity of silica exposure than granite workers and exposure to high concentrations is effected in confined spaces over a short period.

Basic and clinical scientists have studied silicosis extensively, yet little is known about the crucial cellular and molecular mechanisms that initiate and propagate the process of inflammation and scarring.[54] Recent in vivo, in vitro, and human studies have focused on several main areas of investigation into the causes and processes of the development of silicosis. These areas of investigation include the variability of pathogenic potential of different varieties of silica; the role of activated alveolar macrophages products in the development and progression of silicosis; and the direct role played by the silica particle surface in triggering adverse biologic reactions, such as generating ROS (Reactive Oxygen species) and RNS (Reactive Nitrogen Species). The generation of oxidants by silica particles and by silica-activated cells results in cell and lung damage; increased expression of inflammatory cytokines, including TNF-alpha, IL 1 beta, and TGF-beta; activation of cell signaling pathways, including the MAP kinase pathways; and phosphorylation and activation of specific transcription factors (e.g. NFkB). The ROS, RNS, and NO generated by the silica particles also induce apoptosis in macrophages and other cells. To fully understand these pathogenetic mechanisms, further research on the molecular mechanisms involved in the inflammatory processes important for progression to fibrotic diseases is needed for the development of effective treatment of silicosis. Potential therapeutic strategies include inhibition of cytokines such as IL-1, TNF-alpha, the use of antioxidants, and the inhibition of apoptosis.[55]

Inhalation of crystalline (CS) and amorphous silica (AS) results in human pulmonary inflammation. However, silicosis develops only following CS exposure, and the pathogenic mechanisms are poorly understood. Recent reports describe the differential abilities of CS and AS to directly upregulate the early inflammatory mediator COX-2, the recently identified prostaglandin E (PGE) synthase and the downstream mediator PGE2 in primary human lung fibroblasts. Increased cyclooxygenase (COX)-2 gene transcription and protein production were demonstrated by ribonuclease protection assay, Western blot analysis, and immunocytochemistry. In each case the ability of AS to induce COX-2 exceeded that of CS. Similarly, downstream of COX-2, production of the antifibrotic prostaglandin PGE2 was induced in a dose-dependent fashion, but AS was significantly more potent. These increases in COX-2 and PGE2 were preceded by induction of the PGE2 synthase protein, demonstrating the potential role of this novel molecule in silica-mediated inflammation. There was specificity of induction of prostaglandins, as PGF2-alpha, but not PGD2, was induced. Using specific COX-2 inhibitors, and it was concluded that increased PG production to be dependent on the COX-2 enzyme. Furthermore, stimulation of fibroblasts was particle specific, as silica but not carbon black resulted in fibroblast activation. These results demonstrate that silica can directly stimulate human lung fibroblasts to produce key inflammatory enzymes and prostaglandins. Moreover, the findings suggest a mechanism to explain the differing fibrogenic potential of CS and AS. The molecules COX-2, PGE synthase, and PGE2 are identified as effectors in silicosis.[56]

Silica induces p53 transactivation via induction of p53 protein expression and phosphorylation of p53 protein and that p53 plays a crucial role in the signal transduction pathways of silica-induced apoptosis.[57] This finding may provide an important link in understanding the molecular mechanisms of silica-induced carcinogenesis and pathogenesis in the lung.

There are various theories, which are proposed to explain silicagenesis.

Theory of piezoelectric effect: According to this theory, minute electric currents due to mechanical stresses on quartz crystals damages the tissue cells. Recently, it is postulated that emissions of electrons from the edges of the tetrahedral crystals of silicon dioxide or electric charge-transfer between the crystals and cell membranes initiates the cell damage and fibrogenesis.

Solubility theory: This theory postulates that crystalline silica slowly dissolved in the tissue fluids produces silicic acid, which causes fibrosis. However, this theory is not tenable because of many reasons. A modified solubility theory explains that silicic acid is absorbed onto the protein of collagen precursors and they are polymerized into collagen. However, satisfactory evidence is lacking to support this theory.

Cytotoxic theory: Silicosis begins as a desquamative alveolitis and nodule formation occurs due to proliferation of collagen tissue. Macrophages that ingest silica particles soon rupture or become permeable and release their contents into the cytoplasm. After that the macrophages die discharging the ingested silica particles, enzymes and other constituents. The particles are re-ingested by other macrophages and the cycle is repeated. Quartz particles damage macrophages within an hour in a serum-free medium due to interaction with the plasma membrane, and lysosomal and cytoplasmic enzymes are released. In the presence of serum, however, the cytotoxic process is delayed because of coating of silica particles due to proteins. Only when the coating is digested in secondary lysosomes, the interaction occurs with the lysosomal membrane. This reaction occurs due to numerous strong hydroxyl (silanol) groups of silicic acid act' as hydrogen donors in hydrogen bonding reactions with the membranes of the secondary lysosomes causing irreversible injury.

The killed and damaged macrophages secrete a factor, which stimulates fibroblasts to synthesize collagen. One of the factors stimulates an increased production of hydroxyproline. Free silica inside the macrophages also produces or activates a relatively soluble substance, which is capable of stimulating collagen formation, and may act in low concentrations. It appears that this substance is a lipid-free material from the dust-laden macrophages that provokes fibrosis. The lipid substance from type II cells, which is also stimulated by substances released from macrophages, are probably protective.

All these observations are not able to fully explain all the events in silicosis. It appears that the effects of quartz are biphasic, and alter the proportions of both stimulating and inhibiting factors released from macrophages, so that their proportion is important in the development of fibrosis.

Immunological theory: Free silica particles cause immunological reactions in three possible ways; by acting as antigens; by producing autoantigens; and by acting as adjuvants. Experimental observations suggest that lung reactive antibodies might participate, at least in some cases. Possibly, these antibodies stimulate macrophages to release a fibrogenic factor, which enhances synthesis of collagen. To support the immunological basis of lung injury, an unusually high prevalence of antinuclear antibodies have been demonstrated with a good correlation with increasing radiological severity. Rheumatoid factor may be present in high titers in some patients with unexpectedly sudden progression or enhanced activity. Although the significance of these antibodies is not known, they may reflect the severity of macrophage damage/death and release of various substances. Other immunological alterations observed in silicosis include a deficiency of suppressor T cells, although the total numbers of lymphocytes and the number of T cells and B cells is normal. This deficiency could explain the development of autoantibodies and the occasional association of autoimmune disorders like systemic sclerosis. Other indirect evidence of immunological participation comes from the fact that silicotic lesions contain plasma cells and immune globulins and gamma globulins are increased in plasma of silicotics.

The role of genetic influence is not certain. A preliminary study of the HLA antigens indicates a decrease in B7, which could be linked to a greater risk of silicosis.

Pathology

Three types of tissue reactions have been described in silicosis.

1. Chronic, in which moderate exposure extends for a period of 20 to 40 years
2. Accelerated, increased dose for a period of 5 to 15 years
3. Diffuse, in which there is a heavy alveolar deposition of particles for a period of less than 5 years.

Chronic Silicosis

Nodules are easily felt over the lung, and vary from 2 to 6 mm in size, rounded in appearance, and have a whorled pattern and are gray-green to dark gray in color. Similar lesions are seen in the hilar nodes. The pleura is thickened and often adherent. The discrete and conglomerate nodules are more common in the upper lobes and more in the posterior than in the anterior segments. When the conglomerate nodules calcify and fuse with the fibrotic pleura the condition is called as "cuirasse."

Microscopic study recognizes the presence of dust particles in the macrophages or in the naked state in the alveolar walls. The particles can reach the supporting tissue of the finer air spaces either through macrophages or due to movement of the lungs. They also pass towards the hilum. Nodule formation occurs in the interstitial tissue containing free silica near the respiratory bronchioles. Here the nodules lie in relation to bronchioles and small arteries, lymphatics, and venules. The nodules surround a central hyaline zone that contains a variable amount of dust. A concentric zone of cellular connective tissue that contains no particles surrounds this. In turn, this zone is surrounded by a halo of dust containing crystalline silica in a zone of irregularly dispersed connective tissue, which also contains crystalline silica also. It is from the peripheral zone that silica is carried to enlarge the nodules and to start new nodules.

Silicosis is often complicated by formation of massive fibrotic lesions, most commonly in the upper lobes. These consist of matted nodules by fibrosis and obliterated blood vessels and bronchi. Small cystic lesions can be identified in the fibrotic areas. In coalminers with rheumatoid arthritis, the massive fibrosis is more common (discussed subsequently).

Accelerated Silicosis

The changes described in chronic silicosis are similar in accelerated silicosis, but the rate of progression is more rapid and the radiological changes are apparent after 4 to 8 years of exposure. The nodules have a tendency to occur near the alveolar walls in contrast to that in chronic silicosis, where nodules occur near the respiratory bronchioles. Development of massive fibrosis is more common and mostly located in the middle and basal portions of the lungs. Cavitations are common due to Mycobacterial infections.

Acute Silicosis

This is a relatively rare entity related to exposure to heavy concentrations of respirable free silica in enclosed spaces with inadequate protection. The development of disease is very rapid, and clinical features appear within 1 to 3 years of exposure. The lungs usually show massive consolidation with normal lung volumes. Although there is evidence of fibrosis, nodules and massive changes like that of chronic silicosis are lacking, at least grossly. Pulmonary edema develops terminally and exudation of fluid is seen flowing from the cut surfaces. The disease is usually complicated by mycobacterial or other infections. The characteristic microscopic change is the presence of acidophilic fluid, fine granules, macrophages, and type 2 cells within the alveolar spaces. The fluid contains both lipids and proteins, which is PAS positive. The alveolar cells undergo cuboidal transformation. Interstitial fibrosis is prominent, but silicotic nodules are poorly demarcated and are very small. Quartz crystals are present in the lungs and hilar lymph nodes.

Typically the pathological changes in silicosis can be described as follows. Three types of lesions are typically seen in individuals who are exposed to dusts containing a mixture of crystalline silica and silicates. These include macules, mixed-dust fibrotic lesions (MDF), and silicotic nodules.[58] Macules are nonpalpable lesions consisting of interstitial accumulations of dust-laden macrophages. These typically show a peribronchiolar or perivascular distribution and are associated with a delicate meshwork of reticulin fibers without obvious collagenization. MDF is a palpable, irregularly contoured, stellate-shaped lesion with varying degrees of collagenization. Macules and MDF have a tendency to spread diffusely into the adjacent lung tissue (diffuse interstitial fibrosis pattern)[59]. Centrilobular emphysema may accompany macules and MDF, and in some cases, it may be a dominant pathologic feature even in the absence of a history of smoking. Silicotic nodules are well-delineated, firm, almost acellular fibrotic nodules composed of whorled hyalinized collagen. When viewing these various lesions by polarizing microscopy, numerous birefringent particulates are typically observed. Crystalline silica usually shows a weak birefringence in contrast to most silicates, which are intensely double refractile.[58] The presence of particles compatible with crystalline silica under polarized light helps to distinguish silicotic nodules from similar fibrous nodules of other etiologies. In any individual case, macules, MDF, and silicotic nodules may be observed to varying degrees and in various combinations. Progressive massive fibrosis or conglomerate lesions may be observed in some cases.

Mixed-dust pneumoconiosis (MDP) is a recently described entity[60] that is defined pathologically as a pneumoconiosis showing dust macules or mixed-dust fibrotic nodules (MDF), with or without silicotic nodules (SN), in an individual with a history of exposure to mixed dust. The authors defined the latter arbitrarily as a mixture of crystalline silica and nonfibrous silicates. According to their definition of MDP, therefore, MDF should outnumber SN in the lung to make a pathologic diagnosis of MDP. In the absence of confirmation of exposure, mineralogic analyses can be used to support the pathologic diagnosis. The clinical diagnosis of MDP requires the exclusion of other well-defined pneumoconioses, including asbestosis, coal workers' pneumoconiosis, silicosis, hematite miners' pneumoconiosis, welders' pneumoconiosis, berylliosis, hard metal disease, silicate pneumoconiosis, diatomaceous earth pneumo-

coniosis, carborundum pneumoconiosis, and corundum pneumoconiosis. Typical occupations associated with the diagnosis of MDP include metal miners, quarry workers, foundry workers, pottery and ceramics workers, and stonemasons. Irregular opacities are the major radiographic findings in MDP (ILO 1980), in contrast to silicosis, in which small rounded opacities predominate. Clinical symptoms of MDP are nonspecific. MDP must be distinguished from a variety of nonoccupational interstitial pulmonary disorders.

Cases of pneumoconiosis that do not show typical clinicopathologic features of silicosis or other well-defined pneumoconiosis are frequently encountered in Japan and elsewhere. The term *mixed-dust pneumoconiosis* (MDP) originated in European countries to describe the lung lesions of ferrous and nonferrous foundry workers[61-63] where concomitant exposure to silica and nonfibrogenic dusts occurred. However, some confusion and ambiguity remain in terms of its definition. The term is chosen arbitrarily to focus on a narrow definition of MDP, based on the pathologic descriptions of the lungs of patients exposed occupationally to a mixture of crystalline silica and mainly, nonfibrous silicates. Silicates represent relatively weakly fibrogenic dusts and modify the intense fibrogenic response to crystalline silica, as do other dusts such as iron.[64] Iron oxide and non-coal carbon particles are considered to be minor constituents of mixed dust in certain situations. Crystalline silica plays a key role in this definition of MDP, and this definition would constitute the basis for further attempts to evaluate diverse biologic effects of combinations of *nonsiliceous* dust mixture in general.[65]

Mineralogic Analysis

The silica content of the lungs is also increased. The normal lungs contain free silica up to a maximum of 0.2 g, whereas in disease states the content may be as high as 15 to 20 gm. Similarly, in normal persons, the average percentage of silica in ash is 14.7 percent, but in silicosis the range varies from 29.4 to 48 percent. The silicon percentage of dry matter is usually 2 to 3 percent, but may be as high as 20 percent in severe cases, while that in the normal lungs without industrial exposure is 0.1 to 0.2 percent and that of normal hilar lymph nodes range from 0.23 to 0.60 percent. The silica content has a direct bearing on the fibrosis produced in the lungs.

Mineralogic analysis of tissue specimens may be performed in a number of different ways. One approach is the ashing of the tissue and analysis of recovered dust gravimetrically and by X-ray diffraction.[66,67] To obtain accurate identification of the mineral species, the X-ray diffraction analysis is required, employing the X-ray absorption correction.[68,69] Unfortunately, this approach requires a large sample of lung tissue. Another approach involves *in situ* analysis of tissue sections by analytical electron microscopy (scanning, transmission, or scanning transmission electron microscopy). A convenient and frequently employed technique is the examination of 5 μm-thick sections in a scanning electron microscope equipped with a backscattered electron detector and an energy dispersive spectrometer.[70,71] An advantage of this technique is that it can be performed on a section serial to the one used to make the pathologic diagnosis. Another detailed and rather complete technique is the examination of particles directly transferred to electron microscopic grids after ashing 5 to 20 μm-thick lung tissue sections.[65] This provides comprehensive data on particle shape, crystal structure, and chemical composition.[72,73] Electron-microscopic particle analysis can also be performed on particles isolated from lung tissue including transbronchial lung biopsy material,[74] bronchoalveolar lavage fluid, or even lymph nodes after ashing or digestion of the organic components.[75-77] These data contribute to defining the characteristics such as chemistry, crystallinity, size and concentration of the particles. The advantages and disadvantages of these methods are many.[78] Analysis typically shows the presence of silica, silicates, and various metal particles. These dust levels usually exceed by orders of magnitude the levels of such particles that are found in a background, unexposed population.[71]

Clinical Features

The diagnosis is aided by a well-documented occupational history of concomitant exposure to mixed dust as defined above. Typical occupations associated with a diagnosis of silicosis include metal miners, quarry workers, foundry workers, pottery and ceramics workers, and stonemasons.

Silicosis is a *chronic disease,* and the main symptoms develop late and not until after 20 years of exposure, although earlier changes occur in some forms of silicosis.[79-82] There may be no symptoms even though the radiographic appearances may be surprisingly advanced. The earliest symptoms in chronic cases are cough and expectoration. However, the principal symptom in chronic silicosis is progressive dyspnea. Hemoptysis, and chest pain may be present due to infection. Weight loss is marked due to tuberculosis and other types of infections. Fungal infections due to nocardiosis, cryptococcosis, and sporotrichosis complicate this pneumoconiosis and they are common, particularly in accelerated

or acute forms of silicosis. Respiratory failure is the most important sequel of complicated silicosis. Pneumothorax is another important complication and difficult to manage because of poor expansion of the shrunken, fibrotic lung. This may further aggravate respiratory failure.

There is an increased prevalence of connective tissue disorders in silicosis. This association is seen in about 10 percent of cases. The common associations are scleroderma, rheumatoid arthritis, and systemic lupus erythematosus. These diseases are usually associated with a rapid progression of the radiologic and functional abnormalities.

In *accelerated silicosis*, the main features of the disease are similar to that in chronic silicosis, but the chest X-ray findings are apparent within 4 to 8 years of first exposure. The course of the disease is rapid. About 25 percent of the cases are secondarily infected by Mycobacteria, and about half of these cases are due to atypical organisms. The common atypical organisms are *M. intracellulare* and *M. kansasii.*

Exposure to smaller amount of silica particles produces mild form of the disease over a long period of time. This may occur in patients exposed to minor amounts of quartz contaminating other minerals.

Silicoproteinosis

It is very rapidly progressing silicosis in which there are characteristic histological changes. Silicoproteinsosis is a rare disorder. It usually occurs after prolonged exposure to silica dust. The association of silicosis with rheumatoid arthritis (RA) is possible, although rare. This occurs due to heavy exposure to respirable silica dust. Exertional dyspnea develops within 6 months of exposure. There is weight loss, weakness, cyanosis, and diffuse crepitations in the chest. Mycobacterial infection occurs invariably. The disease progresses very rapidly, with some temporary benefit from steroids. Death results from intractable hypoxemia.[83,84]

Silicosis and Tuberculosis

The association of silicosis and tuberculosis has been recognized since a long time ago. In earlier studies, coexistent tuberculosis was reported in 65 to 75 percent of cases of silicosis.[48,85-87] Over the years, the incidence has fallen dramatically, but still may be high in areas of high prevalence of tuberculosis. Although the incidence of tuberculosis may be declining in chronic silicosis, it is still high in accelerated and acute forms of the disease and in the elderly. Nowadays, silicotuberculosis may represent a geriatric problem. In the elderly, recognition of tuberculosis associated with silicosis is often difficult. Occupational history, radiology (conventional chest radiography and computed tomography) and microbiology (identification of *Mycobacterium tuberculosis* in sputum and pleural exudate) are helpful for the correct diagnosis, which, in turn, is important for prognosis and treatment, as well as in relation to medicolegal issues and occupational-related compensation claims. The chest radiographic findings may show cavities, infiltrations, or in the presence of fibrosis, tuberculous elements may be difficult to distinguish. Sputum positive cases may show reversion with treatment, but fibrosis will progress despite antitubercular therapy. The disease is more common in the lower lobes, and more advanced the silicosis, the greater is the incidence of active tuberculosis. The effect of silica dust on tuberculosis infection has also been proved in experimental animals. This is possibly affected through the action of silica on macrophages, which are important in defenses against tuberculous infections. On the other hand, tuberculosis enhances the fibrotic reaction in silicosis and the progression of the disease is very rapid.

Although there appears to be no relationship between silicosis and lung cancer,[88-90] recent reports indicate an increased incidence of this malignancy. Workers from the stone and quarry industry compensated for silicosis are at an increased risk of developing lung cancer. In order to reduce that risk, the exposure has to be lowered, with a peak exposure below 0.15 mg/m³ and an average exposure below 0.10 mg/m³. Other studies also support a causal relationship between lung cancer and quartz exposure after allowance for cigarette smoking, in the absence of other known carcinogens. However some investigators thought it failed to find similar evidence to explain the excess mortality from either chronic renal disease or kidney cancer. Further results support the hypothesis that high exposure to insoluble particulates such as silica in the metal, glass, ceramics, and stone industries promotes bronchial cancer and chronic obstructive pulmonary disease. An increased incidence of stomach cancer is reported in this population that might be related to particles swallowed after clearance from the airways.

Diagnosis

The diagnosis of silicosis is mainly based on the history and radiological findings like any other pneumoconiosis. A history of significant exposure to free silica is required for the diagnosis. In the simple form of the disease, rounded nodules are the basic features. In com-plicated silicosis, massive densities predominate. Radiologic findings of on plain chest radiographs include a mixture of small rounded and irregular opacities as defined by the 1980 International Labor Office International Classification of Radiographs of Pneumoconioses. In some cases with pathologically proven macular pneumoconiosis, the chest radiograph may be within normal limits. If small rounded opacities predominate and siderosis is excluded, the appropriate diagnosis is silicosis. In cases in which irregular opacities predominate or are found exclusively, a diagnosis of mixed dust pneumoconiosis can be made with the appropriate occupational history. Large opacities may or may not be present. Areas of emphysema are often seen. In the emphysematous lungs, ^{99m}Tc macroaggregated human serum albumin scintigrams clearly show a marked reduction of the pulmonary arterial perfusion. The grading of pneumoconiosis in chest X-rays is discussed earlier. The lesions in silicosis are more prominent in the upper lung zones. Presence of massive changes may indicate a complication by mycobacterial infection, or in association with rheumatoid arthritis. Massive changes are usually apparent as masses in the upper lobes with contraction of lung volumes and hyperinflation at the bases. Calcification of silicotic nodules is rare. However, lymph nodes may calcify producing an "eggshell" appearance of the hilar nodes. Extreme enlargements of nodes within the mediastinum may compress the superior vena cava or esophagus. Varying degrees of pleural thickening is not uncommon. The acute form of the disease is characterized radiologically by involvement of both lungs diffusely with airspace shadows. Although infection is common, cavities are rare. Mixed exposure to silica and asbestos can have features of both.

X-ray changes of patients with "late silicosis" that occurred in 5 to 20 years after they had retired from dust-related occupation, have been described. Follow-up over 4 to 25 years demonstrated progression of nodular pneumosclerosis up to macronodular forms or silicotuberculoma formation.[91] The diseases mostly developed gradually, usually were diagnosed by casual X-ray examination and were long considered as tuberculosis, sarcoidosis or other disseminated lesion. Thus, taking occupational history is very essential.

The disease must be differentiated from other conditions, which produce similar changes in chest X-ray. These include sarcoidosis, malignancy, tuberculosis, histoplasmosis, pulmonary alveolar microlithiasis, and calcified lung lesions secondary to chickenpox.

The most common of the pneumoconioses are silicosis, coal workers pneumoconiosis, and asbestosis.

The former two are characterized by the presence of small nodular opacities predominantly distributed in the upper zones of the lung. The small nodular opacities are classified into two patterns on HRCT: (a) ill-defined fine branching lines and (b) well-defined discrete nodules. Asbestosis demonstrates thickened interlobular and intralobular lines, subpleural dot-like or curvilinear opacities, and honeycombing on HRCT, predominantly distributed in the bases of the lungs. Although HRCT findings of other pneumoconioses are variable and nonspecific, there are predominant and characteristic findings for each type of pneumoconiosis. HRCT is useful in achieving more accurate categorization of the parenchymal changes in each type of pneumoconiosis. Profusion of opacities on HRCT correlates with functional impairment. The presence of branching centrilobular structures may be helpful in early recognition of silicosis. Uniformly calcified and hyperdense LNs are common in silicosis, and eggshell LN calcification is rare. There are associations between LN attenuation and lung function impairment, and CT grades of nodular profusion and PMF (Figs 27.1 to 27.4).

Qualitative and quantitative CT parameters can be used as indirect measures of functional impairment in silicosis. PMF and emphysema are independently related to airflow obstruction, whereas mean lung attenuation is related to clinical dyspnea and reduced lung volume.[92-96]

Pulmonary function changes In the early stages of the disease there is no change in the lung function parameters except in few cases a slight reduction in vital capacity and arterial oxygen tension. Pulmonary function tests can be normal or show an obstructive, restrictive, or mixed pattern. With advanced stages, impairments in one or more parameters are abnormal but to a lesser extent than that would be suggested by radiographs. There is a decrease in vital capacity, total lung capacity, residual volume, functional residual capacity, and compliance without evidence of airway obstruction. In some cases, diffusing capacity may be decreased slightly, but it is usually normal till a very late stage of the disease. Arterial hypoxemia is only evident on exercise.

Smoking, dust exposure, and emphysema are three important factors that can confound the association between silicosis and lung function. Despite the importance of smoking in relation to lung function, some studies did not control for smoking, or smoking was controlled inadequately. The data suggest a weak association between lung function (mainly obstruction) and dust exposure, although some studies had crude measures of exposure. In general, the lung function of those with radiographic silicosis in category 1 was indistinguishable from those in category 0. Those in category 2 had small reductions in lung function relative to those with category 0 and little difference in the

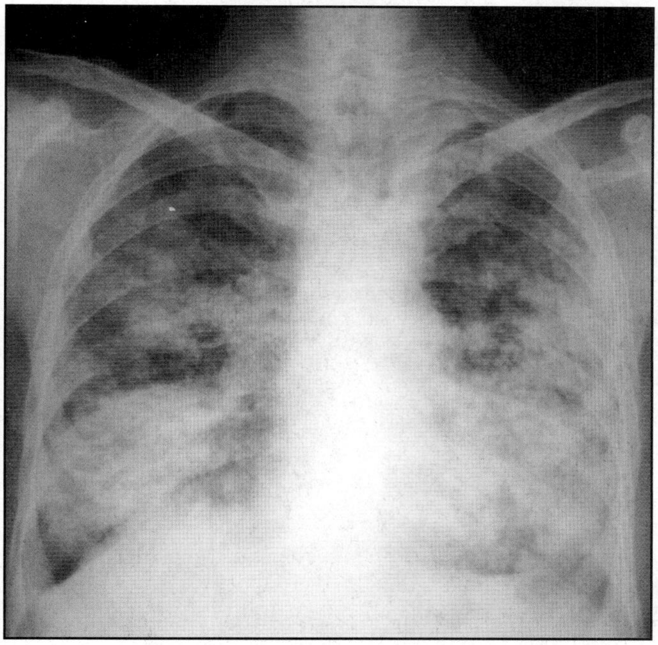

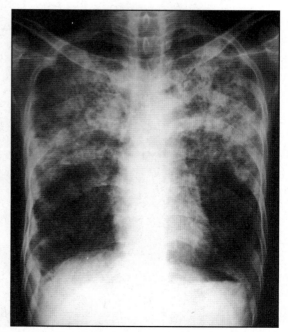

FIGURE 27.1: Sillicosis in a polishing worker

FIGURE 27.2: A case of sillicosis. Note dense opacities with upper zone involvement

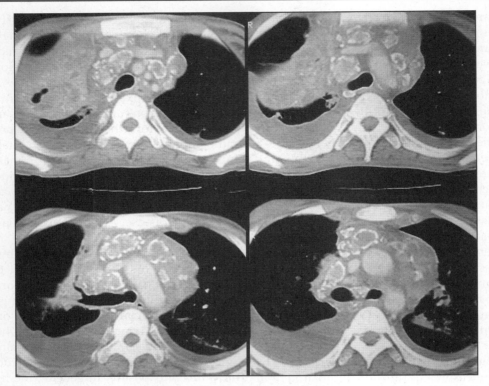

FIGURE 27.3: CT Chest - Right upper lobe consolidation. Right pleural effusion and mediastinal lymphnodes with eggshell calcification-silico-tuberculosis

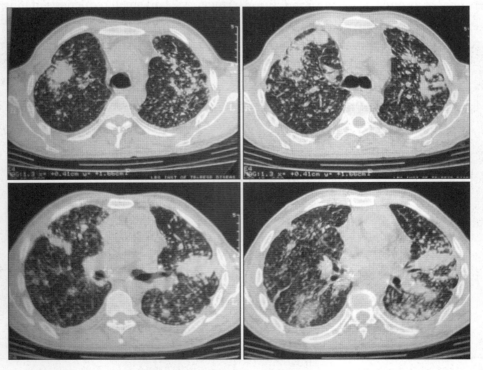

FIGURE 27.4: CT Scan of the previous patient. Note changes of progressive massive fibrosis

prevalence of emphysema. There were slightly greater decrements in lung function with category 3 and more significant reductions with progressive massive fibrosis. Emphysema was related to higher categories of silicosis, as well as to smoking. Silica exposure was often inadequately controlled in studies examining silicosis and lung function. A few studies suggested that emphysema is an independent risk factor associated with significant reductions in lung function.[97-101]

Lung biopsy: Very rarely a lung biopsy is required to diagnose a case of silicosis. Sometimes, this may be undertaken, if the radiological changes are atypical. Such situations include diffuse alveolar filling or diffuse interstitial reactions, complicating autoimmune disease, progressive and rapid deterioration, and when there is history of exposure to more than one type of dust. When a lung biopsy is required, an open biopsy is preferable, because of inadequate tissue sampling in closed biopsy procedures.

When histological patterns are not specific enough, examination under polarized light will demonstrate doubly refractile particles of silica. When further characterization is necessary, fine particles of quartz can be demonstrated by scanning electron microscopy. Excess silica can also be demonstrated by X-ray energy spectrometry. High silicon-sulphur ratios determined by this method are diagnostic of pneumoconiosis and are strongly suggestive of silicosis. Presence of other elements like calcium, magnesium, or iron can also be detected by X-ray energy spectrometry.

Miscellaneous tests: Gallium-67 lung scanning is positive in all stages of silicosis. Similarly, Technetium leveled inhalation tests will be positive in all stages of the disease.

Bronchoalveolar lavage has been used recently in the diagnostic workup of silicosis. Total cell counts are increased with alterations of lymphocytes. The predominant cell in the bronchoalveolar lavage fluid (BALF) in silicosis is macrophage. Various enzymes including LDH, p-glucuronidase, and alkaline phosphatase are increased in the bronchoalveolar lavage fluid. Compared with control subjects, increased TNF-alpha, IL-1beta, IL-8, and IL-6 levels are found in the BALFs in silicosis. Furthermore, IL-6 levels in the BALF of silicosis subjects are significantly higher than that seen in other diseases.[102-104]

Both thin section and high resolution CT scan are helpful in detecting early disease when plain chest X-ray and conventional CT scans are normal. The latter is particularly helpful in detecting subpleural nodules.

Differential diagnosis should include asbestosis, berylliosis, carborundum (silicon carbide) pneumoconiosis, coal workers' pneumoconiosis, corundum pneumoconiosis, diatomaceous earth pneumoconiosis, hematite miners' pneumoconiosis, hard metal (lung) disease (tungsten carbide pneumoconiosis), silicate pneumoconiosis (silicatosis), Fuller's earth, Kaolin, Mica, Talc, mixed dust pneumoconiosis and Welders' pneumoconiosis. They can be differentiated with appropriate occupational history, biopsy and mineral analysis.

Complications

Infections: As already mentioned, tuberculosis is the most common infection in silicosis. The usual organisms are *M.tuberculosis* and other atypical mycobacteria. Fungal infections are also common. The fungal infections include Aspergillosis, Nocardiosis, Cryptococcosis, and Sporotrichosis. *Cor pulmonale* Right ventricular hypertrophy and pulmonary hypertension leading to heart failure is clinically uncommon despite extensive fibrotic changes in the lungs. However, in some cases, death due to heart failure is possible.

Bronchitis: Acute or subacute bronchitis is quite common due to secondary infections. Chronic bronchitis however, is unrelated to silica exposure, unless there is concurrent smoking history.

Emphysema: Scar emphysema are occasionally observed around nodules and larger bullous areas of the same type of emphysema may be related to conglomerate lesions.

Spontaneous pneumothorax: Spontaneous pneumothorax is an uncommon complication due to rupture of a bleb or bulla and the resulting pneumothorax is loculated due to pleural adhesions. However, treatment of pneumothorax is difficult because of poor expansion of the lungs, which may aggravate respiratory failure.

Miscellaneous: Collagen vascular diseases are more common in silicosis. Bronchogenic carcinoma occasionally occurs in silicotic lungs, and the risk of development of such malignancy is controversial. Irreversible abductor paralysis of the left vocal cord is a rare sequel due to involvement of the left recurrent laryngeal nerve in a mass of silicotic lymph nodes. Similarly compressions of the esophagus and superior vena cava obstruction may rarely be possible. A nephropathy has been described in association with silicosis, although adequate explanation for its occurrence is not provided. It is possible that it is just a chance association.

Broncholiths

This is a rare complication.[105] Sartorelli[106] was the first to describe broncholithiasis in patients with silicosis in

1957. Eggshell calcification of the lymph nodes is a common finding in patients with this pneumoconiosis, but these calcified lymph nodes rarely erode into the bronchial lumen. This physiopathological mechanism was reported in cases where the association of silicosis and broncholithiasis was present, leading to bronchial obstruction,[107] bronchoesophageal fistula[108] and hemoptysis.[109] The clinical presentation of broncholithiasis depends primarily on its location and its obstruction level. Some patients may be asymptomatic. The main symptom is a dry cough with eventual expectoration. Hemoptysis may vary from mild to severe. Fever and chills are often related to infectious complications. Wheezing may occasionally occur due to mechanical obstruction of the airways. According to the 15 case series studied by Conces et al,[110] lithoptysis is not frequent, but the present authors' patient presented recurrent lithoptysis with expectoration of multiple broncholiths.

The most important radiological manifestations are signs of bronchial obstruction and changing position or disappearance of a calcified focus on repeat radiographs, this being a significant aspect in the present case. CT allows a better visualization of the lesions and it is especially useful for establishing the relationship between the calcification and the bronchi.[111] Since bronchoscopy was normal, the CT scans provided essential information for the diagnosis of broncholithiasis in this patient, by clearly showing broncholiths closely related to the involved bronchi.

The prognosis of broncholithiasis is usually favorable and its treatment is restricted to clinical follow-up. Some invasive procedures may be necessary, depending on location, size and associated complications. In addition to its diagnostic role in central lesions, bronchoscopy may be useful for the removal of broncholiths. Surgery might be indicated in some selected cases and when there is risk of bleeding.[112]

Treatment

There is no treatment available to halt the progress or cause resolution of silicosis in humans. Although PVPNO and related substances and polybetaine effectively prevent silicosis in animal models, they are not suitable for human use. A related compound, poly-2-vinylpyridine-l-oxide, is under trial since it is neither carcinogenic nor toxic like the other compounds. 3-amino-proprionitrile (BAPN) inhibits or reverts cross linkage of collagen and helps in preventing progression of silicosis in experimental animals and controls scar tissues in human surgery. However, its usefulness in silicosis has not been proved. Corticosteroids do not influence or halt the progress of disease, although recent studies have shown some benefit.[116] Their use is obviously dangerous in the presence of unrecognized tuberculosis, which is not uncommon in silicosis. Appropriate treatment is necessary for, bronchitis, congestive heart failure, cough, and pneumothorax, etc.

Treatment of complicating tuberculosis needs use of most effective drugs for longer periods of time. As mentioned, although sputum conversion is possible, rapid progression of fibrosis is not prevented. In some cases, drug resistance develops rapidly and management becomes difficult.

Prevention of silicosis depends upon recognition of such hazards and should consist of dust control and disposal measures. Continuous and random analysis of atmospheric dust in the work environment is desirable. Adequate ventilation and wet techniques should be used to reduce the quantity of free silica. Whenever possible, materials are to be substituted for free silica. Respirators are required when the concentrations of respirable free silica exceeds the threshold limit value by 5 times. Use of masks at workplace is another simple means of reduction of quantity of dust inhalation.

Prognosis

The overall prognosis of uncomplicated silicosis is invariably good with a normal life span, although some respiratory symptoms may be present. In a small proportion of cases the progression is very rapid with respiratory disability and death. The chances of cor pulmonale and heart failure are increased if there is associated tuberculosis. The presence of rheumatoid arthritis or rheumatoid factor is an indicator of progression. Presence of chronic obstructive disease is another poor prognostic indicator.

Prevention of Silicosis

To control silicosis, one needs to understand how change happens in occupational health. Science alone does not drive policy, because the causes of silicosis are well known, and how to prevent it for decades, yet the disease persists.[113-115] To control occupational disease, the social realm of work is to be understood. In a classical example to investigate the determinants of a successful silicosis control program, the social history of the Vermont Granite Industry from 1938 to 1960, were examined through union journals, newspapers, industry journals, scientific literature and government documents, and interviewing key informants. The crucial factor of the successful program was a strong public health movement to control tuberculosis, rather than pressure to control the occupational disease. Using this lesson, to protect workers from silica exposure, regulation of silica under an environmental law is essential, as is enacted as the Massachusetts Toxics Use Reduction Act. Possibly a stronger movement, currently the environmental movement, is essential to increase the awareness as well control measures. Unions are too weak to demand safe technologies; experts need to emphasize to enforce them.

REFERENCES

1. Parks WR. Occupational Lung Disorders (2nd edn), Butterworths: London, 1982.
2. Fink JN, Ortega HG, Reynolds HY, Cormier YF, Fan LL, Franks TJ, Kreiss K, Kunkel S, Lynch D, Quirce S, Rose C, Schleimer RP, Schuyler MR, Selman M, Trout D, Yoshizawa Y. Needs and opportunities for research in hypersensitivity pneumonitis. Am J Respir Crit Care Med 2005;171:792-98.
3. Moore JE, Convery RP, Millar BC, Rao JR, Elborn JS. Hypersensitivity pneumonitis associated with mushroom worker's lung: An update on the clinical significance of the importation of exotic mushroom varieties. Int Arch Allergy Immunol 2005;136:98-102.
4. Krewski D, Burnett RT, Goldberg M, Hoover K, Siemiatycki J, Abrahamowicz M, Villeneuve PJ, White W. Reanalysis of the Harvard Six Cities Study, part II: Sensitivity analysis. Inhal Toxicol 2005;17:343-53.
5. Sorahan T, Kinlen LJ, Doll R. Cancer risks in a historical UK cohort of benzene exposed workers. Occup Environ Med 2005;62:231-36.
6. Meldrum M, Rawbone R, Curran AD, et al. The role of occupation in the development of chronic obstructive pulmonary disease (COPD). Occup Environ Med 2005;62:212-14.
7. Kennedy SM. Agents causing chronic airflow obstruction. In Harber P, Schenker MB, Balmes JR (Eds): Occupational and environmental respiratory disorders. St Louis: Mosby, 1996;443-49.
8. Christiani DC, Wang XR, Pan LD, et al. Longitudinal changes in pulmonary function and respiratory symptoms in cotton textile workers. Am J Respir Crit Care Med 2001;163:847-53.
9. Chan-Yeung M, Enarson D, Kennedy S. The impact of grain dust on respiratory health. Am Rev Respir Dis 1992;145:476-87.
10. Christiani DC. Organic dust exposure and chronic airway disease. Am J Respir Crit Care Med 1996;154:833-34.
11. Hnizdo E, Sullivan PA, Bang KM, et al. Association between chronic obstructive pulmonary disease and employment by industry and occupation in the US population: A study of data from the Third National Health and Nutrition Examination Survey. Am J Epidemiol 2002;156:738-46.
12. Balmes J, Becklake M, Blanc P, et al. American Thoracic Society Statement: Occupational contribution to the burden of airway disease. Am J Respir Crit Care Med 2003;167:787-97.
13. Barcenas CH, Delclos GL, El-Zein R, Tortolero-Luna G, Whitehead LW, Spitz MR. Wood dust exposure and the association with lung cancer risk. Am J Ind Med. 2005;47:349-57.
14. Ross MH, Murray J. Occupational respiratory disease in mining. Occup Med (Lond) 2004;54:304-10.
15. Mapp CE. Genetics and the occupational environment. Curr Opin Allergy Clin Immunol 2005;5:113-18.
16. Kleeberger SR, Peden D. Gene-environment interactions in asthma and other respiratory diseases. Annu Rev Med 2005;56:383-400.
17. Brunekreef B, Forsberg B. Epidemiological evidence of effects of coarse airborne particles on health. Eur Respir J 2005;26:309-18.
18. Wilson WE, Su HH. Fine particles and coarse particles: Concentration relationships relevant to epidemiologic studies. J Air Waste Manag Assoc 1997;47:1238-49.
19. Claiborn CS, Finn D, Larson TV, Koenig JQ. Windblown dust contributes to high PM2.5 concentrations. J Air Waste Manag Assoc 2000;50:1440-45.
20. Schwartz J, Dockery DW, Neas LM. Is daily mortality associated specifically with fine particles? J Air Waste Manag Assoc 1996;46:927-39.
21. Klemm RJ, Mason RM Jr, Heilig CM, Neas LM, Dockery DW. Is daily mortality associated specifically with fine particles? Data reconstruction and replication of analyses. J Air Waste Manag Assoc 2000;50:1215-22.
22. International Labour Office. Meeting of experts on the international classification of ragiographs of the pneumoconioses. Occupational Safety and Health 9. Geneva: International Labour Office, 1959.
23. ILO. Guidelines for the use of the ILO international classification of radiographs of pneumoconiosis revised edition. ILO 1980.
24. d' Mannetje A, Steenland K, Attfield M, et al. Exposure-response analysis and risk assessment for silica and silicosis mortality in a pooled analysis of six cohorts. Occup Environ Med 2002;59:723-28.
25. IARC. Monographs on the evaluation of carcinogenic risks to humans: Silica, some silicates, coal dust and para-aramid fibrils. Lyon: World Health Organisation, International Agency for Reseach on Cancer 1997;68.
26. Elmes PC. Inorganic dusts. In Raffle PAB, Adams PH, Baxter PJ, Lee WR (Eds): Hunter's diseases of occupations (8th edn). Boston, MA: Little, Brown, and Co. 1994.
27. Palmer K. Silicosis Mortality, Prevention, and Control—United States, 1968-2002. Occup, Environ, Med 2004; 61: 77.
28. National Institute for Occupational Safety and Health. NIOSH criteria for a recommended standard: occupa-

tional exposure to respirable coal mine dust. Cincinnati, OH: US Department of Health and Human Services, CDC, National Institute for Occupational Safety and Health; 1995;(NIOSH) publication no. 95-106.

29. National Institute for Occupational Safety and Health. NIOSH criteria for a recommended standard: Occupational exposure to crystalline silica. Cincinnati, OH: US Department of Health, Education, and Welfare, Public Health Service, CDC, National Institute for Occupational Safety and Health (NIOSH) 1974;75-120.

30. Cherniack M. The Hawks' Nest incident: America's worst industrial disaster. New Haven, CT: Yale University Press 1986.

31. Antao VC, Pinheiro GA, Kavakama J, Terra-Filho M. High prevalence of silicosis among stone carvers in Brazil. Am J Ind Med 2004;45:194-201.

32. Cohen R, Velho V. Update on respiratory disease from coal mine and silica dust. Clin Chest Med 2002;23:811-26.

33. Churchyard G J, Ehrlich R, teWaterNaude J, Pemba L, Dekker K , Vermeijs M , White N, Myers J. Silicosis prevalence and exposure-response relations in South African goldminers. Occup Environ Med 2004;61:811-16.

34. Singh SR. Concentration of free silica and heavy metals in respirable suspended particulate matter in small scale foundries in Chandigarh: India. Ind J Occupat Environ Med 2001;5:196-200.

35. Mukherjee AK, Bhattacharya SK, Saiyed HN. Assessment of respirable dust and its free silica contents in different Indian coalmines. Ind Health 2005;43:277-84.

36. Tiwari RR, Sathwara NG, Saiyed HN. Serum copper levels among quartz stone crushing workers: A cross sectional study. Indian J Physiol Pharmacol 2004;48: 337-42.

37. Malik SK, Behera D, Awasthi GK, Singh JP. Pulmonary silicosis in emery polish workers. Ind J Chest Diseas Alli Scien 1985;27:116-21.

38. Whig J, Sandhu BS, Mahajan R, Sachar RK, Gupta SK, Gupta B, Jain S, Gupta A. Prevalence of silicosis among emery polish workers in cycle industry. Lung India 2004;21:1-4.

39. Tiwari RR, Sharma YK, Seiyad HN. Peak expiratory flow: A study among silica-exposed workers India. Ind J Occupat Environ Med 2004;8:7-10.

40. Sundram P, Kamat R, Joshi JM. Flourmill lung: A pneumoconiosis of mixed aetiology. Indian Journal of Chest Diseases and Allied Sciences 2002;44:199-201.

41. Mathur ML, Murli Lal Mathur. Silicosis among sand stone quarry workers of a desert district: Jodhpur. Annals of the National Academy of Medical Sciences (India) 1996;32:113-18.

42. Ghotkar VB, Maldhure BR, Zodpey SP. Involvement of lung and lung function tests in stone quarry workers. Indian Journal of Tuberculosis 1995;42:155-60.

43. Mathur ML, Choudhary RC. Mortality experience of sand stone quarry workers of Jodhpur district. Lung India 1996;14:66-68.

44. Sadhu HG, Parikh DJ, Sharma YK, Saiyed HN, Rao PVC, Kulkarni PK, Kashyap SK. A follow-up study of health status of small scale agate industry workers. Indian Journal of Industrial Medicine 1995;41:101-05.

45. Saiyed HN. Silicosis: A challenge to industrial physicians. Indian Journal of Industrial Medicine 1994;40:50-55.

46. Tripathy SN, Bhutia RC, Dash DP, Swain SR. Pattern of respiratory disorders among workers of glass and ceramic factories. Indian Journal of Tuberculosis 1992;39:136.

47. Rao NM, Saiyed HN, Kashyap SK, Chatterjee SK, Mohan Rao N. Airway obstruction in silicosis workers. Lung India 1991;9:126-29.

48. Nigam SK, Saiyed HN. Silica dust exposure and its pathogenesis in induction of silicosis, silico-tuberculosis and cancer in man: The recent concept. Ind J Occup Med 2001;5:148-52.

49. Oak JL, Shetty S. Silicoproteinosis with rheumatoid arthritis. JIRA 1997;5:37-39.

50. Rao S, Rau PVP, Rao S. Bilateral spontaneous pneumothorax in silicosis. Indian Journal of Chest Diseases and Allied Sciences 1993;35:47-49.

51. Natarajan AS, Gajalakshmi L, Karunakaran S. Accelerated silicosis in a silica flour mill worker. Lung India 1992;10:33-37.

52. Purohit SD, Gupta PR, Gupta ML, Chauhan A. Acute silicosis in handlers of silica powder bags. Lung India 1992;10:145-48.

53. Pande JN, Khilnani GC. Occupational lung diseases in India. Indian Journal of Community Medicine 1993;18: 136-40.

54. Lugano EM, Daubor JH, Elias JS, et al. The regulation of lung fibroblast proliferation by alveolar macrophages in experimental silicosis. Am Rev Respir Dis 1984;129:767.

55. Rimal B, Greenberg AK, Rom WN. Basic pathogenetic mechanisms in silicosis: Current understanding. Curr Opin Pulm Med 2005;11:169-73.

56. O'Reilly KM, Phipps RP, Thatcher TH, Graf BA, Van Kirk J, Sime PJ. Crystalline and amorphous silica differentially regulate the cyclooxygenase-prostaglandin pathway in pulmonary fibroblasts: Implications for pulmonary fibrosis. Am J Physiol Lung Cell Mol Physiol 2005;288:L1010-16.

57. Wang L, Bowman L, Lu Y, Rojanasakul Y, Mercer RR, Castranova V, Ding M. Essential role of p53 in silica-induced apoptosis. Am J Physiol Lung Cell Mol Physiol 2005;288:L488-96.

58. Craighead JE, Kleinerman J, Abraham JL. Diseases associated with exposure to silica and nonfibrous silicate minerals. Arch Pathol Lab Med 1988;112:673-720.

59. Green FHY, Churg A. Diseases due to nonasbestos silicates. In: Churg A, Green FHY (Eds). Pathology of Occupational Lung Disease. Baltimore: Williams & Wilkins 1998;235-76.

60. Honma K, Abraham JL, Vuyst PD, Dumortier P, Gibbs AR, Green FHY, et al. Proposed criteria for mixed-dust pneumoconiosis: Definition, descriptions, and guidelines

for pathologic diagnosis and clinical correlation. Human Pathol 2004;35:1515-23.

61. Uehlinger E. Über Mischstaubpneumokoniosen. Schweiz Z Pathol Bakt 1946;9:692-700.

62. Harding HE, Gloyne RS, McLaughlin AIG. Industrial lung diseases of iron and steel foundry workers, HMSD, London 1950.

63. Harding HE, McLaughlin AIG. Pulmonary fibrosis in non-ferrous foundry workers. Br J Ind Med 1955;12: 92-99.

64. Gibbs AR, Wagner JC. Diseases due to silica. In: Churg A, Green FHY (Eds) : Pathology of Occupational Lung Disease. Baltimore, MD: Williams & Wilkins; 1998; 209-33.

65. Jederlinic PJ, Abraham JL, Churg A. Pulmonary fibrosis in aluminum oxide workers. Investigation of nine workers, with pathologic examination and micro-analysis in three of them. Am Rev Respir Dis 1990; 142:1179-84.

66. Pooley FD. Tissue mineral identification. In: Weill H, Turner-Warwick M (Eds). Occupational Lung Diseases. Research Approaches and Methods, New York: Marcel Dekker 1981;189-35.

67. Gibbs AR, Pooley FD. Analysis and interpretation of inorganic mineral particles in "lung" tissues. Thorax 1996;51:327-34.

68. Lange BA, Haartz JC. Determination of microgram quantities of asbestos by X-ray diffraction: Chrysotile in thin dust layers of matrix material. Anal Chem 1979;51:520-25.

69. Kohyama N. A new X-ray diffraction method for the quantitative analysis of free silica in airborne dust in working environment. Ind Health 1985;23:221-34.

70. Abraham JL, Burnett BR, Hunt A. Development and use of a pneumoconiosis database of human pulmonary inorganic particulate burden in over 400 lungs. Scanning Microsc 1991;5:95-108.

71. McDonald JW, Roggli VL, Churg A. Microprobe analysis in pulmonary pathology. In Ingram P, Shelburne J, Roggli V, et al (Eds): Biomedical Applications of microprobe analysis. San Diego, CA: Academic Press 1999;201-56.

72. Pooley FD. Electron microscope characteristics of inhaled chrysotile asbestos. Br J Ind Med 1972;29:146-53.

73. Langer AM, Pooley FD. Identification of single asbestos fibers in human tissues. In Bogovski P, Gilson JC, Timbrell V, et al (Eds): Biological effects of asbestos, IARC Sci Publ. No. 8, Lyon, France: IARC 1973;119-25.

74. Kohyama N, Kyono H, Yokoyama K. Evaluation of low-level asbestos exposure by transbronchial lung biopsy with analytical electron microscopy. J Electron Microsc 1993;42:315-27.

75. Mason GR, Abraham JL, Hoffman L. Treatment of mixed-dust pneumoconiosis with whole lung lavage. Am Rev Respir Dis 1982;126:1102-07.

76. Dumortier P, De Vuyst P, Yernault JC. Non-fibrous inorganic particles in human bronchoalveolar lavage fluids. Scanning Microsc 1989;3:1207-18.

77. Dumortier P, De Vuyst P, Yernault JC. Comparative analysis of inhaled particles contained in human bronchoalveolar lavage fluids, lung parenchyma and lymph nodes. Environ Health Perspect 1994;102:257-59.

78. Churg A, Green FHY. Analytic methods for identifying and quantifying mineral particles in lung tissue. In Churg A, Green FHY (Eds): Pathology of occupational lung disease. Baltimore, MD: Williams & Wilkins 1998; 45-55.

79. Ziskind M, Jones RN, Weill H. Silicosis. Am Rev Respir Dis 1976;113:643.

80. Koskinen H. Symptoms and clinical findings in patients with silicosis. Scand J Environ Health 1985;11:101.

81. Irwig LM, Rocks P. Lung function and respiratory symptoms in silicotic and nonsilicotic gold miners. Am Rev Respir Dis 1978;117:429.

82. Occupational lung diseases. Seaton A, Seaton D, Leitch AG. In Crofton and Douglas' Respiratory Diseases (4th edn), Blackwell Scientific Publications, 1989;798.

83. Buchner HA, Ansari A. Acute silicoproteinosis. Dis Chest 1969;55:174.

84. Oak JL, Shetty S. Silicoproteinosis with rheumatoid arthritis. JIRA 1997;5:37-39.

85. Snider DE. The relation between tuberculosis and silicosis. Am Rev Respir Dis 1978;118:455.

86. Scafa F, Minelli CM, Fonte R, Rosso GL, Cappelli MI, Candura SM. Silicotuberculosis in the elderly: Report of two cases. Monaldi Arch Chest Dis 2004;61:241-43.

87. Symposium. Pneumoconiosis and mycobacterial infection. Kekkaku 2003;78:711-15.

88. Ulm K, Gerein P, Eigenthaler J, Schmidt S, Ehnes H. Silica, silicosis and lung-cancer: Results from a cohort study in the stone and quarry industry. Int Arch Occup Environ Health 2004;77:313-8.

89. McDonald JC, McDonald AD, Hughes JM, Rando RJ, Weill H. Mortality from lung and kidney disease in a cohort of north american industrial sand workers: An update. Ann Occup Hyg 2005;49:367-73.

90. Moshammer H, Neuberger M. Lung cancer and dust exposure: Results of a prospective cohort study following 3260 workers for 50 years. Occup Environ Med 2004;61:157-62.

91. Ablamunets KIa, Ornitsan EIu. Results of X-ray follow-up in late silicosis. Tr Prom Ekol 2004;30-32.

92. Akira M. High-resolution CT in the evaluation of occupational and environmental disease. Radiol Clin North Am 2002;40:43-59.

93. Ooi GC, Tsang KW, Cheung TF, Khong PL, Ho IW, Ip MS, Tam CM, Ngan H, Lam WK, Chan FL, Chan-Yeung M. Silicosis in 76 men: Qualitative and quantitative CT evaluation—Clinical-radiologic correlation study. Radiology 2003;228:816-25.

94. Kuschner WG, Stark P. Occupational lung disease. Part 2. Discovering the cause of diffuse parenchymal lung disease. Postgrad Med 2003;113:81-88.

95. Ooi CG, Khong PL, Cheng RS, Tan B, Tsang F, Lee I, Lam VS, Leung KK, Tsang KW. The relationship between mediastinal lymph node attenuation with parenchymal lung parameters in silicosis. Int J Tuberc Lung Dis 2003;7:1199-206.

96. Antao VC, Pinheiro GA, Terra-Filho M, Kavakama J, Muller NL. High-resolution CT in silicosis: Correlation with radiographic findings and functional impairment. J Comput Assist Tomogr 2005;29:350-56.

97. Gamble JF, Hessel PA, Nicolich M. Relationship between silicosis and lung function. Scand J Work Environ Health 2004;30:5-20.

98. Tiwari RR, Narain R, Patel BD, Makwana IS, Saiyed HN. Spirometric measurements among quartz stone ex-workers of Gujarat: India. J Occup Health 2003;45:88-93.

99. Tiwari RR, Sharma YK, Saiyed HN. Peak expiratory flow and respiratory morbidity: A study among silica-exposed workers in India. Arch Med Res 2005;36:171-74.

100. Bahrami AR, Mahjub H. Comparative study of lung function in Iranian factory workers exposed to silica dust. East Mediterr Health J 2003;9:390-98.

101. Hertzberg VS, Rosenman KD, Reilly MJ, Rice CH. Effect of occupational silica exposure on pulmonary function. Chest 2002;122:721-28.

102. Zhai R, Ge X, Li H, Tang Z, Liao R, Kleinjans J. Differences in cellular and inflammatory cytokine profiles in the bronchoalveolar lavage fluid in bagassosis and silicosis. Am J Ind Med 2004;46:338-44.

103. Sharma SK, Pande JN, Verma K, Guleria JS. Broncho-alveolar lavage fluid (BALF) analysis in interstitial lung diseases. Indian Journal of Chest Diseases and Allied Sciences 1989;31:187-96.

104. Sharma SK, Pande JN, Verma K. Bronchoalveolar lavage fluid (BALF) analysis in silicosis. Indian Journal of Chest Diseases and Allied Sciences 1988;30:257-61.

105. Antao VC, Pinheiro GA, Jansen JM. Broncholithiasis and lithoptysis associated with silicosis. Eur Respir J 2002;20:1057-59.

106. Sartorelli E. Broncholithiasis in silicosis. Am Rev Respir Dis 1974;109:687.

107. Cahill BC, Harmon KR, Shumway SJ, Mickman JK, Hertz MI. Tracheobronchial obstruction due to silicosis. Am Rev Respir Dis 1992;145:719-21.

108. Samson IM, Rossoff LJ. Chronic lithoptysis with multiple bilateral broncholiths. Chest 1997;112:563-65.

109. Mulliez P, Darras A, Dabouz R, Smith M. Broncholithiase au cours d'une silico-tuberculose. Rev Pneumol Clin 1990;46:85-87.

110. Conces DJ Jr, Tarver RD, Vix VA. Broncholithiasis: CT features in 15 patients. AJR Am J Roentgenol 1991;157:249-53.

111. Vix VA. Radiographic manifestations of broncholithiasis. Radiology 1978;128:295-99.

112. Case records of the Massachusetts General Hospital. Weekly clinicopathological exercises. Case 46-1991.

113. Mukherjee AK, Bhattacharya SK, Saiyed HN. Assessment of respirable dust and its free silica contents in different Indian coalmines. Ind Health 2005;43:277-84.

114. Rosenberg B, Levenstein C, Spangler E. Change in the world of occupational health: Silica control, then and now. J Public Health Policy 2005;26:192-202; discussion 203-05.

115. Sherson D. Silicosis in the twenty first century. The current permissible exposure limit is inadequate to protect workers. Occupational and Environmental Medicine 2002;59:721-72.

116. Sharma SK, Pande JN, Verma K. Effect of prednisolone treatment in chronic silicosis. Am Rev Respir Dis 1991;143:814-21.

COAL WORKERS' PNEUMOCONIOSIS

Coal mine and silica dust cause significant respiratory diseases in spite of modern dust control regulations. Susceptible individuals in exposed populations may develop fibrosing lung disease, obstructive airways disease, including chronic bronchitis and emphysema, or lung cancer. The inhalation of coalmine dust may lead to the development of following pulmonary conditions:[1-6]

1. Coal workers' pneumoconiosis (CWP)
   - Simple pneumoconiosis
   - Complicated pneumoconiosis or progressive
   - Massive fibrosis (PMF)
   - Caplan's syndrome
2. Industrial bronchitis
3. Emphysema
4. Lung cancer
5. Interstitial fibrosis and
6. Silicosis.

Coal may be found as surface outcrops and as underground seams, the depth of which may vary from few feet to more than a mile below the ground level. Coal is ranked according to certain geological properties like texture, content of volatile matter, and supply of amount of heat when burnt. Anthracite is ranked highest followed by bituminous coal, subbituminous coal, and lignite. The area at which coal is cut is known as the coal surface and is the dusty part of the mine. It is at this face that the cutting machines and the miners are in operation. Thus, workers at the face are exposed to the highest concentrations of coalmine dust. Only slightly less exposed are roof bolters, loading machine operators, and shot-firers. Other groups of workers likely to be exposed to coal dust, although to a lesser extent are the transporters, utilities track maintenance workers, and the men working at the surface.

The data on prevalence, respiratory morbidity and mortality in coal workers have been conflicting, partly because of lack of uniformity in different studies, and partly because most of these workers are smokers, so that an independent effect is difficult to evaluate. However, in general, it is shown that although complicated pneumoconiosis is associated with premature deaths, simple pneumoconiosis has no effect on life expectancy (rather a lower mortality). As a whole, miners have a normal life expectancy. Studies from Britain and United States have concluded that coalminers have a normal life expectancy, and that the excess deaths due to complicated pneumoconiosis are counterbalanced by the lower death rates from lung cancer and coronary artery disease, when deaths due to accidents and injuries are excluded.

In a routine survey of 623 miners in one colliery, 21 men, an unusually high number, showed radiological progression of simple pneumoconiosis in spite of generally low exposures to mixed coalmine dust. Comparison of the dust exposures of the 21 men with those of matched controls without pneumoconiosis showed highly significant differences in the proportion of quartz in the mixed dust to which they had been exposed. Quartz exposure may be an important factor in the development and rapid progression of coalworkers' pneumoconiosis.[4] The quartz exposures experienced by some men in the colliery can cause considerable progression of radiographic abnormalities since exposure ended.[7]

A most recent and reliable exposure-response relations, for damaging respiratory effects, derived from the Pneumoconiosis Field Research (PFR) which collected data over 38 years in the British Coal Industry reported the exposure-response relations and were presented for coal workers' simple pneumoconiosis category II, progressive massive fibrosis, defined deficits of lung function (FEV_1), and category II silicosis.[8] This was a program of prospective research on the respiratory health of coalminers, characterized by regular health surveys and detailed measurements of dust and silica concentrations in the workplace. The most reliable estimates of risks of coal workers' simple pneumoconiosis (CWSP) and progressive massive fibrosis (PMF) were based on about 50,000 observations of men at risk during 25 years of the research. Risks of an attack of PMF rise from about 0.8 percent at 1.5 mg.m^{-3} to about 5 percent at 6 mg.m^{-3}. Risks of category II CWSP are higher, rising from about 1.5 percent at a mean concentration of 1.5 mg.m^{-3} to about 9 percent at 6 mg.m^{-3}. The lung function of miners can be affected adversely by dust exposure, irrespective of the presence of pneumoconiosis. There is strong evidence that emphysema in coalworkers is actually related to lung coal content. The role silica in development of emphysema however remains unclear.[9] Studies of dose-response relationships between respiratory outcomes at autopsy and coal dust exposure from South Africa miners have shown that there are significant dose related associations of disease, including emphysema, with coal dust exposure.[10] The autopsy study showed that the prevalence of silicosis, tuberculosis (TB), coal workers' pneumoconiosis (CWP), and moderate and marked emphysema were 10.7 percent, 5.2 percent, 7.3 percent, and 6.4 percent, respectively. All diseases, except TB, were associated with exposure duration. Black miners had 8.3 and 1.2 fold greater risks for TB and CWP, respectively, than white miners. White miners had an increased risk of 1.4 and 5.4 for silicosis and moderate to marked emphysema, respectively. In models unadjusted for age, and including smoking, moderate to marked emphysema was strongly associated with exposure duration (OR = 3.4; 95% CI = 1.9-5.9 for highest tercile of exposure duration). Exposure-related risk estimates were reduced when age was introduced into the model. However, age and duration of exposure were highly correlated, (r = 0.68) suggesting a dilution of the exposure effect by age.

Reports from USA have shown that since 1997, both number of workers employed in mining and disease and illness rates have decreased; however, the highest disease and illness rates in mining continue to be coal worker's pneumoconiosis and hearing loss.[11] Besides mixed dust pneumoconiosis, coal mining has been shown to be a risk factor for COPD. It is recognized that silicosis is a risk factor for tuberculosis, and there is a well-founded suspicion that those subjects who do not present with silicosis, but have had long exposure to silica, have a greater risk of developing tuberculosis. It has been reported that the risk of tuberculosis does not increase in coalminers who do not have pneumoconiosis, nor does it appear that the presence of pneumoconiosis in coal mine workers increases the risk of infection by mycobacteria, as is the case with silicosis. Mosquera et al[12] found an incidence of tuberculosis of 150 per 10^5 person-years among coalminers in our region, both active or retired, which is a rate that is three times higher than that of the general population of the same area. More than half of the patients presented with complicated pneumoconiosis.

Silica has been classified by the International Agency for Research on cancer as a carcinogen in humans, although it does not seem that the incidence of cancer among coalminers is increased. The different concentrations of silica in this kind of mining, which are related to the type of coal extracted and the rock work required to extract it, may help to explain certain persistent discrepancies and uncertainties about the risk posed by coal mine dust. In our region, coal is extracted from narrow vertical seams embedded in slates and sandstone. To access the coal seams, a great deal of rockwork is required. The coal is bituminous, of low grade, and this fact has been associated with a lesser risk for pneumoconiosis than that posed by high-grade coal.[13] Another study from Spain on working in coalmines has shown that it is a risk factor for pneumoconiosis and COPD.[14] Ninety-nine workers (3.8%) developed round opacities (category 1) that were significantly related to the kind of work in a crude analysis (p = 0.045), with a greater frequency (7.3%) among rockworkers, who have greater exposure to silica, and were almost significantly related to tobacco use (p = 0.092). These round opacities also show a significant relation to smoking, being more frequent (4.9%) among smokers, both in the crude analysis (p = 0.028) and in the multivariable analysis (p = 0.001) controlling for rockwork. In 240 workers (12.7%), accelerated FEV$_1$ decreases were observed with significant relations to tobacco use (p = 0.001) and rockwork (p = 0.044). Pulmonary tuberculosis was diagnosed in four cases, with an incidence of eight in 10^5 person-years. This rate falls within the limits expected for the region. No case of lung cancer was observed. The authors concluded that the round opacities (category 1) were related to smoking and, probably, to rockwork; accelerated FEV$_1$ decreases were related to rockwork and tobacco consumption. There was no identified increase in tuberculosis or lung cancer in this cohort.[14]

Another study made the radiological assessments of coalworkers' simple pneumoconiosis (CWP) in 2600 coalminers at 10 British collieries in relation to the individuals' estimated lifetime (mean 33 years) exposure to respirable coalmine dust. Among men with similar cumulative dust exposures those with longer exposure time had higher prevalence of CWP. In general there was no evidence that the quartz concentrations experienced (average 5% of mixed dust) affected the probability of developing coalworkers' simple pneumoconiosis. Some men reacted unfavorably (two or more steps of change on the 12 point radiological scale) over a 10 year period to coalmine dust with relatively high quartz content.[15] Another British study in a sample of 17738 men who were first examined when working in 24 British collieries in the 1950s has been followed up about 22 years later.

It was possible to examine 61 percent of the survivors, 44 percent of the original sample. Simple pneumoconiosis was more frequent among men (particularly older men) who had left the industry than among those who had stayed in it. A detailed analysis did not show any systematic or statistically significant difference between men who stayed and men who left in the quantitative relations between dust exposure and simple pneumoconiosis. Present estimates of risk of simple pneumoconiosis in relation to exposure to mixed respirable dust in working miners adequately describe the relation found in men who have been miners but have left the industry.[16]

The long-term exposure to dust in the hard coal mining industry can lead to various pathological lung changes, especially to chronic bronchitis without and with obstructive ventilation disorder, lung emphysema, pneumoconiosis (coalminer's pneumoconiosis, in Germany categorized as silicosis) and silicotuberculosis. These health disorders show a close pathogenetic and pathophysiological association and should not necessarily be regarded as individual entities. Most exposed subjects demonstrate more or less all of these pathological disorders. On account of individual (genetic?) susceptibility, their degree differs greatly. Some individuals are largely resistent, other subjects show severe effects like emphysema, progressive massive pneumoconiosis, or the Caplan syndrome. Several studies showed that the pathologically verified degree of lung fibrosis is associated with lung crystalline SiO$_2$ content whereas the emphysema score is inversely correlated with the coal content.[17]

The true prevalence of CWP at any particular time depends upon the environmental condition prevalent 20 to 30 years back and may have little relevance to present working condition. Moreover, because of a lot of inter- and intra-observer variation in the interpretation of chest X-ray changes, the true prevalence may vary. Data from US mines suggest that the prevalence is 10.1 percent, of which 0.4 percent is PMF. The incidence is more in the face and transportation workers than in the maintenance and surface workers. Cutting machine and continuous miner operators and their helpers have the highest prevalence rates, followed by roof bolters, shuttle car operators, and those who work on transportation. The physical and chemical composition of the coal is also important. Certain coals may fragment more easily and produce more harmful particles of 1 to 2 μm, whereas others may tend to generate more particles of 4 to 6 μm. Similarly, the chemical composition or rank of coal influences the prevalence of CWP.

Types of Respiratory Problems in Coalworkers

Coal workers' pneumoconiosis (CWP) is subdivided into *simple* and *complicated* pneumoconiosis, according to the radiographic appearance of the chest film. Simple CWP is further classified into categories 1, 2, and 3 according to the profuseness of small opacities in the lung fields. The role of silica in production of progressive massive fibrosis due to coal dust is uncertain. Although there is some evidence that complicated pneumoconiosis can be produced by pure carbon, as far as coalminers are concerned, there is a fair amount of circumstantial evidence to incriminate silica as the etiologic agent for the initiation of progressive massive fibrosis. Complicated pneumoconiosis or Progressive massive fibrosis (PMF) is diagnosed when there is a larger opacity 1 cm or more in diameter. It is sub classified as A, B, or C according to the size of the larger opacity or opacities. This is a severe form of coal workers' pneumoconiosis (CWP) characterized by severe scarring leading to obliteration of normal lung structures. Although several factors have been implicated, cumulative dust exposure is the most important factor in the pathogenesis of PMF.[18] Recent studies suggest that oxidative stress plays an important role in the pathogenesis of pulmonary fibrosis, affecting fibroblast proliferation, apoptosis, and the cytokine microenvironment.[19,20] This is especially relevant for the lung, which is exposed to oxygen, oxidant pollutants, and endogenous oxidants, produced by inflammatory cells.[21] Many chemical and physical agents in the environment including mineral dusts are potent generators of reactive oxygen species (ROS). In response to these agents, various enzymatic and nonenzymatic defence systems help to protect cells and tissues from oxidative damage, and it is possible that genetically acquired variations in these systems account for interindividual variation in the response to oxidative stress. In this respect, there is substantial evidence that antioxidant genes such as glutathione S-transferases (GST) and manganese superoxide dismutase (*MnSOD*), which is important components of lung defence in response to oxidative stress, are highly polymorphic.[22,23]

Data gathered since 1953 concerning more than 30,000 coalminers while employed at 24 collieries in England, Scotland, and Wales have been used to study the incidence of progressive massive fibrosis (PMF) in working coalminers. Results refer to 52,264 approximately five year intervals when the miners were at risk of an attack of PMF. Film readings, in some cases based on clinical assessments only, showed 462 attacks of PMF over the 5 year risk periods. The men concerned had experienced higher cumulative exposures to dust than their colleagues of similar age at the same collieries, a result found at 65 of the 68 age colliery groups where an attack had occurred. The association was highly significant statistically. Simple pneumoconiosis clearly predisposed to PMF, with 5 year attack rates of 13.9 percent, 12.5 percent, 4.4 percent, and 0.2 percent among men with categories 3, 2, 1, and 0 respectively at the start of the risk periods. Once simple pneumoconiosis category 1 or more had been attained, those with higher cumulative exposure to dust were not at greater risk of an attack of PMF than other men with the same CWSP category. Among most miners, those with category 0, however, the risks of an attack of PMF increased clearly with exposure. Risks of an attack were higher among older men irrespective of CWSP category. In addition, there were large colliery specific variations in incidence related to variations in the carbon content of the coal though not fully explained by them. The authors concluded that cumulative exposure to respirable dust is the decisive central factor in the development of PMF. Its effect is primarily in causing simple pneumoconiosis category 1 or higher, which predisposes to PMF, though the dust related incidence among men with category 0 is not negligible in view of the large numbers at risk. Continuation of the policy to minimize dust concentrations underground therefore seems the only secure strategy to limit, and eventually eliminate, PMF.[24]

Pathogenesis and Pathology of CWP

The coalmine dust is a mixture of coal, kaolin, mica, and silica in varying proportions. The dust is deposited in the alveoli and respiratory bronchioles. As a reaction to this the macrophages increase in number and phagocytose the deposited particles and carry them to the terminal bronchioles, from which the mucociliary blanket removes them. If the load is excessive, the clearance mechanism is ineffective, and the macrophages aggregate in the respiratory bronchioles and alveoli. If this continues for a while, fibroblasts appear and a thin network of reticulin is laid down surrounding the macrophage. If the macrophages contain silica, they undergo lysis, releasing enzymes that stimulate the fibroblasts to produce more collagen. As a result of this reaction, the first and second-generation respiratory bronchioles along with their terminal alveoli are encased in a mixture of coal dust, macrophages, and collagen fibres. This aggregation of debris and fibroblasts form the coal macules, which is the primary lesion of *simple CWP*. They appear as blackish dots on cut section of the lung. They have a predilection for the upper lobes and vary in size and may be as big as 5 mm. As these macules enlarge, the smooth muscles of the respiratory bronchioles atrophy, so that bronchioles dilate, producing *focal emphysema*. The products of such reaction are taken up by the lymphatics that drain into the hilar nodes. The fibrosis may sometimes encroach on the arterioles and gradually occludes it. However, no significant reduction in vascular capillary bed occurs. Development of simple CWP is not influenced by the rank of coal. In coal workers whose lung residue contains 18 percent mine quartz, the classic pathologic lesions of silicosis, rather than CWP are observed. Cor pulmonale is not a complication of simple CWP unless there is associated chronic bronchitis.

The pathologic lesions of progressive massive fibrosis first appear mainly on the posterior segments of the upper lobes or in the apical segment of the lower lobes. The lesions consist of large aggregates of black tissue adherent to the chest wall. The masses are ill defined and rubbery in consistency. In contrast to the conglomerate lesions of silicosis, which are matted aggregates of several silicotic nodules, the lesions of PMF are amorphous, irregular, and relatively homogenous. Cavitation may occur due to ischemic necrosis or tubercular infection. The lesions consist of fibrous tissue with a central core of proteinaceous material, calcium, and mineral dust. The masses affect the blood vessels and bronchi in the affected lobe and ultimately destroy them. Endarteritic changes and occasional thrombus in large pulmonary arteries are seen.

Silicosis and coal workers' pneumoconiosis are complex multifactorial lung diseases whose etiopathogenesis are not well defined. It is generally accepted that fibrotic lung disorders are mediated by macrophage-derived cytokines and growth factors. There is evidence showing a crucial role for tumor necrosis factor-α (TNF-alpha) and interleukin-1 (IL-1) in inflammation caused by silica dust and in the transition from simple to progressive massive fibrosis.[25,26] Oxidative stress plays a major role in the pathogenesis of interstitial lung diseases. The antioxidant enzymes glutathione S-transferases (GST) and manganese superoxide dismutase (MnSOD) are important components of lung defence against oxidative stress, and polymorphisms in the genes, which regulate their expression, may represent important disease modifiers. Polymorphic genotypes within the GST gene cluster and MnSOD do not affect individual susceptibility to PMF.[27] Patients with coal worker's Pneumoconiosis are found to have abnormity of oxyradical reaction, unbalanced oxidation/antioxidation state, and abnormally high expression of cytokine, which might have relations with the occurrence and development of coal worker's Pneumoconiosis.[28] High-resolution

CT scan findings have further suggested that an oxidative stress due to increased free radicals and reactive oxygen metabolite production occurs in early stages and low grades of simple CWP.[29] Bioavailable iron in the coal may induce IL-6 through both ferryl species (via iron autoxidation) and hydroxyl radicals that may contribute to the development of pneumoconiosis.[30] It is further suggested that interactions of genetic background with environmental exposure and intermediate response phenotypes are important components in the pathogenesis of CWP.[31]

Genetic factors that modify the response to oxidative environmental stimuli in humans are largely unknown. The overproduction of reactive oxygen species (ROS) owing to major environmental factors such as cigarette smoking and chronic exposure to particles induces chronic airway inflammation.[32-34] Inflammation is fundamental to the pathogenesis of many chronic lung diseases including asthma, chronic obstructive pulmonary disease (COPD), and pneumoconiosis/fibrosis.[35,36] Coal workers' pneumoconiosis (CWP) is an inflammatory lung disease caused by chronic inhalation of coal dust, and ROS are thought to be important in disease pathogenesis. The source of ROS is proposed to derive directly from the coal dust, and indirectly from activated inflammatory cells such as alveolar macrophages and polymorphonuclear leukocytes.[37]

The specific mechanisms of oxidative injury are becoming increasingly clear. ROS and specific proinflammatory cytokines such as tumor necrosis factor alpha (TNF-α) activate transcription factors including nuclear factor-$\kappa\beta$ (NF-$\kappa\beta$) via specific intracellular signalling pathways. Translocation of transcription factors to the nucleus from the cytoplasm subsequently initiates transcription in genes with multiple inflammatory functions, including cytokines (TNF, IL-4, IL10, etc.), and antioxidant enzymes such as glutathione peroxidase, superoxide dismutases, and catalase.[38,39]

Interestingly, only some people similarly exposed to environmental oxidative stimuli (for example, cigarette smoke and particles) develop lung disease, and the determinants of susceptibility are poorly understood. Intrinsic factors such as genetic background may be important determinants of interpersonal susceptibility to disease pathogenesis. A number of candidate genes for susceptibility to chronic pulmonary diseases have been investigated. The -308 G/A SNP in the promoter region of the gene (*TNF*) for TNF-α has been studied frequently. *TNF* is located in tandem with the lymphotoxin-α gene (*LTA*) in the class III region of the 3.6 Mb human major histocompatibility complex (MHC) on chromosome

6p21.31[40] and the *TNF* gene superfamily plays an important role in inflammation. The −308 promoter polymorphism has been associated with subphenotypes of asthma, COPD, fibrosis, and CWP in some studies[41-44] but not in others. Other genetic factors of CWP have also been studied. Similarly, a functional *Nco*I RFLP polymorphism in *LTA* was associated with sarcoidosis, but it has not been replicated. Discordant results may be related to differences in population characteristics. Differential effects of the same environmental exposure on subjects with different genotypes may change the magnitude or the direction of the associations but, unfortunately, none of the studies mentioned above has considered the effects of gene-environment interactions in the disease etiology or included biological markers of the response to oxidative stress.

The overall hypothesis of the above study was that *TNF*-308 and *LTA Nco*I polymorphisms modify the pulmonary responses to oxidants in coalminers differently exposed to cigarette smoke and coal mine dust. To test this hypothesis, genotype-environment interactions on intermediate quantitative phenotypes of response to oxidative stress were specifically investigated. Further, genotype intermediate phenotype interactions on disease phenotypes were studied. The response to oxidative stimuli (coal dust, cigarette smoke) was assessed by biological intermediate quantitative phenotypes (enzyme activities), and detailed information on coal workers' pneumoconiosis (assessed from computed tomography and twice by chest radiography five years apart). A major strength of this study was the quantitative assessment of environmental exposure to oxidative stimuli that permits evaluation of gene-environment interaction.

A hypothesis for the pathogenesis of progressive massive fibrosis is proposed whereby dust, accumulating in central lymph nodes, leads eventually to spread through the capsule and rupture into bronchi or pulmonary vessels, thereby sending dust laden activated cells back into the lungs to produce progressive massive fibrosis.[45]

A number of immunological and cellular changes have been studied in CWP.[46-49] Men with radiological signs of coalworkers pneumoconiosis (CWP) had significantly raised levels of IgA and IgG with increasing pneumoconiosis category. Even coalworkers with less than category 1 simple pneumoconiosis had raised levels of IgA, suggesting that increased production of this immunoglobulin occurs before radiologically identifiable pathological changes have occurred in the lung tissue. No association between reduced humoral immune competence and radiological category of pneumoconiosis

was found. Whether high Ig levels in men exposed to coal dust are merely a passive response to dusted lung tissue or whether they indicate that an immunological process is important in the development of pneumoconiotic lesions remains uncertain. A significant correlation is found between category of pneumoconiosis and alterations in whole blood cell count, percentage or absolute numbers of lymphocytes, or the presence of antilung antibodies was a decrease in a subgroup of T lymphocytes with increasing severity of pneumoconiosis. The major factor influencing these parameters was the smoking status of the man. Smokers showed increased cell counts and lymphocyte numbers and a higher frequency of antilung antibodies and lymphocyte-mediated cellular cytotoxicity (LMCC) when compared with nonsmokers. It has been shown that collagen is not the major protein material in the lesions of progressive massive fibrosis of coal workers. However, it was demonstrated that a substance similar in composition to fibrin was an important component in these masses. Immunohistochemical studies on the lungs of seven coalworkers have shown that the complex extracellular material in six of the lesions of massive fibrosis contains fibronectin.[49]

In 1953, Caplan described a syndrome characterized by certain peculiar appearances in the chest radiograph of miners that were associated with rheumatoid arthritis.[50] This is now known as *Caplan s syndrome* or rheumatoid pneumoconiosis.[50,51] In contrast to PMF, the opacities in this syndrome are rounded and situated peripherally. They occur mostly in the background of category 0 or 1 simple CWP, and may develop within a few weeks. The nodules are usually 0.5 to 5 cm in diameter and most commonly develop concomitantly with the joint manifestations of rheumatoid arthritis. In some cases, they may precede joint symptoms by several years. Fresh nodules may appear intermittently and herald the exacerbation of the arthritis. There is, however, no association between subcutaneous nodules and those in the lungs.

Cavitations occur commonly in these nodules and burnt out tuberculosis may be present in most cases. Histologically, the nodules consist of necrotic tissue with varying amounts of collagen and dust. Outside the necrotic area, a cellular zone consisting of lymphocytes and plasma cells is present. Endarteritis is a more frequent finding. In many nodules, a peripheral zone of more active inflammation with polymorphonuclear leukocytes is present. Some call this as "rheumatoid zone."

Rheumatoid factor in Caplan's syndrome-like lesions is present in over 70 percent of cases, whereas that in

PMF is present in 30 to 40 percent of cases, and in simple CWP there is still a less number of cases, which are positive for this factor.[52] Immunohistologic studies have shown that vasculitis is a prominent feature in Caplan's syndrome, whereas it is not so in PMF. Similarly, antinuclear antibodies are present in a greater proportion of cases. These nodules differ from silicotid and nodules of CWP in the way that dust lamination, palisading of fibroblasts, cholesterol crystal spaces, central necrosis, and excess peripheral lymphocytes and plasma cells are more marked in these lesions, which are rare or absent in the later types of nodules.

Although the pathogenesis of Caplan's syndrome is not known, presence of immunologically competent cells and rheumatoid factor (IgM) in and around the nodules suggests that it is immunologically mediated. Lungs with Caplan's nodules contain much less dust than those with ordinary PMF. No definite association has been found with HLA as was thought previously.[53,54] HLA typing was performed on 267 Welsh coalworkers with pneumoconiosis (96 cases of simple pneumoconiosis, 115 cases of progressive massive fibrosis and 56 cases of Caplan's syndrome) and 134 coalworkers with no abnormality. The presence or absence of rheumatoid factor was also determined. The results fail to confirm a previously reported increase in HLA-A1 and B18 in coalworkers with no pneumoconiosis. When correction was made for the number of antigens typed (i) HLA-Bw21 was significantly increased from 1.1 percent in the total group with pneumoconiosis to 8.2 percent in coalworkers with no abnormality (P corrected less than 0.032); (ii) HLA-Bw45 was increased in Caplan's syndrome (10.7%) and Caplan's syndrome patients with rheumatoid factor (16.1%) when compared to a non-occupationally exposed control group (0.8%) (P corrected = 0.019 and 0.0064 respectively). These results were not significant when comparisons were made with the coalworker group with no abnormality.[53]

Interesting observations have been made in experimental animals.[55,56] Rats exposed to the inhalation of coal dust from either Utah (low prevalence coalworkers' pneumoconiosis (CWP)) or Pennsylvania (high prevalence CWP) have shown that the number of alveolar macrophages recovered from rats inhaling these two coal dusts (exposures up to 4 months) was not remarkably different from the number recovered from rats inhaling filtered room air. This is in contrast to results obtained after intratracheal intubation of the dust. The capacity of the lavaged cells to phagocytize and kill bacteria decreased after exposure to either dust. The activity of certain enzymes also decreased.[54,55] Further, A comparative immunological and microbiological study of experimental coalworkers' pneumoconiosis (CWP) made in rats and mice subjected to long-term exposures of colamine dust aerosols has shown that both species responded immunologically in a similar manner to humans with CWP in that IgA levels were significantly elevated and lung reactive antibodies were stimulated. Coalmine dust inhalation had little effect on the pulmonary inactivation of inhaled bacteria, but the concomitant occurrence of passively administered lung reactive antibody seemed to enhance the inactivation.[56]

Preliminary pathological and mineralogical studies have been reported on seventy-four sets of lungs from British coalminers who have been employed at the collieries included in the National Coal Boards's Pneumoconiosis Field Research. The degree of lung damage was considered in relation to the lung dust content and to the known dust exposures of the men concerned. Lungs were classified as having soft macules, fibrotic nodules or PMF. Those with soft macules had the lowest dust content but there was no significant difference between the dust contents of the lungs with fibrotic lesions and those with PMF. The percentage of noncoal minerals in the lung dust appeared to increase with the pathological classification from soft macules to PMF, and comparisons with the exposure data indicated a preferential retention of noncoal minerals, and especially of quartz, in the cases with the more severe lesions. Histological examination of the lesions showed the packing of dust was fewer closes and the cellular response more vigorous with the lungs with the highest quartz content.[57] The main variable determining the development of simple pneumoconiosis is exposure to airborne dust, and that this effect is not modified appreciably by whether or not coalminers smoke.[58]

As discussed earlier in the chapter on COPD, emphysema is defined in anatomical terms as enlargement of the gas-exchanging part of the lung (the acinus) accompanied by destruction of respiratory tissue. Emphysema is classified by the way that the acinus is dominantly involved. In proximal acinar emphysema, the proximal part of the acinus-respiratory bronchioles-is dominantly involved and two forms of proximal acinar emphysema are usually recognized: centrilobular emphysema and simple pneumoconiosis of coalworkers. The acinus is more or less uniformly involved in panacinar emphysema, and several clinical associations have been described with this lesion. In distal acinar emphysema, alveolar ducts and sacs are particularly involved, and spontaneous pneumothorax of young adults is associated with this form of emphysema.

Scarring is usually associated with irregular involvement of the acinus (irregular emphysema) and is usually asymptomatic. No uniform agreement exists as to the application of this classification and there is widespread discrepancy of classification of emphysematous lungs between experts, especially when emphysema is severe. The precise definition of destruction of respiratory tissue in emphysema has not been agreed on, and this had led to wide variations in the assessment of prevalence of emphysema in autopsy series. Tobacco smoking is the most important cause of emphysema and is thought to bring it about by imbalance between the protease-antiproteinase mechanisms in the lung. Increasing severity of emphysema is accompanied by increasing frequency of symptoms, but a substantial proportion of subjects with severe emphysema will be apparently free from symptoms. The major functional characteristics of severe emphysema are reduction in expiratory flow, increase in lung volumes, and diminished diffusing capacity. Diminished expiratory flow in emphysema is determined in part by loss of elastic recoil and in part by associated airway disease. Loss of recoil in emphysematous lungs may be brought about by functional changes in the apparently normal intervening lung between the emphysematous spaces.[59] The amounts of emphysema in the smoking and nonsmoking groups with CWP are similar. These findings are true when both the lifelong nonsmokers and the cases with simple pneumoconiosis only were looked at separately. It was found that centrilobular emphysema was much commonest type encountered in both smokers and nonsmokers. The nonsmokers were less disabled in terms of impairment of FEV 1.0 than the smokers, although the difference was not statistically significant.[60] Obliterative bronchitis represents an unusual fibrotic response to free crystalline silica. The process may occur simultaneously in the adjacent lymph node and the bronchial wall; however, it need not be associated with complicated pneumoconiosis. Clinically, obliterative bronchitis may masquerade as bronchogenic carcinoma.[61] The prevalence of right ventricular hypertrophy is low (15%) in the absence of progressive massive fibrosis and appeared to be related to emphysema or airways disease or both, and not to simple pneumoconiosis. It is more evident only in subjects who had smoked. In subjects with progressive massive fibrosis the prevalence of right ventricular hypertrophy is higher (34%) and it is occasionally seen in nonsmokers. The prevalence increases with increasing size of lesion, and for any given size of lesion subjects with right ventricular hypertrophy will have more panacinar emphysema than those without right ventri-cular hypertrophy. There is no relationship, however, between the extent of massive lesions or amount and type of emphysema and the degree of right ventricular hypertrophy.[62]

Clinical Features

Simple pneumoconiosis is symptomless. The presence of cough, expectoration, wheeze, and breathlessness are due to associated smoking. There is little correlation between radiographic changes and clinical symptoms. Larger masses may be associated with minor symptoms to severe disability. Sputum production is mild in cases of PMF. The amount may be large if associated with secondary infection in the dilated and distorted bronchi. The sputum is usually gelatinous and gray colored due to small quantities of coal- or carbon dust. During periods of acute infection it may be dark black because of elimination of larger amounts of coal. Hemoptysis is unusual in the absence of active tuberculosis, although mild blood streaking is not uncommon. Jet-black sputum may be produced if the PMF ruptures into the bronchi due to ischemic necrosis. This may be large in amount and associated with distressing paroxysmal cough. The mucus usually contains large quantities of coal or carbon dust, cholesterol, and blood. Cough in general is due to associated smoking, but in some cases of large PMF lesions cough may be frequent, severe and paroxysmal possibly due to pressure effect on the trachea and bronchi. Pain in the chest may be complained of due to respiratory muscle strain. Recurrent laryngeal nerve palsy may be caused by coalworkers' pneumoconiosis with progressive massive fibrosis (PMF). However, efforts should always be made to exclude more common causes, in particular bronchogenic carcinoma, before attributing the palsy to PMF.[63,64]

Physical signs are minimal or absent. Finger clubbing is very unusual. Central cyanosis may be present in advanced cases. Diffuse crepitation or rhonchi may be heard if associated with chronic bronchitis or emphysema. Massive fibrosis may produce mediastinal shift. Congestive cardiac failure due to cor pulmonale may be present in some cases.[62]

Investigations

Lung function tests: In simple pneumoconiosis all the parameters are within normal limits unless there is an associated lung disease, and such changes are usually minimal. Ventilatory function does not decline with increasing radiographic category of simple pneumoconiosis.

Several studies have shown that miners have a slightly lower ventilatory capacity than nonminers, and that this reduction is related to the number of years spent underground. Some has reported slight reduction in FEV_1, although there was no relationship with the symptoms or radiological category of CWP. Other parameters affected are FVC, FVC/FEV, and FEF 25 to 75 percent. Lung volume changes are also inconspicuous in the coalminers when analyzed independent of smoking. Small increase in RV is however noted with increasing radiographic category. While there are conflicting reports regarding diffusing capacity for carbon monoxide in simple pneumoconiosis, complicated pneumoconiosis in stages B and C is often associated with a decrease in DL_{CO}. In simple pneumoconiosis, the value is normal for the nonsmoking miners, regardless of age and years spent underground. On the other hand, smoking miners usually show a lower DL_{CO} at rest and during exercise. Unequal distribution of ventilation and perfusion manifested by decreased resting PaO_2 increased resting alveolar-arterial difference ($[A-a]PaO_2$), and increased resting $PaCO_2$ has been reported. All these indices show worsening on exercise. Other workers have reported no significant difference between miners and nonminers with regard to pulse rate, oxygen consumption, and minute ventilation at rest and during moderate exercise. Pulmonary artery hypertension has been noted in certain cases with either complicated pneumoconiosis or severe airway obstruction. Pulmonary capillary bed appears to be decreased as measured by perfusion scans correlating well with areas of large opacities or bullae. Reduced lung compliance is reported in patients with complicated pneumoconiosis. Dynamic compliance at quiet breathing frequencies tends to be low in all such cases. Studies of peripheral airways obstruction by mid-flow rates, closing volume, and closing capacity have shown decreased values compared to controls.[65-70]

The lung function of miners can be affected adversely by dust exposure, irrespective of the presence of pneumoconiosis.[71] A study of 7000 miners[72] defined clinically important deficits of forced expired volume in one second (FEV_1) by comparisons with reported symptoms of breathlessness, and then studied the dust related risk of having these deficits. A threefold increase in the odds of reporting "walking slower than other people on level ground because of their chest" was associated on average with a 0.993 litre FEV_1 deficit from predicted. This was defined as a clinically important lung function deficit, and is a substantial deficit by any standard. For nonsmokers, risks are about 10 percent for zero dust concentrations, rising to about 19 percent for

an average concentration of 6 mg.m^{-3}. For smokers, risks were 22 percent and about 36 percent respectively. The slope representing dust related increments in risk is similar to that for category II pneumoconiosis, so reductions in dust levels to protect against pneumoconiosis would protect a similar number of men from this lung function deficit. Smaller deficits of lung function were also examined, showing steeper incremental slopes. For example, a two-fold increase in risk of reporting breathlessness was associated with a 627 ml deficit of FEV_1. The risks of this deficit in nonsmokers were about 25 percent at zero dust concentration, and nearly 40 percent at a mean concentration of 6 mg.m^{-3}. Comparable figures for smokers were 44 percent and nearly 60 percent respectively. A 1.5-fold increase in risk of reporting breathlessness was associated with a 367 ml deficit of FEV_1. The risks of this deficit in nonsmokers were about 41 percent at zero dust concentration, and over 55 percent at a mean concentration of 6 mg.m^{-3}. Comparable figures for smokers were 62 percent and about 75 percent respectively.

Chest Radiographic Features

The earliest abnormality consists of a few ill-defined opacities, which are distinct from the vascular shadows in the outer third of the lung fields and are present mainly in the upper and mid lung fields. Later, they are better defined and more widely distributed. The most common category is the type q, and other categories (r, p) are uncommon. The PMF opacities are also more common in upper zones and may be uni- or bilateral. They vary greatly in shape and size. The opacities may be round, ovoid, sausage-like or linear and well demarcated. The lesions may cavitate with or without fluid level either due to ischemic necrosis or secondary tuberculosis. Bullous emphysema and calcification may be present. *Eggshell* calcification in the hilar nodes, similar to those in silicosis, is seen in a small proportion of cases. Multiple Kerley's B lines are present in some cases of higher category of simple pneumoconiosis and PMF due to dust accumulation in peripheral interlobular septa. When these occur in lower lung fields, they may be confused with interstitial fibrosis. Photo scanning of the lungs after intravenous injection of albumin-[131] correlates well with the vascular pathology.

The radiological features of rheumatoid pneumoconiosis differ from the other two types of pneumoconiosis both in appearance and behavior. The X-ray changes may be classic Caplan type opacities; scanty, large round opacities; mixed, small and large round opacities; multiple small round opacities; one or more of these with those of ordinary or usual types of pneumoconiosis; and sudden appearance of "woolly" opacities. Caplan type opacities are round, fairly dense, and vary from 0.5 to 3.0 cm in diameter, occasionally up to 5 cm, and are moderate in number and scattered irregularly in the lung fields. Calcification in the lesions is fairly common. Cavitation is also possible with fluid levels. Disappearance of the existing ones and appearance of new ones at different sites is usual. The opacities may look like large lobulated masses due to superimposition of a number of nodules in X-ray beam.

The relation between the profusion and predominant type of small rounded opacities on chest radiographs shows that for subjects considered by each reader to present predominantly p type opacities, increasing opacity profusion is exclusively and significantly associated with an increase in the number of pinhead fibrotic nodules. Numbers of nodules measuring 1 to 3 mm and greater than 3 to 9 mm in diameter both shows significant linear associations with opacity profusion category in subjects presenting predominantly q opacities, the closer association being observed with the smaller lesions. Opacities of type r are rarely considered to be the predominant type. The closest association is observed with nodules measuring greater than 3 to 9 mm in diameter. An overall significant linear association between total lung dust content and opacity profusion is found to be due mainly to subjects presenting predominantly p type opacities and to a lesser extent to those with predominantly q opacities.[73]

Studies to document the prevalence of pneumoconiosis among a living South African coal mining cohort, describes dose-response relationships between coal workers' pneumoconiosis and respirable dust exposure, and relationships between pneumoconiosis and both lung function deterioration and respiratory symptoms showed that the overall prevalence of pneumoconiosis was low (2-4%). The degree of agreement between the two readers for profusion was moderate to high (kappa = 0.58). A significant association (P < 0.001) and trend (P < 0.001) was seen for pneumoconiosis with increasing categories of Cumulative respirable dust exposure (CDE) among current miners only. A significant (P < 0.0001) additional 58 mg-years/m³ CDE was seen among those with pneumoconiosis compared to those without. CDE contributed to a statistically significant 0.19 percent and 0.11 percent greater decline in the percent predicted 1 second forced expiration volume (FEV$_1$) and forced vital capacity (FVC), respectively, among current miners with pneumoconiosis than among those without. Logistic regression models showed no significant relationships

between pneumoconiosis and symptoms. The overall prevalence of pneumoconiosis, although significantly associated with CDE, was low. The presence of pneumoconiosis is associated with meaningful health effects, including deterioration in lung function. Intervention measures that control exposure are indicated, to reduce these functional effects.[74]

Radiological opacities of coalworkers' pneumoconiosis are more profuse the more dust is retained in lungs. Among the men who mine low rank coal—that is, with a relatively high proportion of ash—the increase in profusion is most closely related to the ash component of the dust, whereas in men who mine high rank coal both coal and ash increased in the lungs in relation to radiological profusion. The fine p type of opacity is found to be associated with more dust and a higher proportion of coal and less ash than the nodular r opacity, and is also more likely to be associated with emphysema. The pathological basis of the different types of opacity found on the radiographs of coalminers relates to the number, size, and nodularity of the dust lesions. Larger fibrotic lesions are likely to appear as r opacities, whereas fine reticular dust deposition is most likely to present as p opacities, q opacities showing a mixture of appearances. The composition of dust retained in the lung, as well as its amount, makes an important contribution to the radiographic appearances of pneumoconiosis. In particular, the r type of lesion on the radiograph of a low rank coalminer indicates the possibility of a silicotic like lesion.[75] Other interesting findings on plain chest skiagram have been different opacities, fibrotic lesions and emphysematous changes depending upon the quality and duration of dust exposure and retention in the lungs.[76-78]

HRCT findings of CWP have been described recently. The most common of the pneumoconioses are silicosis, CWP, and asbestosis. The former two are characterized by the presence of small nodular opacities predominantly distributed in the upper zones of the lung. The small nodular opacities are classified into two patterns on HRCT: (i) ill-defined fine branching lines and (ii) well-defined discrete nodules. Asbestosis demonstrates thickened interlobular and intralobular lines, subpleural dot-like or curvilinear opacities, and honeycombing on HRCT, predominantly distributed in the bases of the lungs. Although HRCT findings of other pneumoconioses are variable and nonspecific, there are predominant and characteristic findings for each type of pneumoconiosis. HRCT is useful in achieving more accurate categorization of the parenchymal changes in each type of pneumoconiosis.[79] Bronchiectasis is frequent and severe in CWP workers than without. Bronchiectasis is influenced by coal dust exposure.[80] High-resolution computed tomography (HRCT) is more sensitive than chest X-ray (CXR) in the depiction of parenchymal abnormalities. Discordance between CXR and HRCT is often high in pneumoconiosis. Discordance rate is higher in the early pneumoconiosis cases with negative CXR than low-grade pneumoconiosis (60, 36 and 8%, respectively). When coalminers with normal CXR were evaluated by HRCT, six out of 10 cases were diagnosed as positive. In low-grade pneumoconiosis group, the number of patients with positive CXR but negative HRCT was low in comparison to patients with CXR negative and early pneumoconiosis findings. Most of the CXR category 0 patients (10/16) were diagnosed as category 1 by HRCT. Eleven cases diagnosed as CXR category 1 were diagnosed as category 0 (7/11) and category 2 (4/11) by HRCT. In CXR category 2 (eight cases), there were four cases diagnosed as category 1 by HRCT.

Discordance between CXR and HRCT is high, especially for CXR negative and early pneumoconiosis cases. The role of CXR in screening coal workers to detect early pneumoconiosis findings should be questioned. Some suggest using HRCT as a standard screening method instead of CXR to distinguish between normal and early pneumoconiosis.

Other Investigations

The positivity of rheumatoid factor, antinuclear antibody or both is possible in 10 to 24 percent of patients with pneumoconiosis. The highest prevalence occurs in PMF, category B and C.

When the radiograph shows a cavitary PMF or recent development of opacities, sputum should be tested for tubercle bacilli and atypical mycobacteria.

Increased IgA concentrations are noted in coalminers with both simple pneumoconiosis and PMF. Serum levels of IgA, IgG, C3 complement, and α-1 antitrypsin are significantly higher in anthracite compared with bituminous miners with PMF. These components are also increased in Caplan's syndrome. Preliminary reports suggest some impairment of activity of both T and B-lymphocytes, particularly a reduced activity of suppressor T cells, which might explain the presence of autoantibodies (discussed above).

Mild normochromic or slight hypochromic anemia is common in coalminers due to expanded plasma volumes and reduced iron levels.

Diagnosis

Occupational history, and radiology are usually sufficient to diagnose coal worker's pneumoconiosis. Presence of coal tattoo marks is additional evidence of exposure to coal mining. Lung biopsy is not required nor indicated for diagnosis, except to exclude some other pathology.

The radiographic opacities may sometimes be confused with miliary tuberculosis, sarcoidosis, diffuse interstitial fibrosis or connective tissue disorders, which may resemble simple pneumoconiosis, although the quality of the opacities is different and the patient is more sick. CPW may coexist with other types of pneumoconiosis, like asbestosis.

Complications and Prognosis

Pulmonary heart disease is not a common complication and does not occur in simple pneumoconiosis. A small number of cases with PMF when the masses are large, central and bilateral, or when there is concomitant severe airflow obstruction and these patients may develop cor pulmonale and heart failure.

Infections due to mycobacteria and fungi (Aspergillus) are not uncommon, and particularly develop in PMF.

The relationship between lung cancer and coal mining is conflicting. While in British miners there is no evidence of a causal relationship in certain USA miners the incidence is higher. This discrepancy is explained by background ionizing radiation in some mines. The death rate due to this cancer is lower in some studies, although the cause of the lower rate of malignancy is not clear.

Scleroderma is reported to occur with unusual frequency in coalminers as well as in men with silicosis.

Other rare complications include hemoptysis, proximal retrograde spread of a pulmonary artery thrombus adjacent to a PMF lesion, spontaneous pneumothorax, and paralysis of recurrent laryngeal nerve.

Studies on miners and exminers have shown that those with simple pneumoconiosis and category A PMF survive as long as those with no evidence of pneumoconiosis. The life expectancy of miners as a whole is the same as that of the general population. However, EMF curtails life in a minority of cases.

Treatment

No treatment is effective in pneumoconiosis. Symptomatic treatment is required for associated chronic bronchitis, cor pulmonale, or tuberculosis. Rheumatoid pneumoconiosis is unaffected by steroid therapy. The prevention of CPW is based on maintaining permitted dust levels, control of dust production, and regular dust measurements, and medical supervision. The National

Coal Board of Great Britain has recommended the mass concentration of dust should be 7 mg/m³ of air for operations at long wall coal faces; 3 mg/m³ for operations in drivages and headings where the average quartz content exceeds 0.45 mg/m³ and 5 mg/m³ for operations in other localities. Control of dust production is achieved by special attention to mining techniques and the designing of equipment to give rise to a minimum of dust. Periodic medical check up at least once in two years with chest radiograph and pulmonary function tests should be carried out to detect early cases.

Disability and Natural History

A retrospective analysis of the results of serial ventilatory capacity tests (FEV 1-0), which had extended over an average period of almost 15 years, was carried out in 215 miners and exminers who suffer with coalworkers' pneumoconiosis. All were unselected previously diagnosed cases that attend the Cardiff Pneumoconiosis Panel at regular intervals for reassessment examinations. They consisted of 68 miners and 147 exminers and they were divided into three groups according to their radiological category at their most recent examination, carried out in either 1973 or 1974. There were 90 cases of category B progressive massive fibrosis (PMF), 50 cases of category A PMF and 75 cases of simple pneumoconiosis. Findings for the 38 lifelong nonsmokers within the 215 were compared with those for the smokers. All three groups showed progressive impairment of ventilation over the whole period of observation. This was most marked in the category B cases but this group had already acquired a substantial proportion of their eventual impairment while still classified radiologically as category A or as simple pneumoconiosis. These findings are not compatible with the view that coalworkers' pneumoconiosis does not cause significant impairment of ventilation until the category B radiological stage is attained; they suggest rather that cases destined to progress to serious disablement show evidence of progressive impairment of ventilation at very much earlier radiological stages. Nonsmokers showed a pattern of impairment similar to that of the smokers but were less disabled; the differences, however, were slight and not statistically significant.[81]

Bronchitis and Emphysema

An earlier study of the Medical Research Council of Great Britain in 1966, concluded that the intensity of dust exposure did not appear to play a significant role in determining the prevalence of bronchitis and airway obstruction in workers exposed to dust. However, since then a number of studies have related the prevalence of bronchitis to dust exposure. Bronchitis is more common in the group exposed to most dust, mainly those working at the face, and' the least common in surface workers. The effect of increasing exposure to dust on ventilatory capacity is minimal, although some studies have shown a reduction in ventilatory capacity with increasing exposure to dust.

The correlations between progressive massive fibrosis (PMF), emphysema, and impairment of ventilation that both factors are contributory to impairment of ventilation in proportion to their size or extent, but these contributions are in the main independent of one another. Most of the emphysema is of the centrilobular variety, which appears to be unrelated to the PMF.[82]

Although focal emphysema is a frequent accompaniment of the higher degrees of simple CWP and may lead to minor abnormalities in the distribution of expired gas, it does not affect the ventilatory capacity. Some investigators believe that disabling emphysema can present during life, although most people do not believe that simple CWP or coal mining *per se* leads to the development of disabling emphysema in the absence of PMF.

Silicosis

Both simple and complicated silicosis are occasionally seen in coalminers, but only in roof bolters and miners who have worked for long periods on transportation. The simple silicosis is delayed compared to other industries and is seldom seen before 20 years of exposure. It is difficult to differentiate from simple CWP unless eggshell calcification is present in hilar nodes (although this can occur in the latter). Lung biopsy is the only means by which the differentiation can be made with certainty.

REFERENCES

1. Gilson JC, Oldham PD. Coal workers' pneumoconiosis. Br Med J 1970;4:305.
2. Ryder R, Lyons JP, Campbell H, Gough J. Emphysema in coal workers' pneumoconiosis. Br Med J 1970; 3: 481-87.
3. Morgan WK, Lapp NL. Respiratory disease in coalminers. Am Rev Respir Dis 1976;113:531-59.
4. Seaton A, Dick JA, Dodgson J, Jacobsen M. Quartz and pneumoconiosis in coalminers. Lancet 1981;2:1272-75.
5. Cohen R, Velho V. Update on respiratory disease from coal mine and silica dust. Clin Chest Med 2002;23:811-26.
6. Ross MH, Murray J. Occupational respiratory disease in mining. Occup Med (Lond) 2004;54:304-10.

7. Miller BG, Hagen S, Love RG, Soutar CA, Cowie HA, Kidd MW, Robertson A. Risks of silicosis in coalworkers exposed to unusual concentrations of respirable quartz. Occup Environ Med 1998;55:52-58.

8. Soutar CA, Hurley JF, Miller BG, Cowie HA, Buchanan D. Dust concentrations and respiratory risks in coalminers: Key risk estimates from the British Pneumoconiosis Field Research. Occupational and Environmental Medicine 2004;61:477-81.

9. Leigh J, Driscoll TR, Cole BD, Beck RW, Hull BP, Yang J. Quantitative relation between emphysema and lung mineral content in coalworkers. Occup Environ Med 1994;51:400-07.

10. Naidoo RN, Robins TG, Murray J. Respiratory outcomes among South African coalminers at autopsy. Am J Ind Med 2005;48:217-24.

11. Scott DF, Grayson RL, Metz EA. Disease and illness in US mining. 1983-2001. J Occup Environ Med 2004;46:1272-77.

12. Mosquera JA, Rodrigo L, González ZF. The evolution of tuberculosis in coalminers in Asturias, Northern Spain. Eur J Epidemiol 1994;10,291-97.

13. Seaton A. Coal workers' pneumoconiosis. In Morgan WKC, Seaton A (Eds): Occupational lung diseases (3rd edn). WB Saunders Company: Philadelphia, PA 1995,374-406.

14. Montes II, Fernández GR, Reguero J, Mir MAC, García-Ordás E, Martínez JLA, González CA. Respiratory Disease in a Cohort of 2,579 Coalminers Followed Up Over a 20-Year Period. Chest 2004;126:622-29.

15. Hurley JF, Burns J, Copland L, Dodgson J, Jacobsen M. Coalworkers' simple pneumoconiosis and exposure to dust at 10 British coalmines. Br J Ind Med 1982;39:120-27.

16. Soutar CA, Maclaren WM, Annis R, Melville AW. Quantitative relations between exposure to respirable coalmine dust and coalworkers' simple pneumoconiosis in men who have worked as miners but have left the coal industry. Br J Ind Med 1986;43:29-36.

17. Baur X. Effects on the lung due to underground coal mining work. Pneumologie 2004;58:107-15.

18. Green FHY, Vallyathan V. Coal worker's pneumoconiosis due to other carbonaceous dusts. In Churg A, Green FHY, (Eds): Pathology of occupational lung disease. Baltimore: Williams & Wilkins 1998;158-70.

19. Mastruzzo C, Crimi N, Vancheri C. Role of oxidative stress in pulmonary fibrosis. Monaldi Arch Chest Dis 2002;57:173-76.

20. Schins RP, Borm PJ. Mechanisms and mediators in coal dust induced toxicity: A review. Ann Occup Hyg 1999;43:7-33.

21. Nemery B, Bast A, Behr J, et al. Interstitial lung disease induced by exogenous agents: Factors governing susceptibility. Eur Respir J 2001;18:30-42.

22. Kinnula VL, Crapo JD. Superoxide dismutases in the lung and human lung diseases. Am J Respir Crit Care Med 2003;167:1600-19.

23. Hayes JD, Strange RC. Glutathione S-transferase polymorphisms and their biological consequences. Pharmacology 2000;61:154-66.

24. Hurley JF, Alexander WP, Hazledine DJ, Jacobsen M, Maclaren WM. Exposure to respirable coalmine dust and incidence of progressive massive fibrosis. Br J Ind Med 1987;44:661-72.

25. Schins RP, Borm PJ. Epidemiological evaluation of release of monocyte TNF-alpha as an exposure and effect marker in pneumoconiosis: A five year follow up study of coal workers. Occup Environ Med 1995;52:441-50.

26. Yucesoy B, Vallyathan V, Landsittel DP, Simeonova P, Luster MI. Cytokine polymorphisms in silicosis and other pneumoconioses. Mol Cell Biochem 2002;234-35:219-24.

27. Yucesoy B, Johnson VJ, Kashon ML, Fluharty K, Vallyathan V, Luster MI. Lack of association between antioxidant gene polymorphisms and progressive massive fibrosis in coalminers. Thorax 2005;60:492-95.

28. Yao W, Wang ZM, Wang MZ, Wang N. Oxidative injury and serum cytokines in coal workers with pneumoconiosis. Sichuan Da Xue Xue Bao Yi Xue Ban 2005;36:510-12.

29. Altin R, Armutcu F, Kart L, Gurel A, Savranlar A, Ozdemir H. Antioxidant response at early stages and low grades of simple coal worker's pneumoconiosis diagnosed by high resolution computed tomography. Int J Hyg Environ Health 2004;207:455-62.

30. Zhang Q, Huang X. Induction of interleukin-6 by coal containing bioavailable iron is through both hydroxyl radical and ferryl species. J Biosci 2003;28:95-100.

31. Nadif R, Jedlicka A, Mintz M, Bertrand JP, Kleeberger S, Kauffmann F. Effect of TNF and LTA polymorphisms on biological markers of response to oxidative stimuli in coalminers: A model of gene-environment interaction. Tumour necrosis factor and lymphotoxin alpha. J Med Genet 2003;40:96-103.

32. Malech HL, Gallin JI. Neutrophils in human diseases. N Engl J Med 1987;317:687-94.

33. Pryor WA, Stone K. Oxidants in cigarette smoke: Radicals, hydrogen peroxides, peroxynitrate, and peroxynitrite. Ann NY Acad Sci 1993;686:12-28.

34. Petit JC, Boettner JC. Evidence of H_2O_2 formation in the early stage of coal oxidation. In Charcosset H (Ed): Advanced methodologies in coal characterisation. Amsterdam: Elsevier 1990;253-66.

35. Fujimura N. Pathology and pathophysiology of pneumoconiosis. Curr Opin Pulm Med 2000;6:140-44.

36. Jeffery PK. Remodeling in asthma and chronic obstructive lung disease. Am J Respir Crit Care Med 2001; 164:S28-38.

37. Schins RPF, Borm PJA. Mechanisms and mediators in coal dust induced toxicity: A review. Ann Occup Hyg 1999;43:7-33.

38. Barnes PJ, Karin M, Nuclear factor-κβ-A pivotal transcription factor in chronic inflammatory diseases. N Engl J Med 1997;336:1066-71.

39. Rahman I, MacNee W. Regulation of redox glutathione levels and gene transcription in lung inflammation: Therapeutic approaches. Free Radic Biol Med 2000;28: 1405-20.

40. Carroll MC, Katzman P, Alicot EM, Koller BH, Geraghty DE, Orr HT, Strominger JL, Spies T. Linkage map of the human major histocompatibility complex including the tumour necrosis factor genes. Proc Natl Acad Sci USA 1987;84:8535-39.

41. Huang SL, Su CH, Chang SC. Tumor necrosis factor-α gene polymorphism in chronic bronchitis. Am J Respir Crit Care Med 1997;156:1436-39.

42. Whyte M, Hubbard R, Meliconi R, Whidborne M, Eaton V, Bingle C, Timms J, Duff G, Facchini A, Pacilli A, Fabbri M, Hall I, Britton J, Johnston I, Di Giovine F. Increased risk of fibrosing alveolitis associated with interleukin-1 receptor antagonist and tumor necrosis factor-alpha gene polymorphisms. Am J Respir Crit Care Med 2000;162:755-58.

43. Winchester EC, Millwood IY, Rand L, Penny MA, Kessling AM. Association of the TNF-α-308 (GαA) polymorphism with self-reported history of childhood asthma. Hum Genet 2000;107:591-96.

44. Zhai R, Jetten M, Schins RPF, Franssen H, Borm PJA. Polymorphisms in the promoter of the tumor necrosis factor-α gene in coalminers. Am J Ind Med 1998;34: 318-24.

45. Seal RM, Cockcroft A, Kung I, Wagner JC. Central lymph node changes and progressive massive fibrosis in coalworkers. Thorax 1986;41:531-37.

46. Burrel R. Immunological aspects of coalworkers' pneumoconiosis. NY Acad Sci 1972;200:94-105.

47. Robertson MD, Boyd JE, Collins HP, Davis JM. Serum immunoglobulin levels and humoral immune competence in coalworkers. Am J Ind Med 1984;6:387-93.

48. Robertson MD, Boyd JE, Fernie JM, Davis JM. Some immunological studies on coalworkers with and without pneumoconiosis. Am J Ind Med 1983;4:467-76.

49. Wagner JC, Burns J, Munday DE, McGee JO. Presence of fibronectin in pneumoconiotic lesions. Thorax 1982;37:54-56.

50. Caplan A. Certain unusual appearances in the chest film of miners suffering from pneumoconiosis. Thorax 1953;8:29-37.

51. Caplan A, Payne RB, Withey JL. A broader concept of Caplan's syndrome related to rheumatoid factors. Thorax 1962;17:205-12.

52. Lippman M, Eckert HL, Hahon N, Morgan WK. Circulating antinuclear and rheumatoid factors in coalminers. A prevalence study in Pennsylvania and West Virginia. Ann Intern Med 1973;79:807-11.

53. Wagner MM, Darke C. HLA-A and B antigen frequencies in Welsh coalworkers with pneumoconiosis and Caplan's syndrome. Tissue Antigens 1979;14:165-68.

54. Heise ER, Mentnech MS, Olenchock SA, Kutz SA, Morgan WK, Merchant JA, Major PC.HLA-A1 and coalworkers' pneumoconiosis. Am Rev Respir Dis 1979;119:903-08.

55. Bingham E, Barkley W, Murthy R, Vassallo C. Investigation of alveolar macrophages from rats exposed to coal dust. Inhaled Part 1975;4 Pt 2:543-50.

56. Burrell R, Flaherty DK, Schreiber JE. Immunological studies of experimental coalworkers' pneumoconiosis. Inhaled Part 1975;4 Pt 2:519-29.

57. Davis JM, Ottery J, le Roux A.The effect of quartz and other non-coal dusts in coalworkers' pneumoconiosis. Part II. Lung autopsy study. Inhaled Part 1975;4 Pt 2:691-702.

58. Jacobsen M, Burns J, Attfield MD. Smoking and coalworkers' simple pneumoconiosis. Inhaled Part. 1975;4 Pt 2:759-72.

59. Thurlbeck WM. The pathobiology and epidemiology of human emphysema. J Toxicol Environ Health 1984;13: 323-43.

60. Lyons JP, Ryder RC, Seal RM, Wagner JC. Emphysema in smoking and non-smoking coalworkers with pneumoconiosis. Bull Eur Physiopathol Respir 1981;17: 75-85.

61. Kampalath BN, McMahon JT, Cohen A, Tomashefski JF Jr, Kleinerman J. Obliterative central bronchitis due to mineral dust in patients with pneumoconiosis. Arch Pathol Lab Med 1998;122:56-62.

62. Fernie JM, Douglas AN, Lamb D, Ruckley VA. Right ventricular hypertrophy in a group of coalworkers. Thorax 1983;38:436-42.

63. Haffar M, Banks J. Left vocal cord paralysis caused by coalworkers' pneumoconiosis and progressive massive fibrosis. Postgrad Med J 1988;64:143-44.

64. Sherani TM, Angelini GD, Passani SP, Butchart EG. Vocal cord paralysis associated with coalworkers' pneumoconiosis and progressive massive fibrosis. Thorax 1984;39:683-84.

65. Seatton A, Lapp NL, Morgan WKC. Lung mechanics and frequency dependence of compliance in coalminers. J Clin Invest 1972;51:1203-11.

66. Rasmussen DL, Nelson CW. Respiratory function in southern Appalachian coalminers. Am Rev Respir Dis 1971;103:240-48.

67. Zhicheng S. A study of lung function in coalworkers' pneumoconiosis. Br J Ind Med 1986;43:644-45.

68. Huncharek M. Lung function in coalworkers' pneumoconiosis. Br J Ind Med 1987;44:215-16.

69. Cochrane AL, Moore F. Lung mechanics in relation to radiographic category of coalworkers' simple pneumoconiosis. Br J Ind Med 1984;41:284-85.

70. Musk AW, Cotes JE, Bevan C, Campbell MJ. Relationship between type of simple coalworkers' pneumoconiosis and lung function. A nine-year follow-up study of subjects with small rounded opacities. Br J Ind Med 1981;38:313-20.

71. Rogan JM, Attfield MD, Jacobsen M, et al. Role of dust in the working environment in development of chronic bronchitis in British coalminers. Br J Ind Med 1973;30: 217-26.

72. Cowie HA, Miller BG, Soutar CA. Dust-related clinically relevant lung functional defects. Research Report. TM/99/06. Edinburgh: Institute of Occupational Medicine, 1999.

73. Fernie JM, Ruckley VA. Coalworkers' pneumoconiosis: Correlation between opacity profusion and number and type of dust lesions with special reference to opacity type. Br J Ind Med 1987;44:273-77.

74. Naidoo RN, Robins TG, Solomon A, White N, Franzblau A. Radiographic outcomes among South African coalminers. Int Arch Occup Environ Health 2004;77:471-81.

75. Ruckley VA, Fernie JM, Chapman JS, Collings P, Davis JM, Douglas AN, Lamb D, Seaton A. Comparison of radiographic appearances with associated pathology and lung dust content in a group of coalworkers. Br J Ind Med 1984;41:459-67.

76. Amandus HE, Lapp NL, Jacobson G, Reger RB. Significance of irregular small opacities in radiographs of coalminers in the USA. Br J Ind Med 1976;33:13-17.

77. Collins HP, Dick JA, Bennett JG, Pern PO, Rickards MA, Thomas DJ, Washington JS, Jacobsen M. Irregularly shaped small shadows on chest radiographs, dust exposure, and lung function in coalworkers' pneumoconiosis. Br J Ind Med 1988;45:43-55.

78. Cockcroft A, Berry G, Cotes JE, Lyons JP. Shape of small opacities and lung function in coalworkers. Thorax 1982;37:765-69.

79. Akira M. High-resolution CT in the evaluation of occupational and environmental disease. Radiol Clin North Am 2002;40:43-59.

80. Altin R, Savranlar A, Kart L, Mahmutyazicioglu K, Ozdemir H, Akdag B, Gundogdu S. Presence and HRCT quantification of bronchiectasis in coal workers. Eur J Radiol 2004;52:157-63.

81. Lyons JP, Campbell H. Evolution of disability in coalworkers' pneumoconiosis. Thorax 1976;31:527-33.

82. Lyons JP, Campbell H. Relation between progressive massive fibrosis, emphysema, and pulmonary dysfunction in coalworkers' pneumoconiosis. Br J Ind Med 1981;38:125-29.

ASBESTOS RELATED DISEASES

History

The word *asbestos* is derived from a Greek term for inextinguishable or unquenchable, and first appeared in the English language in the late 1300s (Oxford English Dictionary). In the 1700s, asbestos-based items such as wicks for oil lamps, asbestos fabrics for conversion into items of clothing, and the production of asbestos-based papers first appeared, but not until the mid-1850s did industrial production commences. Even from the dawn of the Christian era, there have been sporadic references to objects or materials with unique fire-resistant properties that were considered supernatural. Cloth woven from asbestos fibers known as -"stone wool"- is described in ancient writings as magical because it could be thrown into a fire and removed intact. Subsequently the industrial revolution and the widespread adaptation of steam power caused a dramatic increase in demand. Large deposits of asbestos were first located in Canada and South Africa. In the nineteenth century, additional sources were found in Italy, Russia, China, and the United States. Canada is currently the major supplier in the world. Asbestos (unquenchable) is a fibrous mineral having unique properties of resistance to destruction by a number of physical and chemical means. Therefore, mankind has used it for a variety of purposes.

In 1876, Henry Johns of Brooklyn, NY, patented a stovepipe covering composed of asbestos, paper, and felt. Fire was a major hazard at the time, particularly in crowded urban centers, and the fire-resistant properties of asbestos-based materials made them a desirable commodity and Mr. Johns' (later Johns-Manville) enterprise highly successful. The use of asbestos increased progressively in the first half of the twentieth century with an additional rapid escalation during and following World War II. As the adverse health effects became known, exposure controls were imposed by regulatory agencies. In the United States, the initial exposure limit was established in 1971 at 5 fibers per cubic centimeters, reduced to 2 fibers per cubic centimeter in 1976, to 0.5 fibers per cubic centimeter in 1983, and to 0.1 fibers per cubic centimeter in 1994. Thereafter, the use of asbestos declined in that country almost as dramatically as it had increased, from a peak of 803,000 metric tons in 1973 to 16,000 tons in 1998.[1-3]

Dr Montague Murray, a British physician, is the first person to diagnose a fatal case of asbestos-related disease, a case of asbestosis. Although his observations were made known to various boards of inquiry beginning in 1899, they were not published until 1907,[4] and additional reports began to appear in the 1920s. In 1930, Mereweather and Price[5] published the results of a survey of 363 factory workers in England of whom more than a one fourth had signs of asbestosis. That article firmly established the pulmonary hazards of asbestos exposure. One very significant result of the Merewether report was the adoption of dust-control regulations for Great Britain in 1931.[6] They were not imposed until 1971 in the United States. Although the link between asbestos and lung cancer was acknowledged in Germany in 1943,[7] it was not so recognized in that United States until 1955, and not until 1960 was the connection to mesothelioma well established.[8]

During the twentieth century, asbestos was an integral part of the industrialization process. According to data from the US Geological survey, 182.2 million metric tones (Mt) of asbestos was mined between 1990 and 2003 whereas global production peaked in 1975 at 5 Mt. Despite slight downturn, output remained at over 4 Mt a year until 1991. In 2003, 2.15 Mt ofd chrysotile or white asbestos was mined.

Physical and Chemical Characteristics of Asbestos

Asbestos refers to a group of minerals: crystalline-hydrated silicates that exist in a fibrous form. It is the fiber-like structure, in addition to the chemical composition of the mineral, that is the basis for their extensive commercial use. Asbestos occurs in one of two forms: serpentine and amphibole. The differences between the two are as follows:

Serpentine	Amphibole
• Chrysotile is the only serpentine form of asbestos • Chrysotile fibers are long, curly, and pliable	• There are several forms of the amphiboles • The major amphiboles that have been used commercially are amosite, crocidolite, and to a much lesser degree-anthophyllite • Amphibole fibers are short, straight, and stiff • Noncommercial amphiboles such as *tremolite* and *actinolite*, plus a fibrous zeolite called *erionite*, are morphologically similar but differ chemically from the commercial amphiboles and are present in substantial concentrations in surface soils in various locations

These noncommercial amphiboles are found in areas that include Afghanistan, Bulgaria, Finland, Czechoslovakia, Greece, and Turkey, to cite a few. Significant exposures occur among residents in these regions. In the United States, exposure to tremolite may occur among workers processing, talc, vermiculite, and other products. Ninety to ninety-five percent of all asbestos used in the United States has been chrysotile. Because of its chemical and physical properties, the serpentine form of asbestos is most suitable for making fabrics and other flexible items. The amphiboles have superior chemical and physical stability and have been used to make asbestos-cement pipe, floor tiles, and—

when mixed with chrysotile—a vast array of friction products, gaskets, roofing, insulation, and fireproofing materials. As mentioned, there are mainly two types of asbestos: the *serpentine* and the *amphiboles*. *Chrysotile* or white asbestos belongs to the serpentine mineral and is a magnesium silicate. Amphiboles are straight fibres and do not break into small fibrils, and include *crocidolite* (blue asbestos), *amosite* (brown asbestos), *anthophyllite*, *tremolite* and *actinolite*. Chrysotile is the most widely used form of asbestos, and mainly produced by Canada, and the Commonwealth of Russia. Amosite and crocidolite are mainly produced in South Africa. Asbestos is mainly bound to rocks and is mainly found underground. Asbestos imparts strength to cement, building materials and plastics, and has important fire proofing properties. It is an important insulator and is friction resistant. It is also useful as filler in paints. Various industries/occupations that are likely to expose its workers to hazards of asbestos are shown in Table 27.2.

TABLE 27.2: Occupations with asbestos exposure

- Asbestos cement manufacturing (tiles, corrugated roofing, gutter, water and drain pipes, chimneys, flat sheets, and pressure piping)
- Floor tiling industry
- Insulation and fire proofing (Ship building)
- Asbestos textiles
- Asbestos paper products
- Friction material (Brake lining, clutch facings)
- Gas mask making industries

Because of its durability and tensile strength, asbestos is used in over 3000 products. A number of substitutes to asbestos are used in developed countries, including cellulose polyacrylonitrile, glass fiber and unplasticized polyvinyl chloride (PVC). However many in the developing countries cannot afford to these alternative products. Thus, hazardous working conditions are the norm in developing countries.

It is at the pleural surface where the effect of past asbestos exposure is most often found. There are four types of benign pleural reactions:

A. Benign pleural reactions
- Pleural effusions
- Pleural plaques, local areas of fibrosis of the parietal pleura
- Diffuse pleural fibrosis, extensive visceral pleural fibrosis, often with fusion of both pleural surfaces
- Rounded atelectasis that occurs when an area of visceral pleural fibrosis extends into the parenchyma and renders a portion of the lung airless.

B. Malignant pleural disease
- Mesothelioma, a primary malignancy of the pleura (and occasionally the peritoneum).

C. Other consequences of asbestos exposure
- Asbestosis, which is fibrosis of the lung parenchyma (Diffuse interstitial pulmonary fibrosis)
- Lung cancer associated with asbestosis or without asbestosis
- Carcinoma of the larynx and other neoplasia
- Lung function abnormalities.

Exposure

Asbestos fibers enter the body either by skin contact, ingestion, or inhalation. When raw asbestos fibers were handled with impunity, "asbestos corns" sometimes developed in workers, localized areas on the hands with exuberant epidermal overgrowth due to the intracutaneous deposition of asbestos fibers. This manifestation of asbestos exposure is now solely of historical interest. For the public at large, asbestos is harmless if swallowed. In municipalities with asbestos-cement pipe for water distribution, and a much higher concentration of asbestos fibers in the drinking water than in communities with other types of pipe, no differences in the frequency of asbestos-related diseases were found.[9,10] However, workers with a heavy industrial exposure probably swallow large quantities of asbestos fibers, and this could contribute to the development of peritoneal mesothelioma.

All adverse effects on health from asbestos are due to the inhalation of fibers in concentrations sufficient to overwhelm the normal pulmonary defense and clearance mechanisms. Airborne fibers are carried along in the inspired air stream and impinge on the mucous lining of the smaller bronchioles. Tissue fiber burdens are generally related to cumulative exposure.[11] Chrysotile fibers are less harmful than the amphiboles, in part because they are broken down and removed from the lung.[11] Animal studies[12,13] clearly show that cigarette smoke increases asbestos fiber deposition. Asbestos-related diseases have lengthy latent periods, except for pleural effusions, which can occur within a year to ≥ 20 years after first exposure.[14,15] Brief but intense exposures are quite capable of causing disease, but it may be many years, with either continuing or no further exposure, before they become manifest. The longest latent periods, ≥ 40 years, occur with mesothelioma. Whether or not there is a threshold level of asbestos exposure that does not increase the risk of malignancy is controversial.[16-19] Mesothelioma and lung cancer rates vary by

many orders of magnitude between those with a heavy, lifetime occupational exposure and the unexposed. Low-level exposure, as encountered in public buildings, probably does not represent any additional health hazard beyond what is incurred breathing outdoor air.[20,21] However, reliable information about long-term, low-level exposure is exceedingly difficult to obtain.

Misconceptions about asbestos are legion, and are largely attributable to a lack of awareness of the extended latency—the interval between initial exposure and subsequent biological consequences—that varies from a year or so for some cases of pleural effusion to ≥ 40 years for mesothelioma. Among the public there is widespread anxiety, based on the misunderstanding that a casual exposure, such as walking by a demolition site or entering a schoolhouse that is being repaired, represents a significant health risk to the passerby or to the school child. General concern has been heightened recently by events such as natural disasters or terrorist attacks that produce very high levels of dust. Asbestos diseases are generally dose dependent. Because of difficulties in quantifying exposure, the variable persistence of asbestos fibers in tissue, differences in elapsed time from first exposure to the manifestations of asbestos-related disease, plus interindividual differences in susceptibility to disease, a "safe" exposure level, one that does not cause a specific disease, remains controversial. In the United States, the exposure limit is 0.1 fibers per cubic centimeter.

Asbestos fiber exposure differs by many orders of magnitude between those occupationally exposed and members of their families; those engaged in other types of work in factories, construction, machine maintenance, or mining; and people who reside near asbestos processing facilities or major industrial users. Those who live and work in rural settings are generally considered as not exposed, provided there are no significant asbestos deposits in the local terrain, which may not always be known. These different types of exposure have been categorized as primary (occupational), household (family members of the occupationally exposed,[22] bystander (those working near insulation installers, for example), and environmental (naturally occurring sources). The issue has recently been reviewed.[3]

The aerodynamic behavior of fibrous particles is more important than that of the compact particle. This is important to explain the depth of penetration of the fibre. The free falling speed of fibres is determined by the square of their diameters and is little influenced by the length. Thus, a fibre with a length of 200 μm or more and a diameter of about 3 um has the same free falling speed as a unit density spherical particle of 10 μm diameter, meaning thereby the fiber has an equivalent aerodynamic diameter. The flexural modules or harshness of the fiber is also important. Most amphiboles are harsh and stiff even when they are extremely fine, but most chrysotile fibers are soft or semi-harsh, and curly. The curling of long soft fibers of chrysotile fibers is intercepted higher in the small airways by the mucociliary escalator. On the other hand, more amphiboles such as crocidolite penetrate beyond the mucociliary blanket. But, short chrysotile fibers having short arcs are virtually straight and behave aerodynamically to that of the amphiboles and can reach the periphery of the lungs. Fibers in the alveolar region are less than 3 μm in diameter (usually less than 1 μm). The longest fibers tend to be found in the respiratory bronchioles and alveolar ducts, and shorter fibers in the alveoli. It seems that long fibers in and beyond respiratory bronchioles are responsible for interstitial fibrosis.

It is observed that proportionally higher rates pleural changes occur compared to parenchymal changes, up to almost 13-fold in some work forces. Exposure levels of intermittent, but to higher concentrations, are associated with high rates of pleural changes. Similarly, the biologic dose response of asbestos fiber is important to decide the predominance of pleural or parenchymal disease.

Establishing the relationship of exposure to response is difficult to assess because of the difficulty in quantifying the asbestos fibers and due to the variability in response. However, several studies have suggested that a 1 percent risk of significant functional or radiological abnormalities is associated with exposures of 4 fibers/ml for 50 years. The risk may be also different in different industries. They are lower in mining, milling, and cement production than in textile or insulation work. It is also true that different types of asbestos have different magnitudes of effect. Thus, crocidolites are most dangerous followed by amosite and chrysotile. The risk decreases in proportion to reduction in duration of exposure.[1-3]

Pleural Plaques

Bilateral pleural plaques are associated with exposure to all types of asbestos, especially anthophyllite. It is not clear, how the fibers reach the parietal pleura. It is suggested that sharp fibers from the lung penetrate the visceral pleura during respiration and pass directly into the parietal pleura causing traumatic microhemorrhage and fibrin deposition. It is also possible that they pass through lymphatics. There may be a genetic predisposition to such reaction.

Circumscribed or localized pleural plaques are considered by some as benign markers of prior asbestos exposure, whereas others believe they cause functional impairment, indicate an immunologic deficiency, and are a harbinger of a future malignancy.[23-25] Circumscribed plaques are discrete areas of fibrous tissue limited to the parietal pleura, whereas diffuse pleural thickening or pleural fibrosis is much more widespread and usually extends into the costophrenic angles; additionally the visceral and parietal pleural surfaces are often fused. Both types of pleural thickening are relatively acellular and can coexist.

Plaques are often incidental chest radiographic findings. They occupy irregular, discrete areas on the parietal pleura. The area involved may be barely visible, or plaques may cover much of the parietal pleura and the superior surface of the diaphragm. On gross inspection, plaques have a white, shaggy appearance, originate from the inner surface of a rib, and extend across adjacent intercostal muscles. Asbestos bodies are not generally found in plaque tissue, but asbestos fibers that lack the protein envelope may be visible.[26] Small plaques are often difficult to discern, particularly, if the radiographic technique is less than optimal. Chest radiographs best suited to reveal parenchymal detail are often suboptimal for visualization of the pleura, particularly in obese patients. Some radiologic survey results are based on a single posteroanterior image; others include lateral and/or oblique radiographs that may reveal plaques not visible on the posteroanterior view. Survey results also depend on whether radiographic interpretations were made by a single or by a panel of readers. Current survey results, if based on digital radiology[27] or CT scan of the thorax, cannot be compared with older data based solely on conventional radiographs. Ultrasound has no role in identifying pleural plaques, although it is very useful in locating pleural fluid. MRI can be helpful in identifying rounded atelectasis,[28] but it is of limited value in defining plaques or diffuse pleural fibrosis.

The frequency with which pleural plaques occur in different population groups varies widely. They are invariably found in a much higher proportion of male than female patients, and with increasing frequency with advancing age.[29] In a large autopsy series[29] from a hospital serving a region of Glasgow, Scotland, near major shipyards plaques were identified in 51.2 percent of men ≥ 70 years old. This is in all likelihood due to the extremely slow rate at which plaque formation progresses, the number of years of occupational and possible environmental exposure without the benefit of respiratory protection or air quality controls, and the age of the patient cohort. The dose-response relationship for plaque formation is highly variable given the wide range of fiber levels found in lung tissue and the uncertainties regarding exposures. Plaque detection is uncertain using standard chest radiographs. A substantial proportion of plaques subsequently found postmortem[30] or by CT scanning[31] are missed, and the inverse is also true: plaques reported by the radiologist may not be found on autopsy. This is due in part to the erroneous interpretation of images produced by subpleural fat deposits, old rib fractures, and muscle bundles.[32] Subpleural fat creates uniform, smooth, bilateral, and symmetrical opacities, whereas pleural plaques are irregular and, although often bilateral, are rarely symmetrical. They generally develop in the lower two thirds of the thorax and on the outer two thirds of the diaphragm. Serratus anterior and external oblique muscle slips may be misinterpreted as plaques, but they are oriented in an oblique manner opposite to the usual direction of pleural plaques. Companion shadows due primarily to fat tissue are frequently confused with early, localized pleural plaques. High-resolution CT scans are far superior to any other method for imaging pleural plaques. With digital films, and particularly with CT scans, film contrast and density can be adjusted for optimum visualization of the pleural surfaces.

The lesions are bilateral and consist of elevated areas of hyaline fibrosis, the thickness varying from 1 mm to 1 cm. They are distributed irregularly on the inner surface of the rib cage, mainly in the mid zones anteriorly, laterally, and posteriorly, and tend to follow the rib line. They may pass right angles to the surface also. In advanced cases, they become cuirass-like sheets. The other common locations are along the vertebral gutter and central tendon of the diaphragm. The visceral pleura is not involved. Such changes are not seen in pericardium or peritoneum.

A classification system for rating chest radiographs for the pleural and parenchymal abnormalities of pneumoconiosis, known as the International Labor Organization system, was developed as a tool for epidemiologic studies. Although not intended for the purpose, it is also used for diagnosis. A set of standard reference radiographs, against which a worker's film is compared, is required.[33] An assessment of film quality is also required. Poor quality films are much more likely to be interpreted as abnormal than good quality images.[34] Interobserver agreement is also dependent on the prevalence of abnormalities in the population under surveillance. Agreement is good for normal radiographic findings; variability between readers is increased substantially with abnormal radiographic findings.[34]

Areas of pleural thickening confined to either the anterior or posterior thoracic surfaces differ from lateral chest wall plaques in their radiologic appearance. Plaques on the front or rear thoracic surface are designated *en face* (face on) plaques. They have a maximum density laterally with a gradual diminution and disappearance of their opacity in a medial direction, and may be confused with underlying parenchymal opacities. On a posteroanterior chest radiograph, *en face* plaques that are sufficiently "mature" to have some calcification may have a characteristic coiled or serpentine margin, creating an appearance that has been likened to the edge of a holly leaf and also to the appearance of wax that has hardened after running down the shaft of a burning candle. Diaphragmatic pleural plaques have a variety of contours, but a classic example is a protuberance resembling a mushroom cap, shown in which is virtually diagnostic of prior asbestos exposure. On the other hand a thickened interlobar pleura, primarily between the right upper and middle lobes, has a similar appearance whether it is due to asbestos, prior infection, or any other cause.

Calcium deposition occurs in pleural plaques of long-standing. It is unusual among workers with a < 30 year interval from time of first exposure.[35] Fine, punctate, irregular nodules are early signs. The flecks of calcium gradually coalesce with the formation of dense streaks or platelike deposits. Calcification may be limited to a 1 to 2 cm strand or extend over large areas including the diaphragm. In the absence of an alternative explanation such as previous trauma, surgery, or significant pulmonary infections, a calcified plaque on the diaphragm is virtually pathognomonic of prior asbestos exposure.

The impact of circumscribed plaques, with or without calcification, on lung function has been the subject of numerous reports and conflicting findings. Multiple reasons, including differences in radiologic methods and variability in lung function testing, were cited as explanations for the disparate outcomes. Furthermore, confounding factors such as cigarette use, prior pulmonary ailments, and other occupational exposures were sometimes either overlooked or not known. Although more sophisticated techniques for identifying pleural plaques and for measuring lung function have been used in most of the recent surveys, and there has been better control for potential confounders, the outcome variation persists.[36] Chest CT scanning, now a part of almost all radiologic studies provides better identification of pleural abnormalities, and an alternative method (other than the carbon monoxide diffusing capacity) for determining if some lung fibrosis (asbestosis) is present. A restrictive ventilatory impairment, attributed to a mechanical limitation of lung motion, was reported in some studies of patients with circumscribed plaques. However, studies using high-resolution CT scan and evidence of lymphocytic alveolitis identified by BAL, parenchymal inflammation and fibrosis are considered the basis of the restrictive impairment.[37] Since extensive plaques may obscure underlying fibrosis that can only be visualized with CT scans, conclusions based on studies done prior to the availability of this imaging modality may be questioned. However, CT scan interpretations are subjective, the subtle changes that occur with minimal asbestosis are ill defined, and conclusions based on CT scan findings have also been questioned.[38,39] Limited or circumscribed pleural plaques have no clinically significant adverse impact on pulmonary function.[36] However others believe that impaired lung function can be detected by a combination of CT imaging and the use of exercise tests. The impairment would not be apparent with previously used methods of disability evaluation.[40]

Whether pleural plaques augment the likelihood of mesothelioma or other malignancy development has been evaluated in numerous studies, but with far from consistent results. While some found a two-fold–greater risk of dying from lung cancer among 425 exposed workers with plaques than in the population at large,[41] a contrary result was reported by others[42] who found no link between plaques and asbestos-associated malignancies among 1,500 asbestos-exposed workers followed up for 4 years. A review of 13 reports; among the 10 reports deemed suitably designed to reach a meaningful result, increased rate of lung cancer risk was not found when pleural plaques were present.[43] However, plaques are markers of asbestos exposure, and asbestos is a recognized carcinogen. Lung injury that is not discernible on the chest radiograph, or by other means, could exist and thereby increase the likelihood that a malignant disease will develop.

Pleural thickening unrelated to asbestos exposure is commonplace. It is frequently seen at the lung apices, generally due to prior fungal and/or tuberculous infections. It is unusual for asbestos to cause apical pleural thickening.[44] Obliteration of the costophrenic angle is also commonplace, and is indicative of prior infection, cardiac failure, trauma, other causes, or a previous pleural effusion, possibly an asbestos effusion. At the present time, the preponderance of the evidence indicates that plaques do not increase the cancer risk, but this is far from a universal view.

Pleural plaques alone are symptomless and produce no functional abnormalities except in advanced cases when they are cuirass-like. The plaques may not be visible radiologically unless the amount of fibrous tissue or amount of calcium deposition is sufficiently radiodense. Calcified plaques are seen as very opaque, discontinuous thick illness along the chest wall, diaphragm or cardiac borders. They neither have a segmental or lobar distribution.

Diffuse Pleural Thickening and Diffuse Pleural Fibrosis

Diffuse pleural thickening, unlike circumscribed thickening or plaques, can cause significant restrictive ventilatory impairment.[36,37,45] Respiratory failure occurs because of[46] severe restrictive ventilatory deficiency. The hallmark of diffuse pleural thickening is involvement of the visceral pleura, with blunting of the costophrenic angle the most frequent radiologic clue. Localized or circumscribed plaques do not extend into this region. The pleural shadows often extend up both chest walls, usually with some irregularity. Methods for measuring the area and thickness of abnormal pleura using CT scans and correlating those results with abnormal lung function have revealed an inverse relationship with the FVC depending on the method used to define pleural thickening.[47] In a number of these patients, and also among some of the subjects in other[48] there was a reduction in the carbon monoxide diffusing capacity, which suggests that the reported reductions of lung volumes were not due solely to an abnormal pleura but also to some parenchymal fibrosis.

Rounded Atelectasis

An unique form of pleural thickening is known as *rounded atelectasis*, (*folded lung, Blesovsky syndrome*), and by its major radiologic feature: ***the comet tail sign***. This type of pleural involvement is much less frequent than circumscribed plaques or diffused pleural fibrosis. It has the appearance of a round, mass-like opacity and develops at one, occasionally at several, locations in the pleura with a characteristic curvilinear "tail" extending toward the hilum (the comet tail).[49] Because it may resemble a peripheral tumor, a thorough evaluation of the patient may be necessary. The chest CT and MRI are very useful for visualizing what often presents as an indistinct pleural based mass. If serial chest radiographs are available, the nature of the mass should be apparent. How rounded atelectasis develops is unclear, but a possible mechanism whereby this occurs is a low-grade inflammatory pleural reaction at one site, fusion of the two pleural surfaces with progressive thickening at the fused region. This results in compression of the underlying lung and bronchial occlusion that renders the underlying lung airless. The bronchus and adjacent blood vessels contribute the "tail" or comet sign of this unusual form of pleural fibrosis.[50] Other mechanisms have been suggested and include the regional shrinkage of connective tissue fibrous strands at one location in the visceral pleura[51] and the subsequent development of adhesions between two parts of the lung following an effusion or infection. When the acute process subsides, the adhesion persists with distortion and obstruction of the bronchus resulting in atelectasis of the distal lung. Most patients with rounded atelectasis are asymptomatic, but they may become symptomatic if the atelectatic volume is large and lung function is compromised.

Pleural Effusion

Pleural effusions due to asbestos exposure vary from a completely asymptomatic event, with either total resolution or a blunted costophrenic angle as the only residual evidence, to an active, inflammatory pleuritis with fever, pleuritic type pain, and a substantial accumulation of bloody pleural fluid. The symptoms do not differ from those associated with other forms of acute pleuritis, including some dyspnea. The erythrocyte sedimentation rate is often elevated, but an elevated body temperature is unusual.[52] The effusions are usually unilateral, but may be bilateral and occasionally subside on one side only to recur on the other.[53] Pleural fluid eosinophil counts exceed the normal in about one third of the patients.[53] The fluid usually conforms to the criteria of Light[54] for an exudate. Asbestos bodies (asbestos fibers enveloped by an iron-containing protein coat) are seldom[55] or never[56] found in the pleural fluid, may be seen occasionally in pleural tissue, and are frequently present in the underlying lung tissue.[55]

The most sensitive imaging modality for visualizing pleural fluid is the CT scan of the chest. MRI is useful for distinguishing lesions of the chest wall and visceral pleura from fluid accumulations, but it is of limited use in the evaluation of patients with free-flowing pleural fluid.[57] An unexplained pleural effusion should be sampled for chemical, bacteriologic, and cytologic analysis. Pleural biopsy is indicated unless the findings are diagnostic, and absent contraindications. A pleural effusion can be attributed to asbestos only when there is a history of asbestos exposure and all other causes, particularly a malignancy, have been excluded. This requires an observation period of 2 to 3 years. A left-side predominance has been noted in 11 of 15 cases in one report[58] and in 40 of 73 effusions that occurred in 60 patients in another report.[53] The effusions usually subside slowly and spontaneously over a period of several months.[59]

Asbestos pleural effusions have no specific prognostic implications with respect to the subsequent development of pleural plaques or mesothelioma. Effusions are frequent in the early stage of mesothelioma, and can be very difficult to distinguish from a benign effusion. In one series of 22 patients with an asbestos pleural effusion and follow-up intervals of as long as 17 years, there were no cases of mesothelioma.[52] In another group of 12 patients, mesothelioma developed in only 1 patient 9 years after his first documented effusion.[60]

Asbestosis
(Diffuse Interstitial Pulmonary Fibrosis, DIPF)

Asbestosis is a form of bilateral diffuse interstitial pulmonary fibrosis due to fibrous asbestos. The disease is common in those engaged in milling, and disintegrating ore, in heat and sound insulation, and in shipyards.[61,62]

Although all types of asbestos are capable of producing asbestosis, chrysotile is most active in this respect. The most important factor that determines the development of asbestosis is the product of level and duration of asbestos exposure experienced by the subject. Between 1940 and 1979, it has been estimated that 40 percent of the workforce or almost 27 million individuals were exposed to asbestos.[63,64] After 1980, industrial use of asbestos was curtailed in the United States by government-imposed exposure regulations. The development of asbestos-exposure induced lung disorders is associated with a latency period between date of first exposure and the time when the disease becomes clinically apparent. Typically, benign pleural effusions are the first manifestations of asbestos exposure, followed by pleural plaques, interstitial fibrosis, bronchogenic cancer, and mesothelioma. Any one of these asbestos-related lung diseases may be the first and only sequelae of asbestos exposure that a worker may acquire. Therefore, given a sufficient latency period, a worker may acquire mesothelioma as the initial and only result of asbestos exposure.

The development and severity of asbestos-induced lung disease is related to intensity of exposure (dose) and latency. Asbestos exposure for workers today is remote in time and more limited than described in previous studies.[65-73] Very few patients are exposed in an industry where asbestos is incidental to the enterprise's operation, while most cases arise from exposure in primary asbestos industries, i.e. companies selling, distributing, refining, milling or using raw asbestos to manufacture products. The mean reported duration of exposure is 17.5 years. About 15 percent report less than 5 years' exposure. Few cases will have a latency period from first exposure to diagnosis of less than 6 years.[74]

Pathogenesis and Pathology

A. Pleural Disease

How asbestos fibers that have impacted the airway wall migrate to the pleural surface and, in the case of circumscribed pleural plaques, ignore the visceral pleura in the process is quite obscure. Why asbestos fibers that reach the pleural space induce an effusion in one patient, plaque or diffuse pleural fibrosis in another, or mesothelioma in yet another is equally obscure. Probably in some combination of yet-to-be-determined mechanical, biochemical, and genetic events play roles.[75-78]

One traditional explanation for the formation of circumscribed plaques—mechanical irritation by asbestos fibers protruding from the visceral pleura causing continuous mechanical irritation of the overlying parietal pleura—is very likely incorrect. Inflammatory reactions are not seen at the site of plaque formation, nor are the two pleural surfaces adherent, which would be expected following a local inflammatory process.[79] Alternate routes by which asbestos fibers may reach the parietal pleura include the path of lymph flow and the systemic blood stream. Plaques are said to develop along pathways of lymphatic drainage at sites where there is an uptake into parietal pleural lymphatics.[80] Experimental studies[81] in rabbits indicate that cell recruitment and interaction are important determinants of pleural reactions to asbestos fibers.

There are many features of asbestos fibers that could account for their genotoxic effects on certain cell types. For example, amphibole fibers have a high iron content that can generate reactive oxygen species (ROS) by iron-catalyzed reactions over prolonged periods on the surface of the fiber that is lodged within the lung. ROS can also be generated during frustrated phagocytosis of long asbestos fibers and dissolution of macrophages. In contrast, short asbestos fibers can be successfully phagocytized and incorporated into lysosomes. This phenomenon may explain in part why long thin fibers, i.e. > 8 μm in length, are more carcinogenic after inhalation or injection into the pleura or peritoneum of rodents.[82,83] Asbestos fibers activate inducible nitric oxide synthase in alveolar macrophages and in lung epithelial cells that may generate reactive nitrogen species (RNS).[84,85] Both ROS and RNS can cause mutagenic oxidative lesions.[84] Other indicators of genetic damage, including chromosomal changes, alteration of cell cycle progression, formation of aneuploid and polyploid cells,

and nuclear disruption by long fibers, have been demonstrated in cell culture.[86] However, it is difficult to determine whether these signs of genetic damage are relevant to asbestos-associated carcinogenesis or to cell death, since in some studies high levels of asbestos exposure were utilized.

Apoptosis, regulated physiologic cell death, is crucial for organ development and host defense.[87,88] All forms of asbestos can induce DNA damage, which is a potent stimulus for apoptosis. ROS derived from asbestos fibers induce DNA damage and apoptosis in relevant lung target cells including mesothelial cells.[89,90] There are multiple additional sources of ROS once cells are exposed to apotogenic stimuli.[91] The antioxidant catalase and deferoxamine—an iron chelator—reduce mesothelial cell apoptosis, which is additional support for the role of iron-derived ROS in tumor formation.[90]

The inhibition of normally functioning tumor suppressor genes and/or activation of proto-oncogenes are considered a prerequisite to subsequent tumor promotion, characterized by perpetuation of genetically altered cells and establishment of a tumor. Proto-oncogenes and tumor suppressor genes have been implicated in the development of mesotheliomas, although none have as yet been shown to be essential to tumor formation in humans. p53 is an important transcription factor that regulates the cellular response to DNA damage, and in turn determines whether cells undergo apoptosis or a proliferation blockage, thereby allowing time for DNA repair and cell survival. An important role for p53 in the pathogenesis of mesothelioma is suggested by the finding that heterozygous $p53^{+/-}$ mice have a greater number and earlier onset of asbestos-induced mesotheliomas compared with wild-type mice.[92] Cell-signaling events may be linked to the advent of cell proliferation preceding tumor promotion and establishment. Cell signaling is initiated by asbestos fibers either through the generation of ROS/RNS, or by an interaction of asbestos fiber and growth factor receptors on the cell membrane. Fibers that are highly carcinogenic (erionite, crocidolite) are potent inducers, contrary to a number of other nonpathogenic fibers and particles, of early response proto-oncogene expression such as c-fos and c-jun.[93] How these proto-oncogenes interact with various growth factors is under active investigation.[75] Some growth factor antagonists are presently being assessed in lung cancer treatment clinical trials in the United States and in other countries.

Exposure to asbestos fibers is found to have several effects on immune system. Alterations of these immune parameters may indicate hypersensitivity (increased levels of IgE, increased expression of activation markers CD66b and CD69 on eosinophils) and an elevated inflammatory status (increased levels of interleukins— IL-6, IL-8) in exposed workers.[94]

B. Asbestosis

The inhalation of asbestos is followed by deposition of fibers in the respiratory bronchioles and alveoli with proliferation of type (II cells, desquamation of type I cells, and an influx of alveolar macrophages. The macrophages, which are activated, show an increase in surface membrane receptors for the C3 component of complement and that for IgG. Both the classic and alternate complement pathways are also activated. The macrophages liberate neutrophil chemotactic factor (NCF) for the peripheral polymorphonuclear leukocytes. A number of lysozymes and other substances like fibronectin, platelet-derived growth factors (PDGF), alveolar macrophage-derived growth factor (AMDGF), and interstitium growth factors (IGF) are also produced. The interstitium growth factor-binding proteins (IGFBP) are the major serum binding proteins that modulate fibroblast proliferation. A network of reticulin is formed and is subsequently converted into collagenous fibrosis that lines and later occupies the alveoli. It is the long fiber that are not completely engulfed and transported by macrophages, which are responsible for fibrogenesis rather than short fibers. Fibers shorter than 5 μm are cleared more efficiently by the bronchial route, whereas those longer than 50 μm are not removed by this way. The presence of shorter fibers in areas of fibrosis is due to insufficient clearing from the diseased areas.

There is also an increased prevalence of antinuclear antibodies and rheumatoid factor in patients of asbestosis suggesting the role of immunological reactions in the pathogenesis. Reduction in the proportion and absolute number of circulating T lymphocytes, but not of B-lymphocytes, and impairment of T cell function has also been reported in patients with radiologic evidence of asbestosis.

There is a trend towards an increased frequency of HLA B27 among asbestos workers with radiographic evidence of DIPF. HLA B5 on the other hand, may play a protective role.

Platelet-derived growth factor (PDGF) isoforms and PDGF receptor-alpha are upregulated in fibroproliferative lesions in response to asbestos exposure. PDGF-B overexpression can stimulate increased collagen deposition and vascular smooth muscle hyperplasia following asbestos inhalation and that a limited exposure (8 times) to chrysotile aerosol can produce long-lasting

fibrotic lesions. The 8-week exposure regimen provides an animal model that encompasses an important aspect of human asbestosis, i.e. persistence of fibrosis for long periods after cessation of asbestos exposure.[95]

The fibrosis, whether slight or advanced, is distributed mainly in the proximity of diaphragmatic and posterolateral visceral pleura of both lower lobes, and to a lesser extent of the middle lobe or lingula. In advanced disease, the subpleural zones of the bases of the upper lobes may be involved in addition to the more extensive fibrosis of the lower lobes. The extent of involvement is equal in both lungs. The basal distribution is so characteristic and common that it is said that reversal of this predominantly basal distribution, points to some other lung pathology and not asbestosis. Emphysema may be associated with asbestosis. Hilar nodes are not commonly involved.

Asbestos bodies, intact or fragmented, are usually numerous and often occur in clusters within and adjacent to areas of fibrosis. Asbestos bodies are coated asbestos fibers and are elongated structures, 20 to 50 μm in length and 3 to 5 μm in diameter. They are golden yellow or brown in color and are partly or completely coated with iron-containing protein. The formation of such bodies involves partial digestion of the fiber by alveolar macrophages, accumulation of endogenous iron (ferritin) within the cells and compaction of iron onto the fibers, which appear to be coated with a hyaline layer containing mucopolysaccharides. This coat stains blue with Perl's reagent and is usually segmented giving a 'string of beads' appearance. Both ends are bulbous or swollen. They degenerate ultimately and various stages of disintegration is not usual under the microscope. Uncoated fibers far outnumber the asbestos bodies as seen under electron microscope. The ratio of coated fibers counted by light microscopy, to uncoated fibres counted by electron microscopy ranges from 1:50 to 1:400. Thus, counting of asbestos bodies under the light microscope gives a rough idea of the extent of asbestos exposure. All types of fibers can give rise to asbestos bodies although chrysotile fibers do so rarely because of their rapid clearance. In general, bodies form on fibers longer than 40 μm and rarely on fibers less than 10 μm.

Asbestos bodies can also be detected in sputum, bronchoalveolar lavage fluid and feces. Such bodies in sputum have been found in 57 percent of patients with heavy exposure and in 18 percent in those with mild exposure. One body found in sputum is said to correspond to 1000 bodies/cm^3 of lung. The finding of asbestos bodies in sputum does not prove the presence of asbestos related disease and signifies only previous exposure to asbestos. Similarly, failure to find them does not rule out the presence of asbestosis.

Pseudo-asbestos bodies or *curious bodies* are found in lungs with coal, graphite, and talc pneumoconiosis. Asbestos bodies are commonly found in lung fluids at autopsy in 20 to 48 percent of adults in urban areas with no known exposure to asbestos. Their number, however, is small compared to that in asbestos workers. Similar bodies form on filamentous ceramic aluminium silicate fibers, sheet silicates, and fine glass fibers under experimental conditions. Thus, the term ferruginous bodies are sometimes used for such structures.

Clinical Features

The clinical symptoms and signs are not different from that due to interstitial fibrosis of other causes. The symptoms are of insidious onset. The duration of exposure is variable with few years to many years so that the patient might have forgotten the history of exposure. Progressive dyspnea, cough, and chest pain are usual symptoms.

Clubbing may be present in about a half of the cases. Increasing clubbing and hypertrophies pulmonary osteo-arthropathy indicate onset of malignancy. Crepitations are present in almost all cases, and are important clinical signs in asbestos workers to indicate the development of asbestosis.

Investigations

The examination of sputum for asbestos bodies is of no practical help except they collaborate with other findings.

Bronchoalveolar lavage fluid shows a neutrophilic type of response with increased IgG, IgA, and α-1 antitrypsin. Asbestos fibers, which are similar in length to that in the sputum but shorter than that in the lung tissue, may be recovered in the fluid.

A raised ESR and positive ANA and rheumatoid factor are found in some cases.

Lung function tests in asbestosis have four important applications: *(i)* as an important diagnostic aid; *(ii)* in the evaluation of the progression of the disease; *(iii)* as a monitoring device for healthy asbestos worker; and *(iv)* in epidemiological surveys. Like any other physiological test, lung function test does not confirm the diagnosis of asbestosis, but only indicates the functional abnormality present. A restrictive pattern of ventilatory function is the characteristic disorder found in asbestosis as in any other DIPF. The earliest detectable abnormality is possibly a decrease in compliance. Reduced vital capacity with preserved airflow parameters is the most sensitive and easiest way of following the course of the disease. Other abnormalities include a decreased TLC, RV, and FRC, and diffusing capacity for carbon monoxide.[96] Cumulative doses of asbestos and the presence of radiographic asbestosis are often associated with lower levels of FEV_1 and FVC and a steeper decline during the period of observation. Subjects exposed to asbestos at a younger age had lower levels of FEV_1 and FVC. Current smokers had lower levels and a steeper decline in lung function than never smokers. However some studies have reported no significant interactions between crocidolite exposure and smoking on the levels or rates of change of lung function were found. The deleterious effects of crocidolite exposure on lung function can persist, despite asbestos exposure having ceased more than 30 years ago. No significant inter-actions are found in this population between asbestos and smoking at the first visit or longitudinally according to some authors.[97]

By contrast to silicosis and coal worker's pneumo-coniosis, radiological changes in asbestosis are predo-minant in the lower lung fields. The earliest changes are found in the costophrenic angles. Fine linear opacities, which progresses to reticulo-nodular shadows are common. Honeycombing is an exception rather than a rule. Associated pleural thickening may be seen. Abnormalities reported in a survey in The US Navy Asbestos Medical Surveillance Program included bullae (0.68%), cancer (0.56%), cardiac size/shape abnorma-lities (1.36%), emphysema (0.74%), subpleural fat (2.62%), fractured ribs (1.24%), hilar adenopathy (0.13%), ill-defined diaphragm (0.46%), ill-defined heart border (0.29%), Kerley lines (0.06%), pleural thickening (2.35%), and tuberculosis (0.27%). The rates by age cohort for pleural abnormalities decreased significantly and this suggests that sequential age cohorts in the program are developing fewer pleural abnormalities.[98] Increasing age, blood hemoglobin value and erythrocyte sedimentation rate correlates positively with several HRCT signs. Increasing BMI (Body mass index) is associated with a decrease in several signs, especially parenchymal bands, honeycombing, all kinds of emphysema and bronchiec-tasis. The latter finding might be due to the suboptimal image quality in obese individuals, which may cause suspicious findings to be overlooked. Background data, including patient's age and body constitution, should be considered when CT/HRCT images are interpreted.[99]

Exposure to asbestos is another occupational factor, as is silica exposure that is associated with ANCA positivity. The influence of asbestos appears stronger than that of silica because ANCA positivity is found among subjects who had histories of exposure to asbestos but who did not exhibit typical radiographic signs of asbestosis on their chest X-rays. Additional stimuli may be necessary to induce systemic vasculitis in asbestos-exposed persons.[100]

Treatment

There is no treatment known which can arrest or retard the progress of the disease. Corticosteroids may temporarily be helpful in reducing dyspnea, but practically of no help. The advice to leave the job is not warranted if adequate precautions are taken to prevent further exposure of asbestos and the working environment contains fibers within permissible limits, smoking should be stopped since the combination of smoking and exposure to asbestos increases the risk of lung cancer. Mortality in subjects with asbestosis was inversely related to plasma levels of retinol and Vitamin E concentrations and to their rate of increase during the follow-up. Carotene concentrations at first visit were associated with lower mortality but not during the follow-up period. Chronically low levels of these vitamins are associated with an increased risk of dying with asbestosis. However, their role in the treatment is not clear.[101]

The development of pleural fibrosis follows severe pleural space inflammation, which is typically associated with an exudative pleural effusion. The response of the mesothelial cell to injury and its ability, along with the basement membrane, to maintain its integrity, is vital in determining whether there is normal healing or pleural fibrosis. The formation of a fibrinous intrapleural matrix is critical to the development of pleural fibrosis. This matrix is the result of disordered fibrin turnover, whereby fibrin formation is up regulated and fibrin dissolution is down regulated. Cytokines, such as TGF-beta and TNF-alpha, facilitate the fibrin matrix formation as discussed earlier. A complete understanding of the pathogenesis of pleural fibrosis and why abnormal pleural space remodeling occurs in some and not in others remains unknown. Clinically, significant pleural fibrosis requires involvement of the visceral pleura. Isolated parietal pleural fibrosis, as with asbestos pleural plaques, does not cause restriction or respiratory impairment. The causes of visceral pleural fibrosis include asbestos-associated diffuse pleural thickening, coronary bypass graft surgery, pleural infection (including tuberculous pleurisy), drug-induced pleuritis, rheumatoid pleurisy, uremic pleurisy, and hemothorax. Systemic and intrapleural corticosteroids administered during the initial presentation of rheumatoid pleurisy in

small series may decrease the incidence of pleural fibrosis. Several randomized control trials using corticosteroids in tuberculous pleurisy have not shown efficacy in reducing residual pleural fibrosis. Decortication is effective in treating symptomatic patients regardless of the cause of pleural fibrosis as long as chronicity has been documented and significant underlying parenchymal disease has been excluded.[102] Pleural fibrosis resembles fibrosis in other tissues and can be defined as an excessive deposition of matrix components that results in the destruction of normal pleural tissue architecture and compromised function. Pleural fibrosis may be the consequence of an organized hemorrhagic effusion; tuberculous effusion, empyema or asbestos-related pleurisy and can manifest itself as discrete localized lesions (pleural plaques) or diffuse pleural thickening and fibrosis. Although, the pathogenesis is unknown, it is likely that the complex interactions between resident and inflammatory cells, profibrotic mediators and coagulation, and fibrinolytic pathways are integral to pleural remodeling and fibrosis. It is generally considered that the primary target cell for pleural fibrosis is the subpleural fibroblast. However, increasing evidence suggests that mesothelial cells may also play a significant role in the pathogenesis of this condition, both by initiating inflammatory responses and producing matrix components. A greater understanding of the interactions between pleural and inflammatory cells, cytokines and growth factors, and blood derived proteins is required before adequate therapies can be developed to prevent pleural fibrosis from occurring.[103]

Pulmonary Function Changes and Asbestos Exposure

Exposure to asbestos causes not only cancers and frank asbestosis, but also more subtle changes in the structure and function of the lungs. Thickening of the alveolar-capillary membrane and fibrosis of the interstitium impair oxygen transport and reduce the compliance of the lungs.[104,105] Further, some reports have suggested a positive interaction between smoking and asbestos exposure on the development of interstitial fibrosis.[106,107]

The single-breath carbon monoxide diffusing capacity (D_{LCO}) test is clinically useful in diagnosing pulmonary vascular and interstitial lung diseases and in detecting emphysema. The measurement of D_{LCO} is determined by the diffusing capacity of the alveolar-capillary membrane and the volume of blood in the alveolar capillaries, the former being predominantly affected by diffuse interstitial pulmonary fibrosis (as seen in asbestosis).[105,108] The D_{LCO} measurement is not substantially influenced by airway caliber. It is therefore an easy, noninvasive means of examining the integrity of the lung parenchyma *in vivo* and of monitoring the course of obstructive and restrictive lung diseases. Previous cross-sectional studies have shown that asbestos exposure reduces D_{LCO}.[109,110] A recent study has analyzed the effects of crocidolite (blue asbestos) and tobacco smoking on changes in D_{LCO} over time. The results confirm a continuous deleterious effect of crocidolite on D_{LCO}, especially on people with asbestosis. Smoking was associated with lower D_{LCO} levels, but was not a significant predictor of rate of change in D_{LCO}. Smoking status did not affect the relationships between crocidolite exposures and the level or rate of change of D_{LCO} in this population.[111] The gas diffusion capacity falls by an average of 0.19 to 1.02 units decrement in D_{LCO} per year. The average rate of decline of D_{LCO} in people without asbestosis is about 1.3 percent per year (0.33/24.8), compared with about 2.2 percent per year (0.55/24.8) in people with asbestosis, a rate similar to the rate of decline in a small series of patients with chronic obstructive pulmonary disease (2.7% per year) and a small series of asbestos-exposed workers (2.5% per year).

The presence of a restrictive pattern has been reported in the literature, for asbestosis[67,69,70,112-118] as well as for diffuse pleural thickening in the absence of asbestos-induced parenchymal abnormalities.[119] Many of these reports, however, evaluated small numbers of subjects and failed to measure lung volumes; one large study failed to report FEV_1 in nearly half of the patients analyzed. Workers evaluated in these reports had greater intensity and duration of exposures to asbestos, shorter latencies, were younger, and smoked more than the subjects in this study. Latency in previous reports ranged between 15 years and 35 years. The subjects mean ages in these studies were between 34 years and 62 years, and the frequency of current smokers was 21 to 73 percent. In contrast to these reports, the mean latency in this study was 41.4 ± 10.1 years, the mean age was 65.1 ± 9.9 years, and the frequency of current smokers was 19 percent.

Other investigators[120-128] have also reported an obstructive pulmonary function pattern as the dominant finding in asbestos-related lung disease. The results of these studies, however, have been disputed because of small numbers of subjects evaluated. Furthermore, a standardized definition of obstruction has not been universally applied for each of these investigations. Several factors have fueled the controversy as to whether asbestos-related lung disease causes restriction or airways obstruction.[128-130] These factors include the use of different tests to assess obstruction with different levels of specificity and sensitivity as well as confusion in terminology, failure to measure lung volumes, differences in demographics of subjects, and small numbers of patients evaluated in previous studies.

In a recent analysis it has been shown that airways obstruction is more common than restriction in asbestos-exposed individuals currently undergoing evaluation.[62] Asbestos exposure results in small airways disease. Furthermore, it has been[126-131] demonstrated that mononuclear peribronchiolar inflammation occurs in a sheep model of early asbestosis, a precursor to the peribronchiolar fibrosis of the respiratory bronchioles as seen in humans;[132] they support the hypothesis that asbestos fibers impact on small airway carinae. Fibers are phagocytosed by macrophages initiating an inflammatory response that results initially in bronchitis and subsequently to peribronchial fibrosis. In some cases, this inflammatory response extends to the pulmonary parenchyma to cause interstitial fibrosis (asbestosis). Cigarette smoking-induced chronic bronchitis is in many ways similar to asbestos-induced bronchitis, and in this study the effects of exposure to both cigarette smoke and asbestos acted additively to induce airways obstruction. An animal model[133] demonstrates synergy between cigarette smoke and asbestos exposure in the causation of airway and parenchymal lung disease, possibly through cigarette smoke-induced reduction of mucociliary clearance of asbestos fibers. The synergistic effects of exposure to both cigarettes smoke and asbestos in the induction of lung cancer are well known.

Lung Cancer

Asbestos exposure has been taken as an important risk factor for the development of lung cancer that can develop alone or can be in association with other asbestos-related lung diseases.[63,134] Lung cancer can develop many years after the exposure is over. The question of whether lung cancer can be attributed to asbestos exposure in the absence of asbestosis remains controversial. Recently nine key epidemiological papers are reviewed in a point/counterpoint format, giving the main strengths and limitations of the evidence presented[135] Of the nine papers, two concluded that asbestosis was necessary and seven that it was not. However, the study design, nature and circumstances of exposure and method of analysis of the studies differed considerably, and none was considered definitive. However, because of the relative insensitivity of chest radiography and the uncertain specificity of findings from histological examinations or computed tomography, it is unlikely that epidemiology alone can put either the strict scientific or practical medicolegal questions beyond doubt. It is probable that the issue may depend critically on asbestos fiber type, an aspect not so far addressed. The medicolegal question of whether fibrosis should be required—and, if so, how defined and detected—for attribution of a causal role to asbestos in relation to lung cancer is a matter for debate. This should take into account the strengths and weaknesses of the epidemiological and other medical evidence, and social considerations concerning the level of proof of causation to be required from those developing lung cancer after occupational exposure to asbestos.[136-146] Thus, despite an extensive literature, the relationship between asbestos exposure and lung cancer remains the subject of controversy, related to the fact that most asbestos-associated lung cancers occur in those who are also cigarette smokers: because smoking represents the strongest identifiable lung cancer risk factor among many others, and lung cancer is not uncommon across industrialized societies, analysis of the combined (synergistic) effects of smoking and asbestos on lung cancer risk is a more complex exercise than the relationship between asbestos inhalation and mesothelioma. As a follow-on from previous reviews of prevailing evidence, another recent review critically evaluated more recent studies on this relationship—concentrating on those published between 1997 and 2004—including lung cancer to mesothelioma ratios, the interactive effects of cigarette smoke and asbestos in combination, and the cumulative exposure model for lung cancer induction as set forth in The Helsinki Criteria and The AWARD Criteria (as opposed to the asbestosis—>cancer model), together with discussion of differential genetic susceptibility/resistance factors for lung carcinogenesis by both cigarette smoke and asbestos. The authors concluded that: (i) the prevailing evidence strongly supports the cumulative exposure model; (ii) the criteria for probabilistic attribution of lung cancer to mixed asbestos exposures as a consequence of the production and end-use of asbestos-containing products such as insulation and asbestos-cement building materials—as embodied in The Helsinki and AWARD Criteria—conform to, and are further consolidated by, the new evidence, (iii) different attribution criteria (e.g. greater cumulative exposures) are appropriate for chrysotile mining/milling and perhaps for other chrysotile-only exposures, such as friction products manufacture, than for amphibole-only exposures or mixed asbestos exposures; and (iv) emerging evidence on genetic susceptibility/resistance factors for lung cancer risk as a consequence of cigarette smoking, and potentially also asbestos exposure, suggests that genotypic variation may represent an additional confounding factor potentially affecting the strength of association and hence the probability of causal contribution in the individual subject, but at present there is insufficient evidence to draw any meaningful conclusions concerning variation in asbestos-mediated lung cancer risk relative to such resistance/susceptibility factors.[147]

MALIGNANT MESOTHELIOMA

Malignant mesothelioma of the pleura and peritoneum are rare tumors of the mesothelial tissues and recognized to be associated with asbestos exposure. Although a variety of physical and chemical agents have been implicated in their causation from time to time, aside from therapeutic irradiation, no specific causative factor apart from amphibole asbestos has been established. Chrysotile asbestos is very rarely associated with malignant mesothelioma. The diagnosis and management of malignant pleural mesothelioma are major challenges that often frustrate both patient and clinician alike. Occupational asbestos exposure to crocidolite or amosite forms of the fiber is the most important known risk factors. Other mineral fibers such as erionite, a naturally occurring fibrous zeolite crystal, are associated with mesothelioma in volcanic tuffs of the Cappadocia region of central Anatolia in Turkey. In addition, other possible factors such as the presence of simian virus 40 and genetic susceptibility have been associated recently with the development of mesothelioma in animal models. These latter findings are increasing the understanding of this disease. In addition, the discovery of elevated levels of various markers such as folic acid receptor-α, cyclooxygenase 2, and multidrug resistance proteins 1 and 2 in mesothelioma tissue have opened up new areas of potential diagnostic and therapeutic importance.[148]

Wagner et al[149] initially reported 33 cases of mesothelioma in a South African asbestos mining community in 1960. Since then, data have been collected through various databases in the United States, Western Europe, some Eastern European countries, and the United Kingdom. Mesothelioma is usually diagnosed in the fifth to seventh decades of life, with a strong male predominance where occupational exposure to asbestos is involved.[150] There are approximately 2,500 new cases of mesothelioma annually in the United States, of which 2,000 are in men and 500 are in women.[150,151] The incidence in the United States appears to be rising, mainly in men aged ≤ 75 years, with the maximum lifetime risk in the from 1925 to 1929 birth cohort of men.[150] The incidence in women and in men < 75 years of age appears to have been stable since 1983.[150] This coincides with restrictions and regulations of the US Occupational Safety and Health Administration and the Environmental Protection Agency, enacted in the 1970s, regarding uses and permissible exposure limits for asbestos in the workplace.[150] The incidence of mesothelioma is also rising in Europe, from 5,000 men dying in 1998 to a projected 9,000 men dying by 2018, with the highest incidence in the from 1945 to 1950 birth cohort of men.[152]

ETIOPATHOGENESIS

I. Asbestos

Mesothelioma is usually, but not always, related to the cumulative dose, to the specific mineral form of asbestos fiber, and to the elapsed time from first exposure. The incidence of this tumor has been increasing for many years, roughly parallel with the increase in the use of asbestos, but with a lag time of 25 to 40 years. The incidence among female subjects is 2 per million per year, but between 10 per million per year and 30 per million per year in unselected male populations. Among heavily exposed workers, the mesothelioma rate is as high as 366/100,000 person-years, whereas the rate in low-to-moderately exposed workers is almost 80 percent less (67/100,000 person-years). Whether a minimal threshold exists below which exposures are harmless is uncertain. Exposure to amphibole fibers is much more likely to produce a mesothelioma than chrysotile fibers. Mesotheliomas following exposure thought to be limited to chrysotile have been attributed to tremolite contamination. The greater carcinogenicity of the amphiboles may be due in part to their greater biopersistence and their iron content, which can catalyze the production of reactive oxygen radicals (H_2O_2 and OH^-).

Although significant past asbestos exposure can be identified in many if not most cases of mesothelioma, the tumor also occurs in the absence of known exposure. Mesothelioma has been reported in patients following radiation therapy, chronic pleural inflammation, and chemical carcinogens. From 10 to 20 percent of all mesotheliomas are primary in the peritoneum. It occurs rarely in unusual locations, such as the pericardium, tunica vaginalis testis, and female genital tract. Familial malignant mesotheliomas have been described.

These observations have prompted investigators to seek causes, other than asbestos, such as a genetic component or viral exposure (see below).

Exposure to asbestos, a family of naturally occurring silicate minerals, is the main risk factor for the development of MPM. The association between asbestos exposure and cancer was first established in a case-control study of lung cancer patients in 1955.[153] Several varieties of asbestos fibers occur naturally; those that are narrow and needlelike (amphiboles such as crocidolite and amosite) appear to be more carcinogenic and mutagenic in animal models and tissue culture than those that are curled and more pliable (chrysotile). In addition, asbestos fibers are commonly seen in excised surgical specimens from patients with MPM. Similar to coal dust in coalminers, asbestos fibers are trapped in distal parts of the lung and concentrate to form black spots in the parietal pleura, the main anatomic site of mesothelioma in the chest.[154] The latency period between initial exposure and death has been reported up to 72 years (mean, 48.7 years; range, 14-72 years), with wide variability linked to the type of fibers and intensity of exposure.[155]

The attack rate among occupationally exposed individuals, in general, is less than 7 percent. The excess risk of malignant mesothelioma varies according to the type of industrial exposure. Thus, while the insulation workers have a 7 to 9 percent chance of developing malignant mesothelioma, asbestos-using factory workers have a chance of 1 to 7 percent, and miners and milling workers have a chance of 0 to 0.2 percent. The general population has a chance of malignant mesothelioma of 0.001 percent.

Animal experiments have shown that the tumor appears to develop in response to the long-term presence of fibrous foreign bodies in proximity to mesothelial surfaces. Length and breadth of the fiber is critical in the development of the tumor. As mentioned, amphibole asbestos is responsible most, if not all, cases of malignant mesothelioma. These fibers are retained in the lungs for a long time, and possibly lifelong. The fibers are phagocytized by the macrophages. The macrophages release oxygen radicals and growth substances, which affect adjacent cells and tissues. Exposure of this type results in DNA damage, which at times is associated with either karyotypic alterations or minor mutational changes. The occurrence of mutation and production of growth factors in localized areas of the pleura, lead on to a series of events. The damaged cells are stimulated to proliferate. When this process goes on for a long time, malignant transformation could occur in the mesothelial progenitor cells in the lining layers of the pleura and peritoneum. These observations correlate well with those from epidemiological studies. Amphibole asbestos types are retained in the lungs indefinitely and tend to accumulate adjacent to the lungs and pleura. In contrast, chrysotile fibers break down, deteriorate or dissolve further and are eliminated by the lymphatics.

II. Virus

Although approximately 80 percent of patients with MPM have a history of asbestos exposure, only approximately 10 percent of those with asbestos exposure acquire mesothelioma[156,157] suggesting that other factors may be important either independently or as cofactors in the development of this malignancy. Human mesothelioma cells are highly susceptible to infection by simian virus (SV)-40 *in vitro* and in animal models and often express virus sequences.[158,159] Furthermore, studies have demonstrated that SV-40 is a poor prognostic factor in MPM.[160] Some research has shown that asbestos and SV-40 can function as co-carcinogens, since the presence of asbestos fibers leads to an increase in the number of transformation foci that develop with SV-40 in tissue culture. Prior to 1963, simian virus-40 (SV-40) was an unrecognized contaminant of polio vaccine, and therefore it is present in a substantial number of adults.[161] SV-40 large T-cell antigen (Tag) DNA sequences have been found in as many as 20 percent of patients with mesothelioma without known asbestos exposure and in nearly 50 percent of patients with definite exposure.[161-163] The same DNA sequences have also been found in patients with colon cancer, osteosarcoma, brain tumors, and other cancers.[164] Furthermore, mechanistic studies reveal that human mesothelial cells are uniquely susceptible to SV-40–associated infection, transformation, and immortality.[159,165] Mesothelial transformation by SV-40 is in part due to the capacity of SV-40 Tag to inactivate the tumor suppressor proteins, p53, and p-retinoblastoma family members.[161,166] However, the causal role of SV-40 in the pathogenesis of mesothelioma is controversial. The molecular basis of asbestos-mediated disease is under active investigation to determine the interaction between fiber physical characteristics, free radicals, alteration in proto-oncogene/tumor suppressor genes, and SV-40 expression with the formation of a malignant clone of cells. Understanding these interactions may also provide insight into pulmonary fibrosis, bronchogenic lung cancer and other pulmonary diseases.

III. Genetic

Chromosomal abnormalities such as deletions of chromosome regions 1p, 3p, 9p, and 6q, as well as loss of chromosome 22, are commonly found in MPM. These recurrent genomic losses are consistent with the loss of both defined and putative tumor suppressor genes important in the development of MPM, including the *CDKN2A* locus in chromosomal location 9p21 containing p16 and p14[ARF], and neurofibromatosis 2 in chromosome 22.[167,168]

Genetic susceptibility may also contribute to the etiology of malignant mesothelioma. Two small villages in the central Anatolia region of Turkey share a rare environmental pathogen for malignant mesothelioma (erionite exposure). While 50 percent of the men in one village died of malignant mesothelioma, only one case of malignant mesothelioma was reported in the other village, and that case occurred in a woman who was originally from the former village.[169] Six families have been identified with an obvious familial clustering of malignant mesothelioma, and these could be linked to one large six-generation pedigree, suggesting a founder effect and an autosomal dominant pattern of inheritance with incomplete penetrance.

Malignant pleural mesothelioma (MPM) results from neoplastic transformation of mesothelial cells. Past asbestos exposure represents the major risk factor for MPM, as the link between asbestos fibers and MPM has been largely proved by epidemiological and experimental studies. Asbestos fibers induce DNA and chromosome damage linked to oxidative stress following phagocytosis. Recently, simian virus 40 (SV40) has been implicated in the etiology of MPM. The origin of human infection has been associated with SV40-contaminated polio vaccines, although to date, no epidemiological data supports this hypothesis. SV40 may act as a coactivator of asbestos in mesothelial oncogenesis. The transforming potency of SV40 results from the activity of two viral proteins, large T and small t antigens. SV40 infection stimulates production of growth factors elsewhere implicated in autocrine growth of mesothelioma cells and inactivates RASSF1, a gene silenced in MPM. Roles for ionizing radiation, chemicals or genetic factors have also been suggested from the observation of sporadic MPM cases or animal studies. Genetic alterations in the tumor suppressor genes, P16/CDKN2A and neurofibromatosis 2 (NF2), are found both in human MPM and in asbestos-exposed NF2-deficient mice. MPM is still of great international concern. Despite a ban on asbestos use in Western countries, the incidence of MPM is increasing, due to the long delay between asbestos exposure and diagnosis. Moreover, asbestos is still used in developing countries. The implication of other risk factors, especially SV40, supports a need for further research into MPM.[170]

Apoptosis, regulated physiologic cell death, is crucial for organ development and host defense.[171,172] All forms of asbestos can induce DNA damage, which is a potent stimulus for apoptosis. ROS derived from asbestos fibers induce DNA damage and apoptosis in relevant lung target cells including mesothelial cells.[173,174] There are multiple additional sources of ROS once cells are exposed to apotogenic stimuli 9181). The antioxidant catalase and deferoxamine—an iron chelator—reduce mesothelial cell apoptosis, which is additional support for the role of iron-derived ROS in tumor formation.[175]

The inhibition of normally functioning tumor suppressor genes and/or activation of proto-oncogenes are considered a prerequisite to subsequent tumor promotion, characterized by perpetuation of genetically altered cells and establishment of a tumor. Proto-oncogenes and tumor suppressor genes have been implicated in the development of mesotheliomas, although none have as yet been shown to be essential to tumor formation in humans. p53 is an important transcription factor that regulates the cellular response to DNA damage, and in turn determines whether cells undergo apoptosis or a proliferation blockage, thereby allowing time for DNA repair and cell survival. An important role for p53 in the pathogenesis of mesothelioma is suggested by the finding that heterozygous p53$^{+/-}$ mice have a greater number and earlier onset of asbestos-induced mesotheliomas compared with wild-type mice.[176] Cell-signaling events may be linked to the advent of cell proliferation preceding tumor promotion and establishment. Cell signaling is initiated by asbestos fibers either through the generation of ROS/RNS, or by an interaction of asbestos fiber and growth factor receptors on the cell membrane. Fibers that are highly carcinogenic (erionite, crocidolite) are potent inducers, contrary to a number of other nonpathogenic fibers and particles, of early response proto-oncogene expression such as c-fos and c-jun.[177] How these proto-oncogenes interact with various growth factors is under active investigation. Some growth factor antagonists are presently being assessed in lung cancer treatment clinical trials in the United States and in other countries.

PATHOLOGY

Pathologically the tumor is ivory-white, gray, or yellow. The cut surface is gelatinous due to the production of hyaluronic acid. Hemorrhage, necrosis, cavity and fibrosis are possible in the tumor. The tumor may be confused with adenoma of the adjacent lung periphery, or secondaries from other organs. Malignant mesothelioma spreads to the local lymph nodes more commonly. Distant metastasis however, is rare. Microscopically mesothelial tumors are pleomorphic and there is considerable variation between tumor to tumor, and in different areas of the same tumor. Both the epithelial and mesenchymal elements are present. At one end of the spectrum the tumor resembles adenocarcinoma, while at the other end of the spectrum, fibrosarcoma. Electron microscopic studies demonstrate both typical and atypical epithelial and mesenchymal cells with many transitional cells.

Mesothelioma is classified into three types: *epithelial, sarcomatoid,* and *mixed.* The epithelial type (50% of cases) can be further subdivided into subtypes such as tubular, papillary, giant/large cell, small cell, myxoid, and others that reflect morphologic similarities to carcinomas of other origins. The sarcomatoid type (15% of cases) is characterized pathologically by spindle-shaped cells similar to those seen in fibrosarcomas, and clinically by a poorer prognosis compared with epithelial or mixed pathological types. The mixed type contains elements of both the sarcomatoid and epithelial types.[178,179] Tubulopapillary type of mesothelioma is the commonest type and in some cases is very difficult to distinguish from primary or secondary adenocarcinoma of the lungs.

Immunohistochemical assays developed for specific antigens are often helpful in differentiating mesothelioma from metastatic adenocarcinoma of various origins. Such antigens include carcinoembryonic antigen, CD15 (Leu-M1), and epithelial membrane antigen.[180] Carcinoembryonic antigen and CD15 are typically absent in MPM. MPM stains for epithelial membrane antigen with a distinctive membrane-associated staining pattern, contrary to the cytoplasmic pattern seen in adenocarcinomas.[180] Staining for cytokeratin 5, cytokeratin 6, and calretinin are also relatively specific for MPM.[181,182] Electron microscopy remains the "gold standard" and should be used for difficult cases where morphologic assessment by immunostaining is equivocal. Mesothelioma can usually be distinguished from adenocarcinoma by the presence of long and branching microvilli as well as the relatively higher quantity of tonofilaments and desmosomes found in the former.[183] The most valuable asset to the diagnosis of mesothelioma is an experienced pathologist who sees a relatively high volume of this disease.

Clinical Features

Patients with malignant pleural mesothelioma are usually aged between 50 to 80 years of age with a median of 60. They present with dyspnea, nonpleuritic chest pain, or both. The men are affected more than the females (2.5:1), possibly due to occupational exposure being more often in the former. Weight loss, malaise, and lassitude are rarely early symptoms. Because of gradual onset of symptoms the patient usually seeks medical advice about 3 to 4 months after experiencing them.[184-186]

The initial clinical presentations of patients with mesothelioma are usually chest pain and dyspnea.[187] Less often the first symptoms are nonspecific complaints such as malaise, weight loss, cough, and fever. Most patients will be male and 50 to 70 years of age given the latent interval previously noted.[188] The symptom onset is usually insidious but relentlessly progressive, although it may take the rare patient 1 year before a diagnosis can be established.[189,190]

Clubbing is a very unusual feature in malignant mesothelioma. When first seen most will have a large, freely mobile, unilateral pleural effusion. Physical examination and chest radiograph findings consistent with a pleural effusion are found in 80 to 95 percent of patients.[191] Ten to 29 percent of patients have little or no fluid, and fluid accumulation diminishes with advanced disease.[188] On a standard radiograph, the fluid may appear to be free flowing and indistinguishable from an effusion due to heart failure or other nonmalignant diseases, but it eventually becomes loculated. Tumor masses often create a lobular appearance along the margins of the fluid. The tumor may "anchor" the mediastinum so that it fails to shift away from the fluid toward the opposite hemithorax. The CT scan provides much greater sensitivity than the usual posteroanterior chest radiograph for identifying fluid and visualizing pleural-based masses, lymph nodes, blood vessels, and lung parenchyma that may be obscured by the fluid. MRI may be useful for distinguishing between chest wall, pleural, and peripheral parenchymal lesions.[192] Positron emission tomography scanning can be helpful for differentiating benign from malignant effusions, and identifying nodal or other metastases that are not otherwise apparent. Distant metastases are infrequent. The tumor gradually fills the hemithorax compressing the lung and airways.

Biopsy

Patients presenting with a clinical picture consistent with MPM require further investigation to establish a pathologic diagnosis and the stage of disease. It is mandatory that pleural fluid—and in most cases some pleural tissue—be removed to establish a diagnosis. The diagnostic yield from cytology varies from 25 to 33 percent of patients. Thoracentesis is often the initial diagnostic intervention. Cytologic diagnosis of MPM from pleural fluid is, however, unreliable since reactive mesothelial cells and cells from other malignant tumors such as sarcomas and adenocarcinomas are often very difficult to distinguish from malignant mesothelial cells. This is increased modestly with the addition of closed-needle pleural biopsy with 21 to 77 percent positive results.[189,192,194] Exploration of the pleural space with a rigid medical thoracoscope is diagnostic in up to 90 percent of patients with a pleural effusion.[195] Video-assisted thoracoscopic surgery is supplanting other diagnostic procedures because it provides both a high diagnostic yield and partial staging of the tumor.[189,194] As a result, histologic assessment is preferred, with samples obtained either as a CT-guided pleural biopsy or by biopsy under direct vision via thoracoscopy. CT-guided biopsy has a yield of 60 percent with a single attempt and up to 85 percent with repeat biopsies. Thoracoscopic biopsy using video-assisted thoracoscopy has a yield of > 90 percent and carries a relatively low risk of complications (10%), including persistent air leak, hemorrhage, and infection. Seeding of the tumor biopsy tract occurs in up to 40 percent of cases but may be prevented by prophylactic local radiation to the site. Open thoracotomy is the last resort for obtaining adequate tissue for pathologic diagnosis. Tumor tissue extends through the needle tract or thoracoscopy site in approximately 20 percent of patients,[189] but radiation, either prior to the biopsy or subsequently, provides good local control.

Immunohistochemical staining of the biopsy tissue is often necessary for definitive identification because of the visual similarities between adenocarcinoma and mesothelioma. Malignant mesothelioma is characterized by staining for calretinin (88%) and vimentin (58%), while adenocarcinomas typically lack these markers and are positive for carcinoembryonic antigen (84%), CD15 (77%), and Ber-EP4 (82%).[196] Electron microscopic examination of tissue is most useful for making the distinction and also for determining the tumor subtype. There are three histologic types of mesothelioma; their distribution among 819 cases was as follows: epithelioid, 50 percent; sarcomatous or mesenchymal, 16 percent; and mixed, 34 percent.[188] The epithelioid subtype has the best prognosis,[189] Most (60%) present with right sided lesions and fewer than 5 percent only show bilateral pleural effusion. Rarely, the patient is asymptomatic, and the disease is recognized on chest X-ray for some other reason. Pleural plaques or interstitial fibrosis are present radiologically in only about 20 percent of the cases. Shifting of the mediastinum to the opposite side is infrequent unless pleural effusion is acute and massive. Calcification and loss of lung volumes can be detected more frequently with CT scans. Pleurodesis is unsuccessful. Pneumothorax is quite common although small. As the tumor grows and obliterates the pleural space, fluid becomes loculated or ultimately disappears. At this stage, dyspnea is disproportional to the X-ray findings. Hypoxia usually results from shunting of blood through a poorly ventilated lung.

The disease is locally invasive. Painful masses develop at sites of needle punctures for thoracentesis, chest tube drainage, or thoracotomy in about 10 percent of cases. Direct extension to the ribs, esophagus, vertebra, nerves, and superior vena cava cause pain, dysphagia, cord complexion, brachial plexus involvement, Horner's syndrome, or superior vena caval obstruction respectively. Fever, weight loss, anorexia, and poor performance status are common. Clotting abnormalities including disseminated intravascular coagulation (DIG), thrombosis in the extremities, thrombophlebitis, pulmonary embolism, and Coombs positive hemolytic anemia have been described in up to 20 percent of the cases of peritoneal mesothelioma. Patients usually die of respiratory failure and have a median survival of 6 to 18 months with a range of few weeks to years. Inanition and small bowel obstruction from direct extension through the diaphragm occur in about a third of the cases. Pericardial and myocardial infiltration occur in a few cases. Older age, poor performance status (more than 1), mesenchymal histology, and chest pain at diagnosis are poor prognostic indicators. Pleuropneumonectomy and use of chemotherapy are associated with a significantly longer survival. Five separate staging systems for mesothelioma are described in a recent book.[197] The newer schemes include some clinical features in addition to the anatomic site and extent of the tumor. Favorable factors in one study were as follows: no more than 5 percent body weight loss at the time of diagnosis; tumor confined to the parietal pleura, epithelioid cell type, and tumor confined to the ipsilateral pleura, lung, and pericardium.[194] A favorable outlook has been noted among patients with good performance status, young age, and a platelet count < 400,000/µL.[182,189] Median survival time from symptom onset is approximately 1 year, depending on the initial stage and various other prognostic factors. Shortness of breath and chest pain become progressively worse often followed by weight loss, anorexia, and night sweats. Local invasion of the chest wall and surrounding structures can cause increasing pain as well as functional abnormalities including dysphagia, superior vena cava syndrome, Horner syndrome, vocal cord paralysis, and diaphragmatic paralysis. Death is rarely a result of metastatic disease; it is usually due to infection or respiratory failure along with constitutional symptoms associated with progressive malignancy.

Stage of disease is but one of the known variables that may influence survival. Two prognostic scoring systems have been developed for MPM on the basis of data collected from patients entered into large cooperative group trials.[198,199] The Cancer and Leukemia Group B (CALGB) examined the individual and combined effects of a number of pretreatment clinical characteristics on survival of patients with MPM[198] including poor Eastern Cooperative Oncology Group performance status, chest pain, dyspnea, platelet count > 400,000/µL, weight loss, serum lactate dehydrogenase level > 500 IU/L, pleural involvement, low hemoglobin level, high WBC count, and age > 75 years. Multivariate Cox analysis of these variables demonstrated that pleural involvement, lactate dehydrogenase > 500 IU/L, poor performance status, chest pain, platelet count > 400,000/µL, nonepithelial histology, and age > 75 years were independent predictors of reduced survival time. Performance status (0 vs 1, 2) produced the most significant prognostic split in the resulting regression tree. Six distinct prognostic subgroups were subsequently defined using this tree, with survival times ranging from 1.4 to 13.9 months. The best survival time was in patients < 49 years old, with a performance status of 0 and hemoglobin 10 g/dL. The worst survival time was in patients with a performance status of 1 or 2 and a WBC 10,000 µL. In a similar study undertaken by the European Organization for Research and Treatment of Cancer (EORTC), 13 factors were entered into a COX proportional hazards regression model. Poor prognosis was independently associated with poor performance status, a high WBC, a probable/possible histologic diagnosis of mesothelioma, male gender, and sarcomatoid histologic type.[199] Using these factors, the EORTC group then classified patients into two prognostic groups: a good prognosis group (1 year survival of 40%) having two or fewer poor prognostic factors, and a poor prognosis group (1 year survival of 12%) having three or more poor prognostic factors. A subsequent retrospective analysis of an independent cohort of patients confirmed the prognostic value of both the CALGB and EORTC scoring systems.[200]

Certain biological markers have been reported to be elevated in mesothelioma compared with normal mesothelium, including overexpression of the α-folate receptor.[201] cyclooxygenase-2 (COX-2),[202] and the multidrug resistance proteins 1 and 2.[203] Of these, COX-2 has been correlated with other prognostic factors and contributed significantly to both the EORTC and CALGB prognostic scoring systems. These developments are particularly interesting, as these molecules may represent important targets for future therapies.

Staging

A number of staging systems (at least 5 staging systems) have been published for malignant mesothelioma. However, none of them produces a predictable survival of statistical significance. Several staging systems for

MPM have been proposed, and none have been accepted universally. The oldest staging system, introduced by Butchart et al[204] has largely been abandoned due to a lack of prognostic value, in favor of TNM-based systems.[205] Sugarbaker proposed a classification based on a multi-modality approach including extrapleural pneumonectomy.[206] Most of these earlier staging systems do not use the T, N and M descriptors as used in the classical TNM-classifications of all tumors. For this reason, recently, the International Mesothelioma Interest Group (IMIG) proposed a TNM-based staging system based on an analysis of information about the impact of tumor and node status on survival, shown in Table 27.3.[211] CT scan or MRI is necessary for accurate clinical staging. However, using the IMIG system, surgical staging has been shown to be superior to clinical staging where feasible.[207] 18F-fluorodeoxyglucose based PET scans are helpful in identifying the extent of disease.[208]

The recently proposed International Mesothelioma Interest Group (IMIG) classification is shown in Table 27.4.[205]

Treatment

Treatment of MPM with more than palliative intent remains inadequate at all stages of presentation.[209] Generally, surgery as a single modality has failed to improve survival, and several investigators[210,211] have explored the use of combined modality therapy incorporating radiation and chemotherapy in conjunction with surgery. In advanced disease, chemotherapy remains the main therapeutic modality, although either surgical intervention or local radiation therapy may be useful for the local control of pain or symptoms often associated with pleural fluid accumulation.[212,213] Chemotherapy has generally failed to significantly impact survival.[209] This has been due both to the lack of control subjects in most studies and the lack of statistical power in those randomized trials that have been done. However, recently presented data from a large, well-powered phase III trial[214] comparing the combination of pemetrexed and cisplatin with cisplatin alone are encouraging, and may represent a standard chemotherapeutic regimen against which future treatments can be measured.

Surgery

Three procedures are used in the surgical management of MPM: thoracoscopy with pleurodesis, pleurectomy/decortication (P/D), and extrapleural pneumonectomy (EPP). EPP is the most aggressive procedure. It involves

TABLE 27.3: Previous staging system of malignant mesothelioma

Butchart et al[204]
Ipsilateral pleura, lung, pericardium, diaphragm
Invasion of chest wall or mediastinum (esophagus, heart, opposite pleura, or + lymph node within the chest).
Extension through diaphragm to peritoneum or involvement of opposite pleura, or + lymph node outside the chest.
Distant blood borne metastasis

Dimitrov and McMohan classification
I Ipsilateral pleura ± effusion
  a. Longest diameter < 5 cm
  b. Longest diameter > 5 cm
II Ipsilateral pleura + endothoracic fascia/lung
III Ipsilateral pleura, endothoracic fascia, chest wall, lung, or pericardium
IV Hilar or mediastinal lymph nodes, opposite pleura, or extrathoracic sites

Mattson
I Ipsilateral pleura and lung
II Chest wall, mediastinum or pericardium, contralateral lung or pleura
III Extrathoracic extension
  a. Nodes outside chest
  b. Through diaphragm to peritoneum
IV Distant metastases

Staging system by Sugarbaker[206]

Stage Description
I Disease confined to within capsule of the parietal pleura; ipsilateral pleura, lung, pericardium, diaphragm, or chest wall disease limited to previous biopsy sites
II All of stage I with positive intrathoracic (N_1 or N_2 lymph nodes
III Local extension of disease into chest wall or mediastinum; heart or through diaphragm, peritoneum with or without extrathoracic or contralateral (N_3) lymph node involvement
IV Distant metastatic disease

Chahinian et al

I	TI	NO	MO
II	TI-2	NI	MO
	T2	NO	MO
III	T3	NO-3	MO
IV	T4	NO-3	M1

T-primary tumor; TI-ipsilateral pleura only; T2-superficial (diaphragm, thoracic fascia, ipsilateral lung, fissures); T3-deep local (chest wall beyond endothoracic fascia); T4-extensive direct (opposite pleura, peritoneum, retroperitoneum); N-lymph nodes; NO-no lymph nodes; NI-ipsilateral hilar nodes; N2-mediastinal nodes; N3-contralateral hilar nodes; M-metastases; MO-no metastasis; Mi-blood borne or lymphatic metastasis.

TABLE 27.4: New International TNM Staging System for Diffuse MPM according to the IMIG*

T1	
T1a	Tumor limited to the ipsilateral parietal pleura, including mediastinal and diaphragmatic pleura No involvement of the visceral pleura
T1b	Tumor involving the ipsilateral parietal pleura, including mediastinal and diaphragmatic pleura; scattered foci of tumor also involving the visceral pleura
T2	Tumor involving each of the ipsilateral pleural surfaces (parietal, mediastinal, diaphragmatic, and visceral pleura) with at least one of the following features: • Involvement of diaphragmatic muscle • Confluent visceral pleural tumor (including the fissures) or extension of tumor from visceral pleura in the underlying pulmonary parenchyma
T3	Describes locally advanced but potentially resectable tumor Tumor involving all of the ipsilateral pleural surfaces (parietal, mediastinal, diaphragmatic, and visceral pleura) with at least one of the following features: • Involvement of the endothoracic fascia • Extension into the mediastinal fat • Solitary, completely resectable focus of tumor extending into the soft tissues of the chest wall • Nontransmural involvement of the pericardium
T4	Describes locally advanced technically unresectable tumor Tumor involving all of the ipsilateral pleural surfaces (parietal, mediastinal, diaphragmatic, and visceral) with at least one of the following features: • Diffuse extension or multifocal masses of tumor in the chest wall, with or without associated rib destruction • Direct transdiaphragmatic extension of tumor to the peritoneum • Direct extension of tumor to the contralateral pleura • Direct extension of tumor to one or more mediastinal organs • Direct extension of tumor into the spine • Tumor extending through to the internal surface of the pericardium with or without a pericardial effusion, or tumor involving the myocardium.
N, lymph nodes	
NX	Regional lymph nodes cannot be assessed
N0	No regional lymph node metastases
N1	Metastases in the ipsilateral bronchopulmonary or hilar lymph nodes
N2	Metastases in the subcarinal or the ipsilateral mediastinal lymph nodes, including the ipsilateral internal mammary nodes
N3	Metastases in the contralateral mediastinal, contralateral internal mammary, ipsilateral, or contralateral supraclavicular lymph nodes
M, metastases	
MX	Presence of distant metastases cannot be assessed
M0	No distant metastasis
M1	Distant metastasis present
Stage I	
Ia	T1aN0M0
Ib	T1bN0M0
Stage II	T2N0M0
Stage III	Any T3M0
	Any N1M0
	Any N2M0
Stage IV	Any T4
	Any N3
	Any M1

the *en bloc* resection of the visceral and parietal pleura, lung, pericardium, and ipsilateral diaphragm.[215] Patient selection for EPP is critical, as is the experience of the surgeon and institution at which the procedure is performed. Early series showed a prohibitively high mortality rate.[216] However, more recently, the 30 day postoperative mortality and morbidity in a center with extensive experience with the procedure are 3.8 percent and 50 percent, respectively.[210]

Thoracoscopy is useful not only in obtaining tissue for a diagnosis but also for pleurodesis to palliatively treat recurrent or symptomatic pleural effusions. Several sclerosing agents can be used (i..e. bleomycin, tetracycline, and talc) with no significant differences in efficacy.[213,217] Talc is generally the least expensive and can be administered via a thoracoscope or instilled as slurry through a chest tube.[218]

Radiation

To encompass all known disease and areas at high risk, radiation therapy usually requires a prohibitively large field, as the entire pleural surface is at risk. In addition to the lung parenchyma itself, other thoracic structures can be dose limiting, further complicating treatment planning. Retrospective reviews[209] have shown no suggestion of a clear survival benefit for extensive radiation therapy. A report from the Joint Center for Radiation therapy in Boston suggests a minimum effective dose of 40 Gy in order to achieve palliation.[212] In the post-EPP setting, higher doses of radiation therapy can be delivered safely and are associated with a very low risk of local recurrence, with distant metastasis being the most common form of relapse.[211] In a study by Boutin et al[219] dosing to small fields was found to be highly effective at decreasing malignant seeding along biopsy tracts.[219] Radiation therapy, therefore, seems to have a role in disease palliation but has no real impact on survival.

Chemotherapy

Most single agents have been tested in MPM.[220] In general, single-agent response rates are < 20 percent, and survival benefit for single-agent chemotherapy has not been suggested in single cohort studies. In the past, doxorubicin was regarded as the standard for single-agent chemotherapy for malignant mesothelioma. However, this anthracycline and other anthracycline analogues and formulations, including epirubicin and liposomal doxorubicin, have achieved response rates of < 20 percent as single agents. Platinum analogues have been extensively studied in MPM both as single agents and in combined regimens. Cisplatin demonstrated an overall response rate of 14 percent and 36 percent when administered at a dose of 100 mg/m² every 21 days and 80 mg/m² weekly, respectively. Carboplatin, a better tolerated and easier-to-deliver analog of cisplatin, demonstrated response rates similar to cisplatin when used with a conventional dosing regimen (7-16%). Taxanes, such as paclitaxel and docetaxel, also have very low response rates and therefore do not appear to be effective as single-agent treatments of MPM. Vinorelbine is unique among the vinca alkaloids for its single-agent activity in MPM. Weekly vinorelbine treatment at standard doses had a partial response rate of 24 percent and an improvement in overall quality of life in 41 percent of patients examined in a single cohort phase II study. Gemcitabine appears to have limited activity as a single agent in MPM based on a single phase II study showing a response rate of only 7 percent among 27 patients. Antifolates have demonstrated single-agent activity in MPM; such activity may be related to the overexpression of the α-folate receptor gene in up to 72 percent of MPM tumors. High-dose methotrexate demonstrated a response rate of 37 percent in a phase II trial; this result requires confirmation in a randomized, controlled clinical trial. CALGB demonstrated a response rate of 25 percent for edatrexate but with a considerable degree of toxicity. A single-agent phase II trial of raltitrexed has been completed but not yet reported. Raltitrexed is also currently being evaluated in combination with oxaliplatin and cisplatin in two separate randomized trials. Pemetrexed is a novel multitargeted antifolate that has been studied as a single agent in a phase II study and in a combination regimen with cisplatin compared to cisplatin alone in a phase III trial.

Combination chemotherapy regimens have been extensively evaluated in MPM[220] and some of them are shown in Table 27.5. The majority of these regimens are anthracycline based, platinum based, or both. With few exceptions, however, response rates are 20 percent, and median survival remains largely unaffected in the range of 6 to 12 months.

Reports of activity with other agents in combination have been highly variable. Response rates as high as 48 percent have been reported with the combination of gemcitabine and cisplatin; however, a trial of similar design but slightly higher planned dose intensity of gemcitabine failed to duplicate this result, demonstrating

TABLE 27.5: Combination chemotherapy studies for mesothelioma[226]

Drugs	No. of patients	Response rate %,	Median survival, mo
Anthracycline-based combinations			
Doxorubincin plus cyclophosfamide	36	11	8
Doxorubicin plus cisplatin	59	19	8.8, 10
Doxurubicin plus cisplatin plus mitomycin C	24	21	11
Epirubicin plus interleukin-2	21	5	NA
Platinum-based combinations			
Cisplatin plus irinotecan	15	27	7
Cisplatin plus vinblastine	20	25	5-19
Cisplatin plus mitomycin C	35	26	7.7
Cisplatin plus mitomycin C plus Etoposide plus fluorouracil	45	38	16
Cisplatin (weekly) plus etoposide	25	24	9.5
Cisplatin plus gemcitabine (every 4)	21	48	10
Cisplatin plus gemcitabine (every 3)	32	15	10
Cisplatin plus pemetrexed	456	41	12.1
Carboplatin plus pemetrexed	27	32	14.8

NA = not available. The median survival time varies for responders vs nonresponders; no median survival time for the whole group is available a response rate of only 16 percent.[221] Oxaliplatin, a platinum analog available throughout Europe since 1999 and recently approved by the US Food and Drug Administration for the treatment of advanced colon cancer, has been studied in several regimens, including combination with gemcitabine. Schuette et al[222] reported a response rate of 40 percent with this promising combination. Its toxicity profile is reported as favorable, and responses were noted in patients previously identified as platinum refractory. By contrast, preliminary data in 26 patients receiving the combination of vinorelbine and oxaliplatin yielded a response rate of only 23 percent, a result nearly identical to that mentioned above for single-agent vinorelbine.[223] Halme et al[224] studied 26 patients with localized MPM treated with high-dose methotrexate and leucovorin rescue in combination with α-interferon. This regimen was well tolerated and demonstrated a response rate of 29 percent, a median survival of 17 months, and 1 year and 2 year survival rates of 62 percent and 31 percent, respectively. Although the combination of irinotecan and docetaxel in patients with IMIG stage III-IV was slightly efficacious (overall response rate of 15%), its high toxicity profile (50% incidence of neutropenic fever and 40% of grade 3-4 diarrhea) makes it an improbable candidate for the treatment of MPM.[225] Overall, despite the testing of a variety of older and newer agents in combination, treatment for MPM with currently marketed agents remains inadequate. The incorporation of new-targeted therapies into the most promising cytotoxic regimens of presently marketed agents needs to be tested extensively within more novel strategies of drug delivery.

Novel Therapeutic Approaches

Several novel approaches to the treatment of MPM that incorporate new chemotherapeutic, biological, and targeted therapies are under development. Pemetrexed is a multitargeted antifolate that inhibits multiple enzymes important in folate metabolism, including thymidylate synthetase (TS), dihydrofolate reductase (DHFR), glycinamide ribonucleotide formyltransferase (GARFT), and aminoimidazole carboxamide ribonucleotide formyltransferase.[226,227] The key enzyme targets for pemetrexed are TS, DHFR, and GARFT.[228] TS and DHFR are targets of the known antineoplastic agents 5-flurouracil and methotrexate, respectively, while GARFT is not targeted by any currently used chemotherapeutic agent.

Pemetrexed as a single agent administered at a dose of 500 mg/m² every 21 days has demonstrated promising activity in several malignancies, including nonsmall cell lung cancer, breast cancer, previously untreated colorectal cancer, bladder cancer, cervical cancer, and cancer of the head and neck.[227,229-232] In a phase I trial of pemetrexed combined with cisplatin, 5 of 11 evaluable patients (45%) with MPM achieved a partial response,[233] while a second phase I trial of pemetrexed combined with carboplatin in patients with MPM showed partial response in 8 of 25 assessable patients (32%).[234] In the initial stages of development, pemetrexed therapy was complicated by severe toxicities, thought to be due to deficiencies of folate and/or vitamin B_{12} pools.[235,236] Subsequent supplementation of all patients with vitamin B_{12} and folate significantly reduced severe toxicities associated with the drug.[237,238] An open-label, multi-institutional phase II trial of pemetrexed as a single agent involving 64 patients with MPM showed an overall response rate of 16 percent and a median survival of 13 months in patients supplemented with folic acid and vitamin B_{12}.[237] The initial encouraging results of pemetrexed in phase I and II studies led to the largest randomized trial.[214] conducted to date for MPM, comparing pemetrexed/cisplatin vs cisplatin. Pemetrexed/cisplatin was more effective than cisplatin alone in terms of median survival (12.1 months vs 9.3 months, p = 0.020), median time to disease progression (5.7 months vs 3.9 months), and response rate (41% vs 17%). As expected, the pemetrexed/cisplatin arm had a higher incidence of laboratory toxicities than cisplatin alone, including grade 3/4 neutropenia (28%) and leukopenia (18%), and rare nonlaboratory toxicities. Supplementation improved the efficacy and toxicity profiles. Finally, pemetrexed/cisplatin showed significant improvement in both pulmonary function tests and major disease-related symptoms such as dyspnea and pain.[239,240]

As a 10 min infusion administered every 21 days, pemetrexed is easy to administer; when administered with appropriate folate and vitamin B_{12} supplementation, severe toxicity is controlled. Based on these data, pemetrexed in combination with cisplatin should be considered as a major component of standard care of patients with unresectable MPM.

Ranpirnase, a ribonuclease derived from leopard frog eggs, has been extensively studied in mesothelioma. In a phase II trial of 105 patients with MPM, it demonstrated a response rate of only 5 percent but was noted to produce stable disease in 43 percent of patients.[241] Overall survival was 6 months for the intent-to-treat group and 8.3 months in a subset of patients with a good prognosis based on CALGB criteria. A phase III trial[242] suggested that ranpirnase may have higher efficacy than doxorubicin in certain small subgroups of patients with unresectable malignant mesothelioma, but these retrospective observations had insufficient power to draw any reliable conclusions on efficacy. Larger studies of such γ subgroups are needed.

Various cytokines, alone or in combination, also have been studied in MPM.[243-245] A phase II trial investigating γ-2b interferon in combination with cisplatin and doxorubicin showed a response rate of 29 percent and a median survival of 9.3 months in patients with advanced MPM.[243] Severe myelosuppression and fatigue were significant limiting toxicities. Intrapleural interleukin-2 was also examined for the treatment of malignant pleural effusions with promising results.[244,245]

A variety of new approaches are under investigation for the treatment of mesothelioma, based on the targeting of specific markers. SV-40 has been identified as a possible cause of MPM[160] and a candidate vaccine of the SV-40 T-antigen has shown early evidence of efficacy.[246] Vascular endothelial growth factor (VEGF) is an autocrine growth factor important in the pathogenesis of MPM.[252] Three potential inhibitors of VEGF are being investigated for activity against the disease: bevacizumab (rhuMAbVEGF), SU5416, and thalidomide.[247,248] Bevacizumab, a recombinant anti-VEGF antibody, is in phase II trials in combination with chemotherapy (gemcitabine/cisplatin). ZD1839 (gefinitib), an inhibitor of the epidermal growth factor receptor, and STI-571 (imatinib), an inhibitor of the platelet derived growth factor receptor, were unsuccessful as monotherapies in epidermal growth factor receptor-positive malignant mesothelioma and MPM, respectively.[249,250] Since COX-2 is overexpressed in MPM and may constitute a poor prognostic factor, COX-2 inhibitors may have therapeutic potential.[251] Photodynamic therapy has also been investigated, but a randomized trial[252] failed to show any benefit in either survival or local control.

Palliative Care

Given that the prognosis for patients with mesothelioma has been historically poor regardless of the type of anticancer treatment, palliation of symptoms has been the primary goal of most therapy to date. Palliative therapy focuses on two major symptoms, dyspnea and chest wall pain. All previously described modalities may contribute to the palliation of patients with MPM. Radiation has shown palliative benefit in reducing pain and symptoms of dyspnea, surgical pleurodesis can reduce the symptoms associated with recurrent or persistent pleural effusions, and chemotherapy has demonstrated palliative benefit in terms of overall quality of life. Judicious use of these treatments in combination with adequate pain control and attention to respiratory function has formed the basis of effective palliation in MPM.

Despite a long history of therapeutic nihilism in the treatment of MPM, recent advances have renewed enthusiasm for aggressive management of the disease in all stages. The combination of pemetrexed with cisplatin, which demonstrated a positive benefit on multiple outcomes including survival, time-to-progressive disease, and quality of life, will likely become a major component of the standard of care for patients with advanced disease, and has provided renewed hope for the development of other effective standards of care for this disease. This regimen should now be tested in clinical trials in the adjuvant and neoadjuvant setting as well. Based on a rapidly emerging understanding of the biology of MPM, continued research on novel molecular targets and their respective targeted therapies will be very important for further advances to occur in the treatment of this disease.

Prognostic Factors in Mesothelioma

Review of the best-known prognostic scoring systems from the EORTC (European Organization for Research and Treatment of Cancer) and CALGB (Cancer and Leukemia Group B) has shown that the most important predictors of poor prognosis are:[253]
- Poor performance status (1 or 2)
- Presence of chest pain, breathlessness, pleural involvement, significant weight loss
- Age over 75 years

Nonepitheloid histology (sarcomatoid histology or uncertain diagnosis–probable/possible histological diagnosis of mesothelioma):
- Male gender
- Low hemoglobin (< 1 g/dl lower than normal)
- High platelet count
- High white blood cell count (> 8.3 × 10^9/L)
- High lactate dehydrogenase.

Novel molecular predictors like Glucose transporter-1 (Glut-1), COX-2, Cycline-dependent kinase inhibitor p27, MIB-1, Angiogenic cytokines, glycoprotein 90K.

Prognostic factors can help clinicians and patients when deciding a treatment plan. Patients in the best prognostic group can be considered for more intensive or experimental therapy. Alternatively, patients in the best prognostic group might prefer a period of observation prior to commencement of therapy. For patients with mesothelioma, prognostic factors are potentially important because of the lack of a widely applicable anatomical staging system including that of the IMIG syste described above.

Most series have shown that the median survival for a patient with mesothelioma is between 4 and 18 months.[253]

Prevention of Asbestos-related Diseases

Alternative materials can be used for wide variety of applications including the wide range use of glass, rock and slag wools, and PVC, etc. for thermal and acoustic insulation. To ensure conditions of safety codes of practice like proper storage and conveyance of asbestos, factory conditions, other working conditions, and proper waste disposal should be strictly adhered to. Fibers are to be kept in sealed polythene or impermeable paper bags, which prevents spillage. If wet processes are not used in the factory as in milling, dust can be prevented by total or partial enclosures with effective exhaust ventilations or provision of hoods.

As discussed above, asbestos fibers enter the body either by skin contact, ingestion, or inhalation. For the public at large, asbestos is harmless if swallowed. In municipalities with asbestos-cement pipe for water distribution, and a much higher concentration of asbestos fibers in the drinking water than in communities with other types of pipe, no differences in the frequency of asbestos-related diseases were found. However, workers with a heavy industrial exposure probably swallow large quantities of asbestos fibers, and this could contribute to the development of peritoneal mesothelioma. At the present time, essentially all adverse effects on health from asbestos are due to the inhalation of fibers in concentrations sufficient to overwhelm the normal pulmonary defense and clearance mechanisms. Airborne fibers are carried along in the inspired air stream and impinge on the mucous lining of the smaller bronchioles. Tissue fiber burdens are generally related to cumulative exposure. Chrysotile fibers are less harmful than the amphiboles, in part because they are broken down and removed from the lung. Animal studies clearly show that cigarette smoke increases asbestos fiber deposition.

Asbestos-related diseases have lengthy latent periods, except for pleural effusions, which can occur within a year to > 20 years after first exposure. Brief but intense exposures are quite capable of causing disease, but it may be many years, with either continuing or no further exposure, before they become manifest. The longest latent periods, > 40 years, occur with mesothelioma. Whether or not there is a threshold level of asbestos exposure that does not increase the risk of malignancy is controversial.

Mesothelioma and lung cancer rates vary by many orders of magnitude between those with a heavy, lifetime occupational exposure and the unexposed. Low-level exposure, as encountered in public buildings, probably does not represent any additional health hazard beyond what is incurred breathing outdoor air. However, reliable information about long-term, low-level exposure is exceedingly difficult to obtain.

The asbestos fiber exposure limits in the United States was at 5.0 fibers per cubic centimeter in 1971, followed by successive reductions to 0.1 fibers in 1994. Prior to setting and then reducing asbestos fiber exposure limits, there were the customary public hearings; unlike the usual regulatory procedures, general interest in asbestos regulation was intense, aided in part by widespread publicity, Environmental Protection Agency (EPA) pronouncements, and conflicting medical and scientific opinions. At one time it was the position of the EPA that a single asbestos fiber could cause cancer. The ensuing public outcry and demand for the removal of asbestos from public buildings, particularly schools, was intense, costly, and ill advised. A "third wave" of asbestos-related morbidity and mortality among the general public due to asbestos exposure in public buildings was predicted by some, but subsequently rejected following studies demonstrating the similarity of asbestos fiber concentration in the indoor air of buildings with asbestos in place and in outdoor air. Further, long-term occupants of public buildings containing asbestos insulation had no greater prevalence of asbestos-related chest radiographic abnormalities than similar occupants of asbestos-free buildings. Disagreement about the safety of chrysotile fibers also clouded the issue. Asbestos-containing materials, in both public buildings and private homes, should be left in place, covered, or sealed, and examined periodically to ensure physical integrity. Remodeling or demolition of structures with asbestos in place, no matter how well sealed or covered, requires special precautions plus proper containment and disposal of debris.

Many additional factors have contributed to the massive number of asbestos-related cases. Some examples are as follows: radiologic evidence of asbestos exposure in the absence of any clinical or measurable functional impairment; "emotional harm," justified in part on the extended latent interval from time of exposure to manifestation of disease; the costs of future medical monitoring, which has not been proven useful for detecting diseases for which there is no treatment and that may never occur; and conflicting opinions regarding the significance of pleural plaques. A change in the method of compensation—one based on objective measures of lung function and on radiologic findings—was proposed but not adopted. Because the resources available to compensate the disabled are rapidly diminishing, and to relieve the logjam of claims clogging various legal jurisdictions, there have been renewed efforts to develop objective criteria, such as published standards for disability assessment as the basis for settling claims for nonmalignant types of asbestos diseases. Legislation need to be proposed to mandate disability assessment as the basis for settling claims for nonmalignant asbestos diseases. Physicians responsible for the care of patients with asbestos exposures may be drawn into the medical-legal arena. Detailed clinical records, complete laboratory test results, and biopsy or other interventions when appropriate and indicated will enable the treating physician to confidently meet any legal inquiry.

ASBESTOS PROBLEM IN INDIA

Lack of information and data on asbestos-related disease is a common problem like in many other developing countries. Because of its durability and tensile strength, asbestos is used over 3000 products. India consumes about 100,000 tonnes of chrysotile every year, much of which is imported from Canada. Approximately up to 1 million people in India are currently exposed to asbestos because of their occupation. Studies by the National Institute of Occupational Health (NIOH), Ahmedabad, have found lung impairment and radiological abnormalities in asbestos milling workers (54.8%) and miners (19.5%). The work place asbestos fiber concentration in milling facilities was found to be 33 times higher than the Indian standard for chrysotile asbestos of $2f/cm^3$. Numerous instances of high exposure levels to asbestos fiber have also been reported in the work place, which indicates a potential epidemic like situation of asbestos-related diseases in the coming years. The potential hazards are not fully appreciated. There is no enforcement of health and safety regulations in the asbestos sector, the construction industry or at the docks. The Central Pollution Control Board of the Government of India monitored eight major asbestos products manufacturing operations in India. Six of them were not complying with the emission standards, and for the remaining two, compliance or noncompliance status could not be ascertained.[254]

Surveys conducted in 1997 by Government agencies recorded airborne levels of between 2 and 488 f/cm^3 in occupational settings; the Indian standard for permissible airborne concentrations of chrysotile are 2 f/cm^3.

As mentioned, there is no detailed data available to analyze the total number of deaths in India only due to asbestos, as records do not categorize different sources of respiratory symptoms. A general analysis of the data for the last 20 years shows that deaths reported during this period shows a trend similar to asbestos production, import and reexport of asbestos accelerates cause of death over years due to respiratory system and respiratory infection in India.[255] In the State of Jharkhand, abandoned chysotile asbestos mines are a serious health problem for villagers and former miners. A massive pile of asbestos waste mixed with chromite has accumulated atop the hilltops of Roro village for 2 decades. These gradually seep into the land, water, homes and bodies of the tribal communities living at the foothills of Roro.[256] Preliminary health survey of 14 villages around Roro hills with 45 percent responders indicates a link between asbestos mining workers and respiratory difficulty. About 17.6 percent complained of respiratory difficulty. During monsoon, the asbestos waste from the dumping sites gradually runs into the fields, streams, and ponds. In the summer, warm winds carry fine waste material from these dumpsites across the whole area. Children and the elderly are more prone for exposure. Soil samples collected from different sites of one of the northern Indian cities with increasing distance around an asbestos cement factory showed contamination with asbestos fibers. Soil sample from the close vicinity of the factory revealed higher number of fibers in comparison to increasing distance. Size wise pattern of fiber (< 10 mm) was found higher with distance moving away from the factory and the size of the asbestos fibers may cause harm to human, Analysis of pond showed presence of suspended chrysotile fibers with the size < 30 mm and sediments mostly containing coarse chrysotile fibers of size < 50 mm. While most Scandinavian and Western European countries, USA, and Japan has lower cutoff exposure limits, India has permissible exposure levels greater than 1 f/ ml.

For mysterious reasons, mesothelioma is considered to be rare in India and description of its occurrence is mentioned as case reports in Indian literature. The exact cause the rare occurrence is unknown. Studies in India have shown lung impairment and radiological abnormalities in all varieties of asbestos milling workers (54.8%) and miners (19.5%), (n = 633).[257]

Asbestos is being used predominantly in cement products in India. In installation of pipes and boards exposures during sawing or other abrasive actions can be well controlled with the use of appropriate dust collectors or wetting techniques. However, in India these precautions may not be necessary always and workplace monitoring by regulatory agencies is important.

Uncontrolled sawing produces concentrations in the tens of f/ml. During normal use of such asbestos cement products, there is limited release of fibers because of the strong binding of cement. However, abrasion of the cement will lead to fiber release. Current occupational exposure in India is because of substantial; use of asbestos in thermal insulations. Such products become particularly dangerous because asbestos is readily released. Such releases during installation, repair or removal not only expose the insulator, but also many workers in shipyards through import and reexport and construction sites.

Since, this naturally occurring silicate fiber often occurs in high fluoride host rock, such as amphibolite in the Cuddapah district of Andhra Pradesh, Sighbum district of Jharkhand, and Ajmer district of Rajsthan; and the problem faced can be of two-folds—apart from asbestosis-fluorosis.

Although, India banned the import of asbestos waste in 1998, nearly 75,000 kg were imported from Russia between April 2003 and February 2004. Import duties have also been reduced by 15 percent in 2004 on these items. A number of substitutes to asbestos are used in developed countries like cellulose polyacrylonitrile, glass fiber, and unplasticized polyvinyl chloride (PVC). These substitutes are expensive and these alternative products are not in common use in India. However, for the better health of people such alternative products are to be approved, especially for roofing. Chrysotile being established as a mass killer, its use is to be restricted. Different other types of man-made fibers are being used as substitutes for asbestos. The concern for these materials having similar physiochemical properties to asbestos exists because some fibers can cause pulmonary fibrosis. Pneumoconiosis, a chronic inflammatory reaction due to continued presence of dust in the lungs can eventually lead to fibrosis.[258]

REFERENCES

1. Becklek MR. Asbestos and other fiber-related diseases of the lungs and pleura. Distribution and determinants in exposed populations. Chest 1991;100:248-54.
2. Craighead JE. The epidemiology and pathogenesis of malignant mesothelioma. Chest 1989;96(Suppl):92S-93S
3. Cugell DW, Kamp DW. Asbestos and the Pleura-A Review. Chest 2004;125:1103-17.
4. Murray, M Departmental Committee for Compensation for Industrial Diseases, CND 3495 and 3496. 1907 HMSO: London, UK.
5. Merewether ERA, Price CW. Report on effects of asbestos on the lungs and dust suppression in the asbestos industry. HMSO. London, UK 1930.
6. Parkes WR. Occupational lung disorders (2nd edn). Butterworths: London, UK, 1974,249.
7. Enterline PE. Changing attitudes and opinions regarding asbestos and cancer. Am J Ind Med (1934-1965) 1991;20,685-700.
8. Wagner JC, Sleggs CA, Marchand P. Diffuse pleural mesothelioma and asbestos exposure in the North Western Cape Province. Br J Ind Med 1960;17,260-71.
9. Polissar L, Severson RK, Boatman ES. A case-control study of asbestos in drinking water and cancer risk. Am J Epidemiol 1984;119,456-71.
10. Toft P, Meek ME. Asbestos in drinking water: A Canadian view. Environ Health Perspect 1983;53,177-80.
11. Roggli VL, Sanders LL. Asbestos content of lung tissue and carcinoma of the lung: A clinicopathologic correlation and mineral fiber analysis of 234 cases. Ann Occup Hyg 2000;44,109-17.
12. McFadden D, Wright J, Wiggs B, et al. Cigarette smoke increases the penetration of asbestos fibers into airway walls. Am J Pathol 1986;123,95-99.
13. Sekhon H, Wright J, Churg A. Effects of cigarette smoke and asbestos on airway, vascular and meso-thelial cell proliferation. Int J Exp Pathol 1995;76,411-18.
14. Epler GR, McLoud TC, Gaensler EA. Prevalence and incidence of benign asbestos pleural effusion in a working population. JAMA 1982;247,617-22.
15. Hillerdal G, Ozesmi M. Benign asbestos pleural effusion: 73 exudates in 60 patients. Eur J Respir Dis 1987;71,113-121.
16. Camus M, Siemiatycki J, Meek B. Nonoccupational exposure to chrysotile asbestos and the risk of lung cancer. N Engl J Med 1998;338,1565-57.
17. Landrigan PJ. Asbestos: Still a carcinogen. N Engl J Med 1998;338,1618-19.
18. Mossman BT, Bignon J, Corn M, et al. Letter to the editor. Science 1990;248,799-801.
19. Osinubi OY, Gochfeld M, Kipen HM. Health effects of asbestos and nonasbestos fibers. Environ Health Perspect 2000;108,665-74.
20. Asbestos in public and commercial buildings: A literature review and synthesis of current knowledge. Health Effects Institute–Asbestos Research 1991;8-10.
21. Mossman BT, Bignon J, Corn M, et al. Asbestos: Scientific developments and implications for public policy. Science 1990;247,294-301.
22. Sider L, Holland EA, Davis TJ, et al. Changes on radiographs of wives of workers exposed to asbestos. Radiology 1987;164,723-26.
23. Goldsmith JR. Asbestos as a systemic carcinogen: The evidence from eleven cohorts. Am J Ind Med 1982;3, 341-48.
24. Kagan E, Jacobson RJ. Lymphoid and plasma cell malignancies: Asbestos-related disorders of long latency. Am J Clin Pathol 1983;80,14-20.

25. Sprince NL, Oliver LC, McLoud TC, et al. Asbestos exposure and asbestos-related pleural and parenchymal disease: Associations with immune imbalance. Am Rev Respir Dis 1991;143,822-28.

26. Dodson RF, Williams MG Jr, Corn CJ, et al. Asbestos content of lung tissue, lymph nodes, and pleural plaques from former shipyard workers. Am Rev Respir Dis 1990;142,843-47.

27. Greene R, Schaefer CM, Oliver LC. Improved detection of asbestos-related pleural plaques with digital radiography. Ann NY Acad Sci 1991;643,90-96.

28. Knisely BL, Broderick LS, Kuhlman JE. MR imaging of the pleura and chest wall. Magn Reson Imaging Clin N Am 2000;8,125-41.

29. Svenes KB, Borgersen A, Haaversen O, et al. Parietal pleural plaques: A comparison between autopsy and X-ray findings. Eur J Respir Dis 1986;69,10-15.

30. Ren H, Lee DR, Hruban RH, et al. Pleural plaques do not predict asbestosis: High-resolution computed tomography and pathology study. Mod Pathol 1991;4,201-09.

31. Fitzgerald EF, Stark AD, Vianna N, et al. Exposure to asbestiform minerals and radiographic chest abnormalities in a talc mining region of upstate New York. Arch Environ Health 1991;46,151-54.

32. Gilmartin D. The serratus anterior muscle on chest radiographs. Radiology 1979;131,629-35.

33. To B or not to B: A NIOSH B reader. National Institute of Occupational Safety and Health. Available at: http://www.cdc.gov/niosh/pamphlet.html. Accessed February 2004;19.

34. Ducatman AM. Variability in interpretation of radiographs for asbestosis abnormalities: Problems and solutions. Ann N Y Acad Sci 1991;643,108-20.

35. Epler GR, McLoud TC, Gaensler EA. Prevalence and incidence of benign asbestos pleural effusion in a working population. JAMA 1982;247,617-22.

36. Jones RN, McLoud T, Rockoff SD. The radiographic pleural abnormalities in asbestos exposure: Relationship to physiologic abnormalities. J Thorac Imaging 1988;3,57-66.

37. Schwartz DA, Galvin JR, Dayton CS, et al. Determinants of restrictive lung function in asbestos-induced pleural fibrosis. J Appl Physiol 1990;68,1932-37.

38. Bergin CJ. Determinants of restrictive lung function in asbestos-induced pleural fibrosis. J Appl Physiol 1991;70,472-73.

39. Rosenberg DM. Pleural fibrosis and asbestosis. J Appl Physiol 1991;70,473-75.

40. Rockoff SD, Chu J, Rubin LJ. Special report: Asbestos-induced pleural plaques; a disease process associated with ventilatory impairment and respiratory symptoms. Clin Pulm Med 2002;9,113-124

41. Edge JR. Incidence of bronchial carcinoma in shipyard workers with pleural plaques. Ann NY Acad Sci 1979;330,289-94.

42. Harber P, Mohsenifar Z, Oren A, et al. Pleural plaques and asbestos-associated malignancy. J Occup Med 1987;29,641-44.

43. Weiss W. Asbestos-related pleural plaques and lung cancer. Chest 1993;103,1854-59.

44. Hillerdal G. Pleural and parenchymal fibrosis mainly affecting the upper lung lobes in persons exposed to asbestos. Respir Med 1990;84,129-34.

45. McGavin CR, Sheers G. Diffuse pleural thickening in asbestos workers: Disability and lung function abnormalities. Thorax 1984;39,604-07.

46. Lilis R, Miller A, Godbold J, et al. Radiographic abnormalities in asbestos insulators: Effects of duration from onset of exposure and smoking: relationships of dyspnea with parenchymal and pleural fibrosis. Am J Ind Med 1991;20,1-15.

47. Copley SJ, Wells AU, Rubens MB, et al. Functional consequences of pleural disease evaluated with chest radiography and CT. Radiology 2001;220,237-43.

48. Kee ST, Gamsu G, Blanc P. Causes of pulmonary impairment in asbestos-exposed individuals with diffuse pleural thickening. Am J Respir Crit Care Med 1996;154,789-93.

49. Batra P, Brown K, Hayashi K, et al. Rounded atelectasis. J Thorac Imaging 1996;11,187-97.

50. Mintzer RA, Cugell DW. The association of asbestos-induced pleural disease and rounded atelectasis. Chest 1982;81,457-60.

51. Hillerdal G. Rounded atelectasis: Clinical experience with 74 patients. Chest 1989;95,836-41.

52. Robinson BW, Musk AW. Benign asbestos pleural effusion: Diagnosis and course. Thorax 1981;36,896-900.

53. Hillerdal, G, Ozesmi M. Benign asbestos pleural effusion: 73 exudates in 60 patients. Eur J Respir Dis 1987;71, 113-21.

54. Light RW. Pleural diseases (3rd edn). 1995 Williams and Wilkins: Baltimore, MD:

55. Becklake MR, Cowie RL. Pneumoconioses. In Murray J, Nadel J, Mason R (Eds): Textbook of Respiratory Medicine. Saunders: Philadelphia, PA 2000;1839-40.

56. Eisenstadt HB. Letter: Pleural effusion in asbestosis. N Engl J Med 1974;290,1025.

57. Knisely BL, Broderick LS, Kuhlman JE. MR imaging of the pleura and chest wall. Magn Reson Imaging Clin N Am 2000;8,125-41.

58. Ferrer J, Balcells E, Orriols R, et al. Derrame pleural benigno por asbesto: Descripcion de la primera serie en Espana. Med Clin (Barc) 1996;107,535-38.

59. Cohen M, Sahn SA. Resolution of pleural effusions. Chest 2001;119,1547-62.

60. Gaensler EA, Kaplan AI. Asbestos pleural effusion. Ann Intern Med 1971;74,178-91.

61. Gaensler EA, Jederlinic PJ, Churge A. Idiopathic pulmonary fibrosis in asbestos-exposed workers. Am Rev Respir Dis 1991;144:689.

62. Ohar J, David A, Sterling DA, Bleecker E, Donohue J. Changing patterns in asbestos-induced lung disease. Chest 2004;125:744-53.

63. Consensus Report. Finnish Institute. Asbestos, asbestosis, and cancer: The Helsinki criteria for diagnosis and attribution. Scand J Work Environ Health 1977;23, 311-16.

64. Kamp DW, Weitzman SA. Asbestosis: Clinical spectrum and pathogenic mechanisms. Proc Soc Exp Biol Med 1997;214,12-26.

65. Leathart GL. Pulmonary function tests in asbestos workers. Trans Soc Occup Med 1968;18,49-55.

66. Pearle J. Exercise performance and functional impairment in asbestos-exposed workers. Chest 1981;80,701-05.

67. Selikoff IJ, Churg J, Hammond EC. The occurrence of asbestosis among workers in the United States. Ann NY Acad Sci 1965;132,139-55.

68. Demers RY, Neale AV, Robins T, et al. Asbestos-related pulmonary disease in boilermakers. Am J Ind Med 1990;17,327-39.

69. Pavlovic M, Butkovic M, Jezdimirovic D, et al. Pulmonary function in workers with asbestosis [in Russian]. Arh Hig Rada Toksikol 1988;19,441-45.

70. Miller A, Lilis R, Godbold J, et al. Spirometric impairments in long-term insulators. Chest 1994; 105,175-82.

71. Hillerdale G, Malmberg P, Hemmingsson A. Asbestos-related lesions of the pleura: Parietal plaques compared to diffuse thickening studied with chest roentgenography, computed tomography, lung function, and gas exchange. Am J Ind Med 1990;18,627-39.

72. Begin R, Filion R, Ostiguy G. Emphysema in silica- and asbestos-exposed workers seeking compensation. Chest 1995;108,647-55.

73. Chen C, Chang H, Suo J, et al. Occupational exposure and respiratory morbidity among asbestos workers in Taiwan. J Formos Med Assoc 1992;91,1138-42.

74. Kgalamono SM, Rees D, Kielkowski D, Solomon A. Asbestos in the non-mining industry on the Witwatersrand, South Africa. S Afr Med J 2005;95:47-51.

75. Mossman BT, Gruenert DC. SV40, growth factors, and mesothelioma: Another piece of the puzzle. Am J Respir Cell Mol Biol 2002;26,167-70.

76. Mossman BT, Kamp DW, Weitzman SA. Mechanisms of carcinogenesis and clinical features of asbestos-associated cancers. Cancer Invest 1996;14,466-80.

77. Kamp DW, Mossman BT. Asbestosis associated cancers: Clinical spectrum and pathogenic mechanisms. Clin Occup Environ Med 2002;2,753-57.

78. Shukula A, Her T, Kamp DW, et al. Multiple roles of oxidants in the pathogenesis of asbestos-induced diseases. Free Radic Biol Med 2003;34,1117-29.

79. Roberts GH. The pathology of parietal pleural plaques. J Clin Pathol 1971;24,348-53.

80. Bateman ED, Benatar SR. Asbestos-induced diseases: Clinical perspectives. QJ Med 1987;62,183-94.

81. Sahn SA, Antony VB. Pathogenesis of pleural plaques: Relationship of early cellular response and pathology. Am Rev Respir Dis 1984;130,884-87.

82. Mossman BT, Bignon J, Corn M, et al. Asbestos: Scientific developments and implications for public policy. Science 1990;247,294-301.

83. Kamp DW, Weitzman SA. The molecular basis of asbestos induced lung injury. Thorax 1999;54,638-52.

84. Quinlan TR, BeruBe KA, Hacker MP, et al. Mechanisms of asbestos-induced nitric oxide production by rat alveolar macrophages in inhalation and *in vitro* models. Free Radic Biol Med 1998;24,778-88.

85. Chao CC, Park SH, Aust AE. Participation of nitric oxide and iron in the oxidation of DNA in asbestos-treated human lung epithelial cells. Arch Biochem Biophys 1996;326,152-57.

86. Jaurand MC. Mechanisms of fiber-induced genotoxicity. Environ Health Perspect 1997;105,1073-84.

87. Ferri KF, Kroemer G. Organelle-specific initiation of cell death pathways. Nature Cell Biol 2001;3,E255-E263.

88. Bortner CD, Cidlowski JA. Cellular mechanisms for the repression of apoptosis. Annu Rev Pharmacol Toxicol 2002;42,259-81.

89. BeruBe KA, Quinlan TR, Fung H, et al. Apoptosis is observed in mesothelial cells after exposure to crocidolite asbestos. Am J Respir Cell Mol Biol 1996;15, 141-47.

90. Broaddus VC, Yang L, Scavo LM, et al. Asbestos induces apoptosis of human and rabbit pleural mesothelial cells via reactive oxygen species. J Clin Invest 1996;98, 2050-59.

91. Hoidal JR. Reactive oxygen species and cell signaling. Am J Respir Cell Mol Biol 2001;25,661-63.

92. Vaslet VA, Messier NJ, Kane AB. Accelerated progression of asbestos-associated mesotheliomas in heterozygous p53+/- mice. Toxicol Sci 2002;68,331-38.

93. Heintz NH, Janssen YM, Mossman BT. Persistent induction of c-fos and c-jun expression by asbestos. Proc Natl Acad Sci USA 1993;90,3299-3303.

94. Ilavska S, Jahnova E, Tulinska J, Horvathova M, Dusinska M, Wsolova L, Kyrtopoulos SA, Fuortes L. Immunological monitoring in workers occupationally exposed to asbestos. Toxicology 2005;206:299-308.

95. Li J, Poovey HG, Rodriguez JF, Brody A, Hoyle GW. Effect of platelet-derived growth factor on the development and persistence of asbestos-induced fibroproliferative lung disease. J Environ Pathol Toxicol Oncol 2004;23:253-66.

96. Piirila P, Lindqvist M, Huuskonen O, Kaleva S, Koskinen H, Lehtola H, Vehmas T, Kivisaari L, Sovijarvi AR. Impairment of lung function in asbestos-exposed workers in relation to high-resolution computed tomography. Scand J Work Environ Health 2005;31:44-51.

97. Alfonso HS, Fritschi L, de Klerk NH, Olsen N, Sleith J, Musk AW. Effects of asbestos and smoking on the levels and rates of change of lung function in a crocidolite exposed cohort in Western Australia. Thorax 2004;59:1052-56.

98. Muller JG, Bohnker BK, Philippi AF, Litow FK, Rudolph G, Hernandez JE. Trends in pleural radiographic findings in the Navy Asbestos Medical Surveillance Program (1990-1999). Mil Med 2005;1705:375-80.

99. Vehmas T, Kivisaari L, Huuskonen MS, Jaakkola MS. Scoring CT/HRCT findings among asbestos-exposed workers: Effects of patient's age, body mass index and common laboratory test results. Eur Radiol 2005;15: 213-19.

100. Pelclova D, Bartunkova J, Fenclova Z, Lebedova J, Hladikova M, Benakova H. Asbestos exposure and antineutrophil cytoplasmic Antibody (ANCA) positivity. Arch Environ Health 2003;58:662-68.

101. Alfonso HS, Fritschi L, de Klerk NH, Ambrosini G, Beilby J, Olsen N, Musk AW. Plasma concentrations of retinol, carotene, and vitamin E and mortality in subjects with asbestosis in a cohort exposed to crocidolite in Wittenoom, Western Australia. J Occup Environ Med 2005;47:573-79.

102. Huggins JT, Sahn SA. Causes and management of pleural fibrosis. Respirology 2004;9:441-47.

103. Mutsaers SE, Prele CM, Brody AR, Idell S. Pathogenesis of pleural fibrosis. Respirology 2004;9:428-40.

104. Rom WN, Travis WD, Brody AR. Cellular and molecular basis of the asbestos-related diseases. Am Rev Respir Dis 1991;143:408-22.

105. MacIntyre NR. Diffusing capacity of the lung for carbon monoxide. Respir Care Clin N Am 1997;3:221-33.

106. Lilis R, Selikoff IJ, Lerman Y, et al. Asbestosis: Interstitial pulmonary fibrosis and pleural fibrosis in a cohort of asbestos insulation workers: influence of cigarette smoking. Am J Ind Med 1986;10:459-70.

107. Schwartz DA, Davis CS, Merchant JA, et al. Longitudinal changes in lung function among asbestos-exposed workers. Am J Respir Crit Care Med 1994;150:1243-49.

108. Cotes JE. Lung function assessment and application in medicine (5th edn). Oxford: Blackwell Scientific Publications 1993.

109. Wang XR, Yano E, Nonaka K. Pulmonary function of nonsmoking female asbestos workers without radiographic signs of asbestosis. Arch Environ Health 1998;53:292-98.

110. Sansores RH, Pare P, Abboud RT. Effect of smoking cessation on pulmonary carbon monoxide diffusing capacity and capillary blood volume. Am Rev Respir Dis 1992;146:959-64.

111. Alfonso HS, Fritschi L, Klerk N H de, Olsen N, Sleith J, Musk A W. Effects of asbestos and smoking on gas diffusion in people exposed to crocidolite. Med J Austr 2005;183:184-7.

112. Blanc PD, Gamsu G. The effect of cigarette smoking on the detection of small radiographic opacities in inorganic dust diseases. J Thorac Imaging 1988;3,51-56.

113. Lerman Y, Seidman H, Gelb S, et al. Spirometric abnormalities among asbestos insulation workers. J Occup Med 1988;30,228-33.

114. Brodkin CA, Barnhart S, Anderson G, et al. Correlation between respiratory symptoms and pulmonary function in asbestos-exposed workers. Am Rev Respir Dis 1993;148,32-37.

115. Thomson ML, Pelzer AM, Smither WJ. The discriminant value of pulmonary function test in asbestosis. Ann NY Acad Sci 1965;132,421-36.

116. Bader ME, Bader RA, Selikoff IJ, et al. Pulmonary function in asbestosis of the lung, an alveolar-capillary block syndrome. Am J Med 1961;30,235-42.

117. Williams R, Hugh-Jones P. The significance of lung function changes in asbestosis. Thorax 1960;15,109-19.

118. Wright GW. Functional abnormalities of industrial pulmonary fibrosis. Arch Ind Health 1955;11,196-203.

119. Schwartz DA. New developments in asbestos-induced pleural disease. Chest 1991;99,191-97.

120. Pearle J. Exercise performance and functional impairment in asbestos-exposed workers. Chest 1981;80, 701-05.

121. Demers RY, Neale AV, Robins T, et al. Asbestos-related pulmonary disease in boilermakers. Am J Ind Med 1990;17,327-39.

122. Harber P, Tashkin DP, Lew BS, et al. Physiologic categorization of asbestos-exposed workers. Chest 1987;92,494-99.

123. Kilburn KH, Lilis R, Anderson HA, et al. Interaction of asbestos, age, and cigarette smoking in producing radiographic evidence of diffuse pulmonary fibrosis. Am J Med 1986;80,377-381.

124. Kilburn KH, Warshaw RH. Airway obstruction in asbestos-exposed shipyard workers: With and without irregular opacities. Respir Med 1990;81,449-55.

125. Kilburn KH, Warshaw RH, Einstein K, et al. Airway disease in non-smoking asbestos workers. Arch Environ Health 1985;40,293-95.

126. Begin R, Cantin A, Berthiaume Y, et al. Airway function in lifetime-nonsmoking older asbestos workers. Am J Med 1983;75,631-38.

127. Rodriguez-Roisin R, Merchant JEM, Cochrane GM, et al. Maximal expiratory flow volume curves in workers exposed to asbestos. Respiration 1980;39,158-65.

128. Kilburn KH, Warshaw RH. Airways obstruction from asbestos exposure. Chest 1994;106,1061-70.

129. Kilburn KH, Warshaw RH. Airways obstruction from asbestos exposure and asbestosis revisited. Chest 1995;107,1730-31.

130. Jones RN, Glindmeyer HW III, Engr D, et al. Review of the Kilburn and Warshaw Chest article: Airways obstruction from asbestos exposure. Chest 1995;107, 1727-29.

131. Churg A, Wright JL, Wiggs B, et al. Small airways disease and mineral dust exposure. Am Rev Respir Dis 1985;131,139-43.

132. Tron V, Wright JL, Harrison N, et al. Cigarette smoke makes airway and early parenchymal asbestos-induced lung disease worse in the guinea pig. Am Rev Respir Dis 1987;136,271-75.

133. Begin R, Masse S, Bureau MA. Morphologic features and function of the airways in early asbestosis in the sheep model. Am Rev Respir Dis 1982;126,870-76.

134. Hassmanova V. Diseases caused by asbestos dust and the trend of their development in exposed workers in 1951-2003. Acta Medica (Hradec Kralove) Suppl. 2004;472:107-20.

135. Hessel PA, Gamble JF, McDonald JC. Asbestos, asbestosis, and lung cancer: A critical assessment of the epidemiological evidence. Thorax 2005;60:433-36.

136. Sluis-Cremer GK, Bezuidenhout BN. Relation between asbestosis and bronchial cancer in amphibole asbestos miners. Br J Ind Med 1989;46:537-40.

137. Sluis-Cremer GK, Bezuidenhout BN. Reply to Rudd. Br J Ind Med 1990;47:215-16.

138. Hughes JM, Weill H. Asbestosis as a precursor of asbestos related lung cancer: Results of a prospective mortality study. Br J Ind Med 1991;48:229-33.

139. Martischnig KM, Newell DJ, Barnsley WC, et al. Unsuspected exposure to asbestos and bronchogenic carcinoma. BMJ 1977;1:746-49.

140. Liddell FDK, McDonald JC. Radiological findings as predictors of mortality in Quebec asbestos workers. Br J Ind Med 1980;37:257-67.

141. Karjalainen A, Anttila S, Heikkila L, et al. Lobe of origin of lung cancer among asbestos-exposed patients with or without diffuse interstitial fibrosis. Scand J Work Environ Health 1993;19:102-07.

142. Anttila S, Karjalainen A, Taikina-aho O, et al. Lung cancer in the lower lobe is associated with pulmonary asbestos fiber count and fiber size. Environ Health Perspect 1993;101:166-70.

143. Hillerdal G. Pleural plaques and risk for bronchial carcinoma and mesothelioma: A prospective study. Chest 1994;105:144-50.

144. Wilkinson P, Hansell DM, Janssens J, et al. Is lung cancer associated with asbestos exposure when there are no small opacities on the chest radiograph? Lancet 1995;345:1074-78.

145. Finkelstein MM. Radiographic asbestosis is not a prerequisite for asbestos-associated lung cancer in Ontario asbestos-cement workers. Am J Ind Med 1997;32:341-48.

146. de Klerk NH, Musk AW, Glancy JJ, et al. Crocidolite, radiographic asbestosis and subsequent lung cancer. Ann Occup Hyg 1997;41 (Suppl 1):134-36.

147. Henderson DW, Rodelsperger K, Woitowitz HJ, Leigh J. After Helsinki: A multidisciplinary review of the relationship between asbestos exposure and lung cancer, with emphasis on studies published during 1997-2004. Pathology 2004;36:517-50.

148. Pistolesi M, Rusthoven J. Malignant Pleural Mesothelioma. Update, current management, and newer therapeutic strategies. Chest 2004.

149. Wagner JC, Sleggs CA, Marchand P. Diffuse pleural mesothelioma and asbestos in the North Western Cape Province. Br J Industr Med 1960;17,260-71.

150. Price B. Analysis of current trends in United States mesothelioma incidence. Am J Epidemiol 1997;145, 211-18.

151. Connelly RR, Spirtas R, Myers MH, et al. Demographic patterns for mesothelioma in the United States. J Natl Cancer Inst 1987;78,1053-60.

152. Peto J, Decarli A, La Vecchia C, et al. The European mesothelioma epidemic. Br J Cancer 1999;79,666-72.

153. Doll R. Mortality from lung cancer in asbestos workers. Br J Ind Med 1955;12,81-86.

154. Boutin C, Dumortier P, Rey F, et al. Black spots concentrate asbestos fibers in the parietal pleura. Thoracoscopic and mineralogic study. Am J Respir Crit Care Med 1996;153,444-49.

155. Bianchi C, Giarelli L, Grandi G, et al. Latency periods in asbestos-related mesothelioma of the pleura. Eur J Cancer Prev 1997;6,162-66.

156. Chahinian AP, Pajak TF, Holland JF, et al. Diffuse malignant mesothelioma: Prospective evaluation of 69 patients. Ann Intern Med 1982;96,746-55.

157. Selikoff IJ, Hammond EC, Seidman H. Latency of asbestos disease among insulation workers in the United States and Canada. Cancer 1980;46,2736-40.

158. Testa JR, Carbone M, Hirvonen A, et al. A multi-institutional study confirms the presence and expression of simian virus 40 in human malignant mesothelioma. Cancer Res 1998;58,4505-09.

159. Bocchetta M, Di Resta, I Powers A, et al. Human mesothelial cells are unusually susceptible to simian virus 40-mediated transformation and asbestos cocarcinogenicity. Proc Natl Acad Sci USA 2000; 97,10214-219.

160. Procopio A, Strizzi L, Vianale G, et al. Simian virus-40 sequences are a negative prognostic cofactor in patients with malignant pleural mesothelioma. Genes Chromosomes Cancer 2000;29,173-79.

161. Carbone M, Fisher S, Powers A, et al. New molecular and epidemiological issues in mesothelioma: Role of SV40. J Cell Physiol 1999;180,167-72.

162. Mossman BT, Gruenert DC. SV40, growth factors, and mesothelioma: Another piece of the puzzle. Am J Respir Cell Mol Biol 2002;26:167-70.

163. Pass HI, Pogrebniak HW. Malignant pleural mesothelioma. Curr Probl Surg 1993;30,921-1012.

164. Huang H, Reis R, Yonekawa Y, et al. Identification in human brain tumors of DNA sequences specific for SV40 large T antigen. Brain Pathol 1999;9,33-42.

165. Shivapurkar N, Wiethege T, Wistuba II, et al. Presence of simian virus 40 sequences in malignant mesotheliomas and mesothelial cell proliferations. J Cell Biochem 1999;76,181-88.

166. De Luca A, Baldi A, Esposito V, et al. The retinoblastoma gene family pRb/p105, p107, pRb2/p130 and simian virus-40 large T-antigen in human mesotheliomas. Nature Med 1997;3,913-16.

167. Papp T, Schipper H, Pemsel H, et al. Mutational analysis of N-ras, p53, p16^{INK4a}, p14^{ARF} and CDK4 genes in

primary human malignant mesotheliomas. Int J Oncol 2001;18,425-33.

168. Bianchi AB, Mitsunaga SI, Cheng JQ, et al. High frequency of inactivating mutations in the neurofibromatosis type 2 gene (NF-2) in primary malignant mesotheliomas. Proc Natl Acad Sci USA 1995;92,10854-58.

169. Roushdy-Hammady I, Siegel J, Emri S, et al. Genetic-susceptibility factor and malignant mesothelioma in the Cappadocian region of Turkey. Lancet 2001;357,444-45.

170. Jaurand MC, Fleury-Feith J. Pathogenesis of malignant pleural mesothelioma. Respirology 2005;10:2-8.

171. Ferri KF, Kroemer G. Organelle-specific initiation of cell death pathways. Nature Cell Biol 2001;3,E255-E263.

172. Bortner CD, Cidlowski JA. Cellular mechanisms for the repression of apoptosis. Annu Rev Pharmacol Toxicol 2002;42,259-81.

173. BeruBe KA, Quinlan TR, Fung H, et al. Apoptosis is observed in mesothelial cells after exposure to crocidolite asbestos. Am J Respir Cell Mol Biol 1996;15,141-47.

174. Broaddus VC, Yang L, Scavo LM, et al. Asbestos induces apoptosis of human and rabbit pleural mesothelial cells via reactive oxygen species. J Clin Invest 1996;98,2050-59.

175. Hoidal JR. Reactive oxygen species and cell signaling. Am J Respir Cell Mol Biol 2001;25,661-63.

176. Vaslet VA, Messier NJ, Kane AB. Accelerated progression of asbestos-associated mesotheliomas in heterozygous p53$^{+/-}$ mice. Toxicol Sci 2002;68,331-38.

177. Heintz NH, Janssen YM, Mossman BT. Persistent induction of c-fos and c-jun expression by asbestos. Proc Natl Acad Sci U S A 1993;90,3299-3303.

178. Sugarbaker DJ, Richards WG, Garcia JP. Extrapleural pneumonectomy for malignant mesothelioma. Adv Surg 1998;31,253-71

179. Ho L, Sugarbaker DJ, Skarin AT. Malignant pleural mesothelioma. Cancer Treat Res 2001;105,327-73.

180. King JA, Tucker JA. Evaluation of membranous staining of mesothelioma. Cell Vis 1998;5,24-27.

181. Ordónez NG. Value of calretinin immunostaining in differentiating epithelial mesothelioma from lung adenocarcinoma. Mod Pathol 1998;11,929-33.

182. Ordónez NG. Value of cytokeratin 5/6 immunostaining in distinguishing epithelial mesothelioma of the pleura from lung adenocarcinoma. Am J Surg Pathol 1998; 22,1215-21.

183. Oury TD, Hammar SP, Roggli VL. Ultrastructural features of diffuse malignant mesotheliomas. Hum Pathol 1998;29,1382-92.

184. Antman KH. Natural history and staging of malignant mesothelioma. Chest 1989;96(Suppl):93S-95S.

185. Aisner J. Therapeutic approach to malignant mesothelioma. Chest 1989;96(Suppl):95S-97S.

186. Jones RN. The diagnosis of asbestosis. Am Rev Respir Dis 1991;144:477-78.

187. Chang KC, Leung CC, Tam CM, Yu WC, Hui DS, Lam WK. Malignant mesothelioma in Hong Kong. Respir Med 2006:75-82.

188. Hillerdal G. Malignant mesothelioma 1982: Review of 4710 published cases. Br J Dis Chest 1983;77,321-43.

189. Boutin C, Schlesser M, Frenay C, et al. Malignant pleural mesothelioma. Eur Respir J 1998;12,972-81.

190. Mossman BT, Kamp DW, Weitzman SA. Mechanisms of carcinogenesis and clinical features of asbestos-associated cancers. Cancer Invest 1996;14,466-80.

191. Light R. Tumors of the pleura (2nd edn). Saunders. New York, NY 1994 .

192. Muller N. Imaging of the pleura. Radiology 1993; 186,297-309.

193. Beauchamp HD, Kundra NK, Aranson R, et al. The role of closed pleural needle biopsy in the diagnosis of malignant mesothelioma of the pleura. Chest 1992; 102,1110-12.

194. Boutin C, Rey F, Gouvernet J, et al. Thoracoscopy in pleural malignant mesothelioma: A prospective study of 188 consecutive patients; part 2. Prognosis and staging. Cancer 1993;72,394-404.

195. Wilsher ML, Veale AG. Medical thoracoscopy in the diagnosis of unexplained pleural effusion. Respirology 1998;3,77-80.

196. Kamp DW, Mossman BT. Asbestosis associated cancers: Clinical spectrum and pathogenic mechanisms. Clin Occup Environ Med 2002;2,753-57.

197. Shrager JSD, Kaiser L. Surgery and staging of mesothelioma. Martin Dunitz. London: UK 2002.

198. Herndon JE, Green MR, Chahinian AP, et al. Factors predictive of survival among 337 patients with mesothelioma treated between 1984 and 1994 by the Cancer and Leukemia Group B. Chest 1998;113,723-31.

199. Curran D, Sahmoud T, Therasse P, et al. Prognostic factors in patients with pleural mesothelioma: The European Organization for Research and Treatment of Cancer experience. J Clin Oncol 1998;16,145-52.

200. Edwards JG, Abrams KR, Leverment JN, et al. Prognostic factors for malignant mesothelioma in 142 patients: Validation of CALGB and EORTC prognostic scoring systems. Thorax 2000;55,731-35.

201. Bueno R, Appasani K, Mercer H, et al. The α folate receptor is highly activated in malignant pleural mesothelioma. J Thorac Cardiovasc Surg 2001;121(2),225-33.

202. Edwards JG, Faux SP, Plummer SM, et al. Cyclooxygenase-2 expression is a novel prognostic factor in malignant mesothelioma. Clin Cancer Res 2002;8,1857-62.

203. Soini Y, Jarvinen K, Kaarteenaho-Wiik R, et al. The expression of P-glycoprotein and multidrug resistance proteins 1 and 1 (MRP1 and MRP2) in human malignant mesothelioma. Ann Oncol 2001;12,1239-45.

204. Butchart EG, Ashcroft T, Barnsley WC, et al. Pleuropneumonectomy in the management of diffuse malignant mesothelioma of the pleura: Experience with 29 patients. Thorax 1976;31,15-24.

205. International Mesothelioma Interest Group. A proposed new international TNM staging system for malignant pleural mesothelioma. Chest 1995;108,1122-28.

206. Sugarbaker DJ, Strauss GM, Lynch TJ, Richards W, Mentzers SJ, Lee TH, et al. Nodec status has prognostic significance in the multimodality therapy of diffuse malignant mesothelioma. J Clin Oncol 1993;11:1172-78.

207. Heelan RT, Rusch VW, Begg CB, et al. Staging of malignant pleural mesothelioma: Comparison of CT and MR imaging. AJR Am J Roentgenol 1999;172,1039-47.

208. Melloni B, Monteil J, Vincent F, Bertin F, Gaillard S, Ducloux T, Verbeke S, Maubon A, Vandroux JC, Bonnaud F. Assessment of 18F-fluorodeoxyglucose dual-head gamma camera in asbestos lung diseases. Eur Respir J 2004;24:814-21.

209. Selikoff IJ, Hammond EC, Seidman H. Latency of asbestos disease among insulation workers in the United States and Canada. Cancer 1980;46,2736-40.

210. Sugarbaker DJ, Flores RM, Jaklitsch MT, et al. Resection margins, extrapleural nodal status, and cell type determine postoperative long-term survival in trimodality therapy of malignant pleural mesothelioma: Results in 183 patients. J Thorac Cardiovasc Surg 1999;117,54-65.

211. Rusch VW, Rosenzweig K, Venkatraman E, et al. A phase II trial of surgical resection and adjuvant high-dose hemithoracic radiation for malignant pleural mesothelioma. J Thorac Cardiovasc Surg 2001;122, 788-95.

212. Gordon W Jr, Antman KH, Greenberger JS, et al. Radiation therapy in the management of patients with mesothelioma. Int J Radiat Oncol Biol Phys 1982;8,19-25.

213. Viallat JR, Rey F, Astoul P, et al. Thoracoscopic talc poudrage pleurodesis for malignant effusions: A review of 360 cases. Chest 1996;110,1387-93.

214. Vogelzang NJ, Rusthoven J, Symanowski J, et al. A phase III study of pemetrexed in combination with cisplatin versus cisplatin alone in patients with malignant pleural mesothelioma. J Clin Oncol 2003; 21,2636-44.

215. Sugarbaker DJ, Richards WG, Garcia JP. Extrapleural pneumonectomy for malignant mesothelioma. Adv Surg 1998;31,253-71.

216. Butchart EG, Ashcroft T, Barnsley WC, et al. Pleuro-pneumonectomy in the management of diffuse malignant mesothelioma of the pleura: Experience with 29 patients. Thorax 1976;31,15-24.

217. Martinez-Moragón E, Aparico J, Rogado MC, et al. Pleurodesis in malignant pleural effusions: A randomized study of tetracycline versus bleomycin. Eur Respir J 1997;10,2380-83.

218. Yim APC, Chan ATC, Lee TW, et al. Thoracoscopic talc insufflation versus talc slurry for symptomatic malignant pleural effusion. Ann Thorac Surg 1996;62,1655-58.

219. Boutin C, Rey F, Viallat JR. Prevention of malignant seeding after invasive diagnostic procedures in patients with pleural mesothelioma: A randomized trial of local radiotherapy. Chest 1995;108,754-58.

220. Baas P. Chemotherapy for malignant mesothelioma: from doxorubicin to vinorelbine. Semin Oncol 2002; 29,62-69.

221. van Haarst JMW, Baas P, Manegold CH, et al. Multi-centre phase II study of gemcitabine and cisplatin in malignant pleural mesothelioma. Br J Cancer 2002; 86,342-45.

222. Schuette W. A phase II trial of gemcitabine/oxaliplatin combination chemotherapy in stage II-IV malignant pleural mesothelioma. Proc Am Soc Clin Oncol 2002; 21,334a.

223. Steele JPC, Shamash J, Evans MT, et al. Phase II trial of vinorelbine and oxaliplatin ('VO') in malignant pleural mesothelioma (MPM). Proc Am Soc Clin Oncol 2001; 20,335a

224. Halme M, Knuuttila A, Vehmas T, et al. High-dose methotrexate in combination with interferons in the treatment of malignant pleural mesothelioma. Br J Cancer 1999;80,1781-85.

225. Knuuttila A, Ollikainen T, Halme M, et al. Docetaxel and irinotecan (CPT-11) in the treatment of malignant pleural mesothelioma: A feasibility study. Anti-Cancer Drugs 2000;11,257-61.

226. Shih C, Chen VJ, Gossett LS, et al. LY231514, a pyrrolo[2,3-d]pyrimidine-based antifolate that inhibits multiple folate-requiring enzymes. Cancer Res 1997; 57,1116-23.

227. Adjei AA. Pemetrexed: A multitargeted antifolate agent with promising activity in solid tumors. Ann Oncol 2000;11,1335-41.

228. Calvert H, Bunn PA Jr. Future directions in the development of pemetrexed. Semin Oncol 2002; 29(suppl 5),54-61.

229. Rusthoven JJ, Eisenhauer E, Butts C, et al. Multitargeted antifolate LY231514 as first-line chemotherapy for patients with advanced non-small-cell lung cancer: A phase II study. J Clin Oncol 1999;17,1194-9.

230. Spielmann M, Martin M, Namer M, et al. Activity of pemetrexed (ALIMTA, multitargeted antifolate, LY231514) in metastatic breast cancer patients previously treated with an anthracycline and a taxane: An interim analysis. Clin Breast Cancer 2001;2,47-51.

231. John W, Picus J, Blanke CD, et al. Activity of multi-targeted antifolate (pemetrexed disodium, LY231514) in patients with advanced colorectal carcinoma: Results from a phase II study. Cancer 2000;88,1807-13.

232. Hanauske AR, Chen V, Paoletti P, et al. Pemetrexed disodium: A novel antifolate clinically active against multiple solid tumors. Oncologist 2001;6,363-73.

233. Thodtmann R, Depenbrock H, Dumez H, et al. Clinical and pharmacokinetic phase I study of multitargeted antifolate (LY231514) in combination with cisplatin. J Clin Oncol 1999;17,3009-16.

234. Hughes A, Calvert P, Azzabi A, et al. Phase I clinical and pharmacokinetic study of pemetrexed and carbo-platin in patients with malignant pleural mesothelioma. J Clin Oncol 2002;20,3533-44.

235. Niyikiza C, Baker SD, Seitz DE, et al. Homocysteine and methylmalonic acid: Markers to predict and avoid toxicity from pemetrexed therapy. Mol Cancer Ther 2002;1,545-52.

236. Calvert H. Folate status and the safety profile of antifolates. Semin Oncol 2002;29(suppl 5),3-7.

237. Scagliotti GV, Shin DM, Kindler HL, et al. Phase II study of pemetrexed with and without folic acid and vitamin B_{12} as front-line therapy in malignant pleural mesothelioma. J Clin Oncol 2003;21,1556-61.

238. Bunn P, Paoletti P, Niyikiza C, et al. Vitamin B_{12} and folate reduce toxicity of Alimta™ (pemetrexed disodium, LY231514, MTA), a novel antifolate/antimetabolite [abstract 300]. Proc Am Soc Clin Oncol 2001; 20,76a.

239. Paoletti P, Pistolesi M, Rusthoven JJ, et al. Correlation of pulmonary function tests with best tumor response status: Results from the phase III study of pemetrexed + cisplatin vs. cisplatin in malignant pleural mesothelioma [abstract 2651]. Proc Am Soc Clin Oncol 2003;22,659.

240. Pistolesi M, Symanowski J, Gatzemeier U, et al. Improving pulmonary function in patients with malignant pleural mesothelioma: Results of the phase III trial of pemetrexed + cisplatin vs cisplatin [abstract P-513]. Lung Cancer 2003;41(suppl 2),S220.

241. Mikulski SM, Costanzi JJ, Vogelzang NJ, et al. Phase II trial of a single weekly intravenous dose of ranpirnase in patients with unresectable malignant mesothelioma. J Clin Oncol 2002;20,274-81.

242. Vogelzang N, Taub R, Shin D, et al. Phase III randomized trial of onconase (ONC) vs doxorubicin (DOX) in patients (Pts) with unresectable malignant Mesothelioma (UMM): Analysis of survival [abstract 2274]. Proc Am Soc Clin Oncol 2000;19,577a.

243. Parra HS, Tixi L, Latteri F, et al. Combined regimen of cisplatin, doxorubicin, and γ-2b interferon in the treatment of advanced malignant pleural mesothelioma: A phase II multicenter trial of the Italian Group on Rare Tumors (GITR) and the Italian Lung Cancer Task Force (FONICAP). Cancer 2001;92,650-56.

244. Astoul P, Viallat JR, Laurent JC, et al. Intrapleural recombinant IL-2 in passive immunotherapy for malignant pleural effusion. Chest 1993;103,209-13.

245. Astoul P, Picat-Joossen D, Viallat JR, et al. Intrapleural administration of interleukin-2 for the treatment of patients with malignant pleural mesothelioma: A phase II study. Cancer 1998;83,2099-2104.

246. Prospects for an SV40 vaccine. Semin Cancer Biol 2001;11(1),81-85.

247. Kindler HL. Systemic therapy for malignant mesothelioma. American Society of Clinical Oncology 2002 educational book. Orlando, FL: American Society of Clinical Oncology, 38th Annual Meeting 2002;359-67.

248. Nowak AK, Lake RA, Kindler HL, et al. New approaches for mesothelioma: Biologics, vaccines, gene therapy, and other novel agents. Semin Oncol 2002;29, 82-96.

249. Govindan R, Kratzke RA, Herndon JE, et al. Gefitinib in patients with malignant mesothelioma (MM): A phase II study by the Cancer and Leukemia Group B (CALGB 30101). Proc Am Soc Clin Oncol 2003;22.

250. Millward M, Parnis F, Byrne M, et al. Phase II trial of imatinib mesylate in patients with advanced pleural mesothelioma [abstract 912]. Proc Am Soc Clin Oncol 2003;22.

251. Edwards JG, Faux SP, Plummer SM, et al. Cyclooxygenase-2 expression is a novel prognostic factor in malignant mesothelioma. Clin Cancer Res 2002;8, 1857-62.

252. Pass HI, Temeck BK, Kranda K, et al. Phase III randomized trial of surgery with or without intraoperative photodynamic therapy and postoperative immunotherapy for malignant pleural mesothelioma. Ann Surg Oncol 1997;48,628-33.

253. Steele JPC, Klabasta A, Fennel DA, Pallaska A, Sheaff MT, Evans MT, Shamash J, Rudd RM. Prognostic factors in mesothelioma. Lung Cancer 2005;49S1:S49-S52.

254. Kazan-Allen L. Asbestos and mesothelioma: Worldwide trends. Lung Cancer 2005;49S1:S3-S8.

255. Data from Government of India (2004). Health Information of India 2000-2001, Ministry of Health and Family Welfare; Government of India (2004), monthly statistics of foreign trade in India, volume I and II, Ministry of Commerce and Industry; Government of India (2003), Monthly abstract of Statistics. Ministry of Planning and Programme Implementation.

256. Dutta M, Sreedhar R, Basu A. The blighted hills of Roro, Jharkhand, India: A tale of corporate greed and abandonment. Int J Occup Environ Health 2003;9:254-59.

257. Joshi TK, Gupta RK. Asbestos-related morbidity in India. Int J Occup Environ Health 2003;9:249-53.

258. Subramanian V, Madhavan N. Asbestos problem in India. Lung Cancer 2005;49S1:S9-S12.

OTHER MINERAL PNEUMOCONIOSES

Other minerals that produce pneumoconioses are shown in the beginning.

BYSSINOSIS

Byssinosis was recognized and described in detail a half century ago, but the chronic effects of long-term exposure on workers' health have not been elucidated clearly.[1,2] Byssinosis includes a gradation of respiratory symptoms produced by exposure to cotton dust, flax, soft hemp, and to a lesser extent, sisal. The symptoms vary from acute dyspnea with cough and reversible breathlessness and chest tightness on one or more days of a working week to permanent respiratory disability due to irreversible airflow obstruction. Other symptoms, which are distinct from byssinosis, can occur due to exposure to cotton, flax or hemp and are referred to as *mill fever, weavers cough, and mattress makers fever*, respectively.[3-6]

Numerous studies have investigated the respiratory health effects of exposure to cotton dust.[7-11] The most conspicuous effects of exposure are clinical symptoms of bronchoconstriction together with a decline in expiratory flow over the work-shift. Byssinosis, characterized by a feeling of chest tightness on the first day of the working week that improves as week progresses, has been used to describe the acute and reversible response to exposure to cotton dust. The disease, however, may progress to a stage in which symptoms are present throughout the work week, and may eventually result in severe pulmonary disability as exposure continues.[7,8]

Previous cross sectional studies have reported a wide range in the prevalence of byssinosis. Length of exposure, cumulative or average dust concentration, past levels of dust exposure, and the "mill effect" that may be caused by grade of cotton, or degree of contamination with Gram negative microorganisms, have all been identified as possible causes of the development of byssinosis.[9-14] Gender, age, and ethnic group seem not to be important factors,[15] although gender and ethnicity may be associated with job and length of exposure. In some studies, smoking was found to be an important risk factor for byssinosis, but this has not been established clearly. Exposure to cotton dust has also been reported to be associated with chronic bronchitis, cough, and dyspnea, which are regarded as nonspecific respiratory symptoms.[10,16,17] A limited number of longitudinal studies have assessed the relation between long-term exposure to cotton dust and chronic changes in pulmonary function.[18-21] Fewer data exist with regard to the longitudinal occurrence of respiratory symptoms among populations occupationally exposed to cotton dust. A recent 15 year prospective follow-up study undertaken among a group of Chinese cotton textile workers reported that chronic exposure to cotton dust is related to both work specific and nonspecific respiratory symptoms. Byssinosis is more strongly associated with exposure to endotoxin than to dust. It was suggested that cessation of exposure may improve the respiratory health of cotton textile workers; the improvement appears to increase with time since last exposure.[22]

Few studies have estimated the incidence of byssinosis; most studies reported only prevalence. The prevalence of byssinosis varies widely in the literature on cotton textile workers, from 1.7 to 47 percent.[23,24] This inconsistency in the results can be explained, in part, by great differences in environmental dust levels, grade of cotton being used, and degree of contamination with Gram negative microorganisms, referred to as the "mill effect".[14] In addition, selection bias or healthy worker effect may operate more strongly in some studies. Another potential reason for varying estimates is different criteria for diagnosing byssinosis used in different countries and across studies, as there is no universally acceptable diagnostic criterion for byssinosis. In this study, we applied a more commonly used criterion—that is, typical first day or "Monday" symptoms to define byssinotics.[25]

The above mentioned 15 years follow-up study reported that the cumulative incidence over the 15 years was 24 percent for byssinosis and 23 percent for chest tightness. In other words, as many as 40 percent of the cotton workers experienced work specific disorders during this period, taking 8 percent overlap of the two symptoms into account. The true incidence of byssinosis in these workers might actually be higher since the analysis showed that continued participation depended on the absence of byssinosis. The authors also found that 11 percent and 9 percent of cotton workers reported byssinosis and chest tightness, respectively, in two or more surveys among those who took part in all of the four surveys, whereas 2 percent of silk workers reported chest tightness twice. Among those who missed at least one of the follow-up surveys, 15 percent of cotton workers reported byssinosis once and 4 percent twice; 20 percent reported chest tightness once and 4 percent twice. These proportions were also significantly higher in comparison with silk workers in whom 8 percent of the non-participants reported chest tightness once.[22]

Cotton fiber inhalation can cause diffuse lung disease, though rarely.[26] The clinical features of the disease were entirely different from those of byssinosis.

In India the scenario is slightly different. More than 20 million workers are involved in the textile industry, which is a dye dominant industry in India. In 1995 with interventions of a nongovernmental organization, byssinosis was first recorded in Indian history of 150 years textile industry. Out of 273 in whom the respiratory system was examined; 54 (30%) of the 179 individuals working in the dusty sections of a textile mill had byssinosis. In the nondusty departments, 16 (17%) out of the 94 workers were affected.[27] Similar study in Pondicherry reveals 6-fold risk of byssinosis among workers of spinning section and 2-fold increase among workers of weaving section.[28] In earlier studies, from Ahmedabad and Krishangarh, similar results have been reported.[29,30] In the study from Krishangarh, 616 cotton textile workers were studied; out of which 149 had byssinosis; 37 (24.7%) had grade-1/2, 78 (52.7%) grade-1, 25 (16.6%) grade-2 and 9 (6.0%) of grade-3 byssinosis. Majority of the byssinotics were of age group between 36 to 40 years and had developed disease after 16 years of exposure. Disease was more common among smokers and severe, in whom consumption was more than 15 cigarettes/bidis per day for more than 10 years. Ventilatory function tests were markedly abnormal compared with nonbyssinotic. On clinical examination and laboratory investigation (specially eosinophilia) and, radiological investigation (X-ray chest) no positive finding was detected. The high prevalence rate of the disease in this study was apparently due to poor working conditions of the workers.[29] In another epidemiological study carried out in three textile mills at Ahmedabad, 929 workers were examined from the spinning departments. The mean prevalence of byssinosis in the blow section was 29.62 percent, whereas in the card section it was 37.83 percent. The concentrations of cotton dust (dust less fly) were high in the blow and card sections (4.00 mg/m^3 in the blow and 3.06 mg/m^3 in the card section). This study suggests that the prevalence of byssinosis is not low in the textile mills of India as reported in many earlier Indian studies.[30] In another study, multiple logistic regression model was used considering byssinosis as an independent variable, and dustiness, smoking, exposure years and age as explanatory variables. Dustiness and length of exposure to the dust were found to be the most important contributory factors to byssinosis prevalence. The risk of byssinosis among workers in card room, blow room and waste plant sections and those who had exposure of more than 5 years was nearly three times than that among workers of other sections of the mill and/or with less than 5 years of exposure.[31] Although byssinosis in jute mill workers remains controversial, studies in a few jute mills in West-Bengal, revealed typical byssinotic syndrome associated with acute changes in FEV_1 on the first working day after rest. A study on 148 jute mill workers revealed work related respiratory symptoms. Further, acute and chronic pulmonary function changes studied among exposed workers on the basis of standard questionnaire and spirometric method along with dust level, particle mass size distributions and gram-negative bacterial endotoxins showed typical byssinotic symptoms along with acute post shift FEV_1 changes (31.8%) and chronic changes in FEV_1 (43.2%) among exposed workers. The group with higher exposure showed significantly lower FVC, FEV_1, PEFR and FEF25-75 percent values. Size distribution showed that about 70 to 80 percent dust in

diameter of < 10 micron, 40 to 50 percent, < 5 micron and 10 to 20 percent, < 2 micron. Mean endotoxin levels found in hatching, spinning and weaving, and beaming were 2.319 microg/m^3, 0.956 microg/m^3, 0.041 microg/m^3 respectively and are comparable to the values obtained up to date in Indian cotton mills. Respiratory morbidity study reported The study thus revealed the findings of the earlier studies and clearly indicated that the Indian jute mill workers are also suffering from byssinosis as observed in cotton, flask and hemp workers.[32] Thus, in developing countries, the problem of byssinosis may be more.[33]

OCCUPATION

The chief source of cotton dust production occur (i) in the 'ginnery' where seeds are removed from cotton after picking in a special machine, called the gin; (ii) in the 'mixing room' during opening of bales of cotton; (iii) in the 'blow room' where the cotton is thrashed and blown to eliminate dust and undesirable fibers; (iv) in the 'card room' where carding machines comb the fibers and remove dirt and defective material; (v) during stripping, which consist of removing dust and cotton fibers adherent to the wire teeth of the carding engine, and (vi) during grinding or sharpening the teeth.

Flax is used to produce linen. Opening the bales, hackling, carding and spinning of flax produce dust, and particularly carding are very dusty.

Soft hemp, a stem fiber, is mainly used for production of rope and yarn. Batting and hackling are very dusty procedures, which are harmful and can produce byssinosis.

Sisal is used to produce ropes. Decorticating and brushing the leaves, produce a lot of dust. Similarly, bailing and carding are dusty procedures.

Various occupations where one can be exposed to cotton dust are the following:

Agriculture

- Cotton ginning
- Classing
- Cotton compresses and warehouses
- Cotton seed oil mills.

Yarn Manufacturing

- Broad woven fabric mills, cotton
- Broad woven fabric mills, fiber, silk
- Circular knit fabric mills
- Yarn spinning mills
- Texurizing, throwing, twisting and winding mills.

Thread Mills

- Tire cord and fabric.

Fabric Manufacturing

- Broad woven fabric mills, cotton
- Broad woven fabric mills, man made-fiber, silk
- Narrow fabrics
- Knitting mills.

Textile Waste

- Paddings and upholstery fillings
- Processed waste
- Mattresses and bedsprings.

Pathogenesis

Although a number of hypotheses have been advocated to explain the pathogenesis of byssinosis, mainly there are three mechanisms: (a) *Pharmacological theory*; (b) *Microorganism etiology*; and (c) *Immunological mechanisms*. The mechanism by which cotton and other fibers produce airways obstruction is not clear. A number of hypotheses are put forth. They are: nonimmunologic local release of histamine, an antigen-antibody reaction, bacterial toxins, and fungus enzymes. Byssinosis can be considered as a form of extrinsic asthma produced by exposure to the above substances in some individuals. Bract, the leaf likes structure, which enfolds the cotton ball and the wood fragments are the most friable and produce the most respirable particles. They contain a large range of chemicals including carbohydrates, proteins, lipids, amines, lignins, tannins, phenolic pigments, terpenes, terpenoid alcohols, carbonyl compounds, and epoxides. Many bacteria, fungi, and many fragments of other plants and soil are also present. The active sensitizing agent or agents are contained in the bract, and produce byssinosis.

Endotoxin is derived from Gram-negative bacterial membranes, and its inflammatory effects following inhalation are well characterized. The significance of this fact becomes apparent when the wide-ranging environments containing high levels of this microbial product are considered. Endotoxin is present in numerous industrial environments, especially where organic fibers are processed. Microbial contamination of these fibers mainly occurs at the agricultural stage. Materials such as flax and hemp are affected in this way, but the most important product in this context is cotton, from which chronic dust inhalation causes the disease byssinosis.[34-37]

Pathology

The classical descriptions of lung pathology in byssinosis have been those of nonspecific chronic bronchitis and emphysema. The histopathological features characteristic of byssinosis is mucus gland hyperplasia and infiltration of neutrophils into the bronchi.[38,39] There may also be eosinophilic infiltration (reflecting allergy) in the biopsy specimens. "Byssinosis bodies" have been described. These bodies are essentially consist of a core of black dust surrounded by yellowish material which stains positive for iron. These bodies are oval or round and can be up to 10 microns in size. Right ventricular hypertrophy and changes of cor pulmonale are present in a number of cases. There have been only a few reports of pulmonary fibrosis and pneumoconiosis due to organic dust.[26,40-43]

Clinical Features

The hall mark of byssinosis is chest tightness that is experienced on the first day of the work after an weekend after being away for work. The most common respiratory symptom is chest tightness (20.3%). About a third will have symptoms on the 1st day of the week, and the rest will have symptoms on all days of the week. An acute effect may be seen in 53.6 percent of the workers with byssinosis.[44] The "Monday feeling" consists of chest tightness occurring on some Mondays or on the first day back at work, Subsequently, breathlessness, fatigue, and cough occurs on each Monday and cease completely on Tuesdays. Acute symptoms occur in the afternoons, although in severe cases they occur few hours after work. Symptoms may be more severe in smokers. Wheezing may be present in some cases.

The clinical stages of byssinosis are subdivided into 4 grades on clinical grounds and are as follows:[45]

Grade 0   No symptoms of chest tightness or breathlessness on Mondays

Grade ½   Occasional chest tightness and/or difficulty in breathing or mild symptoms such as irritation of the respiratory system on Mondays (each first day only of the working week).

Grade 1   Chest tightness and/or difficulty in breathing on Mondays only (the first working day).

Grade 2   Chest tightness and/or difficulty in breathing on Mondays and other days.

Subsequently, these grades were modified as follows:

Grade C0   Occasional chest tightness on the first day of the working week.

Grade C1   Chest tightness and/or difficulty in breathing on each first day only of the working week.

Grade C2   Chest tightness and/or difficulty in breathing on the first and other days of the working week.

Grade C3 Symptoms of Grade C2 with evidence of permanent respiratory disability from reduced ventilatory capacity.

C, denotes Clinical grading to distinguish from functional grading.

Grade C3 byssinosis and chronic obstructive bronchitis are often associated, although at this stage it is difficult to separate the two. There may not be, any abnormal finding on physical examination, although scattered rhonchi may be heard in some.

Various other nonspecific symptoms described are the irritation of the eyes, mucous membranes, sneezing and hoarseness as cotton dust is an irritant. Dry cough and exertional dyspnea can be experienced. New workers and those who go to the cotton processing area for a few hours may experience "mill fever" – otherwise called as weavers fever, card room fever, dust chills, dust fever, cotton cold, cotton fever and flax workers as heckling fever. Symptoms that occurs within 12 hrs of exposure consist of chill, rigor, headache, thirst, malaise, thirsting, nausea, and vomiting, with transient fever. With repeated exposures these symptoms may be repeated till the person is seasoned and develops tolerance. Tobacco intolerance may be experienced by some. A second group of febrile syndromes associated with cotton dust exposure include Mattress makers fever or weavers cough. These occur in more experienced workers and consist of fever, chronic cough and dyspnea and is thought to be due to an endotoxin of *Aerobacter cloacae*.

The early symptoms may be stopped if the worker is removed from the source of fiber exposure. The progression to higher stages is variable. In some it does not proceed, while in others respiratory disability occurs within a few years. Some experience no symptom of respiratory airway obstruction. These variations largely depend on the smoking habit of the individual.

Diagnosis

Lung Function Tests

A decreasing lung function, and increasing airway responsiveness are early pulmonary responses to cotton dust. In addition, the occurrence of respiratory symptoms and increasing airway responsiveness, as well as atopy, may be important predictors for acute changes in lung function among cotton textile workers. A gradual reduction in FEV_1, FVC, MMFR, occurs in cases of byssinosis. There is an increase in the airway resistance and closing volume. Earlier changes include small airways obstruction. The most practical tests for routine use in the industry are FEV_1 and PEFR.[46-51]

The acute effects of dust can be determined by measuring FEV_1 before and at the end of a working shift on the first working day after a period away from work. A functional grading is based on the difference between these values and is shown below. An FEV_1 of less than 80 percent predicted is taken as abnormal. The bronchodilator test should be carried out if an abnormal result is obtained. The functional grades are as follows:

Grade FO   No demonstrable acute effect of the dust on ventilatory capacity and no evidence of chronic ventilatory impairment

Grade $F^{1/2}$ Slight acute effect of dust. No chronic ventilatory impairment

Grade Fl   Moderate acute reduction of ventilatory function

Grade F2   Slight to moderate irreversible ventilatory impairment

Grade F3   Moderate to severe irreversible ventilatory impairment

F denotes functional grading.

A more detailed classification is as follows in Table 27.6:[52]

Chest X-ray is usually normal or associated changes of emphysema may be seen.

Ideally, the diagnosis of byssinosis depends upon (i) a history of industrial exposure to cotton, flax, or soft hemp dust; (ii) a typical history of the various clinical grades; and (iii) fall in FEV_1 or MMFR during the working day or the working week.

Treatment

Workers with Grades Cl and C3 byssinosis should be removed from areas of dust exposure. The use of drugs like antihistamines, salbutamol, beclomethasone, and sodium cromoglycate are necessary for symptomatic patients. However, drugs are no substitute for prevention.

Prevention of byssinosis depends upon both engineering and medical methods of dust control. The most effective method is the replacement of the natural fibers by synthetic ones. Water washing reduces dust production significantly during carding. General ventilation should be adequate with recirculated air, which must be adequately filtered. Workers in areas of high dust production should use efficient respirators. Spraying of ripening cotton with bactericides and fungicides, and treatment of raw cotton with gaseous hydrogen chloride or acetic acid have been found to inactivate the active components in cotton bracts and dusts.

In early studies, research to control byssinosis focused on methods to reduce the trash in the textile mill

TABLE 27.6: Classification of byssinosis

Functional severeity	FEV$_1$ (%) predicted	FEV$_1$ (% changes)*	Interpretation of FEV$_1$	Reccomodation for employment
F0	> 80 No evidence of ventilatory impairment	a. −4 to 0, or more; effect of dust on ventilatory function	a. Minimal or no acute	No change; annual FEV$_1$ and questionnaire
		b. − 5 to −9 or more	b. Moderate acute effect of dust on ventilatory function;	No change; biannual FEV$_1$ and questionnaire
		c. −10 or more	c. Definite and marked acute effect of dust on ventilatory function;	Move to low risk area and biannual FEV$_1$ and questionnaire
F1	60-79 (Evidence of mild to moderate irreversible ventilatory impairement)	a. −4 to 0, or more	As (a) above	No change; biannual FEV$_1$ and questionnaire
		b. − 5 or more	As (b) above	Move to low risk area; biannual FEV$_1$ and questionnaire
F2	< 60 (Evidence of moderate to severe irreversible ventilatory impairment)	— —	—	Work requiring no cotton dust exposure, detailed pulmonary function assessment and questionnaire

* *Difference between FEV$_1$ before and after 6+ hrs of cotton dust exposure on a first working day.*

environment. Dust control has been effective in reducing the prevalence of byssinosis, but simple reduction in dust levels does not always assure its prevention. Also, bacteria and fungi present in cotton do not in themselves cause byssinosis, but the endotoxins-heat-stable lipopolysaccharide-protein complexes contained in the cell wall of Gram-negative bacteria are responsible for the development of this respiratory disease of workers on cotton, flax, and some other fibers. Recently experimental work was carried out in cotton fields in different cotton growing countries. Opened cotton capsules were treated by spraying them with bactericidal water solutions of benzododecinium bromide to avoid the growth of bacteria by bacteriostatic effect during transportation and storage and thus to prevent the formation of endotoxins. To simulate transport conditions, treated and nontreated cotton samples were incubated under high air humidity. The endotoxin contents were determined by Limulus amebocyte lysate assay depending on the duration of incubation. In nontreated samples the endotoxin content grew to over 5,000 ng/mg. In comparison, in treated samples the endotoxin content grew extremely slowly. Thus, the bactericidal treating of raw cotton showed high efficiency as a potential method of byssinosis prevention. The irradiation by γ-rays is also efficient, but it is not realistic in cotton growing areas of developing countries at the present time.[53]

Medical surveillance of worker like pre-employment examination and periodic examination should be carried out. Pre-employment examination will exclude atopic subjects and smokers and persons with chronic respiratory problems from working in dusty areas. Periodic medical examination will help in detecting early stages of the disease including deterioration of lung function parameters.

REFERENCES

1. Schilling RS. Byssinosis in cotton and other textile workers. Lancet 1956;2:261-65.
2. Schilling RS, Vigliani EC, Lammers B, Valic F, Gilson JC. A report on a conference on byssinosis. 1963; Int Congr Series No 62, Amsterdam, 1963, Excerpta Medica. pp 137.
3. Bouhuys A, Gilson JC, Schilling RSF. Byssinosis in the textile industry. Arch Environ Health 1970;21:475-78.
4. Lee WR. Clinical diagnosis of byssinosis. Thorax 1979;34:287.
5. Morgan WK, Vesterlund J, Burrel R, Gee JB, Willoughby WF, et al. Byssinosis: Some unanswered questions. Am Rev Respir Dis1982;126:354-57.
6. Lee WR, Stretton TB. Byssinosis: A disease or a symptom? Thorax 1986;41:1-4.
7. Bouhuys A, Beck GJ, Shoenberg JB. Priorities in prevention of chronic lung disease. Lung 1979;156:129-48.
8. Tockman JA, Baser M. Is cotton dust exposure associated with chronic effects? Am Rev Respir Dis 1984;130:1-3.

9. Schilling RSF. Epidemiological studies of chronic respiratory disease among cotton operatives. Yale J Biol Med 1964;37:55-74.

10. Berry G, Molyneux MKB, Tombleson JBL. Relationships between dust level and byssinosis and bronchitis in Lancashire cotton mills. Br J Ind Med 1974;31:18-27.

11. Imbus HR, Suh MW. Byssinosis. A study of 10,133 textile workers. Arch Environ Health 1973;26:183-91.

12. Wang XR, Pan LD, Zhang HX, et al. Follow-up study of respiratory health of newly-hired female cotton textile workers. Am J Ind Med 2002;41:111-18.

13. Jones RN, Diem JE, Glindmeyer H. Mill effect and dose-response relationships in byssinosis. Br J Ind Med 1979;36:305-13.

14. Glindmeyer HW, Lefante JJ, Jones RN, et al. Exposure-related declines in the lung function of cotton textile workers. Relationship to current workplace standards. Am Rev Respir Dis 1991;144:675-83.

15. Fishwick D, Fletcher AM, Pickering CAC, et al. Respiratory symptoms and dust exposure in Lancashire cotton and man-made fiber mill operatives. Am J Respir Crit Care Med 1994;150:441-47.

16. Bouhuys A, Shoenberg JB, Beck GJ, et al. Epidemiology of chronic lung disease in a cotton mill community. Lung 1977;154:167-86.

17. Christiani DC, Eisen EA, Wegman DH, et al. Respiratory disease in cotton textile workers in the People's Republic of China. I. Respiratory symptoms. Scand J Work Environ Health 1986;12:40-45.

18. Berry G, Mckerrow CB, Molyneux MKB, et al. A study of the acute and chronic changes in ventilatory capacity of workers in Lancashire cotton mills. Br J Ind Med 1973;30:25-36.

19. Larson RK, Barman ML. A longitudinal study of pulmonary function in cotton gin workers in the San Joaquin Valley. Chest 1989;96:819-23.

20. Zuskin E, Valic F. Change in the respiratory response to coarse cotton dust over a ten-year period. Am Rev Respir Dis 1995;112:417-21.

21. Christiani DC, Ye TT, Wegman DH, et al. Cotton dust exposure, across-shift drop in FEV_1, and five-year change in lung function. Am J Respir Crit Care Med 1994;150:1250-55.

22. Wang XR, Eisen EA, Zhang HX, Sun BX, Dai HL, Pan LD, Wegman DH, Olenchock SA, Christiani DC. Respiratory symptoms and cotton dust exposure; Results of a 15 year follow up observation. Occupational and Environmental Medicine 2003;60:935-41.

23. Jiang CQ, Lam TH, Kong C, et al. Byssinosis in Guangzhou, China. Occup Environ Med 1995;52:268-72.

24. Zuskin E, Ivankovic D, Schachter EN, et al. A ten-year follow-up study of cotton textile workers. Am Rev Respir Dis 1991;143:301-05.

25. Schilling RSF, Vigiliani EC, Lammers B, et al. A report on a conference on byssinosis. Proceedings of the 14th International Congress on Occupational Health, Madrid, Spain 1963:137-45.

26. Kobayashi H, Kanoh S, Motoyoshi K, Aida S. Diffuse lung disease caused by cotton fibre inhalation but distinct from byssinosis. Thorax 2004;59:1095-97.

27. Murlidhar V, Murlidhar VJ, Kanhere V. Byssinosis in a Bombay textile mill. Natl Med J India 1995;8:204-07.

28. Mishra AK, Rotti SB, Sahai A, Madanmohan, Narayan KA. Byssinosis among male textile workers in Pondicherry: A case-control study. Natl Med J India 2003;16:70-73.

29. Barjatiya MK, Mathur RN, Swaroop A. Byssinosis in cotton textile workers of Kishangarh. Indian J Chest Dis Allied Sci 1990;32:215-23.

30. Parikh JR, Bhagia LJ, Majumdar PK, Shah AR, Kashyap SK. Prevalence of byssinosis in textile mills at Ahmedabad, India. Br J Ind Med 1989;46:787-90.

31. Mathur N, Gupta BN, Rastogi SK. Multivariate analysis of byssinosis risk assessment. Indian J Chest Dis Allied Sci 1993;35:185-90.

32. Chattopadhyay BP, Saiyed HN, Mukherjee AK. Byssinosis among jute mill workers. Ind Health. 2003;41:265-72.

33. Parikh JR. Byssinosis in developing countries. Br J Ind Med 1992;49:217-19.

34. Castellan RM, Olenchock SA, Kinsley KB, et al. Inhaled endotoxin and decreased spirometric values. An exposure-response relation for cotton dust. N Engl J Med 1987;317:605-10.

35. Rylander R, Haglind P, Lundholm M. Endotoxin in cotton dust and respiratory function decrement among cotton workers in an experimental cardamom. Am Rev Repir Dis 1985;131:209-13.

36. Hang J, Zhou W, Wang X, Zhang H, Sun B, Dai H, Su L, Christiani DC. Microsomal epoxide hydrolase, endotoxin, and lung function decline in cotton textile workers. Am J Respir Crit Care Med 2005; 171:165-70.

37. Lane SR, Nicholls PJ, Sewell RD. The measurement and health impact of endotoxin contamination in organic dusts from multiple sources: Focus on the cotton industry. Inhal Toxicol 2004;16:217-29.

38. Rooke GB. The pathology of byssinosis. International conference on byssinosis. Chest 1981;79 (Suppl) :67s-71s.

39. Edwards C, McCartney J, Rooke G, et al. The pathology of the lung in byssinotics. Thorax 1975;30:612-23.

40. Sano T. Pathology and pathogenesis of organic dust pneumoconiosis (Japanese). J Sci Labour 1967;43:3-18.

41. Abe A, Ishikawa T. Studies on pneumoconiosis caused by organic dusts (Japanese). J Sci Labour 1967;43:19-41.

42. Ruttner JR, Spycher MA, Engeler ML. Pulmonary fibrosis induced by cotton fiber inhalation. Path Microbiol (Basel) 1968;32:1-14.

43. Eschenbacher WL, Kreiss K, Lougheed MD, et al. Nylon flock-associated interstitial lung disease. Am J Respir Crit Care Med 1999;159:2003-08.

44. Altin R, Ozkurt S, Fisekci F, Cimrin AH, Zencir M, Sevinc C. Prevalence of byssinosis and respiratory symptoms among cotton mill workers. Respiration. 2002;69:52-56.

45. Schilling RSF. Byssinosis in the British cotton mill industry. Br med J 1950;17:52-56.
46. Krzyzanowski M, Camilli AE, Lebovitz MD. Relationship between pulmonary function and changes in chronic respiratory symptoms. Chest 1990;98:62-70.
47. Rylander R, Haglind P, Lundholm M. Endotoxin in cotton dust and respiratory function decrement among cotton workers in an experimental cardamom. Am Rev Repir Dis 1985;131:209-13.
48. Schwartz DA, Donham KJ, Olenchock SA, et al. Determinants of longitudinal changes in spirometric function among swine confinement operators and farmers. Am J Respir Crit Care Med 1995;151:47-53.
49. Castellan RM, Olenchock SA, Kinsley KB, et al. Inhaled endotoxin and decreased spirometric values. An exposure-response relation for cotton dust. N Engl J Med 1987;317:605-10.
50. Christiani DC, Ye TT, Wegman DH, Eisen EA, Dai HL, Lu PL. Pulmonary function among cotton textile workers. A study of variability in symptom reporting, across-shift drop in FEV1, and longitudinal change. Chest 1994;105:1713-21.
51. Wang XR, Pan LD, Zhang HX, Sun BX, Dai HL, Christiani DC. A longitudinal observation of early pulmonary responses to cotton dust. Occup Environ Med 2003;60:115-21.
52. Merchant JA. Byssinosis. Occupational Respiratory Diseases. DHHS (NIOSH), September 1986;86-102,http://www.cdc.gov/niosh/86-102.html.
53. Hend IM, Milnera M, Milnera SM. Bactericidal treatment of raw cotton as the method of byssinosis prevention. AIHA J (Fairfax, Va). 2003;64:88-94.

OTHER PNEUMOCONIOSES

1. CHRONIC BERYLLIUM DISEASE (CBD)/ BERYLLIOSIS

Beryllium is a ubiquitous element in the environment, and it has many commercial applications. Because of its strength, electrical and thermal conductivity, corrosion resistance, and nuclear properties, beryllium products are used in the aerospace, automotive, energy, medical, and electronics industries. What eventually came to be known as chronic beryllium disease (CBD) was first identified in the 1930s, when a cluster of cases was observed in workers from the fluorescent light industry.[1-4]

The potential hazards from exposure to beryllium or beryllium compounds in the workplace were first reported in the 1930s. Chronic beryllium disease is a granulomatosis mimicking sarcoidosis that predominantly affects the lungs and is due to a hypersensitivity response to beryllium. Exposure to beryllium results in beryllium sensitization, or development of a beryllium-specific, cell-mediated immune response, in 2 to

19 percent of exposed individuals. The physicochemical properties of beryllium (Be) are crucial for high technology industries. The inhalation of beryllium may cause, in certain individuals, a specific sensitization (BeS) and lead, in some of them, to a pulmonary granulomatosis called chronic pulmonary berylliosis (CPB) or chronic beryllium disease—an illness affecting from 2 to 5 percent of workers exposed to beryllium and its compounds. Sensitization usually precedes the development of the scarring lung disease, chronic beryllium disease. The development of granulomatous inflammation in patients with CBD is associated with the production of numerous inflammatory cytokines, including IFN-γ, IL-2, and TNF-α. In some individuals this can result in increased granulomatous inflammation and a more severe form of the disease. Although the exposure response relationship in sensitization and disease is nonlinear, in some studies, higher exposures were associated with higher rates of sensitization and CBD. Machinists usually have higher levels of beryllium exposure and increased risk of developing sensitization and disease. The impact of the physicochemical properties of beryllium, such as form, solubility, and particle size, on the risk of sensitization and disease are less well understood. It is clear from numerous studies that genetic susceptibility affects risk of beryllium-related health effects. The role of HLA-DPB1 Glu69 in the proliferative response to beryllium and risk of sensitization has been the best studied. Some genes, such as Glu69, are important in the development of an antigen-specific, cell-mediated immune response to beryllium or sensitization, whereas others may be important in the development of beryllium-specific granulomatous inflammation or CBD. Two copies of the Glu69 gene may be a disease-specific genetic risk factor. The TNF-α-308 A variant is associated with beryllium-stimulated TNF-α production, which, in turn, is associated with more severe CBD. Whether the TNF-α-308 A is a genetic risk factor in CBD, sensitization, or more severe disease still needs to be determined. It is likely that sensitization and CBD are multigenetic processes, and that these genes interact with exposure to determine risk of disease. However, current genetic markers are not ready for clinical use as a screening test for beryllium-related health effects because of the low specificity of the markers and the low prevalence of BeS and CBD.[5-9] There is growing evidence provided by epidemiological and toxicological studies that chronic beryllium toxicity is also carcinogenic.[10]

"Sarcoidosis"-like syndrome, usually limited to the lungs, may result from exposure to bioaerosols and a number of metals. Exposure to beryllium in the workplace produces a granulomatous lung disease clinically indistinguishable from sarcoidosis, chronic beryllium disease (CBD). Beryllium's ability to produce a beryllium-specific immune response is used in the beryllium lymphocyte proliferation tests to confirm a diagnosis of CBD and exclude sarcoidosis. Exposure to other metals must also be considered in the differential diagnosis of sarcoidosis.[11]

The tritiated thymidine beryllium lymphocyte proliferation test (BeLPT) is an *in vitro* blood test that is widely used to screen beryllium-exposed workers for sensitivity to beryllium. The clinical significance of the BeLPT was described and a standard protocol was developed in the late 1980s. Cell proliferation is measured by the incorporation of tritiated thymidine into dividing cells on two culture dates and using three concentrations of beryllium sulfate. Results are expressed as a 'stimulation index' (SI), which is the ratio of the amount of tritiated thymidine (measured by beta counts) in the simulated cells divided by the counts for the unstimulated cells on the same culture day. Several statistical methods for use in the routine analysis of the BeLPT were proposed in the early 1990s. The least absolute values (LAV) method was recommended for routine analysis of the BeLPT. This report further evaluates the LAV method using new data, and proposes a new method for identification of an abnormal or borderline test. This new statistical-biological positive (SBP) method reflects the clinical judgment that: (i) at least two SIs show a 'positive' response to beryllium; and (ii) that the maximum of the six SIs must exceed a cut-point that is determined from a reference data set of normal individuals whose blood has been tested by the same method in the same serum.[12]

The blood beryllium lymphocyte proliferation test is used in medical surveillance to identify both beryllium sensitization and chronic beryllium disease. Approximately 50 percent of individuals with beryllium sensitization have chronic beryllium disease at the time of their initial clinical evaluation.

Treatment

Chronic beryllium disease shares many of its characteristics with sarcoidosis and is often treated with corticosteroids. The response to long-term corticosteroids in CBD, quite like that in sarcoidosis, is variable. Significant lung function improvement may be seen following cessation of beryllium exposure.[13]

Prevention

The primary beryllium industry has generated a large amount of data on airborne beryllium concentrations that has been used to characterize exposure by task-specific activities, job category, individual worker, and processing area using a variety of methods. These methods have included high-volume breathing zone sampling, high-volume process sampling, high- and low-volume respirable and area sampling, real-time monitoring, and personal sampling. Many of the beryllium studies have used these air sampling methods to assess inhalation exposure and chronic beryllium disease (CBD) risk to beryllium; however, available data do not show a consistent dose-response relationship between airborne concentrations of beryllium and the incidence of CBD. The US Atomic Energy Commission recommended the first 8 hour occupational exposure limit (OEL) for beryllium of 2.0 μ/m^3 in 1949, which was later reviewed and accepted by the American Conference of Governmental Industrial Hygienists (ACGIH), the American Industrial Hygiene Association (AIHA), the American National Standards Institute (ANSI), the Occupational Safety and Health Administration (OSHA), and the vast majority of countries and standard-setting bodies worldwide. The 2.0 μg/m^3 standard has been in use by the beryllium industry for more than 50 years and has been considered adequate to protect workers against clinical CBD. Recently, improved diagnostic techniques, including immunological testing and safer bronchoscopy, have enhanced our ability to identify subclinical CBD cases that would have formerly remained unidentified. Some recent epidemiological studies have suggested that some workers may develop CBD at exposures less than 2.0 μg/m^3. ACGIH is currently reevaluating the adequacy of the current 2.0 μg/m^3 guideline, and a plethora of research initiatives are under way to provide a better understanding of the cause of CBD. The research is focusing on the risk factors and exposure metrics that could be associated with CBD, as well as on efforts to better characterize the natural history of CBD. There is growing evidence that particle size and chemical form may be important factors that influence the risk of developing CBD. These research efforts are expected to provide data that will help identify a scientifically based OEL that will protect workers against CBD.[14,15] Studies of beryllium workers are often not directly comparable because they use a variety of exposure assessment methods that are not necessarily representative of individual worker exposures, and rarely considered respirator use, and have not evaluated changes in work practices. It appears that the current exposure metric for beryllium, total beryllium mass, may not be an appropriate measurement to predict the risk of CBD. Other exposure metrics such as mass of respirable particles, chemical form, and particle surface chemistry may be more related to the prevalence of CBD than total mass of airborne beryllium mass. In addition, assessing beryllium exposure by all routes of exposure (e.g. inhalation, dermal uptake, and ingestion) rather than only inhalation exposure in future studies may prove useful.[16]

In a recent study, a cohort of beryllium-sensitized patients were monitored at 2 year intervals, using bronchoalveolar lavage and repeated transbronchial lung biopsies to determine progression to chronic beryllium disease as evidenced by granulomatous inflammation in lung tissue. Fifty-five individuals with beryllium sensitization were monitored with a range of 2 to 5 clinical evaluations. Disease developed in 17 sensitized individuals (31%) within an average follow-up period of 3.8 years (range, 1.0-9.5 years). Thirty-eight of the 55 (69%) remained beryllium sensitized without disease after an average follow-up time of 4.8 years (range, 1.7-11.6 years). Progressors were more likely to have worked as machinists. The authors found no difference in average age, sex, race or ethnicity, smoking status, or beryllium exposure time between those who progressed to chronic beryllium disease and those who remained sensitized without disease. They conclude that beryllium sensitization is an adverse health effect in beryllium-exposed workers and merits medical follow-up.[17] People exposed to beryllium should be screened routinely for sensitization. Current and former construction workers are also at significant risk for occupational illnesses from work at the nuclear weapons facilities and should be screened regularly.[18]

Little is known about the physicochemical properties of beryllium aerosols associated with increased risk of beryllium sensitization and chronic beryllium disease (CBD). Such information is needed to evaluate whether airborne mass of beryllium is the appropriate metric of exposure or alternatively to provide a scientific basis for using information on particle size, surface area, and chemistry to support an improved exposure limit based on bioavailability through the inhalation and dermal routes of exposure.[19]

REFERENCES

1. Jones-Williams W. A histological study of the lungs in 52 cases of chronic beryllium disease. Br J Ind Med 1958;15:84-91.
2. Hardy HL. Beryllium disease: A continuing diagnostic problem. AmJ Med Sci 1961;142:150-56.
3. Hardy HL, Stoekle JD. Beryllium disease. Chron Dis 1959;9:152-60.
4. Van Ordstrand HS. Diagnosis of beryllium disease. Arch Ind Health 1959;19:157.
5. Rossman MD, Kreider ME. Is chronic beryllium disease sarcoidosis of known etiology? Sarcoidosis Vasc Diffuse Lung Dis 2003;20:104-09.
6. Maier LA. Genetic and exposure risks for chronic beryllium disease. Clin Chest Med 2002;23:827-39.
7. Maier L, Martyny J, Mroz M, McGrath D, Lympany P, duBois R, Zhang L, Murphy J, Newman LS. Genetic and environmental risk factors in Beryllium sensitization and chronic Beryllium disease. Chest 2002;121:81S.
8. Marchand-Adam S, Valeyre D. Chronic pulmonary berylliosis: A model of interaction between environment and genetic predisposition (Part 1). Mineralogy, toxicology, epidemiology and risk factors. Rev Mal Respir 2005;22(Pt 1):257-69.
9. Infante PF, Newman LS. Beryllium exposure and chronic beryllium disease. Lancet 2004;363:415-16.
10. Sieradzki A, Andrzejak R, Sieradzka U. Berylliosis in the work environment: Etiology and medical treatment. Med Pr 2002;53:151-60.
11. Maier LA. Clinical approach to chronic beryllium disease and other nonpneumoconiotic interstitial lung diseases. J Thorac Imaging 2002;17:273-84.
12. Frome EL, Newman LS, Cragle DL, Colyer SP, Wambach PF. Identification of an abnormal beryllium lymphocyte proliferation test. Toxicology 2003;183:39-56. Erratum in: Toxicology 2003;188:335-36.
13. Sood A, Beckett WS, Cullen MR. Variable response to long-term corticosteroid therapy in chronic beryllium disease. Chest 2004;126:2000-07. Comment in: Chest 2004;126:1730-32.
14. Kolanz ME. Introduction to beryllium: uses, regulatory history, and disease. Appl Occup Environ Hyg 2001;16:559-67.
15. Henneberger PK, Goe SK, Miller WE, Doney B, Groce DW. Industries in the United States with airborne beryllium exposure and estimates of the number of current workers potentially exposed. J Occup Environ Hyg 2004;1:648-59.
16. Kolanz ME, Madl AK, Kelsh MA, Kent MS, Kalmes RM, Paustenbach DJ. A comparison and critique of historical and current exposure assessment methods for beryllium: Implications for evaluating risk of chronic beryllium disease. Appl Occup Environ Hyg 2001; 16:593-614.
17. Newman LS, Mroz MM, Balkissoon R, Maier LA. Beryllium sensitization progresses to chronic beryllium disease: A longitudinal study of disease risk. Am J Respir Crit Care Med 2005;171:54-60. Comment in: Am J Respir Crit Care Med 2005;1;171:3-4.
18. Welch L, Ringen K, Bingham E, Dement J, Takaro T, McGowan W, Chen A, Quinn P. Screening for beryllium disease among construction trade workers at Department of Energy nuclear sites. Am J Ind Med 2004;46:207-18.
19. Stefaniak AB, Hoover MD, Day GA, Dickerson RM, Peterson EJ, Kent MS, Schuler CR, Breysse PN, Scripsick RC. Characterization of physicochemical properties of

beryllium aerosols associated with prevalence of chronic beryllium disease. J Environ Monit. 2004;6:523-32.

2. CHROMIUM RELATED LUNG DISEASES

Exposure to chromium can occur as a result of chromate ore processing or paint industry. Spray painters are potentially exposed to aerosols containing hexavalent chromium [Cr(VI)] via inhalation of chromate-based paint sprays. Chromium is an inhaled carcinogen and an important risk factor in the development of lung carcinoma. The workforce of chromite ore processing plant can develop lung cancer. There are no obvious histological or clinical features that could allow differentiation between the occupational and nonoccupational cancers.[1] A continuation of the findings in a study of workers hired in 1931-1937 in a chromate plant, directed at the evaluation of the carcinogenic risk of insoluble, soluble, and total chromium. Chemical analyses of tissues of autopsies, identified by age at hire, cumulative exposure to insoluble, soluble, and total chromium and interval since last exposure are cited for three lung cancer cases. Histological identification of insoluble chromium was demonstrated. Marked deposition and retention of concentrations of chromium was noted 18.0 years since last exposure. In one case with cumulative exposure to insoluble chromium of 10.74 mg versus 0.63 mg for soluble chromium and histological demonstration of insoluble chromium, chrysotile was also identified.[2] In another epidemiologic study, the mortality patterns of commercial painters in The Netherlands were investigated. The hypothesis that painters are at an increased risk of cancer, especially lung cancer, was tested in collaboration with the Dutch Social Fund for painters. The results support previous findings of an increased risk of lung cancer in painters. Although no statement can be made about the actual causal agent, the authors believe that the sanding down of old paint layers may expose painters to particulates that contain carcinogens such as lead chromates and asbestos. The decreased risks of mortality from some neoplasms and circulatory and digestive problems, pneumoconiosis, and "other causes" observed in the painters lack a plausible explanation. Chance or the known limitation of proportionate mortality ratio analysis might play a role.[3] Lung carcinoma with chromate exposure exhibited a variety of genetic abnormalities. Considering genetic aberrations and chromium accumulation in these premalignant lesions leads to the process of carcinogenesis in chromium-induced lung carcinoma.[4] The genetic instability of chromate lung cancer is due to the repression of hMLH1 protein.[5]

REFERENCES

1. Aw TC. Clinical and Epidemiological Data on Lung Cancer at a Chromate Plant. Regul Toxicol Pharmacol 1997;26:S8-S12.
2. Mancuso TF. Chromium as an industrial carcinogen: Part II. Chromium in human tissues. Am J Ind Med 1997;31:140-7. Erratum in: Am J Ind Med 1997;31:669.
3. Terstegge CW, Swaen GM, Slangen JJ, Van Vliet C. Mortality Patterns among Commercial Painters in The Netherlands. Int J Occup Environ Health 1995;1:303-10.
4. Kondo K, Takahashi Y, Ishikawa S, Uchihara H, Hirose Y, Yoshizawa K, Tsuyuguchi M, Takizawa H, Miyoshi T, Sakiyama S, Monden Y. Microscopic analysis of chromium accumulation in the bronchi and lung of chromate workers. Cancer 2003;98:2420-29.
5. Takahashi Y, Kondo K, Hirose T, Nakagawa H, Tsuyuguchi M, Hashimoto M, Sano T, Ochiai A, Monden Y. Microsatellite instability and protein expression of the DNA mismatch repair gene, hMLH1, of lung cancer in chromate-exposed workers. Mol Carcinog 2005;42:150-58.

3. NICKEL AND THE LUNGS

Nickel carbonyl or nickel tetracarbonyl, $(Ni(CO)_4$, is colorless, highly volatile and inflammable liquid that is formed when carbon monoxide comes in contact with active nickel and highly toxic. Nickel carbonyl is used in the extraction of nickel (Mond process), gas planting and as a catalyst and reactant in chemical synthesis, and is usually encountered as a vapor that is rapidly absorbed after inhalation. Nickel compounds are unique in the sense that in vapor form it is highly absorbed compared to other metal compounds in vapor form. In contrast to a rapid absorption and excretion of nickel compounds in the urine, they accumulate within the connective tissues of the lung, which delays its clearance.[1] The slower distribution of nickel compounds result in chronic lung problems like development of lung fibrosis and pneumothorax after the acute presentation is over. Symptoms of nickel carbonyl poisoning may develop insidiously hours or even days after inhalation of vapors. Initial symptoms are usually mild and nonspecific. These include frontal headache, dizziness, and occasionally nausea and vomiting. Acute exposure results in inhalation pneumonitis that may be fatal.[2-7] Delayed symptoms such as chest pain, hemoptysis, and cyanosis, have been reported to occur 12 to 24 hours after exposure. In most cases, nickel carbonyl may not be recognized as the offending agent till several days. The primary injury occurs in the pulmonary alveoli, with maximum severity occurring from the 4th to the 6th days after exposure. In cases of fatal outcomes, the main pathologic changes occur in the lungs, liver, and brain and less commonly the kidneys, liver and adrenal glands. Lung changes include capillary congestion, interstitial edema, interstitial cellular proliferation, fibrinous intra-alveolar exudates, and hypertrophy of the alveolar lining cells.[8] Pulmonary consolidation, edema, hemorrhage, and fibrosis are observed at autopsy in patients who die.[7] Genetic factors have been implicated in the causation of lung injury. Studies have shown that mice deficient in the tyrosine kinase domain (TK-/-) of the receptor Mst1r have an increased susceptibility to nickel-induced acute lung injury. Mst1r TK-/- mice have decreased survival times, alterations in cytokine and nitric oxide regulation, and an earlier onset of pulmonary pathology compared to control mice, suggesting that Mst1r signaling, in part, may regulate the response to acute lung injury.[9]

Both water soluble and insoluble nickel compounds have been implicated in the etiology of human lung and nasal cancers. Water insoluble nickel compounds have been shown to enter cells by phagocytosis and are contained in cytoplasmic vacuoles, which are acidified thus accelerating the dissolution of soluble nickel from the particles. Using Newport Green, a dye that fluoresces when ionic nickel is bound, it has been shown that following exposure (48-72 hr) of human lung (A549) cells to NiS particles, most of the nickel is contained in the nucleus, while cells exposed to soluble $NiCl_2$ exhibit most of the ions localized in the cytoplasm. This effect is consistent with previously published reports showing that short-term exposure of cells to crystalline nickel particles (1-3 days) is able to epigenetically silence target genes placed near heterochromatin, while similar short-term exposure to soluble nickel compounds are not able to induce silencing of genes placed near heterochromatin. However, a 3 week exposure of cells to soluble $NiCl_2$ is also able to induce gene silencing. A similar effect was found in yeast cells where nickel was able to silence the URA-3 gene placed near (1.3 kb) a telomere silencing element, but not when the gene was placed farther away from the silencing element (2.0 kb). In addition to epigenetic effects, nickel compounds activate hypoxia signaling pathways. The mechanism of this effect involves the ability of either soluble or insoluble nickel compounds to block iron uptake leading to cellular iron depletion, directly affect iron containing enzymes, or both. This results in the inhibition of a variety of iron-dependent enzymes, such as aconitase and the HIF proline hydroxylases (PHD1-3). The inhibition of the HIF proline hydroxylases stabilizes the HIF protein and activates hypoxic signaling. Additional studies have shown that nickel and hypoxia decrease histone acetylation and increase the methylation of H3 lysine 9. These events are involved in gene silencing and hypoxia

can also cause these effects in human cells. It is hypothesized that the state of hypoxia either by low oxygen tension or as a result of agents that signal hypoxia under normal oxygen tension (iron chelation, nickel and cobalt) results in low levels of acetyl CoA, which is a substrate for histone and other protein acetylation. This effect may in part be responsible for the gene silencing following nickel exposure and during hypoxia.[10]

REFERENCES

1. Barceloux DG. Nickel. J Toxicol Clin Toxicol 1999;37: 239-58.
2. Correspondent reports: Nickel carbonyl poisoning. Lancet 1903;1:268-69.
3. Jones CC. Nickel carbonyl poisoning. Report of a fatal case. Arch Environ Health 1973;25:245-48.
4. Sunderman FW, Kincaid JF. Nickel poisoning II. Studies on patients suffering from acute exposure to vapors of nickel carbonyl. JAMA 1954:155:889-94.
5. Vuopala U, Huhti E, Takkunen J, et al. Nickel carbonyl poisoning: Report of 25 cases. Ann Clin Res 1970;2:214-22.
6. Shy Z. Nickel carbonyl:toxicity and human health. Sci Total Environ 1994;43:422-24.
7. Seet RC, Johan A, Teo CE, Gan SL, Lee KH. Inhalational nickel carbonyl poisoning in waste processing workers. Chest 2005;128:424-29.
8. Hackett RL. Sunderman FW Jr. Pulmonary alveolar reaction to nickel carbonyl: Ultrastructural and histochemical studies. Arch Environ Health 1968;16: 349-62.
9. Mallakin A, Kutcher LW, McDowell SA, Kong S, Schuster R, Lentsch AB, Aronow BJ, Leikauf GD, Waltz SE. Gene expression profiles of Mst1r deficient mice during Nickel-induced acute lung injury. Am J Respir Cell Mol Biol 2006;34:15-27.
10. Costa M, Davidson TL, Chen H, Ke Q, Zhang P, Yan Y, Huang C, Kluz T. Nickel carcinogenesis: Epigenetics and hypoxia signaling. Mutat Res 2005;592:79-88.

4. WELDER'S LUNG

Welding is an indispensable trade in modern society and has developed rapidly since 1940. Welding is a generic term referring to the union of pieces of metal at joint faces by various processes like heat or pressure or both. There are total almost 200 types of welding methods and even in the twenty-first century, welding is still a common and a highly skilled occupation. The commonest welding technologies used now a days in the industries, particularly the small scale ones, are oxy-fuel gas welding and electric arc welding. Some other occupations include oxy-fuel gas welding, electric welding, resistance welding, plasma arc welding, electron beam welding, and metal arc welding. Approximately 2 percent of work force in developed countries is exposed to the fumes of metallic oxides and oxidant gases, including ozone and oxides of nitrogen. The hazardous agents associated with welding processes are acetylene, carbon monoxide, oxides of nitrogen, ozone, phosgene, tungsten, arsenic, beryllium, cadmium, chromium, cobalt, copper, iron, lead, manganese, nickel, silver, tin, and zinc. Other toxic gases such as carbon monoxide, nitrogen dioxide, ozone, phosgene, etc. are other hazardous substances. All welding processes involve the potential hazards for inhalation exposures that may lead to acute or chronic respiratory diseases. According to literature described earlier it has been suggested that welding fumes cause the lung function impairment, obstructive and restrictive lung disease, cough, dyspnea, rhinitis, asthma, pneumonitis, pneumoconiosis, carcinoma of the lungs. In addition, welding workers suffer from eye irritation, photokeratitis, cataract, skin irritation, erythema, pterygium, nonmelanocytic skin cancer, malignant melanoma, reduced sperm count, motility and infertility. Most of the studies have been attempted previously to evaluate the effects of welding fumes. However, no collectively effort illuminating the general effects of welding fumes on different organs or systems or both in human has not been published. Therefore, the aim of this review is to gather the potential toxic effects of welding fumes documented by individual efforts and provide informations to community on hazards of welding. It is estimated that more than 1 million workers worldwide perform some type of welding as part of their work duties. Epidemiology studies have shown that a large number of welders experience some type of respiratory illness. Respiratory effects seen in full-time welders have included bronchitis, siderosis, asthma, and a possible increase in the incidence of lung cancer. Pulmonary infections are increased in terms of severity, duration, and frequency among welders. Inhalation exposure to welding fumes may vary due to differences in the materials used and methods employed. The chemical properties of welding fumes can be quite complex. Most welding materials are alloy mixtures of metals characterized by different steels that may contain iron, manganese, chromium, and nickel. Animal studies have indicated that the presence and combination of different metal constituents is an important determinant in the potential pneumotoxic responses associated with welding fumes. Animal models have demonstrated that stainless steel (SS) welding fumes, which contain significant levels of nickel and chromium, induce more lung injury and inflammation, and are retained in the lungs longer than mild steel (MS) welding fumes, which contain mostly iron. In addition, SS fumes generated from welding processes using fluxes to protect the resulting weld contain elevated levels of soluble metals, which may affect respiratory health. Recent animal studies have indicated that the lung injury and inflammation induced by SS welding fumes that contain water-soluble metals are dependent on both the soluble and insoluble fractions of the fumem.[1,2]

Mechanism of Action

Welding fumes in particular are respirable in to the distal airways and alveolar spaces of the human lungs. It also means that the metallic oxides crystals may adsorb on their surface molecules of ozone and nitrogen oxide. The target cells, which are the cuboidal epithelial cells of terminal bronchioles and alveolar ducts, are thus exposed to particles, which are chemically active. The march of events are as follows:

Welding fumes (respirable)
⇓
Loss of cilia and mucus burden
⇓
Obstruction of terminal bronchioles
⇓
Distal airways and alveolar spaces
⇓
Target cells (cuboidal epithelial cells)
⇓
Loss of mucociliary escalator
⇓
Loss of cilia and mucus burden
⇓
Obstruction of terminal bronchioles ⇒ ⇓ FVC
⇓
Polypoidal growth and distortion of lumens

There is further evidence that the hexavalent metals may catalyze accidental damage to cell membranes. Thus, we have the most vulnerable part of the tracheobronchial tree exposed to an ideal aerosol, which may stimulate mucous production by causing the epithelium to undergo goblet cell metaplasia. Cilia are lost and thus, a mucus burden is produced in small airways where the mucocilliary escalator is damaged. Mucous production may lead to obstruction of the terminal bronchioles, each of which supplies approximately 5000 alveoli. If damage is prolonged or repeated the subepithelial connective tissue may be stimulated with the production of polypoid masses growing into lumens or the distortion of the lumens by concentric or epicentric scarring. This produces permanent obstruction. The impairment to be looked for is reduction in Forced Expiratory Flow (FEF) 25 to 75 or altered distribution of inspired gas.[3] In a study which is a cross-sectional observational field study, of 126 welders among unorganized sector in Baroda city revealed that Smoke and fumes are common physical hazards present at work places. There is high prevalence of respiratory morbidity (44.4%) among welders. As the duration of exposure increases respiratory morbidity increases. Use of PPE is very poor among welders. The respiratory morbidity is higher in smoker welders but difference between smokers and nonsmokers is statistically not significant.

REFERENCES

1. Antonini JM, Taylor MD, Zimmer AT, Roberts JR. Pulmonary responses to welding fumes: Role of metal constituents. J Toxicol Environ Health A 2004;67:233-49.
2. Meo SA, Al-Khlaiwi T. Health hazards of welding fumes. Saudi Med J 2003;24:1176-82.
3. Jani Umesh, Mazumdar VS. Prevalence of respiratory morbidity among welders in unorganized sector of baroda city. Ind Journal of Occup Environ Med 2004; 8:16-21.

5. TALC WORKER'S PNEUMOCONIOSIS

Talc is mined in many countries and processed in numerous manufacturing industries for use in paints, ceramics, rubber products, roofing materials, paper, insecticides, cosmetics, and pharmaceuticals. Talc ($Mg_3Si_4O_{10}(OH)_2$) is a member of the silicates group of minerals characterized by its structure in sheets which can be separated by slight forces.[1,2] This causes the plate shape of the talc particles and the smoothness in touch. Other characteristics of talc as a mineral are softness, hydrophobic behavior, and insolubility. Given this planar structure of the talc crystal, the term talc fibers are technically not correct. However, when milled, some cleavage fragments (less than 1%) within the talc powder meet the World Health Organization (WHO) definition of fibers, although in fact these fragments are elongated talc platelets.

As talc is formed by alteration or metamorphosis of rocks, it is associated with many types of minerals and may contain other minerals as residues, so that the mined and milled ore hardly ever consists of pure talc. Exposure to talc must therefore be considered bearing in mind the coexposures—among which quartz is the most important—specific to each site. It is noteworthy that, to our knowledge, no asbestos contamination has ever been clearly documented in the talc deposits, at least not in the European sites. Several mortality studies performed among workers from the talc industry reported inconclusive results concerning an increased risk of neoplasms of the respiratory system. Although the risk of nonmalignant respiratory diseases was in excess in most of the study sites, the risk for cancer is different from study to study and may depend on the mineralogy of the exploited mineral or other features of the cohorts. The mortality from nonmalignant respiratory disease is related to high cumulative exposure to talc dust. The small excess in lung cancer does not seem to be attributable to talc.[3-5]

The pathologic appearance of the tissues is similar in primary, secondary, and tertiary exposures, although ferruginous bodies and foreign body giant cells are not always present in cases caused by secondary exposures. Mixed dust fibrotic lesions are found in some cases in which there are substantial quantities of quartz present. There is great variation in the minerals found within the lung tissues. Several cases will show significant quantities of mica and kaolin in addition to talc.[6]

REFERENCES

1. Rohl AN, Langer AM, Selikoff IJ, et al. Consumer talcums and powders: Mineral and chemical characterization. J Toxicol Environ Health 1976;2:255-84.
2. International Agency for Research on Cancer. IARC Monographs on the evaluation of the carcinogenic risk of chemicals to humans: Silica and some Silicates. Lyon, France: IARC, 1987. (IARC Monographs Volume 42).
3. Wild P, Leodolter K, Réfrégier M, Schmidt H, Zidek T. Haidinger G. A cohort mortality and nested case-control study of French and Austrian talc workers. Occupational and Environmental Medicine 2002;59:98-105.
4. Moshammer H, Neuberger M. Lung cancer and dust exposure: Results of a prospective cohort study following 3260 workers for 50 years. Occup Environ Med 2004;61:157-62.
5. Honda Y, Beall C, Delzell E, Oestenstad K, Brill I, Mathews R. Mortality among Workers at a Talc Mining and Milling Facility. Ann Hyg 2002;46:575-85.
6. Gibbs AE, Pooley FD, Griffiths DM, Mitha R, Craighead JE, Ruttner JR. Talc pneumoconiosis: A pathologic and mineralogic study. Hum Pathol 1992;23:1344-54.

6. KAOLIN LUNG

Kaolin is removed from underground seams in the mining area to a processing area, where it is sliced, dried, and pulverized to make the finished product. Parenchymal changes, both simple and complicated pneumoconiosis, have been described in kaolin workers. The presence of ventilatory impairment is related to the presence of complicated pneumoconiosis, employment in clay calcining, and cigarette smoking. In those working with calcined clay, there is an increased prevalence of abnormality of the FEV_1, but not the FVC, when compared to both wet and dry processors. The magnitude of abnormality in the calcined clay workers is, however, unlikely to lead to disabling impairment. In workers with more than 3 year tenure both simple pneumoconiosis and complicated pneumoconiosis can occur, with a prevalence of 3.2 percent and 0.63 percent, respectively. Dry processing is associated with a greater risk of developing pneumoconiosis than wet processing.[1-4] Pleural thickening may be common on chest tomography in workers with kaolinosis and that the exposure to kaolin dust should be considered in the differential diagnosis of pleural thickening.[5]

Considerable pathological lesions are found in the lungs, both nodular and interstitial fibroses being present. Some men have worked with China stone but others have worked entirely with China clay. Nodular fibrosis appeared to be related to high quartz content of the dust recovered from the lung, whereas among those with a high content of kaolinite dust in the lungs interstitial fibrosis was observed. Premortem or preoperative chest roentgenograms demonstrates small irregular shadows and large opacities typical of kaolin pneumoconiosis. On gross examination, there will be firm, gray-brown nodules and masses in the parenchyma and in the hilar lymph nodes. Histologically, there is extensive pulmonary kaolinite deposition associated with formation of peribronchiolar macules and nodules. The latter are comprised of kaolinite aggregates traversed by bands of fibrous tissue rather than dense whorled collagen, as seen in silicosis. Crystallographic studies confirm the presence of kaolinite in the lungs, but silica is not demonstrable by either analytical scanning electron microscopy or X-ray diffractometry. These findings illustrate the pathology of human kaolin pneumoconiosis, confirm the fibrogenic potential of kaolinite, and emphasize differences in pulmonary responses to kaolinite and to silica.[6-8]

Kaolin exposure appeared to have a small but significant effect on ventilatory capacity in those with kaolin pneumoconiosis and in workers with a longer exposure. There was no association between the radiographic appearances of kaolinosis and cigarette smoking or between the presence of radiographic abnormalities and reduced arterial blood gas tensions.[7]

REFERENCES

1. Morgan WK, Donner A, Higgins IT, Pearson MG, Rawlings W Jr. The effects of kaolin on the lung. Am Rev Respir Dis 1988;138:813-20.
2. Levin JL, Frank AL, Williams MG, McConnell W, Suzuki Y, Dodson RF. Kaolinosis in a cotton mill worker. Am J Ind Med 1996;29:215-21.
3. Sheers G. The China clay industry—Lessons for the future of occupational health. Respir Med 1989;83: 173-75.
4. Altekruse EB, Chaudhary BA, Pearson MG, Morgan WK. Kaolin dust concentrations and pneumoconiosis at a kaolin mine. Thorax 1984;39:436-41.
5. Chaudhary BA, Kanes GJ, Pool WH. Pleural thickening in mild kaolinosis. South Med J 1997;90:1106-09.
6. Baser ME, Kennedy TP, Dodson R, Rawlings W Jr, Rao NV, Hoidal JR. Differences in lung function and prevalence of pneumoconiosis between two kaolin plants. Br J Ind Med 1989;46:773-76.
7. Wagner JC, Pooley FD, Gibbs A, Lyons J, Sheers G, Moncrieff CB. Inhalation of China stone and china clay dusts: Relationship between the mineralogy of dust retained in the lungs and pathological changes. Thorax 1986;41:190-96.
8. Lapenas D, Gale P, Kennedy T, Rawlings W Jr, Dietrich P. Kaolin pneumoconiosis. Radiologic, pathologic, and mineralogic findings. Am Rev Respir Dis 1984;130:282-88.
9. Sepulveda MJ, Vallyathan V, Attfield MD, Piacitelli L, Tucker JH. Pneumoconiosis and lung function in a group of kaolin workers. Am Rev Respir Dis 1983;127:231-35.

7. IRON AND THE LUNGS

Iron oxides are present in many occupational atmospheres mainly in iron ore mines and in steel industry. Among these workers, epidemiological studies indicated an excess of lung cancer deaths. In mines, it was difficult to involve iron oxides exposure because there is other possible causes as radon, polycyclic aromatic hydrocarbon (PAH) present in diesel exhausts, silicosis or siderosis. The contradictory results of these studies are due to the differences of exposure levels or to the presence or not of these cofactors or of a sufficient prevention. But generally the results agree with an interaction of iron oxide dusts and smoking habits. It is unclear if this interaction supports an additive or multiplicative risk of lung cancer. Experimental studies with Fe_2O_3 showed that these particles are able to induce lung cancers only in the presence of PAH when administered to animals. *In vitro* studies permitted to observe an interaction in the metabolism of benzo(a)pyrene (BaP) leading to a higher level of precursors of the ultimate carcinogen. This metabolism of BaP is known to be enhanced during lipoperoxidation, and it is possible to involve this mechanism with Fe_2O_3. After phagocytosis and dissolution with production of ferric ions, Fe_2O_3 can enhance the production of reactive oxygen species responsible of damaging both lipidic constituents and DNA. Fe_3O_4 and mainly FeO may be more toxic, introducing directly ferrous ions in the cells after dissolution, but the cancerogenicity of the these compounds is unknown, making necessary to develop research.[1-6]

Extracellular iron present in alveolar structures may contribute to oxidative lung injury induced by toxic mineral dusts by enhancing dust-induced generation of hydroxyl radicals. Alveolar macrophages (AMs) can sequester iron within ferritin and limit generation of hydroxyl radicals. AMs accumulate iron and ferritin in response to both iron loading of the lungs with iron oxide exposure and lung inflammation induced by calcium tungstate exposure.[7]

REFERENCES

1. Haguenoer JM, Shirali P, Hannothiaux MH, Nisse-Ramond C. Interactive effects of polycyclic aromatic hydrocarbons and iron oxides particles. Epidemiological and fundamental aspects. Cent Eur J Public Health 1996;4 Suppl:41-45.
2. Boyd JT, Doll R, Faulds JS, Leiper J. Cancer of the lung in iron ore (haematite) miners. Br Ind Med 1970;27:97-105.
3. Craw J. Pneumoconiosis of the haematite iron oremines of West Cumbria. A study of 45 years of control. J Soc Occup Med 1982;32:53-65.
4. Chen SY, Hayes RB, Liang SR, Li QG, Stewart PA, Blair A. Mortality experience of haematite mine workers in China. Br J Ind Med 1990;47:175-81.
5. Yamada G, Igarashi T, Sonoda H, Morita S, Suzuki K, Yoshida Y, Abe S. Use of bronchopulmonary lavage for eliminating inhaled fume particles from a patient with arc welder's lung. Intern Med 1998;37:962-64.
6. Stokinger HE. A review of world literature finds iron oxides noncarcinogenic. Am Ind Hyg Assoc J 1984; 45:127-33.
7. Wesselius LJ, Smirnov IM, Nelson ME, O'Brien-Ladner AR, Flowers CH, Skikne BS. Alveolar macrophages accumulate iron and ferritin after *in vivo* exposure to iron or tungsten dusts. J Lab Clin Med 1996;127:401-09.

8. BARITOSIS

Baritosis is one of the benign pneumoconioses in which inhaled particulate matter lies in the lungs for years without producing symptoms, abnormal physical signs, incapacity for work, interference with lung function, or liability to develop pulmonary or bronchial infections or other thoracic disease. Owing to the high radiopacity of barium, the discrete shadows in the chest radiograph are extremely dense. Even in the most well marked cases with extreme profusion of the opacities, massive shadows do not occur. When exposure to barium dust ceases the opacities begin slowly to disappear.[1] The radiological and pathological features of the men's lungs may be those of silicosis and high proportions of quartz will be found in these cases at postmortem. The quartz is inhaled from rocks associated with the barytes in the mines. The features of silicosis in barium miners are contrasted with the benign pneumoconiosis, baritosis that occurs in workers exposed to crushed and ground insoluble barium salts. Diagnostic difficulties arise when silicosis develops in workers mining minerals known to cause a separate and benign pneumoconiosis. These difficulties are compounded when, as not infrequently happens, the silicotic lesions develop or progress after exposure to quartz has ceased.[2]

REFERENCES

1. Doig AT. Baritosis: A benign pneumoconiosis. Thorax 1976;31:30-39.
2. Seaton A, Ruckley VA, Addison J, Brown WR. Silicosis in barium miners. Thorax 1986;41:591-95.

9. ALUMINIUM AND LUNGS

Problems due to exposure of workers to dust and fumes of aluminum and its compounds and their toxic effect on the respiratory tract are many. Long-term occupational exposure to the above factors leads to changes in lungs of the pneumoconiotic nature. Other disorders presented in the literature include: Pulmonary fibrosis, pulmonary alveolitis and alveolar proteinosis, asthma, chronic bronchitis, and chronic pneumonia. The respiratory effect depends to some extent on the form of aluminum or the stage of processing in which exposure occurs. Numerous studies of workers occupationally exposed to aluminum dust and fumes have demonstrated the increase in the incidence of pulmonary fibrosis, depending on the air concentration of respirable fraction of dust.[1,2] Airway inflammation is a central feature of potroom asthma and exposure to potroom emissions induces pathological alterations similar to those described in other types of asthma. Cigarette smoking seems to affect the underlying mechanisms involved in asthma, as the cellular composition of airway mucosa appears different in asthmatic smokers and nonsmokers.[3] The early common pathological change of alumina pneumoconiosis is the dust spots. The dust fibrosis has two forms, one is the non-focal fibrous proliferation of interstitial space, and the other is the proliferation of inner-dust-spot fibrosis that finally develops into nontypical pneumoconiosis nodules. The pathological characteristics of the alumina pneumoconiosis may not be all the same to those of aluminium and aluminium oxide pneumoconiosis. Alumina pneumoconiosis is a complex pneumoconiosis. The typical pathological changes are the dust-spot emphysema and dust fibrosis of interstitial tissue. Infection in lung and complication of lung tumor, especially pneumo-tuberculosis would promote dust fibrosis. The pleural thickening, the relationship between lung cancer and alumina dust should be taken seriously.[4]

REFERENCES

1. Mitchell J, Manning JB, Moleneux M, Lane RE. Pulmonary fibrosis in workers exposed to finely powdered aluminium. Br J Ind Med 1961;18:10-23.
2. Nasiadek M, Sapota A. Toxic effect of dust and fumes of aluminium and its compounds on workers' respiratory tract. Med Pr 2004;55:495-500.
3. Sjaheim T, Halstensen TS, Lund MB, Bjortuft O, Drablos PA, Malterud D, Kongerud J. Airway inflammation in aluminium potroom asthma. Occup Environ Med 2004; 61:779-85.
4. Li Y, Wang H. Pathological observation on five autopsies of the alumina pneumoconiosis. Zhonghua Lao Dong Wei Sheng Zhi Ye Bing Za Zhi 2002;20:103-05.

10. RARE METAL RELATED LUNG DISEASES

Other rare metals associated with lung injury include tin (stannosis), polyvinyl chloride, and tungsten. These conditions are rarely encountered in clinical practice.[1-3]

REFERENCES

1. Robertson AJ, Rivers D, Nagelschmidt G, Duncomb P. Stannosis: Benign pneumoconiosis due to tin dioxide. Lancet 1961;1:1089-93.
2. Soutar CA, Copland LH, Thornley PE, et al. Epidemiological study of respiratory disease in workers exposed to polyvinyl chloride dust. Thorax 1980;35:644-52.
3. Coates EO, Watson JHL. Diffuse interstitial lung disease in tungsten carbide workers. Ann Int Med 1971;75:709-16.

INHALATION INJURIES

With increasing industrialization and the use of a wide variety of chemicals, the modern society is threatened with exposure to a large number of noxious gases and fumes, not only to those who work in these industries but also to the rest of the population who live surrounding the industry. Two such worst accidents occurred in 1984: in Bhopal, India, over 5000 people died after about 40 tonnes of methyl isocyanate were discharged on the night of 2nd December,[1,2] and in Mexico City about 500 people were killed and 5000 injured when a liquid petroleum gas plant exploded.[3] In the Bhopal incident, poisonous gases leaked from a fertilizer factory killed 5800 and injured about half a million people. Their injuries ranged from breathlessness, gastrointestinal problems to neurological disorders.[2] The accidental release of chemicals during their distribution either by pipelines, by road or rail or by water can also have serious consequences. Clinical management of patients exposed to various toxic inhalants also poses certain problems. The exposures occur at infrequent intervals and at unpredictable times, large number of individuals may be exposed at the same time and the physician may not know the exact nature of the toxic substance immediately. The lag period between the exposure and the onset of clinical symptoms vary and the long-term effects of many of these substances are poorly understood. Sometimes, even if the identity of the agent is known, knowledge about its human toxicity may be very little. Adequate knowledge exists for only a few percent of over 7000 chemicals in regular commercial use. Antidotes are available for only a handful of chemicals and have no role in most events. Toxic inhalants can be classified by the mechanisms of injury they produce. While irritant gases have direct effects on the epithelial lining of the respiratory tract, **asphyxiant** block oxygen delivery and utilization, and aspirated solids and liquids can cause direct cytotoxic effects, introduce infectious pathogens and cause varying degrees of airways obstruction.[4-6]

The collapse of the World Trade Center (WTC) on September 11, 2001 created a large-scale disaster site in a dense urban environment. In the days and months thereafter, thousands of rescue/recovery workers, volunteers, and residents were exposed to a complex mixture of airborne pollutants. Aerodigestive tract inflammatory injuries, such as declines in pulmonary function, reactive airways dysfunction syndrome (RADS), asthma, reactive upper airways dysfunction syndrome (RUDS), gastroesophageal reflux disease (GERD), and rare cases of inflammatory pulmonary parenchymal diseases, have been documented in WTC rescue/recovery workers and volunteers. In the rescue workers, persistent hyperreactivity associated with exposure intensity, independent of airflow obstruction is reported. One year post-collapse, 23 percent of highly exposed subjects were hyperreactive as compared with only 11 percent of moderately exposed and 4 percent of controls. At 1 year, 16 percent met the criteria for RADS. While it is too early to ascertain all of the long-term effects of WTC exposures, continued medical monitoring and treatment is needed to help those exposed and to improve our prevention, diagnosis, and treatment protocols for future disasters.[6-8]

Smoke Inhalation

Smoke inhalation injuries are the leading cause of fatalities from burn injury. Smoke inhalation is a significant factor in approximately 30 percent of all hospitalized burn patients and this group has a mortality of 50 to 70 percent. It is estimated that presence of significant smoke inhalation in a burn patient will increase the mortality to two to three folds.

The major forms of inhalation injuries are carbon monoxide toxicity, injury to the upper airway, and pulmonary parenchymal damage. The compromised airway is protected by tracheal intubation, and respiratory failure is treated with assisted ventilation. Maintenance of good pulmonary hygiene, optimized fluid resuscitation, and routine invasive hemodynamic monitoring are the mainstays of therapy. The development of acute pulmonary insufficiency, pulmonary edema, or bronchopneumonia requires a comprehensive approach to all aspects of the illness. Acute pathophysiologic responses to inhalation injury are complex. Future therapies will target improved ventilatory strategies and the redundant host inflammatory response.[9] Pediatric burns admitted to the tertiary care burn facility of Kanchi Kamakoti CHILDS Trust Hospital in Chennai (India) revealed that inhalation burns were not very common and were associated only with large flame burns, which occur when a child is burnt while the mother commits suicide, or in cases of abuse of female children in a closed room with lots of inflammable upholstery.[10] In burn patients the incidence of ARDS may be high whereas mortality may be low. A multifactorial origin of ARDS in burns victims as a part of a multiple organ failure event has been suggested.[11] Cytological and biochemical changes of lavage in the upper and lower respiratory system have been described recently.[12]

In fire accidents average CO levels of 40 percent and cyanide (CN) levels of 0.6 ppm may be obtained. The lungs are heavy, hyperemic, and edematous with soot staining the tracheobronchial mucosa. Light microscopy shows soot, pulmonary congestion, and edema. Electron microscopy will confirm the presence of interstitial and intraalveolar congestion and edema. Carbon particles are also present, and occasionally are seen undergoing phagocytosis by alveolar macrophages. Intracellular edema with focal bleb and vesicle formation is prominent within Type I pneumocytes in almost all cases. Endothelial cells will show similar but much less severe changes, lacking the distinct blebs seen in the Type I cells. Thus smoke, like ammonia inhalation and nitric acid instillation, appears to cause pulmonary edema by initial injury to the Type I pneumocyte.[13]

These patients show increased rate of clearance (short $T_{1/2}$) while the retention images will reveal regional lung damage in moderately severe inhalation burns. In patients with abnormal $T_{1/2}$, majority will show abnormal bronchoscopy findings. Lung perfusion scans with Tc-99m MAA (macroaggregated albumin) will show regional defects in perfusion in most patients. When these defects are present, they will generally match with the defects seen on ventilation scans. The Tc-99m DTPA lung clearance measurement and imaging has clinical usefulness in suspected inhalation burns.[14]

Although most subjects continue to inhale smoke in one way or the other, like domestic cooking, pollution and passive smoking with their attendant consequences, acute inhalant injuries are more important in occupational exposures. There are two main causes of lung injury due to acute smoke inhalation: *(i)* thermal injury and *(ii)* inhalation of toxic gases and particulate matter.

Thermal Injury

Although air temperature in a burning room may reach 500 to 1000°F, the low heat capacity of air and the effectiveness of the upper airways in cooling inhaled air protect the lower respiratory tract from the damaging effect of heat. Of course, this mechanism has only a limited protection. However, heat may injure the upper airways and increase the likelihood of airways obstruction, most commonly due to laryngeal edema. In contrast to hot air, inhalation of steam can cause injury to the entire tracheobronchial tree, as steam has 4000 times the heat capacity of air.

Toxic Gases and Particulate Matter

When any material burns, it can either smoulder (pyrolysis) or flame (combustion) in varying combinations. The products of combustion are in general, less harmful than those are released during pyrolysis. As the material burns, oxygen is consumed which decreases the ambient oxygen to as low as 10 percent. This contributes further to asphyxia of individuals in the area and in addition causes the materials that are burning to smoulder. In most fires a number of toxic gases are produced which include carbon dioxide, carbon monoxide, hydrogen cyanide, oxides of nitrogen and sulfur and several organic aldehydes like acrolein. Of these, carbon monoxide (CO) and cyanide cause much of the mortality due to smoke inhalation. The other noxious gases cause direct lung injury, whereas CO primarily affect the oxygen carrying capacity of hemoglobin.

Carbon Monoxide (CO)

It is a colorless, odorless and tasteless gas produced by the combustion of carbon containing materials in the presence of limited oxygen. CO does not injure the lungs directly, but competes for the binding sites for oxygen in the hemoglobin molecule. It has an affinity of 200 times that of oxygen for these binding sites. Moreover, carboxyhemoglobin (COHb) shifts the oxyhemoglobin dissociation curve to the left impairing the unloading of oxygen at the tissue level. This effect is the major cause of tissue hypoxia in CO poisoning. At COHb levels of 30 percent, patients become confused and lethargic and coma ensues at levels greater than 40 to 50 percent. Blood values greater than 60 percent are fatal due to acute cerebral and myocardial hypoxia.

Aldehydes: Inhalation of various noxious aldehydes, which are produced in the fire, causes mucosal damage and loss of ciliary activity. Airways obstruction results from edema and sloughing of the mucosa. The damage also impairs microbial clearance leading on to infections such as bacterial tracheobronchitis and pneumonia. The inflammatory exudative fluid in the respiratory tract and lung parenchyma causes further mismatching of the ventilation and perfusion. Experimental data suggest that the aldehydes in smoke bind irreversibly with hydrogen bonds of amino acids and with the RNA of respiratory tissue perpetuating further damage. Impairment of chemotactic and phagocytic activity of the alveolar macrophages as demonstrated in experimental animals following smoke inhalation will further predispose the individual to infections.

Clinical Management

Most smoke inhalation victims who survive CO asphyxiation, and have no major surface burns, have a relatively mild presentation and a favorable prognosis. However, if smoke inhalation is present in a patient with major burn, mortality is increased. The symptoms of smoke inhalation may include a nonproductive cough and eye irritation to coma and hypoxemia, requiring immediate mechanical ventilation. Cutaneous burns may be evident on the face and other parts of the body. A history of being present in a closed space or the presence of burns to the upper parts should raise the suspicion for possible smoke inhalation. This is one condition where cyanosis is undetected even in the presence of severe hypoxia because of the cherry red color of the blood, which is impacted by COHb. Moreover, the cherry red color and whatever cyanosis is there, become more difficult to detect if there is associated mucosal burn. Physical findings, which strongly correlate with smoke inhalation, include: Hoarseness, expiratory wheezing, severe conjunctivitis and black or sooty sputum. Chest X-ray, arterial blood gas analysis and estimation of blood levels COHb should be performed at admission for all patients who have significant body surface burns.

Establishment of a patent airway is the first step in the management of fire victims with facial burns associated with hoarseness, stridor and hypoxemia. The upper way should be examined with a laryngoscope to assess the degree of mucosal injury and laryngeal edema. Chest X-ray is not sensitive enough in inhalation injury and may be normal in patients with tracheobronchitis and hypoxia in the first few hours. Appearance of diffuse infiltrates may take as long as 24 to 36 hours to develop. If ventilation scanning with ^{133}Xenon, shows abnormal retention of Xe at 90 seconds, it is considered by some to be diagnostic of inhalation injury. However, problem with Xe scanning is that in patients with preexisting disease it will be abnormal, it is expensive, it requires precious time away from the intensive care unit and requires specialized equipments and personnel. The scanning does not add anything to careful clinical evaluation, estimation of COHb levels and laryngeal examination in the diagnosis of smoke inhalation injury- Estimation of blood COHb levels is very important in all cases. Normal nonsmoking individuals have levels of COHb of less than 5 percent while smokers may have levels up to 15 percent. Moreover, in women engaged in cooking and using different cooking fuels, may have levels up to 15 percent (acute exposure). This fact should be borne in mind while evaluating inhalation injury. When COHb levels are high, the arterial tension and the calculated oxygen saturation may be normal. Therefore, it is necessary to measure oxygen saturation of the arterial blood directly using an oximeter. The half-life of COHb is 4 to 6 hours when the patient breathes room air. However, increased alveolar ventilation and high concentrations of inspired oxygen will shorten the half-life. Breathing of 100 percent oxygen at one atmosphere reduces the half-life to approximately 40 minutes. Carbon monoxide can cause myocardial damage and in all victims, an electrocardiogram should be recorded as a routine. Estimation of plasma cyanide levels may be necessary in certain individuals, if they can be readily available. Levels greater than 1 mg per liter are indicative of serious smoke inhalation. On the scene treatment of fire victims consists of removal of the victim from the toxic environment, checking of vital signs and the establishment of an airway if indicated. Supplemental oxygen at moderate to high flow rates via a facemask should be administered if significant smoke inhalation is suspected.

In the emergency room, a quick examination of the nasal and oropharyngeal mucosa should be carried out and definite treatment be started. Laboratory tests including COHb levels, ECG and chest X-ray must be carried out in addition to the usual laboratory tests. A patent airway must be ensured, if necessary, by a tracheostomy if there is severe laryngeal edema. Patients developing acute respiratory failure and adult respiratory distress syndrome should be intubated and mechanical ventilation with positive end expiratory pressure (PEEP) will be required for them. Routine use of antibiotics has no role in the treatment of smoke inhalation victims. There is no convincing data to support the benefit of corticosteroid therapy in these patients. Rather, there is every possibility of infectious complications of such treatment, which will add up to the mortality. Newer guidelines for protection of victims from fire in aircrafts have been suggested.[15] These include the provision of passenger protective breathing equipment (PPBE). Hopcalite filters could provide satisfactory protection against carbon monoxide, hydrogen cyanide, hydrogen fluoride, hydrogen chloride, nitrogen oxides, sulphur dioxide, ammonia, acrolein, and other hydrocarbon compounds, for periods up to 30 min. Filtered levels of carbon dioxide (CO_2) could be maintained within a 5 percent limit (inhaled atmosphere + dead space) against such atmospheres containing up to 4 percent CO_2. Concentrations of oxygen downstream from the filters were up to some 1.0 percent above that present in the challenge atmospheres. Separate lung simulator tests on breathable gas (oxygen) hoods indicate that satisfactory respiratory protection could be provided for periods of up to 31 min.

Chemical Injuries

Chemicals, which are liable to accidental air release, include chlorine, ammonia, sulfuric acid, hydrogen chloride, phosgene, hydrogen sulphide and nitrous fumes. The recent Bhopal incidence adds methyl isocyanate to the list. The water solubility of the gas and the intensity of the exposure decide the primary sites of respiratory tract injury and the acuteness of onset of symptoms. While the more water soluble gases injure the eyes and the mucus membranes of the throat and the upper respiratory tract, the less soluble gases are distributed into the peripheral parts of the lung and cause more diffuse lung injury. The commonly encountered irritant gases with their characteristics and mechanisms of injury are summarized in Table 27.7. Some specific physical properties of the agent such as the pH and chemical reactivity also determine the type of injury besides the water solubility. Cell injury for a

TABLE 27.7: Sources of exposure, water solubility and mechanism of injury of irritant gases and fumes

Agent	Sources of exposure	Water solubility	Mechanism of Injury
Ammonia	Fertilizers, explosives and plastic mining, refrigeration, petroleum refining	High	Alkali burns
Hydrogen chloride	Dyes, fertilizers, textiles	High	Acid burns
Sulphur dioxide	Smelting, paper manufacture, food processing, oil refining	High	Acid burns
Chlorine	Paper and textile manufacture, sewage treatment	Intermediate	Acid burns, free radicals
Oxides of nitrogen	Agriculture (silo) welding, explosives mining dye and lacquer manufacture	Low	Acid burns, free radicals
Phosgene	Welding, paint striping, fire fighting, chemical industry	Low	Acid burns
Isocyanates	Fertilizer, foam factory, adhesives, surface coating, paints, varnish		

variety of these gases is mediated by either the formation of an acid, an alkali or free oxygen radicals. Ammonia (high water solubility), chlorine (intermediate solubility) and nitrogen dioxide (low water solubility) will be discussed as prototypes. Isocyanates, which are not infrequently used, will also be discussed with special reference to methyl isocyanate causing Bhopal gas tragedy."

Ammonia

Ammonia is an important chemical in industry. Because of the widespread use of ammonia in industry and agriculture there is a growing opportunity for ammonia burns to occur. It is a colorless alkaline gas that is highly water soluble and has a pungent odor. Occupational risk of ammonia exposure includes fertilizer and refrigeration industries and the manufacture of explosives, dyes and plastics.

When gaseous ammonia comes into contact with moist mucosal surfaces, it imbibes water and forms ammonia hydroxide (a strong alkali). This causes liquefaction of the mucous membrane exposing the submucosa to more ammonia, formation of more ammonia hydroxide and further liquefaction of the submucosa perpetuating a vicious cycle. The extent of damage depends upon the duration of exposure, concentration of the gas and the depth of inhalation. With mild to moderate exposure (50-150 ppm) the primary effect is irritation of the eyes, skin and upper respiratory tract. Higher exposure will cause extensive mucosal damage of the upper respiratory tract with edema leading to airway obstruction. Massive exposure will result in ARDS and patchy bronchopneumonia. Occasionally, there may be a lag period of up to 48 hours before radiological changes occur. Laryngeal edema should be carefully looked for in those with oral lesions. In the acute phase there may be severe tracheobronchitis and respiratory failure due to burns of the respiratory mucosa. After some improvement there may be fixed airways obstruction. Such acute exposure to high concentrations of ammonia may lead to acute respiratory injury as well as long-term impairment of respiratory function.[16,17] The long-term effects of ammonia exposure have not been characterized well. Some individuals have persistent symptoms of bronchitis and may have evidence of air flow limitations on spirometry. There have been isolated case reports of generalized or segmental bronchiectasis following ammonia exposure. However, bronchiolitis obliterans has not been reported. Other chronic lung problems may include chronic dyspnea, and clinical pictures consistent with restrictive lung dysfunction, obstructive lung disease, and bronchial hyperreactivity and small airways disease.[18] Accidental inhalation of ammonia has resulted in upper airway and bronchoalveolar injury, and even fatal inhalation of anhydrous ammonia has occurred.[19] Thus, ammonia is an extremely irritant gas, capable of producing severe damage to all levels of the respiratory tract, which may result in clinical impairment of respiratory function, ranging from mild to fatal.

Light-microscopic pulmonary findings in the acute ammonia deaths include denudation of the tracheobronchial epithelium, edema of the lamina propria, and marked alveolar edema, congestion, and hemorrhage. Electron microscopy examination of the lungs may show marked swelling and imbitional edema of Type I alveolar epithelial cells; however, alveolar basement membranes and capillary endothelial cells may be as usual. These electron-microscopic findings demonstrate the Type I epithelial cell to be the target cell of acute alveolar wall injury in ammonia inhalation.[20] Autopsy studies will show the recent lesions, which will be discovered in the subjects who die during the first three days. They will consist of some extended cutaneomucous burns, a sharp lung edema sometimes associated with pulmonary emphysema. Deaths are rather caused by the after effects of a pneumopathy (pulmonary infection, bronchiectasis, pulmonary fibrosis). Ammonia belongs to the irritating and caustic gas. The intensity of the lesions and the mortal risk are proportional to the quantity of gas per m³ of air.[21]

Patients having any kind of respiratory symptom should be hospitalized for observation for a day or two. Treatment is largely supportive. Supplemental oxygen, bronchodilators and assisted ventilation should be instituted as and when needed. Prophylactic antibiotic and steroids have not been shown to alter either the course or prognosis of these patients. Prolonged respiratory support may be required. Superinfection may cause a late deterioration in those severely affected.[22] As the injury is thermal as well as chemical, to skin, eyes, airway and lungs, prompt (5-10 seconds) irrigation of the eyes is required, and immediate treatment of airway and pulmonary injuries. Fluid resuscitation and skin wound care are similar to that of other burns. Presence or absence of abnormal chest findings on admission is the best prognostic factor.[23] Corticosteroid inhalation therapy has no proven effect on gas exchange or airway pressure levels in ammonia-induced lung injury.[24]

Chlorine

It is a dense, highly irritant gas with a greenish-yellow color and specific gravity of 2.5 times that of air. It is commonly used as a bleaching agent in the paper and textile industries and also as a disinfectant of water and sewage. For industrial use it is generally transported in liquid form under pressure in steel cylinders. Thus, bursting of a cylinder or fracture of a liquid gas pipe or failure of a road tanker delivery coupling will release the chemical. One liter of liquid chlorine will produce about 434 liters of chlorine gas at 25°C. Chlorine reacts with water to produce hydrochloric acid and other reaction products such as hypochlorous acid and free oxygen radicals. The series of reactions by which unstable oxidizing compounds form hydrates of organic chlorine produce more tissue damage than that produce by equivalent amounts of hydrochloric acid. Since chlorine gas is intermediately soluble, it is capable of causing cellular damage throughout the respiratory tract. Exposure to chlorine gas causes choking, chest pain, cough and dyspnea and the production of white or pink sputum.[25] It can cause rapid death from bronchospasm, laryngeal edema or toxic pulmonary edema. Physical examination will reveal hyperemia of the conjunctiva and oropharynx. On auscultation of the chest, one may hear wheezes and crackles. Pulmonary edema, a common occurrence, develops with severe exposure and may occur immediately or after several hours. Earlier chest X-ray may be normal and subsequently as pulmonary edema ensues, such changes will be apparent. Pathological changes will include focal and confluent areas of edema with protein rich fluid in the alveolar spaces, hyaline membrane formation and denudation of the alveolar epithelium. Intravascular thrombi may be seen in the pulmonary vessels. Bronchial and bronchiolar walls may be denuded or even destroyed. These changes are similar to those seen in other soluble gas poisoning such as sulphur dioxide or ammonia. Pulmonary function tests will demonstrate evidence of airflow obstruction with air trapping. Occasionally, a restrictive defect may be seen.

Treatment of chlorine inhalation injury is mainly supportive including administration of supplemental oxygen. Tracheostomy or intubation may be necessary if the patient has nasopharyngeal or laryngeal edema. Mechanical ventilation will be required if there is pulmonary edema with the use of positive end expiratory pressure. The role of corticosteroid has not been defined clearly although some reports suggest a beneficial effect. Antibiotics should be used for those having overt infection.

Mild airflow obstruction may be seen as long-term sequelae of acute chlorine exposure. However, long function improves over a period of time.

Nitrogen Dioxide (NO₂)

Occupations in which exposure to nitrogen dioxide is possible include: Farm workers exposed to fresh silage (Silo-filler's disease); welders using acetylene during welding and coalminers. Several chemical industries like manufacturing of dyes, lacquers and nitric acid plant may produce NO_2 and the workers are liable to be exposed. Nitrogen dioxide in silo gas is derived from the nitrates in plants and is released as a reddish-brown gas. Although grain plants have low concentrations of nitrates, they are increased by the use of fertilizers. The plant nitrates are fermented into nitrites and oxygen. Nitrites then combine with organic acids to form nitrous acid (HNO_2). As the temperature in the silo rises, this decomposes into nitrous oxide (NO), nitrogen tetroxide (N_2O_4) and nitrogen pentoxide (N_2O_5). Nitrogen dioxide and its dimer nitrogen tetroxide are the gases responsible for the pulmonary injury. Fortunately, large amounts of nitrogen dioxide are only formed for the first five to seven days of filling the silos. During this time concentrations as high as 200 to 4000 ppm may be observed. However, if the silo is adequately ventilated the gases disappear very quickly.[26,27]

The threshold limit for nitrogen dioxide for industrial exposure is 5 ppm. Exposure to 50 ppm concentrations even for brief periods will increase the risk of developing acute respiratory problems. The gas reacts with water in the respiratory tract to form nitric acid which dissociates into nitrates and nitrites which themselves cause extensive damage to the respiratory epithelium. Nitrogen dioxide itself is also a powerful oxidant. All these mechanisms in addition to causing extensive tissue damage may initiate peroxidation of the lung lipids by free oxygen radicals. NO_2 can also cause degradation of collagen.

Clinical Presentation

The clinical stages may be divided into the following: (a) superacute phase. This a consequence of methemoglobin formation and asphyxiation as a result of exposure to very high concentrations of nitrogen dioxide which leads on to severe hypoxemia. These patients are critically ill and most of them die immediately before they can get any medical help. Fortunately its occurrence is very rare (b) acute phase. This is the most common form and the patient often presents with dyspnea, bronchospasm, weakness, nausea, headache and tachycardia. Occasionally there may be pleuritic chest pain. Often, there is a lag period of few hours between exposure and onset of symptoms. Bronchospasm and pulmonary edema are important features in the acute phase. A trial of corticosteroid therapy in the acute phase is advocated. The routine use of antibiotics is not recommended but may be used based on the basis of sputum culture. Some specific treatment such as the use of methylene blue to reverse methemoglobinemia has been proposed but has not been found useful clinically. Since the pulmonary edema is a permeability edema, the treatment essentially consists of that for adult respiratory distress syndrome, which includes supplemental oxygen, intubation in severe cases and ventilatory support with use of PEEP (c) Subacute and chronic phases. If the patient survives, the pulmonary edema clears up within a few days and a secondary phase may develop, which can last for 2 to 5 weeks. During this period the patient is usually asymptomatic or may have exertional dyspnea only with the chest X-ray being normal. Then 3 to 6 weeks after, the patient may experience a relapse and present with fever, progressive breathlessness, cough and cyanosis. The chest skiagram during this period will show multiple discrete nodular opacities or occasionally pulmonary edema. The patient may develop respiratory insufficiency with hypoxemia and carbon dioxide retention. The course may progress to death from chronic respiratory failure or recovery with residual chronic obstructive pulmonary disease. Bronchiolitis obliterans has been noted in patients who die during this period. Some of them may even, develop bronchiectasis. The main treatment in this phase is systemic corticosteroid therapy in an attempt to reduce inflammation. The prognosis is relatively good with prompt treatment. Long-term sequelae of nitrogen dioxide inhalation are related to the extent of exposure and the severity of bronchiolitis obliterans.

Isocyanates

Isocyanates are extensively used in the production of urethane and polyurethane. Products made from these chemicals include adhesives, surface coatings, paints, varnish, rigid and flexible plastic foams and a variety of other products. Although there are different forms of isocyanates used in the industry probably two of them are of considerable importance to human health; Methyl isocyanate (MIC) and toluene di-isocyanate. Nothing much was known about the harmful effects of MIC on human health before the Bhopal incident and this was the principal toxic gas responsible for the high mortality although a combination of toxic materials might have been responsible. MIC gas at a temperature of 170°C undergoes pyrolization and gets converted into HCN, CO and oxides of nitrogen all of which are highly toxic gases. The acute presenting symptoms were irritation of the eyes, dyspnea, cough, pink froth, irritation of throat with choking, chest pain, expectoration, hemoptysis, hoarseness, nausea, anorexia, retching, vomiting, epigastric discomfort, diarrhea, myasthenia like weakness, apathy, coma, listlessness, hypersomnolence, tremor and tetany in varying frequencies. Physical examination revealed tachypnea, tachycardia, rhonchi and crepitations. Cyanosis was conspicuous by its absence (possibly due to high levels of blood COHb). Chest X-rays during the acute phases showed changes consistent with pulmonary edema. The opacities in the X-rays started disappearing at the end of first week of the episode and there was marked clearance in most of the cases by the end of 2 weeks. The mortality was 7.14 percent in the admitted patients. (Most patients had died immediately before any treatment). Lung function studies and blood gas values after four weeks of exposure were normal in most of the patients. In most cases who

showed impaired lung function, the abnormality was of a mild to moderate nature. Long-term effects of the gas exposure are not yet known. The management of the gas victims was mainly symptomatic. Supplemental oxygen, mechanical ventilation, bronchodilators and corticosteroid therapy were instituted to the patients. It seems that high dose corticosteroid (1 gm methyl prednisolone in an intravenous drip) was most effective in controlling symptoms.

TDI

Its toxicity was noted during World War II, but was first reported in 1951 as a cause of persistent respiratory problem. Various respiratory diseases known to be associated with its use are occupational asthma, hypersensitivity pneumonitis and a variety of other nonspecific respiratory symptoms. TDI is highly volatile and hence its danger. Recurrent short-term exposures to high doses may result in respiratory and systemic symptoms resembling acute form of hypersensitivity pneumonitis. Increased mediator release like chemotactic factor and lysozymes of immune complex disease or lymphokines of cellular immunity may be involved in such response. Occupational asthma and in about 5 *percent* of those handling TDI is a long-term effect and has no immediate problem. Acute alterations in pulmonary function like decreased CO transfer and a restrictive defect are observed in some patients. Treatment of acute TDI inhalation injury consists of removal from the site of exposure, oxygen inhalation and corticosteroid therapy.

Aspiration Syndromes

Healthy persons seldom aspirate oropharyngeal or gastric material because of efficient reflex mechanisms and good coordination of various structures in the upper airways area. Risk factors for aspiration include altered levels of consciousness, disorders of esophageal motility and mechanical disruption of the gastroesophageal sphincter. Conditions predisposing to aspiration include general anesthesia, intoxication with alcohol or sedative drugs, seizures, strokes and patients with nasogastric tubes. The character, volume and frequency of the aspirated material decide the extent of lung damage. Small amounts of oropharyngeal secretions by healthy individuals during sleep produce no ill effects. Aspirated material can cause lung disease either due to a direct toxic effect, infectious complications, airways obstruction or a combination of all these.[28]

Toxic Fluids

Acids, animal fat, mineral oil, alcohol and hydrocarbons can initiate an inflammatory reaction in the lung parenchyma independent of a bacterial infection. Gastric acid aspiration is the most common toxic fluid and well studied. The degree of lung damage is inversely related to the gastric pH, with no adverse effect when the pH is above 2.4. Many investigators have equated gastric aspiration with that of chemical burn of the respiratory tract. Within minutes of the aspiration, the patient will develop dyspnea, cough and bronchospasm resulting from peribronchial exudation and hemorrhage. Early in the course of events, chest X-ray may show patchy infiltrates over the lower lobes, which may rapidly progress into noncardiogenic pulmonary edema (ARDS). The treatment is mainly supportive with oxygen supplementation and bronchodilators as and when needed. Steroid may be helpful if given prior to the episode. Antibiotics are indicated only if there is raising temperature, increased white cell counts and purulent sputum.

Mineral oil aspiration in adults produces a syndrome that is termed as "lipoid pneumonia". Since numeral oil is relatively an inert compound, the pneumonia is usually not detected till the aspiration has been going on for several weeks to months. The diagnosis is usually established by detection of lipid-laden macrophages in the sputum, bronchoalveolar fluid or in tissue sections from lung biopsy. Treatment in general is supportive and corticosteroid has no proven benefit. In contrast to mineral oils, aspiration of other more volatile hydrocarbons, such as kerosene and gasolene produces an acute widespread chemical pneumonitis that mimics ARDS. The treatment here is again supportive. Corticosteroids and prophylactic antibiotics have not been shown to alter the course or outcome of the disease.

A large array of potentially toxic substances can cause a variety of lung injuries in a number of ways. There is always the risk that the medical response to the uncommon but major incident might be delayed or mismanaged because the epidemiological, laboratory, and toxicological skills needed rapidly to evaluate and advice on the hazard are not available locally. Hospital protocols should include managing chemical burns of the eyes and skin in addition to the inhalation lung injury. The local population should be advised on the hazards of a release and the protective measures they should adopt in the event of such a mishap. In the emergency room, a quick evaluation of the patient with adequate oxygenation and in most instances an intensive care with ventilatory support is necessary.

REFERENCES

1. Misra NP, Pathak R, Gaur KGBS, Jain SC, Yesikar SS, et al. Clinical profile of gas leak victims in acute phase after Bhopal episode. Ind J Med Res 1987; 86(Suppl):ll-19.
2. Kumar S. Victims of gas leak in Bhopal seek redress on compensation. BMJ 2004;329:366.
3. Baxter PJ. Major chemical disasters. Br Med J 1991; 302:61-62.
4. Flury KE, Dines DE, Rodarte JR, Rodgers R. Airways obstruction due to the inhalation of ammonia. Mayo Cli Proc 1983;58:389-93.
5. Trunkey DD. Inhalation injury. Surg Clin North Am 1978;58:1133-40.
6. Head JM. Inhalation injury in burns. Am Surg 1980; 139:508-12.
7. Banauch GI, Dhala A, Alleyne D, Alva R, Santhyadka G, Krasko A, Weiden M, Kelly KJ, Prezant DJ. Bronchial hyperreactivity and other inhalation lung injuries in rescue/recovery workers after the World Trade Center collapse. Crit Care Med 2005;33(1 Suppl):S102-06.
8. Banauch GI, Dhala A, Prezant DJ. Pulmonary disease in rescue workers at the World Trade Center site. Curr Opin Pulm Med 2005;11:160-68.
9. Latenser BA, Iteld L. Smoke inhalation injury. Semin Respir Crit Care Med 2001;22:13-22.
10. Ramakrishna KM, Sankar J, Venkatraman J. Profile of pediatric burns Indian experience in a tertiary care burn unit. Burns 2005;31:351-53.
11. Liffner G, Bak Z, Reske A, Sjoberg F. Inhalation injury assessed by score does not contribute to the development of acute respiratory distress syndrome in burn victims. Burns 2005;3:263-68.
12. Broz L, Valova M, Vajtr D, Adamek T, Tomasova H, Mocikova H. Inhalation trauma in burns, cytology and biochemical findings. Acta Chir Plast 2004;46:43.
13. Burns TR, Greenberg SD, Cartwright J, Jachimczyk JA. Smoke inhalation: An ultrastructural study of reaction to injury in the human alveolar wall. Environ Res 1986;41:447-57.
14. Sundram FX, Lee ST. Radionuclide lung scanning in the management of respiratory burns. Ann Acad Med Singapore 1992;21:630-34.
15. Trimble EJ. The management of aircraft passenger survival in fire. Toxicology 1996;115:41-61.
16. Leduc D, Gris P, Lheureux P, Gevenois PA, De Vuyst P, Yernault JC. Acute and long term respiratory damage following inhalation of ammonia. Thorax. 1992;47:755-57.
17. de la Hoz RE, Schlueter DP, Rom WN. Chronic lung disease secondary to ammonia inhalation injury: A report on three cases. Am J Ind Med 1996;29:209-14.
18. Montague TJ, MacNeil AR. Mass ammonia inhalation. Chest 1980;77:496-98.
19. Flury KE, Dines DE, Rodarte JR, Rodgers R. Airway obstruction due to inhalation of ammonia. Mayo Clin Proc 1983;58:389-93.

20. Burns TR, Mace ML, Greenberg SD, Jachimczyk JA. Ultrastructure of acute ammonia toxicity in the human lung. Am J Forensic Med Pathol 1985;6:204-10.

21. Woto-Gaye G, Mendez V, Boye IA, Ndiaye PD. Death from ammonia poisoning: Anatomo-pathologic features. Dakar Med 1999;44:199-201.

22. O'Kane GJ. Inhalation of ammonia vapour. A report on the management of eight patients during the acute stages. Anaesthesia 1983;38:1208-13.

23. Arwood R, Hammond J, Ward GG. Ammonia inhalation. J Trauma 1985;25:444-47.

24. Hahn IH, Muhammad A. Does nebulized corticosteroid therapy have an effect on ammonia-induced pulmonary injury? J Toxicol Clin Toxicol 2000;38:79. Comments in: J Toxicol Clin Toxicol 2000;38:81. J Toxicol Clin Toxicol 1999;37:59-67.

25. Tanen DA, Graeme KA, Raschke R. Severe lung injury after exposure to chloramine gas from household cleaners. N Engl J Med 1999;341:848-49.

26. Ramirez JR, Dowell AR. Silofillers disease: Nitrogen dioxide induced lung injury. Ann Int Med 1971;74:569.

27. Dawson SV, Schenker MB. Health effects of inhalation of ambient concentration of nitrogen dioxide. Am Rev Respir Dis 1979;120:281-92

28. Bartlett JG, Gorbach SL. The triple threat of aspiration pneumonia. Chest 1975;68:560-66.

THE BHOPAL GAS TRAGEDY

At 11.00 pm on December 2 1984, while most of the one million residents of Bhopal slept, an operator at the plant noticed a small leak of methyl isocyanate (MIC) gas and increasing pressure inside a storage tank. The vent-gas scrubber, a safety device designer to neutralize toxic discharge from the MIC system, had been turned off three weeks prior.[1,2] Apparently a faulty valve had allowed one ton of water for cleaning internal pipes to mix with 40 tons of MIC.[3] A 30 ton refrigeration unit that normally served as a safety component to cool the MIC storage tank had been drained of its coolant for use in another part of the plant.[4] Pressure and heat from the vigorous exothermic reaction in the tank continued to build. The gas flare safety system was out of action and had been for three months. At around 1.00 am, December 3, loud rumbling reverberated around the plant as a safety valve gave way sending a plume of MIC gas into the early morning air.[5] Within hours, the streets of Bhopal were littered with human corpses and the carcasses of buffaloes, cows, dogs and birds. An estimated 3,800 people died immediately, mostly in the poor slum colony adjacent to the UCC plant.[1,5] Local hospitals were soon overwhelmed with the injured, a crisis further compounded by a lack of knowledge of exactly what gas was involved and what its effects were.[2] It became one of the worst chemical disasters in history and the name Bhopal became synonymous with industrial catastrophe.[6]

Estimates of the number of people killed in the first few days by the plume from the UCC plant run as high as 10,000, with 15,000 to 20,000 premature deaths reportedly occurring in the subsequent two decades.[7] The Indian government reported that more than half a million people were exposed to the gas.[8] Several epidemiological studies conducted soon after the accident showed significant morbidity and increased mortality in the exposed population. Early and late effects on health. These data are likely to under-represent the true extent of adverse health effects[8] are summarized below:

Early effects (0-6 months)	
Ocular	Chemosis, redness, watering, ulcers, photophobia
Respiratory	Distress, pulmonary edema, pneumonitis, pneumothorax
Gastrointestinal	Persistent diarrhea, anorexia, persistent abdominal pain
Genetic	Increased chromosomal abnormalities
Psychological	Neuroses, anxiety states, adjustment reactions
Neurobehavioral	Impaired audio and visual memory, impaired vigilance attention and response time, impaired reasoning

The methyl isocyanate (MIC) gas leak from the Union Carbide plant at Bhopal, India in 1984 was the worst industrial disaster in history. Exposure estimates of gas concentrations in the area range from 85 to 0.12 ppm. Of the approximately 200,000 persons exposed, 3598 deaths have resulted as of November 1989. Chronic inflammatory damage to the eyes and lungs appears to be the main cause of morbidity. Reproductive health problems in the form of increased spontaneous abortions and psychological problems have been reported. Questions about the nature of MIC toxicity have been raised by the persistence of multi-systemic symptoms in survivors. Animal studies using radiolabeled MIC given by the inhalation route have shown that the radiolabel is capable of crossing the lung membranes and being distributed to many organs of the body.[9]

Respiratory symptoms were significantly more common and lung function (percentage predicted forced expiratory volume in one second (FEV$_1$), forced vital capacity (FVC), forced expiratory flow between 25 percent and 75 percent of vital capacity (FEF25-75), and FEV_1/FEV ratio) was reduced among those reporting exposure to the gas leak. The frequency of symptoms fell as exposure decreased (as estimated by distance lived from the plant), and lung function measurements displayed similar trends. These findings were not wholly accounted for by confounding by smoking or literacy, a measure of socioeconomic status. Lung function measurements were consistently lower in those reporting symptoms.[10]

Many studies were subsequently undertaken after the disaster. Sixty patients exposed to methyl isocyanate and presenting with respiratory symptoms were studied using bronchoalveolar lavage (BAL) 1 to 7 years after the accident. Pulmonary function tests included forced vital capacity (FVC) and forced expiratory volume in one second (FEV_1). An index of severity of exposure was derived retrospectively on the basis of the acute symptoms in the victims themselves or the occurrence of death among their family members. Total lung inflammatory cells ($p < 0.01$) and absolute numbers of macrophages ($p = 0.01$) and lymphocytes ($p < 0.05$) increased as severity of exposure increased. FEV_1/FVC percent ($p = 0.05$) was also significantly lower as severity of exposure increased. Moderately exposed subjects had significantly lower FEV_1/FVC percent ($p < 0.05$) compared to those mildly exposed. In nonsmokers, BAL neutrophils, both percentage and absolute numbers, showed significant negative correlations with FEV_1 %predicted (rs = -0.350, $p < 0.05$; and rs = -0.374, $p < 0.01$, respectively). Neutrophil percentage was negatively correlated with FEV_1/FVC % (rs = -0.378; $p < 0.01$). Absolute lymphocytes had significant negative correlations with FVC % pred (rs = -0.318; $p < 0.05$). Macrophages had significant positive correlations with FVC % pred (rs = 0.322; $p < 0.05$) and FEV_1 % pred (rs = 0.433; $p < 0.01$). Radiographic abnormalities [International Labor Organization (ILO) classification] were associated with decline in FEV_1 % pred ($p < 0.05$). This study suggests that pulmonary function abnormalities occur in gas-exposed subjects as a consequence of an abnormal accumulation of lung inflammatory cells (lymphocytes and neutrophils), and that the intensity of lung inflammation and reduction in pulmonary function are greater in severely exposed subjects. As it has been observed that decline in pulmonary function is associated with radiographic abnormalities, there is a suggestion that injury following toxic gas exposure can lead to irreversible lung damage.[11]

Animal toxicologic information was limited prior to the accident, but has since confirmed that the lung is the major target of these lethal injuries, invariably with pulmonary edema.[12] Early concerns regarding acute cyanide intoxication were not supported by subsequent scientific inquiry. Superficial corneal erosions did not result in permanent eye injury. The primary medical (and, presumably, legal) issue which is unresolved, and perhaps unresolvable, is the incidence and determinants of long-term respiratory injury in the survivors. Available evidence, which is limited, suggests that chronic damage, when present, is, or resembles, fibrosing bronchiolitis obliterans, the expected consequence when permanent injury results from acute, high-level irritant gas exposure. Definition of the follow-up population is uncertain, and exposure information is lacking. Dose-response relationships are not likely to emerge from follow-up studies.

The long-term (subacute and chronic) histopathological effects in the lungs of rats subjected to a single exposure to methyl isocyanate (MIC) by both the inhalation and subcutaneous (sc) routes as well as the role of methylamine (MA) and N,N'-dimethyl-urea (DMU), the hydrolytic derivatives of MIC in eliciting the observed changes.[13] At the subacute phase, the intraalveolar and interstitial edema were prominent only in the inhalation group as against the more pronounced inflammatory response in the sc route. With the progress of time the evolution of lesions appeared to be similar, culminating in the development of significant interstitial pneumonitis and fibrosis. MA, one of the hydrolytic derivatives of MIC, also caused interstitial pneumonitis progressing to fibrosis, albeit to a lesser extent than MIC, indicating its contribution to the long-term pulmonary damage. The diffuse interstitial pulmonary fibrosis observed at 10 weeks after a single exposure to MIC by either route is of greater significance in the context of the occurrence of pulmonary fibrosis in the late autopsies of Bhopal gas victims and also clinical sequelae in some of the survivors.

Further, the pathology of acute inhalation exposure to MIC in the tissues of male and female Fischer 344 rats were evaluated immediately after a single 2 hr exposure to 0, 3, 10, or 30 ppm MIC, and through day 91. Early gross pathologic changes in the 30 ppm-exposed rats included a reddish white encrustation around the mouth and nose, a small thymus, and distension of the gastrointestinal tract with gas. Lungs (middle and median lobes) showed consolidation and hemorrhage and failed to deflate when the chest cavity was opened. Microscopic changes in the upper respiratory tract 3 hr after exposure included marked erosion and separation of olfactory and respiratory epithelia from the basement membrane with accumulation of serofibrinous fluid. On day 1, acute inflammation and fibrinopurulent exudate partially blocked the nasal passages. Epithelial cells had sloughed from the nasopharynx, trachea, bronchi, and major bronchioles, leaving the basement membrane covered with fibrin and exudate. Granulomatous inflammation and intraluminal fibrosis of the airways were observed by day 3, with increased intraluminal fibrosis by day 7. Lower airways became blocked by exfoliated cells, mucous plugs, and/or intraluminal fibrosis.[14]

Thus, a series of experimental and clinical studies have highlighted the harful effects of Bhopal Gas Tragedy.

REFERENCES

1. Edward Broughton, The Blopal disaster and its aftermath: A review. Environ Health 2005:4:6
2. Fortun, K. Advocacy after Bhopal. Chicago, University of Chicago Press 2001;259.
3. Shrivastava P. Managing Industrial Crisis. New Delhi: Vision Books 1987;196.
4. Shrivastava P. Bhopal: Anatomy of a Crisis. Cambridge, MA, Ballinger Publishing; 1987;184.
5. Hazardous Installations Directorate. Health and Safety Executive: Accident Summary, Union Carbide India Ltd. Bhopal, India: December 2004;3,1984.
6. MacKenzie D. Fresh evidence on Bhopal disaster. New Scientist 2002;19.
7. Sharma DC. Bhopal: 20 Years On. Lancet. 2005;365:111-112.
8. Cassells J. Sovereign immunity: Law in an unequal world. Social and legal studies. 1996;5:431-36.
9. Dhara VR, Dhara R. The Union Carbide disaster in Bhopal: A review of health effects. Arch Environ Health 2002;57:391-404.
10. Beckett WS. Persistent respiratory effects in survivors of the Bhopal disaster. Thorax 1998;53 Suppl 2:S43-46.
11. Vijayan VK, Sankaran K. Relationship between lung inflamamtion, changes in lung function and severity of exposure in victims of the Bhopal tragedy. Eur Respir J 1996;9:1977-82.
12. Weill H. Disaster at Bhopal: The accident, early findings and respiratory health outlook in those injured. Bull Eurphysiopathol Respir 1987:587-90
13. Sriramachari S, Jeevaratnam K. Comparative toxicity of methyl isocyanate and its hydrolytic derivatives in rats. II. Pulmonary histopathology in the subacute and chronic phases. Epidemiol Prev 1992;52:22-31.
14. Bucher JR, Boorman GA, Gupta BN, Uraih LC, Hall LB, Stefanski SA. Two-hour methyl isocyanate inhalation exposure and 91 day recovery: A preliminary description of pathologic changes in F344 rats. Environ Health Perspect 1987;72:71-75.

OCCUPATIONAL LUNG DISEASES PECULIAR TO INDIA

The main health priorities in India like malnutrition, infections, communicable diseases, poor sanitary conditions takes away the attention from the occupational lung diseases. With change of environment and change in the industrial policy of the Government, occupational diseases pose important challenge to the health care sector. Besides, traditional occupational diseases, Indian situations pose some peculiar problem as regards occupational lung diseases are concerned.[1] With rapid industrialization, there exist the age-old practices of agriculture and plantation. More than half-of the Indian work force is engaged in farming. Besides other occupational hazards like accidents, rice-field dermatitis, high respiratory morbidity has been recorded from a cross-sectional study from Lucknow in mango plantation workers.[2] The farming population attributed this to the prolonged exposure to the organic dust. In a study of respiratory symptoms in farmers from North India, Behera et al[3] reported a high prevalence of respiratory symptoms among different farming practices. About 70 to 115 million children under the age of 14 years form the work force in India. More than 80 percent of this child labor is in the field of agriculture. Most of occupational hazards in them include heat-related problems, mechanical injuries, insect bites and toxic effects of chemicals.[4] Children employed in carpet weaving industry in Jaipur city has a higher prevalence of acute respiratory problems (26.4%) compared to those in the community (15.2%) and these are attributed to cotton dust exposure.[5] In Shivkashi, where about a third of the labor force consists of children in the firecracker industry, cough, cold, throat irritation, dizziness, methemoglobinemia, and anemia are common symptoms besides fire and blasts. These symptoms are due to inhalation or ingestion of chlorate dust by these children.[6] Further, inhalation of sulfates cause cough, asthma, eye irritation, respiratory infections and other chronic lung diseases.[6] HIV infection and related complications are common in commercial sex workers.[7]

There is a rapid growth in the industrialization process and participation of workforce in Industrial sector is on raise since independence in 1947. Occupational health studies in this sector initiated as early as seventies on tobacco workers, among those exposed to tobacco, an elevated level of nicotine was observed in the urine samples that causes several physical problems.[8] Among the tannery workers of Kanpur industrial slums, occupational morbidly was recorded as 28 percent.[9] The lock factory workers of Alighar showed that 73 percent of subjects under study are suffering with respiratory tract problems. Chronic bronchitis and emphysema are frequently diagnosed and increasing with duration of work.[10] Adult carpet weavers in Mirzapur also reported respiratory problems as major occupational risk, the causal factors are carpet dust particles.[11] Epidemiological study in Bangalore by Regional occupation health centre on workers of incense sticks showed the possible inhalation of pollutants and related health hazards.[12] In a retrospective epidemiological study conducted on southeastern coal mine workers revealed the overall prevalence of pneumoconiosis was about 3 percent in India.[13] An increase in the deterioration of lung function was observed in Tamil Nadu among the workers who are exposed to asbestos dust compared to the general workers in a manufacturing unit.[14] Normally workers in the salt industry exposed to sunlight, salt dust and contact with brine. In a knowledge, attitude and practice study it was revealed that there is a huge gap between knowledge and practice of protective devises, despite of universal knowledge about the devises only one-third use them in practice.[15]

More than 20 millions workers are involved in the textile industry in India, which is a dye dominant industry. In 1995, in a survey of 273 respiratory system examinations; 54 (30%) of the 179 individuals working in the dusty sections of a textile mill had byssinosis. In the nondusty departments, 16 (17%) out of the 94 workers were affected.[16] Similar study in Pondicherry reveals 6-fold risk of byssinosis among workers of spinning section and 2-fold increase among workers of weaving section.[17]

Pooled analyses from five units of department of atomic energy seen clearly that the workers in the radiation units are not at extra risk of cancer compared to workers in nonradiation units.[18] In another public sector industry, Indian Oil Corporation limited, prevalence of work related injuries are 35 percent among all injuries reported in their hospital and burn injuries were about 6 percent of all injuries. This study emphasizes causation of industrial burns and importance of prevention of burns in industries.[19] This clearly indicates that the safety measures are in place among organized and premier government and public sector institutes of India. In the similar line a study on heat exposure on glass works industry differs from international standards. It recommends separate standard measures for tropical and subtropical countries like India also suggest on ideal duration of work and duration of rest in the context of Indian glass industry.[20]

Health care providers are at high risk of infection if they ignore safety measures, evidence from cohort study conducted on health care providers in Andhra Pradesh shown an association between occupation (hospital staff) and incidences of malaria. Due to lack of precautions, the risks are 4-fold for nursing students and 2-fold among medical students than well-trained doctors'.[21] Similar study on west Bengal hospital personnel shown elevated risks of Hepatitis B infection.[22] Another interesting study based on traffic policemen from six major town of north India attributed risk of exposure to benzene from fuel exhaust and also discussed how this inhaled benzene metabolized phenol, posing health consequences.[23] Another study from a tertiary care Northern Indian Premier Institute of India had shown a high prevalence of tuberculosis among trainee resident doctors.[24]

Preventive Measures for Occupational Diseases

There are very few professional agencies like National Institute of Occupational Health (NIOH), Industrial Toxicology Research Center (ITRC), Central Labor Institute are working on researchable issues like Asbestos and asbestos related diseases, Pesticide poisoning, Silica related diseases other than silicosis and Musculoskeletal disorders.[25] Indian occupational health is more complex than a health issue, which includes child labor; poor industrial legislation; vast informal sector; less attention to industrial hygiene and poor surveillance data.[26] Due to poor surveillance it is impossible to assess the disease burden in this country due to occupational exposure. There is some sort of awareness or implementation of safety measures and legislation after the Bhopal gas tragedy in 1984.[27] As discussed above, in this incident, poisonous gases leaked from a fertilizer factory killed 5800 and injured about half a million people. Their injuries ranged from breathlessness, gastrointestinal problems to neurological disorders.[28] Most of the industrial laws in this country are only confide to the paper and never seen a reality in implementing their standards. There is always poor investment on industrial safety, labor is cheap and easily replaceable, so employers seen a need for improving occupational safety and health. Labor unions are mostly week, politician driven and lack knowledge about the occupational risks. Under the supervision of Inspector general of India, a small number of three hundred-factory inspectors are responsible to check the industrial safety in this vast country, compared to 3000 factory inspectors in a small country like Japan. This shows the poor concern of the government about industrial safety and subsequently the occupational health.[27] On one hand there is need to understand the risk factors of modern occupations and on other hand the hazards from traditional occupations yet to explore. There is a big gap in the epidemiological evidence from different industry specific, exposure specific areas. Most of the studies mentioned above are very small-scale, community-based studies. They are often concluded from very small sample sizes between 200-300 subjects. The nature of various study-designs, control groups, interview procedures, self-reporting biases and statistical techniques used in those studies made the interpretations very complex, pose difficulties to generalize the conclusions about occupational risks.

Indian doctors and nurses are very poorly trained to deal with occupation health related morbidity. Neither many medical schools were specialized in this faculty nor offer specialized training. There is a big demand and supply equations for Industrial hygienists and occupational professionals and semiprofessionals in the market. A silver line in this training aspect comes from the decision by Indian Medical association to educate all its members in occupational health issues.[26]

Except few major, reputed, public and private industries, other industrialists are not sensitized about the importance of occupational safety in their industries. Occupational health never occupied proper place in their budgets. In some instances worker groups saw occupational safety equipment with negative attitude, and work without safety measures was seen as heroism among illiterate folks. Some of the other problems are from ill equipment, improper checks on fire fighting equipment, lack of training in use the safety equipment and alcoholism during work.

In last decade, there are some environmental activists trying to lobby the government towards ban of some hazardous materials. In the Asian continent, India is emerging as the major user of asbestos where the developed world phasing out its use. Due to poor occupational health and safety systems in India and difficulties in early detection of pulmonary malignancy related to asbestos, Indian government should consider the ban of this material in future.[29] Recently, Indian Association of Occupation Health took a strong and principled stand against the asbestos industry and many of its members requested for the asbestos ban in India.[30]

Occupational and environmental concerns are not two different issues. It is a big task to understand the intensity of environmental deterioration in this county. To mention few examples of environmental problems in India, as many as 42 million people in the West Bengal area may be exposed to arsenic in drinking water at concentrations of health concern. Similarly, as many as 10 million industrial or mine workers in India may be exposed to asbestos or other dusts at concentrations of health concern.[31] Research questions should always need to Integrate concerns of industrial safety, occupational health and environmental health together.

India urgently requires modern Occupational Health Safety (OHS) legislation with adequate enforcement machinery, and establishment of centers of excellence in occupational medicine, to catch up with the rest of the world.[26] To accelerate the process of providing OHS in organized sector, government may initiate local level organizations with industrialists, medical professionals, and researchers and trade unions as partners. Pilot studies are required to address some solutions in informal sectors. Keeping the importance of primary sector in mind, skill training to agricultural units may reduce the accidents and related hazards. A block-level (subdistrict), village levels agricultural workshops and training will help to save our farmers from fatal hazards. The pesticides poisoning may be eliminated with help of latest development of chemical technology. The problem of transferring industries from industrialized world to India has a growing concern. Many of the hazardous industries were pushed from developed countries towards India due to their environmental regulations, increased labor costs and green moments. Due to poor implementation of industrial regulations, cheap labor, poverty and unemployment India welcome these hazardous industries[32] and impose a strict vigilance on all those industries with hazardous materials. Government should also weigh between environment and health costs of our people and cost of importing them from elsewhere.

All health professionals, paramedics and industrial hygienists should be thoroughly trained about occupational health safety and exposure to hazardous material at all levels of hierarchy in the health sector (referral hospitals, primary and urban health centers). Interventions need to be introduced about the awareness of health hazards among public, workers, and trade unions. This effort should also promote universal acceptance of protection material. Many community-based interventions are on going in India (TB, HIV prevention, immunization, etc.), a comprehensive approaches to including occupational health will be cost-effective method to achieve this Himalayan task.

There is a tremendous potentiality for large-scale epidemiological research to determine the exposure and occupational risks. The public-private partnerships are very important to success of this goal. Most difficult part of occupational health research is exposure assessment by recording life time job history, job titles, and information on past occupations, industries, and occupational conditions, and Identification of other causal confounders. Listing all occupational carcinogens were identified and listed by International Agency for Research on Cancer (IARC/WHO), which provides data on carcinogenicity of chemicals, groups of chemicals, industrial process and other complex mixtures.[33] Most of the evidences in these monographs are from developed world; since there are no such studies in India replicate some of the exposure studies in India to test the validity of the similar carcinogencity.

To assess the occupational situation, data from other sources may be streamlined. Record occupation on various data bases of public use (ration cards, driving license, etc.), surveillance of disease occurrence in industrial belts, analyzing occupation on death certificates, using record-linkage techniques between various resources may also improve the research potentiality on occupation health. To start with, some geographical (ecological) correlation studies will helps to generate hypothesis about occupational risks in various parts of India. However, large-scale retrospective cohort studies will address many of the policy questions in this country. Various sophisticated expert assessment tools are needed to validate the occupational exposures and their risk[34] collaborations with international occupational experts will be a quick solution to address these technical difficulties.

Initially we need more focus on epidemiological data for decision-making and setting priorities in the research, pioneering institutes like NIOH and ITRC should be updated with advanced research facilities in epidemiological research. Meanwhile we also need to generate a pool of human resources in occupational health researchers, creation of environmental and occupational health cells at all district levels may help us to develop some databases or information systems across the country. All international treaties and agreements should also address the concerns of occupational health as mandatory.

Some international collaboration are in action for some time for Indo-Dutch Environmental and Sanitary Engineering Project under the Ganga action Plan work working for social health and community improvements in the Industrial slums. Several collaborations are on going in technology of industrial safety. India also signed a bilateral collaborative agreement with United States in terms of emergency preparedness and response; training, education, and technology transfer; and research.[32] To meet local shortage of resources, to address all out-

standing issues in the fields of environmental and occupational health, India should turn towards international community and World Health Organization.[1]

REFERENCES

1. Agnihotram RV. An overview of occupational health research in India. Ind J Occup Environ Med 2005;9:10-14.
2. Gupta BN, Mathur N, Rastogi SK, Srivastava AK, Chandra H, Pangtey BS, et al. Socioeconomic, environmental, and health aspects of farm workers engaged in mango plantations. Biomed Environ Sci 1995;8:301-09.
3. Behera D, Pal D, Gupta D. Respiratory symptoms among farmers in the vicinity of a North Indian City. Lung India 2005;22:43-47.
4. Banerjee SR. Agricultural child labour in west Bengal. Ind Paediatr 1993;30:1425-29.
5. Joshi SK, Sharma U, Sharma P, Pathak SS, Sitaraman S, Verma CR. Health status of carpet weaving children. Ind Paediatr 1994;31:571-74.
6. Sekhar SR. Children at health risks. ICCW New Bulletin 1992;40:53-59.
7. Jana S, Basu I, Rotheram-Borus MJ, Newman PA. The Sonagachi project—A self sustainable community intervention programme. AIDS Edu Prev 2004;16:405-14.
8. Ghosh SK, Parikh JR, Gokani VN, Kashyap SK, Chatterjee SK. Studies on occupational health problems during agricultural operation of Indian tobacco workers: A preliminary survey report. J Occup Med 1979;21:45-47.
9. Shukla A, Kumar S, Ory FG. Occupational health and the environment in an urban slum in India. Soc Sci Med 1991;33:597-603.
10. Hassan MA, Khan Z, Yunus M, Bhargava R. Health profile of lock factory workers in Aligarh. Indian J Public Health 2002;46:39-45.
11. Das PK, Shukla KP, Ory FG. An occupational health programme for adults and children in the carpet weaving industry, Mirzapur, India: A case study in the informal sector. Soc Sci Med 1992;35:1293-302.
12. Rathnakara UP, Krishna Murthy V, Rajmohan HR, Nagarajan L, Vasundhra MK. An enquiry into work environmental status and health of workers involved in production of incense sticks in city of Bangalore. Indian J Public Health 1992;36:38-44.
13. Parihar YS, Patnaik JP, Nema BK, Sahoo GB, Misra IB, Adhikary S. Coal workers' pneumoconiosis: A study of prevalence in coal mines of eastern Madhya Pradesh and Orissa states of India. Ind Health 1997;35:467-73.
14. Gautam AK, Yunus M, Rahman A, Reddy SS. Environmental monitoring of asbestos products manufacturing units—A case study. Indian J Environ Health 2003;45:289-92.
15. Haldiya KR, Sachdev R, Mathur ML, Saiyed HN. Knowledge, attitude and practices related to occu-

pational health problems among salt workers working in the desert of Rajasthan, India. J Occup Health 2005;47:85-88.

16. Murlidhar V, Murlidhar VJ, Kanhere V. Byssinosis in a Bombay textile mill. Natl Med J India 1995;8:204-07.

17. Mishra AK, Rotti SB, Sahai A, Madanmohan, Narayan KA. Byssinosis among male textile workers in Pondicherry: A case-control study. Natl Med J India 2003;16:70-73.

18. Nambi KS, Mayya YS. Pooled analysis of cancer mortality cases among the employees in five units of the Department of Atomic Energy in India. Indian J Cancer 1997;34:99-106.

19. Sarma BP. Epidemiology and man-days loss in burn injuries amongst workers in an oil industry. Burns 2001;27:475-80.

20. Srivastava A, Kumar R, Joseph E, Kumar A. Heat exposure study in the workplace in a glass manufacturing unit in India. Ann Occup Hyg 2000;44:449-53.

21. Rajasekhar M, Nandakumar NV. Occupational malaria and health risk among select occupational health care employee groups in an urban hospital at Tirupati, AP. Indian J Malariol 2000;37:53-60.

22. Bhattacharya S, Dalal BS, Bhattacharya I, Lahiri A. Hepatitis B viral infection amongst hospital personnel in Calcutta. Indian J Public Health 2001;45:135-36.

23. Verma Y, Kumar A, Rana SV. Biological monitoring of exposure to benzene in traffic policemen of north India. Ind Health 2003;41:260-64.

24. Rao KG, Aggarwal AN, Behera D. Tuberculosis among physicians in training. Int J Tuberc Lung Dis 2004; 8:1392-94.

25. Saiyed HN, Tiwari RR. Occupational health research in India. Ind Health 2004;42:141-48.

26. Joshi TK, Smith KR. Occupational health in India. Occup Med 2002;17:371-89.

27. Parekh R. Future occupational health prospection. Indian J Occup Enviorn Med 2004;8:5-6.

28. Kumar S. Victims of gas leak in Bhopal seek redress on compensation. BMJ 2004;329:366.

29. Joshi TK, Gupta RK. Asbestos in developing countries: Magnitude of risk and its practical implications. Int J Occup Med Environ Health 2004;17:179-85.

30. Castleman B. Heroism in occupational health. Int J Health Serv 2001;31:669-72.

31. Allred M, Campolucci S, Falk H, Ganguly NK, Saiyed HN, Shah B. Bilateral environmental and occupational health program with India. Int J Hyg Environ Health 2003;206:323-32.

32. Jeyaratnam J. Occupational Health Issues in developing countries. Environ Res 1993;60:207-12.

33. IARC/WHO (International Agency for Research on Cancer). IARC Monographs on evaluation of carcinogenic risks to humans. Supp l.7. Overall evaluations of carcinogencity: An updating of IARC monographs Vol.1 to 42, Lyon, France: IARC.

34. Siemiatycki J. Risk Factors for cancer in the workplace. Boca Raton, Florida: CRC Press 2000;100-02.

Disorders of Pleura

ANATOMY

The pleura is a serous membrane that covers the lungs, mediastinum, the diaphragm, and the thoracic cage. It is divided into the *visceral* pleura, which covers the entire surface of the lung, including the interlobar fissures, and the *parietal* pleura, which covers the inner surface of the rib cage, mediastinum, and diaphragm. Both the visceral and parietal pleura meet at the lung root. There is a small potential space (*pleural space*) between the two layers, which contains a small amount of fluid (7-14 ml) in normal conditions.[1,2] The areas of two pleural surfaces are approximately 2000 cm^2 in a 70 kg man. The pleura develop from the celomic cavity and both the layers of the pleura from the mesothelial elements of the embryo. The parietal and the visceral pleurae are continuous at the hilum of the lung where they are penetrated by the blood vessels of the lung (pulmonary and bronchial), and the main-stem bronchi along with the lymphatics and nerves accompanying them.

The normal pleura is a smooth, glistening, semi-transparent membrane and on light microscopy consist of five layers: (i) a mesothelial layer; (ii) a thin sub-mesothelial connective tissue layer; (iii) a superficial elastic layer; (iv) a relatively loose subpleural connective tissue layer rich in vessels, nerves, and lymphatics; and (v) a deep fibroelastic layer tightly adherent to or in continuity with the parenchymal structures of the lung, diaphragm, or the thorax.[1] The anatomy of the visceral pleura differs in different species, particularly in its thickness.[3,4] The mesothelial cell although forms a single layer, it may be of different shapes.[5,6] Either it is a flattened cell with an elongated nucleus and a disten-dable cytoplasm or a cuboidal or columnar shaped with round nucleus and indistinct luminal surface. The cell thickness varies from 6 to 12 μ and the surface diameter from 16 to 40 μ. The cell contains surface microvilli with highest density on the visceral pleura and in the lower thorax to decrease friction. There are openings between the mesothelial cells, called as stomata that communicate directly with lymphatic lacunae. The exact function of microvilli is not known, although it was believed that they might increase the surface area to facilitate fluid absorption. Now it is thought that they enmesh glyco-protein rich in hyaluronic acid to lessen friction. The mesothelial cells themselves are very active cells responding to various stimuli and produce a number of factors.[7-9] These cells are capable of transformation into macrophages.[10]

The blood supply to the parietal pleura is from the systemic capillaries. While the costal pleura is supplied by branches of the intercostal and internal mammary arteries, the mediastinal pleura is supplied by branches of the bronchial, upper diaphragmatic, internal mammary, and mediastinal arteries. Branches of the subclavian artery or its tributaries supply the apical portion of the parietal pleura. The diaphragmatic plura is supplied by branches of the internal mammary artery, thoracic and abdominal aorta, and celiac artery. The venous drainage is into the bronchial veins, inferior vena cava and the brachiocephalic trunk.[1] The blood supply to the visceral pleura differs in different species. In humans, the bronchial arteries mainly supply nourish-ment to the visceral pleura.[4,11,12] Pulmonary vessels may supply the convex lung surface and part of the diaphragmatic surface.[13] The terminal branches end in a loose network of large capillaries to form a "starlike "pattern that drain into pulmonary veins. So the pressure in visceral pleural capillaries is little less than that in the parietal pleura.

The visceral pleura have rich lymphatic supply and they run towards the hilum after forming intercommuni-cating plexuses. They also penetrate the lung to join the bronchial lymph vessels. They do not take part in the clearance of proteins or other materials from the pleural space. On the otherhand, lymphatics of the parietal pleura are in direct communication with the pleural space by means of stomas of varying diameters. Lymphatic drainage of the pleural space begins with the stomata, which in turn are connected with lymphatic lacunae that drain into larger lymphatic channels that run along the intercostal space and drain into the mediastinum. The pleura of the anterior thoracic wall and anterior portion of the diaphragm drain to the sternal lymph nodes, the middle portion of the diaphragmatic pleura drains into the middle mediastinal lymph nodes, the anterior portion of the diaphragmatic pleura and mediastinal pleura drain into the anterior mediastinal lymph nodes. The posterior portion drains into the posterior mediastinal lymph nodes, and the costal parietal pleura drains into the intercostal lymph nodes.[1,14,15]

The parietal pleura is richly innervated by sensory nerve endings from the intercostal nerves, and phrenic nerves. While the former supply the costal pleura and peripheral part of the diaphragmatic pleura, the later supply the central part of diaphragmatic pleura. There are no pain fibers in visceral pleura.[16] Therefore, pleuritic chest pain indicates inflammation or irritation of the parietal pleura.

PHYSIOLOGICAL CONSIDERATIONS OF PLEURAL SPACE

The pleural space between the visceral and the parietal pleurae is a potential, but real space and is approximately 10 to 20 μ in width.[17] Normally there is a thin (10-20 μm) layer of fluid between the visceral and parietal pleura and the amount is about 0.1 to 0.2 ml/kg of body weight, i.e. 7 to 14 ml in a 70 kg person.[1,2] The fluid is clear, and colorless with a protein content of less than 1.5 gm/dl and with a cell count of 1500/ml, most of which are mononuclear cells. Leukocytes are rare and there are no red blood cells.[18-22] The mean pleural fluid oncotic pressure is 4.8 cm H_2O in rabbits and 3.2 cm H_2O in dogs.[21] Protein electrophoresis has shown that the pattern of pleural fluid is similar to that of the serum except that low molecular weight proteins like albumin are present in relatively greater quantities in the pleural fluid. However the ionic concentrations in pleural fluid differ significantly from those in serum.

At FRC, the pressure in the pleural space, *the pleural pressure*, is negative in relation to the atmosphere, because of the opposing elastic recoil of the chest wall and the lung. Hydrostatic pressure is not uniform throughout the space. In an upright man, the pleural pressure is approximately -8 cm H_2O at the lung apex and -2 cm H_2O at the lung base, with a mean pleural pressure of 5 cm

H_2O. Although the pressure is negative, fluid does not accumulate in the pleural space. Gases move in and out of the pleural space from the capillaries in the visceral and parietal pleura. The sum of the pressure of all gases in the capillaries is 706 mm Hg ($PH_2O = 47$; $PCO_2 = 46$; $PN_2 = 573$; and $PO_2 = 40$ mm Hg). Fluid will move into the pleural space only if the pleural pressure is below 706 mm Hg, or below (760-706 mm Hg) -54 mm Hg relative to atmospheric pressure. Practically the pleural pressure virtually never occurs to this low level, unless there is a communication with the lungs or the atmosphere or because of a gas-forming organism.

The movement of liquid across the pleural membrane is governed by Starling's law of transcapillary exchange and is as follows:

$$f = L_p \, A[(P_{cap} - P_{pl}) - d_d \, (pcap - ppl)]$$

Where f is the liquid movement; Lp is the filtration coefficient per unit area or the hydraulic water conductivity of the membrane; A is the surface area of the membrane; P and p are the hydrostatic and oncotic pressures, respectively of the capillary (cap) and pleural (pl) spaces, and dd is the solute reflection coefficient of the protein, a measure of the membrane's ability to restrict the passage of large molecules.

Various pressures influencing the movement of fluid in and out of pleural space is shown below.

Parietal pleura		Pleural space	Visceral pleura
28		Hydrostatic Pressre	23
	33 ⇒	-5	28 ⇐
		Oncotic Pressure	30
30	26 ⇐	4	26 ⇒
	30 7 ⇒	NET Pressure	2 ⇐

Pressure gradients across visceral and parietal pleura regulating fluid movement into and out of pleural space

The hydrostatic pressure of the parietal pleura is approximately 28 cm H_2O and that of the pleural space is—5 cm H_2O. This gives a hydrostatic gradient for the parietal pleura of 33 cm H_2O, which favors the movement of fluid from the parietal pleura to the pleural space. The oncotic pressure in the blood is approximately 30 cm H_2O and that of the pleural fluid is about 4 cm H_2O. Thus a net oncotic pressure gradient of 26 cm H_2O across the parietal pleura tries to prevent the hydrostatic gradient of 33, and thus a net gradient of 7 cm H_2O favors the movement of fluid from the capillaries of the parietal pleura to the pleural space. On the otherhand, fluid movement across the visceral pleura is different from that in the parietal pleura. Since the hydrostatic pressure in the visceral pleural capillaries is closer to that of the pulmonary circulation (23 cm H_2O), the net hydrostatic pressure is 28 cm H_2O, which is opposed by the oncotic pressure of 26 cm H_2O (oncotic pressure is not different), causing the net gradient of 28-26 = 2 cm H_2O. This low value allows a very little fluid movement across the visceral pleura and normally most pleural fluid comes from the parietal pleura.

Another important factor that tries to keep the fluid to a minimum is the removal of excess fluid from the pleural space by the lymphatics. Normal fluid formation in the pleural space is about 16.8 ml per day. Whereas about 0.01 ml/kg/hr of fluid enters constantly into the pleural space from the parietal pleura, almost all of these fluid are absorbed by the lymphatics which have a capacity of removal of fluid of at least 0.20 ml/kg/hr, which provides a capacity of 20 times of that is formed. Thus an excess fluid can only accumulate due to any of the six mechanisms:

(1) An increase in the hydrostatic pressure in the microvascular circulation
(2) A decrease in the oncotic pressure in the micro-vascular pressure
(3) Decrease in pressure in the pleural space
(4) Increased permeability of the microvascular circulation
(5) Impaired lymphatic drainage from the pleural space
(6) Movement fluid from the peritoneal space.

I. PLEURAL EFFUSION

A pleural effusion is the accumulation of excess fluid in the pleural space, and results only when the formation of liquid and protein exceeds the removal capacity. Thus, it results from an imbalance between fluid formation and removal. Pleural effusion is divided clinically into *transudative* and *exudative* effusions. The mechanisms of such an excess accumulation of fluid has been described previously. Basically, a transudative pleural effusion occurs when abnormalities in the Starling factors (systemic or pulmonary microvascular hydrostatic pressures, or plasma oncotic pressures) influences the fluid movement as a result of an elevated net hydrostatic pressure gradient. In contrast an exudative pleural effusion occurs when the pleural surfaces themselves are altered in such a way that the conductivity and protein reflection coefficients (see above equation) become abnormal, and an increased quantity of protein rich fluid forms resulting from an increased permeability of pleural vessels. In addition, fluid accumulation will occur due to leakage across the diaphragm from the abdomen, and decreased lymphatic clearance.

An increase in hydrostatic pressure or a decrease in oncotic pressure results in transudative effusion. The limiting factors for fluid accumulation are two: (i) as fluid accumulation increases, the intrapleural pressure increases, which lowers the transpleural hydrostatic gradient and the rate of fluid formation; and the increase in the intrapleural hydrostatic pressure increases the gradient between the pleural space and lymphatics enhancing liquid removal. The most common primary abnormality in exudative effusion is an increased permeability of the pleura to protein. As much as more than 10 gm of protein can be lost this way in some cases each 24 hours (normal protein turnover is 0.25 gm/day), reducing the transpleural oncotic pressure gradient. If lymphatic removal cannot cope with the amount accumulated, the size of effusion increases. The various causes of pleural effusion are summarized in Table 28.1[1,23-34].

CLINICAL CONSEQUENCES OF PLEURAL EFFUSION

The symptoms of pleural effusion depend mainly on the underlying condition causing such effusion. The amount of effusion is also important for the clinical symptomatology and other physiological disturbances. The most common symptom is pleuritic chest pain, indicating the inflammation or irritation of the parietal pleura, since the visceral pleura have no sensory supplies. The pain is usually well localized and corresponds to the area involved because of innervation by intercostal nerves. When the central portion of the diaphragmatic pleura is involved, the pain is referred to ipsilateral shoulder tip because of the involvement of phrenic nerve, which supplies this portion of the pleura. Some experience a dull aching pain that is due to the direct involvement of the parietal pleura, as in a meta-static tumor or an empyema. The pain may be mistaken as that of myocardial infarction in elderly individuals.[35] Dyspnea is probably the other common complaint by the patient with moderate to severe pleural effusion. The exact mechanism of such dyspnea is unclear. It does not depend upon the changes in blood gases nor on the decrease in the pulmonary function. Possibly compres-

TABLE 28.1: Causes of pleural effusion

I. **Transudative pleural effusions**
- Congestive cardiac failure
- Cirrhosis of the liver
- Nephrotic syndrome
- Hypoproteinemia
- Peritoneal dialysis
- Myxedema
- Atelectasis
- Pulmonary embolism
- Urinothorax

II. **Exudative pleural effusion**
- (A) *Infective diseases*
    - Tuberculosis
    - Pyogenic bacterial infections
    - Actinomycosis, Nocardiosis
    - Fungal infections
    - Viral and parasitic infections
    - Hepatitis
- (B) *Malignant diseases*
    - Bronchogenic carcinoma
    - Metastatic disease
    - Mesothelioma
    - Lymphomas
- (C) *Pulmonary embolism*
- (D) *Traumatic*
- (E) *Gastrointestinal diseases*
    - Esophageal perforation
    - Pancreatic disease (Pancreatitis)
    - Intra-abdominal abscesses
    - Amebic liver abscess
    - Postabdominal surgery
    - Sclerotherapy
- (F) *Collagen vascular diseases*
    - SLE,
    - Rheumatoid arthritis
    - Sjögren's syndrome
    - Wegener's granulomatosis
    - Churg-Strauss syndrome
    - Familial Mediterranean fever
- (G) *Postpericardiectomy or postcardiac injury syndrome*

- (H) *Drug induced*
    - Nitrofurantoin
    - Dantrolene
    - Methysergide
    - Bromocriptine
    - Procarbazine
    - Practolol
    - Amiodarone
    - Minoxidil
    - Bleomycin
    - Methotrexate
    - Mitomycin
    - Drug induced lupus
    - Mitomycin
- (I) *Miscellaneous*
    - Yellow nail syndrome
    - Asbestosis
    - Sarcoidosis
    - Uremia
    - Meigs' syndrome
    - Radiation
    - Electric burn
    - Urinothorax
    - Hemothorax
    - Chylothorax
    - Electric burns
    - Immunoblastic lymphadenopathy
    - Trapped lung
    - Lymphangioleiomyomatosis
    - Filariasis

III. **Diseases that can present with transudative or exudative effusions**
- Pulmonary embolism
- Use of diuretics in transudative effusion

IV. **Other rare causes:**
- Post-lung transplantation, sarcoidosis, fetal pleural effusion AIDS, ovarian hyperstimulation, post-partum, amyloidosis, milk of calcium, effusion, interjugular vein catheterization, rupture of germ cell tumor, syphilis

sion of the pulmonary receptors or distortion of respiratory muscle function are responsible. Some patients complain of a dry, nonproductive cough. The mechanism of such cough is not clear; it may be related to pleural inflammation irritating some possible cough receptors in the pleural space (?) or due to lung compression.

Since the effusion acts as a space-occupying lesion in the thoracic cavity, all subdivisions of lung volumes are reduced. Small to moderate effusions displace rather than compress the lungs and affect the ventilatory functions very little. A large effusion on the otherhand reduces lung volumes significantly. The improvement in lung function after thoracentesis is variable.[36-38]

Physical examination of the patient will reveal a shift of the mediastinum to the opposite side with diminished movement of the chest wall on the same side. A stony dull-percussion note, which shifts, is classical of pleural effusion. The exceptions to these findings are too less fluid, loculation, or massive effusion. Grossly diminished or absent breath sounds are usual. A bronchial breathing may be heard above the level of pleural effusion.

Normal amount of fluid present in the pleural space is not visible on plain chest radiographs.[39] However when the amount is excess, radiologically a homogeneous opacity with a rising fluid level is typically seen with evidence of mediastinal shift to the opposite side (Figs 28.1 to 28.3). Small effusions or minimal effusions are seen radiologically as blunting of the costophrenic angle, since free fluid gravitates to the most dependent part of the thoracic cavity, which is the posterior costophrenic sulcus when the patient is upright. The posterior part of the diaphragm is also not visible on lateral chest X-ray. Subpulmonic effusions will present just as an elevation of the diaphragm. Although routine

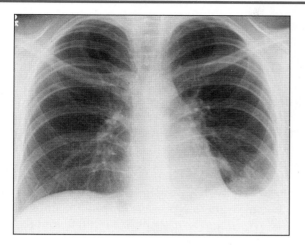

FIGURE 28.1: Left pleural effusion

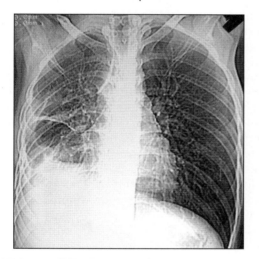

FIGURE 28.2: CXR - Right pleural effusion with intrafissural extension of fluid

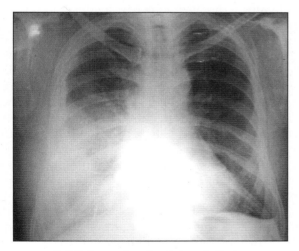

FIGURE 28.3: Loculated pleural effusion

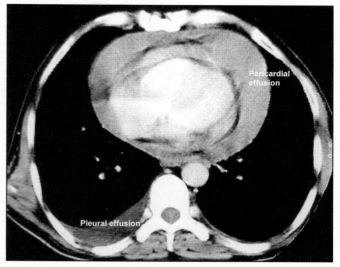

FIGURE 28.4: CT Chest - Pericardial and right pleural effusion

posterior-anterior chest skiagram are routinely used to detect pleural effusions, this may not detect fluid less than 300 ml and sometimes may not differentiate between loculated pleural fluid, intrapulmonary lesions and pleural thickening.[40] Special techniques like decubitus lateral chest radiographs should be obtained to ascertain if free pleural fluid is present and this will detect pleural fluid as little as 100 ml.[41,42] If the distance between the inside of the thoracic cavity and the outside of the lung is less than 10 mm, the pleural effusion is not likely to be clinically significant and is difficult for thoracentesis.[41] At least 175 ml of pleural fluid is necessary to obliterate the lateral costophrenic angle. However, in some cases even more than 500 ml fluid can be present without blunting this angle. As little as 3 to 5 ml of pleural fluid can be demonstrated with properly exposed decubitus radiographs.[43-45] These are however, are complicated methods, need experienced radiologist, and are difficult to perform on serious patients.

Ultrasound, CT scan, (Fig. 28.4) digital radiography, and magnetic resonance imaging (MRI) can also be used to detect pleural effusion. But they are seldom indicated as the conventional chest radiograph is easily obtained, accurate, and inexpensive. However, with an unsuccessful thoracentesis, or loculated effusion, ultrasound guidance is very helpful.[46-51] Ultrasonography will be able to detect the presence of as little as 5 to 50 ml of fluid and is 100 percent sensitive for effusions of 100 ml or more of fluid. Ultrasound is thus superior to plain radiography particularly when effusion is small and loculated. Ultrasound examination is particularly helpful for small or loculated effusions, when both the detection rates and yield of diagnostic thoracentesis are improved. The complication rates are also less. Thus, the usefulness of ultrasonography in pleural effusion can be summarized as follows:

(i) Identification of the location for pleural fluid aspiration, biopsy, or placement of tube
(ii) Identification of pleural fluid loculations
(iii) Distinction of pleural fluid from pleural thickening.[52-54]

Computed tomography is the most superior mode of imaging the pleural space with extra advantage of a simultaneous imaging of the pulmonary parenchyma and mediastinum, and imaging of the whole pleural space is possible.[55-58] This mode is more sensitive than both the conventional radiography and ultrasound in differentiating fluid from pleural thickening and for identification of mass lesions in the region of pleura and chest wall. When there is complete opacification of the hemithorax is present without contralateral mediastinal shift, CT or ultrasound may be helpful in differentiating lung consolidation from pleural effusion. Chylous effusion (density of fat) and pleural nodules due to metastasis may be differentiated easily by these procedures as causes of pleural effusion.

Pleural effusion can be visualized as an area of abnormally low signal intensity. Different types of effusions like transudative fluid collections; chylothorax, hemothorax, or pus may appear somewhat different, although their characteristics are not sufficiently distinct as to be diagnostic. At the present time, it may be said that MRI is less satisfactory than ultrasound or CT in identifying the presence of a pleural effusion and there is no definite clinical indication for MR imaging for management of a patient with pleural effusion.[59-61]

THORACENTESIS AND PLEURAL BIOPSY

Thoracentesis is indicated for both therapeutic and diagnostic purposes.[62-64] It is indicated for any undiagnosed pleural effusion to determine the specific cause of pleural effusion. When the etiology can reasonably be deduced from clinical circumstances, as in congestive cardiac failure, the procedure may be deferred and the response to therapy observed. Besides looking at the gross appearance of the fluid (hemorrhagic, pus, or chylous, etc.), the fluid should be examined for biochemical, cytological, and microbiological parameters; and for malignant cells; and immunological, and other tests should be carried out. Although specific etiology may not be possible from pleural tapping alone, various characteristics of the fluid can be established to guide subsequently diagnostic approach. Thus, based on these characteristics, the fluid can be separated into transu-

dative or exudative (see below) for which there are different causes (see Table 28.1). Repeat thoracentesis and/or biopsy may be required to establish a diagnosis when initial studies fail to do. Therapeutic thoracentesis may be indicated for relief of symptoms due to large effusions. After such a procedure, lung volumes increase by about one third of the volume of fluid removed and arterial blood gas changes are only small, although this can occur in about 50 percent of patients. The fall of PaO_2 may be as much as 20 mm Hg.[65] The relief of dyspnea after therapeutic thoracentesis cannot be explained on these factors only. It is possible that the relief occurs due to a change in the length-tension relationships of the affected diaphragm as a result of a reduction in the size of the thoracic cage allowing the inspiratory muscles to operate on a more advantageous position.[66,67] When frequent or repeated thoracentesis is required for effusions that reaccumulate as in malignancy, tube drainage or pleurodesis can be considered.

Percutaneous pleural biopsy is indicated where malignancy or tuberculosis is suspected, and it should be undertaken in all cases of undiagnosed exudative pleural effusions. All attempts should be made to obtain a histological diagnosis.[68] In cases of transudative effusion, parapneumonic effusions, effusions due to pulmonary embolism pancreatitis or collagen vascular diseases, pleural biopsy is not indicated. It is rather contraindicated in cases of parapneumonic effusion because of increased chance of development of subcutaneous abscesses at the biopsy site. Usually two types of needles are used for this purpose; either a Cope or Abram's needle. Recently some people use Raja needle for this purpose also. Other diagnoses that can be made occasionally (besides malignancy and tuberculosis) include fungal diseases of pleura, rheumatoid pleurisy, and parasitic disease particularly echinococcosis.

In tuberculous pleural effusions the initial needle biopsy is positive for granulomas in 50 to 80 percent of patients and if negative, a second biopsy will yield a positive result in 10 to 40 percent of the time.[69-75] Demonstration of a caseating granuloma is virtually diagnostic of tuberculosis. Fungal pleurisy, rheumatoid arthritis, sarcoidosis, may rarely show granulomatous pathology.[75] It is useful to subject a portion of the biopsy material for mycobacterial examination. Culture positivity to the extent of 76 percent has been reported.[71] Pleural biopsy has been useful in the diagnosis of malignancies also, although in some series cytology gave better result.[69,70,73,74,76-78] The positivity rate ranged from 39 to 75 percent. In a review of 14 publications over 25 years comprising of a total of 2,893 pleural biopsies, the diagnostic yield was 57 percent for carcinoma of the pleura and 75 percent with tuberculous pleurisy.[79] The diagnostic yield will depend upon the stage of malignancy at the time of procedure, experience of the person doing the biopsy, number of sites for biopsy, number of biopsies per site, and location of the biopsy site. Although there is no definite conclusion of the number of biopsies to be taken at a single site, perhaps four or more samples improve the diagnostic yield.[80] False positive pleural biopsies are rare except when mesothelial cells are confused with malignant cells. Although in the presence of thickened pleura, it becomes difficult to undertake the biopsy, it is worth trying whenever possible.

There is no absolute contraindication for thoracentesis and/or pleural biopsy. However, relative contraindications are; (i) insufficient patient cooperation; and (ii) coagulopathy in case of pleural biopsy. Other conditions include small volume of fluid, mechanical ventilation, cutaneous diseases such as herpes zoster infection at the needle entry site. Conditions that are associated with increased risk include: (i) coagulopathy; (ii) inability of the patent to cooperate; (iii) chest wall infection; (iv) very small effusions; (v) removal of large amounts of fluid (> 1.5 L); (vi) performance by inexperienced persons without direct vision; (vii) unstable medical conditions.

The complications of these procedures will depend upon the experience of the person performing the procedure. A decreased rate of serious complications is associated with operator training and experience, use of a smaller needle, ultra sound guidance, and diagnostic (as opposed to therapeutic) thoracentesis. Some of the possible complications include:[64,81]

- Pneumothorax, 3 to 15 percent. Approxi mately 20 percent of them will require tube thoracostomy
- Pain at site
- Bleeding
- Cough
- Vasovagal reactions
- Re-expansion pulmonary edema
- Hypovolemia
- Subcutaneous hematoma
- Pleural infections
- Hemoptysis due to injury to lungs
- Spleen or liver puncture
- Fall in PaO_2
- Transient fever
- Tumor seeding
- Hematoma

- Hydropneumothorax
- Air embolism.

Pneumothorax and *re-expansion pulmonary edema* are more common after therapeutic thoracentesis because of the attempt to remove as much fluid as possible. Some recommend that therapeutic thoracentesis should be stopped after removal of 1000 ml of fluid to prevent re-expansion pulmonary edema. However, if the pleural pressure is monitored during the procedure and this remains more than—20 cm H_2O, procedure can continue as long as the pressure remains above this value. Others however, continue to drain as much fluid as possible. A chest film should be obtained after therapeutic thoracentesis in most cases. Although the exact mechanism of re-expansion pulmonary edema is not known, it is possibly due to a large pressure gradient across the pulmonary vessels created following removal of moderate to large amounts of fluid. This is most commonly seen with carcinoma and with a trapped lung. With carcinoma there is collapse of the lung or tumor and fibrosis trapping the visceral pleura. The trapped lung, due to a remote inflammatory process, does not allow the lung to expand to the chest wall following removal of fluid and usually results in a precipitous fall in intrapleural pressure. A decrease in PaO_2 has been documented in up to 50 percent of patients following therapeutic thoracentesis with the PaO_2 falling as much as 20 mm Hg.

A total of 30 to 50 ml of pleural fluid is necessary for a complete pleural fluid analysis. The tests should be based on the clinical circumstances. The following tests should be routinely ordered for a base line evaluation initially: total protein, lactate dehydrogenase (LDH), total and differential white blood cell count, glucose and pH. A concomitant total serum protein, LDH, and glucose should be measured.[82] The above tests will help to differentiate between a transudate and exudate nature of the effusion and will narrow down the possibility. Further specialized tests like malignant cells, microbiological examination, and immunological tests can be ordered depending upon the basic information and clinical suspicion.

Exudate and transudates are differentiated according to the following criteria described by Light et al.[83-85] Exudates have at least one and transudates none of the following criteria:[86]

(a) Pleural fluid/serum total protein ratio > 0.5
(b) Pleural fluid/serum LDH ratio > 0.6
(c) Pleural fluid LDH > 2/3 the upper limits of normal of the serum or absolute pleural fluid value is > 200.

When exudative criteria are met by LDH only, the diagnosis of malignancy or parapneumonic effusion should be considered. Recently, alternative criteria have been evaluated for distinguishing transudative and exudative effusions.[87,88] It has been suggested that the pleural fluid cholesterol level and pleural: serum cholesterol ratio is perhaps more accurate than the criteria of Light et al.[83-85] A pleural fluid cholesterol level of > 55 mg/dl is 100 percent specific for exudative effusion, although this was not 100 percent sensitive. About 10 percent will have exudative effusion with cholesterol levels of 55 mg/dl or less. However, other studies[89] did not support this contention and believed that Light's criteria are still accurate. Other parameters those are described for separating into these two types of effusion include the gradient between the serum and pleural albumin levels (serum albumin minus pleural fluid albumin) and pleural fluid: serum bilirubin ratio.[90-93] A serum and pleural albumin gradient of < 1.2 mg/dl indicates a transudate and a value more than that indicate an exudate.[90] The pleural fluid: serum bilirubin ratio of equal or more than 0.6 has an accuracy equivalent to, but not superior to the criteria of Light et al. Diuresis can alter the nature of transudates to exudates, although this rarely happens within 48 hours after initiation of diuretic therapy. Thus, it is possible that the longer one waits to obtain pleural fluid after beginning diuresis, the more likely it is that the fluid will show the characteristics of an exudate. In such setting, use of albumin or cholesterol estimation in the pleural fluid may improve diagnostic accuracy. Thus, the differentiating points between a transudate and exudate can be summarized as follows (Table 28.2).

OTHER CHARACTERISTICS OF PLEURAL FLUID

(a) Physical Appearance

The color, odor, and character of the fluid are occasionally helpful in diagnosis.[94,95] Hemorrhagic effusion is

TABLE 28.2: Differentiation between transudative and exudative effusions

Character	Exudates	Transudates
Pleural fluid LDH level*	> 200 or > 2/3rd of serum	< 200 or < 2/3rd of serum
Fluid: Serum LDH*	> 0.6	< 0.6
Fluid: Serum Protein*	> 0.5	< 0.5
Pleural fluid cholesterol	> 55 mg/dl	< 55 mg/dl
Serum pleural albumin gradient	> 1.2 mg/dl	< 1.2 mg/dl
Fluid: Serum bilirubin	=/> 0.6	< 0.6

* Commonly used criteria

due to trauma, malignancy, pulmonary infarction, bleeding disorders, anticoagulant therapy, and post-pericardiectomy or postmyocardial infarction syndromes. A whitish fluid is either due to empyema, chyle, or cholesterol. Brown colored fluid is produced due to a ruptured amebic liver abscess. A yellow-green fluid suggests rheumatoid pleurisy. Malignant pleural mesothelioma produces a viscous fluid due to hyaluronic acid. Putrid odor of the fluid indicated anaerobic infection. Urinothorax impacts an ammonia odor. Food particles can be found in the fluid in case of esophageal rupture.

(b) Cellular Contents[85,96,97]

The total leucocyte counts are not diagnostic of any condition, but counts more than 50,000/ml are seen in parapneumonic effusions/empyema. Transudates usually have a count of less than 1000/ml and exudates above that. Leukocyte counts more than 10,000/ml indicate substantial pleural inflammation and are most commonly due to parapneumonic effusion, although can be seen in pancreatitis, postcardiac injury syndrome, pulmonary infarction, and acute asbestos pleurisy. The measurements of pleural fluid WBC count and differential count are helpful in the diagnosis and management of patients with pleural effusion. In general, a WBC count of > 1,000 cells/µL suggests an exudate, while most transudates have WBC counts of < 1,000 cells/µL. As mentioned above, parapneumonic effusions usually have WBC counts of > 10,000 cells/µL, however, similar WBC counts are also seen in pleural effusions that are related to pancreatitis, pulmonary infarction, collagen vascular diseases, malignancy, and tuberculosis.[98,99]

The differential WBC count is one of the most informative tests performed on pleural fluid samples and can aid significantly in identifying the etiology of many effusions.[99] A predominance of neutrophils in an exudative pleural fluid sample indicates acute inflammation of the pleural surface, as can be seen in pneumonia, pulmonary embolism, subphrenic abscess, early tuberculosis, and also pancreatitis. The discovery of an exudative effusion with > 50 percent small lymphocytes are suggestive of a malignant disease, tuberculous pleuritis, or a pleural effusion after coronary artery bypass graft surgery. If a large percentage of lymphocytes are found, the pleural fluid may be sent for flow cytometry to determine whether a clonal cell population is present, as is seen in lymphoma. Mesothelial cells line the pleural cavity, become dislodged, and are a normal part of pleural effusions. Their presence or absence is useful diagnostically as they are usually absent in tuberculous pleural effusions and complicated parapneumonic effusions. These conditions are associated with a marked inflammatory response that covers the pleura and prevents the shedding of mesothelial cells into the pleural fluid. Eosinophils in the pleural fluid are most often the result of either air or blood in the pleural space. Other unusual diagnoses to consider in the presence of pleural fluid eosinophilia include asbestos-related diseases, drug reactions, or parasitic diseases such as paragonimiasis, hydatid disease, amebiasis, or ascariasis.[100]

No information is available on standards for pleural fluid collection and transport for the determination of the WBC counts and differential cell counts. Moreover, there are no data regarding changes in the measured WBC counts or differential cell counts in pleural fluid specimens over time. Most commonly pleural fluids for WBC count determination and differential cell counts are submitted in tubes that have been anticoagulated with ethylenediaminetetraacetic acid (EDTA), citrate, or heparin, and in plastic or glass tubes without anticoagulants. At most hospitals, cell counts and differential counts of body fluid samples are performed manually. Manual cell counts are dependent on the availability of skilled laboratory personnel, are costly, and often are available only during certain hours, making delays in cell count determinations common. Clearly, an alternative to manual cell counting that is accurate, expeditious, easily obtained, and more cost-efficient is attractive.

A close correlation is found between the WBC counts obtained manually and those obtained with the automated counter from the pleural fluid samples collected in the EDTA tubes (r = 0.92).[101] With the automated counter, the pleural fluid WBC counts are similar among the three tubes containing anticoagulants, but the counts obtained from the tubes without anticoagulants were significantly lower. The differential cell counts obtained manually and those obtained with the automated cell counter differ substantially. Although the percentage of lymphocytes is similar, the automated counter is inaccurate in differentiating neutrophils from large monocytes or mesothelial cells. The WBC counts obtained within 4 hr of collection and 24 hr after collection are virtually identical. Thus the WBC counts obtained manually and with the automated counter from pleural fluid samples in EDTA tubes correlate very closely. The pleural fluid WBC count is lower if the pleural fluids had been collected in tubes without an anticoagulant. Automated WBC counts from pleural fluid specimens are inaccurate, possibly due to difficulty in separating neutrophils from monocyte/mesothelial cells. Refrigerated storage for up to 24 hr has no significant effect on the total WBC count or on the WBC count differential regardless of the tube utilized.

Lymphocytic type of response (85-90%) suggests tuberculosis, lymphoma, sarcoidosis, and chronic rheumatoid pleurisy. Carcinomatous and tuberculous pleurisy will have more than 50 percent of the counts in more than half of the cases. In fact it is suggested that presence of more than 50 percent of small lymphocytes in an exudative pleural effusion are more often (> 90% of the times) either due to tuberculosis or malignancy.[85,102] Separation of lymphocytes into the various subtypes of lymphocytes does not add to any new information. The T:B lymphocyte ratios are increased in malignancy and inflammatory effusions. Transudates and other exudative effusions have similar ratios as in blood. The increased T cells are due to: (i) chemoattraction for these cells; (ii) preferential survival and proliferation of the cells; (iii) lymphatic obstruction by tumor cells; (iv) differences in recirculation kinetics of both the cell types; and (v) immunologically committed T lymphocytes have a tendency to localize in areas of inflammation. The T cells are immunologically important in tuberculosis for granuloma formation and control of mycobacterial growth by releasing lymphokines. In malignancy, the cells are immunologically important to tumor antigens by producing lymphokines, which activate antitumor effects of macrophages. However, the determination of T cell subtypes is not very useful clinically except in chronic lymphatic leukaemia and lymphomas since these are predominantly of B cell types.

Pleural fluid eosinophilia (> 10%) suggests a benign, self-limited diagnosis indicating air or blood in the pleura. The source of eosinophils in pleural fluid appears to be from the bone marrow. These cells have the capacity to form colonies of eosinophils in the bone marrow and prolong the survival of eosinophils. This is mediated by interleukin 5 (IL-5) or IL-3 or GM-CSF.[103,104] The causes are hemothorax, pulmonary infarction, pneumothorax, previous thoracentesis, parasitic diseases like paragonimiasis, hydatid disease, amebiasis, ascariasis, fungal infections (histoplasmosis), drugs (dantrolene, bromocriptine, nitrofurantoin), and asbestos pleurisy. Pleural effusion associated with Churg-Strauss syndrome is also eosinophilic. In about a third of the cases the cause is unknown and they are classified as idiopathic and may be either due to viral infections or occult pulmonary emboli. Eosinophilic pleural effusions have certain clinical significance also. Eosinophilic pleural effusion in parapneumonic effusions indicate good prognosis. In the absence of previous thoracentesis and pneumothorax, eosinophils in the pleural fluid it is highly unlike that the patient has tuberculosis.[105-109] It is also unlikely that he has malignancy except Hodgkin's disease.

Basophilic counts of > 10 percent are suggestive of leukemic infiltrations of the pleura.[108]

Mesothelial cells are common in transudates and present in variable degree in exudates. More than 5 percent of mesothelial cells in an exudative effusion virtually rules out tuberculosis as etiology.[85,102,108,110] Such findings are also common in empyema, rheumatoid pleurisy, malignant effusion of some duration, and pleurodesis. The paucity of such cells indicate that the pleural surface have become extensively involved by the disease process so that the mesothelial cells cannot enter the pleural space. A typical example is the absence of mesothelial cells in complicated parapneumonic effusions and with others where the pleura become coated with fibrin. It is also common with malignant effusions after injection of sclerosing agents have been injected. Another clinical importance of the presence of these cells in the pleural effusion is that they are often confused with malignant cells and in such situations immunohistochemistry is useful.

Macrophages can be found in pleural fluid are found in pleural plaques and granulomatous disorders of pleura. Although the presence of macrophages in pleural fluid has limited diagnostic value, they should not be confused with mesothelial cells since the later is absent in tuberculosis and macrophages can be present in tuberculous pleurisy.

Small number of plasma cells is seen in a number of conditions, but large numbers indicate multiple myeloma involving the pleura.

Only a few drops of blood (5,000 to 10,000 RBC/mm³) in the pleural fluid makes the fluid sanguineous; therefore presence of blood-tinged fluid itself is of no diagnostic value. Up to 50 percent of exudates and 10 to 15 percent of transudates may be sanguineous. Finding of greater than 100,000 red blood cells/mm³ however, is significant.[111-113] A traumatic effusion is differentiated from a true bloody effusion by its nonuniformity of color, clotting within minutes of aspiration, and by the absence of hemosiderin-laden macrophages. In such situations one should obtain a hematocrit on pleural fluid to document the amount of blood in the pleural fluid. If the hematocrit of the pleural fluid is greater than 50 percent of the peripheral hematocrit, a hemothorax is present. Usually, the amount of hematocrit is much less than one would expect from its gross appearance. Such effusions are encountered in the conditions mentioned above for hemorrhagic pleural effusion. When trauma is excluded, malignancy is the most common cause of such effusions. At times, it is necessary to differentiate whether blood is a result of thoracentesis or was present prior to thoracentesis. If the

blood is a result of thoracentesis, the degree of red discoloration of the fluid will not be uniform throughout the course of aspiration. Further, if blood was present prior to thoracentesis, the macrophages in the fluid usually contain hemosiderin/hemoglobin inclusions. Moreover, platelet will be present if it was a traumatic thoracentesis.[114] Crenation of the RBC in the pleural fluid rarely occurs, as the osmotic pressure of the pleural fluid is similar to that of serum.

(c) Biochemical Measurements

i. A low glucose level in the pleural fluid (less than 60 mg/dl or less than 50 percent of the blood level) is common in rheumatoid pleurisy (85%); empyema (80%), malignancy (30%), tuberculosis (20%), lupus pleurisy (20%) and esophageal rupture.[1,115-120] Other rare causes of low glucose levels include paragonimiasis, hemothorax, and Chrurg-Strauss syndrome. The mechanism of such low levels include decreased transport of glucose from blood to pleural fluid because of a selective block to the entry of glucose into the pleural effusion,[121] and increased utilization by constituents of the fluid including polymorphs, malignant cells, and bacteria. The lowest concentrations are found in rheumatoid pleurisy and empyema, with glucose being undetected in some cases. The more the glucose level in pleural fluid is reduced, the more likely it is a complicated parapneumonic effusion and tube insertion is indicated if the level is below 40 mg/dl. The levels in other conditions are usually in the range of 30 to 55 mg/dl. In some cases of malignant pleural effusion glucose levels may be as low as 10 mg/ml. Low glucose levels in malignant pleural effusion indicate greater tumor burden, extent of tumor is higher, cytology for malignant cells and yield of pleural biopsy are more likely to be positive, are less likely to have a successful pleurodesis, and the life expectancy is shortened.[122-124]

ii. Normal pleural fluid pH is approximately 7.60 and is influenced by the arterial pH. With transudative pleural effusions, the pH is usually higher than the simultaneous blood pH because of active transport of bicarbonate from the blood into the pleural space. A pleural fluid pH of less than 7.20 is found in the following conditions: (a) complicated parapneumonic effusions; (b) esophageal rupture; (c) rheumatoid pleurisy; (d) tuberculous pleurisy; (e) malignancy; (f) hemothorax; (g) systemic acidosis; (h) paragonimiasis; (i) lupus pleurisy; and (j) urinothorax. The cause of this relative fluid acidosis is because of accumulation of lactic acid from anaerobic glycolysis.

The resultant hydrogen ions combine with bicarbonate to form water and carbon dioxide. This increases the pleural fluid CO_2 and the pH decreases. Further, there is limited diffusion of CO_2 out of the pleural space. Transudates generally have a pH of 7.40 to 7.55 excepting urinothorax, while in most of the exudates the range is 7.30 to 7.45. A pH of less than 7.30 to 7.20 is found in esophageal rupture in almost all cases after 24 hours. A pleural fluid of less than 6.0 is highly suggestive of esophageal rupture.[125] This low pH may be due to reflux of acid into the pleural space or secondary to infection, which invariably follows oesophageal rupture. The mechanisms responsible for such low levels in various other conditions mentioned above include increased acid production by cells and bacteria, and decreased acid efflux from pleural space. In parapneumonic effusion, a pleural fluid pH of less than 7.0 with a low glucose and high LDH (> 1000 U/L), is an indication of chest tube insertion for adequate resolution. If the ph is above 7.20, chest tube drainage will probably not be required. On the otherhand, if the value is between 7.0 and 7.20, the patient may or may not require a tube.[126] If the infection is due to Proteus organisms, the pH will be high because of production of ammonia by the organism. In malignant effusions, pH of less than 7.30 is a poor prognostic indicator[124]—an indicator of an increased yield on pleural biopsy, and the response to sclerosing agents is poor.[122,124]

iii. Elevated amylase levels in pleural fluid (> the upper limit for serum, or pleural fluid/serum ratio of > 1) can occur in acute pancreatitis, pancreatic pseudocyst, oesophageal rupture, malignancy, and ruptured ectopic pregnancy.[127,128] About 10 percent of patients with inflammatory pancreatic disease will have pleural effusion.[129] In some cases the pleural problem (chest pain and dyspnea) may overshadow abdominal symptoms. The highest amylase levels, usually above 100,000 U, are found in fistulous communications between the pseudocyst and pleura.[130] High amylase values in pleural fluid is also present in about 10 percent of patients with malignant pleural effusion and the elevation is only moderate in contrast to pancreatic diseases. Strangely, the primary site of the tumor in such situations is not the pancreas.[131] The amylase in malignant effusions is of salivary types, and estimation of isoenzymes will distinguish between malignant and pancreas-related pleural effusions. The source of amylase in pleural fluid in esophageal rupture is again of the salivary type that passes on into the pleural space.[132] and the elevation can occur within 2 hours of esophageal rupture.

iv. Pleural fluid lactic dehydrogenase (LDH) level is used to separate transudates from exudates. When exudative pleural effusion is diagnosed only with elevated LDH levels and not with protein levels, either it is due to parapneumonic effusion or malignant effusion. LDH is elevated in almost all exudative effusions.[83,133] The level of LDH in pleural fluid is a good indicator of ongoing pleural inflammation and serial measurements can be useful to know the ongoing inflammation or otherwise. Presence of blood in the pleural fluid does not adversely affect the levels of LDH. Estimation of isoenzymes may be useful indicators of the cause of exudative pleural effusion. All benign effusions with elevated LDH and most malignant effusions are characterized by a higher percentage of LDH-4 and LDH-5 in the fluid than in the corresponding serum values and the source is from the inflammatory cells in the fluid.[134,135] About a third of malignant effusion patients have large amounts (more than 35%) of LDH-2 and less LDH-4 and LDH-5. Most of the LDH as LDH-1 are due to blood.

(d) Immunological Markers[136-141]

These in the pleural fluid are helpful in the diagnosis of rheumatoid pleurisy and lupus pleuritis. A rheumatoid factor of 1:320 or more or equal to or more than the serum concentration is suggestive of rheumatoid pleurisy.[138] RA cells may also be seen in pleural fluid in this condition. LE cells in the pleural fluid are diagnostic of lupus pleurisy.[139] Similarly a pleural fluid antinuclear antibody (ANA) titre of 1:160 or more or when the concentration is equal more than that in serum, it is suggestive of lupus pleuritis.[116] Very low concentrations of complements are found in the two connective tissue diseases.[136,138,140,141] Patients with pleural effusion secondary to RA or SLE will have higher pleural fluid levels of immune complexes than patients with effusions due to other causes.[136-138]

(e) Lipid Studies

When a milky or opalescent pleural fluid is obtained, it should be centrifuged to exclude a large number of leukocytes. If the supernatant is clear, then it is empyema. If still the fluid is opaque, it is either chylous (chylothorax) or chyliform or pseudochylothorax due to cholesterol, or lecithin-globulin complexes.[142,143] While the former is due to disruption of the lymphatic duct so that chyle accumulates in the pleural space, the later is due to unknown causes. The two can be differentiated by measurement of pleural fluid triglycerides. In chylothorax, the triglyceride level is usually more than 110 mg/dl. If the level is less than 50 mg/dl, chylothorax is excluded. Concentrations between 50 to 110 mg/dl are indeterminant,[144] and the presence of chylomicrons should be sought by lipoprotein electrophoresis. The presence of chylomicrons is diagnostic of chylothorax.[144,145] Most patients with chylothorax and triglyceride levels below 110 mg/dl are malnourished. Secondly, chyliform effusions often are chronic and long-standing and will present more with thickened pleura against more acute presentation of chylothorax. Other tests useful for diagnosing turbid pleural fluids are total lipid content, the cholesterol content and microscopic examination of the sediment to cholesterol crystals.

(f) Diagnosis of Pleural Malignancy

The diagnostic yield of malignant pleural effusion for malignant cells is 40 to 87 percent.[146-148] All effusions in malignancy are not due to direct involvement, but may be paramalignant either because of postobstructive atelectasis and impaired lymphatic drainage or because of associated congestive heart failure, pulmonary embolism, pneumonia, hypoproteinemia or superior vena caval obstruction. The yield also varies with the type of malignancy (adenocarcinoma giving a high yield and Non-Hodgkin's lymphoma having a low yield); squamous cell carcinoma is not usually diagnosed in pleural fluid number of specimens examined; and the expertise of the cytologist. Pleural fluids should be placed in sterile containers with an anticoagulant like heparin of 200 units per 20 ml of fluid. The fluid should be examined immediately, although a delay of up to 24 hours is not deleterious unless there is bacterial contamination.

Further studies like electron microscopy,[149,150] scanning electron microscopy[151] and histochemical studies[152] are used to differentiate between adenocarcinoma and mesothelioma in the pleural fluid. With development of monoclonal antibodies, newer technologies are applied in the diagnosis of pleural malignancy.[153-155] The antibodies that are found useful include anticarcinoembryonic antigen, B72.3, Leu-M1, BER-EP4, EMA, MFG, antikeratin, etc. Another approach to the diagnosis of malignant pleural effusions is to measure various cancer-associated antigens using monoclonal antibodies,[1-55,158] expression of oncogenes,[159] and measurement of carcinoembryonic antigen. Flow cytometry provides a method for the rapid quantitative measurement of nuclear DNA and this can be utilized to differentiate between benign and malignant cells. The later possess cells abnormal number of chromosomes (aneuploidy), and abnormal DNA content, DNA aneuploidy.[160] Abnormalities can also be detected in the chromosome number and structure in some cases.[161,162]

Adenosine deaminase (ADA) is an enzyme, important for degradation of purines and is necessary for lymphoid cell differentiation and is involved in monocyte-macrophage maturation. The level is increased in pleural fluid in tuberculosis, rheumatoid arthritis, and empyema. ADA activity in pleural fluid of > 50 U/l differentiates between tuberculosis and malignancy. Beta 2-macroglobulin is high in tuberculosis and rheumatoid arthritis compared to other exudates including malignancy and lupus pleurisy. High levels are also reported in lymphoma. Lysozyme levels are found to be high in tuberculosis, rheumatoid pleurisy, and empyema. Pleural fluid lysozyme levels of > 20 mg/ml and pleural fluid/serum ratios of > 2.0 may separate tuberculosis from malignancy.

Sialic acid estimation in the pleural fluid is increased in malignant pleural effusions.[163]

Some important characteristics of pleural fluid that may be of value to suggest etiology are given in Table 28.3.

TABLE 28.3: Differential diagnosis of exudative pleural effusion based on certain characteristics[1,15]

Parameter	Conditions
pH (< 7.2)	-Empyema
	-Complicated parapneumonic effusion
	-Rheumatoid pleurisy
	-Esophageal perforation
	-Tuberculosis
	-Malignant effusions
	-Parasitic (Paragonimus) effusion
	-Hemothorax
	-Acidosis
Glucose (< 60 mg/dl)	-Complicated parapneumonic effusion
	-Rheumatoid pleural effusion
	-Malignant pleural effusion
	-Tuberculous pleural effusion
	-Parasitic (Paragonimus) effusions
Amylase (more than upper limit of serum value)	-Esophageal rupture
	-Pancreatitis
	-Malignancy
RBC (>100,000/cmm)	-Traumatic effusion
	-Malignant pleural effusion
	-Pulmonary embolism
Hematocrit (> 50% of blood)	-Hemothorax
Hematocrit (<1%)	-No specific pathology
Lymphocytes (>50%)	-Lymphoma
	-Malignancy
	-Tuberculosis
	-Fungal infections
	-Postpericardiotomy syndrome
	-Sarcoidosis
Eosinophils	-Presence of air and blood in the pleural space
	-Drug induced effusions (Nitrofurantoin, dantrolene)
	-Asbestosis
	-Malignancy
	-Paragonimiasis

Pleural fluid analysis will yield a definitive or presumptive diagnosis in about 70 percent of cases and useful information in majority of cases.[164,165] However, the cause of exudative effusion may not be forthcoming after initial thoracentesis, where malignancy and tuberculosis are the main contenders. In such a situation, repeated thoracentesis, pleural biopsy, and cytology studies will increase the chances of a particular etiology.[166] Pleural biopsy is particularly helpful for tuberculosis and the chances of picking up malignancy are also slightly increased.[167-169]

In cases of undiagnosed exudative pleural effusion with nonspecific pleural biopsy, Leslie and Kinasewitz[167] have suggested the following six criteria by which such cases can be followed up without any further work up and in the presence of these criteria; a possibility of tuberculosis or malignancy is highly unlikely. These criteria are:

(i) The patient must be clinically stable
(ii) There should not be any weight loss
(iii) He should have a negative PPD
(iv) He should be afebrile (temperature < 38°C)
(v) Pleural fluid should have < 95 percent of lymphocytes
(vi) The effusion should occupy < 50 percent of the hemithorax.

Pulmonary thromboembolism should be considered and the clinical presentation be reviewed with this possibility in mind[170] before concluding the effusion to be "undiagnosed". Other rare causes as mentioned in Table 28.1 should also be thought of.

(g) Fiberoptic Bronchoscopy

If the patient with an exudative effusion is still undiagnosed then fiberoptic bronchoscopy may be undertaken. This however, has a low diagnostic yield in pleural effusion without concomitant parenchymal shadows or hemoptysis.[171] Blind bronchoscopy produces only very few positive results in about 5 percent of such cases. Therefore, it should not be undertaken in a case of suspected malignancy but only if there are radiological abnormalities in the lungs.

(h) Thoracoscopy

Thoracoscopy is rarely needed in the evaluation of a case of pleural effusion, although it was performed more frequently in the first half of 20th century. It fell out of favor because of the use of more and more open thoracic surgical techniques.[172] The specific indications are controversial. The positive yield with malignancy or tuberculous pleurisy is increased with improved thoraco-

scopy procedures and advances in instrumentation. The diagnosis of tuberculosis and malignancy can be made in 92 and nearly 100 percent of cases respectively. However, it adds little to the other diagnostic methods. Moreover, the procedures produces more morbidity and costly. Barter et al[164] recommend thoracoscopy for evaluation of undiagnosed pleural effusions under local anesthesia, conscious sedation, and without sedation, which is to be separated from thoracoscopic surgery under general anesthesia. Under these circumstances, the complication of thoracoscopy will be the same as that of a pleural biopsy. If this is not possible, repeat pleural biopsy and thoracentesis may be tried before proceeding to thoracoscopy under general anesthesia or open thoracotomy.[167,169] Nevertheless, this technique has not been popularized among physicians.

(i) Open Pleural Biopsy

Open pleural biopsy has the advantage of being combined with open lung biopsy, and thus increasing the diagnostic yield. The main usefulness perhaps is in mesothelioma to obtain large tissue specimens for histological examination. However, because of the high morbidity, mortality and cost, other methods should be tried first before trying open pleural biopsy.

After the above line of investigations, it is possible to arrive at a cause of exudative pleural effusion in more than 90 percent of cases.[173,174] Sixty percent of patients with undiagnosed exudative effusion even after open thoracotomy will have no progression of the disease and most of the remainder will have an underlying malignancy.[175]

TRANSUDATIVE PLEURAL EFFUSIONS

Transudative pleural effusions usually occur when systemic factors influence the formation and absorption of pleural fluid in such a way that fluid accumulates in the pleural cavity.

CONGESTIVE CARDIAC FAILURE

Congestive cardiac failure is the most common cause of transudative pleural effusion.[176] Although the precise incidence is unknown, about 58 percent patients with left ventricular failure will have pleural effusion.[177] Large autopsy series showed that the majority of pleural effusions were bilateral (88%) and that the incidence of unilateral effusions was small with the right side being involved twice (8%) as common as the left side (4%). More than 70 percent of patients with congestive heart failure will have pleural effusion of more than 250 ml.[178]

The mechanisms causing such effusions are controversial. Autopsy studies have generally shown that both left and right heart diseases are associated with pleural effusion as opposed to right ventricular disease alone except mitral valve disease. It was reported that systemic venous hypertension was the single most important factor in fluid accumulation and isolated pulmonary venous hypertension was not associated with such effusion. The effusion was the greatest when both are combined with the volume being more on the right pleural cavity. However, it was subsequently shown that in the subacute or chronic state, pulmonary venous hypertension is the most important determinant for the development of pleural effusion in congestive heart failure. The current theories of pleural effusion in congestive heart failure say that such accumulation occurs when there is left ventricular failure. This increases the pulmonary capillary pressure with accumulation of fluid in the interstitial space of the lung. This increased interstitial pressure result in an increased interstitial pressure in the subpleural interstitial spaces. The fluid then moves from the pulmonary interstitial spaces across the visceral pleura into the pleural space. Elevated systemic venous pressure decreases lymphatic clearance further favoring fluid accumulation.[179-182]

The fluid is a transudate with the usual symptoms and signs of pleural effusion. Mesothelial cells and lymphocytes account for most of the cells. Polymorphonuclear cells rarely exceed 10 percent. In chronic cardiac failure, the protein content may be more than 3.0 gm/dl. Treatment consists of decreasing venous hypertension and control of heart failure. In rare cases, pleurodesis with minocycline or tetracycline or talc will be helpful.[183,184]

Pleural effusion due to pericardial disease is usually left sided, with bilateral effusion occurring in about a third of the cases. Unilateral right-sided effusion is very rare.

HEPATIC HYDROTHORAX

The incidence of pleural effusion in cirrhosis of liver is about 6 percent.[185,186] Pleural effusion usually occurs only when ascites is also present in association with cirrhosis. Even when ascites is not evident clinically, the same will be demonstrated by ultrasonography.[187] The pleural effusion in association with ascites and cirrhosis is usually right-sided in two-thirds of cases and occasionally, it can be left-sided or bilateral.[185,186]

Although plasma oncotic pressure is decreased in cirrhosis because of hypoalbuminemia, this mechanism does not appear to be the dominant cause of pleural effusion. Most probably it is caused by the movement of ascitic fluid through diaphragmatic defects. Diaphragmatic defects may be noted as blebs, which are usually small and less than 1 cm in diameter. This has been demonstrated by injection of India ink into the peritoneal fluid when it appeared in the pleural fluid whereas cells in the peripheral blood contained none. Similarly after injection of radiolabeled albumin intravenously, the albumin first appeared in the peritoneal fluid and then in the pleural fluid.[186] Further evidence of passage of fluid from peritoneum to pleura came from studies by Liberman et al[185] who introduced air into the peritoneal cavity in patients with cirrhosis and ascites and pneumothorax developed after 1 to 48 hour's injection. Thoracoscopy detected air bubbling through diaphragm in one of their patients. Other workers also have demonstrated such defects on thoracoscopy.[188] From these studies, it seems that fluid passes directly into the pleural space through defects in the diaphragm. In the presence of tense ascites and increased intra-abdominal pressure, the diaphragm is stretched causing microscopic defects. The increased hydrostatic pressure in the ascitic fluid results in a one-way transfer of fluid into the pleural cavity. In some patients, transfer of ascitic fluid across the diaphragm may occur by the lymphatic vessels.

The pleural fluid is transudative, although protein content may be higher than that of the ascitic fluid. It may occasionally be blood tinged perhaps due to defective coagulation disorders. Underlying pancreatic disease needs to be excluded. Spontaneous bacterial empyema analogous to the spontaneous bacterial peritonitis may occur in such patients. In that event, the polymorphonuclear cell count will exceed 500 cells/mm³.[189]

The management of pleural effusion in such situations should be directed towards the treatment of ascites. Low salt diet, and diuretics are to be administered. The best diuretic therapy is the combination of furosemide and spironolactone in a starting dose of 40 mg and 100 mg respectively. The doses can however be increased to as much as 4 folds for proper control of ascites and effusion.[190] Serial and rapid thoracentesis will not help because of rapid re-accumulation and this will lead on to hypovolemia and depletion of body proteins. Some patients are refractory to the above management with salt restriction and diuretic therapy. In such patients one may try to do tube thoracostomy followed by the injection of a sclerosing agent; implantation of a peritoneal-to-venous shunt; thoracoscopic insufflation of talc or thoracotomy with surgical repair of the diaphragmatic leak.[191-193]

NEPHROTIC SYNDROME

Pleural effusion is found in about a fifth of the cases.[194] The mechanism of fluid accumulation is decreased oncotic pressure in the pleural microvasculature due to hypoalbuminemia and increased hydrostatic pressure from salt and water overload. Thromboembolic episodes of pulmonary vessels due to increased renal vein thrombosis or due to protein S deficiency may be another cause of pleural effusion.[195] While nephrotic syndrome generally produces bilateral effusions, unilateral pleural effusion or disproportionate fluid in one side in bilateral effusion, should arouse the suspicion of the later condition.

The treatment should aim at decreasing the protein loss in the urine to increase plasma protein. This can be achieved by the use of angiotensin-converting enzyme inhibitors and other treatment of nephrotic syndrome.[196]

OTHER CAUSES OF TRANSUDATIVE PLEURAL EFFUSIONS

Urinothorax is a pleural effusion due to obstructive uropathy. The causes of such obstruction may be carcinoma of the genitourinary system; nephrolithiasis; trauma; surgery; renal transplantation; retroperitoneal inflammation; failed nephrostomy; and renal biopsy.[197,198] This is a very rare cause of pleural effusion. With urinary tract obstruction and hydronephrosis, perirenal and retroperitoneal fluid accumulation occurs. The fluid is then forced into the pleural cavity through the retroperitoneal route or through diaphragmatic lymphatics. Rapid accumulation can occur through the diaphragmatic defect or hiatus. The effusion disappears rapidly once the obstruction is relieved. Characteristically the fluid will have a urine odor, low glucose, and low pH. The pleural fluid/serum creatinine ratio is more than 1.[199,200]

Peritoneal dialysis, particularly continuous ambulatory peritoneal dialysis (CAPD), may be associated with small pleural effusions. Most often they are right-sided. This is due to the movement of the dialysate from the peritoneal cavity due to a mechanism similar to that with cirrhosis and ascites. About 1.6 percent of patients on CAPD develop this complication.[201] Occasionally massive right-sided pleural effusion may be seen.[202] Such effusions usually occur within 30 days of initiation of dialysis. However, this may occur after few months to two years. Changing over to hemodialysis or intermittent peritoneal dialysis in the semierect position will resolve the effusion completely. Once there is development of pleural effusion, the dialysis should be stopped and for further dialysis, pleurodesis or surgical repair will be necessary.

Small pleural effusions are also common in atelectasis, particularly that following upper abdominal surgery. Major bronchial obstruction can also produce such type of effusions. The mechanism of fluid accumulation in the pleural space is due to decreased pleural pressure because of the increased separation of the lung and chest wall. Other rare causes include Fontan procedure performed for tricuspid atresia, or univentricular heart,[203] glomerulonephritis,[204] and myxedema.[205] In superior vena caval obstruction fluid accumulation will occur once the pressure is above 15 mm Hg.[182] Fluid formation occurs either due to lymph leakage. However other causes of pleural effusion, particularly malignancy should be excluded first.

EXUDATIVE PLEURAL EFFUSIONS

Exudative effusions result primarily by pleural inflammation or diminished lymphatic drainage from the pleural space. Thus, a wide variety of causes can cause exudative pleural effusion.

(1) Tuberculous Pleural Effusion[206-214]

Tuberculous pleural effusion is an important and perhaps the most common cause of exudative lymphocytic pleural effusion in countries like India. The effusion occurs on an immunological basis. It may be a sequel to a primary infection 6 to 12 weeks previously or it may represent reactivation tuberculosis.[215] Pleural effusion can occur due to any one of the following mechanisms: (i) rupture of a subpleural focus of *Mycobacterium tuberculosis*,[206,216] (ii) hematogenous dissemination of mycobacteria; and (iii) direct extension of the primary disease.

Both cellular and humoral immunological mechanisms are responsible for the pathogenesis of tuberculous pleurisy, although the former is more important. Delayed hypersensitivity plays a larger role in the pathogenesis of tuberculosis both in the experimental animals and possibly in humans.[209,217-222] Because the host is sensitized to tubercular antigen during early infection, even very few organisms are sufficient to begin an exaggerated immunological response. Tubercular protein or the live bacillus and the antigen interact with sensitized T lymphocytes. The T lymphocytes are predominantly of the helper/inducer subset and are mainly the memory cells that are previously exposed to antigen. *In vitro*, these lymphocytes proliferate when exposed to tuberculin (purified protein derivative, PPD). These lymphocytes produce a number of lymphokines, which alter the permeability of the pleural vessels and affect the activity of mononuclear phagocytes and fibroblasts. Several of these lymphokines are responsible for the development of granulomas. Increased amounts of interferon-gamma serves as a stimulus for further inflammation and this lymphokine increases in the pleural fluid. Experimental studies have shown that when guinea pigs or mice are immunized to tuberculous protein by injecting Freund's adjuvant containing dead tubercles bacilli into their footpads, an intrapleural injection of PPD 3 to 5 weeks later causes rapid appearance of an exudative pleural effusion within 12 to 48 hours. The development of experimental pleural effusion is suppressed when the animals are given antilymphocyte serum.[219] Neutrophils play a key role in the development of such experimental pleurisy.[223] In the BCG model of experimental tuberculous pleurisy, macrophages predominate initially, and subsequently lymphocytes are the predominant cells.[223] Role of delayed hypersensitivity in human pleural effusion is thought to be important because the pleural fluid mycobacterial cultures from most patients are negative.[124,221,222] T lymphocytes specifically sensitized to tuberculous protein are present in the pleural fluid and their number is much larger than that present in the peripheral blood.[224] This local increase of sensitized cells in the pleural fluid may be due to their clonal expansion or due to the migratory inhibition. Rupture of a subpleural caseous focus into the pleural space leads to release of tuberculous protein into the pleural space and hypersensitivity reaction is generated.

Tuberculous pleural effusions contain many potentially immunoreactive cells and substances as enumerated above that lead to vigorous local cell-mediated immune response.[225] Compared to peripheral blood, pleural fluid contains much more T lymphocytes. The helper-inducer CD4 and CD8 (suppressor/cytotoxic) ratio is 3:4 in the fluid compared to 1:7 in blood.[225] Lymphocytes from tuberculous pleural effusion show greater responsiveness to PPD than peripheral blood lymphocytes do.[226-228]

The local inflammatory response in tuberculous pleurisy is mediated partly by a number of inflammatory and immunostimulatory factors that include complement degradation products,[225] interferon-γ,[229] 1,25-dihydroxy-vitamin D,[230] and interleukin-2.[231] These factors attract and activate macrophages and lymphocytes and enhance the elimination of mycobacteria.

Humoral immunity may also play some role in the pathogenesis of tuberculous pleurisy. Tuberculous antigen specific IgG are present in the pleural fluid but not in the peripheral blood indicating their synthesis in the pleural space. The complement system is activated, particularly the C_3, although total complement concentrations in the pleural fluid are normal.

The development of pleural effusion in tuberculous pleurisy is due to the increased permeability of pleural capillaries because of intense inflammation caused by delayed hypersensitivity reaction. This increases the level of proteins in the pleural fluid that further increases further accumulation fluid. In experimental animals this may not be the mechanism however, rather a decreased protein clearance may be important.[218] Lymphatic flow from the pleural space is impaired due to intense inflammation of the parietal pleura, which impedes the lymphatic drainage. The flow is approximately 50 percent that seen in congestive heart failure.[231]

In spite of an increased T lymphocyte function *in vitro*, about one third of the patients with tuberculous pleural effusion are negative to an intermediate strength PPD skin test at the time of presentation. Most will become positive in 6 to 8 weeks. In fact, there is dissociation in the function of the pleural and peripheral blood lymphocytes (see above). While those from the pleural fluid proliferate in response to PPD, autologous lymphocytes from peripheral blood fail to proliferate *in vitro*. Because these lymphocytes from peripheral blood are capable of normal proliferation in response to standard mitogens, they apparently have a specific defect in their ability to respond to tuberculous antigens. Earlier, this lack of response in lymphocytes from peripheral blood was attributed to the sequestration of the majority of responsive cells within the pleural space. Current evidence however demonstrates a circulating population of suppressor cells of the macrophage/monocyte linage that suppresses proliferation of peripheral blood lymphocytes *in vitro*. Thus it may be possible that circulating suppressor cells limit cell-mediated immunity to the pleural compartment, preventing systemic immune effects.[232,233]

Primary tuberculous pleurisy is most commonly seen in children, but recently is seen in increased frequency in adults.[206] This increase may be due to an altered immunological status. Reactivation of tuberculous pleurisy is also possible in the immunologically impaired elderly subjects. In general, patients of tubercular pleural effusion are younger than patients with parenchymal tuberculosis. The mean age is about 28 years.[234] Tuberculous pleurisy most commonly occurs 3 to 7 months after primary infection but may occur at any time during the natural history of the disease. Patients with pleural effusions secondary to reactivation tend to be older than those with postprimary pleural effusion.[215] Tuberculous pleural effusion may present as an acute bacterial pneumonic illness to an indolent disease to be detected on chest radiograph at the first time. About a third of patients will have symptoms less than a week and about two-thirds will have disease less than a month at the time of presentation.[235] The presentations may be acute and can mimic a bacterial pneumonia.[209] Constitutional symptoms like fever, malaise, weight loss, anorexia, and weakness will be present in most of the cases. Nonproductive cough and pleuritic chest pain are two important symptoms at the time of presentation. Dyspnea as a presenting feature depends upon the amount of effusion. Chest pain disappears with onset of effusion and dyspnea becomes a prominent symptom. Cough may be due to compressive effect of effusion irritating cough receptors or may be due to stimulation of cough receptors present in the pleura. Chest radiograph usually shows mild to moderate degrees of pleural effusion.[209,222] Massive effusion can occur although less frequently.[209,236] The effusion is usually unilateral.[185,198] Coexistent parenchymal infiltrates can be detected in about a third of the patients and the effusion is almost always in the same side to that of the infiltrate.[209] The effusion in AIDS patients can have similar presentation to that without AIDS.[237]

The fluid is usually a serous exudate (serosanguinous in less than 10%) with the protein being more than 4 g percent in most cases. The total leucocyte count is generally less than 5,000/ml with a predominance of lymphocytes, which often exceeds 90 to 95 percent.[209,238-241] In fact only 10 percent of tuberculous pleural effusion will have lymphocytes less than 50 percent. In the early stages of effusion following the entry of tubercle bacilli into the pleural space, there may be a predominance of polymorphs,[236] which is rapidly replaced by lymphocytes in the next few days. The common subtypes are the CD4+ and TEC T5.9+ lymphocytes. There is a rise in the CD4+/CD8+ lymphocyte ratio. Mesothelial cells are rare and the absence of these cells is a characteristic feature of tuberculous effusion.[110,206, 239,242,243] Pleural fluid eosinophilia is also rare. If eosinophils are found in significant number in excess of 10 percent, one can exclude the diagnosis of tuberculous pleurisy unless there is concomitant pneumothorax or previous thoracentesis.[109,244] About a fifth of the patients will exhibit a low glucose (< 60 mg/dl) and a low pH (< 7.30). The glucose level is rarely below 20 mg/dl and majority of patients will have glucose levels above 60 mg/dl.[209,234,245,246] The pH is in the range of 7.00 to 7.29. A pleural fluid pH of > 7.40 virtually exclude the possibility of tuberculosis as etiology.[1]

Pleural fluid adenosine deaminase (ADA) and lysozyme levels are helpful diagnostic tests. ADA is an enzyme of purine metabolism. The activity of this enzyme reflects lymphocytic proliferation and differentiation, i.e. it is more in rapidly proliferating and immature lymphocytes. Therefore, whenever there is a cell mediated immune response to antigenic stimuli, the ADA levels are the highest. Adenosine is converted into inosine in the presence of ADA.

$$Adenosine + H_2O + ADA = Inosine + NH_3 + ADA$$

The amount of ammonia so liberated is measured by colorimetric method.[245] Thus, the level may not only be specific in tuberculous effusion, but other lymphocytic conditions like lymphoma. It is suggested that an ADA level of > 50 U/L in the pleural fluid is about 94 percent sensitive and 90 percent specific for tuberculous effusions and an ADA level of 45 U/L is almost 100 percent sensitive and specific for a nontuberculous etiology. A number of investigators have tried to measure ADA levels as an adjunct to the diagnosis of tuberculosis.[246-251] Ocana et al reported that pleural fluid ADA levels above 70 U/L had tuberculosis, whereas no patient with levels below 40 U/L had tuberculosis. Subsequent reports confirmed the same findings.[252,253] Curiously, ADA levels have been reported to be lower in Asian patients,[254-256] therefore the test may not be very useful in those patients. Similarly, immunocompromised patients with tuberculous pleural effusion will have low ADA levels. Elevated levels may be seen in patients with empyema,[253] rheumatoid pleuritis,[257] and neoplasms.[258,259] In questionable cases, the type of ADA may be useful. There are two molecular forms of ADA: A large form; and a small form. The tuberculous effusions contain only the larger form; and other effusions with elevated ADA will have both forms, with the small form being the predominant one.[258,260]

Tuberculostearic acid in pleural aspirates has also been reported to be helpful in the diagnosis.[261]

Pleural fluid interferon-γ can also be used as a marker like that of ADA levels.[253,256,262,263] Mycobacterial antigens in pleural fluid by enzyme-linked immunosorbent assay are a diagnostic test. This substance is produced by CD4+ lymphocytes. About 95 percent of cases with tuberculous effusion will have levels above 140 pg/ml, whereas only 8 percent of nontubercular effusions will have this value.[253] Attempts have been made to establish the diagnosis of tuberculosis by estimation of tuberculous antigens/antibodies in the pleural fluid. However, there is so much overlap that these tests are not considered to be useful at this moment. Similarly, polymerase chain reaction (PCR) is thought to be useful in the diagnosis of pleural effusion of tubercular etiology. But, it appears to be too sensitive to be used as a diagnostic tool.[264] A value of 1.2 for the ratio of the pleural fluid to the serum lysozyme has been proposed as a good indicator for the diagnosis of tuberculous pleuritis.[265] However, this test is inferior to that of interferon or ADA level measurements.

Smear positivity of acid-fast bacillus in the pleural fluid is reported to be less than 10 percent (0-9%) and the culture positivity is in the range of 25 to 70 percent of cases,[1,209,266,267] although most series report a result of culture positivity in fewer than 25 percent of cases.[209, 268] BACTEC system gives better and quicker results. About 7 percent will have sputum cultures for tuberculous bacilli even without concomitant parenchymal infiltrates.[185] Conventional methods for diagnosis of pleural tuberculosis have proven insufficient. Direct examination of pleural fluid by Ziehl-Neelsen staining requires bacillar densities of 10,000/mL and, therefore, has low sensitivity (0-1%).[269,270] Although, culture is more sensitive (11-50%).[266,271] 2 to 6 weeks are required to grow M tuberculosis, and a minimum of 10 to 100 viable bacilli are needed. The sensitivity of pleural biopsy reportedly is higher than thoracentesis whether in terms of culture (39% vs 79%)[269,271] or histologic evaluation (71-80%).[269,270] However, biopsy requires greater expertise, is more invasive, and is subject to sampling error.

A variety of other biological markers have been proposed to aid in the diagnosis of tuberculous pleuritis, including increased pleural fluid concentrations of adenosine deaminase (ADA)[272-274] interferon (INF)-γ,[275-281] immunosuppressive acidic protein (IAP),[285,286] and soluble interleukin 2 receptors (sIL-2Rs).[287-291] However, which of these markers is most useful for diagnosis of tuberculous pleuritis has not been determined. Aoe et al[292] studied 46 patients with pleural effusion to determine whether ADA, INF-γ, IAP, and sIL-2R concentrations in pleural fluid show associations with the cause of pleural effusion. Several previous reports demonstrated that these four markers were significantly higher in tuberculous than in nontuberculous pleural effusions.[272-283] Pleural fluid levels (mean ± SE) of adenosine deaminase (83.3 ± 18.2 U/L vs 25.8 ± 20.4 U/L, $p < 0.0001$), interferon-γ (137 ± 230 IU/mL vs 0.41 ± 0.05 IU/mL, $p < 0.0001$), immunosuppressive acidic protein (741 ± 213 μg/mL vs 445 ± 180 μg/mL, $p < 0.001$) and soluble interleukin 2 receptor (7,618 ± 3,662 U/mL vs 2,222 ± 1,027 U/mL, $p < 0.0001$) were significantly higher for tuberculous pleuritis than for other causes of effusion. Of these, pleural fluid content INF-γ was the best indicator of tuberculous pleurisy among four relevant biological markers. INF-γ in pleural fluid is the most sensitive and specific among four biological markers for tuberculous pleuritis. These results suggest that determination of INF-

γ at the onset of pleural effusion is informative for the diagnosis of tuberculous pleuritis. Whatever roles individual marker may play in development of pleural effusion, these results suggest that the pleural fluid ADA, IAP, sIL-2R, and IFN-γ is a useful indicator for diagnosis of tuberculous pleuritis.

INF-γ is an important immune regulator that exhibits both antiviral and cytotoxic activities.[290-292] INF-γ is produced by T lymphocytes in response to stimulation with specific antigens or nonspecific antigens, and is capable of modifying the response of other cells to the immune system. INF-γ is known to activate macrophages, increasing their bactericidal capacity against M tuberculosis. Therefore, INF-γ detected in pleural fluid may be the result from stimulation of T lymphocytes by tuberculous antigens. INF-γ was found to be the most sensitive and specific indicator for diagnosis of tuberculous pleuritis; an INF-γ assay may prove to be an important screening test for tuberculous pleuritis. Nevertheless, measurement of INF-γ is relatively expensive compared with ADA assays. Pleural fluid concentrations of ADA, INF-γ, IAP and sIL-2R in patients with tuberculous pleural effusions are significantly higher than in other effusions. Most importantly, ROC analysis clearly demonstrated INF-γ to be the most sensitive and specific among four relevant biological markers for diagnosis of tuberculous pleuritis. Determination of INF-γ at the onset of pleural effusion is informative for the diagnosis of tuberculous pleuritis. Further studies including larger numbers of patients should be undertaken confirm this result.

Although the cost of a test can be an important consideration, especially in less-developed countries with a high incidence of disease, the results reported by Aoe et al[289] suggests that INF-γ concentrations in pleural fluid may be helpful in patients strongly suspected to have TB. The levels of TNF-γ were reported to be significantly higher in tuberculous than in malignant pleural effusions.[293-296] Increased levels of pleural fluid TNF-γ appeared to be an important indicator in patients with pleural tuberculosis who might acquire residual pleural thickening.[296,297] Philip-Joët et al[298] indicated that pleural PAI-1 levels were greatly enhanced in exudates due to the inflammatory or infection process.

Pleural biopsy demonstrating granulomas and culture positivity can be seen in 50 to 90 percent of cases.[1,169,268,299-301] The demonstration of granuloma in the parietal pleura is highly suggestive of tuberculosis and further demonstration of caseous necrosis and AFB is not necessary. The yield increases as the number of biopsy pieces increases.[299,300] Other conditions producing such granulomas in the parietal pleura include fungal infections, sarcoidosis, tularemia, and rheumatoid arthritis. Pleural biopsy specimen can be cultured and the result may be positive in 55 to 80 percent of cases. Even when granulomas are not demonstrated in the pleural biopsy, occasionally AFB can be demonstrated. Combining pleural fluid and pleural tissue studies, a diagnosis can be achieved in 90 to 95 percent of cases. In some patients with exudative pleural effusions, no diagnosis can be made in spite of repeated pleural biopsies and cultures. In that situation, some advocate thoracoscopy or open pleural biopsy. However this may not be justified for a benign disease like tuberculosis. In countries like India, an exudative effusion with predominant lymphocytes, positive Mantoux test, and in the absence of any other clinical pointer to another disease, anti-tubercular treatment can be started. However, in the absence of a histological or microbiological confirmation, the patient should strictly be followed up to observe clinical progression or deterioration. The role of Tuberculin skin test in the diagnosis of tubercular pleurisy is discussed elsewhere.

Minor tuberculous effusions may resolve spontaneously with a high likelihood of development of active tuberculosis in later life. However, 50 to 70 percent of the patients with pleural effusions in the setting of primary tuberculosis will develop active pulmonary or extrapulmonary tuberculosis within 5 years. Patiala[302] followed a group of 2816 young Finnish Armed Forces personnel who developed pleural effusion. During a follow-up period of at least 7 years, 43 percent developed tuberculosis. Similar report is available from USA, which showed that while most patients had complete reabsorption the fluid, they became symptomatic within 2 to 4 months and 65 percent developed some form of active tuberculosis subsequently.[303] The incidence of subsequent tuberculosis was 60 percent in those with initially negative pleural fluid cultures for tuberculosis and 65 percent in those with initially positive cultures. The size of the initial effusion, or the presence or absence of any radiological residual pleural disease were not correlated with the subsequent development of active disease.[303] Therefore, all patients with tuberculous effusion should be treated with antituberculous drug therapy. The regimens and duration of such therapy are the same to those of pulmonary tuberculosis. All massive effusions should be tapped. Small effusions will not need any therapeutic thoracocentesis. There is some controversy regarding the role of pleural tapping in moderate effusions. However, it is better to tap these effusions to prevent residual fibrosis in future. With treatment, the patient becomes afebrile within two weeks, although fever

may persist for 6 to 8 weeks. The effusion usually resolves by 6 weeks but may persist for as long as 12 to 16 weeks.[304] The mean duration of complete resolution of pleural fluid is about 6 weeks, but can be as long as 12 weeks.[304] Some authors advocate the use of corticosteroids, particularly in patients with severe symptoms. It has been shown that while prednisolone in a dosage of 0.75 mg/kg/day followed by a tapering dose accelerates the resolution of pleural effusions and symptoms; the incidence of residual pleural fibrosis is not altered.[305] However, most physicians do not use steroids. Approximately 50 percent of patients will have some degree of pleural thickening 6 to 12 months after treatment.[306]

(2) Parapneumonic Effusions

Pleural effusions, even if small, are commonly associated with bacterial pneumonias, lung abscess, and bronchiectasis is known as parapneumonic effusion.[307] Approximately 60 percent of patients with pneumococcal pneumonia and 40 percent of all bacterial pneumonias are associated with pleural effusions, and they are usually very small to be detected radiologically.[308,309] Most parapneumonic effusions resolve with antibiotic therapy and need no specific intervention. However, patients with this complication have a greater morbidity and mortality. From therapeutic point of view *uncomplicated* effusions are those that resolve spontaneously with antibiotic therapy and *complicated* effusions require drainage in addition to antibiotic therapy.[313,314] Complicated effusions are usually purulent (empyema), or have positive Gram stains or cultures. However, it is possible that some patients with complicated parapneumonic effusion may not need chest tube drainage[312] and some patients with uncomplicated parapneumonic effusion will eventually require chest tube drainage.[313] Himelman and Callen reported that presence of loculation is associated with increased morbidity independent of fluid characteristics.[314]

In the earlier inflammatory stage, pneumonia in a subpleural location with abundant polymorphs causes increased pulmonary and pleural capillary permeability resulting in the leakage of sterile, protein rich fluid.[315] The effusion has a moderate number of polymorphs and a glucose content similar to that of the blood with a pH of > 7.30. This can resolve with proper antibiotic therapy. However, if treatment is not instituted at this stage, bacteria invade the pleural space with a further intensification of inflammation and empyema formation (see later for the pathogenesis of empyema). Anaerobic organisms, Gram-negative aerobes, and *Staphylococcus aureus* are the most frequent causes of this complicated pleural effusions.

Parapneumonic effusions are exudates with leukocyte counts in excess of 10,000/ml and a predominance of polymorphs. Pleural fluid glucose, pH, and LDH have been used to differentiate complicated from uncomplicated parapnemonic effusions. In the later the pleural fluid pH is 7.30 or more, the glucose concentration is > 60 mg/dl, and the LDH is < 500 U/l. If the purulent fluid is aspirated or the Gram stain is positive, tube drainage is to be instituted. If the aspirated fluid is not purulent and is negative on Gram stain, biochemical characteristics will provide guidance to therapy. If the pH is less than 7.10 and is associated with a glucose level of, 40 mg/dl with a LDH value > 1000 U/l, tube drainage is indicated.[310,311] pH values between 7.10 to 7.29, may be either complicated or uncomplicated and a second thoracentesis after 8 to 12 hours will resolve the issue. If the pH is dropping or LDH level is raising, then chest tube drainage is warranted.[310] The use of low pH as an indication for chest tube drainage applies only to parapneumonic effusions. Management of empyema is discussed subsequently.

(3) Pleural Effusion Due to Other Organisms[316-339]

Actinomyces israelii, Nocardia asteroides and fungal diseases like aspergillosis, blastomycosis, cryptococcosis, coccidioidomycosis, and histoplasmosis may cause pleural effusion, although they most often are important for causing empyema. Pleural involvement in actinomycosis can occur in over 75 percent of cases either with effusion or pleural thickening. Chest radiograph typically shows consolidation, pleural effusion/thickening, and periosteal proliferation of the ribs, a combination rarely seen in other diseases. Pleural effusions have been reported in 15 to 50 percent of patients with nocardiosis. Aspergillus of the pleura is rare and can occur following lobectomy or pneumonectomy for tuberculosis or lung cancer with bronchopleural fistula or in patients treated in the past with pneumothorax therapy for tuberculosis. Immunocompromised patients can also have Aspergillus pleural disease. The pleural fluid may be serous, serosanguinous, purulent, or black if the infection is due to *Aspergillus Niger*. In blastomycosis the pleural fluid is a serous exudate with typical budding yeasts. Cryptococcal pleural effusion is a serous or serosanguinous exudate with a predominance of lymphocytes. Eosinophils may also increase. Pleural fluid culture may be positive in about 45 percent of the cases. Cryptococcal antigens in high titers can also be demonstrated in pleural fluid. Less than 10 percent of patients with primary coccidioidomycosis will have a serous, lymphocyte predominant exudate with normal glucose concen-

tration. A hydropneumothorax occurs in less than 5 percent of cases. Pleural effusions have been reported in 0 to 5 percent of cases during acute epidemic histoplasmosis and in about 3 percent of cases in patients with culture proven histoplasmosis.

Rarely viral and atypical pneumonias like Mycoplasma, and Q fever and Legionella infections are associated with pleural effusions.[308,309]

(4) Parasitic Pleural Effusions[340]

Amebiasis, echinococcosis, and paragonimiasis are some of the parasitic that cause pleural effusion.

Amebic pleural effusion[341-345] may be caused by diaphragmatic irritation resulting in a sympathetic effusion or due to rupture of a hepatic abscess through the diaphragm into the pleural space. Pleural effusions due to diaphragmatic irritations will result in a pleural rub, with a serous exudative pleural effusion. Chest radiograph will reveal a raised right hemidiaphragm, platelike atelectasis, and small right-sided pleural effusion. The diagnosis is established by ultrasonographic examination of the liver and a positive amebic serology. Pleural involvement due to rupture of the amebic liver abscess usually results in an empyema which may be massive and requires tube drainage besides specific antiamebic therapy.

Echinococcosis can involve pleura[346-352] either due to (i) the rupture of a pulmonary hydatid cyst; or (ii) due the rupture of a hepatic lesion through the diaphragm into the pleural space; or (iii) rarely due to the presence of cyst in the pleura. Pulmonary hydatid rupture produces cough, chest pain, and hemoptysis. Rupture of a hepatic hydatid cyst is associated with an acute presentation with the above features with respiratory distress, fever, and shock. Simultaneous rupture into the bronchial tree is associated with bronchopleural fistula and expectoration of large amounts of cyst membranes and purulent material. Usual findings include an elevated right hemidiaphragm, moderate pleural effusion, right lower lobe pneumonia and hydropneumothorax. Thoracentesis reveals turbid, yellow fluid with a polymorph reaction and increased eosinophil counts. The diagnosis is established by the presence of scolices with hooklets. The Casoni test and hydatid serology are positive in 70 to 75 percent of cases. Treatment is emergency thoracotomy to drain the parasites, and excision of the cysts. Medical therapy with mebendazole has recently been tried.

Pleural effusions due to paragonimiasis[353-358] are usually unilateral small to massive exudates and may be yellow, white or brown in color. Cholesterol crystals are frequently present. The leucocyte count is less than

2000/ml, with eosinophilia. The glucose is low with high LDH values and low pH (< 7.10). High IgE levels may also be present.

Filariasis may involve pleura causing pleural effusion.[359-362] Other parasites that may cause pleural effusion include malaria,[344] Trichomonas,[363] loiasis,[364] and sporotrichosis.[365]

(5) Malignant Pleural Effusion[366-378]

Pleural effusion secondary to malignancy commonly occurs as a result of involvement of the pleura due to metastasis. However paramalignant effusions may occur because of malignancy but do not result from direct pleural involvement. Such paramalignant effusions may occur (i) as a result of direct local effect of the tumor causing lymphatic obstruction of the pleural lymphatics, mediastinal lymph node involvement with decreased pleural lymphatic drainage, thoracic duct interruption (chylothorax), bronchial obstruction with pneumonia, or atelectasis causing decreased pleural pressure; (ii) systemic effect of the tumor causing pulmonary embolism, hypoproteinemia; (iii) venous congestion due to superior vena caval obstruction; and (iv) as a result of therapy (radiation or chemotherapy), or (v) secondary to pericardial involvement. Lymphatic obstruction is the predominant mechanism of pleural effusion. The blockage can occur at any point from the stomata of the parietal pleura to the mediastinum.

Carcinoma from any organ can metastasize to the pleura. However lung cancer is the most common tumor to result in malignant and paramalignant effusions.[379] When patients of lung cancer are first evaluated about 15 to 25 percent have a pleural effusion.[380,381] Pleural effusion can occur with any cell type of lung cancer, but appear to be most frequent with adenocarcinoma.[379,382] Carcinoma of the breast is the second most common cause.[383] With breast carcinoma, the incidence is about 46 to 48 percent and effusions are common with lymphangitic spread (63%) than without lymphangitic spread, and the effusion is usually on the same side as that of the primary disease.[384] The mean interval of the primary tumor and pleural effusion is usually 2 years,[385] but it may be as long as 20 years.[386] In breast cancer, ipsilateral effusion is more common although data is conflicting. Pleural involvement results from chest wall lymphatic invasion causing ipsilateral effusion, and hepatic spread with bilateral, ipsilateral, or contralateral disease by the hematogenous route. Other primary sites include ovary, stomach, prostate, colon, pancreas, uterus, kidneys, and thyroid. A substantial number of cases (6%) with malignant effusion will have an unknown primary site at the time of initial diagnosis. In metastasis the tumor cells either invade the mesothelial or the submucosal layer. With the invasion of the former, a large number of tumor cells can be detected in the pleural fluid. With the involvement of the subserous layer tumor cells are scanty. Reactive changes occur in mesothelium with shedding of mesothelial cells and pleural fibrosis. Increased collagen deposition results in low glucose and pH values. In metastatic lung cancer both layers of the pleura are involved. Visceral pleural metastasis results from pulmonary arterial invasion and embolization.[366,387] Tumor cells spread further or shedding of the cells may adhere to the parietal pleura and multiply. Adenocarcinoma of the lung is the most common cell type to involve the pleura because of its peripheral location and propensity for contiguous spread. Other malignant causes of pleural effusions are lymphomas, sarcomas, and mesotheliomas.

The most common presentation is dyspnea,[382] which is partly due to decreased chest wall compliance, contralateral mediastinal shift, loss of lung volume, and neurogenic factors. Cough is another prominent symptom. The chest radiograph will reveal moderate to large effusions in majority of the cases.[26] The fluid may be serous, serosanguinous, or grossly bloody with the later being more common.[85] Red cell count often ranges from 30,000 to 50,000/ml. When the red cells exceed 100,000/ml, malignancy is the most likely cause (when there is no trauma). The nonhemorrhagic effusion is usually an exudate and lymphocytes are the predominant cell types. Most pleural effusions that meet exudative criteria by the LDH level but not by the protein level are malignant pleural effusions.[83] Eosinophils are distinctly rare. About 30 percent of the cases of malignant pleural effusions have a pH of less than 7.30 with a range of 6.95 to 7.29.[119, 124, 388] The glucose content is low and is usually < 60 mg/dl.[119,122,382] The oxygen tension is also low with a high lactate content and carbon dioxide. Glucose values may be as low as 5 mg/dl. This low pH and glucose contents are usually present in effusions of several months duration and are associated with a large tumor burden and fibrosis of the pleura. The abnormal pleural membranes reduce glucose entry into the pleural space and impair efflux of the end products of glucose metabolism resulting in local acidosis. Further, increased utilization of glucose by the pleural tumor also causes reduced levels in pleural fluid.

Pleural fluid cytology for malignant cells will be positive in two-third of cases and varies from 40 to 87 percent.[146-148,389,390] The yield from pleural biopsy has been below 50 percent, but may vary from 39 to 75 percent.[390-392] When both the tests are combined the diagnostic yield increases to more than 70 percent.[1,166,168] Pleural fluid carcinoembryonic antigen, LDH isoenzymes, and hyaluronic acid levels are increased although themselves they are not diagnostic. Chromosome analysis, immunocytometry, and gene rearrangement analysis on cells from pleural fluid are helpful particularly for lymphomas,[393] and in equivocal cases. Thoracoscopy and open thoracotomy will be indicated when no diagnosis is possible and there is a strong clinical suspicion of malignancy.

Malignancy is a common cause of exudative pleural effusion. Carcinoma arising from any organ can metastasize to the pleura and result in pleural effusion. The patients may present with dyspnea and nonproductive cough when their pleural effusions increase to significant amount. To relieve respiratory distress caused by malignant pleural effusion, therapeutic thoracentesis is usually indicated. Malignant pleural effusion, however, may reaccumulate rapidly, and repeated thoracenteses are needed.[394] Clinically, the presence of fibrin strands in pleural fluid shown on chest ultrasonography is suggestive of an inflammatory exudate.[395] The fibrin strands, nevertheless, could also be found in malignant pleural effusion.[396] Repeated thoracenteses may induce the generation of fibrin strands in malignant effusion and result in loculation of the pleural spaces.[395] As a result, the drainage of malignant effusion may become more difficult. Although this phenomenon is not uncommon, the underlying mechanisms of fibrin formation in malignant effusion induced by repeated thoracenteses remain unknown.

By and large, fibrin turnover in the pleural cavity is greatly affected by the activity of fibrinolysis. The formation of key enzyme in fibrinolysis, plasmin, is based mainly on the equilibrium between plasminogen activators and plasminogen activator inhibitors (PAIs).[397] Agrenius et al[398] indicated that intrapleural injection of quinacrine, an irritative agent, in patients with malignant pleural effusions could increase the concentrations of PAI type 1 (PAI-1) and reduce fibrinolytic activity in pleural fluid. The levels of proinflammatory cytokines such as tumor necrosis factor (TNF)-γ and interleukin (IL)-1β in pleural fluid were reported to be elevated markedly after intrapleural injection of quinacrine in patients with malignant pleural effusions.[399,400] These findings suggest a strong relationship between the fibrinolytic activity and proinflammatory cytokines in the pleural cavity.

The levels of TNF-γ were reported to be significantly higher in tuberculous than in malignant pleural effusions.[293-296] Increased levels of pleural fluid TNF-γ appeared to be an important indicator in patients with pleural tuberculosis who might acquire residual pleural thickening.[296,297] Philip-Joët et al[298] indicated that pleural PAI-1 levels were greatly enhanced in exudates due to the inflammatory or infection process; however, the levels of plasminogen activators were increased in malignant effusions. Significantly higher levels of tissue type plasminogen activator (tPA) and lower values of PAI-1 are found in malignant than in tuberculous effusions.[296,298]

Taken together, these findings suggest that the enhanced release of TNF-γ and/or IL-1β caused by pleural inflammation may result in an imbalance between PAI-1 and tPA in the pleural cavity, which may subsequently lead to fibrin formation and loculation of the pleural effusion. Clinical observations[395] indicated that repeated thoracenteses might induce generation of fibrin strands in malignant effusion, it is speculated that repeated thoracenteses may cause pleural inflammation, enhanced release of proinflammatory cytokines, and an imbalance between PAI-1 and tPA, which may lead to formation of fibrin strands in malignant pleural effusion. Chung et al conducted a prospective study to evaluate the effect of repeated thoracenteses on the fluid characteristics, the levels of cytokines related to inflammation and fibrinolytic activity in malignant pleural effusion and its clinical significance.[401]

The values of TNF-α, PAI-1, IL-8, and neutrophil count in pleural fluid increased significantly during repeated thoracenteses that may cause pleural inflammation and induce local release of proinflammatory cytokine as TNF-α, which may subsequently enhance the release of PAI-1 and lead to fibrin formation in malignant effusion. The presence of fibrin strands after repeated thoracenteses may be of considerable value in predicting the success of subsequent pleurodesis in patients with malignant pleural effusions.[401] Bronchoscopy is of use in some cases of malignant pleural effusion.[402]

Patients with malignant pleural effusions have a poor prognosis particularly in those with low glucose (< 40 mg/dl) and pH (< 7.30). Further, they indicate more extensive involvement of pleural surface with the tumor, a higher yield on fluid cytology, decreased success rates for pleurodesis, and shorter survival times.[403-405] Pleural effusion associated with lung cancer is an indicator of nonoperability. However, about 5 percent of the cases the effusion is a paramalignant one and itself is not a contraindication of surgery. Other patients should receive palliative therapy. Asymptomatic patients need not be treated. Progressive dyspnea needs to be treated with palliative therapy. Pleurectomy and pleural abrasions are virtually 100 percent effective due to complete obliteration of the pleural space. However, they are major surgical procedures and as the patient is generally sick, pleurectomy should be reserved in patients who are in relatively good health and have an expected survival of at least several months. Other indications for this procedure are in those where thoracotomy is done in an undiagnosed pleural effusion and is found to have malignancy; that have a trapped lung; and when pleurodesis have failed.[406]

The other methods of controlling malignant pleural effusion are the use of sclerosing agents. A wide range of sclerosants has been used after chest tube drainage, including tetracycline, bleomycin, quinacrine, nitrogen mustard, adriamycin, talc, and mitoxantrone. Other agents used in the past included silver nitrate, kaoline, lipidol, cyanoacrylate, dicetyl phosphate, and radioactive substances. Talc has been used successfully over many years as a sclerosing agent in the treatment of pleural effusion and pneumothorax. Because of high success rates and low cost, Talc has received substantial attention recently.[407] This can be administered via poudrage or slurry in either pleural effusion or pneumothorax. Success rates are comparable in either form and the overall success rate is around 91 percent. The short-term side effects include fever, pain, infection, systemic embolization (cerebral embolism), hemodynamic compromise, and respiratory failure, which is dose related. Long-term complications include altered pulmonary function, land risk of malignancy, particularly when it contains asbestos and is dose dependent. A dose of 5 gm of Talc has been recommended for use as a pleurodesis agent to avoid some of these complications.[407-411] Quinacrine pleurodesis requires frequent injections and has been associated with central nervous system side effects. Currently, tetracycline hydrochloride appears to be the most widely used sclerosing agent because of high success rates with minimum toxicity.[412-418] Although the exact mechanism of tetracycline pleurodesis is unknown, the initial pH of the tetracycline solution instilled into the pleural space is probably important. The acidic fluid together with the chemical nature of the tetracycline is presumably the cause of destruction and sloughing of the mesothelial cells. With the resparative process, pleural fibrosis develops. The usual dose is 15 mg/kg or 1 gm of tetracycline hydrochloride diluted with 50 mg of lignocaine to reduce pain. Drainage of the pleural fluid as completely as possible should be obtained most often by chest tubes, before instillation of the drug. Because of recent unavailability of this preparation in many countries, new tetracycline agents like minocycline and doxycycline have been used with similar results.[419-421] Alternatively, bleomycin can be used in a dose of 1.25 mg/kg, not to exceed 40 mg in the elderly, or nitrogen mustard 20 mg, can be used. Control of effusion is expected in 70 to 80 percent of cases for at least one month.

Although pleurodesis is reserved by and large for malignant effusions, in rapidly accumulations, massive effusions due to benign causes, this method is also recommended[422].

Biological agents like Corynebacterium parvum[423,424] and β interferon[425,426] have also been proposed. Other experimental drugs that are tried for pleurodesis include OK-432,[427] attaching chemotherapeutic agents to particles that would remain in the pleural space for a longer period, like adsorbing mitomycin C to activated carbon particles,[428] intrapleural transfer of autologous or allogenic lymphokine-activated killer (LAK) cells,[429,430] administration of tumor-associated monoclonal antibodies radiolabeled with iodine-131,[431] and trimidyne Nd: YAG Optilaser.[432] Intrapleural recombinant IL-2 has been used as passive immunotherapy for malignant pleural effusion.[433]

Alternatives to pleurodesis include symptomatic treatment like pleuro-peritoneal shunt, repeated pleurodesis, pleural radiotherapy and pleurectomy.[434]

(6) Lymphoma[435-438]

Lymphomas constitute about 10 percent of all pleural effusions,[439] and 16 percent of the patients with Hodgkin's disease will have radiological evidence of pleural effusion,[440] Pleural effusion is a rare cause of Hodgkin's disease at the time of presentation, but not uncommon as the presenting feature of non-Hodgkin's lymphoma. About 12 to 45 percent of cases of the later are associated with pleural effusion. Lymphomatous infiltration of the pleura occurs rarely and is a late feature of Hodgkin's disease. However, this appears to be common in non-Hodgkin's lymphoma,[436,438,441,442] As the Hodgkin's disease progresses, the incidence of pleural effusion increases and occurs in about a third of cases. The incidence is still higher in autopsy series, which showed 39 percent having pleural effusion and 29 percent having involvement of the parietal pleura and 74 percent with mediastinal or hilar node involvement,[440,443] The pleural effusion associated with lymphoma may be a chylothorax.[444]

The cause of early pleural effusion in lymphoma appears to be due to either impaired lymphatic drainage because of mediastinal adenopathy, infiltration of the pleura or thoracic duct obstruction. While in Hodgkin's disease the primary mechanism is impaired lymphatic obstruction, which in the non-Hodgkin's lymphoma appears to be due to direct pleural infiltration.[438,442]

The most common clinical manifestations of lymphomatous pleural effusion are; dyspnea, chest pain, cough, and orthopnea.[438] About a fifth of the cases, it is asymptomatic. Pleural effusion is usually unilateral and is a serous exudate, but can be hemorrhagic, chylous, transudative, and bilateral.[436,438] The cell count is usually low with predominance of atypical lymphocytes.[102] The glucose content and pH is usually normal, but may be low.[441] Diagnosis of lymphomatous pleural effusion is established more easily in non-Hodgkin's lymphoma than Hodgkin's disease because of different mechanisms in both conditions. Cytological positivity is low, usually in the range of 10 to 25 percent in lymphoma.[445,446]

Presence of pleural effusion is a bad prognostic indicator of lymphoma.[122,357,436,442] However, the survival varies from few months to several years depending on response to therapy. If there is mediastinal adenopathy without parenchymal or pleural nodules, effusion is easily controlled following radiotherapy or chemotherapy. In the later, chemotherapy may be more effective. Pleurodesis should be attempted if these measures are not effective. Chylous lymphomatous effusions respond well to radiotherapy.

(7) Malignant Mesothelioma[447-459]

Pleural mesothelioma is more common in males in the 6th to 7th decade, and two-thirds of the patients are between the ages of 40 and 70 years.[447,448] The manifestation in the late age is due to a long latent period. The onset is insidious with localized chest pain being the most common feature in addition to dyspnea.[449] Rarely the patient is asymptomatic at the time of presentation and it is suggested that an asymptomatic patient with a pleural effusion to have malignant mesothelioma. Dyspnea, cough, and weight loss are the other features. Right-sided pleural effusion is more common occurring in about two-thirds of the patients.[450] The effusion may be large and massive causing contralateral shift of the mediastinum. However, as the tumor progresses, it encases the lung growing along the mediastinum, and inhibits mediastinal shift despite of massive effusion, a characteristic radiological finding in about 42 percent of the cases.[450] Pleural thickening or nodularity near the diaphragm may be the first feature. Other signs of asbestosis in the form of interstitial fibrosis and pleural plaques may be noted in the contralateral lung. Mediastinum may be widened later in the course of the disease with cardiomegaly because of pericardial infiltration of

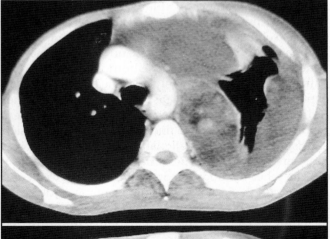
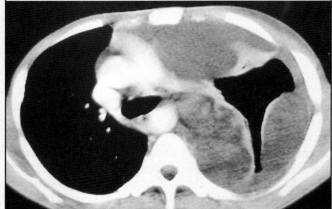

FIGURE 28.5: CT Chest - Multifocal left pleural mass - malignant pleural mesothelioma

the tumor. CT scan is useful in defining the disease extent beyond pleura and often reveals intrapulmonary nodules (Fig. 28.5).[451]

During thoracentesis, marked resistance to the needle may be encountered as one enters into the pleural space. The fluid may be serous, serosanguinous, or frankly hemorrhagic. The fluid is an exudate with low LDH levels. The total cell count is usually less than 5,000/ml. The pH **is** also low in most of the cases. The pleural fluid glucose will be below 50 mg/dl and the pleural fluid pH is below 7.20.[452] Cytological diagnosis of pleural malignant mesothelioma is controversial since it is very difficult to differentiate between benign and malignant mesothelial cells.[453,454] Use of histochemical staining with periodic acid-Schiff stain, immunoperoxidase studies with monoclonal antibodies, and electron microscopy may help in differentiating mesothelioma and metastatic adenocarcinoma. Increased levels of hyaluronic acid are found more often in mesothelioma than with other exudative pleural effusions. Tissue biopsy is the most reliable method of diagnosis. Percutaneous pleural biopsy will not provide adequate tissue sample for diagnosis and thoracotomy will usually be required to establish the diagnosis.[455-457] Infiltration of the surgical scars with mesothelioma is more frequent.

(8) Immunologically Mediated Pleural Effusions[393-472]

In these disorders the alterations in the endothelial barrier may result from humoral or cell-mediated immunologic mechanisms. Humoral mechanisms are important in systemic lupus erythematosus and rheumatoid arthritis. In these disorders, circulating immune complexes, when deposited in the pleural capillaries, are capable of fixing complement. Activated products of the complement cascade (C3a and C5a) increase vascular permeability resulting in pleural fluid formation. Presence of both immune complexes and complement components in the pleural fluid supports this argument.

Systemic lupus erythematosus (SLE). Pleural effusion occurs in about a third of cases of systemic lupus erythematosus, although reported figures vary from 16 to 44 percent and more than 50 percent of the cases complain of pleuritic chest pain some times during the course of the disease and the incidence may be as high as 50 to 70 percent in the course of the illness.[464,473,474] Although pleural disease usually accompanies other manifestations of SLE, pleural effusion may occur in the absence of other systemic manifestations, and may even precede the development of antinuclear antibodies. In autopsy series, about 40 percent of cases will have evidence of pleural inflammation and in about 30 percent of cases there will be pleural fibrosis.[475,476] The pleural inflammation may not be entirely due to SLE, but may be secondary to nonimmunologic mechanisms including intercurrent pneumonia, pulmonary thromboembolism, viral infections, or congestive cardiac failure. The presentation may be indistinguishable clinically from other causes of pleural effusion. Most patients are females and any age group can be affected[474,477] and are symptomatic at the time of presentation with complaints of chest pain, cough, and dyspnea. Fever, and pleural rub may be present on clinical examination. The most common radiological manifestation of lupus pleurisy is small to moderate bilateral pleural effusions, although unilateral effusion can occur.[474] Other pulmonary manifestations of SLE may also be present. The presenting symptoms, signs, and radiographic features are same in both primary and drug induced SLE. Pleural effusions in SLE may also be due to other causes like nephrotic syndrome,

congestive cardiac failure, pulmonary embolism, parapneumonic effusions, and uremia.

The fluid may be serous, turbid, or hemorrhagic. Total cell count varies from several hundred to 20,000/ml with the cellular predominance of polymorphs or mononuclear cells depending upon the stage of inflammation.[139] Pleural fluid eosinophilia has also been reported. Pleural fluid glucose is normal in contrast to that in rheumatoid arthritis. The pH is also normal. However, they may be low as in rheumatoid arthritis. It is reported that pleural fluid glucose, LDH, and pH measurements may be helpful in distinguishing SLE from rheumatoid arthritis.[477] IN SLE, the pleural fluid glucose is above 80 mg/dl; LDH level is below 500 IU/L, and the pH is above 7.20, whereas in rheumatoid arthritis the glucose level is below 25 mg/dl; LDH is above 700 IU/L, and the pH is below 7.20. However, they are not always helpful to distinguish the two. Presence of LE cells in the pleural fluid is diagnostic and at times they may be present in the pleural fluid before they are demonstrated in the peripheral blood.[478,479] The positivity is increased if the fluid is allowed to remain in room temperature for several hours. Total hemolytic complement or complement components are usually low when corrected for protein concentration and immune complexes can be found in the fluid. Determination of pleural fluid antinuclear antibody (ANA) titers has been recommended as the best test for establishing SLE as the cause of a pleural effusion. The pleural fluid ANA is usually positive. In lupus pleurisy, the pleural fluid ANA titer is usually 1:160 or more and the pleural fluid to serum ANA ratio is 1 or more. However, it is important to know the source of substrate antigens. When the substrate antigens are derived from animal cell lines such as the liver or kidney from rats or mice, the ANA positivity used to be nearly 100 percent[139,480] with excellent sensitivity and specificity. However, with the recent use of substrate antigens derived from human cell lines, such as HEp-2 ANA that incorporates the human HEp-2 cell lines derived from human epithelial cell cancer, the positivity can be upto 75 percent. About 11 percent of patients with pleural effusion other than due to SLE can have a positive pleural fluid ANA with speckled pattern.[481] Immune complexes and complements may be identified by immunofluorescence, both in the walls of pleural vessels and in the nuclei of mesothelial cells.[482,483]

Active lupus pleuritis should be treated with corticosteroids. The response is dramatic, in contrast to rheumatoid pleurisy, with relief of symptoms over several days and the fluid disappears over the next 2 weeks.

Spontaneous resolution usually does not occur, although possible.[474,484] Some times other immunosuppressants like cyclophosphamide or azathioprine may be needed. Unresponsive effusions and repeated massive effusions can be treated symptomatically by doing pleurodesis.

Rheumatoid arthritis. Pleural effusion is an uncommon clinical manifestation of rheumatoid arthritis and occurs in about 3 to 5 percent of the cases,[461,485] although at autopsy approximately 50 percent of the patients have evidence of active or previous pleural inflammation. This clinicopathological discrepancy is partly due to the fact that a number of patients are asymptomatic. There may be patchy areas of fibrosis in the visceral pleura, numerous visceral pleural nodules, or extensive fibrosis with pleural symphysis. The nodules have the characteristic features of other rheumatoid nodules like fibrinoid necrosis, palisading cells, and lymphocytic or plasma cell infiltrations.[486-488]

Patients of rheumatoid pleural disease do not reflect the usual characteristics of rheumatoid arthritis patients. Pleural effusion is more common in middle-aged males with long-standing rheumatoid arthritis and does not parallel with the course of articular manifestations of the disease. The typical patient with rheumatoid pleurisy is a male in the 6th decade that develops pleural effusion within 5 years after the onset of rheumatoid disease. Effusions, however, can develop before or even 20 years after the onset of articular disease. Patients with pleurisy will usually have moderate to severe arthritis and subcutaneous nodules.[461,462,485,489] The rheumatoid factor titer is generally high in the serum and is usually in equal or high titers in the pleural fluid. The presentation is usually with pleuritic chest pain or dyspnea or the disease may be discovered on a routine chest radiograph. Fever is not a common manifestation in contrast to lupus pleurisy. The effusion is usually small to moderate and unilateral.[462] It is an exudative effusion. The effusion may appear turbid with a yellow-green tinge or occasionally it may be milky because of high cholesterol. The most characteristic and consistent features of rheumatoid pleural effusions are a low pleural fluid glucose and pH and a high LDH. About two-thirds of the patients will have a glucose value of less than 30 mg/dl and in about 80 percent of cases it will be less than 50 mg/dl. The pH runs parallel to the glucose concentration. It is possibly related to glucose metabolism and retention of glucose metabolism end products in the pleural space due to abnormal pleura. There is a selective blockage of glucose transport from the blood into the pleura. The low value may be due to a combination of impaired transport and increased metabolism by the inflamed pleura. Accumu-

lation of CO_2, the end products of glucose metabolism and lactic acid in the pleural space result in decreased pleural fluid pH. Other changes observed in the pleural fluid include a decreased total hemolytic complement and complement components, a rheumatoid factor of equal to or more than 1:320 or at least as high as the serum titer, and higher levels of immune complexes. Another interesting feature of rheumatoid pleural effusions is the presence of cholesterol crystals or high levels of cholesterol. Nosanchuk and Naylor have described the characteristic cytological picture in pleural fluid.[463] This consisted of a background of orange or red granular material, large, elongated cells, and giant, round or oval multinucleated cells. These pleomorphic cells may be misinterpreted as malignant cells. The other characteristic cytological picture with rheumatoid pleural effusion is characterized by three distinct features; (a) slender, elongated multinucleated macrophages; (b) round giant multinucleated macrophages; and (c) necrotic background material. The pleural fluid will have at least one of the above three characteristics.[490] The fluid may also contain "ragocytes" or rheumatoid arthritis (RA) cells. These are small. Spherical, cytoplasmic inclusions in neutrophilic leukocytes, and can be seen occasionally in monocytes.[491] Diagnostic yield from pleural biopsy is usually low because most of the pathological changes occur in the visceral pleura.

The course of pleural effusion is variable and resolution occurs over several months. Some patients will have a protracted course lasting for several years with marked pleural thickening.

Treatment of rheumatoid pleural effusion with corticosteroids has been controversial as regards their usefulness. Some believe that nonsteroidal anti-inflammatory drugs are of equal value in preventing the development of progressive pleural fibrosis with either a trapped lung or fibrothorax requiring surgery. These drugs should be used for sufficiently longer periods and be continued till the inflammation subsides. The drugs should be continued for at least 2 to 3 months. Some advocates moderate doses of prednisolone for several weeks.

Other connective tissue /Immunological diseases. In Wegener's granulomatosis, the incidence of pleural effusion has been reported to vary from 5 to more than 50 percent of the patients.[468,469] Effusions have not been observed in the absence of parenchymal lesions and the effusions are usually small, and unilateral. Lesions when close to the pleura, they often induce deposition of fibrin on the surface. Moreover, hemorrhagic infarctions with thrombi-occluded vessels may be responsible for pleural effusion. In mixed connective tissue disease, pleural effusion has been observed in 6 percent of cases. Rarely, pleural effusion precedes other evidences of disease. Pleural effusion is a rare finding in Sjögren's syndrome.[470] It occurs in 0 to 1 percent of the cases.[492,493] Pleural effusion is not a feature of dermatomyositis and polymyositis although they may produce interstitial pneumonitis.

(9) Drug Induced Pleural Effusions

A number of drugs have been reported to result in pleural effusion.[494-508] Although there a innumerable case reports implicating drugs in causing pleural effusion, establishment of a causal relationship is difficult. In many instances repeated challenge has not been done. The characteristics of these effusions are rarely reported and the exact mechanisms, whether localized or systemic immunological functions, have rarely been documented. However, there a specific group of drugs for which repeated documentations exist and some immunological information regarding their immunological mechanisms have been reasonably established. While a multitude of drugs have been implicated in causing lung disease, a much smaller number of agents produce pleural effusion. These drugs may incite a pleural reaction alone or in combination with parenchymal disease. The presentation may vary from acute pleurisy to fluid accumulation and pleural thickening.

Drug-induced lupus-like syndrome. The drugs associated with this syndrome and characterized by pleural and pericardial effusions, arthritis, and arthralgias are many. They are:[495]

Hydralazine*
Phenytoin*
D-penicillamine
Isoniazid*
Procainamide*
Methysergide
Chlorpromazine*
Quinidine
Methyldopa
Tetracycline
Penicillin

(* *These drugs are definitely associated*)

The lupus syndrome is indistinguishable from the native lupus, although there are several characteristic features. The age and sex are important for the underlying disease for which the drug is being given in contrast to the typically young, female patients who develop idiopathic systemic lupus erythematosus. Both renal and central nervous system manifestations, common in the idiopathic variety, are distinctly rare in drug-induced lupus. Improvement or resolution of the symptoms with discontinuation of the agent suggests further drug-induced lupus. Further, drug-induced lupus is not associated with the presence of antibodies against native DNA, and serum complement levels are normal. Although withdrawal of the offending agent brings about resolution, in few cases corticosteroid therapy may be necessary.

Nitrofurantoin. Both acute and chronic pleuropulmonary reactions have been reported associated with the use of this drug. In acute reactions about a third of the patients develop both pulmonary infiltrates and pleural effusion, where as pleural effusion alone can occur in about 8 percent of the cases. In contrast, in chronic reactions, pleural reaction alone is rare. Such reactions account for a small percentage of cases (7%). The exact pathogenesis is unknown, but data support an immunological basis for acute lung injury and a toxic reaction in the more chronic cases. Specific IgG antibodies against nitrofurantoin are present in both symptomatic and asymptomatic patients receiving this drug, but are in higher titer in symptomatic cases. Proliferation of peripheral lymphocytes in response to the drug challenge has been observed. In acute reactions, there is a history of previous drug intake. Within hours to days following the initiation of therapy, there is an acute onset of fever, dyspnea, and cough. Blood eosinophilia and leukocytosis are common. Symptoms subside in a few days of stopping the drug. About half of the cases are symptom free within 24 hours and most within 72 hours.

Procainamide. The average duration of procainamide therapy prior to development of symptoms is 12 months with a range of one month to 8 years with a maintenance dose of 1.5 gm/day (range 0.75-3.75 gms/day). Antinuclear antibodies are common in patients treated with this drug, appearing in about 50 percent of asymptomatic patients after 2 months of therapy. Pulmonary involvement is more common than pleural effusion. Serological tests are same as those of idiopathic systemic lupus erythematosus except that the serum complement is not decreased. The patients usually have antibodies to denatured DNA and nucleohistone, but not to native DNA, in contrast to the idiopathic variety. The fluid may contain classic LE cells.

Hydralazine. Although antinuclear antibodies develop in about a third of the patients taking hydralazine, development of drug-induced lupus is uncommon. Genetic differences in drug metabolism may be important in the pathogenesis with an increased frequency of the HLA-DRw4 haplotype. The reaction is more common in women and is dose dependent. The drug induced pleural reaction is uncommon with a dose of less than 50 mg/

day and occurs in about 10 percent of the cases taking 200 mg/day over a period of 4 years.

Other drugs reported to cause pleural effusion include bromocriptine, dantrolene, methysergide, procarbazine, methotrexate, practolol, amiodarone, mitomycin, bleomycin, and minoxidil. Pleural effusions, sometimes with pleural fibrosis, have been associated with long-term *bromocriptine* therapy but occur in less than 10 percent of the cases receiving the drug. The reaction can also occur with moderate doses of the drug and as few as 9 months after therapy. The fluid is usually an exudate with lymphocytosis, and sometimes with pleural eosinophilia. The effusion disappears with discontinuation of therapy. *Dantrolene* is a skeletal muscle relaxant with a structural similarity to that of nitrofurantoin. This may cause an eosinophilic pleural effusion. The usual duration of therapy before pleural involvement occurs varies from 2 months to 3 years with a dose range of 225 to 400 mg/day. Eosinophilia in the fluid and blood suggests an allergic reaction, but immunofluorescent studies of the pleural tissue show only nonspecific immunoglobulin deposition. *Methysergide* induced pleuropulmonary disease is commonly seen in patients between 40 to 60 years of age who have been treated with the drug in a dose of 1 to 6 mg/day for 1 month to 6 years. The effusion may be either unilateral or bilateral. Unusual tumor like nodules has been seen radiology representing areas of inflammation. The fluid is generally either straw-colored or serosanguinous and is an exudate. There are only few case reports of pleural effusion associated with *procarbazine* therapy. Intermittent, low or high dose, and maintenance *methotrexate* therapy have been associated with pleural effusion. A single intramuscular methotrexate of 50 mg has been associated with pleurisy in 4 percent of the cases. In high dose therapy (8-12 gm/m^2) about 9 percent of the cases develop pleuritis. *Practolol* is a beta-adrenergic agent used in the early seventies has been withdrawn following toxicity of the skin, eyes, ears and peritoneum. Pleuropulmonary disease occurs following doses of 300 to 600 mg/day for 1 to 3 years. Insidious, progressive dyspnea is the most common presenting symptom. Characteristic radiographic picture of the chest shows thickened pleura in the lower hemithorax and unilateral or bilateral pleural effusions. The radiological changes most often precede clinical symptoms. *Amiodarone* pulmonary toxicity may occurs in up to 6 percent or more of cases. Pleural thickening is found in a lower percentage of cases and pleural effusion appears to be rare. Although interstitial pneumonitis is the most common pulmonary toxicity of *mitomycin* therapy,

several studies have reported pleural inflammation, thickening, and effusion. The effusion is either unilateral or bilateral. Occasional reports of pleural effusion has described in *bleomycin* pulmonary toxicity, although interstitial fibrosis occurs in about 6 percent of the cases receiving a total dose of > 450 Units.

Other rare drugs that are reported to produce pleural effusion include: ergotamine, metronidazole, isotretinoin, propylthiouracil, interleukin-2, ethosuximide, ethylphenacemide, guanoxan, griseofulvin, mephenytoin, methylthiouracil, oral contraceptives, PAS, phenylbutazone, primidone, reserpine, streptomycin, sulphonamides, tetracyclines, and troxidone.

(10) Postcardiac Injury Syndrome (Dressler's Syndrome)

This syndrome is characterized by inflammation of the pericardium, pleura, and pulmonary parenchyma, occurring 1 to 6 weeks after myocardial infarction.[466,467,509] Subsequently this syndrome has also been reported after any cardiac injury including cardiac surgery, blunt chest trauma, myocardial infarction, percutaneous left ventricular puncture, pacemaker implantation, and angioplasty.[510,511] The incidence has been reported to vary from less than 1 percent to 15 percent following myocardial infarction and perhaps reflects the extent and degree of myocardial injury. The incidence is high following cardiac surgery and may be as high as 30 percent. Pleural effusion is a common presentation occurring in about 80 percent of the cases. Other features are pericardial effusion, fever, pleuritic chest pain, and leucocytosis. The syndrome may be confused with infection, pulmonary embolism, or congestive cardiac failure. The pleural fluid is usually an exudate, with normal glucose and pH values. The fluid may be serosanguinous or hemorrhagic. Initial reactions may show an influx of polymorphs, but subsequently the effusion is classically a lymphocytic one.

Several mechanisms have been proposed to explain the pathogenesis of this syndrome. They include the development of cytotoxic antibodies directed against myocardial antigens, an immune response to a coincidental viral infection, and an acquired defect in cell-mediated immunity. Therapy for the syndrome consists of symptomatic treatment with nonsteroidal anti-inflammatory agents. Steroids may be necessary in severe cases. In patients who have coronary artery bypass surgery, early corticosteroid therapy may be considered because of the danger of postoperative graft occlusion due to continued inflammation.

(11) Gastrointestinal Causes of Pleural Effusion

(i) *Esophageal rupture.* Esophageal perforation[512-518] due to endoscopy or dilatation is the most common cause in the majority of cases (39%). 0.15 to 0.70 percent of all esophagoscopic procedures are complicated by esophageal perforations. Other causes include foreign body, spontaneous rupture (Boerhaave's syndrome), malignancy and trauma.[519] Clinical presentation, radiological findings, and prognosis depend on the etiology, location and extent of perforation. Chest pain is a prominent symptom in most cases, particularly so in cervical perforations. Persistent chest pain or epigastric pain within several hours of the procedure is indicative of a rupture. Patients with spontaneous rupture of the esophagus usually have a history of vomiting followed by chest pain and the patient typically describes a sensation of tearing or bursting in the lower part of the chest or the epigastrium. The pain is excruciating and is unrelieved by analgesics including opiates. In mid-esophageal and distal perforations dyspnea and dysphagia are more prominent symptoms. Almost all patients will have a febrile reaction. About half of the cases will have subcutaneous emphysema.

Spontaneous rupture (*Boerhaave s syndrome*) is commonly associated with severe retching or vomiting or an effort to control vomiting. In some, the perforation may be silent. Radiological changes may depend upon several factors including the time of X-ray taken, the site of perforation, and the integrity of the mediastinal pleura. The chest radiograph is usually normal if taken within minutes of the actual injury and may remain so in about 10 percent of the cases. It takes about 1 to 2 hours for the mediastinal emphysema to develop. This sign is seen in less than 50 percent of the cases. It may several hours for mediastinal widening to develop. Subcutaneous emphysema in the neck is common with rupture of cervical esophagus, where as mediastinal emphysema occurs early due to that of the intrathoracic esophagus. Radiological appearance of air occurs early in the soft tissue of the neck than it can be detected clinically. Pneumothorax is common in spontaneous rupture of the esophagus and occurs in 75 percent of the cases. Most of the time the pneumothorax occurs in the left (70%), less commonly on the right (20%), and rarely bilateral (10%). Pleural effusion is common in association with pneumothorax.

In iatrogenic perforation the diagnosis is more obvious than that of the spontaneous rupture where a high degree of suspicion is required. In the former, the radiological changes can occur in either hemithorax depending on the level and location of trauma. With minor perforations, the mediastinal pleura are intact and the pleural effusion is a sterile, PMN predominant exudate.

The tear is most common distally just above the esophagogastric junction on the left because of deficient striated muscle and lack of extramural support. Rupture generally occurs due to an acute rise of pressure in the esophageal lumen because of the generation of high intra-abdominal pressure against closed glottis during vomiting. The acuteness of the rise of pressure is more important than the absolute pressure generated for the perforation.

Either by barium sulfate or a water-soluble contrast compound study usually accomplishes confirmation of the rupture. Early thoracentesis will reveal a serous, sterile exudate with a predominance of polymorphs, and the pleural amylase and pH being normal.[520] If the mediastinal pleura tears, amylase of salivary origin will be very high in the fluid. Soon, anaerobic organisms from the mouth will contaminate the fluid with a rapid and progressive fall of pH. Further fall in pH is contributed by the leucocyte glucose metabolism, and perhaps to some extent because of gastric acid reflux. Other characteristic findings of esophageal rupture are the presence of food particles and squamous epithelial cells in pleural fluid.

Because of delayed diagnosis, patients with spontaneous rupture have poor survival. Immediate operative treatment is needed once the diagnosis is made. If diagnosed within 24 hours, primary closure should be attempted and such repair results in > 90 percent survival. However, if treatment is delayed beyond 24 hours from time of symptoms, the survival is reduced with any form of therapy. Other therapeutic modalities besides primary closure include antibiotic treatment covering anaerobes, drainage of the pleural and mediastinal spaces, and parenteral nutrition. In some iatrogenic ruptures, a conservative approach can be adopted.

(ii) *Upper abdominal abscess.* This is a serious illness with mortality up to 40 percent with a pleural effusion being frequently present in 70 to 80 percent of cases.[521-525] Subphrenic space is the most common site of containment of infection. Most often, this follows upper abdominal surgery including splenectomy, gastric, duodenal, or pancreatic, and biliary tract surgery. Hepatic and appendicular surgery is the other causes. Nonoperative causes like perforation of abdominal organs are the other causes. The usual presentation is fever, respiratory distress, and abdominal tenderness. The classical chest X-ray will show an elevated hemidiaphragm, pleural effusion, and often gas under the diaphragm. CT scanning is highly accurate in the diagnosis, which will also show the anatomical extent of the abscess. The effusion is usually shows a predominant polymorph response. Empyema occurs in about 20 percent of the cases. Early diagnosis, drainage, and antibiotic therapy remain the mainstay of treatment.

(iii) *Diseases of liver.* Pleural effusion has been reported to occur in about 0.16 percent of cases in a large series of 25,000 cases of *viral hepatitis.*[526] Some investigators have reported a very high incidence of 70 percent even when the pleural effusion is very small.[527] The fluid is a dark, yellow exudate with a small number of lymphocytes. The glucose is normal, but amylase levels are low. Hepatitis B surface antigen, and "e" antigen have been detected in the fluid. It has been suggested that the fluid may be immunologic in origin.[528,529] *Pyogenic abscess* of the liver may involve pleura either by direct rupture through the diaphragm, due to development of a fistulous tract or as a sympathetic effusion. Pleural effusion may occur in about 20 percent of the cases. Resolution of hepatic hydrothorax occurs after transjugular intrahepatic portosystemic shunt.[530]

(iv) *Diseases of the spleen.* Splenic abscess is a rare cause of pleural effusion and carries a high mortality if undetected.[522] A left sided pleural effusion is present in about 20 to 45 percent of the cases. Infarction of the spleen can also result in a left sided pleural effusion. Other rare causes of such effusion include hematomas of the spleen.

(v) *Pancreatic diseases.* Pleural effusion is seen in 3 to 17 percent of cases of pancreatitis either acute or chronic.[531,532] The mechanisms of such effusions include: (a) direct contact of pancreatic enzymes with the diaphragm resulting in a sympathetic effusion; (b) transfer of ascitic fluid through the diaphragmatic defects or the trans-diaphragmatic lymphatics; (c) fistulous communication between a pseudocyst and pleural space; and (d) retroperitoneal movement of fluid into the mediastinum.

The pleural effusion associated with acute pancreatitis is usually small and left sided (60%). In about a third of the cases it is right sided and in about 10 percent of the cases the effusion is bilateral. Although a normal pleural fluid amylase is observed initially, it increases on serial measurements with the concentration being greater than serum. The exudative fluid contains an excess of polymorphs with leucocyte counts reaching as high as 50,000/ml. In chronic pancreatitis, the effusion is usually large to massive and recurrent, and the patient presents with dyspnea, chest pain, or cough. Sometimes the history of pancreatitis may not be forthcoming, although majority of them are alcoholics. In contrast to acute pancreatitis, the amylase level is always elevated and may exceed > 10,000 U/L. The serum amylase level may be elevated due to back diffusion, or it may be normal. Other causes of high amylase level include rupture of oesophagus, malignancy, ruptured ectopic pregnancy, and rarely pneumonia. The effusion may be hemorrhagic. Ultrasound and CT are helpful in the diagnosis.

Treatment is not necessary for effusions due to acute pancreatitis since they are usually small and resolve completely as pancreatic inflammation subsides. However, if the effusion does not subside within 2 to 3 weeks, pancreatic abscess or pseudocyst should be suspected. Treatment of pleural effusion in chronic pancreatitis is not standardized. While conservative approach with repeated thoracentesis or chest tube drainage along with bowel rest and nutritional support by intravenous hyperalimentation may be successful in 50 percent of the cases, surgery will be indicated in the remaining where the effusion is refractory. Pancreatic abscess will need surgical intervention.

Approximately 5 percent of the patients with a pancreatic pseudocyst will have a pleural effusion.[533] The mechanism of pleural effusion in such a situation is the development of a direct sinus tract between the pancreas and the pleural space.[534,535]

There are some rare causes of pleural effusion described recently[536] associated with Fanconi's syndrome (renal tubular acidosis).

(12) Diseases of the Lymphatics

When one gets a milky or sometimes turbid pleural fluid and this persists even after centrifugation, this is almost always due to a high lipid content of the pleural fluid. High levels of lipid accumulates in pleural fluid either due to accumulation of chyle or when large amounts of cholesterol or lecithin-globulin complexes accumulate in long standing pleural effusion. The term *chylothorax* is used when the pleural effusion contains chyle. Chyle is the lymph that is found in the thoracic duct. The content spills over to the pleural space when the thoracic duct ruptures. The later is called a *chyliform pleural effusion* or a *pseudochylothorax.* The causes of chylothorax can be.[537-545]

(a) Malignancy (50%) involving the mediastinum usually lymphoma
(b) Thoracic surgery (20%)
(c) Trauma (< 5%)
(d) Acute hyperextension injury of the neck

(e) Noonan's syndrome/Down's syndrome/Turner's syndrome
(f) Lymphangiomyomatosis
(g) Thoracic lymphangiectasia
(h) Idiopathic/congenital
(i) Thrombosis of the superior vena cava/subclavian vein.

Over 50 percent of the cases of lymphoma are due to a tumor and out of these, in 75 percent of the cases it is lymphoma. Therefore, in a case of nontraumatic chylothorax, a diligent search for lymphoma should be made. Chylothorax may be a presenting feature of lymphoma. The second common cause of chylothorax is trauma and the development of chylothorax depends upon the integrity of the mediastinal pleura. Because of close proximity of the thoracic duct with aorta, left subclavian artery, and esophagus, the duct may be injured during mobilization of these organs. Thrombosis of the superior vena cava or subclavian vein is one of the common causes of chylothorax particularly in children and the new borne. Other rare causes include coronary artery surgery, heart transplant, high translumbar aortography, sclerotherapy for esophageal varices, and cervical node dissection. Penetrating chest trauma or neck by gunshot or knife wounds may lead to chylothorax. Chances of chylothorax are high in trauma in which the spine is hyperextended or vertebra is fractured, more so when this occurs following a fatty meal. Chylothorax secondary to closed trauma like fall from a height, motor vehicle accidents, compression injuries to the trunks, heavy blows to the stomach or back, and child birth, usually on the right side and in the region of 9th or 10th thoracic vertebra. Even, chylothorax has been reported following coughing, vomiting, weight lifting and vigorous stretching whiling yawning. Before diagnosing a case of chylothorax as congenital or idiopathic all possible causes including lymphoma should be excluded. Chylothorax is the most common form of pleural effusion in the first few days of life,[546] although neonatal chylothorax is very uncommon.

The presentation depends upon the underlying etiology. The most common presenting symptom is dyspnea like any other pleural effusion. Fever and chest pain are uncommon as chyle is nonirritant to the pleura. Traumatic chylothorax occurs 2 to 10 days after the trauma when lymph collects extrapleurally in the mediastinum forming a chyloma, which produces a posterior mediastinal mass. Rupture of the chyloma into the pleural space may cause hypotension, cyanosis, and extreme dyspnea. In nontraumatic chylothorax the onset is insidious. The radiology usually shows a large unilateral pleural effusion with or without mediastinal adenopathy.

The main danger to life from chylothorax is malnutrition and immunodeficiency. This is due to the fact that the thoracic duct carries about 2500 ml fluid daily which contains a substantial amount of carbohydrates, proteins, fat, electrolytes and lymphocytes. The patient can become cachectic very rapidly particularly if the chyle is aspirated through a chest tube or repeated thoracentesis. The protein content of the chyle is usually above 3 g/dl, and the electrolyte composition is similar to that of the serum.[518] Further, rapid oncoming lymphopenia and a compromised immunological status develop due to removal of a large number of lymphocytes. This is because the primary cell in the chyle is the small lymphocytes and the lymphocyte count ranges from 400 to 6800/cmm.[547] Almost all the lymphocytes are T cell variety. Unless the thoracic duct is successfully ligated, the mortality rate is 50 percent.

The pleural fluid is usually milky and white in appearance, although it may not be so in as high as 50 percent of the cases. Similarly all milky effusions are not due to chylothorax. This could be either due to a cholesterol effusion or due an effusion with large number of leukocytes. The chylous effusion can be bloody, serous, or turbid. A chylothorax characteristically is an odorless exudate with predominant lymphocytes. The glucose is normal and the pH is > 7.40. The cholesterol/triglyceride ratios are usually < 1, whereas in nonchylous effusions the ratio is > 1. However, overlaps do occur. Cholesterol concentrations are not different in chylous and nonchylous effusion. If the turbidity is due to high levels of cholesterol, it will clear when 1 to 2 ml ethyl ether is added to a test tube of the fluid; if the turbidity is due to chylomicrons or lecithin complexes, the turbidity will not clear.[548] The difference lies in the content of triglycerides and the best way to establish the diagnosis of chylothorax is by measuring the triglyceride levels in the pleural fluid.[142-145] Whereas the content is very high in the chylous effusions (range of 49-2270 mg/dl with a median of 249 mg/dl), in nonchylous effusions the value is low (range of 13-207 mg/dl, with median value of 33 mg/dl). It is estimated that fluids with a triglyceride of > 110 mg/dl are highly suggestive of a chylous effusion with less than 1 percent chance of not being so. Fluids with levels < 50 mg/dl are unlikely to be chylous and have no more than 5 percent chance of being so. Values between 50 to 110 mg/dl require lipoprotein electrophoresis to diagnose or exclude chylothorax. Low levels may be explained by malnutrition or dilution due to concomitant bleeding.

The management consists of pleural drainage, which relieves dyspnea, majors to diminish the rate of chyle formation, and maintenance of adequate nutrition.[548] Tube drainage is perhaps the best method of to empty the pleural fluid. Empyema formation is rare because the chylous fluid is relatively sterile. Chyle formation is minimized by intravenous hyperalimentation, discontinuation of oral feedings, and repeated gastric aspiration. Medium chain triglycerides can be used as substitutes for oral fat as they are directly absorbed into the portal vein and then into the circulation. Most traumatic chylothoraces will respond within 7 to 10 days with these measures. However, if these fail, pleurodesis or thoracic duct ligation can be carried out.[549] In malignant conditions, mediastinal radiation or chemotherapy is generally helpful in controlling chylothorax. If these measures fail, chemical pleurodesis will be necessary. The mortality from congenital chylothorax is quite high and the child usually dies of infection or malnutrition.

Gorham's syndrome is a rare disease of children or young adults that consists of hemangiomatosis, disappearing bone disease, and massive osteolysis because of interosseous proliferation of vascular or lymphatic channels. Usually the maxilla, shoulder girdle, and pelvis are commonly involved. The syndrome has a high incidence of chylothorax.[550] In this situation rib, or scapula, clavicle or the thoracic vertebrae are involved.

A chyliform pleural effusion is due to high lipid content not due to interruption of thoracic duct.[551] Pseudochylothorax with cholesterol crystals is called as *pseudochylous effusions*; and those without cholesterol crystals are designated as *chyliform effusions*. Chyliform effusions will have history of long standing pleural effusion and have thickened and even calcified pleura. In chronic cases the cholesterol is associated with HDL in contrast to acute effusions, which is mostly bound to LDL. This is because of certain changes in the trapped cholesterol. The origin of cholesterol and other lipids is not definitely known, but they come from degenerating red blood cells in the pleural fluid.[552] Two common causes of such effusions are rheumatoid pleurisy and tuberculosis. Similarly artificial pneumothoraces and paragonimiasis can produce such like effusions.

(i) *Yellow Nail Syndrome* (YNS). The triad of this syndrome was described by Emerson in 1966 and consists of yellow nails, lymphedema, and pleural effusion.[553] Subsequently it was recognized that the syndrome is also associated with chronic, recurrent pleural effusions, bronchiectasis, and sinusitis. All the components of the syndrome may not necessarily be present in the same patient. This is a rare syndrome and till now a little over 100 cases have been reported. In a review of a large series of 62 cases, it was observed that yellow nail was present in 85 percent of the cases, 72 percent had lymphoedema, 40 percent had pleural effusion, 32 percent had chronic pulmonary infection, and 11 had sinus infection.[554] One or more of these components may be present. The basic defect in the syndrome is impaired lymphatic drainage. The lymphangiographic findings will typically reveal the number of lymphatics to be decreased. The vessels may be hypoplastic or dilated. Electron microscopic studies shows dilated but otherwise normal lymphatics. This suggests that the obstruction of lymph flow is either in the major vessels or at the lymph nodes. A slow albumin turnover and impaired lymphatic removal of pleural fluid have also been observed.

The median age of onset is 40 years. However lymphedema may be present at birth or may start as late as 65 years. Yellow nails and lymphedema are commonly the first to appear. The nails grow slowly with a yellow to yellow-green discoloration, thickening, onycholysis, and altered curvature in either plane. Respiratory symptoms may be the first to appear in about a third of the cases.

The effusion may be unilateral, bilateral, and small or massive. The pleural effusion is usual recurrent. The fluid is a straw colored exudate with no special characteristics. Pleurectomy and pleurodesis are the treatments of choice.

(ii) Pleural effusion may rarely be seen in the uncommon condition of *lymphangiomyomatosis*, where the main features are interstitial lung disease with preserved or increased lung volumes, chylothorax, and pneumothorax. The characteristics of this rare condition are widespread proliferation of immature smooth muscle throughout the peribronchial, perivascular, and perilymphatic regions of the lung.[555-557] This disease occurs exclusively in women of reproductive age.[536] Most patients are between the ages of 25 to 50 years. Dyspnea, hemoptysis, pneumothorax or chylothorax may be the presenting features. It may at times be a part of the syndrome of pulmonary tuberous sclerosis. Treatment is symptomatic. This is a disease of the women of the reproductive age group.

(13) Miscellaneous Causes of Pleural Effusion

(i) *Pulmonary embolism*. Pleural effusions occur in 30 to 50 percent of patients with pulmonary embolism,[558-560] although most large series reports an incidence of around 5 percent.[561,562] The mechanism of such effusions may be due to increased pleural capillary permeability, imbalanced microvascular and pleural space hydrostatic pressures secondary to right-sided heart failure, and pleuropulmonary hemorrhage. The fluid is commonly an exudate that is due to capillary leak as a result of ischemia from pulmonary vascular obstruction or due to release of inflammatory mediators from platelet-rich thrombi. The fluid can be a transudate in approximately 20 percent of the cases possibly due to atelectasis with increased intrapleural negative pressure. Very rarely, massive pulmonary embolism results in increased systemic venous pressure because of acute cor pulmonale, which may cause transudative effusion. If there is pulmonary infarction, the fluid is hemorrhagic in over 80 percent of cases. Even without radiological evidence of infarction, the effusion may be bloody in 35 percent of cases. Chest pain is usual in almost all cases developing pleural effusion secondary to pulmonary embolism. Chest radiograph typically shows a small, unilateral pleural effusion. Associated pulmonary infiltrates are seen in about 50 percent of the cases.[563] Presence of a bloody effusion is not a contraindication to full dose anticoagulation therapy as hemothorax is a rare complication of heparin therapy and is associated with excess anticoagulation. If the effusion is increasing, a thoracocentesis is necessary to exclude such a bleed, empyema, or another etiology. If there is active bleeding, then anticoagulation therapy is to be discontinued.

(ii) *Meigs syndrome*. This syndrome consists of ovarian fibromas associated with ascites and hydrothorax. Meigs and Cass described it in 1937,[564] which described 7 patients with this syndrome. When the ovarian tumor was removed, the ascites and the pleural effusion were resolved. The syndrome can occur with other tumors like granulosa cell tumors, cystadenomas, and other benign cystic tumors of ovary, benign uterine fibroids and low-grade ovarian malignancies without metastasis.[565,566] Substantial amounts of fluid secreted by large ovarian tumors into the peritoneal cavity that moves into the pleural space through trans-diaphragmatic defects or lymphatics. The syndrome is commonly seen shortly after menopause but can at extremes of age. Patients with this syndrome will have a chronic illness weight loss, pleural effusion, ascites, and a pelvic mass.[567] The effusion is small to massive and common in right side (70%). Bilateral effusions occur in 20 percent of cases an only left sided effusion can be seen in 10 percent of the cases.[568] The fluid is usually a straw colored exudate with a paucity of mononuclear cells and a low WBC count (below 1000/cmm). Many authors have described the effusion to be a transudate, possibly based on gross

appearance only. Most of cases the protein level is more than 3 g/dl. Once the pelvic tumor is operated the pleural effusion and ascites disappears completely and do not recur.

(iii) *Benign asbestos pleural effusion*. Pleural effusions are the most common manifestations of asbestos pleuro-pulmonary disease occurring in the first 20 years after asbestos exposure.[569] Prevalence of the effusion is dose related and varies from 0.2 to 7 percent. The latent period may vary from a short exposure of 1 year to as long as after 50 years. The patients have very few symptoms. The fluid is an exudate and usually serosanguinous or may be serous or frankly bloody. The WBC count in the fluid can be as high as 28,000/cmm. Pleural fluid eosinophilia is characteristic of asbestos related pleural effusion.[570-572] The fluid also contains mesothelial cells. It is not certain whether benign asbestos pleurisy is a predisposing factor for the development of malignant mesothelioma.

(iv) *Uremic pleural effusion*. Autopsy studies have shown that about one-fifth of the cases of uremia have fibrinous pleurisy, when causes like congestive cardiac failure, hypoproteinemia, nephrotic syndrome, and tuberculosis are excluded.[581] Patients on chronic hemodialysis who are uremic for more than one year are more prone to develop this complication. Usually the effusion is moderate and unilateral, although bilateral effusions have been described. The fluid is usually serosanguinous to bloody and is an exudate.[574-576] It is predominantly a lymphocytic effusion. The creatinine concentration is high but less than that in the serum. The effusion usually subsides over several weeks with continued dialysis but may recur.

(v) *Trapped lung*. A trapped lung occurs following a number of conditions including a remote pneumonia with a complicated parapneumonic effusion that was inadequately drained, following hemothorax, pneumothorax, uremia, and rheumatoid arthritis. A fibrous membrane covers a portion of the visceral pleura that prevents that part of the lung from expanding to the chest wall.[577-579] This result in a more negative intrapleural pressure and a constant volume, recurrent pleural effusion results. This is termed as "effusion ex vacuo". The effusion is usually a borderline exudate. Measurement of pleural pressure during thoracentesis will show a more negative pleural pressure. On decortication, the lung expands fully to occupy the hemithorax.

(vi) *Radiation induced pleural effusion*. Pleural effusion may occur following radiation therapy by two mechanisms: (a) radiation pleuritis, and (b) from mediastinal fibrosis resulting in systemic venous hypertension, constrictive pericarditis or lymphatic obstruction. The incidence has been reported to be 6 percent.[580] The effusion occurs within 6 months (range 2-6 months) following radiation therapy, although effusions secondary to radiation induced mediastinitis can occur 1 to 2 years after therapy. The effusion is usually hemorrhagic with multiple reactive mesothelial cells with vacuole formation.[581,582]

(vii) *Esophageal sclerotherapy.* Pleural effusions can occur within 72 hours following sclerotherapy in about 48 percent of the cases.[583] The effusions may be either right sided, left sided, or bilateral in almost equal frequency. Possible the incidence depends upon the volume of sclerosant used. The effusion is mostly exudative. The pleural reaction results from an intensive inflammatory reaction following infiltration of the sclerosant into the esophageal mucosa resulting in mediastinal and pleural inflammations. The effusion is coincidental, and is of little consequence and resolves spontaneously over several days to weeks.

(viii) *Misplacement of enteral feeding tubes.* Pleuro-pulmonary complications have been described following insertion of enteral feeding tubes and result from perforation of the esophagus and right main stem bronchus and penetration into the lung parenchyma.[584-586] Use of stylets for easy insertion is a major risk factor for perforation. Other predisposing factors include depressed sensorium, impaired gag reflex, recent endotracheal intubation, decreased laryngeal sensitivity, esophageal stricture, cardiomegaly, and neuromuscular blocking drugs.

(ix) Other rare conditions which are associated with pleural effusion include (a) lung transplantation because of severing of lymphatics;[587] (b) sarcoidosis which is occasionally complicated by pleural effusion in 1 to 2 percent of cases;[471,588,589] (c) fetal pleural effusion;[590] (d) ovarian hyperstimulation syndrome which occurs in about 2 percent of patients undergoing ovulation induction with HCG;[591] (e) postpartum pleural effusions;[591-593] (f) amyloidosis;[594-596] (g) milk of calcium pleural effusion;[597] (h) ARDS associated pleural effusion;[598] (i) internal jugular and subclavian vein catheterization;[599,600] (j) rupture of benign germ cell tumor into the pleural space;[601] and (k) syphilis.[602]

(x) *Pleural effusion in AIDS.* Pleural effusions are uncommon with AIDS and the incidence was 1.7 percent from one large series reported from New York,[603] although it varies from series to series. The causes of pleural effusion in AIDS are varied and may include parapneumonic effusions or empyema, tuberculosis, Kaposi's sarcoma, end stage renal disease with volume overload, *Pneumocystis* carinii pneumonia and hypoalbuminemia.[604-607]

II. EMPYEMA THORACIC

The word empyema denotes the presence of pus in the pleural cavity.[608,609] When frankly purulent material is present, there is no doubt regarding the diagnosis. However, when the fluid is not turbid, the diagnosis may be uncertain. Under these circumstances confirmation of diagnosis will depend upon the presence of predominantly polymorphonuclear cells or the presence of organisms either on Gram's stain or culture. Certain other biochemical characteristics also imply empyema, and it may be termed as *'incipient empyema'* (see below). Empyemas may be described as acute or chronic, although the division between the two is arbitrary and indistinct. Chronic empyemas may be used in those conditions where organization has occurred in an advanced case and a pleural rind is formed. This usually takes 4 to 6 weeks.

Etiology. The etiology of empyema varies. While tuberculosis remains to be an important cause in the developing countries, nontubercular causes are more frequent in the developed countries. In recent years there is a change in the bacterial causes associated with the use and misuse of antimicrobials as well as alterations in the host associated with increased longevity and chronic disease.[610,611] The most common cause remains to be pneumonia, the parapneumonic empyema. Penetrating trauma is another important cause of empyema. The infectious causes are now more complex with the increasing incidence of anaerobic and hospital-acquired infections, and with an increasing population of immunocompromized patients. Before the availability of antibiotics, streptococci, pneumococci, and mixed group of mouth organisms were the most frequent causative organisms. In recent years, staphylococci, Gram-negative organisms, fungi, and enterococci are being recognized as the more common etiologic agents.[612]

Tuberculosis is still an important cause of empyema in India. In a study of 108 cases, Singh et al[613] reported that 65.22 percent cases of simple empyema were nontubercular and 34.78 percent were of tubercular etiology. However, in cases of bronchopleural fistulae tuberculosis is the cause in 98.83 percent of cases. Tubercular etiology was found in 85.16 percent cases of empyema thoracic. Similar predominance of tubercular etiology has also been reported in various other Indian studies.[614-619]

A number of factors predispose to the development of empyema.[620-632] Pneumonia (tubercular/nontubercular) is the most common factor responsible for more than 60 percent of the cases. Others include: obstruction to a bronchus either due to bronchogenic carcinoma, or foreign body; suppurative lung diseases like bronchiectasis or lung abscess; surgical trauma including instrumentation and rupture of esophagus, leakage from esophageal surgery, bronchopleural fistula following pneumonectomy or segmental resections. Less frequent causes include abdominal sepsis forming a subphrenic abscess; hepatic abscess including that caused by *Entamoeba histolytica*; sepsis in the thoracic spine or chest wall. Nonsurgical penetrating trauma to the chest due to gunshot wounds and stabbing may also be associated with empyema. Chances of developing empyema are increased if there is a hemopneumothorax compared to only hemothorax.

The likely infecting organisms causing empyema vary according to (i) the prior use of antibiotics, (ii) the underlying predisposing factor, and (iii) the age of the patient. The common ones are Gram-negative and anaerobic organisms in adults and Staphylococci in children. Other uncommon microbial causes of empyema include those caused by *Aspergillus* species, *Cryptococcus neoformans*, *Blastomycosis*, *Coccidioides immitis*, *Actinomyces*, *Nocardia*, *Clostridium perfringens*, *Bacillus cereus*, *Pasturella multocida*, *Salmonella enteritidis*, *Ecchynococcus granulosus* (Hydatid disease), *Trichomonas*, and *Entamoeba histolytica*. Recently, pulmonary infections and empyema caused by *Rhodococcus equi* have been reported increasingly in patients with AIDS and other causes of impaired immunity. This pathogen usually causes suppurative infections in farm and ranch animals. It is a Gram-positive bacterium with a coccobacillary shape and clubbed features that can easily be misidentified as a diphtheroid. The disease follows a subacute course with cough, fever, and weight loss. The chest X-ray shows a dense upper lobe consolidation with cavitation, pleural thickening and empyema.

Pathogenesis and pathology. The pleura may become infected by direct extension of an inflammatory process such as pneumonia, lung abscess, or subphrenic abscess. The pleurae may also be infected by either the lymphatics or by the hematogenous routes. Direct inoculation can also occur from penetrating wounds. Underlying bronchopleural fistula is another important source of infection of the pleurae.

The pathologic response is divided into three phases.[633] These phases are not sharply defined but gradually merge one into the other. The progression largely depends on the infecting organism.

(i) *Exudative phase* (Inflammatory phase). This is an immediate response with outpouring of fluid. The inflammatory process in the vicinity causes an abundance of polymorphs, which causes increased pulmonary and pleural capillary permeability. The cellular content of this exudate is relatively low. During this phase the fluid is relatively thin and the lung is relatively expandable.

(ii) *Fibrinopurulent phase* (Loculation phase). If treatment is not instituted, bacteria invade the pleural space and multiply causing a further influx of polymorphs and plasma clotting factors. The result is a gelatinous coagulum. There will be accumulation of large quantities of frank pus with large numbers of cells (mainly polymorphs) and fibrin. The purulent fluid tends to accumulate laterally and posteriorly. The fibrin coagulum is deposited in a continuous sheet, covering both the parietal and visceral pleura in the involved areas. There is an increased tendency towards loculation. A limiting membrane is also formed, which prevents extension of empyema and begins to fix the lung. Clinically, this represents a transition between the exudative and the chronic phase of empyema. The fluid becomes thicker and the lung becomes progressively less expansile.

(iii) *Stage of organization*. During this final phase fibroblasts grow into the exudate. The clottable pleural fluid serves as a latticework for stimulated fibroblasts to attach and lay down collagen. This grows on both the parietal and visceral pleural surfaces and produces an inelastic membrane, called as "the peel." With increasing fibrosis, the process becomes chronic and the lung is fixed more firmly. The stage is characterized by a very thick exudate with heavy sediment, a thick peel that will be felt by the aspirating needle and can be demonstrated by roentgenographic techniques and the development of a negative intrapleural pressure. If untreated the empyema may drain spontaneously through the chest wall (empyema necessitates) or into the lung (bronchopleural fistula).

Clinical manifestations. The clinical presentation of empyema may be variable depending upon the underlying predisposing factor, the causative organism, prior use of antibiotics, the age of the patient and the immunological competence of the patient. There may be complete absence of symptoms to severe systemic toxaemia. Fever is a common symptom, although this may be absent in the elderly and if the empyema wall is well walled-off. Dyspnea, pleuritic chest pain, general malaise, and loss of weight are common. Cough is frequent and expectoration of large volumes of sputum is common if there is a bronchopleural fistula. The clinical presentation of patients with aerobic bacterial pneumonia and pleural effusion is no different from that of patients with bacterial pneumonia[126,634,635] with high WBC counts. In contrast, patients with anaerobic infections, presents with a subacute illness, leukocytosis and mild anemia in majority of the patients.

The physical signs of empyema are same as those of a pleural effusion. There may be tenderness in the chest wall. Clubbing of fingers is common if the process is chronic. There may be associated features of complications (Figs 28.6 to 28.9).

Diagnosis of empyema is relatively easy when there is frank pus. Complicated parapneumonic effusions or incipient empyema are difficult to diagnose, particularly to decide whether to put in a chest tube or not. Some authors use much less stringent criteria to diagnose empyema. For example Weese et al[636] defined empyema

as pleural fluid with specific gravity greater than 1.018, WBC count more than 500/cmm, or a protein level greater than 2.5 g/dl. On the other hand, Vianna[637] defined an empyema as pleural fluid on which the bacterial cultures are positive or the WBC count is greater than 15,000/cmm and the protein level is more than 3 g/dl. These criteria may be too liberal. In effusions with negative Gram stains, a pH lower than 7.3 or glucose less than 60 mg/dl are highly suggestive of empyema in effusions associated with pneumonias. However, large prospective studies have not supported this.[638] Two other tests have been found to be more specific: polymorphonuclear neutrophil elastase and inter-alpha-trypsin

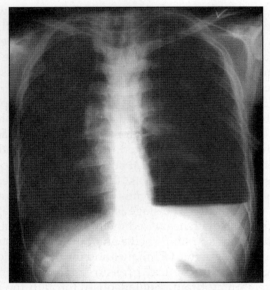

FIGURE 28.6: Hydropneumothorax in a case of COPD

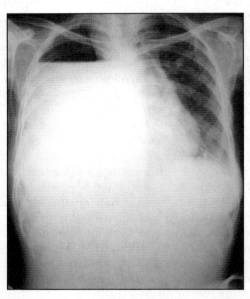

FIGURE 28.7: Right hydropneumothorax. Note the mediastinal shift

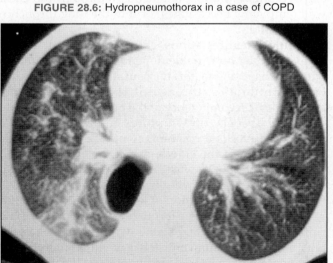

FIGURE 28.8: CT Chest - Loculated pyopneumothorax posterio-medially

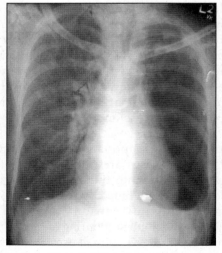

FIGURE 28.9: Air and fluid. But it is not a case of hydropneumothorax as there is no shifting of mediastinum. This is infection in a lung cyst

inhibitor. Polymorphonuclear neutrophil elastase is a marker of inflammation and is elevated in the pleural fluid (average 1,793 mg/dl) in all empyema patients and averaged less than 500 mg/dl in other causes of pleural effusion like malignancy, tuberculosis, and nonspecific pleuritis. Inter-alpha-trypsin inhibitor is degraded into the fragment HI-30 when acted upon by elastase. HI-31 is excreted in the urine and in empyema, it is about 21.6 mg/mg creatinine on an average and in other cases it is less than 4 mg/mg of creatinine.

Complications. Complications of empyema are responsible for significant morbidity. The complications include bronchopleural fistula, trapped or destroyed lung, empyema necessitans, fibrothorax, chondritis and osteomyelitis of the ribs, pericarditis, amyloidosis, spread of infection into the pericardium, mediastinum, peritoneum, or meninges. Pleural calcification is common. When pleural calcification is extensive and there is severe fibrothorax, cor pulmonale and respiratory failure are not uncommon. Patients with long-term empyema are often anemic, malnourished, and have electrolyte abnormalities.

Various complications described above occur when the initiation of treatment is delayed or the treatment is ineffective. The failure of antibiotics alone to treat empyema results from starting antibiotics too late after the empyema has organized at which time effective drainage is mandatory, relying only on antibiotics when there is already encapsulation of the infection inaccessible to drainage, or choosing a wrong antibiotic.

Bronchopleural fistula is a common complication of empyema when there is a delay in the treatment. It is frequently seen in empyemas of tubercular or fungal in origin and in AIDS patients.[639] Very rarely amoebic liver abscess can present as BPF.[619,620,629] The symptoms are characterized by expectoration of a large amount of sputum, the volume sometimes depending on the position the patient adopts and on the pressure of the surrounding atmosphere as in air flights. One may hear an amphoric type of bronchial breath sound. Bronchopleural fistula is evident from the bubbling in the chest tube bottle when the patient is asked to cough. The presence of a fistula can be confirmed by instilling 2 percent methylene blue into the pleural cavity and by observing the blue discoloration of the sputum when the patient is asked to expectorate. Similarly bronchographic dye can be observed in the pleural cavity when injected into the bronchial tree. Very rarely one may see the bronchial rent through the bronchoscope. Presence of the bronchopleural fistula is a common cause of poor response of treatment of empyema and very often,

surgical management will be required. Autologous "blood-patch" pleurodesis for persistent pulmonary air leak has been tried with some success.[640]

Empyema necessitatis. When empyema is long-standing and the suppurative process continues uncontrolled, pus will point through the intercostal space close to the sternum, which is often the thinnest portion. Eventually, it will burst through the skin producing a discharging sinus. Rarely, the pus will track down posterior to the diaphragm and will point at the lumbar region or the groin. Such an occurrence is rare now adays with availability of many potent antibiotics. However, this is possible with tubercular or fungal infections.

Management. Management of empyema essentially consists of drainage of the pus and appropriate antibiotic.[613,617-619,621,628,630,631,641,642] The antibiotic of choice will depend upon whether the associated pneumonia is community acquired or hospital acquired. Empyema following community-acquired pneumonia in an immunocompetent host should consist of penicillin, gentamycin with addition of metronidazole to cover anaerobic organisms. If that fails or patient does not improve within 48 to 72 hours, the ideal agents are the second- or third-generation cephalosporins or a beta-lactam/beta-lactamase inhibitor. With severe form a third generation cephalosporin with anti-pseudomonas activity such as ceftazidime or cefoperazone should be used. Hospital acquired pneumonias leading on to empyema should be treated with antibiotics that cover most Gram-negative organisms, Pseudomonas, or Staphylococci. In addition to the third generation cephalosporin or beta-lactams or beta-lactamase inhibitors, an aminoglycoside antibiotic needs to be added. Controversy exists as to the timing of intervention in empyema, especially the operative intervention. If purulent fluid is aspirated, or the Gram stain is positive, tube drainage should be instituted immediately. If the aspirated fluid is not purulent and the Gram stain is negative, biochemical characteristics will guide therapy. If the pH is < 7.10 and is associated with a glucose value of < 40 mg/dl and a LDH value of > 1000 U/l, tube drainage should be instituted without delay. An undefined area exists between a pH of 7.10 and 7.29. This can be either empyema or simple effusion. Thoracentesis should be repeated after 8 to 12 hours to determine the pH again. If the pH is stable or rising, the clinical course is satisfactory, and the fluid remains free flowing, drainage is not indicated. On the other hand, if the pH is falling substantially or to < 7.10, tube drainage becomes necessary. Since pH value is the deciding factor, it should be determined meticulously, as is done for arterial pH.

Complicated parapneumonic effusions are classified into 7 classes depending on the amount, thickness on chest X-ray, pH values, glucose levels, LDH values, and Gram stain results. The classification and treatment scheme for parapneumonic effusions and empyema are outlined below:[643]

Class 1:

Nonsignificant pleural effusion	Small Less than 10 mm thick on decubitus radiograph No thoracentesis required

Class 2:

Typical parapneumonic pleural effusion	More than 10 mm thick Glucose 40 mg/dl; pH > 7.20 Gram stain and culture negative Antibiotics alone sufficient

Class 3:

Borderline complicated pleural effusion	pH > 7.00 but < 7.20 and/or LDH >100 and glucose > 40 mg/dl Gram stain and culture negative Antibiotics and repeated thoracentesis

Class 4:

Simple complicated pleural effusion	pH < 7.00 and/or glucose < 40 mg/dl and/or Gram stain or culture positive No loculation, no frank pus Tube thoracostomy and antibiotics

Class 5:

Complex complicated pleural effusion	pH < 7.00 and/or glucose < 40 mg/dl and/or Gram stain or culture positive Multiloculated Tube thoracostomy plus thrombolytics (Thoracoscopy or decortication rarely required)

Class 6:

Simple empyema	Frank pus present Single locule or free flowing Tube thoracostomy ± decortication

Class 7:

Complex empyema	Frank pus, multiple loculi Tube thoracostomy and thrombolytics Often thoracoscopy or decortication required

Once a decision is taken to put in a chest tube, it should be done without delay since the morbidity and mortality increases as time to appropriate drainage lengthens.[637,644] A standard chest tube should be placed in the most dependent portion of the pleural space. Failure of thoracostomy is due largely to having the tube placed in the wrong place.[645] The tube should be connected to an underwaterseal drainage system. If the visceral pleura are covered with a fibrinous peel, application of slow negative pressure suction to the chest tube may help to expand the underlying lung. Small-bore catheters should be avoided, although it is easier to insert and is less painful to the patient (26-30). Others have used large bore chest tubes (28-32 French). Percutaneous smaller catheters (8.3-16 French) have recently been used through ultrasound or CT and they are particularly helpful in loculated empyemas.[645,646] Defervescence should occur 48 to 72 hours after placement of the chest tube. If fever persists, either the drainage is inadequate, or the patient is on inappropriate antibiotic therapy. Position of the chest tube should be checked with both posteroanterior and lateral skiagrams of the chest. Some even recommend the use of CT scan for localization of the tube if plain films are uncertain. Thoracic ultrasound and empyema grams also assist chest tube placement. In the later procedure, contrast is injected into the pleural space during thoracentesis. A radiograph or fluoroscopic examination can then identify loculations and the most dependent regions of empyema. The chest tube should be taken out once the drainage is less than 50 ml/day. Complications like bleeding, pneumothorax, and secondary infection are possible with insertion of the chest tube. Chronic complications like frozen shoulder can be prevented by regular exercise using the arm.

Small collections of pus can be managed by repeated aspirations and chest tube may not be required in these circumstances. Repeat chest radiographs and/or ultrasound can determine presence of loculations. Options for such inadequately drained pleural space are the placement of an additional tube, and the use of lytic therapy, or a more invasive surgical procedure. New modalities of treatment like lytic therapy will be necessary for the intermediate phase and are more effective in empyemas of less than 4 weeks duration. Intrapleural streptokinase or urokinase has been used recently with success.[647-654] Intrapleural urokinase can be used in the treatment of loculated pleural effusion. These techniques require multiple instillations of lytic agents with irrigation of the cavity over several days. These procedures are particularly useful in poor risk patients. The instillation of 250,000 units of streptokinase in

100 ml of saline increases the drainage. The dose may be repeated daily for 10 days. Another indication for lytic therapy is as an adjunct to the use of thoracoscopic procedures. Thoracoscopy.[646,655-657] helps in determining the extent of empyema and to break up loculations to allow better drainage, particularly in conjunction with lytic agents. Thoracoscopy has recently been used successfully to treat bronchopleural fistulae and pulmonary air leaks.

Short of surgical therapy, an open drainage procedure involving removal of parts of 1 to 3 ribs at the dependent portion of the empyema cavity establishes more complete drainage and avoids the need for a chest bottle.[658,659] After localizing the dependent zone of the empyema a segment of 2 to 3 cm of overlying rib is resected. The parietal pleura are incised, fibrinous exudate is peeled off the visceral pleura with forceps, and loculations are broken down. It is the preferred drainage procedure in the debilitated patient who cannot tolerate an empyemectomy and decortication. The disadvantage of this procedure is a prolonged time for chest wound closure taking several months.

A practical problem occurs to decide the etiology of empyema at presentation, whether it is of tubercular or bacterial in origin. Most often the presentation will be pointing towards the etiology. However, there are situations when tubercular empyema may present acutely and the pus will not grow the organism. Moreover, a tubercular empyema may be secondarily infected. Thus isolation of a microorganism other than mycobacteria may not always reflect the causative agent. In such a situation, one has to treat empirically with the antibiotics first, and if there is no response, then with antitubercular drugs. However, if there is associated parenchymal lesion, suggestive of tuberculosis, one should start antituberculous drug therapy. Since antibiotics penetrate the pleura well, usual doses are sufficient to treat empyema. Penicillin has traditionally been used against anaerobic infections. Clindamycin is the alternative choice when the organisms are suspected to be resistant to penicillin. Other appropriate antibiotics for anaerobic organisms include chloramphenicol, imipenem-cilastatin, metronidazole, and α β-lactam antibiotic combined with α β-lactamase inhibitor. Simultaneously an antibiotic should be chosen which is effective against Gram-negative organisms. Thus a combination of penicillin, metronidazole, and an aminoglycoside, is an ideal one to start with. The antibiotics can be changed after getting the culture and sensitive report. The choice of antibiotics in different situations is discussed above.

The goals of therapy of chronic empyema are: (i) control of systemic and pulmonary sepsis; (ii) drainage of pus; (iii) expansion of the lung and improvement of the lung function; and (iv) restoration of chest wall and diaphragmatic mobility. Previously, treatment of chronic empyema consisted of closed chest-tube drainage, open drainage with rib resection and irrigation of the empyema cavity. After control of infection, decortication or thoracoplasty would then be performed. This plan of treatment may be valid in extremely ill patients who will not be able to tolerate a thoracotomy as the initial procedure.

With improvement of perioperative care, there is a change in the approach to the treatment of chronic empyema. The above-mentioned staged treatment with multiple procedures over a period of time that is usually lengthy is no more recommended in most patients. Factors those determine the initial choice of an operative procedure in chronic empyema include: (i) nutritional status and immunocompetence of the patient; (ii) presence or absence of a bronchopleural fistula; (iii) the capability of the remaining normal lung to fill the thoracic cavity; and (iv) whether or not muscle is available for thoracoplastic procedures.

In patients with adequate lung volume to fill the lung cavity, decortication is now recommended as the primary procedure. With modern antibiotics and perioperative care the mortality has been negligible with this procedure. The only patients now needing open drainage are those too sick to tolerate a major thoracotomy. It is important to consider early decortication to reduce morbidity and mortality. It is perhaps a mistake to rely on antibiotics only for the treatment of an organized empyema. Delay in surgical therapy will lead to prolonged morbidity.[660-662]

A special problem arises when the lung does not have adequate volume to fill the thoracic cavity. Three choices are available: (i) open drainage with rib resection (the Clagett procedure), irrigation of the cavity with antibiotics until the infection is controlled, followed by wound closure of the antibiotic filled cavity; (ii) thoracoplasty with collapse of the thoracic chest wall into the cavity; or (iii) filling the remainder of the cavity with extrathoracic muscle or an omental flap. Open drainage followed by thoracoplasty has been the procedure of choice in the past. Currently, early decortication and filling the cavity with either thoracic muscle such as latissimus dorsi or with omentum has been the choice.[659,660] This decreases the morbidity and hospital stay. This procedure is preferable to thoracoplasty because of better functional and cosmetic results (Fig. 28.10).

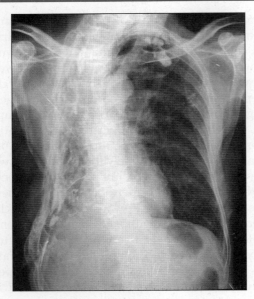

FIGURE 28.10: Thoracoplasty

In some patients and in most patients with broncho-pleural fistula, particularly of tubercular etiology, pneumonectomy may be necessary.[663] Postpneumonectomy empyemas are suspected when the characteristic evolution of radiological findings are absent. In a normal course, immediately after pneumonectomy, the ipsilateral pleural space contains air, and the mediastinum is shifted to the same side and the hemidiaphragm are elevated. The space then begins to fill with serosanguinous fluid at a rate of approximately 2 rib spaces a day. In most cases, the pleural space becomes 80 to 90 percent fluid-filled within 2 weeks and completely filled within 2 to 4 months.[664] During this period the mediastinum progressively shifts to the ipsilateral side. Failure of the shifting of mediastinum to the same side in the post-operative period indicates abnormality and if it is either shifted to the midline or to the opposite side, then postpneumonectomy empyema is to be suspected. This complication is very difficult to manage since it will be virtually impossible to eliminate the space. All such patients should be treated with a chest tube and appropriate antibiotics. If there is a bronchopleural fistula one may try intrathoracic transposition of extrathoracic skeletal muscle,[665] or to use a fibrin sealant through a thoracoscope[666] or a tissue adhesive may be instilled via a bronchoscope,[667] or by an omental pedicle.[668]

III. PNEUMOTHORAX

Pneumothorax is the presence of air in the pleural cavity.[669] Once air enters the pleural cavity that is negative throughout the respiratory cycle, the intrapleural pressure becomes less negative with respect to atmospheric pressure. If a communication develops between the alveolus and the pleural cavity, air will flow from the alveolus into the pleural space until the pressure equalizes or until the communication is sealed. Because the thoracic cavity is below its resting volume and the lung is above its resting volume, with a pneumothorax the thoracic cavity enlarges and the lung becomes smaller. This results in the lung to move away from the thoracic wall due to deflation till the pressure within the pleural cavity is sufficiently negative to prevent further collapse. This is called a *partial* pneumothorax. *Complete* pneumothorax is said to occur when the pressure in the pleural cavity reaches that of the atmosphere. The partial or total pressure equilibration between the intrapleural cavity and the ambient air results in partial or total collapse of the lung. The rupture in the lung tissue is often so small that the point of elastic contraction of the lung tissue can stop further air leakage at the point of partial collapse. If the intrapleural pressure exceeds that of the atmosphere, in addition to the pneumothorax being complete, mediastinal structures are compressed and are shifted to the opposite side. This is a medical emergency and is known as *tension* pneumothorax. Besides tension pneumothorax, there are two other clinically important forms of pneumothorax: the *open* pneumothorax, and the *closed* pneumothorax. If the breach in either of the pleura remains patent then a fistula exists and it is an open pneumothorax. More often the breach is sealed, resulting in a closed pneumothorax. A tension pneumothorax occurs when there is a check-valve like defect, allowing air to pass into the pleural cavity on inspiration or during coughing, but preventing its exit.

The alveolar-arterial oxygen difference also increases.[670] The main physiological consequences of a pneumothorax are a decrease in the vital capacity and a decrease in PaO_2. This is mainly due to ventilation/perfusion mismatch. If the patient is otherwise healthy, these changes may be well tolerated. But, if he has preexisting lung disease this may lead to serious consequences including respiratory failure.

CLASSIFICATION AND ETIOLOGY

Various causes of pneumothorax are shown in Table 28.4.[671-692]

Primary Spontaneous Pneumothorax

This occurs most commonly in otherwise healthy young adult males without any preexisting lung disease. The peak incidence occurs in the third decade. The disease

TABLE 28.4: Causes of pneumothorax

I. Spontaneous pneumothorax

Primary
• Apical blebs

Secondary
• Pulmonary tuberculosis
• Chronic bronchitis and emphysema
• Bronchial asthma
• Suppurative pneumonias (Lung abscess, bronchiectasis)
• Bronchogenic carcinoma
• Cystic fibrosis
• AIDS related due to *Pneumocystis carinii* (jerovicii) pneumonia.

Rare causes
• Cryptogenic fibrosing alveolitis
• Occupational lung diseases (acute silicosis, Shaver's disease)
• Granulomatous diseases (sarcoidosis in the late fibrotic stage, histiocytosis X, Wegener's granulomatosis), rheumatoid disease
• Systemic lupus erythematosus
• Hemosiderosis
• Pulmonary alveolar proteinosis
• Inherited connective tissue disorders (Marfan's syndrome, Ehlers-Danlos syndrome, Marfnoid hypermobility syndrome)
• Hereditary conditions (neurofibromatosis, tuberous sclerosis)
• Coccidioidomycosis
• Parasitic infections of the lung (Hydatid disease)
• Intrathoracic tumors (metastatic sarcomas, metastatic Wilm's tumor, germ cell tumors)
• Cavitating pulmonary infarction
• Catamenial pneumothorax

II. Traumatic

Noniatrogenic
• Chest injuries (open and closed)
• Barotrauma

Iatrogenic
• Thoracentesis
• Pleural biopsy
• Transbronchial biopsy
• Lung biopsies
• Transthoracic needle aspiration
• Central venous canulations
• Mechanical ventilation
• Rupture of esophagus
• Artificial pneumothorax

Pneumothorax is basically classified into two varieties: spontaneous, and traumatic. Any pneumothorax occurring in the absence of trauma is described as *spontaneous* pneumothorax. There are many synonyms for the term such as primary simple pneumothorax, primary pneumothorax, idiopathic pneumothorax, and pneumothorax simplex. The term *primary* spontaneous pneumothorax is used when there is no clinically apparent preexisting pulmonary disease and *secondary* spontaneous pneumothorax denotes a clinically recognizable coexisting structural or functional abnormality in the lung.

predominantly occurs in males with a male:female ratio varying from 4:1 to 12:1. The incidence has been reported to be 7.4 per 100,000 per year for males with the corresponding figure being 1.2 for females in the United States with a similar figure in the United Kingdom.[693] Both lungs are equally affected.

Earlier the etiology of primary spontaneous pneumothorax was thought to be due to pulmonary tuberculosis. However, it was subsequently realized that pneumothorax could occur in the absence of any lung disease. This result from the rupture of a small air filled space usually located in the apices of the lung,[671,672] usually less than 1 to 2 cm in diameter, known as a *subpleural bleb*, into the pleural space. The bleb is a localized collection of air in the cellular layer of the visceral pleura that is continuous with the lung parenchyma. Blebs may arise as a result of congenital weakness in the connective tissue of the subpleural alveoli and may start as interstitial emphysema. The blebs are very frequent and occur in about 90 percent of the cases. They are often multiple, and common in the apices. The occurrence in the apices may be explained on the basis of the fact that there is a regional difference in mechanical stresses, which exists in the lungs, the distending forces being greatest over the apices. Relative ischemia of the lung apices has been put forth as an alternative explanation for their occurrence because of more likelihood of infection and inflammation in these regions of maximal stress.[694-697] Spontaneous pneumothoraces commonly occur following days when there are broad fluctuations in the atmospheric pressure. It is possibly due to the fact that apical blebs are not in free communications with the airways. When the atmospheric pressure falls, the distending pressures of the blebs may increase and results in rupture.[698,699]

Individuals with a tall and thin body habitus and those having longer lungs are more susceptible to develop spontaneous primary pneumothorax.[700,701] The gradient in pleural pressure is greater from the lung base to the apex in taller individuals, so the alveoli at the apices are subjected to greater mean distending pressure. Over a long period this may lead to bleb formation. Although not proved conclusively, familial occurrence of spontaneous pneumothorax has been reported[702] and an association of specific HLA antigen (haplotype A_2B_{40}) and antitrypsin phenotypes has been suggested.[703] The mode of inheritance has been either autosomal-dominant with incomplete penetrance, or X-linked recessive.[704] An association of smoking, and presence of sharp inner borders of the first or second ribs are also noted in primary spontaneous pneumothorax. High concentrations of hydroxyproline, a degradation product of collagen, have been observed in the lungs of these patients. Rupture of these congenital or acquired subpleural blebs is the main cause of spontaneous pneumothorax described as early as 1932.[671] There is a high prevalence of bronchial abnormalities to the tune of 96 percent of the patients.[705] These include disproportionate bronchial anatomy, an accessory bronchus, or a missing bronchus.

There is a significant relationship of spontaneous pneumothorax and weather conditions. The incidence is increased after falls in the atmospheric pressure of at least 10 millibars/24 hours. Upon ascent, or at rapid decompression, divers are prone to develop pneumothorax. It is also observed that pulmonary cavities of previous patients of spontaneous pneumothorax increased corresponding to the nominal altitude in a hypobaric chamber. Pilots suffer pneumothorax in flight with decreased ambient pressure.

Rupture of pulmonary tissue is due to higher intrapulmonary pressure in at least one region of the lung than in other lung regions and the intrapleural space. This is possible only if the intrapulmonary gas cannot find an escape via either the airways or the circulation. Thus, pressure in the closed intrapulmonary region cannot decrease especially when the ambient atmospheric pressure falls. This results in an increased pressure difference between the intrapulmonary and ambient spaces, leading to barotrauma. Smoking increases the risk of developing spontaneous pneumothorax 22 folds in men and 9 folds in women. Thus quitting smoking is an effective preventive measure. This also confirms the theory of obstruction-check valve mechanism of development of spontaneous pneumothorax. This mechanism is enhanced by several factors such as intraluminal factors like inflammation, granulation, blood clot, tumor, and accumulation of exudate, mucus, or meconium; parietal factors like thickening of the bronchial wall due to smoking, inflammation, low atmospheric humidity, inhaled, intravenously administered drug particles, gas and tumor; and peribronchial factors like interstitial pneumonia, fibrosis, drug abuse, and *P. carinii* pneumonia.

Secondary Spontaneous Pneumothorax

Spontaneous pneumothorax occurring as a result of lung disease is called as secondary. Pulmonary tuberculosis is the most common cause in developing countries where it is more common. In cases of tuberculosis pneumothorax result from rupture of a cavity or the subpleural focus of tubercular lesion giving way into the pleural cavity. About 1.4 percent of cases of active pulmonary tuberculosis are complicated by pneumothorax.[706] Over 90 percent of these cases are cavitary. Tubercular pneumothorax is frequently associated with empyema and/or bronchopleural fistula if not treated early. Occurrence of pneumothorax in miliary tuberculosis is extremely uncommon, although can occur.

Chronic bronchitis and emphysema are the other important causes of this type of pneumothorax.[653] Emphysema leading on to pneumothorax may or may not be associated with bullae, although they are more frequently present. Trapped air leaks through the weakened walls of the dilated and distended alveoli assisted by high intrabronchial pressure. Coughing is an aggravating factor. More severe is the COPD; more is the chance of developing pneumothorax.[707-712] Bronchial asthma is a rare cause of pneumothorax occurring in less than 1 percent of adults and in about 2.5 percent of children.[713]

Infective causes like staphylococcal pneumonia in children and klebsiella pneumonia in adults are more commonly associated with pneumothorax.[714,715] In the former, multiple cystic areas, called pneumatoceles, can rupture into the pleural space. Staphylococcal pneumonia continues to be the leading cause of pneumothorax in children and infants beyond the neonatal group.

Catamenial pneumothorax described first by Maurer et al in 1958,[716] is a rare cause of secondary pneumothorax. In 1972, it was called catamenial (catamenial in Greek is monthly). Fewer than 100 cases have been reported.[717] This is characterized by recurrent pneumothorax associated with menstruation occurring within 48 to 72 hours of the onset of menses. It is almost always right sided. It is strongly related to parity. About one third of the patients will have associated pelvic endometriosis. The syndrome has several characteristics compared with that of the spontaneous pneumothorax.[718] This occurs in females only in the age group of 30 to 50 years, in 95 percent of cases they are right sided, onset is within 48 to 72 hours of menstruation, and there is a tendency to recur with menses. Implants of endometrial tissue may be found in the diaphragm. Air possibly passes from the peritoneal cavity into the pleural cavity through diaphragmatic fenestrations. Other speculations include pleural endometriosis, and alveolar rupture secondary to high levels of PGF_2 during menstruation. The symptoms usually regress during a menstrual intervals such as pregnancy, menopause, or following surgical castration. Hormonal therapy like danazol, and GnRH has also been tried.

Other causes of secondary pneumothorax enumerated in the Table 28.4 are very unusual and in these conditions such a complication occurs very rarely.[719-729]

Traumatic Pneumothorax

Both closed and open chest injuries may cause pneumothorax.[679,730-735] These include gunshot or stab injuries, road traffic accidents, and blast injuries. They are more frequently associated with rib fractures and bronchial disruption leading on to hemopneumothorax. With penetrating chest trauma the wound allows air to enter the pleural space directly through the chest wall. Further, if the visceral pleura are penetrated, air enters pleural cavity from the alveoli. In nonpenetrating type of chest trauma there is frequent association of rib fracture or displacement lacerating the nearby pleura. Pneumothorax can also occur in nonpenetrating chest trauma in the absence of obvious rib fractures. Development of such pneumothorax is a due to sudden chest compression and a resultant increase in alveolar pressure causing rupture of alveoli. Air then enters the interstitial space and dissects towards the visceral pleura or mediastinum and rupture of mediastinal pleura, and pneumothorax. Pneumothoraces seen only on CT scan are called *Occult* and overall about 5 percent of multiple trauma patients have a pneumothorax and about 40 percent of such pneumothoraces are occult.[573] Ultrasonography can be of use in diagnosing hydropneumothorax.[736] Recently traumatic pneumothorax has been reported in drug abusers when they attempt to inject the drug into the subclavian or internal jugular vein.

Iatrogenic causes of pneumothorax include defective aspiration of pleural effusions, needle biopsy of the pleura, percutaneous insertion of central venous cannulas, percutaneous lung biopsy, trephine biopsy of the lung, transbronchial lung biopsies, and laser treatment of intrabronchial lesions (*see* Table 28.4). The incidence of pneumothorax under these circumstances has been discussed in the respective chapters.

Barotrauma can cause pneumothorax. Subjects who are at risk for barotrauma include aircrew that is likely to be exposed to accidental decompression.[737] Other groups with similar risk include caisson workers, divers, and submariners. This is because of change of volume with change of pressure resulting in sudden rupture of the bleb. Subjects on mechanical ventilators, particularly with suppurative pneumonia and use of high inflation pressure, are liable to barotrauma and subsequent pneumothorax.

Pneumomediastinum or **mediastinal emphysema** is a condition when air is present in the mediastinal tissue.[738-745] Pneumomediastinum may be classified, as that of pneumothorax and the causes is identical. The condition arises subsequent to the rupture of alveoli and air tracks along the interstitial and perivascular tissue to reach mediastinum. Air may also directly enter the mediastinal tissue from the **surrounding** air containing hollow structures like that of trachea, esophagus, or bronchial ruptures.

CLINICAL FEATURES

The most common clinical symptom is a sudden onset of chest pain. This is invariably associated with breathlessness. The pain may be continuous, and is exacerbated by deep inspiration or with change of posture. Small pneumothoraces may be found only as accidental radiological findings. There may be an associated history of physical exertion. However, in most patients, this is not the case. Tension pneumothorax presents with severe dyspnea with cardiopulmonary compromise. The patient is usually anxious, tachypneic, restless, and may be cyanosed. Tachycardia (heart rate > 140/min), hypotension, cyanosis, and electromechanical dissociations are indicative of tension pneumothorax. If tension is not relieved rapidly, rapid low-volume pulse with hypotension and pulsus paradoxus may develop. Spontaneous left sided pneumothorax may be associated with electrocardiographic changes that may include right axis deviation, diminished R voltage, decreased QRS amplitude, and precordial T-wave inversion.[746]

Small pneumothoraces are missed on physical examination. The classical findings of a pneumothorax include a prominent chest wall with diminished movement with respiration, hyperresonant note, a positive coin test (*bruit de air in*), diminished or absent vocal fremitus, signs of mediastinal shift to the opposite side, and a diminished or absent breath sounds on the side of pneumothorax. A mediastinal crunch or a crepitus sound may be heard over the precordium and sometimes the patient may be aware of this. The sound is present throughout the cardiac cycle and the intensity is influenced by posture and the phase of respiration. Earlier it was thought to be due to free air in the mediastinum and was known as Hamman's sign. However, it can occur in both pneumothorax (left sided) and pneumomediastinum. The mechanism of the sound is perhaps due to the close proximity of trapped air and the moving cardiac musculature.

Mediastinal emphysema may be mild or severe and in the former, it may be undetected. Central chest pain is the most frequent clinical presentation, which may be very mild to very severe mimicking an myocardial infarction. Any maneuver that disturbs the mediastinal structures like deep breathing, and swallowing may aggravate pain. Neck pain may be accompanied by dysphagia. Surgical emphysema is palpable in the neck. The air may track down or up in the soft tissue plane to involve the face, arms, trunk and the groin. The cardiac dullness may be obliterated. Rarely air may entrap vital structures like heart, and trachea to produce serious life threatening situations like cardiac tamponade, hypotension, and shock. Upper airways obstruction will result in cyanosis and respiratory failure. Esophageal rupture may be missed easily.

The characteristic radiological findings of a pneumothorax are a lucent zone devoid of any lung markings with the lung being compressed towards the hilum (Figs 28.11 to 28.15). A sharply defined lung edge will be present with the convexity outwards. Small pneumothoraces not detected by standard inspiratory films can be detected by either taking a film during full expiration[747,748] or by taking a lateral decubitus film with the side of suspected pneumothorax uppermost. In the expiratory film the small pneumothorax appears enlarged because the process reduces the volume of the lung and thorax. However, the volume of the gas contained in the pleural cavity is incompressible at physiological pressure and therefore the volume remains unchanged. It thus gives an apparent enlargement of the pneumothorax since the same volume is now accommodated in a reduced thorax. In the lateral decubitus view a small pneumothorax becomes visible as the air/lung interface becomes clearly visible underneath the lateral chest wall. In infants, this is the preferred view. In complete pneumothorax the lung is compressed towards the hilum and appears globular. Opposite side will show exaggerated bronchovascular markings because of increased blood flow to that lung. In tension pneumothorax, the mediastinum is shifted to the opposite side. Radiographic findings are characteristic of pneumomediastinum. Free air as sharp outlines may be seen as lucent areas running along the cardiac borders with a clear outline. This may extend to the superior mediastinum that will appear widened. Lucent

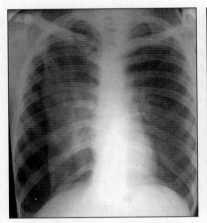

FIGURE 28.11: Left pneumothorax

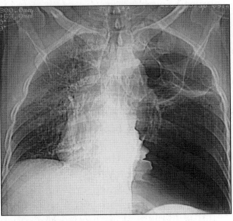

FIGURE 28.12: CXR - Multiloculated left pneumothorax

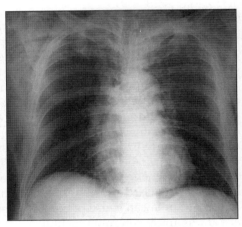

FIGURE 28.13: Pneumomediastinum

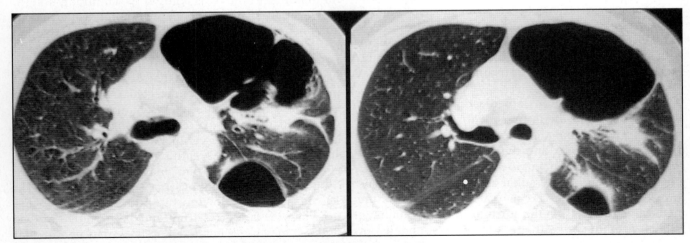

FIGURE 28.14: CT Chest - Multiloculated left pneumothorax

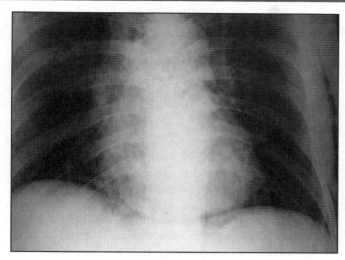

FIGURE 28.15: Pneumomediastinum

areas will be easily marked in the neck and soft tissues because of the presence of air in these areas. Measuring an average diameter of the hemithorax and the lung and finding the ratio of their cubes can measure the amount of lung collapse. For example, if the average diameter of the hemithorax is 10 cm and the distance between the lung and the chest wall is 4 cm (i.e. collapsed lung is 6 cm), then the ratio of their cubes is $6^3/10^3 = 22$ percent, and thus 78 percent pneumothorax is present. Another method has been described to calculate the percentage of collapse.[749] In this method, the average interpleural distance is calculated, which is the mean of the maximum apical interpleural distance and two measurements of interpleural distances in the mid points of the upper and lower halves of the lung. Then a nomogram is used to calculate the percentage of lung collapsed. Neither of the two methods is very accurate, and the best way is to use CT scans in conjunction with computer programs.[750]

A restrictive type of ventilatory impairment is classically seen in pneumothorax with reduced vital capacity, functional residual capacity, and total lung capacity. There may be small reduction in diffusion capacity. Hypoxemia is commonly seen soon after pneumothorax if it is more than 20 percent. This is gradually improved. The initial hypoxemia is due to the collapsed lung causing less blood flow to that side. With time however, arterial blood gas returns to normal because of compensatory hypoxic vasoconstriction that corrects gross ventilation/perfusion imbalance.

MANAGEMENT

The management of pneumothorax[751-763] may be conservative or by intercostal tube drainage depending upon the amount of air in the pleural cavity and the underlying physiological disturbance (i.e. tension pneumothorax).

(i) CONSERVATIVE APPROACH

The basic principle in this approach is that there is a natural tendency for the gas to be absorbed. This is indicated in (a) otherwise healthy adults who is not dyspneic and (b) in whom the volume of pneumothorax is very small, i.e. less than 20 percent of the hemithoracic volume. It is estimated that on an average there is re-expansion at the rate of 1.25 percent hemithoracic volume per day. Thus a 10 percent pneumothorax will re-expand approximately within 10 days; and a 20 percent pneumothorax in 16 days. The absorption is hastened by giving 100 percent supplemental oxygen. The mechanism by which 100 percent oxygen enhances absorption is based on the principle that the rate of transfer of gases across the alveoli is directly proportional to the difference in partial pressure of the gas constituents across the alveoli and pulmonary capillaries. As 100 percent oxygen is breathed, partial pressure of nitrogen in the alveoli falls and nitrogen is gradually washed out of the tissues as oxygen is taken up resulting in a substantial fall of the total end-capillary pressures from approximately 706 mm Hg to 146 mm Hg. This results in a large gradient between the tissue capillary with low partial pressure of nitrogen and in the air in the pleural space, which is almost atmospheric of about 760 mm Hg with a relatively high partial pressure of nitrogen. Thus, the absorption of gas from the pneumothorax is enhanced several folds. Although one should be careful in situations where high oxygen concentration is harmful as in cases of COPD with carbon dioxide retention, in other conditions this is quite helpful, so that a chest tube may not be required. This is true particularly true in situations like a coexisting bleeding diathesis.

(ii) ACTIVE MANAGEMENT

Active management consists of removing the air from the pleural cavity either by simple aspiration or by inserting a chest tube through the intercostal spaces. The indications of such active management are: (i) a tension pneumothorax; (ii) a pneumothorax of > 20 percent of the hemithorax; (iii) coexisting lung disease; (iv) presence of dyspnea; (v) increasing pneumothorax; (vi) previous pneumothorax in the opposite lung; (vii) bilateral pneumothorax; (viii) associated pleural effusion or empyema; and (ix) institution of intermittent positive pressure ventilation.

The most commonly accepted initial method of treatment of pneumothorax is insertion of an intercostal tube connected to an underwater seal, which allows gradual re-expansion of the lung. In the past a red rubber tube was used for this purpose, but recently disposable plastic ones have been used more commonly. It is argued that irritation of the pleura by the tube causes adhesions, which helps preventing the pneumothorax to recur. However, it is doubtful if adhesion in a smaller area of the lung surface is effective in preventing recurrence. If the lung fails to expand then suction may be applied, although it may not be effective always. The problem with this method is the risk of a hemothorax and thrombo-embolism because of confinement to bed. The later complication can be prevented if the patient becomes mobile as early as possible.

One alternative to the chest tube drainage is a drain connected to some sort of a valve mechanism such as the Heilmlich flutter valve, which is cheap and allows the patient to be mobile. The patient can be treated as an outpatient. The method is not, however very popular because of mechanical problems with the valve.

Simple manual aspiration is an alternative procedure that spares the patient discomfort of the commonly used intercostal tube with an under water seal drain. The aspiration method is also simple. A 16-gauge plastic cannula can be inserted into an appropriate site in the chest wall and is to be connected to a large syringe by a three-way tap. If there is no success then a chest tube can be inserted. The disadvantages of the needle aspiration are that there is a risk of laceration of the lung and possibility of other complications like empyema and chronic pneumothorax.

The risk for a second spontaneous pneumothorax is 20 to 25 percent and for a fourth, after a third, is 80 percent. Thoracotomy with pleural abrasion or pleurec-tomy is the current standard method for inducing pleurodesis and preventing recurrent pneumothorax. However, such a pleurodesis is possible without the need for a thoracotomy by chemical pleurodesis, especially in patients who are poor risks for surgery. The use of sclerosing agents to cause pleurodesis is not new and numerous agents have been used in the past. They are discussed in the previous section on pleural effusion. Tetracycline in acidic solutions causes destruction of mesothelial cells when injected into the pleural space of laboratory animals. Most mesothelial cells are sloughed one hour after 100 mg of tetracycline is injected into the rabbit's pleural space. Other animal studies also have proved that tetracycline is the most reliable in developing pleural adhesions. Usually a solution of tetracycline hydrochloride in a dose of 1 gm in 50 ml normal saline with 10 ml of 1 percent lignocaine is injected into the chest tube and where possible is allowed to remain like that for several hours before drainage. It causes less pain than silver nitrate, diminished exudation, and a shorter hospital stay. Lignocaine helps to diminish pain. Talc is another sclerosing agent helpful in pleurodesis for pneumothorx.[764-770]

If the patient's condition permits and the lung fails to expand fully within 7 to 10 days despite a good chest tube, a parietal pleurectomy is carried out through a posterolateral thoracotomy. The parietal pleura is stripped off the chest wall and mediastinum leaving a raw area that becomes adherent to the remaining visceral pleura. Similar purpose can be served by pleural abrasion by producing extensive scars in the parietal pleura with a dry gauze sponge. Such surgical procedures are indicated in cases with persisting pneumothorax, ipsilateral recurrence, contralateral first occurrence, bilateral simultaneous pneumothorax, persistent pleural effusion, special risk groups like air crews, divers, seafarers, and in hose where the first episode was life threatening. Any bleb or bullae identified are resected.

Over the past few years thoracoscopy,[771] particularly video-assisted thoracic surgery (VATS) has been used more commonly in the management of pneumothorax. The visibility of the entire hemithorax through VATS is similar to that obtained by direct view through a limited thoracotomy.[772-775] Thoracoscopy is useful in the treatment of pneumothorax in two ways: (a) to treat the bleb or bullous disease either by endoscopic stapling device, or through a Nd-YAG laser or by ligating the apical bullae with a Roeder loop;[776,777] and (b) to create a pleurodesis.

Tension pneumothorax is an acute medical emergency requiring urgent attention and treatment. This is said to be present when the intrapleural pressure exceeds atmospheric pressure throughout expiration and often during inspiration as well. As explained earlier, this occurs as a result of a check-valve mechanism. With the development of tension pneumothorax there is a sudden deterioration of the cardiopulmonary status of the patient. This is due to a combination of decreased cardiac output because of impaired venous return and marked hypoxemia. This condition can develop in spontaneous pneumothorax, but is more commonly associated with mechanical ventilation or during cardiopulmonary resuscitation. Clinically the patient appears distressed with rapid labored breathing, cyanosis, profuse dia-phoresis, and marked tachycardia. Arterial blood gas analysis will reveal marked hypoxemia and at times respiratory acidosis. The physical findings are that of a large pneumothorax with marked mediastinal shifting.

The diagnosis of tension pneumothorax is to be suspected in any patient receiving mechanical ventilation, in those with a pneumothorax, or in patients whose condition suddenly deteriorates after a procedure known to cause pneumothorax. The diagnosis should also be suspected if there is difficulty in ventilating the patient during cardiopulmonary resuscitation or the patient is having a electromechanical dissociation. Other situations of tension pneumothorax include hyperbaric oxygen therapy, or misfitted Heimlich valves. Radiography will show a severely shifted mediastinum to the other side with a depressed diaphragm on the side of pneumothorax along with other findings. When the diagnosis is suspected, (a) the patient should be given a high concentration of supplemental oxygen; (b) then a large-bored needle should be inserted into the pleural space through the second anterior intercostal space. The needle should be attached to a three-way stopcock or can be directly attached through a water seal. Sudden rush of air through water as soon as the needle is pushed confirms the diagnosis. Once the tension is relieved, a usual chest tube can replace it.

Pneumomediastinum most often require no specific treatment except reassurance, and use of simple analgesics for relief of pain. 100 percent oxygen may be helpful. Multiple nicks may be given in cases where the neck swelling is increasing although the outcome is not changed substantially.[779,780] Rarely in life threatening situations, mediastinal decompression may be tried.

Re-expansion pulmonary edema is a condition when unilateral pulmonary edema develops in the lung that has been rapidly reinflated following a variable period of collapse secondary to pleural effusion or pneumothorax.[780,781] The condition is associated with variable degrees of hypoxia and hypotension, occasionally needing intubation and mechanical ventilation and sometimes can cause death. The exact mechanism of development of unilateral pulmonary edema is not known. But it occurs when the pleural effusion or pneumothorax is present for at least three days and a negative pressure is applied which may vary from—10 to 20 mm Hg pleural pressure, although application of negative pressure is not a must always. It is possibly caused due to increased permeability of the pulmonary vasculature[782] that is because of the fact that the mechanical stress applied to the lung during re-expansion damages the capillaries.[783] Recently, it is hypothesized that re-expansion pulmonary edema is due to a reperfusion injury.[784] With collapsed lung, hypoxia becomes severe in the atelectatic lung, and when this area is reperfused, oxygen free radical formation is promoted and lung injury results. Clinically, the patient will complain of severe coughing and chest tightness immediately following thoracentesis or placement of a chest tube. The symptoms progress for 24 to 48 hours and chest radiograph reveals pulmonary edema throughout the ipsilateral lung. Pulmonary edema may also develop in the contralateral lung. The occurrence of this condition is of course very rare. This can be prevented by withdrawing smaller amount of fluid (less than 1000 ml) unless pleural pressures are monitored. Some authors advocate pleural pressure monitoring during thoracentesis. Similarly, when a pneumothorax is drained, the chest tube should be attached to an under waterseal drainage apparatus.

IV. TUMORS OF PLEURA[785-791]

Pleural tumors are most commonly secondaries from another primary site. Such sites include the lungs, gastrointestinal tract, breast, prostate, and genitourinary tract. The most common and important primary pleural tumor, malignant mesothelioma is discussed previously. Benign mesothelioma[792] or pleural fibroma and sarcoma of the pleura are rare tumors.

Pleural fibroma or benign mesothelioma may be discovered accidentally in a chest X-ray or because of symptoms. Direct pressure effects are more common like breathlessness. Other indirect effects include fever, weight loss, hypoglycemia, and hypertrophic pulmonary osteoarthropathy. The usual age is above 40 years. Clinical signs will depend on the size of the tumor like a mass lesion with prominence of the chest wall and other features of a space occupying lesion or massive pleural effusion. Radiologically a spherical or lobulated mass may be recognized in the periphery. Usually the mass is attached to the pleura by means of a pedicle. The tumor is well capsulated and surrounded by compressed lung tissue. Histology picture will reveal interlaced fibrous tissue with some mitotic figures and areas of myxomatous degeneration. Pleomorphic features may also be present making the distinction from a sarcoma more difficult. The origin of the tumor is from the mesothelial cells, but in some cases it may be from the submesothelial mesenchymal tissue.

Surgical resection is the treatment of choice for the tumor. Presence of a hemorrhagic pleural effusion is not a contraindication for surgery. Surgery is so effective that pain and fever disappears by the time the patient recovers from anesthesia. Clubbing and hypertrophic pulmonary osteoarthropathy takes few months to disappear.

Pleural sarcoma is a very rare and uncommon tumor of the pleura. It is a very highly malignant tumor and commonly occurs in young adults. It metastasizes early both blood-borne, and, local invasion to the lungs and chest wall.

REFERENCES

1. Sahn SA. The pleura. State of the art. Am Rev Respir Dis 1988;136:184-234.
2. Agostoni E. Mechanics of the pleural space. Physiol Rev 1972;52:57-128.
3. Albertine KH, Weiner-Kronish JP, Staub NC. The structure of the parietal pleura and its relationship to pleural fluid dynamics in sheep. Anat Rec 1984;208:401-09.
4. Albertine KH, Weiner-Kronish JP, Roos PJ, Staub NC. Structure, blood supply and lymphatic vessels of the sheep's visceral pleura. Am J Anat 1982;165:227-94.
5. Gaudio E, Rendina EA, Pannarale L, et al. Surface morphology of the human pleura: A scanning electron microscopic study. Chest 1988;92:149-53.
6. Wang NS. The regional difference of pleural mesothelial cells in rabbits. Am Rev Respir Dis 1974;110:623-33.
7. Antony VB, Sahn SA, Mossman B, Gail DB, Kalica A. Pleural cell biology in health and disease. Am Rev Respir Dis 1992;145:1236-39.
8. Idell S, Zuieb C, Kumar A, Koenig KB, Johnson AR. Pathways of fibrin turnover of human pleural mesothelial cells in vivo. Am J Respir Cell Mol Biol 1992;7:414-26.
9. Bermudez E, Everitt J, Walker C. Expression of growth factor and growth factor RNA, in rat pleural mesothelial cells in culture. Expt Cell Res 1990;190:91-98.
10. Efrati P, Nir E. Morphological and cytochemical investigation of human mesothelial cells from pleural and peritoneal effusions. Isr J Med Sc 1976;12:662-73.
11. McLaughlin RF, Tyler WS, Canada RO. A study of the gross pulmonary anatomy in various animals and humans. Am J Anat 1961;108:149-65.
12. McLaughlin RF, Tyler WS, Canada RO. Subgross pulmonary anatomy of the rabbit, rat, and guinea pig, with additional notes on the human lung. Am Rev Respir Dis 1966;94:380-87.
13. Von Hayek H. The human lung. New York: Hafner Publishing, 1960;34-39.
14. Miller WS. The Lung (2nd edn). Springfield, II: Charles C Thomas 1947;89:118.
15. Wang NS. The preformed stomas connecting the pleural cavity and the lymphatics in the parietal pleura. Am Rev Respir Dis 1975;111:12-20.
16. Light RW. Pleural diseases (3rd edn). Williams and Wilkins 1995;1-6.
17. Agostoni E, D'Angelo E. Thickness and pressure of the pleural fluid at various heights and with various hydrothoraces. Respir Physiol 1969;6:330-42.
18. Stauffer JL, Potts DE, Sahn SA. Cellular contents of the normal rabbit pleural space. Acta Cytol 1978;22:570-74.
19. Stewart PB, Burgen ASV. The turnover of fluid in the dog's pleural cavity. J Lab Clin Invest 1958;52:212.
20. Staub NC, Weiner-Kronish JP, Albertine KH. Transport through the pleura. Physiology of the normal liquid and solute exchange to the pleural space. In Chretien J, Bignon J, Hirsch A (Ed): The pleura in health and disease, New York: Marcel Dekker, 1985;169:93.
21. Miserocchi G, Agostoni E. Contents of the pleural space. J Appl Physiol 1971;30:208-13.
22. Sahn SA, Wilcox MI, Good JT, et al. Characteristics of normal rabbit pleural fluid: Physiologic and biochemical implications. Lung 1979;156:63-69.
23. Celikoglu F, Teirstein AS, Krellenstein DJ, Strauchen JA. Pleural effusion in non-Hodgkin's lymphoma. Chest 1992;101;1357-60.
24. Marel M, Stastny B, Melinova L, Svandova E, Light RW. Diagnosis of pleural effusions—Experience with clinical studies 1986-1990. Chest 1995;107:1598-1603.
25. Joseph J, Strange C, Sahn SA. Pleural effusion in hospitalized patients with AIDS. Ann Intern Med 1993;118:856-59.
26. Maher GG, Berger HW. Massive pleural effusions: Malignant and nonmalignant causes in 46 patients. Am Rev Respir Dis 1972;105:458.
27. Beck JM. Immunologically mediated pleural effusions. Semin Respir Med 1991;12:238.
28. Mellins RB, Levine OR, Fishman AP. Effects of systemic and pulmonary venous hypertension on pleural and pericardial fluid accumulation. J Appl Physiol 1970;29:564.
29. Jayes RL, Kamerow HN, Hasselquist SM, et al. Disseminated pneumocystosis presenting as a pleural effusion. Chest 1993;103:306-07.
30. Kollef MH, McCormack MT, Kristo DA, Reddy VBB. Pleural effusion in patients with systemic cholesterol embolization. Chest 1993;103:792-95.
31. Celikoglu F, Teirstein AS, Krellenstein DJ, Strauchen JA. Pleural effusion in non-Hodgkin's lymphoma. Chest 1992;101:1357-60.
32. Vernon AN, Sheeler AR, Biscotti CV, Stoller JK. Pleural effusion resulting from metastatic papillary carcinoma of thyroid. Chest 1992;101:1448-49.
33. LaRoche CM, Wells F, Shneerson J. Massive hemothorax due to enlarging arterio-enous fistula in pregnancy. Chest 1992;103:1452-53.
34. Coodley EL, Yoshinaka R. Pleural effusion as the major manifestation of actinomycosis. Chest 1994;106:1615-17.
35. Manthous CA, Schmidt GA, Hall JB. Pleural effusion masquerading as myocardial infarction. Chest 1993;103:1619-20.
36. Yoo OH, Ting EY. Effects of pleural effusion on pulmonary function. Am Rev Respir Dis 1964;89:55-63.
37. Anthonisen NR, Martin RR. Regional lung function in pleural effusion. Am Rev Respir Dis 1977;116:201-07.
38. Pati AR, Pande JN, Guleria JS. Mechanical properties of the lung in pleural effusion. Ind J Chest Dis All Sc 1983;25:120-26.
39. Rudikoff JC. Early detection of pleural fluid. Chest 1980;77:109.

40. Gryminski J, Krakowka P, Lypacewicz G. The diagnosis of pleural effusion by ultrasonic and radiology techniques. Chest 1976;70:33-37.
41. Fraser RG, Pare JAP. Diagnosis of diseases of the chest. (2nd edn). Philadelphia: WB Saunders Company; 1979;184-274.
42. Reigler LG. Roentgen diagnosis of small pleural effusion. J Am Med Ass 1931;96:104-08.
43. Muller R, Lofstedt S. the reaction of pleura in primary tuberculosis of the lungs. Acta Med Scand 1945;122:105.
44. Hessen I. Roentegen examination of pleural fluid. Acta Radiol 1951;152:1-80.
45. Woodring JH. Recognition of pleural effusion on supine radiographs. How much fluid is required? Am J Radiol 1984;142:59.
46. Doust BD, Baum JK, Makland NF, Doust VL. Ultrasonic evaluation of pleural opacities. Radiology 1975;114;135.
47. Matalon TA, Neiman HL, Mintzer RA. Non-cardiac chest sonography: The state of the art. Chest 1983;83:675-78.
48. Ravin CE. Thoracocentesis of loculated pleural effusions using grey scale ultrasound guidance. Chest 1977;71;666-68.
49. Yang PC, Sheu JL, Kyo SH, Yang SP. Clinical application of real time ultrasonography in pleural and subpleural lesions. J Foronoson Med Asso 1984;83:646.
50. Forsberg L, Tylen U. Ultrasound examination of lesions in thorax. Acta Radiol 1980;21:375-78.
51. Mathur RB, Sharma VK, Jain NK, et al. Ultrasonic evaluation of pleural opacities. Ind J Chest Dis All Sc 1994;36:21-25.
52. McLoud TC, Flower CD. Imaging the pleura: Sonography, CT, and MR imaging. Am J Radiol 1991;156:1145-53.
53. Yang PC, Luh KT, Chang DB, et al. Value of sonography in determining the nature of pleural effusion: Analysis of 320 cases. Am J Radiol 1992;159:29-33.
54. Wu RG, Yuan A, Liaw YS, et al. Image comparison of real-time gray-scale ultrasound and colour Doppler ultrasound for use in diagnosis of minimal pleural effusion. Am J Respir Crit Care Med 1994;150:510-14.
55. Henscheke CI, Yankelevitz DF, Davis SD. Pleural disease: Multimodal imaging and clinical management. Cur Prob Diagnost Radiol 1991;20:155-81.
56. Pugatch RD, Spirn PW. Radiology of the pleura. Clin Chest Med 1985;6:17-32.
57. Paling MR, Griffin GK. Lower lobe collapse due to pleural effusion: A CT analysis. J Comput Assist Tomogr 1985;9:1079-83.
58. Proto AV, Ball JB Jr. Computer tomography of the major and minor fissures. Am J Radiol 1983;140:439-48.
59. Gamsu G, Sostman D. Magnetic resonance imaging of the thorax. Am Rev Respir Dis 1989;95:166-73.
60. Fisher MR. Magnetic resonance for the evaluation of the thorax. Chest 1989;95:166-73.
61. Bartter TC, Santarelli RJ, Akers SM, Pratter MR. The evaluation of pleural effusion. Chest 1994;106:1209-14.
62. Sahn SA. Pleural fluid analysis: Narrowing the differential diagnosis. Semin Respir Med 1987;9:22.
63. Good JT Jr, Tryle DA, Maulitz RM, Kaplan RL, Sahn SA. The diagnostic value of pleural fluid pH. Chest 1980;78:55.
64. Collins TR, Sahn SA. Thoracentesis: Complications, patient experience and diagnostic value. Chest 1987;91:817-22.
65. Brandstetter RD, Cohen RP. Hypoxemia after thoracentesis: A predictable and treatable condition. JAMA 1959;242:1060-61.
66. Estenne M, Yernault JC, DeTroyer A. Mechanism of relief of dyspnoea after thoracentesis in patients with large pleural effusions. Am J Med 1983;74:813-19.
67. Wang JS, Tseng CH. Changes in pulmonary mechanics and gas exchange after thoracentesis on patients with inversion of a hemidiaphram secondary to large pleural effusion. Chest 1995;107:1610-14.
68. Noppen MM, Mey JD, Meysman M, et al. Percutaneous needle biopsy of localized pulmonary, mediastinal, and pleural disease with an automatic disposable guillotine soft-tissue needle: Preliminary results. Chest 1995;107:1615-21.
69. Scerbo J, Keltz H, Stone DJ. A prospective study of closed pleural biopsies. JAMA 1977;218:377-80.
70. Mestitz P, Purves MJ, Pollard AC. Pleural biopsy in the diagnosis of pleural effusion. Lancet 1958;2:1349-53.
71. Levine H, Metzger W, Lacera D, Kay L. Diagnosis of tuberculous pleurisy by culture of pleural biopsy specimen. Arch Intern Med 1970;126:269-71.
72. Poppius H, Kokkola K. Diagnosis and differential diagnosis in tuberculous pleurisy. Scand J Respir Dis 1968;63(Suppl):105-10.
73. Von Hoff DD, LiVolsi V. Diagnostic reliability of needle biopsy of the parietal pleura. Am J Clin Pathol 1975;64:200-03.
74. Levine H, Cugell DW. Blunt end needle biopsy of the pleura and rib. Arch Intern Med 1971;109:516-25.
75. Nelson O, Light RW. Granulomatous pleuritis secondary to blastomycosis. Chest 1977;71:433-34.
76. Bueno CE, Clemente G, Castro BC, et al. Cytologic and bacteriologic analysis of fluid and pleural biopsy specimens with Cope's needle. Arch Intern Med 1990;150:1190-94.
77. Salyer WR, Eggleston JC, Erozan YS. Efficacy of pleural needle biopsy and pleural fluid cytopathology in the diagnosis of malignant neoplasms involving the pleura. Chest 1975;67:536-39.
78. Frist B, Kahan AW, Koss LG. Comparison of the diagnostic values of biopsies of the pleura and cytologic evaluation of pleural fluids. Am J Clin Pathol 1979;72:48-51.
79. Tomlinson JR, Sahn SA. Invasive procedures in the diagnosis of pleural disease. Semin Respir Med 1987;9:30-36.
80. Mungall IPF, Cowen PN. Cooke NT, Roach TC, Cooke NJ. Multiple pleural biopsy with the Abrams needle. Thorax 1982;35:600-02.

81. Ali J, Summer WR. Hemothorax and hyperkalemia following pleural biopsy in a 43-year-old woman on hemodialysis. Chest 1994;106:1235-36.

82. Akkurt I, Copur AS, Samurkasoglu AB, Seyfkli Z, Ugur P. Serum-effusion albumin gradient. Chest 1993; 103:1634-35.

83. Light RW, MacGregor MI, Luschinger PC, Ball WC. Pleural effusions: The diagnostic separation of transudates and exudates. Ann Intern Med 1972;77:507-13.

84. Light RW, Ball WC Jr. Glucose and amylase in pleural effusions. JAMA 1973;225:257.

85. Light RW, Erozan RS, Ball WC Jr. Cells in pleural fluid; Their value in differential diagnosis. Arch Intern Med 1973;132:854-60.

86. Broaddus VC, Light RW. What is the origin of pleural transudates and exudates? Chest 1992;102:658-59.

87. Ham H, Brohan U, Bohmer R, Missmal HP. Cholesterol in pleural effusions. Chest 1987; 92:296-302.

88. Valdes L, Pose A, Suarez J, Gonzalez-Juanate JR, Sarandeses A, San Jose E, et al. Cholesterol: A useful parameter for distinguishing between pleural exudates and transudates. Chest 1991;99:1097-102.

89. Romero S, Candela A, Martin C, Hernandez L, Trigo C, Gil J. Evaluation of different criteria for the separation of pleural transudates from exudates. Chest 1993;104:399-404.

90. Roth BJ, O'Meara TF, Cragun WH. The serum-effusion albumin gradient in the evaluation of pleural effusions. Chest 1990;98:546-49.

91. Miesel S, Shamiss A, Thaler M, Nussinovitch N, Rosenthal T. Pleural fluid to serum bilirubin ratio for the separation of transudates from exudates. Chest 1990;98:141-44.

92. Marel M, Stastny B, Melinova L, Svandova E, Light RW. Diagnosis of pleural effusions: Experience with clinical studies, 1986-1990. Chest 1995;107:1598-603.

93. Burgess LJ, Maritz FJ, Taljaard JJF. Comparative analysis of the biochemical parameters used to distinguish between pleural transudates and exudates. Chest 1995;107:1604-09.

94. Light RW. Pleural diseases. Philadelphia; Lee and Febiger 1983.

95. Sahn SA. Pleural fluid analysis: Narrowing the differential diagnosis. Semin Respir Med 1987;9:22-29.

96. Albera C, Mabritto I, Ghio P, Scagliotti GV, Pozzi E. Lymphocyte subpopulations analysis in pleural fluid and peripheral blood in patients with lymphocytic pleural effusions. Respiration 1991;58:65.

97. Herbert A. Pathogenesis of pleurisy, pleural fibrosis, and mesothelial proliferation. Thorax 1986;41:176.

98. Light RW, Macgregor MI, Luchsinger PC, et al. Pleural effusions: The diagnostic separation of transudates and exudates. Ann Intern Med 1972;77,507-13.

99. Light RW, Erozan YS, Ball WC, Jr. Cells in pleural fluid: Their value in differential diagnosis. Arch Intern Med 1973;132,854-60.

100. Light R. Pleural diseases (4th edn). Lippincott Williams & Wilkins. Philadelphia, PA 2001,413.

101. Conner BD, Gary Lee YC, Branca P, Rogers JT, Michael Rodriguez R, Light RW. Variations in pleural fluid WBC count and differential counts with different sample containers and different methods. Chest 2003;123:1181-87.

102. Yam LT. Diagnostic significance of lymphocytes in pleural effusions. Ann Intern Med 1967;66:972-82.

103. Nakamura Y, Ozaki T, Kamei T, et al. Factors that stimulate the proliferation and survival of eosinophils in eosinophilic pleural effusion: Relationship to granulocyte/macrophage colony-stimulating factor, interleukin-5, and interleukin-3. Am J Respir Cell Mol Biol 1993;8:605-11.

104. Schandene L, Namias B, Crusiaux A, et al. IL-5 in post-traumatic eosinophilic pleural effusion. Clin Exper Immunol 1993;93:115-19.

105. Johonson RJ, Johonson JR. Paragonimiasis in Indo-chinese refugees: Roentgenographic findings with clinical correlations. Am Rev Respir Dis 1983;128;534-38.

106. Yacoubian HD. Thoracic problems associated with hydatid cyst of the dome of the liver. Surgery 1976; 79:544-48.

107. Erzurum SE, Underwood GA, Hamilos DL, Waldron JA. Pleural effusion in Churg-Strauss syndrome. Chest 1989;95:1357-59.

108. Spriggs AI, Boddington MM. The cytology of effusions. 2nd Ed. New York: Grune and Stratton 1968.

109. Adelman M, Albelda SM, Gottlieb J, Haponik EF. Diagnostic utility of pleural fluid eosinophilia. Am J Med 1984;77:915-20.

110. Hurwitz S, Leiman G, Shapiro C. Mesothelial cells in pleural fluid: TB or not TB? S Afr Med J 1980;57: 937-39.

111. Yung CM, Bessen SC, Hingorani V, et al. Idiopathic hemothorax. Chest 1993;103:638-39.

112. Ravindran P, Raj RJ, Parameswaran K. Concurrent catamenial hemothorax and hemopneumothorax. Chest 1993;103:646-47.

113. Kupferschmid JP, Shahian DM, Villanueva AG. Massive hemothorax associated with intrathoracic extra-medullary haematopoiesis involving pleura. Chest 1993;103:974-75.

114. Judson MA, Lazarchick J, Sahn SA. Pleural fluid platelets: Can they help identify traumatic thoracenteses. Am J Respir Crit Care Med 1994;149:A1104.

115. Barber LM, Mazzadi L, Deakins DO, et al. Glucose level in pleural fluid as a diagnostic aid. Dis Chest 1957;31:680-81.

116. Berger HW, Maher G. Decreased glucose concentrations in malignant pleural effusions. Am Rev Respir Dis 1971;103:427-29.

117. Carr DT, Power MH. Pleural fluid glucose with special reference to its concentration in rheumatoid pleurisy with effusion. Dis Chest 1960;37:321-24.

118. Vianna NJ. Nontuberculous bacterial empyema in patients with and without underlying diseases. JAMA 1971;215:69-75.

119. Rodriguez-Panadero F, Lopez MJ. Low glucose and pH levels in malignant pleural effusions. Am Rev Respir Dis 1989;139:663-67.

120. Lillington GA, Carr DT, Mayne JG. Rheumatoid pleurisy with effusion. Arch Int Med 1971;128:764-68.

121. Dodson WH, Hollingsworth JW. Pleural effusion in rheumatoid arthritis. N Engl J Med 1966;275:1337-42.

122. Sahn SA, Good JT Jr. Pleural fluid pH in malignant effusions. Ann Int Med 1988;108:345-49.

123. Sanchez-Armengol A, Rodriguez-Panadero F. Survival and talc pleurodesis in metastatic pleural carcinoma, revisited. Report of 125 cases. Chest 1993;104:1482-85.

124. Rodriguez-Panadero F, Lopez MJ. Survival time of patients with pleural metastatic carcinoma predicted by glucose and pH studies. Chest 1989;95:320-24.

125. Dye RA, Laforet EG. Esophageal rupture: Diagnosis by pleural fluid pH. Chest 1974;66:454-56.

126. Light RW, Girard WM, Jenkinson SG, George RB. Parapneumonic effusions. Am J Med 1980;69:507-11.

127. Light RW, Ball WC. Glucose and amylase in pleural effusions. JAMA 1973;225:257-60.

128. Joseph J, Viney S, Beck P, et al. A prospective study of amylase-rich pleural effusions with special reference to amylase isoenzyme analysis. Chest 1992;102:1455-59.

129. Kaye MD. Pleuropulmonary complications of pancreatitis. Thorax 1968;23:297-306.

130. Rockey DC, Cello JP. Pancreaticopleural fistula. Report of 7 cases and review of literature. Medicine 1990;69:332-44.

131. Ende N. Studies of amylase activity in pleural effusions and ascites. Cancer 1960;13:283-87.

132. Sherr HP, Light RW, Merson MH, et al. Origin of pleural fluid amylase in oesophageal rupture. Ann Intern Med 1972;76:985-86.

133. Wroblewski F, Wroblewski R. The clinical significance of lactic dehydrogenase activity of serous effusions. Ann Intern Med 1958;48:813-22.

134. Light RW, Ball WC. Lactate dehydrogenase isoenzymes in pleural effusions. Am Rev Respir Dis 1973;108:660-64.

135. Raabo E, Rasmussen KN, Terkildsen TC. A study of the isoenzymes of lactic dehydrogenase in pleural effusions.Scand J Respir Dis 1966;47:150-56.

136. Hunder GG, Mcduffie FC, Huston KA, et al. Pleural fluid complement, complement conversion, and immune complexes in immunologic and nonimmunologic diseases. J Clin Lab Med 1977;90:971-80.

137. Andrews BS, Arora NS, Shadforth MF, et al. The role of immune complexes in the pathogenesis of pleural effusions. Am Rev Respir Dis 1981;124:115-20.

138. Halla JT, Schrohenloher RE, Volanakis JE. Immune complexes and other laboratory features of pleural effusions. Ann Intern Med 1980;92:748-52.

139. Good JT Jr, King TE, Antony VB, Sahn SA. Lupus pleuritis: Clinical features and pleural fluid characteristics with special reference to pleural fluid antinuclear antibodies. Chest 1983;84:714-18.

140. Hunder GG, McDuffie FC, Hepper NGG. Pleural fluid complement in systemic lupus erythematosus and rheumatoid arthritis. Ann Intern Med 1972;76:357-62.

141. Glovsky MM, Loui JS, Pitts WH Jr, Alenty A. Reduction in pleural fluid complement activity in patients with systemic lupus erythematosus and rheumatoid arthritis. Clin Immunol Immunopathol 1976;6:31-41.

142. Bruneau R, Rubin P. The management of pleural effusions and chylothorax in lymphoma. Radiology 1965;85:1085-92.

143. Hughes RL, Mintzer RA, Hidvegi DF, et al. The management of chylothorax. Chest 1979;76:212-18.

144. Staats BA, Ellefson RD, Budahn LL, et al. The lipoprotein profile chylous and nonchylous pleural effusions. Mayo Clin Proc 1980;55:700-04.

145. Seriff NS, Cohen ML, Samuel P, Schulster PL. Chylothorax: Diagnosis by lipoprotein electrophoresis of serum and pleural fluid. Thorax 1977;32:98-100.

146. Jarvi OH, Kunnas RJ, Laitio MC, Tyrkko JES. The accuracy and significance of cytologic cancer diagnosis of pleural effusions. Acta Cytol 1972-16:152-57.

147. Grunze H. The comparative diagnostic accuracy, efficiency, and specificity of cytologic techniques used in the diagnosis of malignant neoplasms in serous effusions of the pleural and pericardial cavities. Acta Cytol 1964;8:150-64.

148. Bueno CE, Clemente G, Castro BC, et al. Cytologic and bacteriologic analysis of fluid and pleural biopsy specimens with Cope's needle. Arch Intern Med 1990;150:1190-4.

149. Warhol MJ, Hickey WF, Corson JM. Malignant mesothelioma: Ultrastructural distinction from adenocarcinoma. Am J Surg Pathol 1982;6:307-14.

150. Gondos B, McIntosh KM, Renston RH, King EB. Application of electron microscopy in the definitive diagnosis of effusions. Acta Cytol 1978;22:297-304.

151. Jandik WR, Landas SK, Bray CK, Lager DJ. Scanning electron microscopic distinction of pleural mesothelioma from adenocarcinoma. Modern Path 1993;6:761-64.

152. Warnock ML, Stoloff A, Thor A. Differentiation of adenocarcinoma of the lung from mesothelioma. Periodic-acid-Schiff, monoclonal antibodies B72.3, and Leu M1. Am J Pathol 1988;133:30-38.

153. Wirth PR, Legier J, Wright GL Jr. Immunohistochemical evaluation of seven monoclonal antibodies for differentiation of pleural mesothelioma from adenocarcinoma. Cancer 1991;67:655-62.

154. Frisman DM, McCarthy WF, Schleiff P, Buckner SB, Nocito JD Jr, O'Leary TJ. Immunocytochemistry in the differential diagnosis of effusions: Use of logistic regression to select a panel of antibodies to distinguish adenocarcinomas from mesothelial proliferations. Modern Pathol 1993;6:179-84.

155. Brown RW, Clark GM, Tandon AK, Allred DC. Multiple marker immunohistochemical phenotypes distinguishing malignant pleural mesothelioma from pulmonary adenocarcinoma. Huan Pathol 1993;24:347-54.

156. Shimokata K, Totani Y, Nakanishi K, et al. Diagnostic value of cancer antigen 15-3(CA15-3) detected by monoclonal antibodies (115D8 and DF3) in exudative pleural effusions. Eur Respir J 1988;1:341-44.

157. Niwa Y, Kishimoto H, Shimokata K. Carcinomatous and tuberculous pleural effusion. Comparison of tumor markers. Chest 1985;87:351-55.

158. Klockars M, Petterson T, Froseth B, Selroos O, Stenman UH. Concentration of tumor associated trypsin inhibitor (TATI) in pleural effusions. Chest 1990;98:1159-64.

159. Tawfik MS, Coleman DV. C-myc expression in exfoliated cells in serous effusions. Cytopathol 1991;2:83-92.

160. Croonen AM, van der Valk P, Herman CJ, Lindeman J. Cytology, immunopathology and flow cytometry in the diagnosis of pleural and pericardial effusion. Lab Invest 1988;58:725-32.

161. Dewald G, Dines DE, Weiland LH, Gordon H. Usefulness of chromosome examination in the diagnosis of malignant pleural effusions. N Engl J Med 1976;295:1494-1500.

162. Korsggard R. Chromosome analysis of malignant human effusions in vivo. Scand J Respir Dis 1979; 105 (Suppl):1-100.

163. Imecik O, Ozer F. Diagnostic value of sialic acid in malignant pleural effusions. Chest 1992;102:1819-22.

164. Bartter T, Santarelli R, Akers S, Pratter MR. The evaluation of pleural effusion. Chest 1994;106:1209-14.

165. Collins TR, Sahn SA. Thoracocentesis: Clinical value, complications, technical problems, and patient experience. Chest 1987;91:817-22.

166. Light RW, Erozan YS, Ball WC. Cells in pleural fluid. Arch Int Med 1973;132:854-60.

167. Leslie WK, Kinasewitz GT, Clinical characteristics of the patient with nonspecific pleuritis. Chest 1988;94:603-08.

168. Prakash UBS, Reiman HM. Comparison of needle biopsy with cytologic analysis for the evaluation of pleural effusion: Analysis of 414 cases. Mayo Clin Proc 1985;60:158-64.

169. Bueno CE, Clement MG, Castro BC, Martin LM, Ramos SR, Panizo AG, et al. Cytologic and bacteriologic analysis of fluid and pleural biopsy specimens with Cope's needle. Arch Intern Med 1990;150:1190-94.

170. Bynum LJ, Wilson JE III. Characteristics of pleural effusions associated with pulmonary embolism. Arch Intern Med 1976;136:159-62.

171. Chang S, Perng R. The role of fiberoptic bronchoscopy in evaluating pleural effusions. Arch Intern Med 1989;149:855-57.

172. Colt HG, Harrell JH. Diagnostic thoracoscopy: New look at an old technique. J Respir Dis 1992;13:1246-51.

173. Menzies R, Charbonneau M. Thoracoscopy for the diagnosis of pleural disease. Ann Intern Med 1991;114:271-76.

174. Boutin C, Viallat JR, Cargnino P, Farisse P. Thoracoscopy in malignant effusions. Am Rev Respir Dis 1981;124:588-92.

175. Ryan CJ, Rodgers RF, Unni KK, Hepper NG. The outcome of patients with pleural effusion of indeterminate cause at thoracotomy. Mayo Clin Proc 1981; 56:145-49.

176. Marel M, Satstny B, Light RW. Incidence of pleural effusion in the Central Bohemia Region. Chest 1993;104:1486-89.

177. Logue RB, Rogers JV Jr, Gay BB Jr. Subtle roentgenographic signs of left heart failure. Am Heart J 1963;65:464-73.

178. Race GA, Scheiffey CH, Edwards JE. Hydrothorax in congestive heart failure. Am J Med 1957;22:83-89.

179. Weiner-Kronish JP, Broaddus VC. Interrelationship of pleural and pulmonary interstitial liquid. Annu Rev Physiol 1993;55:209-26.

180. Bhattacharya J, Gropper MA, Staub NC. Interstitial fluid pressure gradient measured by micropuncture in excised dog lung. J Appl Physiol 1984;56:271-77.

181. Broaddus VC, Weiner-Kronish JP, Staub NC. Clearance of lung edema into the pleural space of volume loaded anesthetized sheep. J Appl Physiol 1990;68:2623-30.

182. Allen SJ, Laine GA, Drake RE, Gabel JC. Superior vena caval pressure elevation causes pleural effusion formation in sheep. Am J Physiol 1988;255:H492-H495.

183. Webb WR, Ozmen V, Moulder PV, Shabahang B, Breaux J. Iodized talc pleurodesis for the treatment of pleural effusions. J Thorac Cardiovasc Surg 1992;103:881-85.

184. Vargas FS, Wang NS, Lee HM, Gruer SE, Sassoon CSH, Light RW. Effectiveness of bleomycin in comparison to tetracycline as pleural sclerosing agent in rabbits. Chest 1993;104:1582-84.

185. Lieberman FL, Hidemura R, Peters RL, Reynolds TB. Pathogenesis and treatment of hydrothorax complicating cirrhosis with ascites. Ann Intern Med 1966;64:341-51.

186. Johnston RF, Loo RV. Hepatic hydrothorax: Studies to determine the source of the fluid and report of thirteen cases. Ann Intern Med 1964;61:385-401.

187. Rubinstein D, McInnes IE, Dudley FJ. Hepatic hydrothorax in the absence of clinical ascites: Diagnosis and management. Gastroenterology 1985;88:188-91.

188. Mouroux J, Hebuterne X, Perrin C, et al. Treatment of pleural effusion of cirrhotic origin by videothoracoscopy. Br J Surg 1994;81:546-47.

189. Xiol X, Castellote J, Baliellas C, et al. Spontaneous bacterial empyema in cirrhotic patients: Analysis of eleven cases. Hepatology 1990;11:365-70.

190. Runyon BA. Care of the patients with ascites. N Engl J Med 1994;330:337-42.

191. Falchuk KR, Jacoby I, Colucci WS, Rybak ME. Tetracycline-induced pleural symphysis for recurrent hydrothorax complicating cirrhosis. Gastroenterology 1977;72:319-21.

192. Runyon BA, Greenblatt M, Ming RHC. Hepatic hydrothorax is a relative contraindication to chest tube insertion. Am J Gastroenterol 1986;81:566-67.

193. Ikard RW, Sawyers JL. Persistent hepatic hydrothorax after peritoneo-jugular shunt. Arch Surg 1980;115: 1125-27.

194. Cavina C, Vichi G. Radiological aspects of pleural effusions in medical nephropathy in children. Ann Radiol Diagn 1958;31:163-202.

195. Llach F, Arieff AI, Massry SG. Renal vein thrombosis and nephrotic syndrome: A prospective study of 36 adult patients. Ann Intern Med 1975;83:8-14.

196. Palmer BF. South Western medicine conference: Nephrotic edema-pathogenesis and treatment. Am J Med Sc 1993;306:53-67.

197. Belie JA, Millan D. Pleural effusion secondary to ureteral obstruction. Urology 1979;14:27-29.

198. Sulcate JR. Urinothorax: Report of 4 cases and review of the literature. J Urol 1986;135:805-08.

199. Stark D, Shades J, Baron RI, Koch D. Biochemical features of urinothorax. Arch Intern Med 1982;142:1509-11.

200. Miller KS, Wooden S, San SA. Urinothorax: A cause of low pH transudative pleural effusions. Am J Med 1988;85:448-49.

201. Nomoto Y, Suga T, Nakajima K, et al. Acute hydro-thorax in continuous ambulatory peritoneal dialysis—A collaborative study of 161 centers. Am J Nephrol 1989;9:363-67.

202. Milutinovic J, WU WS, Lindhold DD, Lapp NL. Acute massive unilateral hydrothorax: A rare complication of chronic peritoneal dialysis. South Med J 1980;73:827.

203. Laks H, Milliken JC, Perioff JK, et al. Experience with the Fontana procedure. J Thorac Cardiovasc Surg 1984;88:939-51.

204. Kirkpatrik JA Jr, Fleisher DS. The roentgen appearance of the chest in acute glomerulonephritis in children. J Pediatr 1964;64:492-98.

205. Gottechrer A, Roa J, Stanford GG, Chernow B, Sahn SA. Hypothyroidism and pleural effusions. Chest 1990;98:1130-32.

206. Epstein DM, Kline LR, Albelda SM, Miller WT. Tuber-culous pleural effusions. Chest 1987;91:106.

207. Ocana I, Martinez-Vazquez JM, Ribera E, et al. Adenosine deaminase activity in the diagnosis of lymphocytic pleural effusions of tuberculous, neoplastic and lymphomatous origin. Tubercle 1986;67:141.

208. Petterson T, Kaarina O, Weber TH. Adenosine deami-nase in the diagnosis of pleural effusion. Acta Med Scand 1984;215:299.

209. Berger HW, Mejia E. Tuberculous pleurisy. Chest 1973;63:88-92.

210. Malik SK., Behera D, Gilhotra R. Treatment of pleural effusion and lymphadenitis with rifampicin containing regimen. Chest 1987;92:904.

211. Lee CH, Wang WJ, Lan RS, et al. Corticosteroids in the treatment of tubercular pleurisy. A double-blind, placebo-controlled, randomized study. Chest 1988;94:1256.

212. Scharer L, McClement JH. Isolation of tubercle bacilli from needle biopsy specimens of parietal pleura. Am Rev Respir Dis 1968;97:466.

213. Levine H, Metzger W, Lacera D, Kay L. Diagnosis of tuberculous pleurisy by culture of pleural biopsy specimen. Arch Intern Med 1970;126:269.

214. Enarson DA, Dorken E, Gzybowsky S. Tuberculous pleurisy. Can Med Assoc J 1982;1216:493.

215. Moudgil H, Sridhar G, Leitch AG. Reactivation disease: The commonest form of tuberculous pleural effusion in Edinburgh, 1980-1991. Respir Med 1994;88:301-04.

216. Stead WW, Eichenholz A, Stauss HK. Operative and pathologic findings in twenty four patients with syndrome with idiopathic pleurisy with effusion, presumably tuberculous. Am Rev Respir Dis 1955; 71:473-502.

217. Allen JC, Apicella MA. Experimental pleural effusion as a manifestation of delayed hypersensitivity tuberculin PPD. J Immunol 1968;101:481-87.

218. Apicella MA, Allen JC. A physiological differentiation between delayed and immediate hypersensitivity. J Clin Invest 1969;48:250-59.

219. Leibowitz S, Kennedy L, Lessof MH. The tuberculin reaction in the pleural cavity and its suppression by antilymphocyte serum. Br J Exp Pathol 1973;54:152-62.

220. Yamamoto S, Dunn CJ, Willoughby DA. Studies on delayed hypersensitivity pleural exudates in guinea pigs: II. The interelationship of monocytic and lymphocytic cells with respect to migration activity. Immunology 1976;30:513-19.

221. Bueno CE, Clements G, Castro BC, et al. Cytologic and bacteriologic analysis of fluid and pleural biopsy specimens with Cope's needle. Arch Intern Med 1990;150:1190-94.

222. Chan CH, Arnold M, Chan CY, Mak TW, Hoheisel GB. Clinical and pathological features of tuberculous pleural effusion and its long-tern consequences. Respiration 1991;58:171-75.

223. Antony VB, Sahn SA, Antony AC, Repine JE. Bacillus-Calmette-Guerin-stimulated neutrophils release chemotoxins for monocytes in rabbit pleural space *in vitro*. J Clin Invest 1985;76:1514-21.

224. Fujiwara H, Tsuyguchi I. Frequency of tuberculin - reactive T-lymphocytes in pleural fluid and blood from patients with tuberculous pleurisy. Chest 1986;89:530-32.

225. Ellner JJ, Barnes PF, Wallis RS, Modlin RL. The immunology of tuberculous pleurisy. Sem Respir Infect 1988;3:335-42.

226. Ribera E, Espanol T, Martinez-Vazquez, Ocana I, Encabo G. Lymphocyte proliferation and gamma-interferon production after "in-Vitro" stimulation with PPD. Differentiation between tuberculous and non-tuber-culous pleurisy in patients with positive tuberculin test. Chest 1990;97:1381-85.

227. Lorgat F, Keraan MM, Lukey PT, Ress SR. Evidence for in vivo generation of cytotoxic T-cells. PPD-stimulated lymphocytes from tuberculous pleural effusions demons-trate enhanced cytotoxicity with accelerated kinetics of induction. Am Rev Respir Dis 1992;145:418-23.

228. Kurasawa T, Shimokata K. Cooperation between accessory cells and T lymphocytes in patients with tuberculous pleurisy. Chest 1991;100:1046-52.

229. Shimokata K, Saka H, Murate T, Hasegawa Y, Hasegawa T. Cytokine content in pleural effusion. Chest 1991;99:1103-07.

230. Barnes PF, Modlin RL, Bikle DD, Adams JS. Transpleural gradient of 1,25-dihydroxy vitamin D in tuberculous pleuritis. J Clin Invest 1989;83:1527-32.

231. Leckie WJH, Tothill P. Albumin turn over in pleural effusions. Clin Sci 1965;29:339-52.

232. Ellner JJ. Pleural fluid and peripheral blood lymphocyte function in tuberculosis. Ann Intern Med 1978;89:932-33.

233. Rossi GA, Balbi B, Manca F. Tuberculous pleural effusions: Evidence for selective presence of PPD-specific T-lymphocytes at site of inflammation in the early phase of infection. Am rev Respir Dis 1987;136:575-79.

234. Aho K, Brander E, Patiala J. Studies of primary drug resistance in tuberculous pleurisy. Scand J Respir Dis 1968;63(Suppl):111-14.

235. Levine H, Szanto PB, Cugell DW. Tuberculous pleurisy: An acute illness. Arch Intern Med 1968;122:329-32.

236. Mahr GG, Berger HW. Massive pleural effusion: Malignant and nonmalignant causes in 46 patients. Am Rev Respir Dis 1972;105:458-60.

237. Richter C, Perenboom R, Mtoni I, et al. Clinical features of HIV-seropositive and HIV-seronegative patients with tubetrculous pleural effusiion in Dar es salaam, Tanzania. Chest 1994;106:1471-75.

238. Kramer F, Modilevsky T, Waliany AR, Leedon JM, Barnes PF. Delayed diagnosis of tuberculosis in patients with human immunodeficiency virus infection. Am J Med 1990;89:451-56.

239. Yam LT. Diagnostic significance of lymphocytes in pleural effusions. Ann Intern Med 1967;66:972-82.

240. Kapila K, Pande JN, Garg A, Verma K. T lymphocyte subsets and B lymphocytes in tubercular pleural effusion. Ind J Chest Dis All Sc 1987;29:90-93.

241. De Oliveira HG, Rossatto ER, Prolla JC. Pleural fluid adenosine deaminase and lymphocyte proportions: Clinical usefulness in the diagnosis of tuberculosis. Cytopathology 1994;5:27-32.

242. Spriggs AI, Boddington MM. The cytology of effusions: (2nd Ed). New York; Grune and Straton 1968.

243. Spriggs AI, Boddington MM. Absence of mesothelial cells from tuberculous pleural effusions. Thorax 1968;15:169-71.

244. Lakhotia M, Mehta RS, Mathur D, Baid CS, Verma AR. Diagnostic significance of pleural fluid eosinophilia during initial thoracocentesis. Ind J Chest Dis All Sc 1989;31:259-64.

245. Guisti G. Adenosine deaminase. In Bergmeyer HU (Ed): Method of enzymatic analysis. New York: Academic Press 1974;2:1092-99.

246. Ocana I, Martinez-Vazquez JM, Segura RM, Fernadez-Desilva T, Capdevila JA. Adenosine deaminase in pleural fluid. Chest 1983;84:51-53.

247. Sulochana G, Khallifullah PA, Padmanabhan L. Adenosine deaminase, alpha-1-antitrypsin, alpha-1-acid glycoprotein, ceruloplasmin and protein in the diagnosis of tuberculous pleural effusion. Ind J Chest Dis All Sc 1988;30:15-18.

248. Shah A. Tuberculous pleural effusion: A diagnostic problem. Ind J Chest Dis All Sc 1992;34:115-16.

249. Prasad R, Tripathy RP, Mukerji PK, Singh M, Srivastava VML. Adenosine deaminase activity in pleural fluid: A diagnostic test of tuberculous pleural effusion. Ind J Chest Dis All Sc 1992;34:123-26.

250. Gupta A, Sharma SK, Pande JN. Diagnostic methods for tuberculosis. Ind J Chest Dis All Sc 1992;35:63-84.

251. Gilhotra R, Sehgal S, Jindal SK. Pleural biopsy and adenosine deaminase enzyme activity in effusions of different aetiologies. Lung India 1989;7:122-24.

252. Fontan BJ, Verea HH, Garcia BJP, et al. Diagnostic value of simultaneous determination of pleural adenosine deaminase and pleural lysozyme/serum lysozyme ratio in pleural effusion. Chest 1988;93:303-07.

253. Valdes L, San Jose E, Alvarez D, et al. Diagnosis of tuberculous pleurisy using biologic parameters adenosine deaminase, lysozyme, and interferon gamma. Chest 1993;103;458-65.

254. Niwa Y, Kishimoto H, Shimokata K. Carcinomatous and tuberculous pleural effusion. Comparison of tumor markers. Chest 1985;87:351-55.

255. Tamura S, Nishigaki T, Moriwaki Y, et al. Tumor markers in pleural effusion diagnosis. Cancer 1988;61:298-302.

256. Aoki Y, Katoh O, Nakanishi Y, Kuroki S, Yamada H. A comparison study of IFN-gamma, ADA, and CA125 as the diagnostic parameters in tuberculous pleuritis.

257. Ocana I, Ribera E, Martinez-Vazquez JM, et al. Adenosine deaminase activity in rheumatoid pleural effusion. Ann Rheum Dis 1988;47:394-97.

258. Ungerer JP, Brobler SM. Molecular forms of adenosine deaminase in pleural effusion. Enzyme 1988;40:7-13.

259. Rodriguez E, Martinez JA, Buges J, Torres M. High adenosine deaminase level in pleural effusion due to bronchoalveolar carcinoma. Chest 1993;103:978-79.

260. Gakis C. Adenosine deaminase in pleural effusions. Chest 1995;107:1772-73.

261. Pang J. Diagnosis of tuberculous pleural effusion by the detection of tuberculostearic acid in pleural aspirates. Chest 1992;102:1635.

262. Riberra E, Ocana I, Martinez-Vazquez JM, et al. High level of interferon gamma in tuberculous pleural effusion. Chest 1988;93:308-11.

263. Barnes PF, Mistry SD, Cooper CL, et al. Compartmentalization of a CD4+ T lymphocyte subpopulation in tuberculous pleuritis. J Immunol 1989;142:1114-19.

264. De Wit D, Maartens G, Steyn L. A comparative study of the polymerase chain reaction and conventional procedures for the diagnosis of tuberculous pleural effusion. Tubercle Lung Dis 1992;73:262-67.

265. Verea HHR, Masa JJF, Dominguez JL, et al. Meaning and diagnostic value of determining the lysozyme level of pleural fluid. Chest 1987;91:342-45.

266. Sibley JC. A study of 200 cases of tuberculous pleurisy with effusion. Am Rev Tuberc 1950;62:314-23.

267. Falk A. Tuberculous pleurisy with effusion: Diagnosis and result of chemotherapy. Postgrad Med 1965;38: 631-35.

268. Scharer L, McClement JH. Isolation of tubercle bacilli from needle biopsy specimens of parietal pleura. Am Rev Respir Dis 1968;97:466-68.

269. Escudero-Bueno C, Garcia-Clemente M, Cuesta-Castro, B, et al. Cytologic and bacteriologic analyzes of fluid and pleural biopsy with Cope's needle. Arch Intern Med 1990;150,1190-94.

270. Wai W, Yeung CH, Yuk-Lins, et al. Diagnosis of tuberculous pleural effusion by the detection of tuberculostearic acid in pleural aspirates. Chest 1991;100,1261-63.

271. Barbas C, Cukier A, de Varvalho CR, et al. The relationship between pleural fluid findings and development of pleural thickening in patients with pleural tuberculosis. Chest 1991;100,1264-67.

272. Banales JL, Pineda P. Mark J, et al. Adenosine deaminase in the diagnosis of tuberculous pleural effusions: A report of 218 patients and review of the literature. Chest 1991;99,355-57.

273. Burgess LI, Maritz FJ, Le Roux I, et al. Use of adenosine deaminase as a diagnostic tool for tuberculous pleurisy. Thorax 1995;50,672-74.

274. Valdes L, Alvarez D, San Jose E, et al. Tuberculous pleurisy: Study of 254 patients. Arch Intern Med 1998;158,2017-21.

275. Ribera E, Ocana I, Martinetz-Vasquez JM, et al. High level of interferon gamma in tuberculous pleural effusion. Chest 1988;93,308-11.

276. Shimokata K, Saka H, Murata T, et al. Cytokine content in pleural effusion: Comparison between tuberculous and carcinomatous pleurisy. Chest 1991;99, 1103-07.

277. Aoki Y, Katoh O, Nakanishi Y, et al. A comparison study of INF-α, ADA, and CA125 as the diagnostic parameters in tuberculous pleuritis. Respir Med 1994;88,139-43.

278. Ogawa K, Koga H, Hirakata Y, et al. Differential diagnosis of tuberculous pleurisy by measurement of cytokine concentrations in pleural effusion. Tuber Lung Dis 1997;781,29-34.

279. Wongtim S, Silachamroon U, Ruxringtham K, et al. Interferon a for diagnosing tuberculous pleural effusions. Thorax 1999;54,921-24.

280. Villegas MV, Labrada LA, Saravia NG. Evaluation of polymerase chain reaction, adenosine deaminase, and interferon-a in pleural fluid for the differential diagnosis of pleural tuberculosis. Chest 2000;118,1355-64.

281. Chen YM, Yang WK, Whang-Peng J, et al. An analysis of cytokine status in the serum and effusions of patients with tuberculous and lung cancer. Lung Cancer 2001;31,25-30.

282. Niwa Y, Kishimoto H, Shimokata K. Carcinomatous and tuberculous pleural effusions: Comparison of tumor markers. Chest 1985;87,351-55.

283. Tamura S, Nishigaki T, Moriwaki Y, et al. Tumor markers in pleural effusion diagnosis. Cancer 1988; 61,298-302.

284. Ito M, Kojiro N, Shirasaka T, et al. Elevated levels of soluble interleukin-2 receptors in tuberculous pleural effusions. Chest 1990;97,1141-43.

285. Sarandakou A, Poulakis N, Rizos D, et al. Pleural fluid and serum soluble interleukin-2 receptors in pleural effusions. Anticancer Res 1991;11,1365-68.

286. Chang SC, Hsu YT, Chen YC, et al. Usefulness of soluble interleukin 2 receptor in differentiating tuberculous and carcinomatous pleural effusions. Arch Intern Med 1994;154,1097-101.

287. Chiang CS, Chiang CD, Huang PL, et al. Neopterin, soluble interleukin-2 receptor and adenosine deaminase levels in pleural effusions. Respiration 1994;61,150-54.

288. Porcel JM, Gazquez I, Vives M, et al. Diagnosis of tuberculous pleuritis by the measurement of soluble interleukin 2 receptor in pleural fluid. Int J Tuberc Lung Dis 2000;4,975-79.

289. Aoe K, Hirak A, Murakami T, Eda R, Maeda T, Sugi K, Takeyama H. Diagnostic significance of interferon-g in tuberculous pleural effusions. Chest 2003;123:740-4.

290. Metz CE. Basic principles of ROC analysis. Semin Nucl Med 1978;8,283-98

291. Green JA, Cooperband SR, Kibrick S. Immune specific induction of interferon production in cultures of human blood lymphocytes. Science 1969;164,1415-17.

292. Baron S, Tyring SK, Fleischmann WR, Jr, et al. The interferons: Mechanisms of action and clinical applications. J Am Med Assoc 1991;266,1375-83.

293. Gürsel G, Gökcora N, Elbeg S, et al. Tumor necrosis factor-α (TNF-α) in pleural fluids. Tuberc Lung Dis 1995;76,370-71.

294. Söderblom T, Nyberg P, Teppo AM, et al. Pleural fluid interferon-g and tumor necrosis factor-a in tuberculous and rheumatoid pleurisy. Eur Respir J 1996;9,1652-55.

295. Orphanidou D, Gaga M, Rasidakis A, et al. Tumor necrosis factor, interleukin-1 and adenosine deaminase in tuberculous pleural effusion. Respir Med 1996;90,95-98.

296. Hua CC, Chang LC, Chen YC, et al. Proinflammatory cytokines and fibrinolytic enzymes in tuberculous and malignant pleural effusions. Chest 1999;116,1292-96.

297. de Pablo A, Villena V, Echave-Sustaeta J, et al. Are pleural fluid parameters related to the development of residual pleural thickening? Chest 1997;112,1293-97.

298. Philip-Joët F, Alessi MC, Philip-Joët C, et al. Fibrinolytic and inflammatory processes in pleural effusions. Eur Respir J 1995;8,1352-56.

299. Deshmukh MD, Virdi SS. Pleural punch biopsy in tubercular pleural effusion-to find out comparative value of single and multiple specimens. Ind J Tuberc 1972;19:95-100.

300. Jain SK. Diagnostic yield of multiple pleural biopsies in tubercular pleural effusion. Ind J Chest Dis All Sc 1983;25:242-43.

301. Levine H, Metzger W, Laccera D, Kay L. Diagnosis of tuberculous pleurisy by culture of pleural biopsy specimens. Arch Intern Med 1970;126:269-71.

302. Patiala J. Initial tuberculous pleuritis in the Finnish Armed Forces in 1939-1945 with special reference to eventual post pleuritic tuberculosis. Acta Tuberc Scand 1954;36(Suppl):1-57.

303. Roper WH, Waring JJ. Primary serofibrinous pleural effusion in military personnel. Am Rev Respir Dis 1955;71:616-634.

304. Tani P, Poppius H, Makipaja J. Cortisone therapy for exudative tuberculous pleurisy in the light of the follow up study. Acta Tuberc Scand 1964;44:303-09.

305. Lee CH, Wang WJ, Lan RS et al. Corticosteroids in the treatment of tuberculous pleurisy: A double blind, placebo-controlled, randomized study. Chest 1988;94: 1256-59.

306. Barbas CSV, Cukier A, de Varvalho CRR, Barbas-Fiho JV, Light RW. The relationship between pleural fluid findings and the development of pleural thickening in patients with pleural tuberculosis. Chest 1991;100:1264-67.

307. Light RW, MacGregor MI, Ball WC Jr, Luchsinger PC. Diagnostic significance of pleural fluid pH and PCO_2. Chest 1973;131:516-20.

308. Taryle DA, Potts DE, Sahn SA. The incidence and clinical correlates of parapneumonic effusions in pneumococcal pneumonia. Chest 1978;74:170.

309. Fine NL, Smith LR, Sheedy PF. Frequency of pleural effusions in mycoplasma and viral pneumonias. N Engl J Med 1970;283:790.

310. Light RW, Girard WM, Jenkinson SG, George RB, Parapneumonic effusions. Am J Med 1980;69:985-86.

311. Sahn SA, Light RW. The sun should never set on a parapneumonic effusion. Chest 1989;95:945-47.

312. Berger HA, Morganroth ML. Immediate drainage is not required for all patients with complicated parapneumonic effusions. Chest 1990;97:731-35.

313. Poe RH, Marin MG, Israel RH, Kallay MC. Utility of pleural fluid analysis in predicting tube thoracostomy/decortication in parapneumonic effusions. Chest 1991;100:963-67.

314. Himmelman RB, Callen PW. The prognostic value of loculations in parapneumonic pleural effusions. Chest 1986;90:852-56.

315. Heffner JE, Brown LK, Barberi C, DeLeo J. Pleural fluid chemical analysis in parapneumonic effusion: A meta analysis. Am J Respir Crit Care Med 1995;151:1700-08.

316. Bates M, Cruikshank G. Thoracic actinomycosis. Thorax 1957;12:99-24.

317. Brown JR. Human actinomycosis. A study of 181 subjects. Hum Pathol 1973;4:319-30.

318. Harrison RN, Thomas DJB. Acute actinomycotic empyema. Thorax 1979;34:406-07.

319. Frazier AR, Roseno EC III, Roberts GD. Nocardiosis: a review of 25 cases occuring during 24 months. Mayo Clin Proc 1975;50:657-63.

320. Feigin DS. Nocardiosis of the lung; Chest radiographic findings in 21 cases. Radiology 1986;159:9-14.

321. Palmer DL, Harvey RL, Wheeler JK. Diagnostic and therapeutic considerations in *Nocardia asteroides* infection. Medicine 1974;53:391-401.

322. Krakowaka P, Rowinska E, Halweg H. Infection of the pleura by *Aspergillus fumigatus*. Thorax 1970;25:245-53.

323. Hillerdal G. Pulmonary Aspergillus infection invading the pleura. Thorax 1981;36:745-51.

324. Wex P, Utta E, Drozdz W. Surgical treatment of pulmonary and pleuro-pulmonary Aspergillus disease. Thorac Cardiovasc Surg 1993;41:64-70.

325. Blastomycosis Cooperative Study of the Veterans Administration: Blastomycosis. A review of 198 collected cases in Veterans Administration: Hospitals. Am Rev Respir Dis 1964;89:659-72.

326. Cush R, Light RW, George RB. Clinical and roentgenographic manifestations of acute and chronic blastomycosis. Chest 1976;69:345-49.

327. Sarosi GA, Davis SF. Blastomycosis. Am Rev Respir Dis 1979;120:911-38.

328. Salyer WR, Salyer DC. Pleural involvement in cryptococcosis. Chest 1974;66:139-40.

329. Chechani V, Kamholz SL. Pulmonary manifestations of disseminated cryptococcosis in patients with AIDS. Chest 1990;98:1060-65.

330. Epstein R, Cole R, hunt KK Jr. Pleural effusion secondary to pulmonary cryptococcosis. Chest 1972;61:296-98.

331. Cadranel JL, Chouaid C, Denis M, et al. Causes of pleural effusion in 75 HIV-infected patients. Chest 1993;104:655.

332. Lonky SA, Catanzaro A, Moser KM, Einstein H. Acute coccidiodal pleural effusion. Am Rev Respir Dis 1976;114:681-88.

333. Drutz DJ, Catanzaro A. Coccidioidomycosis. Am Rev Respir Dis 1978;117:727-71.

334. Pinkney L, Parker BR. Primary coccidioidomycosis in children presenting with massive pleural effusion. Am Rev Respir Dis 1979;120:1393-97.

335. Cunningham RT, Einstein H. Coccidioidal pulmonary cavities with rupture. J Thorac Cardiovasc Surg 1982;84:172-77.

336. Goodwin RA Jr, DesPrez RM. Histoplasmosis. Am Rev Respir Dis 1978;117:929-56.

337. Randhawa HS, Khan ZU. Histoplasmosis in India: Current status. Ind J Chest Dis All Sc 1994;36:193-214.

338. Connel JV Jr, Muhm JR. Radiographic manifestations of pulmonary histoplasmosis: A 10 years review. Radiology 1976;121:281-85.

339. Brewer Pl, Himmelwright JP. Pleural effusion due to infection with *Histoplasma capsulatum*. Chest 1970;58:76-79.

340. Barrett-Conner E. Parasitic pulmonary disease. Am Rev Respir Dis 1982;126:558-63.

341. Ibarra-Perez C. Thoracic complications of amoebic abscess of liver: Report of 501 cases. Chest 1981;79: 672-76.

342. Reed SL. Amebiasis: An update. Clin Infect Dis 1992;14:385-93.

343. Lyche KD, Jensen WA, Kirsch CM, et al. Pleuropulmonary manifestations of hepatic amebiasis. West J Med 1990;153:275-8.

344. Sharma OP, Maheswari A. Lung diseases in the tropics. Part 2: Common tropical lung diseases. Diagnosis and management. Tubercle Lung Dis 1993;74:359-70.

345. Verghese M, Eggleston FC, Handa AK, Singh CM. Management of thoracic amoebiasis. J Thorac Cardiovasc Surg 1979;78:757-60.

346. Rakower J, Milwidsky H. Hydatid pleural disease. Am Rev Respir Dis 1964;90:623-31.

347. Agarwal RL, Jain SK, Gupta Sc, Agarwal DK, Ahmed KR, Nandi D. Hydropneumothorax secondary to hydatid lung disease. Ind J Chest Dis All Sc 1993;35: 93-96.

348. von Sinner WN. Ultrasound, CT, and MRI of ruptured and disseminated hydatid cysts. Eur J Radiol 1990;11: 31-37.

349. Jerry M, Benzarti M, Garrouche A, Klabi N, Hayouni A. Hydatid disease of the lung. Am Rev Respir Dis 1992;146:185-89.

350. Xanthakis DS, Katsaras E, Efthimiadis, et al. hydatid cyst of the liver with intrathoracic rupture. Thorax 1981; 36:497-501.

351. Jacobson ES. A case of secondary echinococcosis diagnosed by cytologic examination of pleural fluid and needle biopsy of pleura. Acta Cytol 1973;17:76-79.

352. Yacobian HD. Thoracic problems associated with hydatid cyst of the dome of the liver. Surgery 1976;79: 544-48.

353. Yokogawa M, Kojima S, Araki K, et al. Immunoglobulin E: Raised levels in sera and pleural exudates of patients with paragonimiasis. Am J Trop Med Hyg 1976;25: 581-86.

354. Eikas J, Kim PK. Clinical investigation of paragonimiasis. Acta Tuberc Scand 1960;39:140-47.

355. Im JG, Whang HY, Kim WS, Han MC, Shim YS, Cho SY. Pleuropulmonary paragonimiasis: Radiologic findings in 71 patients. AJR 1992;159:39-43.

356. Ikeda T, Oikawa Y, Owhashi M, Nawa Y. Parasitic specific IgE and IgG levels in the serum and pleural effusion of Paragonimiasis westermanii patients. Am J Trop Med Hyg 1992;47:104-07.

357. Singh YI, Singh NB, Devi S, Mohan Y, Razaque M. Pulmonary paragonimiasis in Manipur. Ind J Chest Dis All Sc 1982;24:304-06.

358. Singh NB, Singh KC. Pulmonary paragonimiasis in childhood: A cause of recurrent haemoptysis and pneumonia. Ind J Chest Dis All Sc 1989;31:211-5.

359. Seth GP, Mukherjee S. Filarial, pleurisy with effusion. Ind J Chest Dis 1969;9:213-17.

360. Arora VK, Gowrinath K. Pleural effusion due to lymphatic filariasis. Ind J Chest Dis All Sc 1994;36:159-61.

361. Singh RSJ, Sridhar MS, Bhaskar CJ. Tropical pulmonary eosinophilia presenting as eosinophilic pleural effusion. Ind J Chest Dis All Sc 1992;34:225-29.

362. Shrivastva MP, Grover AK, Madhu SV, Pandey ON, Arora VK. Filarial pleural effusion with constrictive pericarditis. Ind J Chest Dis All Sc 1994;36:87-90.

363. Walzer PD, Rutherford I, East R. Empyema with trichomonas species. Am Rev Respir Dis 1978;118:415-18.

364. Klion AD, Einstein EM, Smirniotopoulos TT, Neumann MP, Nutman TB. Pulmonary involvement in loiasis. Am Rev Respir Dis 1992;145:961-63.

365. Morrissey R, Caso R. Pleural sporotrichosis. Chest 1983;84:507.

366. Meyer PC. Metastatic carcinoma of the pleura. Thorax 1966;21:427-33.

367. Sahn SA. Malignant pleural effusions. Clin Chest Med 1985;6:113.

368. Sahn SA. Malignant pleural effusions. Semin Respir Med 1987;9:43

369. Hausheer FH, Yarbo JW. Diagnosis and treatment of malignant pleural effusion. Semin Oncol 1985;12:54.

370. Leff a, Hopewell PC, Costello J. Pleural effusion from malignancy. Ann Intern Med 1978;88:532.

371. Boutin C, Viallat JR, Cargnino P, Farisse P. Thoracoscopy in malignant effusions. Am Rev Respir Dis 1981;124:588.

372. McKenna JA, Chandrasekhar AJ, Henkin RE. Diagnostic value of carcinoembryonic antigen in exudative pleural effusions. Chest 1980;78:587.

373. Gravelyn TR, Michelson MK, Gross BH, Sitrin RG. Tetracycline pleurodesis for malignant pleural effusions. A 10 years retrospective study. Cancer 1987;59:1973.

374. Anderson CB, Philpott GW, Ferguson TB. The treatment of malignant pleural effusions. Cancer 1974; 33:916.

375. Millar JW, Hunter AM, Horne NW. Intrapleural immunotherapy with *Corynobacterium* parvum in recurrent malignant pleural effusions. Thorax 1979; 35:856.

376. Rosso R, Rimoldi R, Salvati L, et al. Intrapleural natural beta interferon in the treatment of malignant pleural effusions. Oncology 1988;45:253.

377. Martini N, Bains MS, Beattie EJ. Indications for pleurectomy in malignant effusion. Cancer 1975;35:734.

378. Tattersfield MHN, Boyer MJ. Management of malignant pleural effusions. Thorax 1990;45:81.

379. Johnston WW. The malignant pleural effusion: A review of cytopathologic diagnoses of 584 specimens from 472 consecutive patients. Cancer 1985;56:905-09.

380. Cohen S, Hossain S. Primary carcinoma of the lung: A review of 417 histologically proved cases. Dis Chest 1966;49:67-73.

381. Jindal SK, Behera D. Clinical spectrum of primary lung cancer: Review of Chandigarh experience of 10 years. Lung India 1990;8:94-98.

382. Chernow B, Sahn SA. Carcinomatous involvement of pleura. Am J Med 1977;63:695-702.

383. Fracchia AA, Knapper WH, Carey JT, Farrow JH. Intrapleural chemotherapy for effusion from metastatic breast carcinoma. Cancer 1970;26:626-29.

384. Goldsmith HS, Bailey HD, Callahan EL, Beattie EJ Jr. Pulmonary lymphangitic metastases from breast carcinoma. Arch Surg 1967;94:483-88.

385. Banerjee AK, Willetts I, Robertson JF, Blamey RW. Pleural effusion in breast cancer: A review of the Nottingham experience. Eur J Surg Oncol 1994;20:33-36.

386. Raju RN, Kardinal CG. Pleural effusion in breast carcinoma: Analysis of 122 cases. Cancer 1981;48:2524-27.

387. Rodriguez-Panadero F, Borderas NF, Lopez MJ. Pleural metastatic tumors and effusions. frequency and pathogenic mechanisms in a postmortem series. Eur Respir J 1989;2:366-69.

388. Mahr GG, Berger HW. Massive pleural effusion: Malignant and non-malignant causes in 46 patients. Am Rev Respir Dis 1972;105:458-60.

389. Light RW, Erozan YS, Ball WC. Cells in pleural fluid: Their value in differential diagnosis. Arch Intern Med 1973;132:854-60.

390. Prakash URS, Reiman HM. Comparison of needle biopsy with cytologic analysis for the evaluation of pleural effusion: Analysis of 414 cases. Mayo Clin Proc 1985;60:158-64.

391. Scrbo J, Keltz H, Stone DJ. A prospective study of closed pleural biopsies. JAMA 1971;218:377-80.

392. von Hoff DD, Livolsi V. Diagnostic reliability of needle biopsy of the parietal pleura. Am J Clin Pathol 1975;64:200-03.

393. Kavuru MS, Tubbs R, Miller ML, Wiedmann HP. Immunocytometry and gene re-arrangement analysis in the diagnosis of lymphoma in an idiopathic pleural effusion. Am Rev Respir Dis 1992;145:209-11.

394. Light RW. Pleural diseases (4th edn), Lippincott Williams & Wilkins. Philadelphia, PA: 2001;108-34.

395. McLoud TC, Flower CDR. Imaging the pleura: Sonography, CT, MR imaging. AJR Am J Roentgenol 1991;156,1145-53.

396. Yang PC, Luh KT, Chang DB, et al. Value of sonography in determining the nature of pleural effusion: Analysis of 320 cases. AJR Am J Roentgenol 1992;159, 29-33.

397. Bithell TC. Blood coagulation. In Lee GR Bithell, TC Foerster J, et al (Eds): Wintrobe's clinical hematology (9th edn). 1993,566-615 Lea and Febiger. Philadelphia, PA.

398. Agrenius V, Chmielewska J, Widström O, et al. Pleural fibrinolytic activity is decreased in inflammation as demonstrated in quinacrine pleurodesis treatment of malignant effusion. Am Rev Respir Dis 1989;140,1381-85.

399. Agrenius V, Gustafsson LE, Widström O. Tumor necrosis factor-α and nitric oxide, determined as nitrate, in malignant pleural effusion. Respir Med 1994;88, 743-48.

400. Agrenius V, Ukale V, Widström O, et al. Quinacrine-induced pleural inflammation in malignant pleurisy: Relation between drainage time of pleural fluid and local interleukin-1β. Respiration 1993;60,366-72.

401. Chung CI, Chen YC, Chang SC. Effect of repeated thoracenteses on fluid characteristics, cytokines, and fibrinolytic activity in malignant pleural effusion. Chest 2003;123:1188-95.

402. Robinson GR II, Gleeson K. Diagnostic flexible fiberoptic pleuroscopy in suspected malignant pleural effusions. Chest 1995;107:424-29.

403. Sahn SA, Good TJ. Pleural fluid pH in malignant effusions. Ann Intern Med 1988;108:345-49.

404. Rodriquez-Panadero F, Lopez-Mezias J. Survival time of patients with pleural metastatic carcinoma predicted by glucose and pH studies. Chest 1989;95:320-25.

405. Rodriquez-Panadero F, Lopez-Mezias J. Low glucose and pH levels in malignant pleural effusions. Am Rev Respir Dis 1989;139:663-67.

406. Waller DA, Morritt GN, Forty J. Video-assisted thoracoscopic pleurectomy in the management of malignant pleural effusion. Chest 1995;107:1454-56.

407. Kennedy L, Sahn SA. The pleurodesis for the treatment of pneumothorax and pleural effusion. Chest 1994;106:1215-22.

408. Harris RJ, Kavuru MS, Mehta AC, et al. The impact of thoracoscopy in the management of pleural diseases. Chest 1995;107:845-52.

409. Kennedy L, Vaughan LM, Steed LL, Sahn SA. Sterilization of talc for pleurodesis: Available techniques, efficacy and cost analysis. Chest 1995;107:1032-34.

410. Light RW, Wang NS, Sasson CSH, et al. Talc slurry is an effective pleural sclerosant in rabbits. Chest 1995;107:1702-06.

411. Kennedy L, Harley RA, Sahn SA. Talc slurry pleurodesis: Pleural fluid and histologic analysis. Chest 1995;107:1707-12.

412. Guzman C, Quijada C. Tetracycline pleurodesis. Chest 1993;103:984.

413. Costabel U. Adieu, tetracycline pleurodesis (but not in Germany). Chest 1993;103:984.

414. De Vries BC, Bitran JD. On the management of malignant pleural effusions. Chest 1994;105:1-2.

415. Hurewitz AN, Wu CL, Mancuso P, Zucker S. Tetracycline and doxycycline inhibit pleural fluid metalloproteinasess a possible mechanism for chemical pleurodesis. Chest 1993;103:1113-17.

416. Hurewitz AN, Lidonicci K, Liang C, et al. Histologic changes of doxycycline pleurodesis in rabbits: Effect of concentration and pH. Chest 1994;106:1241-45.

417. Vargas FS, Telxeira LR, Coehlo IJC, et al. Distribution of pleural injectate: Effect of volume injectate and animal rotation. Chest 1994;106:1246-49.

418. Vargas FS, Milanez JRC, Felomeno LTB, Fernadez A, Jatene A, Light RW. Intrapleural talc for the prevention of recurrence in benign or undiagnosed pleural effusions. Chest 1994;106:1771-75.

419. Light RW, Sassoon VCSH, Vargas FS, Gruer SE, Despars JA, Wang NS. Comparison of the effectiveness of tetracycline and minocycline as pleural sclerosing agents in rabbits. Am Rev Respir Dis 1992;145:A868.

420. Kitamura S, Sugiyama Y, Izumi T, Hayashi R, Kosaka K. Intrapleural doxycycline for control of malignant pleural effusion. Curr Thera Res 1981;30:515-21.

421. Mansson T. Treatment of malignant pleural effusion with doxycycline. Scand J Infect Dis 1988;53:29-34.

422. Sudduth CD, Sahn SA. Pleurodesis for nonmalignant pleuraleffusions. recommendations. Chest 1992;102:1855-60.

423. Feletti R, Ravazonni C. Intrapleural *Corynebacterium parvum* for malignant pleural effusion. Thorax 1983;38:22-24.

424. Hillerdal G, Kiviloog J, Nou E, Steinholtz L. *Corynebacterium parvum* in malignant pleural effusion: A randomized prospective study. Eur J Respir Dis 1986;69:204-06.

425. Rosso R, Rimoldi R, Salvati F, et al. Intrapleural natural beta interferon in the treatment of malignant pleural effusions. Oncology 1988;45:253-56.

426. Bhatia A, Rice TW, McLain D, et al. A phase I trial of intrapleural recombinant human interferon alpha (rHuINFalpha 2b) in patients with malignant pleural effusions. J Cancer Res Clin Oncol 1994;120:169-72.

427. Luh KT, Yang PC, Kuo SH, Chang DB, Yu CJ, Lee LN. Comparison of OK-432 and mitomycin C pleurodesis for malignant pleural effusion caused by lung cancer. a randomized trial. Cancer 1992;69:674-79.

428. Ike O, Shimizu Y, Hitomi S, Wada R, Ikada Y. Treatment of malignant pleural effusions with doxorubicin hydrochloride containing poly(L-lactic acid) microspheres. Chest 1991;99:911-15.

429. Liu X, Li d, Zhang C, et al. Treatment of 121 patients with malignant effusion due to advanced lung cancer by intrapleural transfer of autologous or allogenic LAK cells combined with rIL-2. Chinese Med Sc J 1993;8:186-89.

430. Yashumoto K, Mivazaki K, Nagishma A, et al. Induction of lymphokin-activated killer cells by intrapleural instillation of recombinant interleukin-2 in patients with malignant pleurisy due to lung cancer. Cancer Res 1987;47:2184-87.

431. Pectasides D, Stewart S, Courtenay LN, et al. Antibody-guided irradiation of malignant pleural and pericardial effusions. Br J Cancer 1986;53:727-32.

432. Jensen MO, Matthees DJ, Antonenko D. Laser thoracoscopy for pleural effusion. Am Surg 1992;58:667-69.

433. Astoul P, Viallat JR, Laurent JC, Brandely MB, Boutin C. Intrapleural recombinant IL-2 in passive immunotherapy for malignant pleural effusion. Chest 1993;103:209-13.

434. Walter DA, Morritt GN, Forty J. Video-assisted thoracoscopic pleurectomy in the management of malignant pleural effusion. Chest 1995;107:1454-56.

435. Blank N, Castellino RA. The intrathoracic manifestations of the malignant lymphomas and leukaemia. Semin Roentgenol 1980;12:227-45.

436. Xaubet A, Diumenzo MC, Marin A, et al. Characteristics and prognostic value of pleural effusions in non-Hodgkin's lymphomas. Eur J Respir Dis 1985;66:135-40.

437. Wong FM, Grace WJ, Rottino A. Pleural effusions, ascites, pericardial effusions, and oedema in Hodgkin's disease. Am J Med Sci 1963;246:678-82.

438. Weick JK, Kieley JM, Harisson EG Jr, Carr DT, Scanlon PW. Pleural effusion in lymphoma. Cancer 1973;31:848-53.

439. Sahn SA. Malignant pleural effusions. In: Fishan A (Ed): Pulmonary diseases and disorders (2nd edn). New York, Mcgraw Hill.

440. Vieta JO, Craver LF. Intrathoracic manifestations of the lymphomatoid diseases. Radiology 1941;37:138-58.

441. van de Molengraft FJ, Vooijs GP. The interval between the diagnosis of malignancy and the development of effusions with reference to the role of cytological diagnosis. Acta Cytol 1988;32:183-87.

442. Jenkins PF, Ward MJ, Davies P, Fletcher J. Non-Hodgkin's lymphoma, chronic lymphatic leukaemia and the lung. Br J Dis Chest 1981;75:22-30.

443. Stolberg HO, Patt NL, MacEwen KF, et al. Hodgkin's disease of the lung: Roentgenologic-pathologic correlation. AJR 1964;92:96-115.

444. Staats BA, Ellefson RD, Budahn LL, et al. The lipoprotein profile of chylous and nonchylous pleural effusions. Mayo Clin Proc 1980;55:700-04.

445. Celikoglu F, Teirstein AS, Krellenstein DJ, Strauchen JA. Pleural effusion in non-Hodgkin's lymphoma. Chest 1992;101:1357-60.

446. Melamed MR. The cytological presentation of malignant lymphomas and related diseases in effusions. Cancer 1963;16:413-31.

447. Antman KH. Clinical presentation and natural history of benign and malignant mesothelioma. Semin Oncol 1981;8:313-20.

448. Branscheid D, Krysa S, Bauer E, Bulzebruck H, Schirren J. Diagnostic and therapeutic strategy in malignant pleural mesothelioma. Br J Cardiothorac Surg 1991;5: 466-72.

449. Pisani RJ, Colby TV, Williams DE. Malignant mesotheliomas of the pleura. Mayo Clin Proc 1988;68:1234-44.

450. Kawashima A, Libsitz HI. Malignant pleural mesothelioma: CT manifestations in 50 cases. Am J Roentgenol 1990;155:965-69.

451. Kreel L. Computed tomography in mesothelioma. Semin Oncol 1981;8:302-12.

452. Gottehrer A, Taryle DA, Reed CF, Sahn SA. Pleural fluid analysis in malignant mesothelioma. Chest 1991;100:1003-06.

453. Law MR, Hodson ME, Turner-Warwick M. Malignant mesothelioma of the pleura. Clinical aspects and symptomatic management. Eur J Respir Dis 1984;65:162-68.

454. Stevens MW, Leong AS, Fazzalari NL, Dowling KD, Henderson DW. Cytopathology of malignant mesothelioma.: A stepwise logistic regression analysis. Diag Cytopathol 1992;8:333-42.

455. Menzies R, Charbonneau M. Thoracoscopy for the diagnosis of pleural diseases. Ann Intern Med 1991;114: 271-76.

456. Hucker J, Bhatnagar NK, Al-Jilaihawi AN, Forrester-wood CP. Thoracoscopy in the diagnosis and management of recurrent pleural effusions. Ann Thorac Surg 1991;52:1145-47.

457. Boutin C, Rey F. thoracoscopy in pleural malignant mesothelioma:a prospective study of 188 consecutive patients. Part I.: Diagnosis. Cancer 1993;72:389-93.

458. Oels HC, Harrison EG, Carr DT, Bernatz PE. Diffuse malignant mesothelioma of the pleura; A review of 37 cases. Chest 1971;60:564-70.

459. Legha S, Muggia FM. Pleural mesothelioma: Clinical features and therapeutic implications. Ann Intern Med 1977;87:613.

460. Talbott JA, Calkins E. Pulmonary involvement in rheumatoid arthritis. JAMA 1964;189:911.

461. Horler AR, Thompson M. The pleural and pulmonary complications of rheumatoid arthritis. Ann Intern Med 1959;51:1179-203.

462. Lillington GA, Carr DT, Mayne JG. Rheumatoid pleurisy with effusion. Arch Intern Med 1971;128:764-68.

463. Nosanchuk JS, Naylor B. A unique cytologic picture in pleural fluid from patients with rheumatoid arthritis. Am J Clin Pathol 1968;50:330.

464. Alarcon-Segovia D, Alarcon DG. Pleuropulmonary manifestations of systemic lupus erythematosus. Dis Chest 1961;39:7-17.

465. Reda MG, Baigelman W. Pleural effusion in systemic lupus erythematosus. Acta Cytol 1980;24:553.

466. Dressler W. The postmyocardial infarction syndrome: A report of 44 cases. Arch Intern Med 1959;103:28-42.

467. Stelzner TJ, King TE Jr, Antony VB, Sahn SA. The pleuropulmonary manifestations of the post-cardiac injury syndrome. Chest 1983;84:383.

468. Fauci AS, Wolff SM. Wegener's granulomatosis: Studies in 18 patients and review of literature. Medicine 1973;52:535.

469. Bambery P, Sakhuja V, Behera D, Deodhar SD. Pleural effusion in Wegener's granulomatosis. Report of five cases and a brief review of literature. Scand J Rheumatol 1991;20:445.

470. Strimlan CV, Rosenow EC, Divertie MB, Harrison EG. Pulmonary manifestations of Sjögren's syndrome. Chest 1976;70:354.

471. Chusid EL, Siltzbach LE. Sarcoidosis of the pleura. Ann Intern Med 1974;81:190.

472. Beekman JF, Zimmet SM, Chun BK, Mirranda AA, Katz S. Spectrum of pleural involvement sarcoidosis. Arch Intern Med 1976;136:323.

473. Harvey AM, Shulman LE, Tumulty PA, et al. Systemic lupus erythematosus. review of literature and clinical analysis of 138 cases. Medicine 1954;33:291-37.

474. Winslow WA, Ploss LN, Loitman B. Pleuritis in systemic lupus erythematosus: Its importance as an early manifestation in diagnosis. Ann Intern Med 1958;49: 70-88.

475. Purnell DC, Baggenstoss AH, Olsen AM. Pulmonary lesions in disseminated systemic lupus erythematosus. Ann Intern Med 1955;42:619-28.

476. Gueft B, Laufer A. Further cytochemical studies in systemic lupus erythematosus. Arch Pathol 1954;57: 201-26.

477. Halla JT, Schronhenloher RE, Volanakis JE. Immune complexes and other laboratory features of pleural effusions. Ann Intern Med 1980;92:748-52.

478. Naylor B. Cytological aspects of pleural, peritoneal and pericardial fluids from patients with systemic lupus erythematosus. Cytopathology 1992;3:1-8.

479. Carel RS, Shapiro MS, Shoham D, Gutman A. Lupus erythematosus cells in pleural effusion. Chest 1977; 72:670-72.

480. Leechawengwong M, Berger HW, Sukumaran M. Diagnostic significance of antinuclear antibodies in pleural effusion. Mt Sinai J Med 1979,46:137-39.

481. Khare V, Baethge B, Lang S, Wolf RE, Campbell D Jr. Antinuclear antibodies in pleural fluid. Chest 1994; 106:866-71.

482. Pertschuk LP, Moccia LF, Rosen Y, et al. Acute pulmonary complications in systemic lupus erythematosus. Immunofluorescence and light microscopic study. Am J Clin Pathol 1977;68:553-57.

483. Andrews BS, Arora NS, Shadforth MF, et al. The role of immunecomplexes in the pathogenesis of pleural effusions. Am Rev Respir Dis 1981;124:115-20.

484. Hunder GG, McDuffie FC, Hepper NGG. Pleural fluid complement in systemic lupus erythematosus and rheumatoid arthritis. Ann Intern Med 1972;76:357-62.
485. Walker WC, Wright V. Rheumatoid pleuritis. Ann Rheum Dis 1967;26:467-74.
486. Faurschou P, Francis D, Faarup P. Thoracoscopic, histological, and clinical findings in nine cases of rheumatoid pleural effusion. Thorax 1985;40:371-75.
487. Feagler JR, Sorensen JD, Rosenfeld MG, Osterland CK. Rheumatoid pleural effusion. Arch Pathol 1971;92:257-66.
488. Ferguson GC. Cholesterol pleural effusion in rheumatoid lung disease. Thorax 1966;21:577-82.
489. Halla JT, Schronhenloher RE, Volanakis JE. Immune complexes and other laboratory features of pleural effusions. Ann Intern Med 1980;92:748-52.
490. Naylor B. The pathognomonic cytologic picture of rheumatoid pleuritis. Acta Cytol 1990;34:465-73.
491. Sahn SA. Immunological diseases of the pleura. Clin Chest Med 1985;6:103-12.
492. Strimlan CV, Rosenow AC, Divertie MG, Harrison EG. Pulmonary manifestations of Sjögren's syndrome. Chest 1976;70:354-61.
493. Bloch KJ, Buchanan WW, Wohl MJ, Bunim JJ. Sjögren's syndrome. Medicine 1965;44:187-31.
494. Miller KS. Drug induced pleural disease. Semin Respir Med 1987;9:86.
495. Harpey JP. Lupus like syndrome induced by drugs. Ann Allergy 1974;33;256-61.
496. Hailey FJ, Glascock HW Jr, Hewitt WF. Pleuropulmonary reactions to nitrofurantoin. N Engl J Med 1969;281:1087-90.
497. Holmberg L, Boman G. Pulmonary complications to nitrofurantoin: 447 cases reported to the Sweden adverse drug reaction committee, 1966-1976. Eur J Respir Dis 1981;62:180-89.
498. Petusevsky ML, Faling LJ, Rocklin RE, et al. Pleuropericardial reaction to treatment with antrolene. JAMA 1979;242:2772-74.
499. Graham JR. Cardiac and pulmonary fibrosis during methysergide therapy for headache. Am J Med Sci 1967;254:1-12.
500. Jones SE, Moore M, Blank N, Castellino RA. Hypersensitivity to procarbazine (Matulane) manifested by fever and pleuropulmonary reaction. Cancer 1972;29:498-500.
501. Ecker MD, Jay B, Keohane MF. Procarbazine lung. Am J Radiol 1978;131:527-28.
502. Everts CS, Westcott JL, Bragg DG. Methotrexate therapy and pulmonary disease. Radiology 1973;107:539.
503. Rinne UK. Pleuropulmonary changes during long term bromocriptine treatment for Parkinson's disease. Lancet 1981;1:44.
504. Dyer NH, Varley CC. Practolol induced pleurisy and constrictive pericarditis. Br Med J 1975;1:443.
505. Rakita L, Sobol SM, Mostow N, Vrobel T. Amiodarone pulmonary toxicity. Am Heart J 1983;106:906.
506. Gunstream SR, Seidenfeld JJ, Sobonya RE, McMohan LJ. Mitomycin-associated lung disease. Cancer Treat Rep 1983;67:301-04.
507. Webb DB, Whale RJ. Pleuropericardial effusion associated with minoxidil administration. Postgrad Med J 1982;58:319.
508. Middleton KL, Santella R, Couser JI. Eosinophilic pleuritis due to propylthiouracil. Chest 1995;103:955-56.
509. Khan AH. The post cardiac injury syndromes. Clin Cardiol 1992;15:67-72.
510. Wiener-Kronish JP. Postoperative pleural and pulmonary abnormalities in patients undergoing coronary artery bypass grafts. Chest 1992;102:1313-14.
511. Vargas FS, Cukier A, Terra-Fihlo M, et al. Relationship between pleural changes after myocardial revascularization and pulmonary mechanics. Chest 1992;102:1333-36.
512. DeMeester TR. Perforation of the oesophagus. Ann Thorac Surg 1986;42:231-32.
513. O'Connell ND. Spontaneous rupture of the oesophagus. Am J Roentgenol 1967;99;186.
514. Maultiz RM, Good JT Jr, Kaplan RL, Reller LB, Sahn SA. The pleuropulmonary complications of oesophageal rupture: an experimental model. Am Rev Respir Dis 1979;120:363.
515. Abbott OA, Mansour KA, Logan WD Jr, Hatcher CR Jr, Symbas PN. Atraumatic so-called "spontaneous" rupture of the oesophagus. J Thorac Cardiovasc Surg 1970;59:67-83.
516. Michel I, Grillo HC, Malt RA. Operative and non-operative management of oesophageal perforations. Ann Surg 1981;194:57-63.
517. Bladergroen MR, Lowe JE, Postlethwait RW. Diagnosis and recommended management of oesophageal perforations and rupture. Ann Thorac Surg 1986;42:235-39.
518. Graeber GM, Niezgoda JA, Albus RA, et al. A comparison of patients with endoscopic esophageal perforations and patients with Boerhaave's syndrome. Chest 1987;92:995-98.
519. Jenkins IR, Raymond R. Boerhaave's syndrome complicated by a large bronchopleural fistula. Chest 1994;105:964-65.
520. Drury M, Anderson W, Heffner JE. Diagnostic value of pleural fluid cytology in occult Boerhaave's syndrome. Chest 1992;102:976-78.
521. Vander Sluis RF. Subphrenic abscess. Surg Gynaecol Obstet 1984;158:427-30.
522. Sarr MG, Zuidema GD. Splenic abscess-presentation, diagnosis, and treatment. Surgery 1982;92:480.
523. Carter R, Brewer LA. Subphrenic abscess: A thoraco-abdominal clinical complex. Am J Surg 1964;108:165-74.
524. deCosse JJ, Poulin TI, Fox PS, Condon RE. Subphrenic Abscess. Surg Gynaecol Obstet 1974;138:841-46.

525. Sanders RC. Post-operative pleural effusion and subphrenic abscess. Clin Radiol 1970;21:308-12.

526. Katsilabros L, Triandafillou G, Kontoytannis P, Katsilabros N. Pleural effusion and hepatitis. Gastroenterology. 1972;63:718.

527. Gross PA, Gerding DN. Pleural effusion associated with viral hepatitis. Gastroenterology 1971;60:898-902.

528. Cocchi P, Silenzi M. Pleural effusion in HBsAg-positive hepatitis. J Paediatr 1976;89:329-30.

529. Tabor L, Russel RP, Gerety RJ, et al. Hepatitis B surface antigen and e antigen in pleural effusion—A case report. Gastroenterology 1977;73:1157-59.

530. Haskal ZJ, Zuckerman J. Resolution of hepatic hydrothorax after transjugular intrahepatic portosystemic shunt. Chest 1994;106:1293-94.

531. Kaye MD. Pleuropulmonary complication of pancreatitis. Thorax 1968;23:297-306.

532. Gumaste V, Singh V, Dave P. Significance of pleural effusion in patients with acute pancreatitis. Am J Gastroenterol 1992;87:871-74.

533. Rockey DC, Cello JP. Pancreaticopleural fistula. Report of 7 cases and review of literature. Medicine 1990;69:332-34.

534. Tombroff M, Loicq A, Dekoster JP, et al. Pleural effusion with pancreatico pleural fistula. Br Med J 1973;1:330-31.

535. Anderson WJ, Skinner DB, Zuidema GD, Cameron DL. Chronic pancreatic pleural effusions. Urg Gynecol Obstet 1973;137:827-30.

536. Hayes JP, Wiggins J, Ward K, Muldowney F, Fitzgerald MX. Familial cryptogenic fibrosing pleuritis with Fanconi's syndrome (renal tubular acidosis): A new syndrome. Chest 1995;107:876-78.

537. Bower GC. Chylothorax: Observations in 20 cases. Dis Chest 1964;46:464-8.

538. Williams KR, Burford TH. The management of chylothorax. Ann Surg 1964;160:131-40.

539. Staats BA, Ellefson RW, Budahn LL, et al. The lipoprotein profile of chylous and non-chylous pleural effusions. Mayo Clin Proc 1980;55:700-04.

540. Roy PH, Carr DT, Payne WS. The problem of chylothorax. Mayo Clin Proc 1967;42:457-67.

541. Bresser P, Kromhout JG, Reekers JA, Verhage TL. Chylous pleural effusion associated with primary lymphedema and lymphangioma-like malformations. Chest 1993;103:1916-18.

542. Mason PF, Thorpe JAC. Chylothorax—A new surgical strategy. Chest 1993;103:1929.

543. Rosenblum HM, Schrader JB. Chylothorax due to benign lymphangioma. Chest 1992;101:1737.

544. Delgado C, Martin M, de la Portilla F. Retrosternal goiter associated with chylothorax. Chest 1994;106:1924-25.

545. Strausser JL, Flye MW. Management of non-traumatic chylothorax. Ann Thorac Surg 1981;31:520-26.

546. Chernick V, Reed MH. Pneumothorax and chylothorax in the neonatal period. J Pediatr 1970;76:624-32.

547. Teba L, Dedhia HV, Bowen R, Alexander JC. Chylothorax review. Crit Care Med 1985;13:49-52.

548. Hughes RL, Mintzer RA, Hidvegi DF, et al. The management of chylothorax. Chest 1979;76:212-18.

549. Zoetmulder FAN, Rutgers EJT, Bass P. Thoracoscopic ligation of a thoracic duct leakage. Chest 1992;106:1233-34.

550. Tie MLH, Poland GA, Rosenow EC III. Chylothorax in Gorham's syndrome. A common complication of a rare disease. Chest 1994;105:208-13.

551. Valentine VG, Raffin TA. The management of chylothorax. Chest 1992;102:586-91.

552. Coe JE, Aikawa JK. Cholesterol pleural effusion. Arch Int Med 1961;108:763-74.

553. Emerson PA, Yellow nails, lymphedema and pleural effusion. Thorax 1966;21:247-53.

554. Pavlidakey GP, Hashimoto. K, Blum Blum D. Yellow nail syndrome. J Am Acad Dermatol 1984;11:509-12.

555. Silverstein EF, Ellis K, Wolff M, Jaretzki A. Pulmonary lymphangiomyomatosis. AJR 1974;120:832-50.

556. Corrin B, Leibow AA, Friedman PJ. Pulmonary lymphangiomyomatosis. Am J Pathol 1975;79:348-67.

557. Carrington CB, Cugell DW, Gaenseler EA, et al. Lymphangioleiomyomatosis. Am Rev Respir Dis 1977;116:977-95.

558. Bynum LJ, Wilson JE III. Radiographic features of pleural effusions in pulmonary embolism. Am Rev Respir Dis 1978;117:829-34.

559. Worseley DF, Alavi A, Aronchick JM, Chen JTT, Greenspan RH, Ravin CE. Chest radiographic indings in patients with acute pulmonary embolism: Observations from the PIOPED study. Radiology 1993;189:133-36.

560. Stein PD, Athanasoulis C, Greenspan RH, Henry JW. Relation of plain chest radiographic findings to pulmonary arterial pressure and arterial blood oxygen levels in patients with acute pulmonary embolism. Am J Cardiolo 1992;69:394-96.

561. Storey DD, Dines De, Coles DT. Pleural effusion: A dilemma. JAMA 1976;236:2183-86.

562. Bynum LJ, Wilson JE III. Characteristics of pleural effusions associated with pulmonary embolism. Arch Int Med 1976;136:159-62.

563. Dalen JE. Pulmonary embolism, pulmonary haemorrhage and pulmonary infarction. N Engl J Med 1977;296:1431-34.

564. Meigs JV, Cass JW. Fibroma of the ovary with ascites and hydrothorax. Am J Obstet Gynecol 1937;33:249-67.

565. Meigs JV, Armstrong SH, Hamilton HH. A further contribution to the syndrome of fibroma of ovary with fluid in the abdomen and chest, Obstet Gynecol 1954;3:471-86.

566. Meigs JV. Pelvic tumors other than fibromas of ovary with ascites and hydrothorax. Obstet Gynecol 1954;3:471-86.

567. Meigs JV. Fibromas of the ovary with ascites and hydrothorax. Meig's syndrome. Am J Obstet Gynecol 1954;67:962-87.

568. Majzlin G, Stevens SL. Meig's syndrome: case report and review of literature. J Int Coll Surg 1964;42:625-30.

569. Epler GR, McLoud TC, Gaensler EA. Prevalence and incidence of benign asbestos pleural effusion in a working population. JAMA 1982;247:617-22.

570. Hillerdal G, Ozesmi M. Benign asbestos pleural effusion: 73 exudates in 60 patients. Eur Respir J 1987;71:113-21.

571. Gaensler EA, Kaplan AI. Asbestos pleural effusions. Ann Intern Med 1971;74:187.

572. Mattson SB. Monosymptomatic exudative pleurisy in persons exposed to asbestos dust. Scand J Respir Dis 1975;56:263-72.

573. Hopps HC, Wissler RW. Uremic pneumonitis. Am J Pathol 1955;31:261-73.

574. Nidus BD, Matalon R, Cantacuzino D, Eisinger RP. Uremic pleuritis: A clinicopathological entity. N Engl J Med 1969;281:255-56.

575. Berger HW, Rammohan G, Neff G, Buhain WJ. Uremic pleural effusion: A study in 14 ptients on chronic dialysis. Ann Intern Med 1975;82:362-64.

576. Galen MA, Steinberg SM, Lowrie EG, et al. Haemorrhagic pleural effusion in patients undergoing chronic haemodialysis. Ann Intern Med 1975;82:359-61.

577. Moore PJ, Thomas PA. The trapped lung with chronic pleural space, a cause of recurring pleural effusion. Milit Med 1967;132:998-1002.

578. Dernevik L, Gatzinsky P, Hultman E, Selin K, et al. Shrinking pleuritis with atelectasis. Thorax 1982;37:252.

579. Light RW, Jenkinson SG, Minh V, George RB. Observations on pleural pressure as fluid is withdrawn during thoracentesis. Am Rev Respir Dis 1980;121:799-804.

580. Bachman AL, Macken K. Pleural effusions following supervoltage radiation for breast carcinoma. Radiology 1959;72:699-709.

581. Fentanes de Torres E, Guevara E. Pleuritis by radiation. Acta Cytol 1981;25:427-29.

582. Whitecomb ME, Schwarz MI. Pleural effusion complicating intensive mediastinal radiation therapy. Am Rev Respir Dis 1971;103:100.

583. Bacon BR, Bailey-Newton RS, Connors AF Jr. Pleural effusions after endoscopic variceal sclerotherapy. Gastroenterology 1985;88:1910-14.

584. Miller KS, Tomilnson JR, Sahn SA. Pleuropulmonary complications of enteral tube feedings. Two reports, review of literature, and recommendations. Chest 1985;88:230-33.

585. Vaughan ED. Hazards associated with narrow-bore nasogastric tube feeding. Br J Oral Surg 1981;19:151-54.

586. Muthuswamy PP, Patel K, Rajendran R. "Isocal pneumonia" with respiratory failure. Chest 1982;81:390.

587. Medina LS, Siegel MJ, Bejarano PA, et al. Pediatric lung transplantation: Radiographic -histopathologic correlation. Radiology 1993;187:807-10.

588. Wilen SB, Rabinowitz JG, Ulreich S, Lyons HA. Pleural involvement in sarcoidosis. Am J Med 1974;57:200-09.

589. Sharma OP, Gordonson J. Pleural effusion in sarcoidosis: A report of six cases. Thorax 1975;30:95-101.

590. Hagay Z, Reece A, Roberts A, Hobbins JC. Isolated fetal pleural effusion; A prenatal management dilemma. Obstet Gynecol 1993;81:147-52.

591. Rizk B, Aboulghar M. Modern management of ovarian hyperstimulation syndrome. Human Reprod 1991; 6:1082-87.

592. Wallis MG, Mchugo JM, Carruthers DA, Selwyn CJ. The prevalence of the pleural effusions in pre-eclampsia: An ultrasound study. Br J Obstet Gynecol 1989;96:431-33.

593. Udeshi UL, Mchugo JM, Selwyn CJ. Postpartum pleural effusion. Br J Obstet Gynecol 1988;95:894-97.

594. Knapp MJ, Roggli VL, Kim J, et al. Pleural amyloidosis. Arch Pathol Lab Med 1988;112:57-60.

595. Graham DR, Ahmad D. Amyloidosis with pleural involvement. Eur Respir J 1988;1:571-72.

596. Kavuru MS, Adamo JP, Ahmad M, Mehta AC, Gephardt GN. Amyloidosis and pleural disease. Chest 1990;98:20-23.

597. Im JG, Chung JW, Han MC. Milk of calcium pleural collections: CT findings. J Comp Assist Tomography 1993;17:613-16.

598. Taglibue M, Casella TC, Zincone GE, Fumagalli R, Salvini E. CT and chest radiography in evaluation of adult respiratory distress syndrome. Acta Radiol 1994;35:230-34.

599. Hopkinson RB, Parkin CE. Hydrohemothorax following percutaneous internal jugular vein cannulation recognized by intravenous pyelography. Anesth Analg 1978;57:507-12

600. Holt S, Kirkman N, Myerscough E. Hemothorax after subclavian vein cannulation. Thorax 1977;32:101-03.

601. Hiraiwa T, Hayashi T, Kaneda M, et al. Rupture of a benign mediastinal teratoma into the right pleural cavity. Ann Thorac Surg 1991;51:110-32.

602. Impens N, Warson P, Roels P, Schandevyl W. A rare cause of pleurisy. Eur Respir Dis 1986;68:388-89.

603. Lababidi HMS, Gupta K, Newman T, Fuleihan FJD. A retrospective analysis of pleural effusion in human immunodeficiency virus infected patients. Chest 1994;106:86S.

604. Cadranel JL, Chouaid C, Denis M, Lebeau B, Akoun GM, Mayaud CM. Causes of pleural effusion in 75 HIV-infected patients. Chest 1993;104:655.

605. Batungwanayo J, Taelman H, Allen S, Bogaerts J, Kagame A, Van de Perre P. Pleural effusion, tuberculosis, and HIV-1 infection in Kigali, Rwanda. AIDS 1993; 7:73-79.

606. Gill V, Cordero PJ, Greses JV, Soler JJ. Pleural tuberculosis in HIV-infected patients. Chest 1995;107:1775.

607. Joseph J, Strange C, Sahn SA. Pleural effusions in hospitalized patients with AIDS. Ann Intern Med 1993;118:856-69.

608. Willsle-Ediger SK, Salzman GA, Reisz GR. Empyema thoracis. Chest 1992;101:1475-76.

609. Read CA, Sporn TA, Yeager H Jr. Parapneumonic empyema: A pitfall in diagnosis. Chest 1992;101: 1712-13.

610. Strange C, Sahn SA. The clinicians perspective on parapneumonic effusions and empyema. Chest 1993; 103:259-61.

611. Alfageme I, Munoj F, Pena N, Umbria S. Empyema of the thorax in adults: Aetiology, microbiological findings and management. Chest 1993;839-43.

612. Brook I, Frazier FH. Aerobic and anaerobic microbiology of empyema: A retrospective review in two military hospitals. Chest 1993;103:1502-07.

613. Singh RP, Katiyar SK, Singh KP. Conservative management of empyema thoracis and bronchopleural fistula. Ind J Chest Dis All Sc 1994;36:15-19.

614. Jha VK, Singh RB. Empyema of thorax. Ind J Chest Dis All Sc 1972;14:243-48.

615. Aggarwal SK, Ray DC, Jha N. Empyema thoracis: A review of 70 cases. Ind J Chest Dis All Sc 1985;27: 17-22.

616. Tandon RK, Patney NL, Srivastava VK, Wadhawan VP. Empyema thoracic in infancy and childhood. Ind J Chest Dis All Sc 1972;14:254-58.

617. Sarma K, Ramchandran V, Thoreja RN, Aga HM, Ahuja AM. Surgical excision of empyema. Id J Chest Dis All Sc 1972;14:249-53.

618. Jain SK, Mishra RM, Gupta RK, Aggarwal RL. Treatment of empyema thoracic by different conservative methods. Ind J Chest Dis All Sc 1981;23:134-47.

619. Tandon RK. Management of spontaneous bronchopleural fistula in children. Ind J Chest Dis All Sc 1974;16:108-12.

620. Raj B, Janmeja AK, Bihari K, Mittal RC, Chawla RK. Broncho-pleuro-biliary fistula - A rare manifestation of pleuropulmonary amobiasis. Ind J Chest Dis All Sc 1987;29:56-59.

621. Sharma TN, Jain NK, Madan A, Sarkar SK, Durlbhji P. Tubercular empyema thoracic: A diagnostic and therapeutic problem. Ind J Chest Dis All Sc 1983;25:127-31.

622. Gupta SK, Kishan J, Singh SP. Review of one hundred cases of empyema thoracis. Ind J Chest Dis All Sc 1989;31:15-20.

623. Singla R, Singh P, Bhagi RP, Singh PR. Pleuropulmonary complications of staphylococcal pulmonary infections in children. Ind J Chest Dis All Sc 1989;31:151-58.

624. Bartlett JG, Gorbach SL, Thadepalli H, Finegold SH. Bacteriology of empyema. Lancet 1974;1:338.

625. Varkey B, Rose HD, Kutty CPK, Politis J. Empyema thoracic during a ten-year period. Arch Intern Med 1981;141:1771.

626. Bartlett JG, Finegold SM. Anaerobic infection of the lung and pleural space. Am Rev Respir Dis 1974;110:56.

627. Samson PC. Empyema thoracic: Essentials of present day management. Ann Thorac Surg 1971;11:210.

628. Sherman MM, Subramanian V, Berger RL. Management of thoracic empyema. Am J Surg 1977;133:474.

629. Iseman MD, Madsen LA. Chronic tuberculous empyema with bronchopleural fistula resulting in treatment failure and progressive drug resistance. Chest 1991;100:124-27.

630. Swain JA. Empyema: An update on diagnosis and management. Pulmonary Perspectives. American College of Chest Physicians 1992;9:6.

631. Heffner J. A successful approach to empyema. Contemporary Int Med 1991; June:95.

632. Mill N, Auckenthaler R, Nicod LP. Chronic brucella empyema. Chest 1993;103:620-21.

633. American Thoracic Society. Management of nontuberculous empyema. Am Rev Respir Dis 1962;85:93.

634. Taryle DA, Potts DE, Sahn SA. The incidence and clinical correlates of parapneumonic ffusions in pneumococcal pneumonia. Chest 1978;74:170-3.

635. Van de Water JM. The treatment of pleural effusion complicating pneumonia. Chest 1970;57:259-62.

636. Weese WC, Shindler ER, Smith IM, Rabinovich S. Empyema of the thorax then and now. Arch Int Med 1973;131:516-20.

637. Vianna NJ. Nontuberculous bacterial empyema in patients with and without underlying diseases. JAMA 1971;215:69-75.

638. Ebert W, Bauer HG, Bauer E, Trefz G. Significance of microbiological and biochemical analyses in empyema thoracis. Thorac Cardiovasc Surg 1990;38:348-51.

639. Travalline JM, Criner GJ. Persistent bronchopleural fistula in an AIDS patient with *Pneumocystis carinii* pneumonia: Successful treatment with pleurodesis. Chest 1993;103:981.

640. Mallen JK, Landis JN, Frankel KM. Autologous "blood-patch" pleurodesis for persistent pulmonary air leak. Chest 1993;103:326-27.

641. Moores DWO. Management of acute empyema. Chest 1992;102:1316-17.

642. LeMense GP, Strange C, Sahn SA. Empyema thoracis: Therapeutic management and outcome. Chest 1995; 107:1532-37.

643. Light RW. Parapneumonic effusions and empyema. In; Pleural Diseases (3rd edn); Williams and Wilkins, Baltimore 1995;129-53.

644. Landay MJ, Christensen EE, Bynum IJ, Goodman C. Anerobic pleural and pulmonary infections. AJR 1980;134:233-40.

645. Kerr A, Vasudevan VP, Powell S, Ligenza C. Percutaneous catheter drainage for acute empyema. Improved cure rate using CAT scan, fluoroscopy, and pigtail drainage catheter.s. NY State J Med 1991;91:4-7.

646. Shields TW. Parapneumonic empyema. In: Shields TW (Ed). General Thoracic Surgery (4th edn), Baltimore, Williams and Wilkins 1994;684-93.

647. Bergh NP, Ekroth R, Larsson S, Nagy P. Intrapleural streptokinase in the treatment of haemothorax and empyema. Scand J Thorac Cardiovasc Surg 1977;11; 265-68.

648. Henke CA, Leatherman JW. Intrapleurally administered streptokinase in the treatment of acute loculated nonpurulent parapneumonic effusions. Am Rev Respir Dis 1992;145:680-84.

649. Lee KS, Im JG, Kim YH, et al. Treatment of thoracic multiloculated empyemas with intracavitary kinase: A prospective study. Radiology 1991;179:771-75.

650. Aye RW, Froese DP, Hill LD. Use of purified strepto-kinase in empyema and haemothorax. Am J Surg 1991;161:560-62.

651. Moulton JS, Moore PT, Mencini RA. Treatment of loculated pleural effusions with transcatheter intracavitary urokinase. AJR 1989;153:941-45.

652. Robinson LA, Moulton AL, Fleming WH, Alonso A, Galbraith TA. Intrapleural fibrinolytic treatment of multiloculated thoracic empyemas. Ann Thorac Surg 1994;57:803-13.

653. Pollak JS, Passik CS. Intrapleural urokinase in the treatment of loculated pleural effusions. Chest 1994;105:868-73.

654. Rosen H, Nadkarni VM, Theroux M, Padman R, Klein J. Intrapleural streptokinase as adjuvant treatment for persistent empyema in paediatric patients. Chest 1993;103:1190-93.

655. Ferguson MK. Thoracoscopy for empyema, bronchopleural fistula and chylothorax. Ann Thorac Surg 1993;56:644-45.

656. Moores DWO. Management of acute empyema. Chest 1992;102:1316-17.

657. Ridley PD, Braimbridge MV. Thoracoscopic debride-ment and pleural irrigation in the management of empyema thoracic. Ann Thorac Surg 1991;51:461-64.

658. Sherman MM, Subramanian V, Berger RL. Management of thoracic empyema. Am J Surg 1977;133:474-79.

659. Samson PC. Empyema thoracic: essentials of present day management. Ann Thorac Surg 1971;11:210-20.

660. Morin JE, Munro DD, MacLean LD. Early thoracotomy for empyema. J Thorac Cardiovasc Surg 1972;64:530-36.

661. Hoover EL, Hsu HK, Ross JM, et al. Reappraisal of empyema thoracis: Surgical intervention when the duration of illness is unknown. Chest 1986;90:511-15.

662. Pothula V, Krellenstein DJ. Early aggressive surgical management of parapneumonic empyemas. Chest 1994;105:832-36.

663. Lan RS. Treatment of bronchopleural fistulas. Chest 1992;101:1737-38.

664. Fraser RG, Pare JAP, Pare PD, Fraser RS, Genetreux GP. Diagnosis of diseases of chest (3rd edn). Phila-delphia: Saunders 1991;2520-23.

665. Pairolero PC, Arnold PG, Trastek VF, Meland NB, Kay PP. Postpneumonectomy empyema. The role of intrathoracic muscle transposition. J Thorac Cardiovasc Surg 1990;99:958-68.

666. Onotera RT, Unruth HW. Closure of a postpneu-monectomy bronchopleural fistula with fibrin sealant (Tisseel). Thorax 1988;43:1015-16.

667. Menard JW, Prejean CA, Tucker WY. Endoscopic closure of bronchopleural fistula using a tissue adhesive. Am J Surg 1988;155:415-16.

668. Martini G, Widmann J, Perkman R. Treatment of bronchopleural fistula after pneumonectomy by omental pedicle. Chest 1994;105:957-58.

669. Judson JP, Hill C. Describing a pneumothorax. Chest 1995;107:583.

670. Norris RM, Jones JG, bishop JM. Respiratory gas exchange in patients with spontaneous pneumothorax. Thorax 1968;23:427-33.

671. Gobbell WG Jr, Rhea WG Jr, Nelson IA, Daniel RA Jr. Spontaneous pneumothorax. J Thoracic Cardiovasc Surg 1963;46:331-45.

672. Lesur O, Delorme N, Fromaget JM, Bernadac P, Polu JM. Computed tomography in the aetiologic assess-ment of idiopathic spontaneous pneumothorax. Chest 1990;98:341-47.

673. O'Rourke JP, Yee ES. Civilian spontaneous pneumo-thorax. Treatment options and long term results. Chest 1989;96:1302-06.

674. Wait MA, Estrera A. Changing clinical spectrum of spontaneous pneumothorax. Am J Surg 1992;164:528-31.

675. Lillington GA, Mitchell SP, Wood GA. Catamenial pneumothorax. J Am Med Assoc 1972;219:1328-32.

676. Chernick V, Reed MH. Pneumothorax and chylothorax in the neonatal period. J Pediatr 1970;76:624-32.

677. Sasoon CSH, Light RW, O'Hara VS, Moritz TE. Iatrogenic pneumothorax: Aetiology and morbidity. Respiration 1992;59:215-20.

678. Despars JA, Sasoon CSH, Light RW. Significance of iatrogenic pneumothoraces. Chest 1994;105:1147-50.

679. Bridges KG, Welch G, Silver M, Schinco MA, Esposito B. CT detection of occult pneumothorax in multiple trauma patients. J Emerg Med 1993;11:179-86.

680. Waller DA, Morritt GN, Forty J. Video-assisted thoracoscopic pleurectomy in the management of malignant pleural effusion. Chest 1995;107:1454-56.

681. Dogra VS, Smeltzer JS. Risk of pneumothorax and percutaneous needle biopsy. Chest 1995;107:1477.

682. Lacayo L, Taveras JM III, Sosa N, Ratzan KR. Tension fecal pneumothorax in a postpartum patient. Chest 1993;103:950-51.

683. Sheehan GJ, Miedzinski LJ, Schroeder DG. Pneumo-thorax complicating BiPAP therapy for *Pneumocystis carinii* pneumonia. Chest 1993;103:1310.

684. Matsumoto MA, Rockoff SD, Aaron BL. Tension pyopneumothorax: Rare presentation of ruptured Barrett's oesophagus. Chest 1993;103:1604-06.

685. Bense L. Spontaneous pneumothorax. Chest 1992;101:891-92.

686. Tunon-de-Lara JM, Constans J, Vincent MP, Receveur MC, Conri C, Taytard A. Spontaneous pneumothorax associated with *Pneumocystis carinii* pneumonia. Chest 1992;101:1177-78.

687. Russomanno JH, Brown LK. Pneumothorax due to ball-valve obstruction of an endotracheal tube in a mechanically ventilated patient. Chest 1992;101:1444-45.
688. Sider L, Field LR, Courser JI, Yolandis AV, Martin GJ. Recurrent pneumothorax and adenopathy. Chest 1995;107:860-62.
689. Renzi PM, Corbell C, Chasse M, Braldy J, Matar N. Bilateral pneumothoraces hasten mortality in AIDS patients receiving secondary prophylaxis with aerosolized pentamidine. Chest 1992;102:491-96.
690. Gammon RB, Shin MS, Buchalter SE. Pulmonary barotrauma in mechanical ventilation: patterns and risk factors. Chest 1992;102:568-72.
691. O'Coner BM, Ziegler P, Spaulding MB. Spontaneous pneumothorax in small cell lung cancer. Chest 1992;102:628-29.
692. Reich JM. Pneumothorax due to pleural perforation of the pseudocavity contsaining aspergilloma in a patient with allergic bronchopulmonary aspergillosis. Chest 1992;102:652-53.
693. Melton IJ, Hepper NGG, Offord KP. Incidence of spontaneous pneumothorax in Olmsted County, Minnesota: 1950 to 1974. Am Rev Respir Dis 1979;120:1379-82.
694. O'Hara VS. Spontaneous pneumothorax. Milit Med 1978;143:32-35.
695. Jansveld CAF, Dijkman JH. Primary spontaneous pneumothorax and smoking. Br Med J 1975;4:559-60.
696. Seremetis MG. The management of spontaneous pneumothorax. Chest 1970;57:65-68.
697. Bense L, Eklund G, Wiman IG. Smoking and the increased risk of contracting spontaneous pneumothorax. Chest 1987;92:1009-12.
698. Scott GC, Berger R, McKean HE. The role of atmospheric pressure variation in the development of spontaneous pneumothoraces. Am Rev Respir Dis 1989;139:659-62.
699. Bense L. Spontaneous pneumothorax related to falls in atmospheric pressure. Eur J Respir Dis 1985;65:544-46.
700. Withers JN, Fishback ME, Kiehl PV. Spontaneous pneumothorax: Suggested aetiology and comparison of treatment methods. Am J Surg 1964;108:772-76.
701. Kawakami Y, Irie T, Kamishima K. Stature, lung height and spontaneous pneumothorax. Respiration. 1982;43:35.
702. Abolnik IZ, Lossos IS, Gillis D, Breuer R. Primary spontaneous pneumothorax in men. Am J Med Sci 1993;305:297-303.
703. Sharpe IK, Ahmed M, Braun W. Familial spontaneous pneumothorax and HLA antigens. Chest 1980;78:264-68.
704. Abolnik IZ, Lossos IS, Zlotogora J, Brauer R. On the inheritance of primary spontaneous pneumothorax. Am J Med Genetics 1991;40:155-58.
705. Bense L, Eklund G, Wiman LG. Bilateral bronchial anomaly. A pathologic factor in spontaneous neumothorax. Am Rev Respir Dis 1992;146:513-16.
706. Wilder RJ, Beacham EG, Ravitch MM. Spontaneous pneumothorax complicating cavitary tuberculosis. J Thorac Cardiovasc Surg 1962;43:561-73.
707. Light RW, O'Hara VS, Moritz TE, et al. Intrapleural tetracycline for the prevention of recurrent spontaneous pneumothorax. JAMA 1990;264-2224-30.
708. George RB, Herbert SJ, Shames JM, et al. Pneumothorax complicating emphysema. J Am Med Assoc 1975;234:389.
709. Ohata M, Suzuki H. Pathogenesis of spontaneous pneumothorax with special reference to the ultrastructure of emphysematous bullae. Chest 1980;77:771.
710. Watt AG. Spontaneous pneumothorax. A review of 210 consecutive admissions to Royal Perth Hospital. Med J Aust 1978;1:186.
711. Hart GJ, Stokes TC. Couch AHC. Spontaneous pneumothorax in Norfolk. Br J Dis Chest 1983;77:164.
712. Getz SB, Beasley WE. Spontaneous pneumothorax. Am J Surg 1983;145:183.
713. Jorgensen JR, Falliers CJ, Bukantz SC. Pneumothorax, and mediastinal and subcutaneous emphysema in children with bronchial asthma. Paediatrics 1963;31:824.
714. Rebhan AW, Edwards HE. Staphylococcal pneumonia. Can Med Asso 1960;82:513.
715. Lichter I, Gwynne JF. Spontaneous pneumothorax in young subjects- A clinical and pathological study. Thorax 1971;26:409.
716. Maurer ER, Schaal JA, Mendez FL Jr. Chronic recurring spontaneous pneumothorax due to endometriosis of the diaphragm. J Am Med Assoc 1958;13:168:2013-14.
717. Jamal S, Maurer JR. Pulmonary disease and the menstrual cycle. Pulmonary Perspective.1994;11(3):3-5.
718. Schoenfeld, et al. Obstet Gynecol Surg 1986;41:20.
719. Ross RJM, Empey DW. Bilateral spontaneous pneumothorax in sarcoidosis. Postgrad Med J 1983;59:106.
720. Davidson AR. Eosinophilic granuloma of the lung. Br J Dis Chest 1976;70:125.
721. Jaspan T, Davison AM, Walker WC. Spontaneous pneumothorax in Wegener's granulomatosis. Thorax 1982;37:774.
722. Anton HC, Gray B. Pulmonary alveolar proteinosis presenting as spontaneous peumothorax. Clin Radiol 1967;18:428.
723. Wood JR, Bellamy D, Child AH, Citron KM. Pulmonary disease in patients with Morfan syndrome. Thorax 1984;39:780.
724. O'Neill S, Sweeney J, Walker F, et al. Pneumothorax in the Ehlers-Danlos syndrome. Irish J Med Sci 1981;150:43.
725. Handa AK, Eggleston FC. Pneumothorax caused by hydatid cysts. Ind J Chest Dis 1982;24:47.
726. Torrington KG, Ashbaugh DG, Stackle EG. Recklinghausen's disease. Occurrence with intrathoracic vagal and contralateral spontaneous pneumothorax. Arch Intern Med 1983;143:568.
727. Harris JO, Waltuk BL, Swenson EW. The pathophysiology of the lungs in tuberous sclerosis. A case report and literature review. Am Rev Respir Dis 1969;100:379.

728. Yeung K, Bonnet JD. Bronchogenic carcinoma presenting as spontaneous pneumothorax. Case report with review of literature. Cancer 1977;39:2286.

729. Hall FM, Salzman EW, Burton IE, Kurland GS. Pneumothorax complicating aseptic cavitating pulmonary infarction. Chest 1977;72:232.

730. Mukart DJ, Luvuno FM, Baker LW. Penetrating injuries of the pleural cavity. Thorax 1984;39:789.

731. Pierce AK. Pleural disease. In: Guenter CA, Welch MH (Ed). Pulmonary Medicine, Philadelphia: JB Luppincott 1977.

732. Garramone RR Jr, Jacobs LM, Sahdev P. An objective method to measure and manage occult pneumothorax. Surg Gynecol Obstet 1991;173:257-61.

733. Shorr RM, Crittenden M, Indek M et al. Blunt thoracic trauma: Analysis of 515 patients. Ann Surg 1987;206: 200-05.

734. Ordog GJ, Wasserberger J, Balsubramanium S, Shoemaker W. Asymptomatic stab wounds of the chest. J Trauma 1994;36:680-84.

735. Wolfman NT, Gilpin JW, Bechtold RE, Meredith JW, Ditesheim JA. Occult pneumothorax in patients with abdominal trauma: CT studies. J Comp Assist Tomog 1993;17:56-59.

736. Targhetta R, Bourgeois JM, Chavagneux R, Marty-Double C, Balmes P. Ultrasonographic approach to diagnosing hydropneumothorax. Chest 1992;101:931-34.

737. Douglas JDM. Medical problems of sport diving. Br Med J 1985;291:1224.

738. Hamman L. Spontaneous mediastinal emphysema. Bull John Hopkins Hosp 1939;64:1.

739. Yellin A, Gapany MG, Lieberman Y. Spontaneous pneumomediastinum: Is it a rare cause of chest pain? Thorax 1983;38:383.

740. Gray JM, Hanson GC. Mediastinal emphysema. aetiology, diagnosis and treatment. Thorax 1966;21:325.

741. Lau KY. Pneumomediastinum caused by subcutaneous emphysema in the shoulder: A rare complication of arthroscopy. Chest 1993;103:1606-07.

742. Flattey ME, Schapira RM. Hydropneumomediastinum and bilateral hydropneumothorax as delayed complications of central veinous catheterization. Chest 1993;103:1614-16.

743. Lee HC, Dewan N, Crosby L. Subcutaneous emphysema, pneumomediastinum, and potentially life threatening tension pneumothorax: Pulmonary complication from arthroscopic shoulder decompression. Chest 1992;101:1265-67.

744. Yellen A. Spontaneous pneumomediastinum. Chest 1992;101:1742-43.

745. Schwartz M, Rossoff LJ. Pneumomediastinum and bilateral pneumothoraces in a patient with hyperemesis gravidarum. Chest 1994;106:1904-06.

746. Walston A, Brewer DL, Kitchens CS, Krook JE. The electrocardiographic manifestations of spontaneous left pneumothorax. Ann Intern Med 1974;80:375-79.

747. Aitchison F, Bleetman A, Munro P, McCarter D, Reid AW. Detection of pneumothorax by accident and emergency officers and radiologist on single chest films. Arch Emerg Med 1993;10:343-46.

748. Beres RA, Goodman LR. Pneumothorax: Detection with upright versus decubitus radiography. Radiology 1993;186:19-22.

749. Rhea JT, DeLuca SA, Green RE. Determining the size of pneumothorax in the upright patient. 1982;144: 733-36.

750. Engdahl O, Toft T, Boe J. Chest radiograph: A poor method for determining the size of a pneumothorax. Chest 1993;103:26-29.

751. Horne NW. Spontaneous pneumothorax; Diagnosis and management. Br Med J 1966;1:281.

752. Anonymous. Spontaneous pneumothorax. Br Med J 1976;2:1407.

753. Seaton A, Seaton D, Leitch AG. Pneumothorax. In: Crofton and Douglas's Respiratory Diseases. Oxford: Blackwell, 1989;761.

754. Seaton D, Yoganathan K, Coady T, Barker R. Spontaneous pneumothorax: Marker gas technique for predicting outcome of manual aspiration. Br Med J 1991;302:262.

755. Hamilton AAD, Archer GJ. Treatment of spontaneous pneumothorax by simple aspiration. Thorax 1983; 38:934.

756. Sy So, Dye WU. Catheter drainage of spontaneous pneumothorax: Suction or no suction, early or late removal. Thorax 1982;37:46.

757. Bernstein A, Waqarudin M, Shah M. Management of spontaneous pneumothorax using a Heimlich flutter valve. Thorax 1973;28:386.

758. Gaensler EA. Parietal pleurectomy for recurrent spontaneous pneumothorax. Surg Gynec Obstet 1956;102:293.

759. Northfield TC. Oxygen therapy for spontaneous pneumothorax. Br Med J 1971;4:86:142.

760. Thompson HT, Baily RR,. Management of spontaneous pneumothorax. NZ Med J 1966;65:101.

761. Macoviac JA, Stephenson LW, Oachs R, Edmunds LH. Tetracycline pleurodesis during active pulmonary-pleural leak for prevention of recurrent pneumothorax. Chest 1982;81:78.

762. Weeden D, Smith GH. Surgical experience in the management of spontaneous pneumothorax 1972-82. Thorax 1983;38:737.

763. Noyes BE, Orenstein DM. Treatment of pneumothorax in cystic fibrosis in the era of lung transplantation. Chest 1992;101:1187-88.

764. Kennedy S, Vaughan LM, Steed LL, Sahn SA. Sterilization of talc for pleurodesis: Available techniques, efficacy and cost analysis. Chest 1995;107:1032-34.

765. Mauris GL. Pleurodesis for spontaneous pneumothorax. Chest 1995;107:1183-84.

766. van de Brekel JA, Duurkens VAM, Vanderschueren RGJRA. Pneumothorax; results of thoracoscopy and pleurodesis with talc poudrage and thoracotomy. Chest 1993;103:345-47.

767. Aelony Y. Thoracoscopic talc poudrage. Chest 1992; 102:1922.

768. Berger R. Pleurodesis for spontaneous pneumothorax: Will the procedure of choice please stand up? Chest 1994;106:992-94.

769. Milanez JR, Vargas FS, Paulo S, et al. Intrapleural talc for the prevention of recurrent pneumothorax. Chest 1994;106:1162-65.

770. Kennedy L, Sahn SA. Talc pleurodesis for the treatment of pneumothorax and pleural effusion: A review of literature. Chest 1994;106:1215-22.

771. Slabbynck H, Kovitz KL, Vialette JP, Kasseyet S, Boutin C. Thoracoscopic findings in spontaneous pneumothorax in AIDS. Chest 1992;106:1582-86.

772. Landreneu RJ, Hazelrigg SR, Mack MJ, Keenan RJ, Ferson PF. Video-assisted thoracic surgery for pulmonary and pleural disease. In Shields TW (Ed): General Thoracic Surgery. Malvern, PA: Williams and Wilkins, 1994;4:508-28.

773. Liu HP, Lin PJ, Hsieh MJ, Chang JP, Chang CH. Thoracoscopic surgery as a routine procedure for spontaneous pneumothorax: Results from 82 patients. Chest 1995;107:559-62.

774. Harris RJ, Kavuru MS, Mehta AC, et al. The impact of thoracoscopy on the management of pleural disease. Chest 1995;107:845-52.

775. Melvin WS, Krasna MJ, McLaughlin JS. Thoracoscopic management of spontaneous pneumothorax. Chest 1992;102:1877-79.

776. Takeno Y. Thoracoscopic treatment of spontaneous pneumothorax. Ann Thorac Surg 1993;56:688-90.

777. Inderbitzi RGC, Leiser A, Furrer M, Althaus U. Three years experience in video-assisted thoracic surgery (VATS) for spontaneous pneumothorax. J Thorac Cardiovasc Surg 1994;107:1410-15.

778. Terada Y, Matsunobe S, Nemoto T, et al. Palliation of severe subcutaneous emphysema with use of a trocar-type chest tube as a subcutaneous drain. Chest 1993; 103:323.

779. Herlan DB, Landreneau RJ, Ferson PF. Massive spontaneous subcutaneous emphysema: Acute management with infraclavicular "blow-holes". Chest 1992; 102:503-05.

780. Pavlin J, Cheney FW Jr. Unilateral pulmonary oedema in rabbits after re-expansion of collapsed lung. J Appl Physiol 1979;46:31-35.

781. Davis SW, Bailey JW, Wilkinson P. Reexpansion pulmonary oedema. Chest 1992;102:1920-21.

782. Sprung CL, Loewenherz JW, Baier H, Hauser MJ. Evidence for increased permeability in re-expansion pulmonary oedema. Am J Med 1981;71:497-500.

783. Pavlin DJ, Nessly ML, Cheney FW. Increased pulmonary vascular permeability as a cause of re-expansion Oefdema in rabbits. Am Rev Respir Dis 1981;124:422-27.

784. Pavlin DJ. Lung re-expansion: For better or worse. Chest 1986;89:2-3.

785. Dalton WT, Zolliker AS, McCaughey W, et al. Localized primary tumours of pleura. Cancer 1979;44:1465.

786. Le Roux BT. Pleural tumours. Thorax 1962;17:111.

787. Briselli M, Mark EJ, Dickersin GR. Solitary tumours of the pleura. Eight new cases and review of 360 cases in the literature. Cancer 1981;47:2678.

788. Clagett OT, Mcdonald JR, Schmidt HW. Localised benign mesothelioma of the pleura. JThoracic Surg 1952;24:213.

789. Nwafo DC, Adi FC. Giant fibromyxoma of the parietal pleura. Thorax 1978;33:520.

790. Spry CJF, Williamsom DH, James ML. Pleural mesothelioma and hypoglycaemia. Proc Royal Soc Med 1968;61:1105.

791. Price-Thomas C, Drew CE. Fibroma of visceral pleura. Thorax 1953;8:180.

792. Robinson LA, Reilly RB. Localized pleural mesothelioma: The clinical spectrum. Chest 1994;106:1611-14.

Chapter 29

Mediastinal Diseases

Mediastinum is that portion of the thoracic cavity, which lies between the *two* pleural cavities and extends from the thoracic inlet to the diaphragm. The sternum bound it anteriorly, and it is bounded posteriorly by the thoracic vertebrae, and laterally by the parietal layers of the mediastinal pleura. It contains important structures including that of the heart. The mediastinum is divided into 4 identifiable compartments. They are the superior, anterior, middle, and the posterior mediastinum. Superior and anterior mediastinum are conveniently grouped together as the anterosuperior mediastinum. The superior mediastinum is the portion, which lies above the level of pericardium, and is bounded posteriorly by the first four thoracic vertebrae. Manubrium sterni is situated anteriorly and mediastinal pleural layers form its lateral boundaries. Anterior mediastinum is the portion that is anterior to the pericardium, inferior to superior mediastinum, and posterior to the sternum. The posterior mediastinum is the area that lies posterior to the heart and anterior to 5th to 12th thoracic vertebrae. Anatomically, if an imaginary line is drawn in the mediastinum from the fourth thoracic intervertebral disc to the sternal angle, the area so bounded constitutes the superior mediastinum. The remaining area if subdivided vertically by the heart, anterior, middle, and posterior mediastinum is recognized. Thus, in a lateral chest skiagram, anterior mediastinum is bounded by the sternum, the first rib, and an oblique line drawn from the diaphragm along the anterior border of the heart until it meets the boundaries of the posterior mediastinum. The posterior mediastinum is bounded by the posterior ribs and paravertebral gutter posteriorly. Its anterior boundary is formed by a line drawn along the anterior surface of the vertebral bodies from the diaphragm to the first rib. The remaining area constitutes the middle mediastinum and is triangular in shape.[1,2]

The contents of various compartments of the mediastinum are as follows: *Superior* thymus, upper portion of esophagus, trachea, thoracic duct, aortic arch with the three major branches of the aorta, upper portion of superior vena cava the innominate veins, phrenic nerve, recurrent laryngeal nerve, vagus nerve, and the upper sympathetic ganglia with tributaries: *Anterior* — fibro fatty tissue; *Middle* — bifurcation of trachea, right and left main bronchi, phrenic nerves, pericardial sac, ascending aorta, pulmonary arteries, lower portion of superior vena cava, and the pulmonary veins; *Posterior* descending aorta, thoracic duct, azygous veins, and the vagus nerves.

MEDIASTINAL TUMORS/CYSTS

Major changes have recently occurred in the presentation, diagnosis, and management of primary mediastinal tumors and cysts. New diagnostic techniques and availability of better therapeutic modalities have led to more objective preoperative diagnosis and better long-term results. Recent advances in radiographic techniques like computed tomography, magnetic resonance imaging (MRI), and improved radioisotopic scanning, have improved the ability to exactly delineate the nature and extent of the mass preoperatively. Application of monoclonal antibody techniques to immunohistochemistry has helped in more accurate histological diagnosis. Measurement of various secretory products by radioimmunoassays has further enhanced the diagnostic clue as well as indicators of the disease activity and response to therapy. Electron microscopy helps more precise diagnosis of the lesion. Advances in surgical and anesthesia techniques have led to improved surgical results.

The differential diagnosis of a mediastinal mass by anatomic location is shown in Table 29.1.[3] The likelihood of malignancy is influenced primarily by the following three factors: mass location; patient age; and the presence or absence of symptoms. Although more than two thirds of mediastinal tumors are benign, masses in the anterior compartment are more likely to be malignant.

TABLE 29.1: Mediastinal mass by anatomic location

Anterior	Middle	Posterior
Thymoma	Lymphoma	Neurogenic tumor
Teratoma, seminoma	Pericardial cyst	Bronchogenic cyst
Thyroid (Intrathoracic goiter)	Bronchogenic cyst	Enteric cyst
Lymphoma	Metastatic cyst	Xanthogranuloma
Carcinoma	Systemic granuloma	Diaphragmatic hernia
Parathyroid adenoma		Meningocele
Lipoma		Paravertebral abscess
Lymphangioma		
Aortic aneurysm		

A review of 2399 patients (1952-1986) with primary mediastinal tumors and cysts revealed that neurogenic tumors and thymomas are the most frequent forms of mediastinal lesions. The incidence of various tumors, of course varies from series to series. The overall occurrence of such lesions is shown in Table 29.2.

TABLE 29.2: Incidence of mediastinal tumors

Type of lesion	Incidence (%)
Tumors	
Neurogenic tumors	20.7
Thymoma	19.1
Lymphoma	12.5
Germ cell neoplasm	10.0
Primary carcinoma	4.6
Mesenchymal tumor	6.0
Endocrine tumor	6.4
Others	2.4
Cysts	
Pericardial	6.0
Bronchogenic	6.3
Enteric	2.3
Other	3.7

In the study by Davis et al in 400 patients from the Duke University Medical Centre, with mediastinal masses, malignancy was seen in 59 percent, 29 percent, and 16 percent, respectively, of anterior, middle, and posterior mediastinal masses. Age was an important predictor of malignancy as well with many of the lymphomas and germ cell tumors (GCTs) presenting between the second and fourth decade of life. Last, symptomatic patients are more likely to have a malignancy. Eighty-five percent of patients with a malignancy were symptomatic at presentation, compared to 46 percent of patients with benign neoplasms.[4] In that series, different lesions with their subtypes are shown in Table 29.3.

TABLE 29.3: Primary mediastinal tumors and cysts in 400 patients[4]

Type	% of patients
Thymic tumors	17
Thymoma (Benign)	8
Thymoma (Malignant)	6.5
Thymic cysts/hyperplasia	2.5
Neurogenic tumors	
Benign	11
Ganglioneuromas	
Neurofibroma	
Neurilemmomas	
Paragangliomas	
Malignant	3
Ganglioneuroblastoma	
Neuroblastoma	
Neurosarcoma	
Lymphomas	16
Non-Hodgkin's	10
Hodgkin's	6
Germ cell tumors	11
Benign teratoma	5
Malignant teratoma	2.5
Seminoma	2
Embryonal tumor	1
Carcinoma	9
Mesenchymal tumors	6
Benign	4
Malignant	2
Endocrine tumors	3
Benign and malignant thyroid tumors	2
Parathyroid	1
Miscellaneous tumors	1
Cysts	25
Bronchogenic	10
Pericardial	9
Enteric	3
Others	3

Symptoms and Signs

About one-thirds of patients with mediastinal tumors or cysts are asymptomatic. In these cases the lesion is detected on routine skigram. However, about 85 percent of cases with malignant neoplasm are symptomatic at presentation. On the contrary, only 46 percent of patients with benign lesions are symptomatic. Absence of symptoms correlates well with benign neoplasm. More than eighty percent of cases that are symptomatic at presentation are usually benign. Patients who are symptomatic have equal chance of having malignant or benign lesions. In symptomatic patients, the most common symptoms at presentation were as follows: cough (60%); chest pain (30%); fevers/ chills (20%); and dyspnea (16%). Most symptoms can be categorized into the following two groups: localizing symptoms (Table 29.4) and systemic symptoms. Localizing symptoms are secondary to tumor invasion. Common localizing symptoms include respiratory compromise; dysphagia; paralysis of the limbs, diaphragm, and vocal cords; Horner syndrome; and superior vena cava syndrome. Systemic symptoms are typically due to the release of excess hormones, antibodies, or cytokines. A classic example is hypercalcemia, which is caused by a parathyroid adenoma.[5,6]

TABLE 29.4: Localizing symptoms

Involved anatomic structure	Localizing symptom
Bronchi/trachea	Dyspnea, postobstructive pneumonia, atelectasis, hemoptysis
Esophagus	Dysphagia
Spinal cord/vertebral column	Paralysis
Recurrent laryngeal nerve	Hoarseness, vocal cord paralysis
Phrenic nerve	Diaphragmatic paralysis
Stellate ganglion	Horner syndrome
Superior vena cava	Superior vena cava syndrome

Clinical syndrome	Type of tumor
Myasthenia gravis, RBC aplasia, Hypogammaglobulinemia, Good syndrome, Whipple disease, Megaesophagus, Myocarditis	Thymoma
Multiple endocrine adenomatosis	
Cushing syndrome	Carcinoid,
Hypertension	Pheochromocytoma, Ganglioneuroma, Chemodectoma
Diarrhea	Ganglioneuroma
Hypercalcemia	Parathyroid adenoma, Lymphoma
Thyrotoxicosis	Intrathoracic goiter
Hypoglycemia	Mesothelioma, Teratoma, Fibrosarcoma, Neurosarcoma
Hypertrophic osteoarthropathy	Neurofibroma, Neurilemmoma, Mesothelioma
Vertebral abnormalities	Enteric cysts
Pyrexia of unknown origin	Lymphoma
Alcohol-induced pain	Hodgkin's disease
Opsomyoclonus	Neuroblastoma

Diagnostic Approach to Mediastinal Tumors

Diagnostic evaluation of mediastinal tumors and cysts has improved greatly due to recent advances in imaging techniques.[4] The initial workup of a suspected mediastinal mass involves obtaining posteroanterior and lateral chest radiographs. This can provide information pertaining to the size, anatomic location, density, and composition of the mass. Anatomic localization of the mass on the basis of chest radiograph is an important first step to acertain about the tumor (*see* Table 29.1). The consistency of the tumor, whether cystic or solid and the presence or absence of calcification are further clues to the nature of the mass. For example, the presence of a tooth is diagnostic of a dermoid teratoma. Computed assisted tomography (CT) scanning is used to further characterize mediastinal masses and their relationship to surrounding structures as well as to identify cystic, vascular, and soft-tissue structures. With bolus contrast injection, one can easily distinguish a vascular lesion like an aneurysm. Additional information is obtained concerning the extent of the neoplasm and its relationship with other structures in the mediastinum. An accurate diagnosis is occasionally possible depending on attenuation values and classic location of the tumor within the mediastinum. Pericardial cyst is one such example. Similarly lipomas will have the attenuation values of fat. Limitations of a CT scan, however, are the false positive result particularly in recognizing tissue invasion and metastatic spread. Local desmoplastic reaction and reactive hyperplasia of the lymph nodes may be responsible for these false positive results. Angiocardiography was previously used to evaluate mediastinal masses, but with the advent of contrast enhanced CT scans, this procedure is no more being used. In rare circumstances, fluoroscopy, barium swallow, angiography, CT angiography, and three-dimensional reconstruction may provide additional information[5] (Figs 29.1 to 29.26).

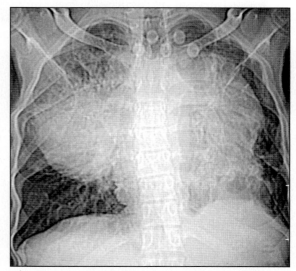

FIGURE 29.1: CXR - Mediastinal widening with aneurysm of arch of aorta

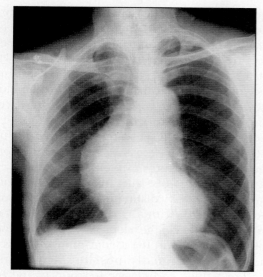

FIGURE 29.2: Mediastinal mass - Aortic aneurysm

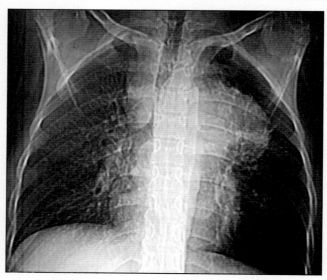

FIGURE 29.3: CXR - Aneurysm of arch of aorta

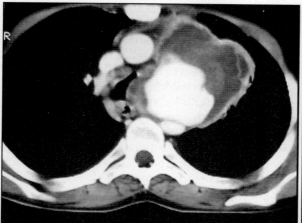

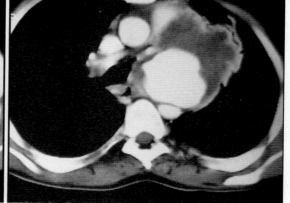

FIGURE 29.4: CT Chest - Aneurysm of arch of aorta

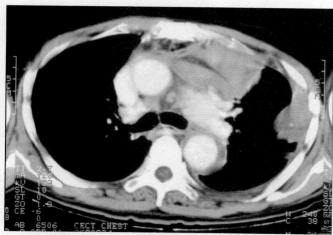

FIGURE 29.5: Ruptured aortic aneurysm

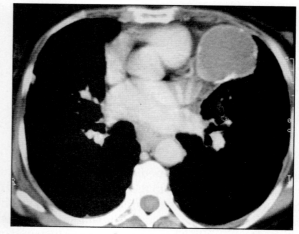

FIGURE 29.6: CT Chest - Pericardial cyst at left cardiophrenic angle

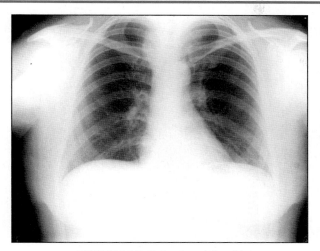

FIGURE 29.7: Retrosternal thyroid

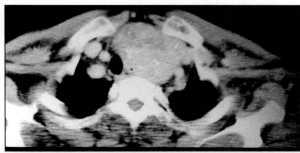

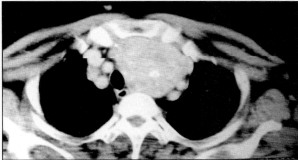

FIGURE 29.8: CT Chest - Retrosternal thyroid

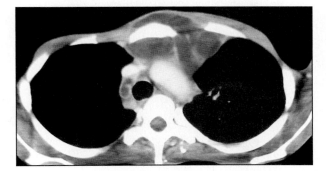

FIGURE 29.9: CT Chest - Right paratracheal and anterior mediastinal lymphadenopathy

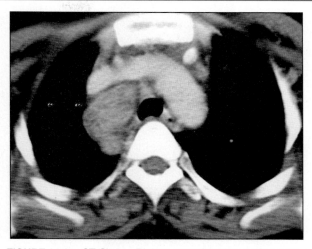

FIGURE 29.10: CT Chest - Right paratracheal lymphadenopathy without any caseation

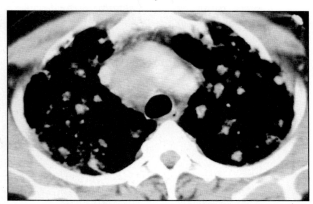

FIGURE 29.11: CT Chest - Right pretracheal malignant lymphadenopathy with SVC obstruction

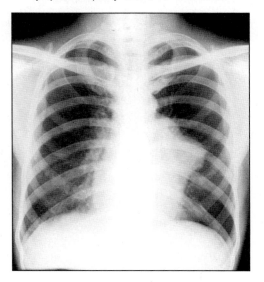

FIGURE 29.12: Thymoma

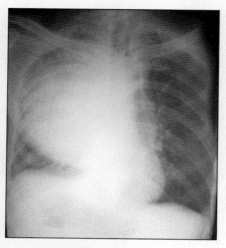

FIGURE 29.13: Large mediastinal mass - Malignant thymic tumor

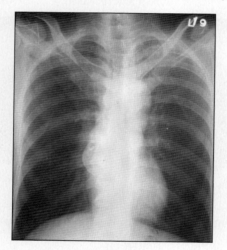

FIGURE 29.14: Thymic cyst

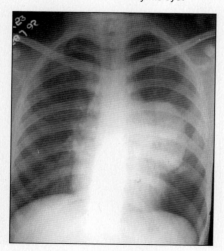

FIGURE 29.15: Middle mediastinal tumor obliterating the cardiac border

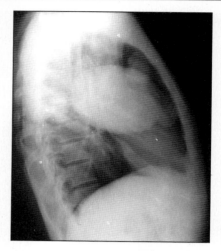

FIGURE 29.16: Middle mediastinal mass

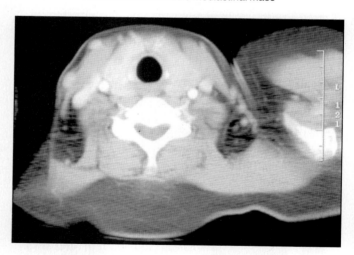

FIGURE 29.17: CT scan of retrosternal thyroid

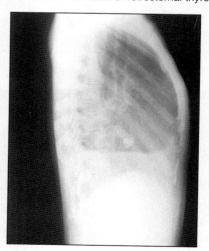

FIGURE 29.18: Mediastinal dermoid

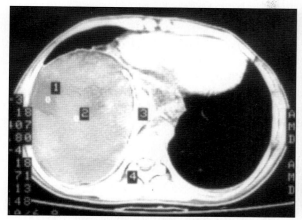

FIGURE 29.19: CT scan of mediastinal dermoid

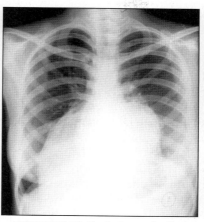

FIGURE 29.20: Posterior mediastinal teratoma

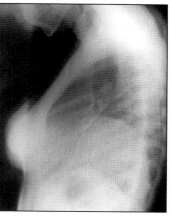

FIGURE 29.21: Posterior mediastinal teratoma - Leteral view

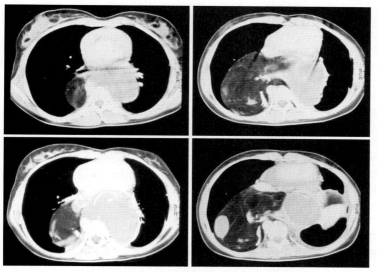

FIGURE 29.22: CT scan of posterior mediastinal teratoma

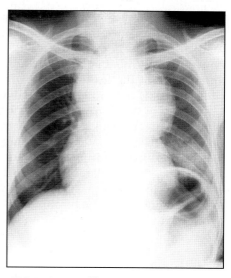

FIGURE 29.23: Metastatic carcinoma in the mediastinum (small cell carcinoma)

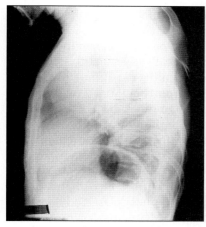

FIGURE 29.24: Lateral view - Metastatic carcinoma in the mediastinum (small cell carcinoma)

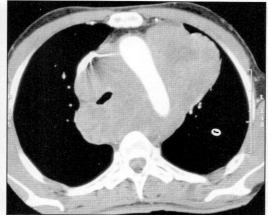

FIGURE 29.25: CT scan - Metastatic carcinoma in the mediastinum (small cell carcinoma)

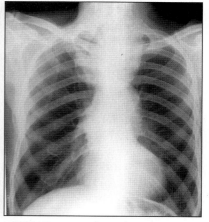

FIGURE 29.26: Superior mediastinal mass - Goiter with retrosternal extension

MRI is a new noninvasive technique that has the advantage of defining the anatomical extent of disease without the potential risk of contrast media. Respiratory compensation and cardiac gating techniques have improved the overall quality of the image. The role of MRI is primarily in ruling out or evaluating a neurogenic tumor. MRI is also valuable to evaluate the extent of vascular invasion or cardiac involvement. Disadvantages of the technique are the long scanning timings with its expenses and its limited availability.[6,7] Further, it is contraindicated in persons with metallic stents in the heart. Although nuclear scans and biochemical studies can be used to further characterize a lesion, tissue diagnosis is almost always required. If a mass is likely to be benign after initial workup, it can be removed surgically without biopsy. Otherwise, a diagnostic biopsy specimen can be obtained by transthoracic or transbronchial needle aspiration, mediastinoscopy, anterior mediastinotomy, or video-assisted thoracic surgery, depending on the anatomic location and radiographic appearance of the lesion.

Fine needle aspiration cytology biopsy, usually under CT guidance has improved preoperative histological diagnosis. Even plain skiagram of the chest with both posteroanterior and lateral views, are sufficient for fine needle aspiration biopsy in centers where CT scan facilities are not available, particularly when the tumor is too anterior or posterior. Although exact histopathological diagnosis cannot be obtained in some cases with cytological biopsies alone, it should be sufficient to distinguish between a malignant or benign lesion in most cases. It is particularly useful in the diagnosis of mediastinal metastasis with an accuracy of over 90 percent of cases.

Radioimmunoassays of a number of tumor secretory products using monoclonal antibodies have helped further in the diagnosis, evaluation of response to therapy, and monitoring of tumor recurrence. Measurements of alpha-fetoprotein (AFP) and β-human chorionic gonadotropin (β-hCG) are particularly helpful in the evaluation of patients with malignant germ cell tumors. Some even recommend that male patients in their second through fifth decades of life with anterior mediastinal masses should have their β-hCG measured as a routine. Other secretory products that can be measured using monoclonal antibody techniques include catecholamines, ACTH, 5-HIAA, T_3, T_4, and carcinoembryonic antigen (CEA). Immunohistochemical stains using monoclonal antibodies coupled to immunoperoxidases increase the precision of histological diagnosis.

Application of electron microscopy on a routine basis further improves the accuracy of histological diagnosis. For example, carcinoid tumors have dense core granules, fewer tonofilaments, and desmosomes; lymphomas lack junctional attachments, and epithelial features are absent; germ cells have even chromatin, prominent nuclei, scanty desmosomes, and rare tonofilaments; and neuroblastomas will show neurosecretory granules and synaptic endings.

I. THYMOMAS

Thymoma is a rare epithelial tumor of the thymus[8] and is the most common neoplasm of the anterior mediastinum with an incidence of 0.15 cases per 100,000.[9-12] Although rare in children, thymomas represent 20 percent of anterior mediastinal neoplasms in adults.[13,14]

The thymus gland is a lymphoreticular organ, which develops as a pair of solid buds arising from the third bronchial pouch at the 6th week of intrauterine life. It migrates caudally during development and takes up a retrosternal position. It consists of two lobes bound by fatty tissue. The gland is encapsulated. It is divided into lobules by loose connective tissue. Each lobule has a cortex and a medulla. The former consists of small lymphocytes and the latter comprises of reticular cells and Hassall's corpuscles. These are zones of squamous cells and epithelial cells. The thymus is relatively large in size during infancy and may weigh as much as 15 gm. It grows in size subsequently, so that by puberty it is about twice in size. Thereafter, it undergoes involution returning to its original infantile size.

As the thymus is composed of heterogeneous admixture of lymphoid and epithelial elements, tumors originating in the thymus may be of varied histologic types. Thymomas are the most common thymic tumor in adults. Thymoma classification has historically been controversial, but a system put forth by the World Health Organization (WHO) in 2004 has been generally accepted as a reproducible and clinically relevant classification. In addition to histologic subtype, tumor stage and resection status are important factors in determining outcome in thymomas. Thymomas are neoplasms that arise from epithelial cells of the thymus.[15,16] Because of their low incidence, wide range of histologic appearance, and unique biologic behavior, they have been a source of controversy for many years. The histologic classification of thymoma in particular is still a topic of dispute.[17-20] Bernatz and colleagues[21] classified thymoma into 4 histologic subtypes according to the relative proportion of epithelial cells and lymphocytes: predominantly lymphocytic, mixed, epithelial, and spindle cell. In many studies, no significant correlation was observed between this histologic subtype and clinical behavior, and probably the only important prognostic determinant was invasion.[22-25] In 1985, Marino and Müller-Hermelink[26] developed a new histologic classification of thymic epithelial neoplasm based on the morphologic and functional resemblance of neoplastic epithelial cells to normal thymic cortical and medullary epithelial cells: medullary, mixed, predominantly cortical, and cortical. In addition, they proposed well-differentiated thymic carcinoma as an organotypic low-grade carcinoma of the thymus.[27] Some studies showed that this classification was useful for predicting clinical behavior,[28-31] whereas others disputed its clinical relevance.[24,32] On the other hand, Moran and Suster[33] presented 3 categories of thymic epithelial tumor based simply on the grade of histologic atypia: thymoma, atypical thymoma, and thymic carcinoma. Thus, several histologic classifications for thymoma have been published, but the prognostic significance of such histologic classification is still controversial. Recently, the World Health Organization (WHO) histologic typing of tumors of the thymus was published[34-39] based on cytologic differences, which may be helpful in determining treatment regimens and predicting survival (Table 29.5).

The types of tumors can be described in short as:

Type A — Spindle cell, medullary
Type AB — Mixed
Type B1 — Lymphocyte rich, lymphocytic, predominantly cortical
Type B2 — Cortical
Type B3 — Epithelial, atypical, squamous, well-differentiated thymic carcinoma

There is a strong association between histologic subtype and invasiveness as well as prognosis.[40-42] Most thymomas are solid tumors, but up to one third may have components that are necrotic, hemorrhagic, or cystic. Thirty-four percent of thymomas invade through their own capsules, extending into surrounding structures.[43-50] Likewise, trans-diaphragmatic extension into the abdomen and metastasis into the ipsilateral pleura and pericardium can occur, although lymphogenous and hematogenous spread is rare.

The Masaoka clinical staging system[51] is based on the degree of invasion of the tumor through the capsule into the surrounding structures, which has important implications for prognosis (Table 29.6). The Masaoka staging system is shown to be useful as an independent predictor of survival in patients with thymoma.

TABLE 29.5: World Health Organization classification of thymomas

Class of thymoma	Cytologic features
Type A	A tumor composed of a population of spindle or oval neoplastic thymic epithelial cells lacking nuclear atypia and accompanied by few or nonneoplastic lymphocytes.
Type AB:	A tumor in which foci with the features of type A thymoma are admixed with foci rich in lymphocytes.
Type B1:	A tumor that resembles the normal functional thymus in that it combines large expanses with an appearance practically indistinguishable from normal thymic cortex with areas resembling thymic medulla.
Type B2	A tumor in which the neoplastic epithelial component appears as scattered plump cells with vesicular nuclei and distinct nucleoli among a heavy population of lymphocytes, perivascular spaces are common and sometimes very prominent, and a perivascular arrangement of tumor cells resulting in a palisading effect may be seen.
Type B3	A type of thymoma predominantly composed of round or polygonal epithelial cells exhibiting no or mild atypia admixed with a minor component of lymphocytes, resulting in a sheet-like growth of the neoplastic epithelial cells.

TABLE 29.6: Masaoka staging system of thymoma

Stage	Degree of Invasion	5 yr survival rate, %
1	Complete encapsulation macroscopically and no capsular invasion microscopically	96–100
2	Invasion into the surrounding fatty tissue or mediastinal pleura macroscopically or invasion into the capsule microscopically	86–95
3	Invasion into neighboring organs macroscopically	56–69
4a	Pleural or pericardial dissemination	11–50
4b	Lymphogenous or hematogenous metastasis	0

Typically, a thymoma is an incidental finding on a chest radiograph. Such symptoms consist of chest pain, dyspnea, dysphagia, and hoarseness of voice, superior vena caval syndrome, and other mediastinal compression symptoms. Metastasis is uncommon; however, parathymic syndromes, which include myasthenia gravis, hypogammaglobulinemia, and pure RBC aplasia, may develop. Other rare manifestations can also occur.[52-61] Thymomas can occur at any time after the age of 20 years. There is a slight predominance in males. About 60 percent of cases are symptomatic at presentation.

A unique feature is its association with paraneoplastic syndromes, in particular myasthenia gravis.

Myasthenia gravis is most frequent in women and is associated with thymoma. Myasthenia gravis (MG) is an autoimmune disease that affects neuromuscular transmission and determines chronic weakness and fatigue at various levels of the striated muscles. Symptoms range from ocular disturbances characterized by ptosis and diplopia, to mild, moderate, or severe generalized weakness involving respiratory muscles in the final stage. The thymus gland seems to have an important function in the complex pathogenesis of this disorder as it is implicated in mechanisms of self-tolerance and autoimmunity. Since 1941, when Blalock and colleagues first reported results of transsternal thymectomy in patients affected by MG, thymectomy has had a significant role in the treatment of MG. Though thymectomy is currently a widely accepted therapeutic option in the integrated management of MG, the selection of patients, the extent of thymic resection, and the surgical approach remain controversial. As discussed symptoms include diplopia, ptosis, dysphagia, weakness, and fatigue. Thirty percent to 50 percent of patients with thymomas have myasthenia gravis, compared to 10 to 15 percent of patients with myasthenia gravis who have a thymoma.[62,63] Clinical severity of MG is described according to the Osserman classification.

TABLE 29.7: Osserman classification of severity of myasthenia gravis

Stage	Definition
I	Ocular myasthenia gravis: involvement of extra ocular muscles, with diplopia and ptosis.
IIa	Mild generalized myasthenia gravis: ocular symptoms are associate to slow involvement of bulbar (dysarthria and dysphagia) and skeletal muscles (generalized weakness). Respiratory muscles are spared.
IIb	Moderately generalized myasthenia gravis: progressive onset of symptoms with significant manifestation of weakness. Respiratory muscles are spared.
III	Acute myasthenia gravis: rapid onset (within 6 months) of severe bulbar and skeletal muscles involvement with important weakness. Respiratory muscles are involved.
IV	Late severe myasthenia gravis: progressive in severity for 2 or more years.

Pathogenesis of MG is thought to occur via myeloid cell lineages derived from the thymus that recognize antigens on the neuromuscular junction producing autoantibodies.[64] These autoantibodies bind to acetylcholine receptors of the neuromuscular junction, causing muscle fatigue.[64] Thymectomy can alleviate symptoms; however, this benefit is often delayed for months after surgery. Given the association between thymoma and myasthenia gravis, the serum antiacetylcholine receptor

antibody level should be measured in all patients with a suspected thymoma to rule out myasthenia gravis before surgery.[65,66] Hypogammaglobulinemia and pure RBC aplasia are present in 10 percent and 5 percent of patients with a thymoma, respectively.[10] Good syndrome is diagnosed in patients with a thymoma and combined B-cell/T-cell immunodeficiency.[67] Thymoma is also associated with various other autoimmune disorders, such as systemic lupus erythematosus, polymyositis, and myocarditis.[4,10,47,68]

Thymomas appear on a chest radiograph as a well-defined lobulated mass in the anterosuperior mediastinum, typically anterior to the aortic root.[10,47] Further evaluation with contrast-enhanced thoracic CT scanning usually reveals an encapsulated, well-defined, soft-tissue mass, often with hemorrhage, necrosis, or cyst formation.[69] They can also appear predominantly cystic with a nodular component.[70] Further, modalities of investigations as indicated earlier can be useful in the diagnosis of thymoma.[71,72] Diagnosis can be achieved during the time of surgery. However, ultrasound/CT guided FNAC or trucut biopsy can give the diagnosis before surgery.[73,74] Cytogenetic techniques and immunohistochemistry have recently been used to help in the cytopathological diagnosis of thymoma.[75-80]

MANAGEMENT

Surgery, radiotherapy, and chemotherapy, either alone, or in combination, depending upon the tumor type is the approach of managing thymomas.[81-95] Thymic tumors including thymomas, thymic carcinomas, and thymic carcinoid tumors, are relatively infrequent. These tumors with a wide spectrum of histological and biological features may exhibit an indolent clinical course (thymomas) or manifest an aggressive behavior (thymic carcinoma) with a high risk of relapse and metastasis. Successful management of these tumors depends on accurate diagnosis, thorough staging, proper assessment of patient health status, and selection of treatment modality. Surgery remains the mainstay of therapy whereas radiation therapy plays an important role in subtotally resected or unresectable cases. The risk of side effects and late sequelae is generally low when proper radiation technique is employed.[91] Chemotherapy has an important role in the treatment of advanced thymic tumors. Early stage tumors are successfully treated with surgery. Locally advanced tumors (Masaoka stage III and IVA) are often treated with combined modality treatment including surgery, radiation, and chemotherapy. For patients with curable thymic tumors, the ability to attain a complete resection is a critical prognostic factor. Locally advanced tumors have a relatively high risk of recurrence and decreased rates of long-term survival. A multimodality approach including induction chemotherapy and postoperative radiation therapy can improve complete resection rates and long-term outcomes. Thymic tumors are chemoresponsive with optimal responses achieved with cisplatin-based combination chemotherapy. Chemotherapy with radiation can result in long-term progression-free survival for patients with locally advanced disease who remain inoperable following induction therapy. Patients with disseminated (stage IVB) thymic tumors can also have significant disease response and palliation of symptoms when treated with chemotherapy. Octreotide and corticosteroids also have shown efficacy. For best results, it is important that thoracic surgeons, radiation oncologists, and medical oncologists work together to obtain the best local control of tumor and optimal treatment of metastases.[92]

Tumor stage (according to Masaoka)[51] is the most important prognostic factor. Noninvasive tumors (stage I) are usually completely resected and no further therapy is warranted. For incompletely resected tumors and locally advanced invasive thymomas (stage Ill-IV) postoperative radiotherapy with 50-60 Gy is advisable. Chemotherapy, preferably with Cisplatinum, is indicated with inoperable thymomas or metastatic disease. In general thymomas have a fair prognosis even in advanced stage. Long-term follow-up is mandatory up to 10 years.

In a report from Taipei, the records of 20 patients with histologically confirmed thymic carcinoma treated between 1988 and 2002 at the Division of Oncology at Taipei Veterans General Hospital were reviewed. Therapy consisted of surgical debulking, adjuvant radiotherapy, and chemotherapy in six patients (30%), surgical debulking with adjuvant chemotherapy in two patients (10%), surgical debulking with adjuvant radiotherapy in one patient (5%), radiotherapy with adjuvant chemotherapy in eight patients (40%), and chemotherapy alone in three patients (15%). After a median follow-up of 22 months (range, 5-72 months), three patients (15%) were alive. Eighteen patients (90%) experienced disease recurrence after a median of 9 months (range, 2-41 months); 12 (66%) of these patients initially had stage IVa disease, and 6 (33%) had stage IV b disease. Five patients had an undifferentiated type of histology. The median time to progression was 5 months. However, none of these patients was able to receive salvage therapy due to their poor performance status. For those patients with a lymphoepithelioma-like histology, the median survival was 36 months; there was

tumor recurrence in five patients and they all received salvage chemotherapy. The median survival time for these five patients was 51 months. For patients with squamous cell type, the median time to progression was 10 months. Five patients received salvage chemotherapy and the median survival was 28 months. There was a significant difference (P < 0.0001) in the median survival between those who received chemotherapy (18 months) after tumor relapse and those who did not (1 month). These results indicate that multidisciplinary treatment, including surgery, radiotherapy, and chemotherapy, is beneficial in treating primary thymic carcinoma. Chemotherapy plays an important role in both primary and relapsed stage IV thymic carcinoma in terms of prolonging the disease-free survival and median survival of patients with lymphoepithelioma-like or squamous cell histology types. For patients with an undifferentiated histology, multidisciplinary treatment or chemotherapy might not be helpful in either primary or relapsed stage IV thymic carcinoma.[95]

In a 38-year period from 1962 to 2000, 152 patients with thymoma at the National Cancer Center Hospital, Tokyo were treated. The distribution of histologic subtype was type A (n = 18), type AB (n = 56), type B1 (n = 15), type B2 (n = 29), and type B3 (n = 12). A close correlation was seen between the histologic subtype and stage (P = .000). The overall survivals at 5 and 10 years were 92 percent and 91 percent, respectively. The 5- and 10-year survivals according to stage were 100 percent and 100 percent (stage I, N = 40; stage II, N = 54), 81 percent and 76 percent (stage III, N = 25), and 47 percent and 47 percent (stage IV, N = 11), respectively. The difference in survival between stage III and stage IV was significant (P = .000). Patients with type A or AB thymoma demonstrated a 100 percent survival at both 5 and 10 years. Recurrences were seen in 12 patients with complete resection. According to a multivariate analysis, tumor size (P = .001), completeness of resection (P = .002), histologic subtype (P = .011), and stage (P = .00) were significant prognostic factors. The authors concluded that the World Health Organization histologic classification significantly correlated with the clinical stage. Tumor size, completeness of resection, histologic subtype, and stage predicted the prognosis of thymoma.[41] In another study from Italy, the specimens of 69 patients, who underwent surgical treatment between 1983 and 1998, were analyzed, comparing the clinical features of the patients and the histological typing of the neoplasm, according to the WHO classification. A survival analysis of clinical and pathological prognostic factors was carried out. The incidence of thymus-related syndrome was related to the histological subtype and increases progressively from A to B3, while in C subtype the incidence was nil. With a mean follow-up of 108 months (range 54-239 months), there were 6 intrathoracic recurrencies, 3 of those were intrapleuric and 3 mediastinal. At the last follow-up, 52 patients were alive; 1 with disease. Five deaths were related to the tumor (2 mediastinal and 3 intrapleuric relapses). Actuarial five-year and ten-year survival was 95 percent and 88.9 percent. Because of the absence of deaths related to thymomas in most samples it was not possible to perform a comparison among different histological types and different clinical stages. It was concluded that the WHO histologic classification seems to correlate with the incidence of thymus related syndromes and the clinical stage of Masaoka. Despite the higher incidence of recurrences in type B3 and C thymoma the WHO classification did not prove to be a prognostic factor.[35] In another study, thymomas surgically removed from 100 consecutive patients at Juntendo University Hospital between October 1983 and February 2002 was classified according to the WHO histological classification. The overall survival was assessed and recurrence-free rate calculated for each tumor type in the WHO classification compared with those of tumors classified by the Masaoka system. The thymic epithelial tumors in this series comprised 10 type A, 15 type AB, 18 type B1, 21 type B2, 33 type B3, and 3 type C tumors according to the WHO classification. Based on the Masaoka system, the disease was stage I in 53 patients, stage II in 30, stage III in 15, and stage IV in 2. The 15 year recurrence-free rate was 100 percent for type A, AB and B1, while the rates for types B2 and B3 were 66.7 percent and 54.5 percent, respectively. The 10 year recurrence-free rate was 66.7 percent for type C. The 15 year recurrence-free rate of the 64 patients with type A, AB, B1, and B2 thymomas was significantly higher from that of the 33 patients with type B3 thymoma (p = 0.0026). It was concluded that when using the WHO classification, it is critical to distinguish type B3 thymoma from other tumor types.[50]

THYMIC CARCINOMA

Thymic carcinomas are a heterogeneous group of aggressive, invasive epithelial malignancies. Their incidence is rare, occurring predominantly in middle-aged men. Most patients present with cough, shortness of breath, and chest pain. Fatigue, weight loss, and anorexia are common, while superior vena cava syndrome and cardiac tamponade have been described.[94-102] Histologically, thymic carcinomas are large, firm, infiltrating masses with areas of cystic change and necrosis. They are classified as low grade or high grade, with squamous cell-like and lymphoepithelioma-like variants being the most common cell types. In contrast to thymomas, thymic carcinomas are cytologically malignant, with typical features of cellular necrosis, atypia, and mitoses. Radiographically, thymic carcinomas are heterogeneous with necrosis and calcifications and can be associated with pleural and pericardial effusions.

Treatment and prognosis has been discussed above.[103,104]

THYMIC HYPERPLASIA

This is most often difficult to differentiate from thymoma, particularly in children. The definite feature of hyperplasia on histology is the presence of germinal centers in the medulla. Thymic hyperplasia is most often asymptomatic. Whenever symptoms occur, they are mainly respiratory and occur in small children. Such hyperplasia may be common in patients with myasthenia gravis (50%) and other collagen vascular diseases like SLE, and thyrotoxicosis. Steroid therapy is given to differentiate between a hyperplasia and a true tumor. With such a therapy, the former regresses. However, lymphomas do also regress with steroid therapy. Surgery is indicated if there are pressure symptoms. If such a decision is taken, then the hyperplastic should be removed leaving behind the rest.

THYMIC CYSTS

Normal thymic tissue may contain cystic spaces. They occur at all ages. Thymic cysts are rare tumors of unclear etiology.[105-107] The pathogenesis of cysts may be: congenital, due to hemorrhage, or because of cystic degeneration. They can be congenital or acquired, and are associated with inflammation or with an inflammatory neoplasm, such as Hodgkin's disease (HD). Congenital thymic cysts are remnants of the thymopharyngeal duct. Inflammatory cysts probably arise from an inflamed thymic parenchyma. Radiographically, they appear as simple homogenous cysts. Microscopically, thymic cysts may be identical to cystic thymic neoplasms. Thus, thorough sampling and examination are essential. Cavitation in a thymoma may be confused with thymic cysts, which can only be distinguished on histological examination. Surgical excision is curative.

OTHER RARE THYMIC TUMORS

Thymic carcinoid is a malignant tumor, which is histologically similar to carcinoid tumors found at other sites.[108-111] Its highest incidence is in the fourth and fifth decades of life. Thymic carcinoid is associated with Cushing syndrome and multiple endocrine neoplasia syndrome. Thymic carcinoid presents as a large, lobulated, invasive mass of the anterior mediastinum with or without hemorrhage and necrosis. Metastasis is common, with spread to regional lymph nodes as well as distant metastasis developing in two thirds of patients. The treatment is complete surgical resection. For a locally invasive tumor, radiotherapy and chemotherapy are used despite minimal effect. The prognosis of these tumors is poor but difficult to assess.

Thymolipoma is a rare, benign, slowly growing tumor of the thymus gland that occurs in young adults of both sexes.[78,112] CT scans and MRI studies show a characteristic fat density. The treatment of choice is surgical excision.

II. MEDIASTINAL GERM CELL TUMORS (GCT)

These tumors are thought to be either really of gonadal origin and represent spread from an occult or burnt out primary tumor or are of true extragonadal origin with separate clinical and biological behavior. The initial theory regarding the genesis of these tumors was that they represent isolated metastasis from an inapparent gonadal primary. This was strengthened by occasional demonstration of testicular scars in these patients. However, subsequent large autopsy studies have suggested otherwise. Now it is generally accepted that extragonadal germ cell tumors, particularly of pineal and mediastinal sites, are due to malignant transformation of germal elements of these sites without a primary gonadal focus. The location of these tissues in these sites result from abnormal migration of germ cells during embryogenesis. Other suggestions are that there are wide distributions of germ cells in the liver, thymus, bone marrow, and brain during normal embryogenesis, which regulate somatic functions or convey genetic information. Mediastinal GCTs account only a very small percentage of all germinal tumors. However, mediastinal germ cell tumors represent the most common extragonadal site and account for more than 50 percent of all germ cell tumors in adults. Mediastinal GCTs in children occur at all age groups and in both sexes. In adults either sex has equal distribution of these tumors. Malignant GCTs, however, occur predominantly in males. The most common age in adults is in the third decade. In contrast to gonadal GCTs where seminomas occur a decade later than nonseminomatous tumors, primary mediastinal seminoma occurs at a relatively young age similar to mediastinal nonseminomatous germ cell tumors.

However, advanced age does not rule out the possibility of such a tumor. The tumors is more common in whites than Blacks.

Mediastinal GCTs are derived from primitive germ cells that fail to migrate completely during early embryonic development.[113-115] GCTs are found in young adults and represent 15 percent of anterior mediastinal masses found in adults.[112] Malignant GCTs are more common (> 90%) in men. A mediastinal GCT should prompt a search for a primary gonadal malignancy. Mature teratomas are the most common histological type of germ cell tumors, followed by seminomas.[116] Germ cell tumors are predominantly found in gonads, while the anterior mediastinum is the most common extragonadal site.[117] The mediastinal germ cell tumors comprise 15 percent of anterior mediastinal tumors in adults and 25 percent in children.[118] According to the mediastinal germ cell tumor classification system proposed in 1986 by Mullen and Richardson, there are three categories: benign germ cell tumors, seminomas, and nonseminomatous germ cell tumors, also called malignant teratomas.[119] The benign germ cell tumors are also called epidermoid cysts, benign teratomas, or simply teratomas. These tumors can characteristically be cystic or solid or a combination of the two, contain multiple germ cell layers (sometimes all three are recognized, i.e. ectoderm, mesoderm, and endoderm), and are composed of tissue foreign to the organ or anatomic site in which they arise. The embryonal tumors, also called malignant teratomas or nonseminomatous GCTS, are diverse and include choriocarcinomas, yolk sac carcinomas, embryonal carcinomas, and teratocarcinomas.[120] These tumors often produce serologic markers such as α-fetal protein (AFP) and human chorionic gonadotropin (hCG), which can be useful in the diagnostic evaluation.[112]

Thus, all histological varieties of gonadal germ cell tumors are found among mediastinal germ cell tumors. They are:
- Benign teratomas
- Seminomas (dysgerminomas)
- Teratocarcinomas (Malignant teratomas)
- Endodermal sinus tumor (yolk sac tumor)
- Choriocarcinoma (Embryonal cell carcinoma, Trophoblastic teratoma).

Germ cell tumors typically occur in young adults in their second to fourth decade with equal sex distribution. Some authors have reported a female predominance with a 1.27 to 2.05: 1 female: male ratio. Multicompartment extension is observed in 10 to 15 percent of the cases. According to another review, 3 to 8 percent are located in the posterior portion of the visceral compartment or the paravertebral regions, where neurogenic tumors and neoplastic lymphadenopathy commonly exist. In the case reported, the teratoma occupied at least two of the three-mediastinal compartments (the anterior and the middle) exerting compression on relevant vital anatomical structures.[121-129]

Nearly one half of patients (36-62% in various series) have no signs or symptoms when the mass is initially diagnosed. Symptoms commonly present are chest, back or shoulder pain, dyspnea, cough, fever, pleural effusion, and bulging of the chest wall. In a typical case, the patient presents with symptoms from her tumor for 2 months, either due to tumor inflammation or the total atelectasis of the lung, following recurrent pulmonary infections. Such a sizeable tumor was thus asymptomatic for a long period. Hemoptysis or expectoration of hair or sebum can rarely occur when communication between the tumor and the tracheobronchial tree develops. Symptoms can also derive from the pressure exerted on the surrounding tissues (for example superior vena cava syndrome). In spite of the pressure on the mediastinal vessels or the airway, invasion of these anatomical elements does not usually occur. However, erosion of the tumor to the bronchus, as well as to the pleural space, to the skin, and to the aorta has been reported. Occasionally there may be symptoms of metastasis to the liver, bone, and lung parenchyma.

Physical signs will include those of a mass lesion (bulging of mediastinum, impaired percussion note, diminished or absent breath sounds). Tumor extension into the pericardium or pleura will produce signs of pericardial or pleural effusion. Features of extrathoracic spread in the form of supraclavicular lymphadenopathy and hepatomegaly may be present. Testicular swelling is uncommon. Recently, there has been an increasing awareness of associations of mediastinal nonseminomatous germ cell tumors with a variety of clinical conditions such as nongerm cell malignancies and certain karyotypic abnormalities. They are shown in Table 29.8.

Diagnostic assessment is performed with classical X-rays, followed-up by CT. Radiographically most mediastinal germ cell tumors arise in the anterior mediastinum. Only about 3 to 8 percent of these tumors arise in the posterior mediastinum. Presence of a tooth in the plain skiagram is diagnostic of a benign teratoma. Typically, a well-circumscribed anterior mediastinal mass extending to one side of the midline and protruding into one lung field is revealed. CT accurately estimates the density of all included tissues, such as soft tissue (in virtually all cases), fluid (88%), fat (76%), calcification

TABLE 29.8: Disorders associated with mediastinal nonseminomatous germ cell tumors

1. Klinefelter syndrome
2. Malignant nongerm cell elements
   - Embryonal rhabdomyosarcoma
   - Neuroblastoma
   - Small cell undifferentiated cell carcinoma
   - Adenocarcinoma
3. Hematological malignancies
   - Acute megakaryocytic leukemia (M_7)
   - Acute nonlymphocytic leukemia
   - Myelodysplstic syndrome
   - Malignant histiocytosis
   - Myeloproliferative disorder
   - Refractory thrombocytopenia
   - Acute lymphoblastic leukemia
   - Hemophagocytic syndrome

(53%), and teeth and such imaging findings are considered specific. MRI is valuable in detecting the anatomic relations to the mediastinal and the hilar structures, such as vessels and airways.[130-136]

Measurements of serum tumor marker like β-HCG, alpha fetoprotein (AFP), and lactate dehydrogenase are indispensable in the management of mediastinal germ cell tumors. Benign teratoma is negative for these markers and a significant elevation of these markers indicates a malignant component of the tumor.

Mediastinal Teratomas (Benign)

The most common germ cell tumor, particularly in children, is benign teratoma. These tumors exhibit a variety of mature tissues from the three germ cell layers. The term "dermoid cyst" or teratodermoid is commonly used for this tumor because of frequent expression of the ectodermal component. Consisting of tissue from at least two of the three primitive germ layers, benign teratomas are the most common mediastinal GCT.[137] Ectodermal tissues, which usually predominate, include skin, hair, sweat glands, and tooth-like structures. Mesodermal tissues, such as fat, cartilage, bone, and smooth muscle are less common, as are endodermal structures like respiratory and intestinal epithelium.[138] The majority of mediastinal teratomas are mature teratomas that are histologically well defined and benign.[137] If a teratoma contains fetal tissue or neuroendocrine tissue, it is defined as immature and malignant. In children, the prognosis is favorable, but it can often recur or metastasize.[139]

Most patients are completely asymptomatic. Like other mediastinal masses, presenting symptoms include cough, dyspnea, and chest pain. Digestive enzymes secreted by intestinal mucosa or pancreatic tissue found in the teratoma can lead to the rupture of the bronchi, pleura, pericardium, or lung.[112] A rare result of a ruptured mediastinal teratoma is the expectoration of hair or sebum.[140,141] Mature teratomas do have the potential in rare circumstances to undergo malignant transformation into a variety of malignancies. Reports[142] of rhabdomyosarcoma, adenocarcinoma, leukemia, and anaplastic small cell tumors have all been identified as arising from mature or immature teratomas.

Benign teratomas are well-defined, round, or lobulated masses when seen on a chest radiograph. Up to 26 percent are calcified, as they often have elements of bone or teeth.[143] CT scanning and MRI are used to assess resectability, and may identify sebaceous elements and fat, supporting the diagnosis.[144,145] Complete surgical resection is the treatment of choice; however, subtotal resection can relieve symptoms. Adjunctive chemotherapy may be useful after subtotal resection.[146] Complete resection is the treatment of choice for benign mediastinal teratoma and this results in near universal cure. There is no role for radio- or chemotherapy. However, complete removal of the tumor is often difficult. The tumors are more frequently adherent to the adjacent structures such as the pericardium, lung, and great vessels. If it is so, a more extensive surgery like pericardiectomy, resection of the phrenic nerve, or lobectomy will be necessary. In spite of these limitations, excellent outcome is the rule.

Mediastinal Seminoma

Primary mediastinal seminomas, although uncommon, comprise 25 to 50 percent of malignant mediastinal GCTs occurring most frequently in men ages 20 to 40 years. Patients present with dyspnea, substernal pain, weakness, cough, fever, gynecomastia, or weight loss. About 10 percent of patients present with superior vena cava syndrome because of the tumor location.[147] However, tumors can grow to huge sizes (up to 20 to 30 cm) before symptoms develop.[148]

Radiographically, seminomas are bulky, lobulated, homogenous masses. Local invasion is rare, but metastasis to lymph nodes and bone does occur.[112] CT and gallium scanning is used to evaluate the extent of disease.[149]

The initial problem with the management of patients with suspected malignant mediastinal germ cell tumor is the difficulty in establishing the diagnosis. Elevation of beta-HCG and AFP in a young man with a mediastinal mass is highly suggestive of a mediastinal germ cell tumor. Whenever possible, a tissue diagnosis is to be obtained. Mediastinal seminoma was usually treated with mega voltage radiotherapy resulting in 60 to 80 percent long-term survival. Seminomas are uniquely sensitive to radiation therapy. The problem with radiotherapy is that the tumor may be too bulky at presentation with invasion of the surrounding structures. When radiotherapy *is given to* such an extensive area, this can result in excess radiation of the normal lung and other mediastinal structures. Secondly, even *if local* control is obtained, 20 to 40 percent of the patient will relapse at distant sites. Chemotherapy has recently been introduced to treat cases of seminoma. Such chemotherapy regimens consist of cisplatin, bleomycin, etoposide and vinblastin. Although exact regimens are in evolution patients with isolated mediastinal seminoma without metastasis are managed with mediastinal radiation alone. Patients with extramediastinal spread are given cisplatin-containing regimens. Management of patients with residual seminoma after chemotherapy remains controversial. While some advocate surgery, others recommend close watch of the patient. Chemotherapy is the treatment of choice for mediastinal nonseminomatous germ coil tumors. All such patients should receive cisplatin-based chemotherapy. When the tumor markers become normalized, resection of the remaining tumor should be undertaken. However, this group of tumors carries a poor prognosis.

In a study by Bush et al[150] of 13 patients with localized disease who were treated with External beam radiation, the 10 year disease-free survival rate was 54 percent, with an actuarial survival rate of 69 percent. A retrospective study by Bokemeyer et al[151] showed that chemotherapy alone led to a 90 percent 5 year disease-free survival rate and that additional radiation offered only a slight survival advantage, while patients treated with just radiation initially had a much higher rate of disease recurrence. In patients with locally advanced disease, the preferred treatment includes chemotherapy followed by the surgical resection of residual disease.[152]

Mediastinal Nonseminomatous GCTs

Nonseminomatous malignant GCTs comprise a heterogeneous group of masses that includes embryonal cell carcinomas, endodermal thymus tumors, choriocarcinomas, yolk sac tumors, and mixed GCTs with multiple cellular components. These tumors are often symptomatic and malignant, and predominantly affect young men.[112] In addition, they can be associated with hematologic malignancies, and 20 percent of patients have Kleinfelter syndrome.[153,154] At diagnosis, 85 percent of patients are symptomatic, which includes complaints of chest pain, hemoptysis, cough, fever, or weight loss. Gynecomastia can develop as a result of beta-hCG secretion from certain tumor types.[155]

These tumors are large, irregularly shaped, with areas of central necrosis, hemorrhage, or cyst formation.[156] Measuring AFP and beta-hCG levels is important in making the diagnosis. An elevated AFP level is suggestive of an endodermal sinus tumor or embryonal carcinoma and is sufficient, in the presence of a mediastinal mass, to establish the diagnosis.[120,155]

Chemotherapy with bleomycin, etoposide, and cisplatin is the current standard of care for patients with nonseminomatous malignant GCTs.[157] Following chemotherapy, > 5 percent of patients have total resolution of their malignancy with normalized serum markers. Patients with residual tumor undergo surgical resection, although studies have shown that the normalization of tumor markers prior to surgery will have a better prognosis.[157,158] In contrast to pure seminomas, nonseminomatous GCTs carry a poorer prognosis; patients with these tumors have a 5 year overall survival rate of 48 percent, compared to 86 percent in patients with seminomas.[159]

III. NEUROGENIC TUMORS

During embryogenesis, a group of cells of ectodermal origin get separated from the main neural tube and are called the neural crest cells. These cells separate into four categories of neural cells, namely, the peripheral nerve cells or neurocytes; nerve sheath cells; APUD cells; and the melanocytes. Neurogenic tumors are derived from tissue of the neural crest, including cells of the peripheral, autonomic, and paraganglionic nervous systems. Ninety-five percent of posterior mediastinal masses arise in the intercostals nerve rami or the sympathetic chain region.[160] They are classified on the basis of cell type and comprise approximately 12 to 21 percent of all mediastinal masses, although 95 percent occur in the posterior compartment.[161] Seventy percent to 80 percent of neurogenic tumors are benign, and nearly half are asymptomatic; however, they can occasionally cause compressive or neurologic symptoms.[160,162,163] Various neural tumors of the mediastinum are derived from these component cells (no mediastinal melanocytic tumor is described) and are as follows:

1. Tumors from peripheral nerve cells or neurocytes
   - Ganglioneuromas (benign)
   - Ganglioneuroblastomas (malignant)
   - Neuroblastomas
2. Tumors of nerve sheath cells
   - Neurilemmomas (neurinoma; Schwannomas)
   - Neurofibromas
   - Neurosarcomas (malignant neurilemmomas)
   - Granular cell myoblastoma
3. APUD cell tumors (APUDomas)
   - Carcinoid tumors
   - Paraganglionomas (Chemodectomas, aortic body tumors, pheochromocytomas)
   - Small cell carcinomas.

Benign mediastinal tumors of neurocytes arising from the autonomic ganglia are called ganglioneuromas. The malignant counterparts are called ganglioneuroblastomas. In theses tumors, the ganglionic tissue components can still be identified. Neuroblastomas are more aggressive tumors of neurocytes where the ganglionic cell differentiation is lost. Nerve sheath cells give rise to both Schwann cells and the perineural and endoneural fibrous tissue. Neurilemmomas arise from Schwann cells and the neurofibromas arise from the fibrous tissue elements. Some believe that these tumors also arise from Schwann cells. Both the tumors of the nerve sheath cells are considered benign and they have potential of undergoing malignant changes, when they are called neurosarcomas. An extremely uncommon humor, the granular cell myoblastoma, arises from the precursors of Schwann cells. APUD cells have the characteristic histochemical features—high amine content; amine precursor uptake; amino acid decarboxylase. Carcinoid tumors arise commonly in the thorax. Paraganglionomas arise from the paraganglionic tissue and they are in close proximity of the sympathetic ganglion in the posterior mediastinum and in the region of the aortic arch. Hormonally inactive paraganglionomas of the chemoreceptor system are called chemodectomas. Those tumors that arise near the aortic arch are called aortic body tumors. When the paraganglionomas are hormonally active, they are called pheochromocytomas.

Benign nerve sheath tumors (neurilemmomas and neurofibromas) are the largest number of neural neoplasms of the mediastinum and occur almost exclusively in the posterior mediastinum. In children, the nerve cell tumors are the commonest neural tumors. Neurilemmomas are well capsulated, rounded tumors, which arise laterally from their parent nerves, which are usually spinal, but may occasionally the sympathetic chain, or rarely, the vagus. Neurofibromas are similar tumors and mostly arise from the spinal nerves. Neurofibromas may be multiple and may assume a serpentine form. It may be part of the von Recklinghausen's disease or neurofibromatosis. These tumors occur equally in both sexes and the common age of presentation is between 30 to 60 years. The tumor is most often asymptomatic and discovered accidentally. When present, the clinical features are the same as in any other benign mediastinal tumor. Spinal cord compression is a rare but well recognized complication of this tumor, because of the dumbbell or hourglass tumors straddling the intervertebral foramina. Spinal nerve involvement may cause segmental pain. The malignant component of the tumors — neurosarcomas—occurs more frequently in von Recklinghausen's disease. They are rare tumors comprising of less than 5 percent of all neural tumors. Besides the usual symptoms of any mediastinal tumor, and those due to metastatic complications, both local and systemic, nausea, vomiting, and hypoglycemia are other symptoms of this tumor.

Presence of extrathoracic manifestations of neurofibromatosis like cutaneous *cafe au lait* spots may be there. The prognosis is poor because of their tendency to invade locally and metastasize systemically. Neurocytic tumors arise from autonomic ganglia of the sympathetic chain. Ganglioneuromas occur in younger ages and are usually asymptomatic. The tumor is slow growing and well encapsulated. They should be removed surgically because of their malignant potentials. Mediastinal anglioneuroblastomas are rare tumors in adults and are asymptomatic in about 50 percent of cases. The histological features suggest that it is intermediate between the benign ganglioneuroma and the more malignant neuroblastoma. The tumors arise mainly from the sympathetic chain and lie in the posterior mediastinum. The tumor should be removed when diagnosed because it is locally malignant and a 5 year survival is reported in 86 percent of these cases. In about a tenth of cases, the tumor is biologically active producing catecholamines. Neuroblastomas are common.

Tumors in childhood, about a fifth of all neuroblastomas arise in the mediastinum and almost always in the posterior mediastinum from the sympathetic neural cells. The usual age of presentation is early childhood at the age of two. The patient presents with systemic symptoms like anorexia, fever and cough. Symptoms of catecholamine overproduction like diarrhea, sweating, flushing, tachycardia and hypertension may be present in some cases. Spinal cord compression can occur. Microscopically, there are small rounded immature cells arranged in rosettes with varying degrees of differentiation. The mainstay of treatment is surgery followed by postoperative radiotherapy and chemotherapy. The prognosis is very poor.

Mediastinal apudomas are very rare tumors accounting for only 1 to 5 percent of the neural tumors. The treatment of these tumors is surgical and they are relatively radioresistant.

A brief account of each tumor will be discussed below:

Nerve Sheath Tumors

These benign, slowly growing tumors comprise 40 to 65 percent of neurogenic mediastinal masses. Neurilemmomas or schwannomas constitute 75 percent of this group of masses. These tumors are firm, encapsulated masses consisting of Schwann cells. Neurofibromas are nonencapsulated, soft, and friable, and are associated with von Recklinghausen neurofibromatosis.[164,165] They are often asymptomatic and are discovered incidentally.

Radiographically, nerve sheath tumors are sharply marginated spherical masses. Being adjacent to the spine, they can cause erosion and deformity of the ribs and ventral bodies as they increase in size. Low attenuation on CT scans can indicate hypocellularity, cystic changes, hemorrhage, or the presence of lipid within myelin.[112] Ten percent of these tumors grow through the intervertebral foramina and create a dumbbell appearance on radiographs.[166] MRI is used to rule out intraspinal extension.

Surgery is the treatment of choice for removal of these tumors through thoracoscopy, or thoracotomy.[162,163] For tumors invading the vertebral body or foramina, en bloc resection can be achieved.[167] There may be a role for postoperative chemotherapy or radiation therapy when total resection is not possible. Postoperative complications include Horner syndrome, partial sympathectomy, recurrent laryngeal nerve damage, and paraplegia.[163]

Malignant Tumors of Nerve Sheath Origin

Malignant nerve sheath tumors are spindle cell sarcomas of the posterior mediastinum, and include malignant neurofibromas, malignant schwannomas, and neurogenic fibrosarcomas. They affect men and women equally in the third to fifth decade of life and are closely associated with neurofibromatosis, with a 5 percent risk of sarcomatous degeneration.[168] Pain and nerve deficits are common. Complete surgical resection is the optimal treatment, but, in patients with unresectable tumors, adjuvant chemotherapy and radiation are options.

Autonomic Ganglionic Tumors

Tumors of the autonomic nervous system arise from neuronal cells rather than from the nerve sheath. They form a continuum ranging from benign encapsulated ganglioneuroma to aggressive malignant nonencapsulated neuroblastoma. Derived from embryologic origins, these tumors arise in the adrenal glands or in the sympathetic ganglia. However, ganglioneuromas and ganglioneuroblastomas arise mostly in the sympathetic ganglia of the posterior mediastinum.[169] Fifty percent of neuroblastomas arise in the adrenal glands and up to 30 percent in the mediastinum.[169,170]

Ganglioneuroma: Ganglioneuromas are benign tumors composed of one or more mature ganglionic cells. Arising from the nerve ganglion cells, they are the most benign and differentiated of the autonomic ganglionic tumors.[171] Most patients are asymptomatic and receive diagnoses in the second or third decade of life.[172] Radiographically, the tumors are oblong and well margined, occurring along the anterolateral aspect of the spine and spanning three to five vertebrae.[172] CT scanning is not particularly helpful as the mass can be homogenous or heterogeneous. Complete surgical resection is ideal.[173]

Ganglioneuroblastoma: Ganglioneuroblastomas have histologic features of both ganglioneuromas and neuroblastomas. They are the least common type of neurogenic tumor. Prognosis depends on histologic appearance.[112] Both sexes are equally affected in the first decade of life.[174] Symptoms may arise due to large tumor size, intraspinal extension, and metastasis. Staging is similar to that for neuroblastoma, as described in the following section.

Neuroblastoma: Neuroblastoma is a disease of young children, with 95 percent occurring in patients < 5 years of age.[170,175] Neuroblastomas are highly aggressive and readily metastasizing tumors that are composed of small round cells arranged in sheets or pseudorosettes.[176] They are nonencapsulated lesions, often-exhibiting hemorrhage, necrosis, or cystic degeneration. Symptoms include pain, neurologic deficits, Horner syndrome, respiratory distress, and ataxia.[175,176] Neuroblastomas have the highest propensity of any tumors in its class to produce vasoactive substances that can cause hypertension, flushing, and diarrhea.[169]

TABLE 29.9: Staging of neuroblastoma and ganglioneuroblastomas[177]

Stage	Characteristics
I	Well-circumscribed, noninvasive ipsilateral tumors
II	Local invasion without extension across the midline, ipsilateral regional lymph node involvement
III	Tumor extension across the midline and involvement of bilateral regional lymph nodes
IV	Metastatic disease
IVS	Clinical stage I or II and metastatic disease limited to the liver, skin and bone marrow

Grossly, these tumors appear as an elongated paraspinous mass, sometimes impinging on adjacent structures and causing skeletal damage.[178,179] On CT scans, 80 percent of these tumors have calcification.[179] As with all neurogenic tumors, MRI is useful to determine the extent of intraspinal involvement.[173] Radionuclide imaging with[123] metaiodobenzylguanide can also be used to detect primary and metastatic disease.[180]

Treatment for neuroblastoma depends primarily on the stage of diseases out lined in Table 29.9. Treatment for limited-stage disease is surgical resection. For patients with stage I disease, resection is usually curative. For patients with partially respectable stage II and III disease, treatment includes postoperative chemotherapy and radiation. For patients with stage IV disease, there is much controversy over the role of surgery; however, some studies[181] have suggested that delayed surgery after initial treatment with chemotherapy and radiation results in a better outcome than initial surgical intervention. In addition, there are ongoing studies looking at the role of radioactive ^{131}I metaiodobenzylguanide therapy in combination with chemotherapy in patients with advanced-stage disease.[182] Poor prognostic factors in neuroblastoma include large tumor size, poorly differentiated cell type, advanced stage, extrathoracic origin, and presentation in an elderly patient.[165]

IV. MEDIASTINAL CYSTS

These consist of foregut duplication (bronchogenic cyst, enteric cyst, neuroenteric), pericardial cysts, thymic cysts, and cysts associated with thoracic duct. Such congenital cysts account for 15 percent of all mediastinal tumors and cysts.

Mediastinal cysts comprise 12 to 20 percent of mediastinal masses and are found in the middle compartment of the mediastinum.[183-185] Despite a similar incidence, children are more often symptomatic at presentation due to compression on the surrounding structures.[186] The most common type of mediastinal cyst is a foregut cyst, which are derived as an embryonic abnormality, with enterogenous cysts (50 to 70%) and bronchogenic cysts (7 to 15%) being the most common subtypes.[112]

It is the formation of cysts, diverticulae, or fistulae resulting from developmental malformation of the tracheobronchial tree, esophagus, or the stomach. All these structures are derived from the primitive foregut. Defective separation of the tracheobronchial bud from the foregut results in a cystic space between the trachea or bronchi and the esophagus or stomach. There may also be a defective coalescence of chains of vacuoles during epithelial proliferation within the tracheobronchial tree giving rise to bronchogenic or bronchial cysts which may be solitary or multiple. Neuroenteric cysts may result from abnormal development, which runs between the upper gastrointestinal tract and the skin surface over the upper thoracic vertebrae. Intrathoracic foregut duplication may be intra- or extrapulmonary and usually occurs in relation to the esophagus, trachea, or, a major bronchus. They are more common in the right than in the left hemi-thorax. They are often recognized during infancy.

Grossly, they appear as rounded or oval saccular structures. They may be tubular or elongated, containing thick mucus. Microscopically, ciliated columnar or pseudostratified epithelium of the respiratory type, or those of gastrointestinal tract containing parietal cells of the stomach line foregut duplication. The latter may produce acid causing peptic ulcers. Sometimes cartilages, bone tissues, mucous glands, smooth muscles, and even pancreatic tissue may be identified in the cyst wall.

Most of the children with foregut cysts present with dyspnea, stridor, persistent cough, and those with neuroenteric cyst may present with neurological symptoms. In adults most foregut cysts are chance radiographic findings. Complications like recurrent chest infections with abscess formation are common. Peptic ulcers may perforate into the pleura or pericardium. There is an increased risk of adenocarcinoma in a foregut cyst. Chest radiograph usually reveals a rounded opacity with a hairline margin. The cyst is usually large measuring about 5 cm or more in the longest axis. The cyst may contain a fluid level because of communication with either the respiratory tract or the gastrointestinal tract. Fused vertebrae and scoliosis may indicate the presence of a neuroenteric cyst.

Treatment of these cysts is surgical excision. Needle aspiration may improve acute respiratory distress in a child. The prognosis is excellent.

Bronchogenic Cysts

Bronchogenic cysts are formed during embryonic development as an anomalous budding of the laryngotracheal groove.[187] These cysts are lined with ciliated, pseudostratified, columnar epithelium, and contain bronchial glands and cartilaginous plates.[112] Approximately 40 percent of bronchogenic cysts are symptomatic resulting in cough, dyspnea, or chest pain.[188]

Radiographically, bronchogenic cysts can be identified on plain radiographs but are best defined by CT scanning. These cysts are well-defined round masses with a homogenous density similar to water; however, some bronchogenic cysts are mucoid and can give the impression of being as solid mass.[186] Bronchogenic cysts are nonenhancing, and, when there is a direct communication with the tracheobronchial tree, air-fluid levels may be seen.[188] MRI can differentiate the lesion from other masses.

Tissue is often required to make a definitive diagnosis of a bronchogenic cyst. This can be accomplished by tracheobronchial, endoscopic, or thoroscopic needle aspiration. Most bronchogenic cysts are removed surgically or are drained by needle aspiration. The treatment of asymptomatic cysts is controversial as surgery is not without risk, yet these cysts can grow to cause symptoms in the future.[189]

Enterogenous Cysts

Enterogenous cysts arise from the dorsal foregut and are lined by squamous or enteric (alimentary) epithelium and may contain gastric or pancreatic tissue. Esophageal duplication cysts are located in or are attached to the esophageal wall. Twelve percent of patients with esophageal duplication cysts have associated malformations, mostly of the GI tract.[190] Symptoms of enterogenous cysts are similar to those of other mediastinal cysts. They are often asymptomatic, but if they contain gastric or pancreatic mucosa, there is the added risk of hemorrhage or rupture of the cyst from mucosal secretions. Radiographically, it can be difficult to distinguish these from bronchogenic cysts, although they are more often calcified. The presence of cartilage suggests the presence of a bronchogenic cyst.[187] Most cysts should be surgically excised, and video-assisted thoracic surgery is the treatment of choice.[191]

Neuroenteric Cysts

Neuroenteric cysts are characterized by the presence of both enteric and neural tissue in surgical specimens.[192] Most of these cysts form in the posterior mediastinum above the level of the main carina. The close association of the foregut and notochord during embryogenesis possibly explains this anatomic location. Neuroenteric cysts are associated with multiple vertebral anomalies, such as scoliosis, spina bifida, hemivertebra, and vertebral fusion. Almost all are discovered by age 1 year due to symptoms from tracheobronchial compression.[112] Neurologic symptoms may be caused by intraspinal extension. Complete surgical excision is curative.[193]

Pericardial Cysts

Otherwise known as *spring-water cysts*, or the *hydrocele of the mediastinum*, these are the second most common cysts following foregut duplication. The cyst is relatively rare. They are developmental anomalies possibly as a result of persistent ventral parietal recess of the primitive intra-embryonic coelomic cavity from which the pleura, pericardium, and the peritoneum develop. Pericardial cysts are part of a larger group of mesothelial cysts. They form as a result of a persistent parietal recess during embryogenesis.[187] They are estimated to occur in 1 of 100,000 people. Although most are congenital, a few cases of acquired pericardial cysts do exist. Two-thirds of these cysts occurs in the right cardiophrenic angle and is usually situated anteriorly. Other sites, are left cardiophrenic angle, and rarely in the superior or posterior mediastinum. They can occur at any age. The size varies considerably ranging from 5 to 25 cm. The cyst is usually unilocular with a thin lining epithelium. It contains crystal clear fluid (*spring-water cyst*). The fluid is devoid of any cells, but contains proteins and characteristically is a transudate. Most of these cysts are asymptomatic and detected as a chance radiological finding. They are often asymptomatic and are identified in the fourth to fifth decade of life. Rarely, cardiac compression may occur, causing hemodynamic compromise. Radiographically, pericardial cysts are well-marginated spherical or teardrop-shaped masses that characteristically abut the heart, anterior chestwall, and diaphragm.[112] The most common location of pericardial cysts is at the right cardiophrenic angle (70%), followed by the left cardiophrenic angle (22%).[194] Chest pain is more common in symptomatic patients. Compression of right middle lobe bronchus may cause cough and dyspnea. Radiologically, a sharply demarcated smooth edged cystic lesion is on the posteroanterior and lateral skiagram of the chest. They are usually situated in the right and rarely on the left. It is nonpulsatile and may alter shape during respiration on fluoroscopic examination. Echocardiography is confirmatory. CT will classically show a mass, which contains fluid. The differential diagnosis is pericardial fat, eventration of the diaphragm, and a diaphragmatic hernia, and rarely a ventricular aneurysm. On CT scans, these masses appear as unilocular and nonenhancing. As with most mediastinal cysts, surgical removal is the treatment of choice, although clinically asymptomatic patients may be observed without intervention. The cyst should be removed surgically and the prognosis is good following such a procedure.

Lymphatic cysts and tumors like thoracic duct cysts, lymphangioleiomyoma, and cystic hygroma are rarely found in the mediastinum.

Lymphangiomas

Lymphangiomas are rare congenital abnormalities of the lymphatic vessels. Typically, they are isolated solitary masses, but they can be more widespread or associated with chromosomal abnormalities.[195] These lesions are benign in nature and are found in the cervical region 75 percent of the time. In 10 percent of cases, the cysts extend into the mediastinum and are associated with chylothorax and hemangiomas.[195] Although these tumors are commonly identified in children before the age of 2 years, when the mass is isolated to the mediastinum it is often not identified until it has gotten large enough to cause compressive symptoms.[196] Such symptoms include chest pain, cough, and dyspnea. Radiographically, these lesions appear cystic and can be confused with pericardial cysts, although lymphangiomas are more likely to have a loculated appearance.[196] The use of lymphangiographic contrast media combined with CT scanning can also differentiate these lesions.[195] Total resection is optimal; however, in cases complicated by chylothorax, there is some evidence suggesting that additional radiotherapy may be of some benefit.[197] Lymphangiomatosis seen in young women is typically a more progressive form of disease in which multiple tumors are found and invade multiple organ structures, including the lung, heart, and bone.[198]

V. MISCELLANEOUS DISORDERS OF MEDIASTINUM

Primary Mediastinal Lymphoma

Primary mediastinal lymphoma is a rare entity comprising only 10 percent of lymphomas in the mediastinum. Lymphoma usually occurs in the anterior mediastinum and is part of more widespread disease. HD represents approximately 50 to 70 percent of mediastinal lymphomas, while non-Hodgkin lymphoma comprises 15 to 25 percent.[90,91] The three most common types of mediastinal lymphoma include nodular sclerosing HD, large B-cell lymphoma, and lymphoblastic lymphoma.[112]

Mediastinal Goiter

In patients undergoing thyroidectomy, the incidence of mediastinal goiter is 1 to 15 percent.[199] Most goiters are euthyroid and are found incidentally during a physical examination. Radiographically, mediastinal goiters are encapsulated, lobulated, heterogeneous tumors.[112] A classic finding on a CT scan is continuity of the cervical and mediastinal components of the thyroid. If the goiter contains functional thyroid tissue, then scintigraphy with a radioactive isotope of iodine can be diagnostic.[112]

Surgical resection is recommended since these lesions are not usually amenable to needle biopsy, and malignancy develops in a significant number. Nearly all substernal goiters can be removed easily through a cervical incision minimizing surgical morbidity.[200]

Mediastinal Parathyroid Adenoma

The mediastinum is the most common location at which an ectopic parathyroid tumor may develop. Overall, 20 percent of parathyroid adenomas develop in the mediastinum, with 80 percent occurring in the anterior mediastinum.[201] These tumors are encapsulated, round, and usually < 3 cm in size, so that they may not be identified on a CT scan. Thus, MRI or nuclear scans with ^{99m}Tc and ^{201}Ti are more effective for the diagnosis of parathyroid adenomas.[202] Surgical resection is curative.

Mediastinitis

Various causes of acute mediastinitis are as follows:
- Perforation of the esophagus
  — Following endoscopy
  — Following dilatation of a stricture
  — Insertion of a tube for palliative purposes for carcinoma
  — Accidental blunt or penetrating injury
  — Surgery of the esophagus or surrounding structures
  — Ingeston of foreign bodies
  — Following vomiting (Mallory-Weiss syndrome)
- Direct extension of infection from the neck
  — Retropharyngeal space, lung, pleura, or pericardium
  — Osteomyelitis of the ribs, vertebrae
  — Central venous cannulation
- Tuberculosis or fungal infections.

The patient is usually ill with fever, rigors, chest pain, dysphagia, and discomfort on moving the neck. Compression of trachea may produce cough. Mediastinal or subcutaneous emphysema can be present if the esophagus is perforated and pleural effusion, empyema, or pyopneumothorax may be present. Sternal tenderness is common.

Chest radiograph reveals a smooth walled convex opacity, which bulges laterally beyond the mediastinum, with displacement of the trachea, and esophagus. Gas may be present in the mediastinum or in the tissue plane in the neck. There may be evidence of pleural] involvement. The chest X-ray may even be normal. CT scan can confirm presence of mediastinal fluid.

Treatment consists of broad-spectrum antibiotics with anaerobic cover. When there is radiographic evidence of collection of fluid or there is pressure symptoms/signs, surgical drainage is indicated through a low cervical incision. The underlying cause should be tackled simultaneously.

Mediastinal Fibrosis (Fibrosing Mediastinitis)

This is a slowly progressive envelopment of the mediastinal structures due to scar tissues. The exact etiology of the condition is unknown although a number of infectious agents have been implicated. Most often, it is idiopathic or cryptogenic. Other synonyms of the condition are: *Chronic fibrous* or *fibrosing mediastinitis, idiopathic fibrosis of the mediastinum,* and *chronic mediastinal fibrosis.* In this condition, masses of ill-defined scar tissue encase and compress mediastinal structures. Any part of the mediastinum may be involved. They are mainly bundles of interwoven collagenous tissue with plasma cell, lymphocytes, neutrophils, and fibroblast infiltrations.

This is a slowly progressive envelopment of the mediastinal structures due to scar tissues. John Hunter described the condition as early as 1957 due to syphilis when this was a very common condition. Subsequently other conditions were recognized. Fibrosing mediastinitis is an uncommon benign disorder characterized by proliferation of dense fibrous tissue within the mediastinum.[203] This entity is also known as *sclerosing mediastinitis* and as *mediastinal fibrosis.* Affected patients are typically young and present with signs and symptoms related to obstruction of vital mediastinal structures, such as central systemic veins, the esophagus, airways, and pulmonary arteries or veins. The precise cause and pathogenesis of fibrosing mediastinitis in most cases is unknown, and links to infectious and noninfectious causes remain speculative. Recently, Flieder and colleagues[204] proposed the term *idiopathic fibroinflammatory lesion of the mediastinum* to replace the present term *fibrosing mediastinitis.* In doing so, they emphasized that, in most cases, a definite cause cannot be established with certainty and that there is substantial variability in the histopathologic appearance of the lesions.

Various causes of mediastinal fibrosis are as follows:
- Idiopathic
- Infections
  — Tuberculosis
  — Syphilis
  — Histoplasma capsulatum
  — Aspergillosis
  — Mucormycosis
  — Blastomycosis
  — Cryptococcosis.

- Autoimmune disease
- Behçet disease
- Rheumatic fever
- Radiation therapy
- Trauma
- Hodgkin disease
- Drugs (methysergide maleate, protocol)
- Other idiopathic fibroinflammatory disorders
  — Retroperitoneal fibrosis
  — Sclerosing cholangitis
  — Riedel thyroiditis
  — Pseudotumor of the orbit.

Despite extensive investigation, the precise cause and pathogenesis of fibrosing mediastinitis remains unclear. The cause will be different for different countries. Many, cases in the United States have been linked to *Histoplasma capsulatum* infection.[203,205-211] The relationship between fibrosing mediastinitis and the so-called mediastinal granuloma is controversial.[212,213]

Other infections, including tuberculosis,[214] aspergillosis, mucormycosis, blastomycosis,[215] and cryptococcosis,[216] are implicated in some cases of mediastinal fibrosis. Fibrosing mediastinitis has also been reported in the setting of autoimmune disease,[216] Behçet disease,[217] rheumatic fever, radiation therapy,[218] trauma, Hodgkin disease, and drug therapy with methysergide maleate.[216] In addition, fibrosing mediastinitis can occur in association with other idiopathic fibroinflammatory disorders such as retroperitoneal fibrosis, sclerosing cholangitis, Riedel thyroiditis, and pseudotumor of the orbit.[219-229]

Fibrosing mediastinitis is characterized by an ill-defined soft-tissue mass involving the mediastinum in which dense, white fibrous tissue is seen in cut sections. The process may occur as a localized mass or may diffusely infiltrate the mediastinum and, in rare cases, extend into the soft tissues of the neck,[230] the posterior mediastinum,[231] and the lung.

Microscopic examination of biopsy specimens from patients with fibrosing mediastinitis reveals abundant, paucicellular fibrous tissue infiltrating and obliterating adipose tissue. The fibrous tissue can contain patchy infiltrates of mononuclear cells. Flieder and colleagues,[204] in a study of 30 cases of idiopathic fibrosing mediastinitis, described a histopathologic spectrum of changes for which they established a three-step staging system. Stage I lesions are composed predominantly of edematous fibromyxoid tissue. In stage II disease, the lesions contain glassy bands of eosinophilic hyaline material that encircle and infiltrate mediastinal structures. Obliterative lesions of dense paucicellular collagen

characterize stage III disease, and their appearance represents the classic microscopic features of fibrosing mediastinitis. Although Flieder et al found their system useful for describing the variety of histopathologic findings seen in cases of fibrosing mediastinitis, their staging system does not appear to be clinically relevant at this time.

Because fibrosing mediastinitis is associated with a multiplicity of clinical syndromes and diseases, great care must be exercised when one evaluates open or needle biopsy specimens that demonstrate fibrosis. The histologic differential diagnosis of fibrosing mediastinitis includes localized fibrosis associated with infection, most commonly histoplasmosis and tuberculosis, and fibrosis occurring in association with a variety of malignancies. The neoplasms that most frequently produce fibrosis and thus must be included in the differential diagnosis include sclerosing non-Hodgkin lymphoma and the nodular sclerosis variant of Hodgkin disease. Localized fibrous tumors of the pleura and diffuse desmoplastic malignant mesotheliomas should also be considered, although these spindle cell tumors can be readily excluded because of their increased cellularity and the characteristic immunohistochemical staining for CD34 and bcl-2 of the former and keratin of the latter. Metastatic carcinomas with a fibrogenic inflammatory response, thymoma, and thymic carcinoid all show keratin staining of tumor cells. Simple fibrosis, fibromatosis, and low-grade sarcoma are also possibilities in the differential diagnosis. Because all these lesions may exhibit areas of fibrosis, biopsy samples obtained with a percutaneous needle technique may be insufficient to rule out malignancy due to their limited size; an open biopsy with extensive sampling is frequently required to establish a definitive diagnosis.[212,216]

Clinical Features

Patients with fibrosing mediastinitis are typically young at presentation, although the disease is reported to occur over a very wide age range. It affects males and females in roughly equal proportions. A recent study suggested that African-American patients are disproportionately affected,[204] but this predilection has not been reported in other series. Most patients present with signs or symptoms related to obstruction or compression of vital mediastinal structures such as the central airways, superior vena cava, pulmonary veins, pulmonary arteries and esophagus. The heart, pericardium, coronary arteries, aorta, and aortic branch vessels are much less frequently involved. The most common presenting complaints include cough, dyspnea, recurrent pulmonary infection, hemoptysis, and pleuritic chest pain. Patients may present with systemic signs such as fever and weight loss. Fibrosing mediastinitis has been reported to be the most common benign cause of the superior vena cava syndrome.[203] However, this syndrome is unusual in many series of patients with fibrosing mediastinitis, particularly when cases of mediastinal granuloma are excluded. In fact, some authors have concluded that superior vena cava syndrome more typically results from compression of the superior vena cava by a mediastinal granuloma and that superior vena cava obstruction in cases of fibrosing mediastinitis is comparatively rare.[203] Obstruction of the central airways typically manifests with cough and dyspnea. Affected patients can also present with a history of recurrent or persistent pneumonia or exhibit atelectasis in the lung distal to the occluded airway.

Patients with pulmonary venous occlusion can present with progressive or exertional dyspnea as well as with hemoptysis. This pattern of symptoms has been called the "*pseudo-mitral stenosis syndrome.*" Long-standing pulmonary venous occlusion can also result in secondary pulmonary arterial hypertension and cor pulmonale—one of the most important causes of morbidity and mortality in patients with fibrosing mediastinitis. Pulmonary venous occlusion can also lead to pulmonary infarction. Pulmonary arterial stenosis or occlusion less frequently results in pulmonary hypertension.

Fibrosing mediastinitis often has an unpredictable course, with both spontaneous remission and exacerbation of symptoms being reported. Loyd et al[203] reported a mortality rate of greater than 30 percent, which is much higher than that reported in other studies. Causes of death are usually recurrent infection, hemoptysis, or cor pulmonale. The mortality rate among patients with subcarinal or bilateral mediastinal involvement may be higher than that among patients with more localized mediastinal or hilar fibrosis.[203] There are three possible avenues for treatment: systemic antifungal or corticosteroid treatment, surgical resection, and local therapy for complications.

Investigations[232]

Chest Radiography

Although chest radiographs of patients with fibrosing mediastinitis usually appear abnormal, the findings can be quite subtle and the extent of mediastinal involvement is frequently underestimated. Fibrosing mediastinitis usually manifests on chest radiographs as nonspecific widening of the mediastinum, with distortion and obliteration of normally recognizable mediastinal interfaces or lines. The middle mediastinum is affected most often, particularly the subcarinal and right paratracheal regions. The right side of the mediastinum is more commonly involved than the left. Less frequently, a focal hilar mass is observed. Calcification within the mediastinum or hila is seen in up to 86 percent of patients. As expected, the radiographic findings of fibrosing mediastinitis in an individual patient very much depend on the mediastinal structure or structures involved. Patients with superior vena cava obstruction may have bilateral widening of the superior mediastinum on chest radiographs due to engorged collateral veins. Involvement of the central airways can result in segmental or lobar atelectasis or recurrent pneumonia in the affected portions of lung. Less commonly, actual narrowing of the affected airways is seen. The area of narrowing usually occurs at the level of the carina and in the majority of cases involves both main bronchi.[209] Pulmonary arterial obstruction is typically unilateral and can result in an appreciable diminution in size and quantity of vessels and localized regions of oligemia in the affected portions of lung. Pulmonary venous obstruction manifests radiographically with findings of localized pulmonary venous hypertension: peribronchial cuffing, septal thickening, and localized edema.[209] Pulmonary arterial or venous obstruction can also cause pulmonary infarcts that manifest as peripheral, wedge-shaped areas of homogeneous opacity. Pleural effusions are uncommon.

Computed Tomography

Fibrosing mediastinitis typically manifests on CT scans as an infiltrative mass of soft-tissue attenuation that obliterates normal mediastinal fat planes and encases or invades adjacent structures. Fibrosing mediastinitis most commonly affects the middle mediastinal compartment, including the right and left paratracheal and subcarinal regions as well as the hila. The anterior and posterior mediastinum are much less frequently involved.[231]

Two patterns of involvement on CT scans have been described: a *focal pattern* and a *diffuse pattern*. The focal pattern, seen in 82 percent of cases, manifests as a mass of soft-tissue attenuation that is frequently calcified (63% of cases) and is usually located in the right paratracheal or subcarinal regions or in the hila. This type of fibrosing mediastinitis is, in all probability, caused by histoplasmosis in patients from the United States. The diffuse pattern, seen in 18 percent of cases, manifest as a diffusely infiltrating, noncalcified mass that affects multiple mediastinal compartments. The diffuse pattern is probably not related to histoplasmosis but often occurs in the setting of other idiopathic fibrosing disorders such as retroperitoneal fibrosis.

In a relatively large radiologic series, Sherrick and colleagues[233] noted two distinct patterns of mediastinal involvement on CT scan. In 82 percent of affected patients, they observed relatively localized mediastinal disease most commonly affecting the right paratracheal and subcarinal regions. This pattern was frequently (63% of cases) associated with stippled calcification, and affected patients typically had evidence of prior granulomatous infection, either histoplasmosis or tuberculosis. In a minority of patients (18%), they observed a diffusely infiltrating, noncalcified mass that affected multiple mediastinal compartments. These patients did not have evidence of prior granulomatous infection, and half had other associated conditions such as retroperitoneal fibrosis.

MR Imaging

Fibrosing mediastinitis typically manifests on T1-weighted MR images as a heterogeneous, infiltrative mass of intermediate signal intensity. Its appearance on T2-weighted MR images is more variable;[48,57] regions of both increased and markedly decreased signal intensity are frequently seen in the same lesion.

Although careful MR imaging–histopathologic correlation has not been performed, areas of decreased signal intensity are thought to indicate the presence of calcification or fibrous tissue, and areas of increased signal intensity may indicate more active inflammation. Extensive regions of decreased signal intensity within the lesion, when present, help differentiate fibrosing mediastinitis from other infiltrative lesions of the mediastinum, such as metastatic carcinoma and lymphoma that typically have increased signal intensity on T2-weighted images. Heterogeneous enhancement of the mass may be seen after administration of a gadolinium-based contrast medium.

Other Imaging Modalities

Esophageal involvement by fibrosing mediastinitis is best demonstrated by contrast esophagography. The junction of the upper and middle thirds of the esophagus is most frequently affected, although extensive involvement can also occur. The affected segment of the esophagus is usually adjacent to involved regions of the trachea and main bronchi. Typical findings include both circumferential narrowing and long-segment strictures. Findings of "downhill" esophageal varices can be seen in cases of superior vena cava obstruction.

Perfusion scintigraphy performed with technetium-99m–labeled macroaggregated albumin (MAA) can show focal or diffuse perfusion defects in patients with pulmonary arterial or venous obstruction. Complete, unilateral absence of perfusion has also been seen in patients with focal hilar fibrosis. Ventilation scintigraphy, performed with either xenon-133 or aerosolized Tc-99m–DTPA (diethylenetriaminepentaacetic acid), can show ventilation defects in patients with lobar or segmental bronchial occlusion. Delayed washout of Xe-133 can be seen in partially obstructed regions of the lung.

Pulmonary arteriography has traditionally been performed in patients with suspected pulmonary arterial obstruction,[210] and contrast venography has been used to demonstrate central venous obstruction. Typical findings of fibrosing mediastinitis from either study include long-segment, smooth, or funnel-like stenoses of affected vessels. Both techniques are now less commonly used as diagnostic procedures, however, with the advent of contrast-enhanced spiral CT and MR angiography. These older techniques are now primarily reserved for patients in whom percutaneous therapy is performed.

The fluorine-18 fluorodeoxyglucose positron emission tomographic findings of fibrosing mediastinitis have been reported in a single case. In this case, although the majority of the lesion was hypometabolic, focal areas of increased metabolic activity were observed. Biopsy of these metabolically active sites revealed typical findings of fibrosing mediastinitis.

Because the chest radiographic findings of fibrosing mediastinitis are nonspecific and because MR imaging poorly depicts calcification, CT is considered the mainstay for diagnostic evaluation of patients with known or suspected fibrosing mediastinitis. The differential diagnosis of fibrosing mediastinitis at CT includes other infiltrative lesions of the mediastinum, such as lung cancer, metastatic carcinoma, lymphoma, and mediastinal sarcoma or, in rare cases, mediastinal desmoids tumors. When an extensively calcified, infiltrative mediastinal mass is seen on CT scans in a young patient from an area endemic for histoplasmosis, fibrosing mediastinitis is the most likely diagnosis. When the mass is not calcified, however, fibrosing mediastinitis cannot be confidently differentiated from these other lesions, and biopsy and culture of affected tissues is required.[233] It is essential that the lesion is sampled extensively to confidently exclude an underlying neoplasm such as Hodgkin disease that may occur in association with a fibrotic process.[216] For these reasons, surgical sampling performed during mediastinoscopy, thoracoscopy, or open thoracotomy may be preferred to transthoracic fine needle aspiration biopsy.[203] The role of percutaneous large-bore core needle biopsy has not been evaluated in this context.

Treatment

In cases where fungal infections like *H. capsulatum* infection is suspected, particularly in countries like USA with suspicion of an ensuing inflammatory reaction, some investigators will patients with systemic antifungal agents or corticosteroids. Most of the available data in this regard are based on either case reports or small series; prospective, randomized controlled trials have not been performed.[207,208,212] The limited data available suggest that ketoconazole therapy may result in stabilization of the disease process or, in some cases, limited symptomatic improvement.[208] However, given the unpredictable nature of the disorder, the significance of these uncontrolled data is not clear. Most studies have shown little or no beneficial effect of corticosteroid therapy.[212] Similarly, when there is suspicion of other infections is there, treatment should be directed towards that.

If disease is localized, surgical resection of affected tissues may be curative or result in amelioration of signs and symptoms.[205,207,212] A complete resection may require extensive vascular or airway reconstruction, techniques that are available at only a few centers. Bilateral mediastinal involvement is generally thought to preclude a surgical approach. On the whole, the results of surgical therapy have been disappointing, and resection is often associated with high morbidity and mortality.[203]

Increasingly, symptomatic patients are treated with local therapies directed toward reopening occluded or severely stenosed airways, pulmonary arteries, or venae cavae. Laser therapy, balloon dilation, and intravascular or endobronchial stent placement have all been used with some success to treat affected patients Spiral vein grafts to bypass an occluded vena cava have also been used with success.

REFERENCES

1. Fraser RS, Pare JAP, Fraser RG, et al. The normal chest. In: Fraser RS, Pare JAP, Fraser RG (Eds): Synopsis of diseases of the chest. (2nd edn) Philadelphia, PA: WB Saunders 1994;1-116.
2. Duwe BV, Sterman DH, Musani AI. Tumors of the mediastinum. Chest 2005;128:2893-909.
3. Crapo JD, Glassroth J, Karlinsky J, et al. Baum's textbook of pulmonary diseases. Philadelphia, PA: Lippincott Williams & Wilkins, 2004;883-12.
4. Davis RD Jr, Newland Oldham H Jr, Sabiston DC Jr. Primary cysts and neoplasms of the mediastinum: Recent changes in clinical presentation, methods of diagnosis, management and results. Ann Thorac Surg 1987;44:229-37.
5. Silverman NA, Sabiston DC Jr. Mediastinal masses. Surg Clin North Am 1980; 60:757-77.
6. Crapo JD, Glassroth J, Karlinsky J, et al. Baum's textbook of pulmonary diseases. Philadelphia, PA: Lippincott Williams & Wilkins 2004;883-912.
7. Grillo HC, Ojemann RG, Scannell JG, et al. Combined approach to "dumbbell" intrathoracic and intraspinal neurogenic tumors. Ann Thorac Surg 1983;36:402-07.
8. Gripp S, Bolke E, Orth K. Thymoma.Wien Klin Wochenschr 2005;117:620-27.
9. Wychulis AR, Payne WS, Clagett OT, et al. Surgical treatment of mediastinal tumors. J Thorac Cardiovasc Surg 1972;62:379-91.
10. Rosai J, Levine GD. Tumors of the thymus. In: Firminger HI (Ed): Atlas of tumor pathology. Washington, DC: Armed Forces Institute of Pathology 1976;34-212.
11. Lattes R. Thymoma and other tumors of the thymus: An analysis of 107 cases. Cancer 1962;15:1224-60.
12. Engels EA, Pfeiffer RM. Malignant thymoma in the United States: Demographic patterns in incidence and associations with subsequent malignancies. Int J Cancer 2003;105:546-51.
13. Mullen B, Richardson JD. Primary anterior mediastinal tumors in children and adults. Ann Thorac Surg 1986;42:338-45.
14. Gerein AN, Srivastava SP, Burgess J. Thymoma: A ten-year review. Am J Surg 1978;136:49-53.
15. Rosai J, Levine GD. Tumors of the Thymus. In Harlan I, Ferminger MD (Eds): Atlas of tumor pathology, 2nd series, fascicle 13. Washington (DC): The Armed Forces Institute of Pathology 1976;1-221.
16. Shimosato Y, Mukai K. Tumors of the Mediastinum. In: Rosai J, Sobin LH (Eds): Atlas of tumor pathology, 3rd series, fascicle 21. Washington (DC): The Armed Forces Institute of Pathology 1997;40-120.
17. Shimosato Y. Controversies surrounding the subclassification of thymoma. Cancer 1994;74:542-44.
18. Harris NL, Müller-Hermelink HK. Thymoma classification. A Siren's song of simplicity. Am J Clin Pathol 1999;112:299-303.
19. Kornstein MJ. Thymoma classification: My opinion. Am J Clin Pathol 1999;112:304-07.
20. Suster S, Moran CA. Thymoma classification. The ride of the Valkyries? Am J Clin Pathol 1999;112:308-10.
21. Bernatz PE, Harrison EG, Clagett OT. Thymoma: A clinicopathologic study. J Thorac Cardiovasc Surg 1961;42:424–44.
22. Maggi G, Giaccone G, Donadio M, Ciuffreda L, Dalesio O, Leria G, et al. A review of 169 cases, with particular reference to results of surgical treatment. Cancer 1986;58:765-76.
23. Lewis JE, Wick MR, Scheithauer BW, Bernatz PE, Taylor WF. Thymoma. A clinicopathologic review. Cancer 1987;60:2727-43.

24. Kornstein MJ, Curran WJ Jr, Turrisi AT 3rd, Brooks JJ. Cortical versus medullary thymomas: A useful morphologic distinction?. Hum Pathol 1988;19:1335-39.

25. Wick MR. Assessing the prognosis of thymomas. Ann Thorac Surg 1990;50:521-22.

26. Marino M, Müller-Hermelink HK. Thymoma and thymic carcinoma. Virchows Arch A Pathol Anat Histopathol 1985;407:119-49.

27. Kirchner T, Müller-Hermelink HK. New approaches to the diagnosis of thymic epithelial tumors. Prog Surg Pathol 1989;10:167-89.

28. Pescarmona E, Rendima EA, Venuta F. Analysis of prognostic factors and clinicopathological staging of thymomas. Ann Thorac Surg 1990;50:534-38.

29. Quintanilla-Martinez L, Wilkins EW, Ferry JA, Harris NL. Thymoma–morphologic subclassification correlates with invasiveness and immunohistologic features: A study of 122 cases. Hum Pathol 1993;24:958-69.

30. Quintanilla-Martinez L, Wilkins EW, Jr, Choi N, Efird J, Hug E, Harris NL. Thymoma. Histologic subclassification is an independent prognostic factor. Cancer1994;74:606-17.

31. D Lardinois, R Rechsteiner. Prognostic relevance of Masaoka and Müller-Hermelink classification in patients with thymic tumors. Ann Thorac Surg 2000;69:1550-55.

32. Pan CC, Wu HP, Yang CF, Chen WY, Chiang H. The clinicopathological correlation of epithelial subtyping in thymoma: A study of 112 consecutive cases. Hum Pathol 1994;25:893-99.

33. Moran CA, Suster S. Thymoma atypical thymoma, and thymic carcinoma. A novel conceptual approach to the classification of thymic epithelial neoplasms. Am J Clin Pathol 1999;111:826-33.

34. Rosai J. Histological typing of tumors of the thymus. World Health Organization International Histological Classification of Tumors (2nd edn), Springer-Verlag, New York, Berlin (1999).

35. Lucchi M, Basolo F, Ribechini A, Ambrogi MC, Bencivelli S, Fontanini G, Angeletti CA, Mussi A. Thymomas: Clinical-pathological correlations. J Cardiovasc Surg (Torino) 2006;47:89-93.

36. Wright CD, Wain JC, Wong DR, Donahue DM, Gaissert HA, Grillo HC, Mathisen DJ. Predictors of recurrence in thymic tumors: importance of invasion, World Health Organization histology, and size. J Thorac Cardiovasc Surg 2005;130:1413-21.

37. Strobel P, Marx A, Zettl A, Muller-Hermelink HK. Thymoma and thymic carcinoma: an update of the WHO Classification 2004. Surg Today 2005;35:805-11.

38. Uekusa T, Abe H, Suda K. Clinical usefulness of the WHO histological classification of thymoma. Ann Thorac Cardiovasc Surg 2005;11:367-73.

39. Hasserjian RP, Strobel P, Marx A. Pathology of thymic tumors. Semin Thorac Cardiovasc Surg 2005;17:2-11.

40. Okumura M, Ohta M, Tateyama H, et al. The World Health Organization histologic classification system reflects the oncologic behavior of thymoma: A clinical study of 273 patients. Cancer 2002;94:624-32.

41. Nakagawa K, Asamura H, Matsuno Y, et al. Thymoma: A clinicopathologic study based on the new World Health Organization classification. J Thorac Cardiovasc Surg 2003;126:1134-40.

42. Lardinois D, Rechsteiner R, Lang RH, et al. Prognostic relevance of Masaoka and Muller-Hermelink classification in patients with thymic tumors. Ann Thorac Surg 2000;69:1550-55.

43. Rosai J, Levine GD. Tumors of the thymus. In: Firminger HI (Ed): Atlas of tumor pathology. Washington, DC: Armed Forces Institute of Pathology 1976;34-212.

44. Lattes R. Thymoma and other tumors of the thymus: An analysis of 107 cases. Cancer 1962;15:1224-60.

45. Lewis JE, Wick MR, Scheithauer BW, et al. Thymoma: A clinicopathologic review. Cancer 1987; 60:2727-43.

46. Verstandig AG, Epstein DM, Miller WT, et al. Thymoma-report of 71 cases and a review. Crit Rev Diagn Imaging 1992;33:201-30.

47. Zerhouni EA, Scott WW, Baker RR, et al. Invasive thymomas: Diagnosis and evaluation by CT. J Comput Assist Tomogr 1982;6:92-100.

48. Yokoi K, Miyazawa N, Mori K, et al. Invasive thymoma with intracaval growth into right atrium. Ann Thorac Surg 1992;53:507-09.

49. Masaoka A, Monden Y, Nakahara K, et al. Follow-up study of thymomas with special reference to their clinical stages. Cancer 1981;48:2485-92.

50. Sonobe S, Miyamoto H, Izumi H, Nobukawa B, Futagawa T, Yamazaki A, Oh T, Uekusa T, Abe H, Suda K. Clinical usefulness of the WHO histological classification of thymoma. Ann Thorac Cardiovasc Surg 2005;11:367-73.

51. Shamji F, Pearson FG, Todd TR, et al. Results of surgical treatment for thymoma. J Thorac Cardiovasc Surg 1984;87:43-47.

52. Caramori G, Calia N, Pasquini C, Arar O, Ravenna F, Guzzinati I, Boniotti A, Cavazzini L, Ciaccia A, Cavallesco G, Papi A. Ectopic thymoma simulating a pericardial cyst. Monaldi Arch Chest Dis 2005;63:230-33.

53. Durand F, Camdessanche JP, Jomir L, Antoine JC, Cathebras P. Myasthenia in elderly patients: A series of 23 cases. Rev Med Interne 2005;26:924-30.

54. Tseng YL, Chang JM, Shu IL, Wu MH. Myasthenia gravis developed 30 months after resection of recurrent thymoma. Eur J Cardiothorac Surg 2006;29:268.

55. Sonobe S, Miyamoto H, Izumi H, Nobukawa B, Futagawa T, Yamazaki A, Oh T, Deymeer F, Akca S, Kocaman G, Parman Y, Serdaroglu P, Oktem-Tanor O, Coban O, Vincent A. Fasciculations, autonomic symptoms and limbic encephalitis: A thymoma-associated Morvan's-like syndrome. Eur Neurol 2005;54:235-37.

56. Kanayama S, Matsuno A, Nagashima T, Ishida Y. Symptomatic pituitary metastasis of malignant thymoma. J Clin Neurosci 2005;12:954-57.

57. Gray KM, Windsor M. Thymoma presenting with infarction. Heart Lung Circ 2004;13:191-94.

58. Iizuka O, Suzuki K, Ohno T, Soma Y, Mori E. Pure amnesic syndrome with thymoma.Eur Neurol. 2005; 54:123-24.

59. Montella L, Merkabaoui G, Vitiello L, Bulgarelli G, Sinagra G, Masci AM, Racioppi L, Palmieri G. Fatal immunodeficiency in a patient with thymoma and Good's syndrome. Tumori. 2005;91:361-63.

60. Maslovsky I, Gefel D, Uriev L, Ben Dor D, Lugassy G. Malignant thymoma complicated by a megakaryocytic thrombocytopenic purpura. Eur J Intern Med 2005; 16:523-24.

61. McHayleh W, Kressel B, Nylen ES. Thymoma-associated hypocalcemic crisis. South Med J 2005;98:836-38.

62. Osserman KE, Genkins G. Studies in myasthenia gravis: Review of a 20-year experience in over 1200 patients. Mt. Sinai J Med 1971;38:497-37.

63. Marx A, Muller-Hermelink HK, Strobel P. The role of thymomas in the development of myasthenia gravis. Ann NY Acad Sci 2003;998:223-36.

64. Drachmnan DB. Myasthenia gravis. N Engl J Med 1994;330:1797-1810.

65. Lennon VA, Jones G, Howard F, et al. Auto antibodies to acetylcholine receptors in myasthenia gravis. N Engl J Med 1983;308:402-03.

66. Howard FM Jr, Lennon VA, Finley J, et al. Clinical correation of antibodies that bind, block or modulate human acetylcholine receptors in myasthenia gravis. Ann N Y Acad Sci 1987;505:526-38.

67. Souadjian JV, Enriquez P, Silverstein MN, et al. The spectrum of diseases associated with thymoma. Arch Intern Med 1974;134:374-79.

68. Kelleher P, Misbah SA. What is Good's syndrome? Immunological abnormalities in patients with thymoma. J Clin Pathol 2003;56:12-16.

69. Kim JH, Goo JM, Lee HJ, et al. Cystic tumors in the anterior mediastinum: Radiologic-pathological correlation. J Comput Assist Tomogr 2003;27:714-23.

70. Rosado de Christenson ML, Galobardes J, Moran CA. Thymoma: Radiologic-pathologic correlation. Radiographics 1992;12:151-68.

71. Maher MM, Shepard JA. Imaging of thymoma. Semin Thorac Cardiovasc Surg 2005;17:12-19.

72. Ohtsuka T, Nomori H, Watanabe K, Naruke T, Suemasu K, Kosaka N, Uno K. Positive Imaging of Thymoma by 11C-Acetate Positron Emission Tomography. Ann Thorac Surg 2006;81:1132-34.

73. Anderson T, Lindgren PG, Elvin A. Ultrasound guided tumor biopsy in the anterior mediastinum. Acta Radiol 1992;33:310-11.

74. Pantidou A, Kiziridou A, Antoniadis T, Tsilikas C, Destouni C. Mediastinum thymoma diagnosed by FNA and thinprep technique: A case report. Diagn Cytopathol 2006;34:37-40.

75. Suzuki M, Chen H, Shigematsu H, Ando S, Iida T, Nakajima T, Fujisawa T, Kimura H. Aberrant methylation: Common in thymic carcinomas, rare in thymomas. Oncol Rep 2005;14:1621-24.

76. Kojima M, Tanaka M, Nakamura M, Katano M. Immunohistochemical staining of hedgehog pathway-related proteins in human thymomas. Anticancer Res 2005;25:3697-701.

77. Yamazaki H, Tateyama H, Asai K, Fukai I, Fujii Y, Tada T, Eimoto T. Glia maturation factor-beta is produced by thymoma and may promote intratumoral T-cell differentiation. Histopathology 2005;47:292-302.

78. Chateil JF, Pietrera P. Mediastinal thymolipoma. Presse Med 2005;34(Pt 1):1741.

79. Iwasaki T, Nakagawa K, Yasukawa M, Shiono H, Nagano T, Kawahara K. Ectopic cervico-mediastinal thymoma confirmed by flow cytometric analysis of tumor-derived lymphocytes. Jpn J Thorac Cardiovasc Surg 2006;54:35-39.

80. Kim DJ, Yang WI, Kim SH, Park IK, Chung KY. Expression of neurotrophin receptors in surgically resected thymic epithelial tumors. Eur J Cardiothorac Surg 2005;28:611-16.

81. Mineo TC, Ambrogi V, Mineo D, Baldi A. Long-term disease-free survival of patients with radically resected thymomas: Relevance of cell-cycle protein expression. Cancer 2005;104:2063-71.

82. Rea F, Marulli G, Bortolotti L, Feltracco P, Zuin A, Sartori F. Experience with the "da Vinci" robotic system for thymectomy in patients with myasthenia gravis: Report of 33 cases. Ann Thorac Surg 2006;81:455-59.

83. Chen KN, Xu SF, Gu ZD, Zhang WM, Pan H, Su WZ, Li JY, Xu GW. Surgical treatment of complex malignant anterior mediastinal tumors invading the superior vena cava. World J Surg 2006;30:162-70.

84. Chang PC, Chou SH, Kao EL, Cheng YJ, Chuang HY, Liu CK, Lai CL, Huang MF. Bilateral video-assisted thoracoscopic thymectomy vs. extended transsternal thymectomy in myasthenia gravis: A prospective study. Eur Surg Res 2005;37:199-203.

85. Cheng YJ, Kao EL, Chou SH. Videothoracoscopic resection of stage II thymoma: Prospective comparison of the results between thoracoscopy and open methods. Chest 2005;128:3010-12.

86. Tasaki A, Akiyoshi T, Koga K, Nakashima H, Yamanaka N, Kubo M, Matsumoto K, Ayabe T, Matsuzaki Y, Edagawa M, Shimizu T, Hara M, Tomita M, Akiyama Y, Onitsuka T. Surgery for the thymoma combined with pure red cell aplasia and myasthenia gravis. Kyobu Geka 2005;58:1023-29.

87. Pishchik VG, Iablonskii PK, Nuraliev SM. A technique of videothoracoscopic thymectomy in diseases of the thymus. Vestn Khir Im I I Grek 2005;164:46-51.

88. Wright CD, Kessler KA. Surgical treatment of thymic tumors. Semin Thorac Cardiovasc Surg 2005;17:20-26.

89. Bjork-Eriksson T, Bjelkengren G, Glimelius B. The potentials of proton beam radiation therapy in malignant lymphoma, thymoma and sarcoma. Acta Oncol 2005;44:913-17.

90. Cesaretti JA. Adjuvant radiation with modern techniques is the standard of care for stage III thymoma. Ann Thorac Surg 2006;81:1180-81.

91. Eng TY, Thomas CR Jr. Radiation therapy in the management of thymic tumors. Semin Thorac Cardiovasc Surg 2005;17:32-40.

92. Evans TL, Lynch TJ. Role of chemotherapy in the management of advanced thymic tumors. Semin Thorac Cardiovasc Surg 2005;17:41-50.

93. Ciccone AM, Rendina EA. Treatment of recurrent thymic tumors. Semin Thorac Cardiovasc Surg 2005; 17:27-31.

94. Kadowaki T, Hamada H, Yokoyama A, Katayama H, Aramoto T, Ueda N, Tomioka H, Higaki J. Thymic carcinoma originating from the mid-posterior mediastinum. Respirology 2005;10:689-91.

95. Lin JT, Wei-Shu W, Yen CC, Liu JH, Chen PM, Chiou TJ. Stage IV thymic carcinoma: A study of 20 patients. Am J Med Sci. 2005;330:172-75.

96. Hernandez-Ilizaliturri FJ, Tan D, Cipolla D, et al. Multimodality therapy for thymic carcinoma (TCA): Results of a 30-year single-institution experience. Am J Clin Oncol 2004;27:68-72.

97. Truong LD, Mody DR, Cagle PT, et al. Thymic carcinoma: A clinicopathologic study of 13 cases. Am J Surg Pathol 1990;14:151-66.

98. Tamura Y, Kuroiwa T, Doi A, et al. Thymic carcinoma presenting as cranial metastasis with intradural and extracranial extension: Case report. Neurosurgery 2004;54:209-11.

99. Yaqub A, Munn NJ, Wolfer RS. Thymic carcinoma presenting as cardiac tamponade. South Med J 2004;97:212-13.

100. Suster S, Rosai J. Thymic carcinoma: A clinicopathologic study of 60 cases. Cancer 1991;67:1025-32.

101. Blumberg D, Burt ME, Bains MS, et al. Thymic carcinoma: Current staging does not predict prognosis. J Thorac Cardiovasc Surg 1998;115:303-38.

102. Ritter JH, Wick MR. Primary carcinoma of the thymus gland. Semin Diagn Pathol 1999;16:18-31.

103. Loehrer PJ, Kim KM, Aisner SC, et al. Cisplatin plus doxorubicin plus cyclophosphamide in metastatic or recurrent thymoma. J Clin Oncol 1994;12:1164-68.

104. Yoh K, Goto K, Ishii G, et al. Weekly chemotherapy with cisplatin, vincristine, doxorubicin, and etoposide is an effective treatment for advanced thymic carcinoma. Cancer 2003;98:926-31.

105. Graeber GM, Thompson LD, Cohen DJ, et al. Cystic lesions of the thymus. J Thorac Cardiovasc Surg 1984; 87:295-300.

106. Indeglia RA, Shea MA, Grage TB. Congenital cysts of the thymus gland. Arch Surg 1967;94:149-52.

107. Suster S, Rosai J. Multilocular thymic cyst: An acquired reactive process. Am J Surg Pathol 1991;15:388-98.

108. Gibril F, Chen YJ, Schrump DS, et al. Prospective study of thymic carcinoids in patients with multiple endocrine neoplasia type 1. J Clin Endocrinol Metab 2003;88:1066-81.

109. Wick MR, Bernatz PE, Carney JA, et al. Primary mediastinal carcinoid tumors. Am J Surg Pathol 1982;6:195-205.

110. Economopoulos GC, Lewis JW Jr, Lee MW, et al. Carcinoid tumors of the thymus. Ann Thorac Surg 1990;50:58-61.

111. Tiffet O, Nicholson AG, Ladas G, et al. A clinicopathologic study of 12 neuroendocrine tumors arising in the thymus. Chest 2003;124:141-46.

112. Strollo DC, Rosado-de-Christenson ML, Jett JR, et al. Primary mediastinal tumors: Part 1. Tumors of the anterior mediastinum. Chest 1997;112:511.

113. Parker D, Holford CP, Begent RH. Effective treatment for malignant mediastinal teratoma. Thorax 1983; 38:897-902.

114. Bohle A, Studor UK, Sonntag RW, et al. Primary or secondary extragonadal germ cell tumor? J Urol 1986;135:939-43.

115. Recondo J, Libshitz HI. Mediastinal extragonadal germ cell tumors. Urology 1978;11:369-75.

116. Nichols CR. Mediastinal germ cell tumors. Clinical features and biologic correlates. Chest 1991;99:472-79.

117. Moeller KH, Rosado-de-Christenson ML, Templeton PA. Mediastinal mature teratoma: Imaging features. AJR Am J Roentgenol. 1997;169:985-90.

118. Rosado-de-Christenson ML, Templeton PA, Moran CA. From the archives of the AFIP. Mediastinal germ cell tumors: Radiologic and pathologic correlation. Radiographics 1992;12:1013-30.

119. Mullen B, Richardson JD. Primary anterior mediastinal tumors in children and adults. Ann Thorac Surg. 1986;42:338-45.

120. Javadpour N. Significance of elevated serum alpha fetoprotein (AFP) in seminoma. Cancer 1980;45:2166-68.

121. Davis RD Jr Oldham HN Jr, Sabiston DC Jr. The Mediastinum. In Sabiston, Spencer (Ed): Surgery of the chest. 6. I. WB Saunders 1996;596.

122. Takeda S, Miyoshi S, Ohta M, Minami M, Masaoka A, Matsuda H. Primary germ cell tumors in the mediastinum. A 50-year experience at a single Japanese institution. Cancer. 2003;97:367-76.

123. Lewis BD, Hurt RD, Payne WS, Farrow GM, Knapp RH, Muhm JR. Benign teratomas of the mediastinum. J Thorac Cardiovasc Surg 1983;86:727-31.

124. Dulmet EM, Macchiarini P, Suc B, Verley JM. Germ cell tumors of the mediastinum. A 30-year experience. Cancer 1993;72:1894-901.

125. Shirodkar NP, Chopra PS, Marker M, Murphy KD, Dhamoon A, Kwon OJ. Conjoined gastric and mediastinal benign cystic teratomas. Case report of a rare

occurrence and review of literature. Clin Imaging 1997;21:340-45.

126. Sinclair DS, Bolen MA, King MA. Mature teratoma within the posterior mediastinum. J Thorac Imag 2003;18:53-55.

127. Drevelegas A, Palladas P, Scordalaki A. Mediastinal germ cell tumors: A radiologic-pathologic review. Eur Radiol 2001;11:1925-32.

128. Cheng YJ, Huang MF, Tsai KB. Video-assisted thoracoscopic management of an anterior mediastinal teratoma: Report of a case. Surg Today 2000;30:1019-21.

129. Sohn L, Gribbin C, Rizzo N, Nosher JL. Radiology/pathology conference at Robert Wood Johnson Medical School. Benign mediastinal teratoma. N J Med 1995; 92:241-44.

130. Tominaga K, Kadokura M, Saida K, Nakao K, Kushiro H, Ryu K, Yamamoto N. A surgical case of giant mediastinal teratoma. Kyobu Geka. 1994;47:944-47.

131. Zisis C, Rontogianni D, Stratakos G, Voutetakis K, Skevis K, Argiriou M, Bellenis I. Teratoma occupying the left hemithorax. World J Surg Oncol 2005;3:76.

132. Völkl TM, Langer T, Aigner T, Greess H, Beck JD, Rauch AM, Dorr HG. Klinefelter syndrome and mediastinal germ cell tumors. Am J Med Genet A 2006;140:471-81.

133. Chen KN, Xu SF, Gu ZD, Zhang WM, Pan H, Su WZ, Li JY, Xu GW. Surgical treatment of complex malignant anterior mediastinal tumors invading the superior vena cava. World J Surg 2006;30:162-70.

134. Bandyopadhyay SK, Bandyopadhyay R, Moulick A, Dutta A, Saha DK. Benign mediastinal teratoma producing recurrent hemoptysis. J Assoc Physicians India 2005;53:698.

135. McLeod NP, Vallely MP, Mathur MN. Massive immature mediastinal teratoma extending into the left pleural cavity. Heart Lung Circ 2005;14:45-47.

136. Margery J, Le Berre JP, Bredin C, Bordier L, Dupuy O, Mayaudon H, Guigay J, Bauducea B. Klinefelter's syndrome diagnosed three years after surgery for mediastinal teratoma. Presse Med 2005;34:1078-79.

137. Nichols CR. Mediastinal germ cell tumors: Clinical features and biologic correlates. Chest 1991;99:472-79.

138. Crussi-Gonzalez F. Extragonadal teratomas. In: Hartmann WH (Ed): Atlas of tumor pathology. Washington, DC: Armed Forces Institute of Pathology 1982;77–94.

139. Carter C, Bibro MC, Touloukian RJ. Benign clinical behavior of immature mediastinal teratoma in infancy and childhood. Cancer 1982;49:398-402.

140. Adebonojo SA, Nicola ML. Teratoid tumors of the mediastinum. Am Surg 1976;42:361-65.

141. Thompson DP, Moore TC. Acute thoracic distress in childhood due to spontaneous rupture of large mediastinal teratoma. J Pediatr Surg 1969;4:416-23.

142. Donadio AC, Motzer RJ, Bajorin DF, et al. Chemotherapy for teratoma with malignant transformation. J Clin Oncol 2003;21:4285-91.

143. Lewis BD, Hurt RD, Payne WS, et al. Benign teratoma of the mediastinum. J Thorac Cardiovasc Surg 1983; 86:727-31

144. Graeber GM, Shriver CD, Albur RA, et al. The use of computed tomography in the evaluation of mediastinal tumors. J Thorac Cardiovasc Surg 1986;91:662-66.

145. Moeller KH, Rosado-de-Christenson ML, Templeton DA. Mediastinal mature teratoma: Imaging features. AJR Am J Roentgenol 1997;169:985-90.

146. Arai K, Ohta S, Suzuki M, et al. Primary immature mediastinal teratoma in adulthood. Eur J Surg Oncol 1997;23:64-67.

147. Polansky SM, Barwick KW, Revie CE. Primary mediastinal seminoma. AJR Am J Roentgenol 1979; 132:17-21.

148. Hainsworth J. Diagnosis, staging, and clinical characteristics of the patient with mediastinal germ cell carcinoma. Chest Surg Clin N Am 2002;12:665-72.

149. Hosono M, Machida K, Honda N, et al. Intense Ga-67 accumulation in pure primary mediastinal seminomas. Clin Nucl Med 2003; 28:25-28.

150. Bush SE, Martinez A, Bagshaw MA. Primary mediastinal seminoma. Cancer 1981;48:1877-82.

151. Bokemeyer C, Droz JP, Horwich A, et al. Extragonadal seminoma: An international multicenter analysis of prognostic factors and longterm treatment outcome. Cancer 2001;91:1394-401.

152. Bukowski RM, Wolf M, Kulander BG, et al. Alternating combination chemotherapy in patients with extragonadal germ cell tumors: A Southwest Oncology Group Study. Cancer 1993;71:2631-38.

153. Dexeus FH, Logothetis CJ, Chong C, et al. Genetic abnormalities in men with germ cell tumors. J Urol 1988;140:80-84.

154. Nichols CR, Hoffman R, Einhorn LH, et al. Hematologic malignancies associated with primary mediastinal germ cell tumors. Ann Intern Med 1985;102:603-09.

155. Hori K, Uematsu K, Yasoshima H, et al. Testicular seminoma with human chorionic gonadotropin production. Pathol Int 1997;47:592-99.

156. Lee KS, Im JG, Han CH, et al. Malignant primary germ cell tumors of the mediastinum: CT features. AJR Am J Roentgenol 1989;153:947-51.

157. Wright C, Kesler K. Surgical techniques and outcomes for primary nonseminomatous germ cell tumors. Chest Surg Clin N Am 2002;12:707-15.

158. Walsh GL, Taylor GD, Nesbitt JC, et al. Intensive chemotherapy and radical resections for primary nonseminomatous mediastinal germ cell tumors. Ann Thorac Surg 2000;69:337-43.

159. International Germ Cell Consensus Classification. A prognostic factor-based staging system for metastatic germ cell cancers: International Germ Cell Cancer Collaborative Group. J Clin Oncol 1997;15:594-603.

160. Kumar A, Kumar S, Aggarwal S, et al. Thoracoscopy: The preferred approach for the resection of selected

posterior mediastinal tumors. J Laparoendosc Adv Surg Tech A 2002;12:345-53.

161. Reeder LB. Neurogenic tumors of the mediastinum. Semin Thorac Cardiovasc Surg 2000;12:261-67.

162. Shapiro B, Orringer MB, Gross MD. Mediastinal paragangliomas and pheochromocytomas. In Shields TW, LoCicero J III, Ponn RB (Eds): General thoracic surgery (Vol 2) (5th edn). Philadelphia, PA: Williams & Wilkins 2000;2333–55.

163. Saenz NC. Posterior mediastinal neurogenic tumors in infants and children. Semin Pediatr Surg 1999;8:78-84.

164. Wain JC. Neurogenic tumors of the mediastinum. Chest Surg Clin N Am 1992;2:121-36.

165. Shields TW, Reynolds M. Neurogenic tumors of the thorax. Surg Clin North Am 1988;68:645-68.

166. Aughenbaugh GL. Thoracic manifestations of neurocutaneous diseases. Radiol Clin N Am 1984;22:741-56.

167. Mazel CH, Grunenwald D, Laudrin P, et al. Radical excision in the management of thoracic and cervicothoracic tumors involving the spine: Results in a series of 36 cases. Spine 2003;28:782-92.

168. Ducatman BS, Scheithauer BW, Piepgras DG, et al. Malignant peripheral nerve sheath tumors: A clinicopathologic study of 120 cases. Cancer 1986;57:2006-21.

169. Gale AW, Jelihovsy T, Grant AF, et al. Neurogenic tumors of the mediastinum. Ann Thorac Surg 1974; 17:434-43.

170. Davis S, Rogers MAM, Pendergrass TW. The incidence and epidemiologic characteristics of neuroblastoma in the United States. Am J Epidemiol 1987;126:1063-74.

171. Forsythe A, Volpe J, Muller R. Posterior mediastinal ganglioneuroma. Radiographics 2004;24:594-97.

172. Benjamin SP, McCormack LJ, Effler DB, et al. Primary tumors of the mediastinum. Chest 1972;62:297-303.

173. Wang YM, Li YM, Sheih CP, et al. Magnetic resonance imaging of neuroblastoma, ganglioneuroblastoma, and ganglioneuroma. Acta Pediatr Surg 1995;36:420-24.

174. Adams A, Hochholzer L. Ganglioneuroblastoma of the posterior mediastinum: A clinicopathologic review of 80 cases. Cancer 1981;47:373-81.

175. Grosfeld JL, Baehner RL. Neuroblastoma: An analysis of 160 cases. World J Surg 1980;4:29-38.

176. Page DL, DeLellis RA, Hough AJ. Atlas of tumor pathology: Tumors of the adrenal. Washington, DC: Armed Forces Institute of Pathology 1986;219-60.

177. Crapo JD, Glassroth J, Karlinsky J, et al. Baum's textbook of pulmonary diseases. Philadelphia, PA: Lippincott Williams & Wilkins 2004;883–912.

178. Bar-Ziv J, Nogrady MB. Mediastinal neuroblastoma and ganglioneuroma: The differentiation between primary and secondary involvement on the chest roentgenogram. Am J Roentgenol 1975;125:380-90.

179. Stark DD, Moss AA, Brasch RC, et al. Neuroblastoma: Diagnostic imaging and staging. Radiology 1983;148: 101-05.

180. Hoefnagel CA. Radionuclide therapy in children with neuroblastoma. Hell J Nucl Med 2002;2:107-10.

181. Castel V, Tovar JA, Costa E, et al. The role of surgery in stage IV neruoblastoma. J Pediatr Surg 2002;37:1574-78.

182. Mastrangelo S, Tornesello A, Diociaiuti L, et al. Treatment of advanced neuroblastoma: Feasibility and therapeutic potential of a novel approach combining 131-I-MIB Gand multiple drug chemotherapy. Br J Cancer 2001;84:460-64.

183. Pun YW, Moreno BR, Prieto VJ, et al. Multicenter experience of video-assisted thoracic surgery to treat mediastinal cysts and tumors. Archivos de Bronconeumologia 2002;38:410-14.

184. Wychulis AR, Payne WS, Clagett OT, et al. Surgical treatment of mediastinal tumors: A 40-year experience. J Thorac Cardiovasc Surg 1971;62:379-92.

185. Whooley BP, Urschel JD, Antkowiak JG, et al. Primary tumors of the mediastinum. J Surg Oncol 1999;70:95-99.

186. Ahrens B, Wit J, Schmitt M, et al. Symptomatic bronchogenic cyst in a six month old infant: Case report and review of the literature. J Thorac Cardiovasc Surg 2001;122:1021-23.

187. Takeda S, Miyoshi S, Minami M, et al. Clinical spectrum of mediastinal cysts. Chest 2003;124:125-32.

188. Crapo JD, Glassroth J, Karlinsky J, et al. Baum's textbook of pulmonary diseases. Philadelphia, PA: Lippincott Williams & Wilkins 2004;883-912.

189. Kumar A, Aggarwal S, Halder S, et al. Thorascopic excision of mediastinal bronchogenic cyst: A case report and review of literature. Ind J Chest Dis llied Sci 2003;45:199–201.

190. O'Neill JA. Foregut duplications. In: Fallis JC, Filler RM, Lemoine G (Eds): Current topics in general thoracic surgery: An international series. New York, NY: Elsevier 1991;121-23.

191. Cioffi U, Bonavina L, De Simone M. Presentation and surgical management of bronchogenic and esophageal duplication cysts in adults. Chest 1998;113:1492–96.

192. Superina RA, Ein SH, Humphreys RP. Cystic duplications of the esophagus and neurenteric cysts. J Pediatr Surg 1984;19:527-30.

193. Rescorla FJ, Grosfeld JL. Gastroenteric cysts and neurenteric cysts in infants and children. In: Shields TW, LoCicero J III, Ponn RB (Eds): General thoracic surgery (vol 2) (5th edn). Philadelphia, PA: Williams & Wilkins 2000;2415-22.

194. Feigin D, Fenoglio JJ, McAllister HA, et al. Pericardial cysts: A radiologic-pathologic correlation and review. Radiology 1977;125:15-20.

195. Shahriari A, Odell JA. Cervical and thoracic components of multiorgan lymphangiomatosis managed surgically. Ann Thorac Surg 2001;71:694-96.

196. Nakazato Y, Ohno Y, Nakata Y, et al. Cystic lymphangioma of the mediastinum. Am Heart J 1995;129:406-09.

197. Johnson DW, Klazynski PT, Gordon WH, et al. Mediastinal lymphangioma and chylothorax: The role of radiotherapy. Ann Thorac Surg 1986;41:325-38.

198. Rostom AY. Treatment of thoracic lymphangiomatosis. Arch Dis Child 2000;83:138-39.
199. Kathic M, Wang C, Grillo H. Substernal goiter. Ann Thorac Surg 1985;39:391-99.
200. Allo MD, Thompson NW. Rationale for the operative management of substernal goiters. Surgery 1983; 94:969-77.
201. Clark O. Mediastinal parathyroid tumors. Arch Surg 1988;123:1096–100.
202. Oates E. Improved parathyroid scintigraphy with Tc 99m MIBI, a superior radio tracer. Appl Radiol 1994;23:37–40.
203. Loyd JE, Tillman BF, Atkinson JB, Des Prez RM. Mediastinal fibrosis complicating histoplasmosis. Medicine (Baltimore) 1988; 67:295-310.
204. Flieder DB, Suster S, Moran CA. Idiopathic fibroinflammatory (fibrosing/sclerosing) lesions of the mediastinum: A study of 30 cases with emphasis on morphologic heterogeneity. Mod Pathol 1999;12:257-64.
205. Garrett HE Jr, Roper CL. Surgical intervention in histoplasmosis. Ann Thorac Surg 1986;42:711-22.
206. Goodwin RA, Nickell JA, Des Prez RM. Mediastinal fibrosis complicating healed primary histoplasmosis and tuberculosis. Medicine (Baltimore) 1972;51:227-46.
207. Mathisen DJ, Grillo HC. Clinical manifestation of mediastinal fibrosis and histoplasmosis. Ann Thorac Surg 1992;54:1053-1057; discussion 1057-58.
208. Urschel HC, Jr Razzuk MA, Netto GJ, Disiere J, Chung SY. Sclerosing mediastinitis: Improved management with histoplasmosis titer and ketoconazole. Ann Thorac Surg 1990;50:215-21.
209. Wieder S, Rabinowitz JG. Fibrous mediastinitis: A late manifestation of mediastinal histoplasmosis. Radiology 1977;125:305-12.
210. Wieder S, White TJ, Salazar J, Gold RE, Moinuddin M, Tonkin I. Pulmonary artery occlusion due to histoplasmosis. AJR Am J Roentgenol 1982;138:243-51.
211. Peebles RS, Carpenter CT, Dupont WD, Loyd JE. Mediastinal fibrosis is associated with human leukocyte antigen-A2. Chest 2000;117:482-85.
212. Dunn EJ, Ulicny KS Jr, Wright CB, Gottesman L. Surgical implications of sclerosing mediastinitis: A report of six cases and review of the literature. Chest 1990;97:338-46.
213. Dines DE, Payne WS, Bernatz PE, Pairolero PC. Mediastinal granuloma and fibrosing mediastinitis. Chest 1979;75:320-24.
214. Lee JY, Kim Y, Lee KS, Chung MP. Tuberculous fibrosing mediastinitis: Radiologic findings. Am J Roentgenol 1996;167:1598-99.
215. Lagerstrom CF, Mitchell HG, Graham BS, Hammon JW Jr. Chronic fibrosing mediastinitis and superior vena caval obstruction from blastomycosis. Ann Thorac Surg 1992;54:764-65.
216. Mole TM, Glover J, Sheppard MN. Sclerosing mediastinitis: A report on 18 cases. Thorax 1995;50:280-83.

217. Othmani S, Bahri M, Louzir B, Borhan K. Mediastinal fibrosis combined with Behçet's disease: Three case reports. Rev Med Interne 2000;21:330-36.
218. Dechambre S, Dorzee J, Fastrez J, Hanzen C, Van Houtte P, d'Odemont JP. Bronchial stenosis and sclerosing mediastinitis: An uncommon complication of external thoracic radiotherapy. Eur Respir J 1998; 11:1188-90.
219. Bullimore DW, Mascie-Taylor BH, Muers M, Losowsky MS. Combined retroperitoneal and mediastinal fibrosis associated with variceal haemorrhage. Br J Clin Pract 1987;41:1064-65.
220. Bourgault I, Poli F, Roujeau JC, Shaeffer A, Rodier JM, Revuz J. Retroperitoneal and mediastinal fibrosis complicating periarteritis nodosa. Ann Dermatol Venereol 1989;116:824-5[French].
221. Dehner LP, Coffin CM. Idiopathic fibrosclerotic disorders and other inflammatory pseudotumors. Semin Diagn Pathol 1998;15:161-73.
222. Fenner MN, Moran JP, Jr, Dillon JC, Madura JA. Retroperitoneal fibrosis and sclerosing mediastinitis. Indiana Med 1987;80:334-38.
223. Graal MB, Lustermans FA. A patient with combined mediastinal, mesenteric, and retroperitoneal fibrosis. Neth J Med 1994;44:214-19.
224. Hanley PC, Shub C, Lie JT. Constrictive pericarditis associated with combined idiopathic retro-peritoneal and mediastinal fibrosis. Mayo Clin Proc 1984;59:300-04.
225. Klisnick A, Fourcade J, Ruivard M, et al. Combined idiopathic retroperitoneal and mediastinal fibrosis with pericardial involvement. Clin Nephrol 1999;52:51-55.
226. Morad N, Strongwater SL, Eypper S, Woda BA. Idiopathic retroperitoneal and mediastinal fibrosis mimicking connective tissue disease. Am J Med 1987;82:363-66.
227. Morgan AD, Loughridge LW, Calne RY. Combined mediastinal and retroperitoneal fibrosis. Lancet 1966;1:67-70.
228. Pang J, Vicary FR, Beck ER. Coexisting retroperitoneal and mediastinal fibrosis. Postgrad Med J 1983;59: 450-51.
229. Savelli BA, Parshley M, Morganroth ML. Successful treatment of sclerosing cervicitis and fibrosing mediastinitis with tamoxifen. Chest 1997;111:1137-40.
230. Meredith SD, Madison J, Fechner RE, Levine PA. Cervical manifestations of fibrosing mediastinitis: A diagnostic and therapeutic dilemma. Head Neck 1993;15:561-65.
231. Kountz PD, Molina PL, Sagel SS. Fibrosing mediastinitis in the posterior thorax. AJR Am J Roentgenol 1989; 153:489-90.
232. Rossi SE, McAdams HP, Rosado-de-Christenson ML, Franks TJ, Galvin JR. Fibrosing mediastinitis. Radiographics 2001;21:737-57.
233. Sherrick AD, Brown LR, Harms GF, Myers JL. The radiographic findings of fibrosing mediastinitis. Chest 1994;106:484-89.

30
Disorders of the Diaphragm and Chest Wall

CHEST WALL AND THORACIC CAGE ABNORMALITIES

Disorders of the chest wall are a group of conditions affecting the inspiratory pump and potentially leading to respiratory failure.

These disorders may affect all mechanical components of the inspiratory pump, that include the respiratory muscles, bony rib cage, the spine and its articulations, and the soft tissues compromising the abdomen. They may lead to a mechanical disadvantage to the inspiratory pump and an increased work of breathing. This group of disorders is characterized usually by a restrictive defect and share the potential of long-term hypercapnic respiratory failure.

These disorders include:[1-5]

1. Spine and articulations
   - Kyphoscoliosis
   - Ankylosing spondylitis.
   - Previous thoracoplasty
2. Rib cage
   - Flail chest (particularly with pulmonary contusion)
   - Pectus excavatum
   - Pectus carinatum
3. Respiratory muscle involvement
   - Central
   - Peripheral: nerve/neuromuscular junction/muscle
4. Soft tissue
   - Obesity.

KYPHOSCOLIOSIS

Kyphosis may exist as an isolated entity and can follow osteoporosis or radiation. The estimated prevalence of mild deformity is about 1 in 1000 and severe deformity is approximately 1 in 10000 in USA.

Scoliosis invariably associated with kyphosis. Scoliosis is a lateral curvature of the spine and is associated with rotation of the vertebral column. This results in marked disortion of the thoracic cage. Thus, the spinal column is bent having a convexity towards one side and concavity towards the opposite side. The rotation results in anterior displacement of the posterior ribs on one side so that the volume of the hemithorax is decreased. The ribs are hypoplastic because of lack of space to grow. On the opposite side, the ribs will be displaced posteriorly, usually on the convex side, and thus increasing the lung volume on that side.[6-10]

This may be of the following types:

A. Congenital
   — Isolated
   — Associated syndromes: (Neurofibromatosis, Marfan's syndrome, and Ehlers-Danlos syndrome.
B. Paralytic/secondary
   — Neuromuscular: Poliomyelitis/musculardystrophy.
   — Connective tissue related: Erlos-Danlos syndrome and Morquio's syndrome.
   — Vertebral disease: Osteoporosis/osteomalacia/spina bifida.
   Compensatory: Post-thoracoplasty.
C. Idiopathic

There are many causes of scoliosis. The causes are both nonstructural and structural. In the nonstructural group postural, compensatory, and irritation of the sciatic nerve roots are important. In the structural group and perhaps the most common cause of scoliosis, is idiopathic. Other causes are congenital scoliosis, Kippel-Feil anomaly, spondylolisthesis, muscular dystrophies, poliomyelitis, neurofibromatosis, Morfans's syndrome, Friedreich's ataxia, syringomyelia, cerebral palsy, Ehlers-Danlos syndrome, homocystinuria, Turner's syndrome, thoracoplasty, and fibrothorax. Idiopathic scoliosis is seen at all ages and at all spinal levels. It is more common in girls. Higher the curvature, and more is the

Cobb's angle, worse is the prognosis. The patient is substantially shorter because of loss of spine height. There will be marked alteration in the shape of the chest wall. Abnormalities of lower thoracic spine have more ventilatory abnormalities than that in higher thoracic spines. The lung may be hypoplastic with reduced number of alveoli and hypoplastic with reduced number of alveoli and hypoplasia of the bronchial tree and pulmonary vessels.

There may be marked displacement of the mediastinum and lateral movement of thoracic wall with varying degrees of decreased breath sounds. The scoliosis is more apparent during rapid growth years. Cor pulmonale and respiratory failure are the two common and fatal complications of kyphoscoliosis. Respiratory infections are commonly superadded.

Idiopathic Kyphoscoliosis

This variety often begins in late childhood or early adolescence and has a female predominance of 4:1. This may account for as many as 80 percent of cases of kyphoscoliosis. The Cobb angle (see below) is associated with the degree of restriction. Patients with mild to moderate idiopathic kyphoscoliosis may not be restricted or only have mild restrictive dysfunction. However, those with an angle greater than 60 degrees are more likely to exhibit a restrictive defect. Those with angles in the 90 to 100 degree range invariably have pulmonary function impairment proportional to the degree of spinal deformity. Although the Cobb's angle is primarily associated with restriction, and the restriction is proportional to the angle, the relationship is however more complex. Other factors involved are: number of vertebrae affected; location of curve; Patient's age, presence of kyphosis; and the degree of rotation.

Although the exact pathophysiology of kyphoscoliosis is not clear, it is mostly genetic in origin that leads to neurophysiological predisposition and diminished melatonin production, which is possibly regulated via Ca^{++} chelators. That leads to increased production of calmodulin around puberty that causes idiopathic scoliosis. Further, neurophysiological changes around puberty also contribute to the development. Connective tissue abnormalities and abnormal biochemical forces also play important roles in the development of scoliosis. Thus, possible interrelationships of various factors have been shown to have possible role in cause of idiopathic scoliosis.

Congenital Kyphoscoliosis

This may be solated or present as a syndromic entity. This may be genetic and is usually present at birth. This occurs as a result of malformations of vertebrae during ontogeny. The loss of vital capacity greater than in idiopathic scoliosis (~15%).

Paralytic Kyphoscoliosis

This occurs as a result of loss of muscular tone primarily or secondary to unequal resting tone and remodeling. The entity should be ruled before other two categories are considered. The association between this form of scoliosis and restriction is not strong. The reduction of vital capacity is primarily associated with weakness. There is early onset of scoliosis with faster progression.

Physiological Changes Associated with Kyphoscoliosis

Maximum restriction occurs in this condition among all chest wall disorders. Lung function tests will reveal a restrictive pattern.[11] Because of reduced height, the predicted values are calculated on the basis of arm span measurements, which closely correlate with height in normal subjects, or more correctly if 1.03 multiplies the arm span, the accurate height is determined. Pulmonary function testing will show a decreased total lung capacity and vital capacity with reduced FEV_1. The residual volume will be either normal or increased with a reduction in the RV/TLC ratio. Typical of a restrictive defect the FEV_1/FVC ratio is normal. Specific airway conductance is actually increased (radial traction because of recoil). Diffusion capacity (DLCO) is reduced proportionate to the reduction of TLC. Respiratory system compliance is reduced in kyphoscoliosis primarily due to a reduction in chest wall compliance and to a lesser degree, reductions in lung compliance. FRC is at a lower lung volume. PImax and PEmax are normal in young patients with idiopathic scoliosis with Cobb angles of less than 50 degree. With Cobb angles > 50 degrees, both PImax and PEmax are mildly decreased to 70 percent and 80 percent of control values, respectively. In older patients with somewhat more scoliosis, PImax is about 50 percent of predicted in eucapnic patients and 25 percent of predicted in hypercapnic patients.

Hypoxemia may be due to ventilation-perfusion mismatch (under ventilation of lung regions); underlying atelectasis, or alveolar hypoventilation. When hypoventilation supervenes, hypoxemia worsens and hypercapnia develops. Hypercapnia initially appears during sleep and with exercise. Eventually, with further disease progression, it occurs at rest. Pulmonary hypertension develops as a result of persistent hypoxemia that leads to pulmonary vasoconstriction, right ventricular hypertrophy and cor pulmonale. The other causes include proliferation of pulmonary artery smooth muscle and compression of the pulmonary vascular bed by a deflated lung. Exercise capacity significantly impaired in patients with severe kyphoscoliosis.

Maximum oxygen consumption is reduced to about 60 to 80 percent of predicted. These patients develop sleep disorder breathing mainly in the form of hypoventilation.

Clinical Features of Kyphoscoliosis

Five major presentations in the natural history of untreated adolescent idiopathic scoliosis in adults are:
1. Back pain
2. Psychosocial effects
3. Curve progression
4. Cardiopulmonary complications
5. Mortality.

The physician often notes congenital and secondary scoliosis during screening. Congenital kyphoscoliosis may be associated with neuro-deficit due to rapid progression. Secondary kyphoscoliosis is recognized as part of overall diagnosis.

The incidence of low-backache (LBA) in patients with idiopathic scoliosis is comparable (60-80%) to general population. In a long-term follow-up study of over 40 years, it was found that 80 percent of scoliotic patients complained of some backache. Patients with lumbar or thoracolumbar curves, especially those with translatory shifts at the lower end of the curves, had a slightly greater incidence of backache than did patients with other curve patterns. The backache in this population was never disabling and was unrelated to the presence of osteo-arthritic changes on roentgenogram. In a recent 50 year follow-up of same patients, using a validated questionnaire LBA in the scoliosis patients was 77 percent compared with 37 percent in control subjects. The location of pain was variable and generally unrelated to the location or magnitude of the curve.

Measurement of Cobb's angle is very important in assessing the severity of kyphoscoliosis. This is a simple investigation to quantify the degree of Kyphoscoliosis and requires only anteroposterior and lateral X-rays.

This angle is formed by the intersection of two lines, each of which is parallel to the top and bottom vertebra of the scoliotic or kyphotic curves.

The magnitude of the Cobb's angle has been used to predict development of respiratory failure and need for intervention. A Cobb's angle > 100 degrees is considered a severe deformity and more likely to be associated with respiratory failure. In idiopathic kyphoscoliosis, the Cobb's angle is associated with the degree of restriction. Patients with an angle > 60 degrees are more likely to

exhibit a restrictive defect. Those individuals with angles in the 90 to 100 degree range have severe restriction. In secondary kyphoscoliosis reductions in vital capacity correlates closely with muscle weakness than with the degree of spinal curvature. In patients with congenital scoliosis, for any given Cobb's angle, the loss in vital capacity is 15 percent greater than in patients with idiopathic scoliosis.

Progression of the thoracic deformity depends on skeletal immaturity and the degree of deformity at the time of diagnosis. After skeletal maturity, progression will depend upon the degree of deformity. Thoracic deformities < 30 degrees are unlikely to progress, 30 to 50 degrees increase slowly by a 10 to 15 degrees and > 50 degrees increase steadily at a rate of about 1 degree annually. Mild to moderate idiopathic kyphoscoliosis and severe idiopathic kyphoscoliosis < 35 years of age are similar to the general population with regard to symptoms, loss of lung volume with aging, and life expectancy. Factors those affect progression of idiopathic scoliosis in young adolescents in clued Girls > boys; premenarchal; double curves > single curves; thoracic curves > lumbar curves; and more severe curves.

Ventilatory failure commonly occurs in middle-aged patients with > 100 degrees and they tend to develop dyspnea and decreased exercise tolerance, usually have repeated acute respiratory infections. The onset of respiratory failure is insidious and incidence variable. Kyphoscoliosis accounts for less than 5 percent of chronic ventilatory failure in adults. After Cor pulmonale develops, the prognosis is poor; without treatment, death generally occurs within a year. Pregnancy usually poses no added risk for respiratory complications. With severe degrees of kyphoscoliosis and reductions in VC to less than 1 liter the risk for respiratory complications during pregnancy may be increased. Prime factor that has been historical related to progression to respiratory failure has been the degree of kyphoscoliosis. This notion has been challenged by cases of survival into 70s with curves > 100 without any specific therapy. Other Factors predisposing to ventilatory failure in kyphoscoliosis include spinal deformity > 100 degrees; underlying neuromuscular disease; inspiratory muscle weakness; sleep disordered breathing; airway compression; and co-existent pulmonary disease.

Medical Management

This includes both preventive and supportive measures. They include:
1. Immunization
2. Adequate hydration

Disorders of the Diaphragm and Chest Wall **1659**

3. Prompt care of respiratory infections
4. Avoidance of sedatives
5. Carefully monitored supplemental oxygen
6. Abstaining from smoking
7. Maintaining body weight within desirable levels
8. Physical training is encouraged to improve exercise capacity in sedentary patients.

All efforts are to be made to restore normal curvature as early as possible. Such procedures include use of external and internal splints. They are: use of plaster casts, spinal rods, and other traction procedures. Although they have more cosmetic effects, they perhaps do not improve lung function. The most common benefit is an improvement in ventilation perfusion relationship with reduced A-a gradient.[11-15]

Recently, life-threatening respiratory failure has been treated with tank respirators or cuirass shells. IPPB therapy has been useful in some patients. All efforts should be made to treat infections and these patients should be persuaded not to smoke. Appropriate diuretic therapy will be needed in those who develop right heart failure. Nocturnal assisted ventilation or ventilation through a tracheostomy tube may be more beneficial in patients. Chronic respiratory failure treated with chest physiotherapy, bronchodilators, oxygen therapy, and diuretics if needed. Noninvasive ventilation has been useful both as a prophylactic therapy in high-risk patients and as definite therapy for respiratory failure in kyphoscoliosis.[16-29]

Pectus Excavatum or Funnel Chest

Pectus excavatum is characterized by excessive depression of the sternum.[30-37] It may be minimal or extreme, diffuse or local; and symmetrical or asymmetrical. In this condition, although the manubrium is normal, the body of the sternum is angled backwards towards the spine from the manubriosternal joint downwards with maximum recession at the xiphoid. It is usually symmetrical. It is one of the most common chest wall deformities seen by pediatricians and primary care providers affecting between 0.5 percent and 2.0 percent of the population. Occurs in approximately 1 in every 1000 children. Boys are affected about three times more often than girls. It is apparent at birth in over 80 percent of individuals. The natural history is variable; and it usually progresses, especially during the teenage years. The deformity results from defects in the anterior portion of the diaphragm, which alters the balance between the inward, pull of the diaphragm on the xiphisternum. When the posterior displacement of the lower portion of the sternum is severe, the intrathoracic structures may be displaced laterally. The PA film of the chest reveals a broadened cardiac silhouette with some straightening of the left cardiac border. Surgery is rarely required because of symptoms except for cosmetic reasons. Although extremely rare, respiratory failure can occur in adults with severe pectus excavatum.

The etiology is unknown. A defect in the connective tissue surrounding the sternum has been implicated. Frequent association with connective tissue disorders such as Marfan's syndrome has been reported. A genetic predisposition is suggested by one large series in which a family history of pectus deformity was present in 41 percent of the members. In most series, family history is not prominent. Reported associations with pectus excavatum include scoliosis 15 percent, congenital heart disease 4 percent, and functional heart murmurs in 31 percent.

Pectus Carinatum

Pectus carinatum is a disorder in which the sternum is protuberant. It is less common than pectus excavatum. It is a congenital condition in which the sternum is prominent, forming an anterior ridge. The ribs fall away steeply on either side. This deformity occurs during early ages, possibly due to inadequate segmentation during fetal life. The deformity may also occur because of malattachment of the anterior portion of the diaphragm to the posterior portion of the rectus sheath instead of the xiphoid process. It is of unknown etiology and may be associated with congenital heart disease, severe childhood asthma and rickets. There is no functional impairment. The most frequent complaints are cosmetic in nature and arise in patients between the ages of 15 and 20 years.

Psychological problems related to the deformity occur in as many as 85 percent of patients. Dyspnea on exertion also occurs in 30 to 70 percent of patients. Other symptoms include chest pain, palpitations, and frequent respiratory infections.

Objective Assessment of Pectus Disorders

Hollow index is a bedside test used for determination of pectus deformity. It is the ratio between the amount of water that can be held in the chest depression and the body surface area. An index more than 50 mL/m^2 indicates the presence of pectus deformity. The degree of chest wall deformity can also be assessed clinically or radiographically. A distance more than 3 cm between the surface of the anterior chest wall and the deepest sternal depression is taken as significant. A minimal distance of < 10 cm between the posterior border of the sternum and the anterior border of the thoracic vertebra on the lateral chest radiograph is also diagnostic of pectus. This does not account for differences in body size. To take care of this issue, the ratio of the AP to transverse diameters of the rib cage (as seen on the poster anterior and lateral chest radiograph) is calculated. A ratio of less than 0.4 indicates the presence of pectus, and a ratio less than 0.3 indicates a severe deformity. Anatomic definition can be obtained with CT scans. Measurements of transverse and AP chest wall diameters are taken at the level of the deepest sternal depression A ratio of the transverse to AP diameter of the inner chest wall of greater than 3.25 is considered significant for pectus. This ratio has been used to select patients for surgical correction.

Lung volumes are usually normal or mildly reduced. If a restrictive impairment is present, it is positively associated with the degree of sternal depression and is more severe if there is associated scoliosis. The RV may be normal or slightly reduced. FEV_1/FVC ratio is typically within normal limits. FRC is usually within the normal range. Although deformed, the mobility of the rib cage is not impaired during quiet breathing. Lung compliance in pectus excavatum is within normal limits. Cardiopulmonary exercise testing is often normal. Maximal work rate, oxygen consumption, and heart rate, as well as the oxygen pulse are similar to controls. Patients with more severe deformities may have a mild reduction in the maximal work rate or a decrease in the oxygen consumption for a given work.[38-41]

Usually no intervention is required, unless the patient wants this for cosmetic reasons. Candidates for surgical repair are patients with a transverse-to-AP diameter ratio of greater than 3.25 as determined by CT of the chest. The *Ravitch repair* included resection of costal cartilage and sternal osteotomy with or without fixation of the sternum with external or internal supports. However, this is an invasive procedure and complications like sternal necrosis, infection and recurrence of the deformity, especially in younger children in whom sternal supports are not used. Less invasive approaches to pectus excavatum have been developed. Of these, the *Nuss procedure* is widely used as an alternative. In this procedure, a customized, curved metal bar is placed under the sternum at the point of its deepest depression through small incisions made on each side of the chest. The bar is removed after 2 to 4 years when permanent chest wall remodeling has occurred. Surgical repair provides cosmetic benefits and may positively affect the psychosocial well-being of the patient.[42-78]

Rib Abnormalities

Abnormalities like bifid, fused, and absent ribs are a group of congenital disorders. Bifid rib is common in the first 6 ribs. Cervical rib occurs quite commonly and about 0.5 percent of population will have this anomaly. It is bilateral in about 80 percent of the cases. Although it is most often a radiological finding, neurological symptoms like pain, paresthesia, and weakness of the arm may be present. Intrinsic muscle atrophy of the hand will occur.[79,80]

Ankylosing Spondylitis

This is common in young adult males and less frequent in females. There is strong association of this condition with HLA-B27.[81-93] The thoracic cage is fixed because of ankylosis of the costotransverse and costovertebral joints. Diminished chest movement, usually less than 2 inches, is the first abnormality. Deformity of the chest wall with increased kyphosis is noted subsequently. The spine becomes more and more rigid. Typically, there will be a restrictive type of ventilatory defect. The lungs are fixed in an inspiratory position, so that the FRC and RV are increased. Compliance of the chest wall is severely reduced, but that of the lungs is well maintained. Diaphragmatic movements are normal. Although ventilation may be affected because of fixity, overall gas exchange is not altered.[94,95]

It is a systemic disease more commonly seen in males in their thirties and forties. Most patients have low back pain involving the sacroiliac joint that progresses gradually to involve other joints. Dyspnea on exertion may be present. Chest pain is not infrequent. Radiologically, one may see the typical "bamboo spine".

Pulmonary changes occur in about 1.8 percent of cases and those described in ankylosing spondylitis are as follows:[96-108]

- Apical lung fibrosis
- Cavitation and bullae formation
- Aspergillomata in the cavity with hemoptysis
- Transient pleural effusion
- Increased incidence of infection particularly tuberculosis
- Increased incidence of adenocarcinoma
- Bronchocentric granulomatosis associated with Aspergillus colonization
- Increased risk of abdominal surgery
- Acute respiratory failure because of extrathoracic obstruction due to arthritis of the cricoarytenoid joints
- Cor pulmonale, hypoventilation are uncommon unless there is associated parenchymal disease.

There is no specific treatment for this condition except that for the symptoms. Ankylosing spondylitis is a chronic inflammatory disease of unknown cause, characterized by sacroiliitis and spondylitis. To date, treatment of AS has been limited to the alleviation of symptoms, mainly using nonsteroidal anti-inflammatory drugs (NSAIDs). For patients refractory or intolerant to NSAIDs, the disease modifying antirheumatic drugs (DMARDs) have been used as a second line approach. Methotrexate (MTX) is currently one of the most widely used DMARDs and its efficacy in rheumatoid arthritis (RA) has been confirmed. There is uncertainty whether MTX works in the treatment of ankylosing spondylitis. Recently more immunomodulatory drugs have also been tried.[109-121] Surgery is useful only in specific cases.[122]

Flail Chest

Flail chest denotes a condition in which fractures of ribs produce a segment of the rib cage that is disconnected from the rest of the chest wall and deforms markedly with breathing.

Usually, double fractures of three or more contiguous ribs or combined sternal and rib fractures are needed to create the flail segment. The detached part of the rib segment is pulled inward with inspiration and bulges outward with expiration compromising ventilation. It is estimated to occur in up to 25 percent of adults but in only 1 percent of children following blunt chest trauma. This lower incidence in children may be related to their greater chest wall compliance.[123-135]

Etiology

- Trauma
  - Automobile accidents, falls
  - After cardiopulmonary resuscitation.
- Pathologic fractures
  - Multiple myeloma
  - Other rib metastases
- Sternotomy and simple rib fractures
- Corrective rib resection
- Congenital.

Flail chest is a clinical diagnosis made by observing the paradoxical motion of the chest wall in the spontaneously breathing patient with blunt trauma and radiographic documentation of rib or sternal fractures.

Chest radiographs underestimate the presence and extent of rib fractures. Hemothorax and pulmonary contusion are commonly associated with the condition. Special rib views or oblique films can diagnose many rib fractures missed by plain chest radiographs.

Nuclear radionuclide scans are the most accurate in detecting rib fractures.

A three-dimensional reconstruction of a thoracic helical-CT scan done to evaluate the extent of thoracic injuries, can also identify rib fractures. TLC, VC, and FRC can be reduced to 50 percent of predicted. The initial reductions attributed to disordered chest wall motion. VC either returns to its baseline value within 6 months or remains mildly reduced. In contrast, patients with pulmonary contusion complicating flail chest may have persistent reductions in FRC longer periods due to fibrous changes in the contused area.

The multiple rib fractures uncouple the flail segment from the remainder of the chest wall. During inspiration, the subatmospheric pleural pressure is unopposed, and the uncoupled segment of chest wall moves paradoxically inward during inspiration. During expiration, pleural pressure becomes less negative, and the flail segment can be seen moving paradoxically outward. A reduction in lung compliance due to pulmonary contusion or microatelectasis or an increase in airway resistance further lowers pleural pressure during inspiration and worsens the flail.

On the basis of rib fractures and anatomic location of flail segment, flail chest can be of three types:
- Lateral
- Anterior
- Posterior.

Lateral flail chest is the most common. The flail segment is located posteriorly and laterally. Anterior flail chest occurs when there is separation of the sternum from the ribs. Posterior flail chest is associated with less severe clinical derangement because of splinting provided by the back muscles. However, this anatomic classification is merely descriptive and does not provide any information about the actual degree of chest wall distortion in flail chest. Chest wall distortion is better characterized by recording the respiratory changes in the dimensions of not only the rib cage but also the abdomen. Paradoxical motion may occur between the rib cage and abdomen or within the rib cage itself. Abnormal patterns seen include:
1. Inward displacement of the transverse rib cage as the lower anterior rib cage and abdomen are expanding.
2. Inward displacement of the anterior lower rib cage and abdomen as the transverse rib cage is expanding.
3. Inward displacement of the lower rib cage as the transverse rib cage and abdomen are expanding.

A given location of flail segment is not necessarily associated with a specific pattern of distortion. These different flail patterns may therefore reflect not only differences in the location of the rib cage fractures but also differences in respiratory muscle recruitment patterns. Clinical observations and recent experimental data suggest that the pathogenesis is complex.

Flail chest and the pain that invariably accompanies chest trauma lead to cough impairment, regional atelectasis, rib cage muscle spasm, and specific changes in the pattern of muscle activation and recruitment. Paradoxical motion of the flail segment may also increase the degree of muscle shortening during inspiration adding to energetic cost. Inspiratory muscles become inefficient when operating over shorter lengths the paradoxical motion of the flail segment may result in diaphragm inefficiency. Pulmonary contusion or pleural restriction adds to the work of breathing by increasing the negative pressure needed to inhale. The added work of breathing, along with respiratory muscle inefficiency increases the oxygen cost of breathing and predisposes these muscles to fatigue. Atelectasis and lung contusion in conjunction with respiratory muscle fatigue result in hypoxemia, hypercapnia, and ultimately respiratory failure. Hypoxemia is due to either process would contribute to respiratory muscle dysfunction by reducing energy supplies to the muscles. The presence of multiple vicious cycles ensures perpetuation of the process. Traumatic flail chest is a marker of severe chest injury. An independent risk factor for significant respiratory complications, respiratory failure, and death. Flail chest promotes atelectasis. Atelectasis, via its effect on compliance, increases the severity of flail chest and lead to worsening of respiratory failure.

Patients with isolated flail chest developed respiratory failure and required mechanical ventilation almost twice as often (57%) as did patients with isolated pulmonary contusion (31%). The mortality rate from chest wall trauma alone ranges from 7 to 14 percent. The lung may also be injured in patients who sustain chest wall trauma. Pulmonary contusion, hemothorax, and pneumothorax, can occur in up to 60 percent of patients with flail chest. Patients with multiple trauma and lung contusion had a mortality rate (56%) almost as high as those with flail chest (67%). Associated pulmonary contusion is best detected by chest CT scans. If the contusion is seen on the chest radiograph, however, it may be more clinically significant. If the patient survives the initial injury, symptoms of chest tightness, chest pain, or dyspnea on exertion is seen in half of patients. Operative stabilization of the chronic flail chest can correct the defect and dramatically relieve the symptoms. Because of an incompetent chest wall in patients with flail chest, external chest compressions during cardio-

pulmonary resuscitation are ineffective. In such cases, internal cardiac massage may be recommended.

The primary goal of treatment is to restore the anatomic and functional integrity of the chest wall by providing stability of the flail segment. This can be accomplished with conservative management or with surgical intervention. Pain should be adequately controlled in all patients with flail chest. Chest wall pain may cause patients to adopt a rapid, shallow breathing pattern, worsening atelectasis and lead to arteriovenous shunting and hypoxemia. Analgesia reduces splinting, improves tidal volume, and facilitates cough. Oral medications, patient-controlled analgesia pumps, intermittent intercostal nerve blocks, or epidural anesthesia can accomplish pain control. Mechanical ventilation has been used in the treatment of flail chest for more than 40 years. Such "internal pneumatic stabilization" consisted of tracheostomy with a prolonged 3 to 5 week period of mechanical ventilation. Mechanical ventilation failed to improve survival and predisposed patients to several complications such as pneumonia, barotrauma, sepsis, and tracheal stenosis. It is no longer recommended as a primary means of stabilizing the chest wall; it is only recommended when there is concomitant central nervous system or intra-abdominal injury, shock, or a need to operate for other injuries. The role of noninvasive mechanical ventilation in stabilizing the flail segment has not been fully evaluated in patients with flail chest. When mechanical ventilation is needed to treat respiratory failure, the mode of ventilation chosen should minimize the resistive and elastic loads imposed by the ventilator. IMV has been frequently used as a mode of ventilating patients with flail chest. Pressure support ventilation may be an alternate means of reducing the ventilator-imposed loads, but the effects of this mode on chest wall distortion have not been evaluated.

The purpose of surgical stabilization is to achieve a mechanically stable chest to reduce ventilator time, and to avoid ventilator-associated complications. Initial attempts consisted of applying tape, strapping, and external devices to the chest wall with limited success. By externally stabilizing the chest wall, inward displacement of the ribs during the healing phase can be avoided, and the chest wall contour can be restored to normal. No randomized studies have defined the effectiveness of this modality. Possible indications include:

- Ventilator-dependent patients able to protect their upper airways with no need prolonged mechanical ventilation.

- Flail chest patients undergoing thoracotomy for intrathoracic injuries.
- Young patients with severe chest wall deformation and patients with large, unstable segments ("*stove-in chest*").
- Patients with borderline pulmonary function may be candidates for external fixation.

Chest wall external fixation in such patients improves respiratory mechanics, reduces the duration of mechanical ventilation, reduces hospital stay, and decreases the incidence of pulmonary infection and barotraumas.

Tumors of Chest Wall

Tumors of the chest wall can arise from any of its constituents like soft tissue, muscles, nerves, vessels, and bones and cartilages.[136-142] Thus, they may be lipomas, hemangiomas, cystic hygromas, neurofibromata, osteo-chondroma, chondroma, simple bone cyst, osteomas, and fibrous dysplasia. The malignant counterparts include fibrosarcoma, chondrosarcoma, Ewing's tumor, osteo-genic sarcoma, and myeloma.

Other infective conditions of the chest wall include osteomyelitis, tuberculosis of the ribs, cold abscess, septic arthritis, actinomycosis and fungal infections (Figs 30.1 to 30.4).

Costochondritis (Tietze's Syndrome)

This condition is of obscure origin occurring in young adults with pain and swelling in the costal cartilages. Usually the upper six costal cartilages are involved although the sternoclavicular joint may also be involved. The exact etiology of the condition is unknown. A viral

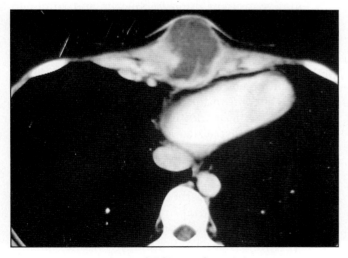

FIGURE 30.1: CT Chest - Sternal abscess

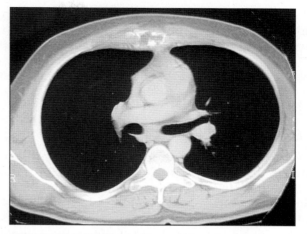

FIGURE 30.2: CT Chest - Bone window showing sternum abscess and erosion

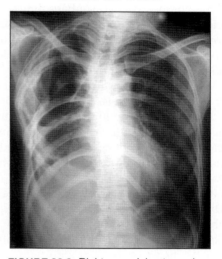

FIGURE 30.3: Right upper lobectomy done

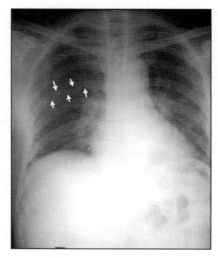

FIGURE 30.4: Rib erosion - Tuberculosis

etiology is suggested. The most common presentation is pain with swelling and tenderness of the costal cartilages. The pain is localized and variously described as aching, sharp, or dull. Most cases respond to analgesics, although the condition is self-limiting. Rarely, local hydrocortisone may be required to relieve local pain.[143-156]

DIAPHRAGM

Diaphragm is the main muscle of respiration. Although intrinsic diseases of the diaphragm are rare, because of its complex development congenital anomalies are common. The development of the diaphragm is complex both anatomically and physiologically. There are six sources of tissues, which join to form the complete diaphragm. They are the septum transversum, pleuro-peritoneal membranes, dorsal esophageal mesentery, and the thoracic myotomes. The ventral septum transversum is the major contributor, which grows dorsally to envelop the gut, inferior vena cava, and aorta. This leaves the abdominal and pleural cavities connected by only the paired posterolateral (pleuro-peritoneal) canals. Normally these canals close during the 8th week of gestation. At this time, the mid gut also returns to the abdomen. Either premature return of the mid gut or delayed closure of the pleuro-peritoneal canals is cited as the cause of congenital posterolateral diaphragmatic hernia (Bochdalek's hernia).

Normally the right hemidiaphragm is higher than the left by about one space. The upper level of right hemidiaphragm lies at the anterior end of the sixth rib. This is because of the underlying liver, but also due to the push of the heart on the left side, which is lower.

Diaphragmatic Disorders

Diaphragmatic Hernias

The common sites of diaphragmatic hernia are through the esophageal hiatus, foramen of Morgagni, foramen of Bochdalek, traumatic tear, central tendon, vena cava, and aorta in that order. In congenital diaphragmatic hernia the abdominal contents herniated into the thoracic cavity through a defect in the diaphragm. Bochdalek's hernia is a condition of infancy (Fig. 30.5). The incidence is reported to be 1 in 22,00 births constituting 1.4 percent of all postmortems in infants and 8.5 percent of all stillbirths and neonatal deaths. Most of the cases the child is usually 24 hours old and rarely only few months of age. The condition is rare in adults. Over a period of more than 100 years from 1853 to 1976 there are only 63 cases of this hernia in adults. The mortality is very high in

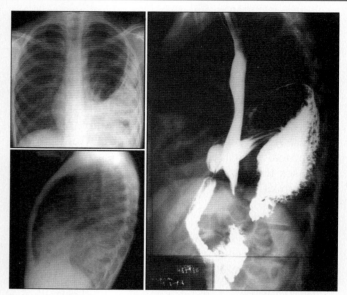

FIGURE 30.5: Bochdalek's hernia - Note the intestines are in the left hemithorax

infants because of associated major anomalies present to an extent of 47 percent. These include pulmonary hypoplasia, anencephalus, Arnold-Chiari malformation, hydrocephalus, alimentary canal defects such as malrotation or atresia of esophagus, or rectum and cardiovascular or genitourinary tract abnormalities. Other minor anomalies associated with this condition include Klippel-Feil anomaly, ventricular septal defect, hydronephrosis, bicornuate uterus, cystic kidney, and cleft palate. The hernia occurs more often on the left side. The contents of the hernia are small bowel (88%), stomach (60%), colon (56%), spleen (54%), liver (51%), pancreas (24%), and kidneys in 12.1 percent.

Clinical symptoms differ in children and adults. In children the onset is catastrophic with respiratory distress, in adults the symptoms develop gradually, occasionally strangulation of the bowel loops have been reported. The abdominal contents when enter the thorax displace the mediastinum. Usually a barium meal follow-through will confirm the diagnosis.

As soon as the condition is recognized, surgical correction is desirable. Both abdominal and/or thoracic approach is advocated. Postoperative recovery is very good in adult patients compared to that in children.

Herniation through the esophageal hiatus is the commonest type of diaphragmatic hernia (Hiatus hernia). The main clinical presentation is retrosternal burning pain which is relieved by semi-recumbent position[157-171] (Fig. 30.6).

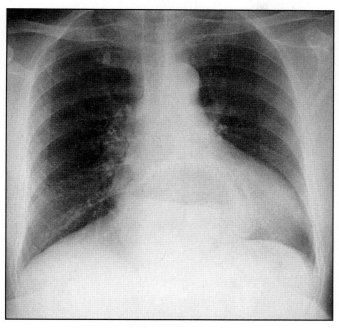

FIGURE 30.6: Hiatus hernia

Morgagni Hernia

This is the herniation of loose connective tissue, omentum, colon, liver, or other infradiaphragmatic structures including gallbladder through the foramen of morgagni and occurs more commonly on the right. Presentation in the childhood is rare. Chest tightness, fullness or pain in the right anterior chest is common symptoms. The chest skiagram usually reveals a rounded density in the cardiophrenic angle. Barium meal examination will demonstrate the presence of intestine. Reduction of the hernia followed by surgical repair is the treatment of choice[172-187] (Fig. 30.6).

Traumatic Hernias

These hernias are common following blunt non-penetrating trauma more commonly as a result of trauma, to the lower chest or abdomen following high velocity accidents or fall from a height.[188-191] This constitutes about 5 percent of all diaphragmatic hernias and the most common cause of strangulation. Traumatic rupture on the left leaf (90%) is common. Omentum, stomach, or colon and rarely the kidneys, may herniated through the defect. The patient usually presents with pain, and dyspnea. Severe vomiting, and retching with abdominal guarding may occur in strangulation. Rarely, acute pancreatitis can occur because of a traumatic broncho-pancreatic fistula. There may be diminished air entry on the side of rupture with shifting of mediastinum.

Radiological features include an elevated diaphragm with multiple air fluid levels. Barium meal examination will reveal the stomach or colon. Surgical repair can be done through thoracic, abdominal, or combined routes.

Eventration of Diaphragm

Enventration of the diaphragm may be complete or partial.[192-195] In this condition, all or part of the diaphragm is mainly composed of fibrous tissue with only a few or no interspersed muscle fibers. The condition is usually congenital but may be acquired. Complete eventration almost invariably occurs in the left side and is characterized by elevation of the hemi-diaphragm. The condition is differentiated from herni-ation by the absence of shifting of the mediastinum to the opposite side. The diaphragm is immobile on screening which moves paradoxically on sniffing. The condition is asymptomatic and is detected only on a screening X-ray. Occasionally there may be upper abdominal discomfort. The stomach may be inverted. In infants the condition produces severe symptoms with respiratory distress and can occur on either side. Cough, dyspnea, wheezing, and recurrent bronchopneumonia are common symptom. Clinically, the hemithorax may be bulged. Diaphragmatic plication is helpful in symptomatic patients (Figs 30.7 to 30.10).

Partial eventration almost always occurs on the right side. It is a chance radiological finding as it is largely asymptomatic and is seen as an anteromedial bulge of the diaphragm which moves paradoxically on

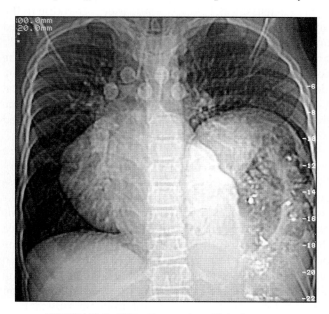

FIGURE 30.7: CXR - Eventration of left diaphragm

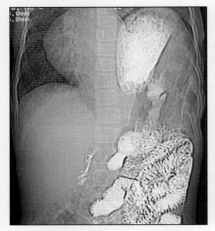

FIGURE 30.8: CXR - Eventration of left dome of diaphragm with barium

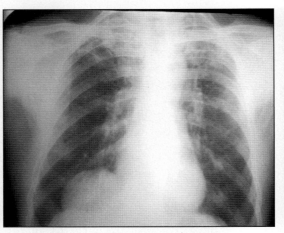

FIGURE 30.9: Eventration of right diaphragm

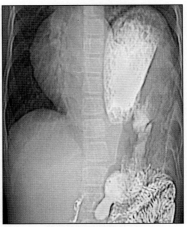

FIGURE 30.10: Eventration of diaphragm

respiration. There is usually corresponding deformity of the liver. Ultrasound is helpful in differentiating eventration from diaphragmatic hernias and pleuro-pericardial cysts, both of which will have similar radiological appearances.

Diaphragmatic Paralysis

The commonest cause of diaphragmatic paralysis is due to the involvement of the phrenic nerve of the same side by bronchogenic carcinoma. Other rare causes of unilateral diaphragmatic paralysis include surgery, trauma, neurological problems, and idiopathic. Very rarely fibrosis due to tuberculosis may entrap the nerve at the hilum. The patient is usually not symptomatic except that due to the underlying cause. The hemidiaphragm may be elevated on the affected side that will be apparent both clinically and radiologically. Paradoxical movement of the paralyzed diaphragm can be demonstrated at bedside by simple inspection. This can be confirmed by radiological examination, when fluoroscopy will demonstrate the same thing and when the patient is asked to sniff, the affected diaphragm will move down.[196-200]

Bilateral diaphragmatic paralysis is a very rare condition and most often it is idiopathic. It usually follows viral infections, trauma, and other neuromuscular diseases including quadriplegia. A similar condition is described in systemic lupus erythematosus because of myopathy of both the diaphragms. Dyspnea in the supine position is the usual symptom. In supine position, the abdomen will show paradoxical motion with inward movements during inspiration. Tachycardia is usual. Both the diaphragms are located higher on chest X-ray and the movement may be sluggish or paradoxical on screening.

REFERENCES

1. Golladay ES, Golladay GJ. Chest wall deformities. Indian J Pediatr 1997;64:339-50.
2. Grillo HC, wright CD, Dertevelle PG, Wain JC, Murakarani S. Tracheal compression caused by straight back syndrome, chest wall deformity, and anterior spinal displacement: Techniques for relief. Ann Thorac Surg 2005;80:2057-62.
3. Donnelly LF, Frush DP, Foss JN, O'Hara SM, Bisset GS 3rd. Anterior chest wall: Frequency of anatomic variations in children. Radiology 1999;212:837-40.
4. Akcali Y, Ceyran H, Hasdiraz L. Chest wall deformities. Acta Chir Hung 1999;38:1-3.
5. Fokin AA, Robicsek F. Acquired deformities of the anterior chest wall. Thorac Cardiovasc Surg 2006;54:57-61.
6. Lowe TG, Edgar M, Margulies JY, Miller NH, Raso VJ, Reinker KA, Rivard CH. Etiology of idiopathic scoliosis: Current trends in research. J Bone Joint Surg Am 2000;82-A:1157-68.
7. Giunta C, Randolph A, Al-Gazali LI, Brunner HG, Kraenzlin ME, Steinmann B. Nevo syndrome is allelic to the kyphoscoliotic type of the Ehlers-Danlos syndrome (EDS VIA). Am J Med Genet A 2005;133:158-64.
8. Kuorilehto T, Poyhonen M, Bloigu R, Heikkinen J, Vaananen K, Peltonen J. Decreased bone mineral density and content in neurofibromatosis type 1: Lowest local values are located in the load-carrying parts of the body. Osteoporos Int 2005;16:928-36.
9. Das MN, Ghorpade A, Mercy P, Pandey TK, Sharma R. Ehlers-Danlos syndrome in two siblings. Indian J Dermatol Venereol Leprol 2005;71:186-88.
10. Tsirikos AI, Ramachandran M, Lee J, Saifuddin A. Assessment of vertebral scalloping in neurofibromatosis type 1 with plain radiography and MRI. Clin Radiol 2004;59:1009-17.

11. Malek MH, Fonkalsrud EW, Cooper CB. Ventilatory and cardiovascular responses to exercise in patients with pectus excavatum. Chest 2003;124;870-82.

12. Ding LX, Qiu GX, Wang YP, Zhang JG. Simultaneous anterior and posterior hemivertebra resection in the treatment of congenital kyphoscoliosis. Chin Med Sci J 2005;20:252-56.

13. Suk SI, Chung ER, Lee SM, Lee JH, Kim SS, Kim JH. Posterior vertebral column resection in fixed lumbosacral deformity. Spine 2005;30:E703-10.

14. Yuan N, Fraire JA, Margetis MM, Skaggs DL, Tolo VT, Keens TG. The effect of scoliosis surgery on lung function in the immediate postoperative period. Spine 2005;30:2182-85.

15. Smith JT, Gollogly S, Dunn HK. Simultaneous anterior-posterior approach through a costotransversectomy for the treatment of congenital kyphosis and acquired kyphoscoliotic deformities. J Bone Joint Surg Am 2005;87:2281-89.

16. Munoz X, Crespo A, Marti S, Torres F, Ferrer J, Morell F. Comparative study of two different modes of non-invasive home mechanical ventilation in chronic respiratory failure. Respir Med 2006;100:673-81.

17. Reddy R, Evans E, Khoo O, Allen MB. Pregnancy in kyphoscoliosis: Benefit of non-invasive ventilatory support. J Obstet Gynaecol 2005;25:267-68.

18. Saraph VJ, Bach CM, Krismer M, Wimmer C. Evaluation of spinal fusion using autologous anterior strut grafts and posterior instrumentation for thoracic/thoracolumbar kyphosis. Spine 2005;30:1594-601.

19. Mohan AL, Das K. History of surgery for the correction of spinal deformity. Neurosurg Focus 2003;15;14(1):e1.

20. Singh K, Samartzis D, An HS. Neurofibromatosis type I with severe dystrophic kyphoscoliosis and its operative management via a simultaneous anterior-posterior approach: A case report and review of the literature. Spine J 2005;5:461-66.

21. Rinella A, Lenke L, Whitaker C, Kim Y, Park SS, Peelle M, Edwards C, Bridwell K. Perioperative halo-gravity traction in the treatment of severe scoliosis and kyphosis. Spine 2005 15;30:475-82.

22. Christodoulou A, Ploumis A, Terzidis J, Tapsis K, Hantzidis P. Surgical management of a congenital kyphotic deformity in an adolescent. Stud Health Technol Inform 2002;91:454-56.

23. McArdle FJ, Griffiths CJ, Macdonald AM, Gibson MJ. Monitoring the thoracic sagittal curvature in kyphoscoliosis with surface topography: A trend analysis of 57 patients. Stud Health Technol Inform 2002;91:199-203.

24. Domanic U, Talu U, Dikici F, Hamzaoglu A. Surgical correction of kyphosis: Posterior total wedge resection osteotomy in 32 patients. Acta Orthop Scand 2004;75:449-55.

25. Mehta S, Hill NS. Noninvasive ventilation. Am J Respir Crit Care Med 2001;163:540-77.

26. Elliott MW, Ambrosino N. Non-invasive ventilation in acute and chronic respiratory failure. Eur Respir J 2002;20:480-87.

27. Chailleux E, Fauroux B, Binet F, Dautzenberg B, Polu JM. Predictors of survival in patients receiving domiciliary oxygen therapy or mechanical ventilation. A 10-year analysis of ANTADIR Observatory. Chest 1996;109:741-49.

28. Gonzalez C, Ferris G, Diaz J, Fontana I, Nunez J, Marin J. Kyphoscoliotic ventilatory insufficiency: Effects of long-term intermittent positive-pressure ventilation. Chest 2003;124:857-62.

29. Duiverman ML, Bladder G, Meinesz AF, Wijkstra PJ. Home mechanical ventilatory support in patients with restrictive ventilatory disorders: A 48-year experience. Respir Med 2006;100:56-65.

30. Goretsky MJ, Kelly RE Jr, Croitoru D, Nuss D. Chest wall anomalies: Pectus excavatum and pectus carinatum. Adolesc Med Clin 2004;15:455-71.

31. Dalton ML. Current overview of pectus excavatum. Curr Surg 2000;57:16-21.

32. Kelly RE Jr, Lawson ML, Paidas CN, Hruban RH. Pectus excavatum in a 112-year autopsy series: Anatomic findings and the effect on survival. J Pediatr Surg 2005;40:1275-78.

33. Kabir ML, Rahman M, Talukder K, Rahman A, Hossain Q, Mostafa G, Mannan MA, Kumar S, Chowdhury AT. Rickets among children of a coastal area of Bangladesh. Mymensingh Med J 2004;13:53-58.

34. Fokin AA, Robicsek F. Acquired deformities of the anterior chest wall. Thorac Cardiovasc Surg 2006;54: 57-61.

35. Williams AM, Crabbe DC. Pectus deformities of the anterior chest wall. Paediatr Respir Rev. 2003;4:237-42.

36. Colombani PM. Recurrent chest wall anomalies. Semin Pediatr Surg 2003;12:94-99.

37. Giant intrathoracic extrapulmonary hydatid cyst manifested as unilateral pectus carinatum. South Med J 2002;95:1207-08.

38. Kinuya K, Ueno T, Kobayashi T, Tuji T, Yamamoto Y, Kinuya S. Tc-99m MAA SPECT in pectus excavatum: Assessment of perfusion volume changes after correction by the Nuss procedure. Clin Nucl Med 2005;30:779-82.

39. Andres AM, Hernandez F, Martinez L, Fernandez A, Encinas JL, Avila LF, Luis AL, Rivas J, Olivares P, Tovar JA. Cardiac function alterations in pectus excavatum. Cir Pediatr 2005;18:192-95.

40. Rowland T, Moriarty K, Banever G. Effect of pectus excavatum deformity on cardiorespiratory fitness in adolescent boys. Arch Pediatr Adolesc Med 2005; 159:1069-73.

41. Welter S, Hinterthaner M, Stamatis G. Heart failure following left-sided pneumonectomy in a patient with known pectus excavatum—Successful treatment using the Ravitch procedure. Eur J Cardiothorac Surg 2006; 29:630-31.

42. Haje SA, Haje DP. Overcorrection during treatment of pectus deformities with DCC orthoses: Experience in 17 cases. Int Orthop 2006;30(4):262-67.

43. Haecker FM, Mayr J. The vacuum bell for treatment of pectus excavatum: An alternative to surgical correction? Eur J Cardiothorac Surg 2006; 29:557-61.

44. Hoel TN, Rein KA, Svennevig JL. A life-threatening complication of the Nuss-procedure for pectus excavatum. Ann Thorac Surg 2006;81:370-72.

45. Krasopoulos G, Dusmet M, Ladas G, Goldstraw P. Nuss procedure improves the quality of life in young male adults with pectus excavatum deformity. Eur J Cardiothorac Surg 2006;29:1-5.

46. Schaarschmidt K, Kolberg-Schwerdt A, Lempe M, Schlesinger F, Bunke K, Strauss J. Extrapleural, submuscular bars placed by bilateral thoracoscopy—A new improvement in modified Nuss funnel chest repair. J Pediatr Surg 2005;40:1407-10.

47. Kim do H, Hwang JJ, Lee MK, Lee DY, Paik HC. Analysis of the Nuss procedure for pectus excavatum in different age groups. Ann Thorac Surg 2005;80:1073-77.

48. Nuss D. Recent experiences with minimally invasive pectus excavatum repair "Nuss procedure". Jpn J Thorac Cardiovasc Surg 2005;53:338-44.

49. Ong CC, Choo K, Morreau P, Auldist A. The learning curve in learning the curve: A review of Nuss procedure in teenagers. ANZ J Surg. 2005;75:421-24.

50. Croitoru DP, Kelly RE Jr, Goretsky MJ, Gustin T, Keever R, Nuss D. The minimally invasive Nuss technique for recurrent or failed pectus excavatum repair in 50 patients. J Pediatr Surg 2005;40:181-86.

51. Lawson ML, Mellins RB, Tabangin M, Kelly RE Jr, Croitoru DP, Goretsky MJ, Nuss D. Impact of pectus excavatum on pulmonary function before and after repair with the Nuss procedure. J Pediatr Surg 2005;40:174-80.

52. Hwang J, Glick PL. Our minimally invasive approach to pectus excavatum. J Pediatr Surg 2005;40:751.

53. Robicsek F. Surgical treatment of pectus excavatum. Chest Surg Clin N Am 2000;10:277-96.

54. Backer CL, Mavroudis C. Congenital Heart Surgery nomenclature and Database Project: Vascular rings, tracheal stenosis, pectus excavatum. Ann Thorac Surg 2000;69(Suppl):S308-18.

55. Engum S, Rescorla F, West K, Rouse T, Scherer LR, Grosfeld J. Is the grass greener? Early results of the Nuss procedure. J Pediatr Surg 2000;35:246-51.

56. Kosumi T, Yonekura T, Owari M, Hirooka S. Late-onset hemothorax after the Nuss procedure for funnel chest. Pediatr Surg Int 2005;21:1015-17.

57. Fox ME, Bensard DD, Roaten JB, Hendrickson RJ. Positioning for the Nuss procedure: Avoiding brachial plexus injury. Paediatr Anaesth 2005;15:1067-71.

58. Robicsek F. Innovative single-stage repair of severe asymmetric pectus excavatum defects. Ann Thorac Surg 2005;80:2419.

59. Grillo HC, Wright CD, Dartevelle PG, Wain JC, Murakami S. Kikuchi S, Ingu A, Ito M. Simultaneous repair of pectus excavatum and tetralogy of fallot: Report of a case. Ann Thorac Cardiovasc Surg 2005; 11:320-23.

60. Leonhardt J, Kubler JF, Feiter J, Ure BM, Petersen C. Complications of the minimally invasive repair of pectus excavatum. J Pediatr Surg 2005;40:e7-9.

61. Wang LS, Kuo KT, Wang HW, Yang CH, Chin T. A novel surgical correction through a small transverse incision for pectus excavatum. Ann Thorac Surg 2005;80:1951-54.

62. Boia ES, Susan-Resiga R, Raicov PC, Popoiu CM, Iacob RE. Determination of the mechanical requirements for a progressive correction system of pectus excavatum in children. J Laparoendosc Adv Surg Tech A 2005; 15:478-81.

63. Schwabegger AH, Piza H. Free sternum turnover flap for correction of pectus excavatum deformity. Plast Reconstr Surg 2005;116:1182.

64. Schaarschmidt K, Kolberg-Schwerdt A, Lempe M, Schlesinger F. New endoscopic minimal access pectus carinatum repair using subpectoral carbon dioxide. Ann Thorac Surg 2006;81:1099-103.

65. Frey AS, Garcia VF, Brown RL, Inge TH, Ryckman FC, Cohen AP, Durrett G, Azizkhan RG. Nonoperative management of pectus carinatum. J Pediatr Surg 2006;41:40.

66. Davis JT, Weinstein S. Repair of the pectus deformity: Results of the Ravitch approach in the current era. Ann Thorac Surg 2004;78:421-26.

67. Fonkalsrud EW, Anselmo DM. Less extensive techniques for repair of pectus carinatum: The undertreated chest deformity. J Am Coll Surg 2004;198:898-905.

68. Fonkalsrud EW. Management of pectus chest deformities in female patients. Am J Surg 2004;187:192-97.

69. Serafin J, Swiatkowski J, Majkusiak R, Nowakowski P. 40-year experience in surgical treatment of congenital chest deformations—Ethiopathogenesis, operative techniques and clinical results. Acta Chir Orthop Traumatol Cech 2003;70:207-13.

70. Fonkalsrud EW. Pectus carinatum: The undertreated chest malformation. Asian J Surg 2003;26:189-92.

71. Mansour KA, Thourani VH, Odessey EA, Durham MM, Miller JI Jr, Miller DL. Thirty-year experience with repair of pectus deformities in adults. Ann Thorac Surg 2003;76:391-95.

72. Mouroux J, Venissac N, Alifano M, Padovani B. Morgagni hernia and thoracic deformities. Thorac Cardiovasc Surg 2003;5:44-45.

73. Fonkalsrud EW, DeUgarte D, Choi E. Repair of pectus excavatum and carinatum deformities in 116 adults. Ann Surg 2002;236:304-12.

74. Fonkalsrud EW, Beanes S. Surgical management of pectus carinatum: 30 years' experience. World J Surg 2001;25:898-903.

75. Schoenmakers MA, Gulmans VA, Bax NM, Helders PJ. Physiotherapy as an adjuvant to the surgical treatment of anterior chest wall deformities: A necessity? A prospective descriptive study in 21 patients. J Pediatr Surg 2000;35:1440-43.

76. Robicsek F. Surgical treatment of pectus carinatum. Chest Surg Clin N Am 2000;10:357-76.

77. Saxena AK, Willital GH. Surgical repair of pectus carinatum. Int Surg 1999;84:326-30.

78. Robicsek F, Fokin A. Surgical correction of pectus excavatum and carinatum. J Cardiovasc Surg (Torino) 1999;40:725-31.

79. Tsirikos AI, McMaster MJ. Congenital anomalies of the ribs and chest wall associated with congenital deformities of the spine. J Bone Joint Surg Am 2005;87:2523-36.

80. Marks MW, Iacobucci J. Reconstruction of congenital chest wall deformities using solid silicone onlay prostheses. Chest Surg Clin N Am 2000;10:341-55.

81. Salaffi F, De Angelis R, Grassi W. MArche Pain Prevalence; Investigation Group (MAPPING) study. Prevalence of musculoskeletal conditions in an Italian population sample: Results of a regional community-based study. I. The MAPPING study. Clin Exp Rheumatol 2005;23:819-28.

82. Harjacek M, Ostojic J, Djakovic Rode O. Juvenile spondyloarthropathies associated with Mycoplasma pneumoniae infection. Clin Rheumatol 2006;25(4):470-75.

83. Amroun H, Djoudi H, Busson M, Allat R, El Sherbini SM, Sloma I, Ramasawmy R, Brun M, Dulphy N, Krishnamoorthy R, Toubert A, Charron D, Abbadi MC, Tamouza R. Early-onset ankylosing spondylitis is associated with a functional MICA polymorphism. Hum Immunol 2005;66:1057-61.

84. Masi AT, Sierakowski S, Kim JM. Jacques Forestier's vanished bowstring sign in ankylosing spondylitis: A call to test its validity and possible relation to spinal myofascial hypertonicity. Clin Exp Rheumatol 2005;23:760-66.

85. Zink A, Thiele K, Huscher D, Listing J, Sieper J, Krause A, Gromnica-Ihle E, von Hinueber U, Wassenberg S, Genth E, Schneider M. German Collaborative Arthritis Centres. Healthcare and burden of disease in psoriatic arthritis. A comparison with rheumatoid arthritis and ankylosing spondylitis. J Rheumatol 2006;33:86-90.

86. Spencer DG, Hick HM, Dick WC. Ankylosing spondylitis—The role of HLA-B27 homozygosity. Tissue Antigens 1979;14:379-84.

87. Woodrow JC. HLA typing in clinical rheumatology. Acta Rhumatol 1979;3:191-94.

88. Veys EM, Mielants H, Poriau S, Verbruggen G, van der Jeught J, Dhondt E, Goethals L. Rheumatic disorders in a HLA B27 positive population. Acta Rhumatol 1979;3:176-89.

89. Dequeker J, Decock T, Walravens M, van de Putte I. HLA B27 prevalence in spondylo-arthropathy syndromes. Acta Rhumatol 1979;3:144-53.

90. Huaux JP, De Bruyere M, Nagant de Deuxchaisnes C. Study of the phenomenon of discordance of HLA-B27 during the course of ankylosing spondylitis. Acta Rhumatol 1979;3:128-42.

91. Chappel R, Muylle L, Mortier G, Peetermans M, Brusselaers H. Risk of developing ankylosing spondylitis in "healthy" persons positive for HLA-B27 antigen. Acta Rhumatol 1979;3:319-28.

92. Toussirot E, Saas P, Pariset J, Chabod J, Tiberghien P, Wendling D. Decreased levels of serum soluble HLA class I antigens in HLA-B27 positive spondyloarthropathies. Ann Rheum Dis 2006;65:279-80.

93. Kohler S, Thiel A, Rudwaleit M, Sieper J, Braun J. CD27+ memory and CD27-effector CD8+ T cells are responsible for a decreased production of proinflammatory cytokines in HLA B27-positive subjects. Clin Exp Rheumatol 2005;23:840-46.

94. Fisher LR, Cawley MI, Holgate ST. Relation between chest expansion, pulmonary function, and exercise tolerance in patients with ankylosing spondylitis. Ann Rheum Dis 1990;49:921-25.

95. Davis D. Ankylosing spondylitis and lung fibrosis. QJ Med 1972;41:395-417.

96. Rosenow EC, Strimlan CV, Muhn JR, Ferguson RH. Pleuropulmonary manifestations of ankylosing spondylitis. Mayo Clin Proc 1977;52:641-49.

97. Dudly HE, Emerson PA, Greg I. Thorax in ankylosing spondylitis. Ann Rheumatol Dis 1963;22:11-15.

98. Luthra HS. Extra-articular manifestations of ankylosing spondylitis. Mayo Clin Proc 1977;52:655-56.

99. Leventhal MR, Maguire JK Jr, Christian CA. Atlanto-axial rotary subluxation in ankylosing spondylitis. A case report. Spine 1990;15:1374-76.

100. Gilvarry J, Keeling F, Fielding JF. Sibship Crohn's disease and ankylosing spondylitis. J Clin Gastroenterol 1990;12:711-12.

101. Will R, Palmer R, Bhalla AK, Ring F, Calin A. Bone loss as well as bone formation is a feature of progressive ankylosing spondylitis. Br J Rheumatol 1990;29:498-99.

102. Will R, Edmunds L, Elswood J, Calin A. Is there sexual inequality in ankylosing spondylitis? A study of 498 women and 1202 men. J Rheumatol 1990;17:1649-52.

103. Khan MA, van der Linden SM. A wider spectrum of spondyloarthropathies. Semin Arthritis Rheum 1990;20:107-13.

104. Rudwaleit M, Metter A, Listing J, Sieper J, Braun J. Inflammatory back pain in ankylosing spondylitis: A reassessment of the clinical history for application as classification and diagnostic criteria. Arthritis Rheum 2006;54:569-78.

105. Kaya T, Gelal F, Gunaydin R. The relationship between severity and extent of spinal involvement and spinal mobility and physical functioning in patients with ankylosing spondylitis. Clin Rheumatol 2006;1-5.

106. Davis Jr JC, Dougados M, Braun J, Sieper J, van der Heijde D, van der Linden S. The definition of disease duration in ankylosing spondylitis: Reassessing the concept. Ann Rheum Dis 2006;65(11):1518-20.

107. Rashid T, Ebringer A, Wilson C, Bansal S, Paimela L, Binder A. The Potential Use of Antibacterial Peptide Antibody Indices in the Diagnosis of Rheumatoid Arthritis and Ankylosing Spondylitis. J Clin Rheumatol 2006;12:11-16.

108. Kiris A, Kaya A, Ozgocmen S, Kocakoc E. Assessment of enthesitis in ankylosing spondylitis by power Doppler ultrasonography. Skeletal Radiol 2006;10:1-7.

109. Haibel H, Rudwaleit M, Brandt HC, Grozdanovic Z, Listing J, Kupper H, Braun J, Sieper J. Adalimumab reduces spinal symptoms in active ankylosing spondylitis: Clinical and magnetic resonance imaging results of a fifty-two-week open-label trial. Arthritis Rheum 2006;54:678-81.

110. Ferraz MB, Tugwell P, Goldsmith CH, Atra E. Meta-analysis of sulfasalazine in ankylosing spondylitis. J Rheumatol 990;17:1482-86.

111. Ozer HT, Sarpel T, Gulek B, Alparslan ZN, Erken E. Evaluation of the Turkish version of the Bath Ankylosing Spondylitis Patient Global Score (BAS-G). Clin Rheumatol 2006;25(2):136-39.

112. Ritchlin C. Newer therapeutic approaches: Spondyloarthritis and uveitis. Rheum Dis Clin North Am 2006;32: 75-90.

113. Aletaha D, Smolen JS. The definition and measurement of disease modification in inflammatory rheumatic diseases. Rheum Dis Clin North Am 2006;32:9-44.

114. Alberding A, Stierle H, Brandt J, Braun J. Efectiveness and safety of radium chloride in the treatment of ankylosing spondylitis. Results of an observational study. Z Rheumatol 2006;65(3):245-51.

115. Smith MD, Ahern MJ. Pharmaceutical Benefits Scheme criteria for the use of tumour necrosis factor-alpha inhibitors in the treatment of ankylosing spondylitis in Australia: Are they evidence based? Intern Med J 2006;36:72-76.

116. Kobelt G, Andlin-Sobocki P, Maksymowych WP. Costs and quality of life of patients with ankylosing spondylitis in Canada. J Rheumatol 2006;33:289-95.

117. Methotrexate for ankylosing spondylitis. Cochrane Database Syst Rev 2004;(3):CD004524.

118. Pham T, Landewe RB, van der Linden S, Dougados M, Sieper J, Braun J, et al. An International Study on Starting TNF-blocking agents in Ankylosing Spondylitis (ISSAS). Ann Rheum Dis 2006; Feb 7.

119. Keeling S, Oswald A, Russell AS, Maksymowych WP. Prospective observational analysis of the efficacy and safety of low-dose (3 mg/kg) infliximab in ankylosing spondylitis: 4-year followup. J Rheumatol 2006;33: 558-61.

120. Borenstein D. Inflammatory Arthritides of the Spine: Surgical versus Nonsurgical Treatment. Clin Orthop Relat Res 2006;443:208-21.

121. Gossec L, Henanff AL, Breban M, Vignon E, Claudepierre P, Devauchelle V. Continuation of treatment with infliximab in ankylosing spondylitis: 2-yr open follow-up. Rheumatology (Oxford) 2006;45(7):859-62.

122. Payer M. Surgical management of cervical fractures in ankylosing spondylitis using a combined posterior-anterior approach. J Clin Neurosci 2006;13:73-77.

123. Farooq U, Raza W, Zia N, Hanif M, Khan MM. Classification and management of chest trauma. J Coll Physicians Surg Pak 2006;16:101-03.

124. Weening B, Walton C, Cole PA, Alanezi K, Hanson BP, Bhandari M. Lower mortality in patients with scapular fractures. J Trauma 2005;59:1477-81.

125. Yee WY, Cameron PA, Bailey MJ. Road traffic injuries in the elderly. Emerg Med J 2006;23:42-46.

126. Borrelly J, Aazami MH. New insights into the pathophysiology of flail segment: The implications of anterior serratus muscle in parietal failure. Eur J Cardiothorac Surg 2005;28:742-49.

127. Bragg S. A 44-year-old woman with multiple blunt trauma related to horseback riding. J Emerg Nurs 2005;31:458-59.

128. Gamblin TC, Dalton ML. Flail chest caused by penetrating trauma: A case report. Curr Surg 2002;59:418-19.

129. Stahel PF, Schneider P, Buhr HJ, Kruschewski M. Emergency management of thoracic trauma. Orthopade 2005;34:865-79.

130. Balci AE, Balci TA, Eren S, Ulku R, Cakir O, Eren N. Unilateral post-traumatic pulmonary contusion: Findings of a review. Surg Today. 2005;35:205-10.

131. Yamamoto L, Schroeder C, Morley D, Beliveau C. Thoracic trauma: The deadly dozen. Crit Care Nurs Q 2005;28:22-40.

132. Engel C, Krieg JC, Madey SM, Long WB, Bottlang M. Operative chest wall fixation with osteosynthesis plates. J Trauma 2005;58:181-86.

133. Balci AE, Kazez A, Eren S, Ayan E, Ozalp K, Eren MN. Blunt thoracic trauma in children: Review of 137 cases. Eur J Cardiothorac Surg 2004;26:387-92.

134. Athanassiadi K, Gerazounis M, Theakos N. Management of 150 flail chest injuries: Analysis of risk factors affecting outcome. Eur J Cardiothorac Surg 2004;26: 373-76.

135. Gunduz M, Unlugenc H, Ozalevli M, Inanoglu K, Akman H. A comparative study of continuous positive airway pressure (CPAP) and intermittent positive pressure ventilation (IPPV) in patients with flail chest. Emerg Med J 2005;22:325-29.

136. Haraguchi S, Hioki M, Hisayoshi T, Yamashita K, Yamashita Y, Kawamura J, Hirata T, Yamagishi S, Koizumi K, Shimizu K. Resection of sternal tumors and reconstruction of the thorax: A review of 15 patients. Surg Today 2006;36:225-29.

137. Thongngarm T, Lemos LB, Lawhon N, Harisdangkul V. Malignant tumor with chest wall pain mimicking Tietze's syndrome. Clin Rheumatol 2001;20:276-78.

138. Haraguchi S, Hioki M, Hisayoshi T, Yamashita K, Yamashita Y, Kawamura J, Hirata T, Yamagishi S, Koizumi K, Shimizu K. Resection of sternal tumors and reconstruction of the thorax: A review of 15 patients. Surg Today 2006;36:225-29.

139. Pandiyan MS, Kavunkal AM, Cherian VK, Christopher DJ. Chest wall mass with double pathology. Eur J Cardiothorac Surg 2006;29(4):625-26.

140. Orta L, Suprun U, Goldfarb A, Bleiweiss I, Jaffer S. Radiation-associated extraskeletal osteosarcoma of the chest wall. Arch Pathol Lab Med 2006;130:198-200.

141. Kim L, Park IS, Han JY, Kim JM, Chu YC. Aspiration cytology of fibrosarcomatous variant of dermato-fibrosarcoma protuberans with osteoclastlike giant cells in the chest wall: A case report. Acta Cytol 2005;49: 644-49.

142. Kawasaki T, Watanabe G, Hasegawa G, Naito M. Multiple extranodal follicular dendritic cell tumors initially presenting in the soft tissue in the chest wall. Pathol Int 2006;56:30-34.

143. Rumball JS, Lebrun CM, Di Ciacca SR, Orlando K. Rowing injuries. Sports Med 2005;35:537-55.

144. Freeston J, Karim Z, Lindsay K, Gough A. Can early diagnosis and management of costochondritis reduce acute chest pain admissions? J Rheumatol 2004;31:2269-71.

145. Moses MA, Banwell PE, Murphy JV, Quinlan MJ, Coleman DJ. Infective costochondritis following breast reconstruction. Plast Reconstr Surg 2004;114:1356-57.

146. Pijning JM, de Boeck H, Desprechins B, Ernst C. Tietze's syndrome in a 2-year old boy. Ned Tijdschr Geneeskd 2003;147:2134-36.

147. Uthman I, El-Hajj I, Traboulsi R, Taher A. Hodgkin's lymphoma presenting as Tietze's syndrome. Arthritis Rheum 2003;49:737.

148. No authors listed. Costochondritis: Not a heart attack but it feels like one. Harv Womens Health Watch 2003;10:6-7.

149. Hiramuro-Shoji F, Wirth MA, Rockwood CA Jr. Atraumatic conditions of the sternoclavicular joint. J Shoulder Elbow Surg 2003;12:79-88.

150. Lee JK. Tc-99m MDP and Ga-67 citrate images in suppurative costochondritis. Clin Nucl Med 2002;27:665.

151. Lin EC. Costochondritis mimicking a pulmonary nodule on FDG positron emission tomographic imaging. Clin Nucl Med 2002;27:591-92.

152. Fioravanti A, Tofi C, Volterrani L, Marcolongo R. Malignant lymphoma presenting as Tietze's syndrome. Arthritis Rheum 2002;47:229-30.

153. Young JE, Miller JD, Urschel JD. Costal chondritis after thoracoabdominal esophagectomy: How to prevent it. J Surg Oncol 2002;80:61-62.

154. Gregory PL, Biswas AC, Batt ME. Musculoskeletal problems of the chest wall in athletes. Sports Med 2002;32:235-50.

155. Saltzman DA, Schmitz ML, Smith SD, Wagner CW, Jackson RJ, Harp S. The slipping rib syndrome in children. Paediatr Anaesth 2001;11:740-43.

156. Jensen S. Musculoskeletal causes of chest pain. Aust Fam Physician 2001;30:834-39.

157. Grethel EJ, Nobuhara KK. Fetal surgery for congenital diaphragmatic hernia. J Paediatr Child Health 2006; 42:79-85.

158. Casaccia G, Mobili L, Braguglia A, Santoro F, Bagolan P. Distal 4p microdeletion in a case of Wolf-Hirschhorn syndrome with congenital diaphragmatic hernia. Birth Defects Res A Clin Mol Teratol 2006;76(3):210-13.

159. Mousa A, Sanusi M, Lowery RC, Genovesi MH, Burack JH. Hand-assisted thoracoscopic repair of a bochdalek hernia in an adult. J Laparoendosc Adv Surg Tech A 2006;16:54-58.

160. Behera D, Malik SK, Jindal SK, Kataria RN, Kataria S. Congenital diaphragmatic hernia of Bochdalek's type in an adults. Ind J Chest Dis All Sci 1982;24:43-46.

161. Robb BW, Reed MF. Congenital diaphragmatic hernia presenting as splenic rupture in an adult. Ann Thorac Surg 2006;81:e9-10.

162. Fisher JC, Bodenstein L. Computer simulation analysis of normal and abnormal development of the mammalian diaphragm. Theor Biol Med Model 2006;3:9.

163. Jesudason EC. Small lungs and suspect smooth muscle: Congenital diaphragmatic hernia and the smooth muscle hypothesis. J Pediatr Surg 2006;41:431-35.

164. Kitano Y, Lally KP, Lally PA. Congenital Diaphragmatic Hernia Study Group. Late-presenting congenital diaphragmatic hernia. J Pediatr Surg 2005;40:1839-43.

165. Deprest J, Jani J, Van Schoubroeck D, Cannie M, Gallot D, Dymarkowski S, Fryns JP, Naulaers G, Gratacos E, Nicolaides K. Current consequences of prenatal diagnosis of congenital diaphragmatic hernia. J Pediatr Surg 2006;41:423-30.

166. Larson JE, Cohen JC. Improvement of pulmonary hypoplasia associated with congenital diaphragmatic hernia by In utero CFTR gene therapy. Am J Physiol Lung Cell Mol Physiol 2006;291(1):4-10.

167. Crankson SJ, Al Jadaan SA, Namshan MA, Al-Rabeeah AA, Oda O. The immediate and long-term outcomes of newborns with congenital diaphragmatic hernia. Pediatr Surg Int 2006;1-6.

168. Scott DA, Cooper ML, Stankiewicz P, Patel A, Potocki L, Cheung SW. Congenital diaphragmatic hernia in WAGR syndrome. Am J Med Genet A 2005;134:430-33.

169. Shehata SM, Sharma HS, Mooi WJ, Tibboel D. Pulmonary hypertension in human newborns with congenital diaphragmatic hernia is associated with decreased vascular expression of nitric-oxide synthase. Cell Biochem Biophys 2006;44:147-55.

170. Trachsel D, Selvadurai H, Bohn D, Langer JC, Coates AL. Long-term pulmonary morbidity in survivors of congenital diaphragmatic hernia. Pediatr Pulmonol 2005;39:433-39.

171. Holcomb GW 3rd, Ostlie DJ, Miller KA. Laparoscopic patch repair of diaphragmatic hernias with Surgisis. J Pediatr Surg 2005;40:E1-5.

172. Caprotti R, Mussi C, Scaini A, Angelini C, Romano F. Laparoscopic repair of a Morgagni-Larrey hernia. Int Surg 2005;90:175-78.

173. Rogers FB, Rebuck JA. Case report: Morgagni hernia. Hernia 2006;21;1-3.

174. Bouzouita A, Bouchiba N, Ghodhbane W, Hmida A, Mighri MM, Touinsi H, Sassi S. Morgagni hernia in elderly patients: A study about two cases. Tunis Med 2005;83:631-34.

175. Colakoglu O, Haciyanli M, Soyturk M, Colakoglu G, Simsek I. Morgagni hernia in an adult: Atypical presentation and diagnostic difficulties. Turk J Gastroenterol 2005;16:114-16.

176. Sirmali M, Turut H, Gezer S, Findik G, Kaya S, Tastepe Y, Cetin G. Clinical and radiologic evaluation of foramen of Morgagni hernias and the transthoracic approach. World J Surg 2005;29:1520-24.

177. Knight CG, Gidell KM, Lanning D, Lorincz A, Langenburg SE, Klein MD. Laparoscopic Morgagni hernia repair in children using robotic instruments. J Laparoendosc Adv Surg Tech A 2005;15:482-86.

178. Barut I, Tarhan OR, Cerci C, Akdeniz Y, Bulbul M. Intestinal obstruction caused by a strangulated Morgagni hernia in an adult patient. J Thorac Imaging 2005;20:220-22.

179. Percivale A, Stella M, Durante V, Dogliotti L, Serafini G, Saccomani G, Pellicci R. Laparoscopic treatment of Morgagni-Larrey hernia: Technical details and report of a series. J Laparoendosc Adv Surg Tech A 2005;15:303-07.

180. Lau ST, Kim SS, Ledbetter DJ, Healey PJ. Fraternal twins with Morgagni hernias. J Pediatr Surg. 2005;40:725-27.

181. Loong TP, Kocher HM. Clinical presentation and operative repair of hernia of Morgagni. Postgrad Med J 2005;81:41-44.

182. Erdem LO, Erdem CZ, Comert M. Intrapancreatic lipoma and Morgagni hernia: A previously unrecognized association. Dig Dis Sci 2004;49:1962-65.

183. Ceylan E, Onen A, Sanli A, Yilmaz E, Ucan ES. Morgagni hernia: Late diagnosis in a case with Down syndrome. Respiration 2004;71:641.

184. Lanteri R, Santangelo M, Rapisarda C, Di Cataldo A, Licata A. Bilateral Morgagni-Larrey hernia: A rare cause of intestinal occlusion. Arch Surg 2004;139:1299-300.

185. Naveed-ur-Rehman, Ahmad Z, Anwar-ul-Haq, Abbas KA. Down syndrome with morgagni hernia and hypothyroidism. J Coll Physicians Surg Pak 2004;14:689-90.

186. Soylu H, Koltuksuz U, Kutlu NO, Sarihan H, Sen Y, Ustun N, Baki A, Sonmezgoz E, Dogrul M, Akinci A. Morgagni hernia: An unexpected cause of respiratory complaints and a chest mass. Pediatr Pulmonol 2000;30:429-33.

187. Tarim A, Nursal TZ, Yildirim S, Ezer A, Caliskan K, Torer N. Laparoscopic repair of bilateral morgagni hernia. Surg Laparosc Endosc Percutan Tech 2004;14: 96-97.

188. Abboud B, Jaoude JB, Riachi M, Sleilaty G, Tabet G. Intrathoracic transverse colon and small bowel infarction in a patient with traumatic diaphragmatic hernia. Case report and review of the literature. J Med Liban 2004;52:168-70.

189. Rattan KN, Magu S, Agrawal K, Ratan S. Traumatic diaphragmatic herniation. Indian J Pediatr 2005;72: 985-86.

190. Hsu YP, Chen RJ, Fang JF, Lin BC. Blunt diaphragmatic rupture in elderly patients. Hepatogastroenterology 2005;52:1752-58.

191. Khalil MW, Sarkar PK. Late presentation of traumatic rupture of the right hemidiaphragm. Br J Hosp Med (Lond) 2005;66:482-83.

192. Hamano K, Kumada S, Hayashi M, Kurano N, Uchiyama A, Kurata K. An autopsy case of caudate nucleus lobulation accompanied with diaphragmatic eventration. Brain Dev. 2005;28(6)401-04.

193. Salami MA, Adebo OA. Congenital diaphragmatic eventration in a Nigerian child. Niger J Med 2005;14:317-18.

194. Becmeur F, Talon I, Schaarschmidt K, Philippe P, Moog R, Kauffmann I, Schultz A, Grandadam S, Toledano D. Thoracoscopic diaphragmatic eventration repair in children: About 10 cases. J Pediatr Surg 2005;40:1712-15.

195. Yang CK, Shih JC, Hsu WM, Peng SS, Shyu MK, Lee CN, Hsieh FJ. Isolated right diaphragmatic eventration mimicking congenital heart disease *in utero*. Prenat Diagn 2005;25:872-75.

196. Lloyd T, Tang YM, Benson MD, King S. Diaphragmatic paralysis: The use of M mode ultrasound for diagnosis in adults. Spinal Cord 2006;44(8):505-08

197. Lin PT, Andersson PB, Distad BJ, Barohn RJ, Cho SC, So YT, Katz JS. Bilateral isolated phrenic neuropathy causing painless bilateral diaphragmatic paralysis. Neurology 2005;65:1499-501.

198. Xu WD, Gu YD, Lu JB, Yu C, Zhang CG, Xu JG. Pulmonary function after complete unilateral phrenic nerve transection. J Neurosurg 2005;103:464-67.

199. Abbott RA, Hammans S, Margarson M, Aji BM. Diaphragmatic paralysis and respiratory failure as a complication of Lyme disease. J Neurol Neurosurg Psychiatry 2005;76:1306-07.

200. Celli BR. Respiratory management of diaphragm paralysis. Semin Respir Crit Care Med 2002;23:275-81.

Congenital Anomalies of the Respiratory System

Developmental and genetic anomalies of the tracheo-bronchial tree and the lungs are most often congenital and severe forms of the disease may result in intrauterine deaths. As various parts of the system are developed at certain definite times during intrauterine life, defects can be timed accurately. While major structural and functional abnormalities are incompatible with life, more minor forms are recognized during life, either during early in life or late in the adulthood. Present knowledge of genetic science has enabled to diagnose some of these conditions during intrauterine life. Genetically related diseases such as ciliary dysfunction, cystic fibrosis, and alpha antitrypsin deficiency are considered earlier. Some other abnormalities will be discussed in brief in this section.

ANOMALIES OF THE TRACHEOBRONCHIAL TREE

The tracheobronchial tree has a common developmental origin with that of the primitive foregut and all such developments are completed by the 16th week of intrauterine life. Because of this common origin most of the anomalies are associated with that of the foregut.

Tracheal Agenesis and Atresia

Tracheal agenesis is a rare and uniformly lethal congenital malformation. It presents with severe respiratory distress at birth. In this anomaly there is a congenital absence of the trachea and the bronchus communicates with the esophagus. The diagnosis should be suspected in newborn infant with respiratory distress whose intubation is impossible.[1-4] These are very rare anomalies and are incompatible with life. There are three main types of such agenesis. Type 1, in which there is agenesis of the proximal part of the trachea. The distal trachea, which is well developed, is communicated with the esophagus by a fistulous tract. Type 2 agenesis is the commonest type, in which the main bronchi join with the esophagus

in the midline. In type 3, both the bronchi communicate with the esophagus independently.[5] Very rarely, the tracheoesophageal fistula allows enough air to enter into the lungs, so that the newborn can survive long enough to undergo reconstructive surgery.[6]

Tracheoesophageal Fistula

This may be small enough to remain for a long time till the adult life, although symptoms like cough, cyanosis, and choking may be present from time to time because of aspiration of esophageal contents. Recurrent infections are very common. Demonstration of the fistulous tract is possible by the presence of contrast material in the trachea introduced into the esophagus.[7]

Tracheal Stenosis

Tracheal stenosis is defined as cicatricial narrowing of the endotracheal lumen. Endotracheal manipulation remains to be the most common etiology followed by inflammatory and collagen vascular diseases. Predisposing factors include host systemic conditions such as gastroesophageal reflux and tube characteristics mainly the size and composition of the tube.[8,9] This condition includes congenital webs, absent of deformed tracheal cartilages, and extrinsic pressures by various vascular anomalies. Such anomalies are: Double aortic arch, right aortic arch with left ligamentum arteriosum, retro-esophageal right subclavian artery, anomalous innominate and left carotid artery.

The stenosis is of three types; *diffuse*; in which the pars membranacea is absent and cartilages surround the trachea only and the number of cartilages may be more than the usual number of 22. The stenosis may be *segmental*, the commonest variety, and can occur at any part of the trachea. The third variety is the *funnel-like stenosis*, which may be associated with left pulmonary abnormality. The clinical picture may be misleading and ranges from mild decrease in exercise tolerance to severe respiratory distress. The patient is usually investigated radiologically followed by flexible or rigid laryngoscopy and bronchoscopy. Radiographs may demonstrate the defects or contrast material may have to be injected. Computerized tomography is used more often than magnetic resonance imaging and correlates well with the endoscopic findings. The cervical portion of the trachea is usually involved with marked narrowing varying in length and diameter.

Clinically significant benign stenoses of the large airways develop in about 1 percent of patients after intubation. The treatment includes endoscopic repair, laryngotracheal reconstruction or segmental resection with end-to-end anastomosis.[10-26]

Airway obstruction from congenital tracheal stenosis (CTS) in infants and children often presents as a life-threatening emergency. Congenital tracheal stenosis invariably requires interventions, including surgical correction, to relieve an obstruction. Operative procedures widely used to repair this rare condition include cartilage patch tracheoplasty and slide tracheoplasty. Although, historically, this condition was associated with a high risk of mortality, multiple centers have recently reported successful outcomes following the surgical repair of CTS by these techniques. However, few centers have had extensive experience with both techniques, as indicated by the low number of patients reported in most case series. Furthermore, the variabilities in patient presentation, patient features (including the presence of associated congenital anomalies), and patient age at which CTS lesions are repaired have resulted in a paucity of data defining prognostic factors in the surgical management of patients with complex CTS. There is currently no multicenter registry organized to collect data on the surgical outcomes and co-morbid diagnoses of patients with CTS. Therefore, prognostic factors useful for determining patient morbidity and mortality risks in CTS repairs have been difficult to delineate. Congenital tracheal stenosis (CTS) often requires urgent surgical intervention. In a large series reported from Prague, sixty-two patients developed stenoses after endotracheal intubation or tracheostomy, in 18 patients the stenosis was caused by other diseases or pathological situations. Thirty-eight patients were sent for surgical resection of the stenotic part of the airways. 2 surgically treated patients developed recurrence of the stenosis and had to be reoperated on. Narrowing of the trachea at the site of end-to-end anastomosis developed in 6 other patients and was cured by interventional bronchoscopy. The remaining 42 patients were treated by interventional bronchoscopy (Nd-YAG laser, electrocautery, stent), which was curative in 35 patients. Sixty-five patients were alive at the time of evaluation, 15 patients died. Five of them died between 3 and 14 (median 4) months after surgery from a disease other than airway stenosis. Ten nonresected patients also died, with 1 exception, due to a disease other than airway stenosis; the median survival was 9 months.[13] Another large series from Canada reported 68 patients who were treated (cartilage patch tracheoplasty, n = 31; slide tracheoplasty, n = 37), with 19 deaths (overall mortality = 28%). A total of 10 patients who underwent cartilage patch tracheoplasty died (32% mortality), whereas only 9 patients died following slide tracheoplasty (24% mortality). A total of 8 of 11 patients who were repaired at the age of 1 month or younger died (73% mortality), whereas only 11 of 57 patients who were repaired at an age older than 1 month died (19% mortality) (P = .04). A total of 10 of 19 patients with CTS who had comorbid intracardiac anomalies died following CTS repair (53% mortality), whereas only 9 of 49 patients with CTS who did not have intracardiac anomalies died (18% mortality) (P = .02).[14]

Tracheal Diverticuli

Diverticuli of the trachea are usually found during a simple systematic radiological examination, or when an established pulmonary condition is being investigated. Routine bronchography, alone, or associated with a tomograph, can be used to demonstrate its characteristics and precise location. Bronchoscopy may then be carried out in order to study the area surrounding the diverticular orifice more closely, and to establish the condition of its mucous lining. Several evolutive stages are involved in the pathogenesis of tracheal diverticuli, varying from a rudimentary bronchiole to megalotrachea, which, for many authors, is an autonomous condition because of its anatomical and pathological makeup, producing its own well-defined symptomatology. The diverticuli are of clinical curiosities and as such do not produce much problem.

These are outpouchings from the tracheobronchial tree and are of four types: (i) Rudimentary bronchus arising most commonly from the lower right lateral aspect of the trachea; (ii) cystic dilatation of the cystic gland ducts; (iii) tracheocele, or outpouching from the right lower posterior trachea because of structural deficiencies; and (iv) acquired diverticuli associated with the congenital tracheal wall weakness of tracheobronchomegaly.[27-30]

Tracheobronchomegaly (Mounier-Kuhn syndrome)

Tracheobronchomegaly is a rare disorder of uncertain etiology, characterized by marked dilatation of the trachea and major bronchi, associated with tracheal diverticulosis, bronchiectasis and recurrent respiratory tract infection. This is a very rare condition in which the trachea is unusually dilated. The bronchi are also dilated with repeated infections and bronchiectasis.[31-45] This is because of defects in the supporting tissues resulting from an autosomal recessive trait. Tracheobronchomegaly consists in trachea clearance and central bronchi widening, which disturbs air, flow in air-passages and decreases cough effectiveness. The normal diameter of the trachea is 20.2 ± 3.4 mm, the right main bronchus is 16.0 + 2.6, and that of the left main bronchus is 14.5 ± 2.8 mm. In this condition, the size is increased and in tracheo-bronchomegaly the diameter exceeds the normal size by more than three standard deviations. Other radiologic signs include deep corrugations produced by redundant tissue between cartilages (Figs 31.1 to 31.3).

Main symptoms are: paroxysmal cough, recurring bronchi inflammation and pneumonia resulting in mucus residing in air-passages. The clinical spectrum varies from absence of symptoms to severe lower respiratory tract infection with respiratory insufficiency.[46-49] The cough is characteristically loud and booming quality. Airways obstruction in adulthood is common and is a result of expiratory collapse of the poorly supported large airways. Other symptoms include: Wheeze, dyspnea, respiratory distress, stridor, tugging inspiratory effort with retraction of intercostals muscles, cyanosis, and apnea. Tracheobronchomegaly (TBM) occasionally

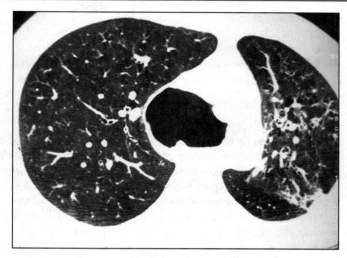

FIGURE 31.2: CT Chest - Extensive tracheomegaly - Mounier Kuhn syndrome

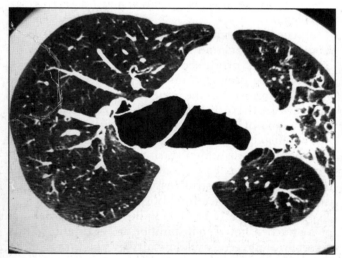

FIGURE 31.3: HRCT Chest - Bronchomegaly

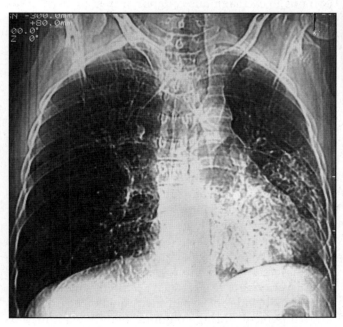

FIGURE 31.1: CXR - Tracheo-bronchomegaly with left cystic bronchiectasis

may progress to extensive tracheomalacia that leads to respiratory failure. Spirometry, dynamic expiratory multidetector computed tomography (CT), bronchoscopy are used to diagnose patients of suspected tracheobron-chomalacia.[50-54] Night-time monitoring of respiratory variables can be used to show the presence of respiratory abnormalities during sleep that may be corrected by applying nasal continuous positive airway pressure (CPAP). It may show the presence of both apnea and hypopneas, which may be obstructive in nature with high apnea-hypopnea index (AHI), no snoring and associated oxygen desaturation. A second overnight study with nasal continuous positive airway pressure at a critical pressure of 8 cm, the AHI will decrease along with no drop in oxygen saturation. This noninvasive technique should be considered as a diagnostic tool in tracheobronchomalacia and to know the outcome of CPAP, surgical or stent therapy in this condition. Lung transplantation may be required in some cases.[55]

Tracheobronchomalacia

Tracheobronchomalacia (TBM) is a pathologic condition in which softening of tracheal and bronchial cartilage causes dynamic narrowing of the transverse or sagittal diameters of the tracheobronchial lumen.[56-66] This condition may or may not be associated with substantial invagination of the posterior membrane of the tracheobronchial tree, an entity referred to as excessive dynamic airway collapse (EDAC). This rare condition implies weakness of the tracheobronchial wall because of soft and pliable cartilages resulting in easy collapsibility. TBM has also been called *tracheobronchial collapse, expiratory tracheobronchial stenosis,* and *tracheobronchial dyskinesia.*

Excessive dynamic airway collapse (EDAC) is frequently associated with this condition. Airways obstruction is produced because high intrathoracic pressures are produced during expiration resulting in excess compression of the upper airways. During normal expiration, there is a physiologic reduction in all dimensions of the intrathoracic airways. In healthy individuals, cinebronchography studies show that the tracheobronchial lumen during coughing is 18 to 39 percent narrower than the maximal inspiratory lumen observed during restful respiration.[67-76] Dynamic CT during forced expiration shows a mean decrease of 35 percent (range 11 to 61%) in the cross-sectional area of the trachea, between inspiration and expiration. Thus, a certain degree of dynamic airway collapse, characterized by invagination of the posterior membrane and narrowing of cross-sectional area of the tracheobronchial tree, is physiologic. This phenomenon is exaggerated, however, in some patients with obstructive pulmonary disease, such as chronic bronchitis, emphysema, asthma, or as an isolated finding in patients during cough and forced expiration. EDAC can also be noted in patients with true malacia (defined as softening of airway cartilage) due to chronic diseases, such as relapsing polychondritis, other cartilage and connecting tissue disorders, chronic infections, and congenital diseases.

The signs and symptoms of TBM and EDAC are nonspecific but may include cough, dyspnea, wheezing resistant to corticosteroids and inhaled bronchodilators, stridor, recurrent bronchitis or pneumonia, atelectasis, difficulty clearing secretions, and respiratory insufficiency. Pulmonary function tests are only helpful when they show diminished expiratory flow, notching on the flow-volume loop, dynamic airway compression (calculated as slow vital capacity minus (FVC), or a biphasic flow-volume loop or flow oscillations. Chest radiographs and fluoroscopy are unsatisfactory for identifying the morphologic aspects of the diseases processes. In fact, determining the true incidence of TBM and EDAC is difficult, because most clinicians have, until recently, been unable to satisfactorily distinguish dynamic abnormalities of the posterior membrane from abnormalities of the cartilaginous airway walls.

Dynamic CT

Dynamic CT, suing rapid electron beam and multislice helical studies, allows volumetric acquisition of data at end-inspiration and during expiration. Simultaneous display of the anteroposterior and lateral walls of the airway allows reconstruction of three-dimensional images and detailed analysis of anatomic detail, adjacent structures, and measurement of the degree of central airway collapse. Studies have shown good correlation of dynamic CT with bronchoscopy findings for extent of collapse, but patients must be able to cooperate with breathing instructions during examinations.

Based on results in normal individuals, a decreased cross-sectional area of 70 percent of more (2 SD from the mean) has been proposed to diagnose malacia, but it is unclear whether this decrease in airway diameter pertains to cartilaginous collapse or invagination of the posterior membrane. The reported shortcomings of electron beam tomography for airway collapse evaluation, which may miss short-length, focal abnormalities, may be irrelevant, because malacia and EDAC are usually more extensive abnormalities.

Cine Magnetic Resonance Imaging

Cine magnetic resonance imaging allows axial, coronal, and sagittal sequences of the tracheobronchial tree during quiet respiration, as well as during cough, deep breathing, and forced expiration, thereby identifying abnormalities present both at rest and during dynamic respiration. Because there is no ionizing radiation, cine magnetic resonance imaging allows repeated assessments of the airway lumen. In at least one, small, controlled study, a collapsibility index was defined as (maximum cross-sectional area—minimum cross-sectional area)/maximum cross-sectional area) × 100(%). Patients with a mean collapsibility index of 50 percent during forced expiration and 75 percent during coughing may be identified as having central airway collapse, but further studies are needed before this technique becomes mainstream.

TABLE 31.1: FEMOS (Functional, Extent, Morphology, Origin and Severity) classification of tracheobronchomalacia

Criteria	Description
Functional class	Refers to degree of functional impairment, as defined by the World Health Organization I. Asymptomatic II. Symptomatic on exertion III. Symptomatic with daily activity IV. Symptomatic at rest
Extent	Defines the length of the tracheobronchial wall affected or the number of cartilaginous rings involved and the location of the abnormal airway segment *Focal*: Abnormality is present in one main, lobar, or segmental bronchus or one tracheal region (upper, mid or lower) *Multifocal*: Abnormality is present in two contiguous or at least two noncontiguous regions *Diffuse*: Abnormality is present in more than two contiguous regions
Morphology	Describes the morphology of the airway lumen that is reduced during expiration and respiratory movements, as assessed by bronchoscopy or radiological studies *Saber-sheath*: Refers to reduction in the transversal (coronal) diameter *Crescent type*: Refers to reduction in the anteroposterior (sagittal) diameter *Circumferential*: Refers to reduction in both transversal and anteroposterior diameters
Origin	Describes the underlying mechanism responsible for the abnormality *Idiopathic*: No underlying etiology is identified (may be congenital) *Secondary*: May be due to known underlying processes
Severity	Describes the degree of the airway collapse during expiration, as documented by bronchoscopic or radiologic studies *Mild*: Expiratory airway collapse of 50 to 75 percent *Moderate*: Expiratory airway collapse of 75 to 100 percent *Severe*: Expiration airway collapse of 100 percent; the airway walls make contact

Dynamic Flexible Videobronchoscopy

Dynamic flexible videobronchoscopy is a minimally invasive procedure in which the airways are visualized while moving the awake or minimally sedated patient into the supine, upright, and lateral decubitus positions. Patients are examined during spontaneous breathing, as well as during forced maneuvers, such as cough, forced expiration, and deep inspiration. Changes in bronchial and tracheal caliber are noted; extent of collapse is measured; cartilaginous weakening can be differentiated from EDAC and the morphologic aspect of malacia-induced airway narrowing can be classified as being of the crescent, saber-sheath, or circumferential type.

Morphometric Videobronchoscopy

Morphometric videobronchoscopy allows video recordings of the collapsing airway during inspiration, passive expiration, and forced expiration. Selected still-frame images are then scanned, and the maximal cross-sectional area is measured using specially designed grid or image-analysis software. Differences in airway caliber during the respiratory cycle are identified and expressed as a percentage of maximum inspiration and expiration.

A classification system, in which degrees of malacia and EDAC are characterized according to clinical symptoms, physiologic impairment, radiographic importance, morphologic type, degree of airway narrowing, origin, and associated airway abnormalities or comorbidities, would also facilitate a comprehensive approach to patient care and assist health-care providers in choosing among appropriate medical, surgical, and minimally invasive therapeutic interventions. Therefore, the FEMOS classification system has been developed (Table 31.1) that addresses functional status, extent of abnormalities noted, morphology of the abnormality, origin (or etiology of the abnormality, and severity of the disease process. FEMOS can be used for the diagnostic approach to patients with TBM and EDAC as well as for comparison of findings after therapeutic interventions. Such a multidimensional classification system would allow clinicians to evaluate functional impairment, accurately identify abnormalities, potentially correlate physiologic impairment with the disease process, and evaluate progression of disease with or without therapy.

Treatment of the condition will include antibiotics and other measures for infection, and various other surgical procedure in symptomatic cases.[77-85]

Tracheopathia Osteoplastica (Tracheobronchopathia Osteochondroplastica)

Tracheobronchopathia osteochondroplastica (TPO) is an uncommon benign disease of unknown etiology characterized by multiple cartilaginous or bony submucosal

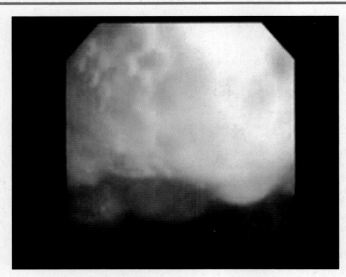

FIGURE 31.4: Fiberoptic bronchoscopic picture in a case of tracheobronchopathia osteoplastica

nodules, which project into the tracheobronchial lumen. The nodules originate in the airway cartilages and thus typically spare the posterior membranous wall of the airways. The disorder is more common in men and the diagnosis is usually made in the fourth through sixth decades of life. There is no relationship to smoking or other systemic disorders. The disease is manifested by chronic cough and wheezing, which frequently lead to the mistaken diagnosis of asthma.[86-92] Other pulmonary symptoms include dyspnea and hemoptysis. One of the complications is the increased incidence of recurrent respiratory infections. The pulmonary symptoms and complications are the consequence of narrowing and thickening of the airway walls. Even though roentgenologic imaging studies may indicate the diagnosis, bronchoscopy is the most definitive diagnostic test (Fig. 31.4). The bronchoscopic appearance alone is diagnostic of the disease, and biopsy of the airway lesions is seldom, if ever, required.[93-97] Although there is no specific therapy for this disorder, management of tracheobronchopathia osteochondroplastica includes bronchodilators, prompt treatment of pulmonary infections, and bronchoscopic dilatation when indicated.

Abnormal Branching

These are more of bronchoscopic or bronchographic curiosities rather than having any clinical significance except when resectional surgery is undertaken. The commonest abnormality is the presence of a supernumerary upper lobe bronchus in the right side that may arise anywhere between the trachea and the right main bronchus. The other abnormalities include absence of a right upper lobe bronchus, double-stem apical lower lobe segmental bronchus, and a supernumerary apical upper lobe bronchus arising from the trachea, absence of the fissures, bilobation of the right lung, trilobation of the left lung, and an accessory inferior lobe on either side.

Bronchogenic Cysts

Bronchogenic or bronchial cysts are due to abnormal budding of the tracheobronchial tree during intrauterine life between the 6th and 16th week of development. A tracheal or bronchial bud gets detached from the parent structure and can occur either in the mediastinum (central type) or in the parenchyma or one of the lobes (peripheral). They are more common in males. The central cysts occur early in the development and the peripheral types occur late in life. The cysts are usually single, but may be multiple. Majority of the peripheral ones occur in the lower lobes. Ectopic sites where such cysts can develop include the pericardium, diaphragm, vertebral column, and the skin.[98-124]

The cysts vary in size but can be as large as 10 cm. They are usually thin walled but become thick once infection supervenes. The characteristic findings are the presence of ciliated epithelium in addition to the intestinal cells, smooth muscles, elastic tissues, and cartilages. However, infection destroys the characteristic histological features making it difficult to distinguish between a chronically infected bronchogenic cyst and an acquired lung abscess.

Most often, they are asymptomatic being detected as an abnormal shadow on chest X-ray. The symptoms are either due to a space-occupying lesion or because of secondary infection behaving as a lung abscess. Compression of trachea may produce cough, dyspnea, stridor and that of the esophagus causing dysphagia. Radiologically one may see a cystic lesion with or without evidence of infection. The treatment of choice is surgical removal.

Agenesis and Hypoplasia of the Lung

Agenesis means absence or complete absence of the lung and hypoplasia mean underdevelopment of the lung, when the lung contain a normal number of lobes but is smaller in size with small number of bronchial branching and reduced number of alveoli. Complete agenesis of both lungs is extremely rare and incompatible with life. Unilateral agenesis is rare.[125-129] The left lung is affected more frequently than the right. The condition is most often associated with often congenital anomalies like patent ductus arteriosus. There are three patterns of

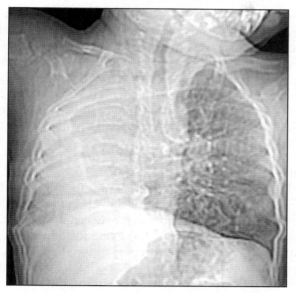

FIGURE 31.5: CXR - Opaque right hemithorax with absent right main bronchus, right lung agenesis

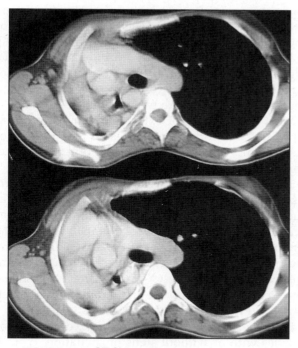

FIGURE 31.6: CT Chest - Absent right lung and right pulmonary artery - Right lung agenesis

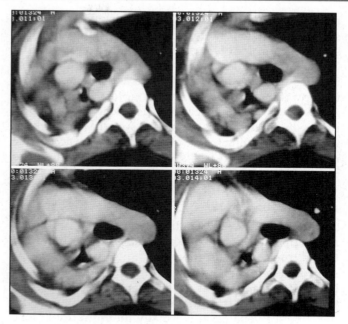

FIGURE 31.7: CT Chest - Absent right pulmonary artery with absent right lung

agenesis of the lung. In the first type, the bronchus is rudimentary and there is complete absence of lung tissue. In the second variety, there is total absence of the bronchial and lung tissue, and in the third, there is a rudimentary bronchus as well as alveoli, which are reduced in number. This is the hypoplastic lung. The exact cause of these malformations is unknown although this may occur in conditions, which cause a decreased space in the thorax as in a congenital diaphragmatic hernia, and vascular anomalies. Oligohydramnios is a predisposing factor for bilateral hypoplasia of the lungs (Figs 31.5 to 31.7).

Congenital Cystic Malformations of the Lung

The condition is otherwise known as adenomatoid malformation of the lung. This malformation results from a developmental failure of the proximal bronchi, which arise from the tracheobronchial bud.[130] There are three types of this malformation. There may be single or multiple large cysts, which are lined with respiratory epithelium, and when single, are indistinguishable from bronchogenic cysts. There may be multiple small cysts of less than 1 cm which may involve almost whole of the lung lobes and are filled with air, fluid or both. Other lung lesions, bronchopulmonary sequestration (BPS), hybrid lesions involving both malformations, congenital lobar emphysema (CLE), This carries a poor prognosis. Congenital bronchiectasis is due to deficiency in the bronchial or bronchiolar tree. It is commonly associated with dextrocardia. In the other type there may be a mass of solid airless tissue, which carries a very poor prognosis.

Prenatal identification of lung abnormalities has increased with prenatal surveillance. Treatment usually requires serial ultrasound observation but in rare situations *in utero* therapy may be required for fetal survival. Outcome of fetuses identified to have congenital cystic adenomatoid malformation (CCAM) lung abnormalities resulting in fetal hydrops and having *in utero* therapy (thoracoamniotic shunting, fetal thoracotomy, EXIT delivery) are the recent developments. In the appropriate situation, this maternal fetal surgery approach for CCAM is life saving for the affected fetus with acceptable maternal morbidity risks in the present and future pregnancies.

Azygos Lobe

An azygos lobe is the medical portion of a bifurcated right upper lobe and is an anatomical variation rather than a true congenital anomaly.[131-141] It is formed at the apex of the right lung during lung development. As the lung grows caudally, it encounters the azygos vein as this vessel arches over the root of the right lung to join the superior vena cava. Normally the right upper lobe as a whole lies lateral to the azygos vain, but in this condition, the vein runs through the right upper lobe so that a portion of this lobe lies on either side of the venous arch. The invagination of the azygos vein is accompanied by that of the pleural layers which form a fissure. The condition is not associated with any morbidity, but is a radiological curiosity. The overall incidence is about 0.25 percent. Very rarely, a similar abnormality may be seen on the left side.

Sequestration of the Lung

A sequestrated lung tissue is a mass of unventilated abnormal lung tissue, having no bronchial communication, and having its arterial blood supply from the systemic rather than from the pulmonary circulation.[142-168] Although the exact cause of lung sequestration is unknown, it is proposed that pulmonary sequestration results from formation of an accessory lung bud on the ventral aspect of the foregut. They have their own bronchial tissue, which develops within them. The sequestration becomes intra or extra depending on the development of the lung bud proximal or distal to the tracheobronchial tree during development. There are mainly two types of sequestration of the lung although many variants do exist. They are; the *intralobar* and *extralobar* sequestrations. In the intralobar sequestration the abnormal lung tissue is contained within the normal lung substance, which completely surrounds it. This is the commonest variety. In the extralobar form, the abnormal lung tissue lies outside the pleural coverings,

although in close proximity of the lung tissue. It has its own pleural coverings. The intralobar form occurs with equal frequency in either males or females. Both types occur more commonly on the left side. Right-sided sequestration is more often due to an intralobar sequestration. The more frequent occurrence of both the types on the left side is thought to be due to the absence of liver on that side providing more space, and the primitive pleuro-peritoneal canal closes later in the left side. Ipsilateral diaphragmatic defect is more common in the extralobar form.

The intralobar sequestration is more common within the posterior basal segment of the left lower lobe. The extralobar form is more common between the lower lobe and the diaphragm. Other ectopic sites include below the diaphragm, within the substance of the diaphragm, in the mediastinum, and in the neck. Both the forms receive their blood supply from the descending thoracic aorta or one of its branches. The supply may be either intra- or supradiaphragmatic. Infra-diaphragmatic supply is more common to the extralobar type. The supply may come from the celiac axis. In such a situation, the artery comes through one of its openings. The venous drainage for both types is through the pulmonary veins. The azygos system drains the extralobar sequestration more frequently. Shunt may be very severe so as to present as congestive cardiac failure early in the childhood.

Most of the cases of extralobar sequestration are associated with other anomalies so that the patient presents early in childhood. On the other hand, such anomalies are uncommon in the intralobar variety.

Therefore, the patient presents late in life. Both forms of sequestration contain ciliated bronchi, which are usually dilated, and areas of alveolar tissue. Cysts form because of bronchial dilatation and infection. The extralobar form is recognized in early childhood while investing other congenital anomalies. In others, they are detected on a routine chest X-ray. Other features include nonspecific infections with pneumonia, lung abscess, cough, and hemoptysis.

Radiologically they are seen as rounded homogenous opacities with or without signs of cavitation, typically located in the posterior basal segments. Bronchography will reveal nonopacification of the sequestrated lung, which is displaced by normal bronchial branches. The diagnosis is confirmed by thoracic aortography, which may also show aberrant blood vessels. Use of MRI angiography has replaced the invasive procedures.[169-171] Prenatal and early neonatal diagnosis is possible by use of ultrasonography.[172,173]

A sequestrated lung should be resected. Precaution is to be taken to identify all the systemic vessels before surgery to avoid disastrous bleeding. Embolization can block the systemic supply preventing fatal hemoptysis. Surgery can be done by the use of laporoscopy or under videoassistance.[174-179]

Anomalies of Pulmonary Vasculature

Various anomalies of the pulmonary vasculature include absent pulmonary artery trunk, absent unilateral pulmonary artery, pulmonary artery stenosis, anomalous origin of the left pulmonary artery, anomalous systemic pulmonary perfusion, anomalous pulmonary venous drainage, and pulmonary arteriovenous malformations.[180-186]

Pulmonary Artery Stenosis

It is rare and may occur at any level from above the pulmonic valve to the segmental arteries or beyond. Central stenoses are common than those occurring in the periphery. This may be associated with rubella syndrome and hypercalcemia. The diagnosis is usually confirmed by pulmonary angiography.

Anomalous Venous Drainage of the Lung

This may result because of persistent communication between the embryonic venous system and the pulmonary venous plexus. The aberrant pulmonary veins drain into the systemic veins like inferior vena cava, instead of returning oxygenated blood into the left heart. This anomalous drainage is usually partial and causes a left-to-right lung by an anomalous scimitar-shaped pulmonary vain which passes through the lung running parallel to, but separate from, the mediastinal structures before joining the inferior vena cava, usually below the diaphragm. Other associations include anomalous systemic arterial supply to the territory drained by the scimitar vain, hypoplasia of the right lung, cardiac dextroposition, and diaphragmatic abnormalities. The condition may run in families with an autosomal dominant inheritance pattern. The chest X-ray shows a characteristic curvilinear vascular density in the right lower lung with features of loss of lung volume in the ipsilateral lung, with mediastinal shift to the right side, and an elevated diaphragm. Tomography, bronchography and pulmonary angiography will demonstrate the anomaly, but are rarely necessary.

Pulmonary Arteriovenous Malformation

Also known a pulmonary arteriovenous fistula, pulmonary arteriovenous aneurysm, pulmonary angioma, pulmonary hemangioma, and pulmonary cavernous angioma, in this condition, there are abnormal communications between arteries and veins within the lung that effectively bypass part of the normal pulmonary capillary bed. The size varies considerably being very small to large thin-walled spaces of lobar proportions. Most often the arterial supply is from the pulmonary artery, but rarely the supplying vessel arises from the aorta, innominate subclavian, internal mammary bronchial and intercostals arteries and the drainage may be via the pulmonary or systemic veins. It is closely associated with hereditary hemorrhagic telangiectasia (Osler-Rendu-Weber syndrome). The condition is slightly more in females and are usually single. About 10 percent of cases are bilateral. The malformation is closely related to the pleura and often occurs in the lower lobes.

Usual age of presentation is in the third decade or beyond. Most often there is no symptom. Respiratory symptoms include dyspnea, hemoptysis, and the presence of a bruit. A systolic murmur can also be heard. Cyanosis may be present. Finger clubbing is usual. The most common complication is hemorrhage into the bronchial tree or into the substance of the lung. Hemopneumothorax, pneumothorax, cerebral ischemia, hypoxemia and secondary polycythemia may occur. Paradoxical embolism, bacterial endoangitis and metastatic brain abscess are other rare complications.

Radiologically, the lesion is recognized as a rounded, lobulated, or tortuous opacity in the periphery of the lower lung field. Feeding vessels can be recognized. The size of the lesion varies according to change in intrathoracic pressure. The size becomes smaller during a Valsalva maneuver and larger during a Muller maneuver. Bilateral pulmonary angiography confirms the diagnosis.

Surgical treatment is indicated if the size is increasing or if the patient is symptomatic. Various nonsurgical techniques including embolization or occlusion procedures, using balloons or steel coils, have been used with success in some patients.

REFERENCES

1. Agarwal S, John S, Latta S, Sahni M, Kumar N. Tracheal agenesis: Two case reports. Int J Pediatr Otorhinol 2006;70:737-39.
2. Bercker S, Kornak U, Buhrer C, Henrich W, Kerner T. Tracheal atresia as part of an exceptional combination of malformations. Int J Pediatr Otorhinolaryngol 2006; 70(6):1137-39.
3. Fraser N, Stewart RJ, Grant J, Martin P, Gibbin KP, Padfield CJ. Tracheal agenesis with unique anatomy. J Pediatr Surg 2005;40:e7-10.

4. Felix JF, van Looij MA, Pruijsten RV, de Krijger RR, de Klein A, Tibboel D, Hoeve HL. Agenesis of the trachea: Phenotypic expression of a rare cause of fatal neonatal respiratory insufficiency in six patients. Int J Pediatr Otorhinolaryngol 2006;70:365-70.

5. Nishino M, Kubo T, Kataoka ML, Gautam S, Raptopoulos V, Hatabu H. Evaluation of thoracic abnormalities on 64-row multi-detector row CT: Comparison between axial images versus coronal reformations. Eur J Radiol 2006;59(1):33-41.

6. Schweizer P, Berger S, Petersen M, Kirschner HJ, Schweizer M. Tracheal surgery in children. Eur J Pediatr Surg 2005;15:236-42.

7. Nagaya M, Kato J, Niimi N, Tanaka S, Iio K. Proposal of a novel method to evaluate anastomotic tension in esophageal atresia with a distal tracheoesophageal fistula. Pediatr Surg Int 2005;21:780-85.

8. Hadi U, Hamdan AL. Diagnosis and management of tracheal stenosis. J Med Liban 2004;52:131-85.

9. Cusack RJ, Seth A, Madden BP. Tracheal stenosis diagnosed on pulmonary ventilation/perfusion scan. Eur J Intern Med 2006;17:53-54.

10. Chiu PP, Rusan M, Williams WG, Caldarone CA, Kim PC. Long-term outcomes of clinically significant vascular rings associated with congenital tracheal stenosis. J Pediatr Surg 2006;41:335-41.

11. Schweinfurth JM. Endoscopic treatment of severe tracheal stenosis. Ann Otol Rhinol Laryngol 2006; 115:30-34.

12. Chen MS, Chia YY, Chiang HL, Liu K, Wang YR, Ye XD, Hsu HK. Bilateral severe bronchial obstruction after metallic tracheal stent insertion for tracheal stenosis—A case report. Acta Anaesthesiol Taiwan 2005;43:231-35.

13. Marel M, Pekarek Z, Spasova I, Pafko P, Schutzner J, Betka J, Pospisil R. Management of benign stenoses of the large airways in the university hospital in Prague, Czech Republic, in 1998-2003. Respiration 2005;72: 622-28.

14. Chiu PPL, Kim PCW. Prognostic factors in the surgical treatment of congenital tracheal stenosis: A multicenter analysis of the literature. J Pediatr Surg 2006;41:221-25.

15. Elliott M, Roebuck D, Noctor C, et al. The management of congenital tracheal stenosis. Int J Pediatr Otorhinolaryngol 2003;(67 suppl 1):S183–S192.

16. Kimura K, Mukohara N, Tsugawa C, et al. Tracheoplasty for congenital stenosis of the entire trachea. J Pediatr Surg 1982;17:869-71.

17. Kamata S, Usui N, Ishikawa S, et al. Experience in tracheobronchial reconstruction with a costal cartilage graft for congenital tracheal stenosis. J Pediatr Surg 1997;32:54-57.

18. Tsang V, Murday A, Gilbe C, et al. Slide tracheoplasty for congenital funnel shaped tracheal stenosis. Ann Thorac Surg 1989;48:632-35.

19. Grillo HC. Slide tracheoplasty for long-segment congenital tracheal stenosis. Ann Thorac Surg 1994; 58:613-21.

20. Lang FJW, Hurni M, Monnier P. Long-segment congenital tracheal stenosis: Treatment by slide-tracheoplasty. J Pediatr Surg 1999;34:1216-22.

21. Koopman J, Bogers A, Witsenburg M, et al. Slide tracheoplasty for congenital tracheal stenosis. J Pediatr Surg 2004;39:19-23.

22. Rutter M, Cotton R, Azizkhan R, et al. Slide tracheoplasty for the management of complete tracheal rings. J Pediatr Surg 2003;38:928-34.

23. Backer C, Mavroudis C, Gerber ME, et al. Tracheal surgery in children: An 18-year review of four techniques. Eur J Cardiothorac Surg 2001;19:777-84.

24. Anton-Pacheco J, Cano I, Garcia A, et al. Patterns of management of congenital tracheal stenosis. J Pediatr Surg 2003;28:1452-58.

25. Kagawa S, Fujiwara T, Nishizaki M, Tokunaga N, Gochi A, Tanaka N. Stenting and radiotherapy for malignant tracheal stenosis due to mediastinal lymph node recurrence from gastric cancer—A case report. Gan To Kagaku Ryoho 2006;33:91-93.

26. Isa AY, Macandie C, Irvine BW. Nitinol stents in the treatment of benign proximal tracheal stenosis or tracheomalacia. J Laryngol Otol 2006;120:32-37.

27. Jegaden O, Boyer J, Guibert B, Devolfe C, Morin A. Tracheal diverticuli: Apropos of a case: Malformation etiopathogenesis? Bull Assoc Anat (Nancy). 1985;69: 291-95.

28. Frenkiel S, Assimes IK, Rosales JK. Congenital tracheal diverticulum: A case report. Ann Otol Rhinol Laryngol 1980;89:406-08.

29. Choffel C, Milleron B, Collot L, Busy F, Wachtel L. Voluminous tracheal diverticulum. One case. J Radiol Electrol Med Nucl 1978;59:53-56.

30. Kennedy RK. Traumatic tracheal separation with diverticuli in a cat. Vet Med Small Anim Clin. 1976; 71:1384-85.

31. Marom EM, Goodman PC, McAdams HP. Diffuse abnormalities of the trachea and main bronchi. Am J Roentgenol 2001;176:713-17.

32. Roig Figueroa V, Herrero Perez A, Rodriguez Carrera E. Mounier-Kuhn syndrome. An Med Interna 1999; 16:265.

33. Al-Mubarak HF, Husain SA. Tracheobronchomegaly-Mounier-Kuhn syndrome. Saudi Med J 2004;25:798-801.

34. Wiesner B, Mader I, Leonhardi J, Strauss HJ. Tracheobronchomegaly—Mounier-Kuhn syndrome—Case report and review of the literature. Pneumologie 1997;51:291-95.

35. Celenk C, Celenk P, Selcuk MB, Ozyazici B, Kuru O. Tracheomegaly in association with rheumatoid arthritis. Eur Radiol 2000;10:1792-94.

36. Jain P, Dave M, Singh DP, Kumawat DC, Babel CS. Mounier-Kuhn syndrome. Indian J Chest Dis Allied Sci 2002;44:195-98.

37. Grunebaum M, Kornreich L, Horev G, Ziv N. Tracheomegaly in Brachmann-de Lange syndrome. Pediatr Radiol 1996;26:184-87.

38. Sundaram P, Joshi JM. Tracheobronchomegaly associated tracheomalacia: Analysis by sleep study. Indian J Chest Dis Allied Sci 2004;46:47-49.

39. Hubbard M, Masters IB, Chang AB. Rapidly progressing case of Mounier-Kuhn Syndrome in early childhood. Pediatr Pulmonol 2003;36:353-56.

40. Adani GL, Baccarani J, Lorenzin D, Benzoni E, Montanardo D, Tulissi P, Groppuzzo M, Risaliti A, Bresadola F. Renal transplantation in a patient affected by Mounier-Kuhn syndrome. Transplant Proc 2005; 37:4215-17.

41. De Pauw I, Smeets P, Verstraete K. Pneumothorax complicating tracheobronchomegaly. JBR-BTR 2004; 87:126-27.

42. Genta PR, Costa MV, Stelmach R, Cukier A. A 26-yr-old male with recurrent respiratory infections. Eur Respir J 2003;22:564-67.

43. Bates CA, Rosenwasser LJ. A 49-year-old male with intractable dyspnea, wheeze, and cough. Ann Allergy Asthma Immunol 2003;91:20-25.

44. Yamakawa T, Tanaka SI, Ito Y, Shoji A, Sekihara H. Recurrent pneumonia with unconsciousness. J Intern Med 2002;251:278-79.

45. Lazzarini-de-Oliveira LC, Costa de Barros Franco CA, Gomes de Salles CL, de Oliveira AC Jr. A 38-year-old man with tracheomegaly, tracheal diverticulosis, and bronchiectasis. Chest 2001;120:1018-20.

46. Banerjee S, Sundaram P, Joshi JM. Chronic pulmonary suppuration. Postgrad Med J 2001;77:272; discussion 282-83.

47. Ker JA, Prinsloo H. Tracheobronchomegaly associated with recurrent pneumonia. Trop Doct 2000;30:242-43.

48. Benesch M, Eber E, Pfleger A, Zach MS. Recurrent lower respiratory tract infections in a 14-year-old boy with tracheobronchomegaly (Mounier-Kuhn syndrome). Pediatr Pulmonol 2000;29:476-79.

49. Haro M, Vizcaya M, Jimenez Lopez J, Nunez A, Loeches N, Mansilla F. Tracheobronchomegaly: An exceptional predisposing factor for pulmonary aspergillomas and massive hemoptysis. Arch Bronconeumol 2000;36:103-05.

50. Haugen G, Jenum PA, Scheie D, Sund S, Stray-Pedersen B. Prenatal diagnosis of tracheal obstruction: Possible association with maternal pertussis infection. Ultrasound Obstet Gynecol 2000;15:69-73.

51. Menon B, Malik A, Chugh A, Vashishat B. Radiological appearances in a rare case of tracheomegaly, tracheal diverticulosis, bronchomegaly and bronchiectasis. Indian J Chest Dis Allied Sci 2005;47:39-41.

52. Blake MA, Clarke PD, Fenlon HM. Thoracic case of the day. Mounier-Kuhn syndrome (tracheobronchomegaly). Am J Roentgenol 1999;173:822,824-25.

53. Dee PM. Chest case of the day. Tracheobronchomegaly—The Mounier-Kuhn syndrome. Am J Roentgenol 1996;167:235,238.

54. Hetzel MR. Commentary: Yet more to see down the bronchial tree? Thorax. 1996;51:226-27.

55. Drain AJ, Perrin F, Tasker A, Stewart S, Wells F, Tsui S, Sivasothy S. Double lung transplantation in a patient with tracheobronchomegaly (Mounier-Kuhn syndrome). J Heart Lung Transplant 2006;25:134-36.

56. Carden KA, Boiselle PM, Waltz DA, Ernst A. Tracheomalacia and tracheobronchomalacia in children and adults: An in-depth review. Chest 2005;127:984-1005.

57. Shinawi M, Boileau C, Brik R, Mandel H, Bentur L. Splicing mutation in the fibrillin-1 gene associated with neonatal Marfan syndrome and severe pulmonary emphysema with tracheobronchomalacia. Pediatr Pulmonol 2005;39:374-78.

58. Segel MJ, Godfrey S, Berkman N. Relapsing polychondritis: Reversible airway obstruction is not always asthma. Mayo Clin Proc 2004;79:407-09.

59. Collard P, Freitag L, Reynaert MS, Rodenstein DO, Francis C. Respiratory failure due to tracheobronchomalacia. Thorax 1996;51:224-26.

60. Tsunezuka Y, Sato H, Hiranuma C, Ishikawa N, Oda M, Watanabe G. Spontaneous tracheal rupture associated with acquired tracheobronchomalacia. Ann Thorac Cardiovasc Surg 2003;9:394-96.

61. Baydur A, Kanel G. Tracheobronchomalacia and tracheal hemorrhage in patients with Duchenne muscular dystrophy receiving long-term ventilation with uncuffed tracheostomies. Chest 2003;123:1307-11.

62. Asai T, Shingu K. Airway obstruction in a child with asymptomatic tracheobronchomalacia. Can J Anaesth 2001;48:684-87.

63. Sundaram P, Joshi JM. Tracheobronchomegaly associated tracheomalacia: Analysis by sleep study. Indian J Chest Dis Allied Sci 2004;46:47-49.

64. Ghanei M, Moqadam FA, Mohammad MM, Aslani J. Tracheobronchomalacia and air trapping after mustard gas exposure. Am J Respir Crit Care Med 2006;173: 304-09.

65. Castillo A, Smith J, Figueroa V, Bertrand P, Sanchez I. Tracheobronchomalacia in pediatric patients: Clinical experience. Rev Med Chil 2002;130:1014-20.

66. Amdekar YK. Emerging issues in pediatric pulmonology in India. Indian J Pediatr 1998;65:347-49.

67. Mok Q, Negus S, McLaren CA, Rajka T, Elliott MJ, Roebuck DJ, McHugh K. Computed tomography versus bronchography in the diagnosis and management of tracheobronchomalacia in ventilator dependent infants. Arch Dis Child Fetal Neonatal Ed 2005;90: F290-93.

68. Baroni RH, Ashiku S, Boiselle PM. Dynamic CT evaluation of the central airways in patients undergoing tracheoplasty for tracheobronchomalacia. Am J Roentgenol 2005;184:1444-49.

69. Baroni RH, Feller-Kopman D, Nishino M, Hatabu H, Loring SH, Ernst A, Boiselle PM. Tracheobronchomalacia: Comparison between end-expiratory and dynamic expiratory CT for evaluation of central airway collapse. Radiology 2005;235:635-41.

70. Boiselle PM, Ernst A. State-of-the-art imaging of the central airways. Respiration 2003;70:383-94.
71. Boiselle PM, Feller-Kopman D, Ashiku S, Weeks D, Ernst A. Tracheobronchomalacia: Evolving role of dynamic multislice helical CT. Radiol Clin North Am 2003;41:627-36.
72. Boiselle PM. Multislice helical CT of the central airways. Radiol Clin North Am 2003;41:561-74.
73. Zhang J, Hasegawa I, Hatabu H, Feller-Kopman D, Boiselle PM. Frequency and severity of air trapping at dynamic expiratory CT in patients with tracheobronchomalacia. Am J Roentgenol 2004;182:81-85.
74. Gilkeson RC, Ciancibello LM, Hejal RB, Montenegro HD, Lange P. Tracheobronchomalacia: Dynamic airway evaluation with multidetector CT. Am J Roentgenol 2001;176:205-10.
75. Gour A, Peters MJ, Gordon I, Petros AJ. Non-invasive diagnosis of tracheobronchomalacia using a modified ventilation radioisotope lung scan. Arch Dis Child 2003;88:1122-23.
76. Garcia-Pachon E. Tracheobronchomalacia: A cause of flow oscillations on the flow-volume loop. Chest 2000;118:1519.
77. Baydur A, Kanel G, Koss M. Tracheobronchomalacia and noninvasive ventilation revisited. Chest 2004;126:1390-92.
78. Bach JR. Tracheobronchomalacia and noninvasive ventilation? Chest 2003;124:2038.
79. Masters IB, Chang AB. Interventions for primary (intrinsic) tracheomalacia in children. Cochrane Database Syst Rev 2005;(4):CD005304.
80. Inan M, Ayvaz S, Basaran UN. Treatment of tracheomalacia with Palmaz stent: A case report. Folia Med (Plovdiv) 2005;47:58-60.
81. Tanino M, Takeuchi M, Iwasaki T, Toda Y, Ohe K, Morita K. Relief of bronchial obstruction using a Fogarty catheter in a patient with bronchomalacia. Anesth Analg 2006;102:85-86.
82. Saito Y, Imamura H. Airway stenting. Surg Today 2005;35:265-70.
83. Sakamoto T, Nagase Y, Hasegawa H, Shin'oka T, Tomimatsu H, Kurosawa H. One-stage intracardiac repair in combination with external stenting of the trachea and right bronchus for tetralogy of Fallot with an absent pulmonary valve and tracheobronchomalacia. J Thorac Cardiovasc Surg 2005;130:1717-18.
84. Anton-Pacheco Sanchez J, Garcia Vazquez A, Cuadros Garcia J, Cano Novillo I, Villafruela Sanz M, Berchi Garcia FJ.Treatment of tracheobronchomalacia with expandable metallic stents. Cir Pediatr 2002;15:135-39.
85. Kamata S, Usui N, Sawai T, Tazuke Y, Nose K, Kawahara H, Okada A. Pectus excavatum repair using a costal cartilage graft for patients with tracheobronchomalacia. J Pediatr Surg 2001;36:1650-52.
86. Prakash UB. Tracheobronchopathia osteochondroplastica. Semin Respir Crit Care Med 2002;23:167-75.
87. Simsek PO, Ozcelik U, Demirkazik F, Unal OF, Orhan D, Aslan AT, Dogru D. Tracheobronchopathia osteochondroplastica in a 9-year-old girl. Pediatr Pulmonol 2006;41:95-97.
88. Shigematsu Y, Sugio K, Yasuda M, Sugaya M, Ono K, Takenoyama M, Hanagiri T,Yasumoto K. Tracheobronchopathia osteochondroplastica occurring in a subsegmental bronchus and causing obstructive pneumonia. Ann Thorac Surg 2005;80:1936-38.
89. Mohan K, Owen S, Yeong C. Tracheobronchopathia osteochondroplastica as an incidental finding. Asian Cardiovasc Thorac Ann 2004;12:280-81.
90. Ennaifer-Jerbi E, Ayadi-Kaddour A, Lagha M, Lassaad Loussaief M, Boubaker S. Tracheopathia osteochondroplastica associated with a liver hydatic cyst broken in bronchi. Ann Pathol 2001;21:425-27.
91. Barthwal MS, Chatterji RS, Mehta A. Tracheobronchopathia osteochondroplastica. Indian J Chest Dis Allied Sci 2004;46:43-46.
92. Doshi H, Thankachen R, Philip MA, Kurien S, Shukla V, Korula RJ. Tracheobronchopathia osteochondroplastica presenting as an isolated nodule in the right upper lobe bronchus with upper lobe collapse. J Thorac Cardiovasc Surg 2005;130:901-02.
93. White BD, Kong A, Khoo E, Southcott AM. Computed tomography diagnosis of tracheobronchopathia osteochondroplastica. Australas Radiol 2005;49:319-21.
94. Pinheiro GA, Antao VC, Muller NL. Tracheobronchopathia osteochondroplastica in a patient with silicosis: CT, bronchoscopy, and pathology findings. J Comput Assist Tomogr 2004;28:801-03.
95. Restrepo S, Pandit M, Villamil MA, Rojas IC, Perez JM, Gascue A. Tracheobronchopathia osteochondroplastica: Helical CT findings in 4 cases. J Thorac Imaging 2004;19:112-16.
96. Hantous-Zannad S, Sebai L, Zidi A, Ben Khelil J, Mestiri I, Besbes M, Hamzaoui A, Ben Miled-M'rad K. Tracheobronchopathia osteochondroplastica presenting as a respiratory insufficiency: Diagnosis by bronchoscopy and MRI. Eur J Radiol 2003;45:113-16.
97. Prince JS, Duhamel DR, Levin DL, Harrell JH, Friedman PJ. Nonneoplastic lesions of the tracheobronchial wall: Radiologic findings with bronchoscopic correlation. Radiographics 2002;22 Spec No:S215-30.
98. Avalos P, Garcia-Hernandez MJ, Rios JJ, Moreno D, Camacho F. Cutaneous bronchogenic cyst. Actas Dermosifiliogr 2005;96:186-87.
99. Liang MK, Yee HT, Song JW, Marks JL. Subdiaphragmatic bronchogenic cysts: A comprehensive review of the literature. Am Surg 2005;71:1034-41.
100. Pedicelli G, Ciarpaglini LL, De Santis M, Leonetti C. Congenital bronchial atresia (CBA). A critical review of CBA as a disease entity and presentation of a case series. Radiol Med (Torino) 2005;110:544-53.
101. Gleizal A, Abouchebel N, Lebreton F, Beziat JL. Dermoid cyst of the tongue: An association of dermoid

cyst with bronchogenic epithelium. J Craniomaxillofac Surg 2006;34:113-16.

102. Ahn SG, Tahk SJ, Shin JH. Images in cardiology. Abnormal left atrial membranous structure in transthoracic echocardiography caused by external compression from a large bronchogenic cyst. Heart 2006;92:200.

103. Anh D, Dudar B, Ananthasubramaniam K. Acquired isolated left pulmonary vein stenosis: A complication of bronchogenic cyst removal diagnosed by transesophageal echocardiography. Echocardiography 2006;23:73-74.

104. Koga Y, Uchiyama A, Noshiro H, Rai M, Miyatake E, Shimizu S, Tanaka M. Complete extirpation of a bronchogenic cyst causing recurrent laryngeal nerve palsy by thoracoscopy: Report of a case. Surg Today 2006;36:79-81.

105. Lokey JS, Palmer RM, Macfie JA. Unexpected findings during thyroid surgery in a regional community hospital: A 5-year experience of 738 consecutive cases. Am Surg 2005;71:911-13.

106. Jo WM, Shin JS, Lee IS. Supradiaphragmatic bronchogenic cyst extending into the retroperitoneum. Ann Thorac Surg 2006;81:369-70.

107. Liang MK, Marks JL. Congenital bronchogenic cyst in the gastric mucosa. J Clin Pathol 2005;58:1344.

108. Hattori H. High prevalence of estrogen and progesterone receptor expression in mediastinal cysts situated in the posterior mediastinum. Chest 2005;128:3388-90.

109. Lin SH, Lee LN, Chang YL, Lee YC, Ding LW, Hsueh PR. Infected bronchogenic cyst due to Mycobacterium avium in an immunocompetent patient. J Infect 2005;51:e131-33.

110. Kim JH, Jang AS, Park JS, Lee JH, Park SW, Koh ES, Park JS, Park CS. Polypoid endobronchial lung cyst with bronchoscopic removal: A case report. J Korean Med Sci 2005;20:892-94.

111. Chen VK, Eloubeidi MA. Endoscopic ultrasound-guided fine-needle aspiration of intramural and extraintestinal mass lesions: Diagnostic accuracy, complication assessment, and impact on management. Endoscopy 2005;37:984-89.

112. Ozel SK, Kazez A, Koseogullari AA, Akpolat N. Scapular bronchogenic cysts in children: Case report and review of the literature. Pediatr Surg Int 2005;21:843-45.

113. Yohena T, Kuniyoshi M, Kono T, Uehara T, Uehara T, Miyahira T, Kawasaki H, Hirayasu T, Ohta M, Kawabata T, Ishikawa K. Novel approach for a pulmonary bronchogenic cyst: A report of a case. Ann Thorac Cardiovasc Surg 2005;11:249-51. Erratum in: Ann Thorac Cardiovasc Surg 2005;11:432.

114. Jakopovic M, Slobodnjak Z, Krizanac S, Samarzija M. Large cell carcinoma arising in bronchogenic cyst. J Thorac Cardiovasc Surg 2005;130:610-12.

115. Fang SH, Dong DJ, Zhang SZ. Imaging features of ciliated hepatic foregut cyst. World J Gastroenterol 2005;11:4287-89.

116. Beall DP, Daley ND, Liu CZ, Fish JR. Paravertebral bronchogenic cyst diagnosed by computed tomography-guided biopsy.Curr Probl Diagn Radiol 2005;34:163-66.

117. Ustundag E, Iseri M, Keskin G, Yayla B, Muezzinoglu B. Cervical bronchogenic cysts in head and neck region. J Laryngol Otol 2005;119:419-23.

118. Cervical bronchogenic cysts in head and neck region. J Laryngol Otol 2005;119:419-23.

119. Lee T, Tsai IC, Tsai WL, Jan YJ, Lee CH. Bronchogenic cyst in the left atrium combined with persistent left superior vena cava: The first case in the literature. Am J Roentgenol 2005;185:116-19.

120. Koontz CS, Oliva V, Gow KW, Wulkan ML. Video-assisted thoracoscopic surgical excision of cystic lung disease in children. J Pediatr Surg 2005;40:835-37.

121. Mampilly T, Kurian R, Shenai A. Bronchogenic cyst-cause of refractory wheezing in infancy. Indian J Pediatr 2005;72:363-64.

122. Paik SS, Jang KS, Han HX, Oh YH, Lee KG, Choi D. Retroperitoneal bronchogenic cyst mimicking pancreatic pseudocyst in a patient with colorectal cancer. J Gastroenterol Hepatol 2005;20:802-03.

123. Wilson RL, Lettieri CJ, Fitzpatrick TM, Shorr AF. Intralobular bronchopulmonary sequestrations associated with bronchogenic cysts. Respir Med 2005;99:508-10.

124. Rubio CA, Orrego A, Willen R. Congenital bronchogenic cyst in the gastric mucosa. J Clin Pathol 2005; 58:335.

125. Abrams ME, Ackerman VL, Engle WA. Primary unilateral pulmonary hypoplasia: Neonate through early childhood—Case report, radiographic diagnosis and review of the literature. J Perinatol 2004;24:667-70.

126. Munro HM, Sorbello AM, Nykanen DG. Severe stenosis of a long tracheal segment, with agenesis of the right lung and left pulmonary arterial sling. Cardiol Young 2006;16:89-91.

127. Gokhan GA, Ozbilim G, Bozova S, Gura A, Ongun H, Mihci E, Arslan G. Unilateral pulmonary agenesis associated with colloidal goiter in a newborn: A case report. Turk J Pediatr 2005;47:295-97.

128. Greenough A, Ahmed T, Broughton S. Unilateral pulmonary agenesis. J Perinat Med 2006;34:80-81.

129. Hamdan MA, Abu-Sulaiman RM, Najm HK. Sildenafil in pulmonary hypertension secondary to unilateral agenesis of pulmonary artery. Pediatr Cardiol 2006; 27(2):0172-0643.

130. Wilson RD, Hedrick HL, Liechty KW, Flake AW, Johnson MP, Bebbington M, Adzick NS. Cystic adenomatoid malformation of the lung: Review of genetics, prenatal diagnosis, and in utero treatment. Am J Med Genet A 2006;140:151-55.

131. Asai K, Urabe N, Takeichi H. Spontaneous pneumothorax and a coexistent azygos lobe. JPN J Thorac Cardiovasc Surg 2005;53:604-6. Cimen M, Erdil H,

Karatepe T. A cadaver with azygos lobe and its clinical significance. Anat Sci Int 2005;80:235-37.

132. Eradi B, Cusick E. Aygos lobe associated with esophageal atresia: A trap for the unwary. J Pediatr Surg 2005;40:e11-12.

133. Internullo E, Migliore M. Pneumothorax and mediastinal emphysema due to an air leak from a bulla in an azygos lobe. Eur J Cardiothorac Surg 2005;28:641.

134. Rakototiana AF, Rakotoarisoa AJ, Hunald F, Laborde Y. Spontaneous pneumothorax and azygos lobe in a child. Arch Pediatr 2005;12:1406.

135. Reisfeld R. Azygos lobe in endoscopic thoracic sympathectomy for hyperhidrosis. Surg Endosc 2005;19:964-66.

136. Sen S, Barutca S, Meydan N. Azygos lobe small cell carcinoma. Eur J Cardiothorac Surg 2004;26:1041.

137. Aziz A, Ashizawa K, Nagaoki K, Hayashi K. High resolution CT anatomy of the pulmonary fissures. J Thorac Imaging 2004;19:186-91.

138. Gill AJ, Cavanagh SP, Gough MJ. The azygos lobe: An anatomical variant encountered during thoracoscopic sympathectomy. Eur J Vasc Endovasc Surg 2004;28: 223-24.

139. Tuzun M, Hekimoglu B. Double accessory fissures in the upper lobe of the right lung (double azygos fissures?): High resolution computed tomography appearance. Acta Radiol 2004;45:109-10.

140. Smith J, Karthik S, Thorpe JA. Pulmonary azygous lobe: A potential obstacle during thoracoscopic sympathectomy. Eur J Cardiothorac Surg 2004;25:137.

141. Munn S. Pseudoazygos lobe caused by lymph node pneumatocele. J Thorac Imaging 2002;17:310-13.

142. Witters L, Moerman P, Brouwers A, Fryns JP. Diaphragmatic hernia with extralobar lung sequestration in the Beckwith-Wiedemann syndrome. Genet Couns 2004; 15:371-74.

143. Sato Y, Endo S, Saito N, Otani S, Hasegawa T, Sohara Y. A rare case of extralobar sequestration with hemoptysis. J Thorac Cardiovasc Surg 2004;128:778-79.

144. Franko J, Bell K, Pezzi CM. Intraabdominal pulmonary sequestration. Curr Surg 2006;63:35-38.

145. Lo W, Hemli JM, Brady PW. Bronchopulmonary sequestration supplied by the coronary circulation associated with a right-sided aortic arch. Heart Lung Circ 2004;13:92-96.

146. Alvarez Suero J, Lanusse C, Mellado Gazquez JM, Venero Gomez J. Pulmonary sequestration with systemic coronary arterial supply. Med Clin (Barc). 2004;123:596-7.Erratum in: Med Clin (Barc) 2004;123:774.

147. Tsitouridis I, Tsinoglou K, Cheva A, Papapostolou P, Efthimiou D, Moschialos L. Intralobar pulmonary sequestration with arterial supply from the coronary circulation. J Thorac Imaging 2005;20:313-15.

148. Hunninghake GM, Kanarek DJ. Pulmonary sequestration supplied by a coronary artery. Thorax 2005; 60:792.

149. Pop D, Venissac N, Perrin C, Leo F, Padovani B, Mouroux J. Extralobar sequestration with anomalous pulmonary artery return or patent ductus arteriosus? J Thorac Cardiovasc Surg 2005;130:903-04.

150. Chen F, Heller DS, Bethel C, Faye-Petersen O. Intrathoracic ectopic lobe of liver presenting as pulmonary sequestration. Fetal Pediatr Pathol 2005;24:155-59.

151. Okamoto T, Masuya D, Nakashima T, Ishikawa S, Yamamoto Y, Huang CL, Yokomise H. Successful treatment for lung cancer associated with pulmonary sequestration. Ann Thorac Surg 2005;80:2344-46.

152. Hofman FN, Pasker HG, Speekenbrink RG. Hemoptysis and massive hemothorax as presentation of intralobar sequestration. Ann Thorac Surg 2005;80:2343-44.

153. Ferretti GR, Jouvan FB, Coulomb M. MDCT demonstration of intralobar pulmonary sequestration of the right upper lobe in an adult. Am J Roentgenol 2005;185:1663-64.

154. Yatera K, Izumi M, Imai M, Ikegami T, Miyazaki N, Kido M. Intralobar sequestration with tuberculous infection confined to the sequestrated lung. Respirology 2005;10:685-88.

155. Armatys SA, Cheng L, Gardner TA, Sundaram CP. Pulmonary sequestration presenting as retroperitoneal cyst: Case report. J Endourol 2005;19:997-99.

156. Andrisani MC, Peschechera R, Reale F, Ciavarrella C, Filograna E, Pinnelli M, Masselli G. Intralobar pulmonary sequestration in an elderly adult. Rays 2005;30:25-29.

157. Lohani S, Varma R, Leahy B. A case of pulmonary sequestration with Aspergillus species infection presenting as an enlarged right paratracheal mass. J Thorac Cardiovasc Surg 2005;129:1459-60.

158. Becker J, Hernandez A, Dipietro M, Coran AG. Identical twins concordant for pulmonary sequestration communicating with the esophagus and discordant for the VACTERL association. Pediatr Surg Int 2005;21:541-46.

159. Sanchez Abuin A, Somoza I, Liras J, Mendez R, Tellado M, Rios J, Pais E,Vela D. Congenital cystic adenomatoid malformation associated with pulmonary sequestration. Cir Pediatr 2005;18:39-41.

160. Shanmugam G. Aspergillosis complicating intralobar sequestration. Eur J Cardiothorac Surg 2005;27: 1132-33.

161. Lin SH, Lee LN, Chang YL, Lee YC, Ding LW, Hsueh PR. Infected pulmonary sequestration caused by *Mycobacterium kansasii*. Thorax 2005;60:355.

162. Sato H, Watanabe A, Yamaguchi T, Harada N, Yamauchi A, Inoue S, Abe T. Pulmonary sequestration associated with asymptomatic aspergillosis. Ann Thorac Cardiovasc Surg 2005;11:41-43.

163. Laberge JM, Puligandla P, Flageole H. Asymptomatic congenital lung malformations. Semin Pediatr Surg 2005;14:16-33.

164. Wilson RL, Lettieri CJ, Fitzpatrick TM, Shorr AF. Intralobular bronchopulmonary sequestrations asso-

ciated with bronchogenic cysts. Respir Med 2005;99: 508-10.

165. Yildiz K, Ozcan N, Cebi M, Kose N, Karakaya F. Intrapericardial extralobar pulmonary sequestration: Unusual cause of hydrops fetalis. J Ultrasound Med 2005;24:391-93.

166. Berna P, Lebied el D, Assouad J, Foucault C, Danel C, Riquet M. Pulmonary sequestration and aspergillosis. Eur J Cardiothorac Surg 2005;27:28-31.

167. Harris K. Extralobar sequestration with congenital diaphragmatic hernia: A complicated case study. Neonatal Netw 2004;23:7-24.

168. Pappa KI, Anagnou NP, Elsheikh A, Bikouvarakis SS, Konstantinidou A, Salamalekis E. Congenital broncho-pulmonary sequestration presenting as a thoracic tumor: A case report. Eur J Gynaecol Oncol 2004;25: 749-51.

169. Platon A, Poletti PA. Image in clinical medicine. Pulmonary sequestration. N Engl J Med 2005;17;353:e18.

170. Remy J. Radiologic diagnosis of pulmonary sequestra-tions. Rev Mal Respir 2005;22:490-91.

171. Deguchi E, Furukawa T, Ono S, Aoi S, Kimura O, Iwai N. Intralobar pulmonary sequestration diagnosed by MR angiography. Pediatr Surg Int 2005;21:576-77.

172. Ruano R, Benachi A, Aubry MC, Revillon Y, Emond S, Dumez Y, Dommergues M. Prenatal diagnosis of pulmonary sequestration using three-dimensional power Doppler ultrasound. Ultrasound Obstet Gynecol 2005;25:128-33.

173. Shimizu T, Tamai H, Owari M, Kosumi T, Yonekura T. Doppler echocardiography and MR angiography for diagnosis of systolic murmurs in pulmonary seques-tration. J Pediatr 2004;145:713.

174. Shanmugam G, MacArthur K, Pollock JC. Congenital lung malformations—antenatal and postnatal evalua-tion and management. Eur J Cardiothorac Surg 2005;27:45-52.

175. van der Zee DC, NMa Bax K. Laparoscopic resection of intra-abdominal extralobar pulmonary seques-tration. Pediatr Surg Int 2005;21:841-42.

176. Nayar PM, Thakral CL, Sajwani MJ. Congenital lobar emphysema and sequestration—Treatment by embo-lization. Pediatr Surg Int 2005;21:727-29.

177. Duan M, Wang L, Cao Y, Li Z, Yang W, Rao X, Xiao K. Results of surgical treatment of congenital cystic lung disease. Thorac Cardiovasc Surg 2005;53:61-64.

178. Tayama K, Eriguchi N, Tanaka A, Futamata Y, Harada H, Yoshida A, Matsunaga A. Video-assisted thoracic surgery lobectomy for extralobar pulmonary seques-tration in a child: Report of a case. Surg Today 2004;34:954-57.

179. Sakuma T, Sugita M, Sagawa M, Ishigaki M, Toga H. Video-assisted thoracoscopic wedge resection for pulmonary sequestration. Ann Thorac Surg 2004; 78:1844-45.

180. Tedoriya T, Date H, Okabe K, Aoe M, Sano Y, Sano S, Shimizu N. Anastomosis of an anomalous segmental vein with the azygos vein in living-donor lobar lung transplantation. J Heart Lung Transplant 2004;23:644-46.

181. Okamoto K, Kodama K, Kawai K, Wakebe T, Saiki K, Nagashima S. An anatomical study of the partial ano-malous pulmonary venous return with special refe-rences to the bronchial vein. Anat Sci Int 2004;79:82-86.

182. Hardin RE, Brevetti GR, Sanusi M, Bhaskaran D, Burack JH, Genovesi MH, Lowery RC, Rafii S, Bondi E. Treatment of symptomatic vascular rings in the elderly. Tex Heart Inst J 2005;32:411-15.

183. Sondakh A, Daenen W, Gewillig M, Devriendt K, Meyns B. Right aortic arch with vascular ring in one mono-zygotic twin. J Thorac Cardiovasc Surg 2005;130: 883-84.

184. Vazquez-Antona CA, Munoz-Castellanos L, Kuri-Nivon M, Vargas-Barron J. Double symmetrical aortic arch: Case report. Arch Cardiol Mex 2005;75:178-81.

185. Ozlugedik S, Ozcan M, Unal A, Yalcin F, Tezer MS. Surgical importance of highly located innominate artery in neck surgery. Am J Otolaryngol 2005;26:330-52.

186. Park JG, Wylam ME. Congenital stridor: Unusual manifestation of coarctation of the aorta. Pediatr Cardiol 2006;27:137-39.

Lung Transplantation

With significant development in the field of solid organ transplant of kidney, liver, and heart, lung transplantation has become a therapeutic reality in many end stage pulmonary diseases, and over the years it has come up tremendously from its infancy about a few years ago. Over the past several decades developments in lung transplantation has changed from being experimental to a realistic treatment option for some patients with end stage lung diseases. Patients with end stage pulmonary and pulmonary vascular disease can now be successfully treated by transplantation. A total of 3,836 lung transplants have taken place worldwide till January 1995 as per the report of the St Louis International Lung Transplant Registry. Of these 2,227 has taken place in USA alone.[1,2] The main problem, however, is the scarcity of organ donors. The decades of the 1980s saw the development of successful heart-lung (HLT), single-lung (SLT), and double-lung (DLT) transplantation and subsequently the re-transplantation. Presently the assessment of success has focused on patient survival and documentation of improved lung function. Reported 2 year actual survival rates are 54 percent for HLT, 72 percent for DLT, and 62 percent for SLT.[3-10]

The Russian Scientist Demikhov had attempted the first lung transplantation in canine models as early as in 1947.[5,9] Till the early sixties, the procedure remained purely experimental and provided deep insight into the problems of such a procedure. While these series of experiments showed that lung transplantation is technically feasible, they raised concern that pulmonary denervation would alter respiratory pattern and can lead to potential respiratory failure. Subsequently, the Hardy et al attempted the first human lung transplantation in 1963 in a 58 year old man having bronchogenic carcinoma of the left side. The patient survived only 18 days.[11] Over the next 20 years, a number of human lung transplantations were carried out in a number of patients without long-term success, except in one patient who survived for 10 months spending most of the time in the hospital. The patient apparently died of rejection, respiratory failure, and shock.[12] Because of these apparent failures, further laboratory investigations were carried out and problems following transplantation like effects of ischemia, denervation, loss of lymphatics, and loss of bronchial circulation to the transplanted lung were sorted out. Subsequent success in heart transplant and knowledge in other organ transplantations increased the enthusiasm in the field of lung transplantation. Development of anti-thymocyte globulin and recognition of the immunosuppressive properties of azathioprine and cyclosporine A were major breakthroughs during this period. The first successful heart-lung transplantation in a young woman with primary pulmonary hypertension in 1981 further determined the desire towards the efforts in single lung transplantation.[6] In the mean time considerable advancement occurred in the field of care of acute respiratory failure, extracorporeal membrane oxygenation, and fiberoptic bronchoscopy. During those periods, it was recognized that the major complications were related to the bronchial anastomosis. It was postulated that this failure of bronchial healing was either due to ischemia, rejection, immunosuppression or a combination of these factors. Steroid therapy during early post-transplantation period was thought to be a major factor in this complication. To obviate this problem, steroids were eliminated during this period.[5,9]

Interest was renewed in single lung transplantation, which has several advantages over combined heart-lung transplantation in the patient in whom a single lung is adequate. In unilateral lung transplantation, there is no worry about the occurrence of premature coronary artery disease and the necessity to monitor cardiac rejection is not there. Cardiopulmonary bypass is usually not required during surgery which avoids the problems associated with heparin therapy and prolonged periods of bypass. Another major benefit is that the other donor lung and heart can be transplanted individually to at least two more patients. The problem of such unilateral transplantation, however, was the dehiscence of the bronchial anastomosis after 2 weeks of surgery. This occurs because such procedures do not re-establish the bronchial arterial circulation. This problem was resolved by the technique of bronchial omentopexy or by an intercostal flap or a pedicle of pericardial fat. Another fact that was realized is the use of high dose prednisolone before the transplantation that may be responsible for bronchial dehiscence. These facts and special procedures helped to revascularize and protect the anastomosis.

Utilizing these technical advances, the Toronto Lung Transplantation Group performed the first clinically successful single lung transplantation in 1983 in a 58 year old man with idiopathic pulmonary fibrosis.[4] The patient survived for more than 6 years before he died of renal failure despite the occurrence of two early rejections. The rest has been the history. Over the years the techniques have been refined and the procedures include double lung transplantation, and bilateral sequential single lung transplantation. Now a number of centers worldwide perform this procedure and the number has risen dramatically over these years.

Lung transplantation has become an acceptable treatment option for end-stage lung disease. As of 1999, > 10,000 lung transplants have been performed in North America.[13]

INDICATIONS OF LUNG TRANSPLANTATION

Although lung transplantation can be undertaken in any untreatable, end stage pulmonary disease, the choice is limited because of shortage of organ donor, the nature of the original disease, and the likelihood of success. Various indications of lung transplantation are shown in Table 32.1.

The main indication of lung transplantation is the presence of irreversible, progressively disabling end-stage pulmonary disease. Although single lung transplantation is easier to perform and there is no need for cardiopulmonary bypass, there are disadvantages also by retaining the remaining opposite native lung. The double lung transplantation as described earlier is technically difficult and is currently done only if there is contraindication for SLT. Currently most centers perform double lung operations, which involves bilateral single lung transplantations, which have eliminated many problems associated with the DLT procedures. Double-lung transplantation is performed in all patients with cystic fibrosis or other suppurative lung diseases,

TABLE 32.1: Indications of lung transplantation[2,3,5,14,15]

A. *Single lung transplantation*
 – Idiopathic pulmonary fibrosis (Restrictive fibrotic lung disease)
 – Chronic obstructive pulmonary disease (α_1-Antitrypsin deficiency, others)
 – Eisenmenger's complex with correctable cardiac lesions
 – Primary pulmonary hypertension with adequate right ventricular function
 – Sarcoidosis
 – Eosinophilic granuloma
 – Bronchiolitis obliterans
 – Lymphangioleiomyomatosis
B. *Bilateral (double) lung transplantation*
 Cystic fibrosis
 Generalized bronchiectasis
C. *Heart-lung transplantation*
 – Eisenmenger's complex with uncorrectable cardiac lesions
 – Pulmonary hypertension with cor pulmonale
 – End-stage lung disease with concurrent severe cardiac disease

while single-lung or double-lung transplantation is used for patients with COPD, idiopathic pulmonary fibrosis, and primary pulmonary hypertension.[16]

Restrictive lung disease of the idiopathic variety was the most common indication of SLT till recently. However, COPD is the commonest indication now.[1] These patients usually show declines in functional status, because of disease progression. Since the most important cause of death in these patients is respiratory failure, transplantation is an attractive form of treatment. Factors considered for transplant selection include:[2,4]

• Severe dyspnea
• Exercise intolerance
• Honey combing or pulmonary hypertension on chest skiagram/CT scans
• Severe physiologic derangement
• Increasing requirements for supplemental oxygen.

Absence of infection, poor chest compliance and high vascular resistance of the remaining native lung results in ventilation-perfusion imbalance that favors the transplanted lung. The native lung is not hyperinflated and therefore does not mechanically compromise the transplanted lung.

Chronic obstructive pulmonary lung disease is currently the most common indication of lung transplantation.[1] Initially it was thought that hyperinflation of the native lung might impair mechanically the ventilation-perfusion of the transplanted lung and it was proposed that DLT is the procedure of choice. However, the procedure is technically complicated and recently SLT has been done successfully in several cases of COPD. Because of simple procedure and being economical in terms of the availability of donor organs, this is the procedure of choice in suitable patients of end stage COPD without infection.[14,17-20] Patients with alpha-1 antitrypsin deficiency and emphysema are excellent lung transplant candidates because of their relatively young age and lack of other organ system involvement. However, it is not yet clear what effect the persistence of the alpha-1 anti-trypsine deficiency state will have on the transplanted lung and whether replacement therapy will be of value. Bilateral lung transplantation may be considered for patients with significant chronic bronchitis and may be preferable in patients with extensive bullae in both lungs.

Single lung transplantation is also indicated in patients with *primary pulmonary hypertension and Eisenmenger s syndrome* with good right ventricular function. Heart-lung transplantation is no longer necessary for these patients. It has been shown that even poor right ventricular function is not a contraindication for SLT in view of the observation that the ventricle might recover function once the chronic pressure is relieved. SLT is most often considered if the right ventricular ejection fraction is more than 20 percent and if echocardiography shows that the ventricle is not severely diseased.[3] In primary pulmonary hypertension, the main cause of death is due to progressive right ventricular failure or sudden death syndrome. Several factors are correlated with mortality and these are currently used for selecting patients for transplantation. These include: cardiac disease resulting in marked limitation of physical activity, Raynaud's phenomenon, and hemodynamic variables.[2,21]

Many consider SLT as the procedure of choice in appropriate patients with nonseptic end stage lung disease. Besides the above-mentioned conditions, many cases of chronic respiratory failure from a variety of causes have been treated with transplantation, although the number is small.

In septic lung diseases, like bronchiectasis or cystic fibrosis single lung transplantation is not the procedure of choice. This is because the infection still remains in the remaining native lung particularly when immuno-suppression will be necessary in the post-transplantation period. In these settings double lung transplantation is the procedure of choice. Because of technical reasons bilateral sequential single lung transplantation is the method of choice in these cases. Another advantage of this procedure is that cardiopulmonary bypass is not required. Heart-lung transplants can also be performed in these subjects. Double lung transplant is the preferred procedure for patients with cystic fibrosis, particularly in North America.[22-25] According to the

International Society for Heart and Lung Transplant registry, this is the most common (61%) indication of all pediatric double lung transplant performed up to the end of 1992 and 38 percent of all adult double lung transplantation.[26] The usual indications for consideration of lung transplantation are (i) FEV_1 is 30 percent predicted or less, (ii) when clinical deterioration is associated with a declining FEV_1 of 40 percent predicted, (iii) frequency of hospitalization and antibiotic use (iv) weight loss.[27-29]

Over the years, several program-related issues have been identified which have important bearings in the success of lung transplants. These include; donor related issues, issues related to the recipient particularly selection of the patient, complications of lung transplantation, their diagnosis, and management, transplant center characteristics, and choice of the procedure.

DONOR SELECTION

There is scarcity of donor lungs because of religious, social, or other reasons. It is estimated that organs could be obtained only from 20 to 30 percent of potential organ donors and about only 5 to 10 percent of available donors have lungs that are currently considered suitable for transplantation. There are some criteria of acceptance of donor lungs that again varies from center to center. Most centers however accept donors if he is less than 55 years; normal chest skiagram, PaO_2 300 mm Hg on FiO_2 1.0, PEEP 5 cm H_2O, for 5 minutes; normal bronchoscopy with no evidence of purulent secretions or aspiration; no significant chest trauma or contusion; and no previous thoracic surgery. As with other organ transplants, lung transplantation requires ABO compatibility. There is no evidence which shows that HLA matching is necessary. The retrieval procedure for the donor lung is quite extensive and the lung can remain viable only for few hours before which it should be utilized. Therefore, in leading centers the organ is flown to the place of transplantation. Usually the cadaver organ is used although in October 1990, the first lung transplant using a living donor has been performed at the Stanford University.[30] However, this is not a usual practice in general because of the potential problem of respiratory insufficiency in the donor because of one remaining lung. The donor selection criteria vary from center to center. The usual guidelines are shown in Table 32.2.

The ABO identity and matched CMV serology between the recipient and the donor are desirable. If there is no ABO identity, there is the possibility of hemolytic anemia mediated by immunocompetent donor cells present in the donor organ. HLA typing is not done in

TABLE 32.2: Usual donor selection guidelines.[2,5,18,31]

- Age < 65 for lung; < 45 for heart-lung (some recent guidelines put the age < 55 years)
- ≤ 20 pack-years of smoking history
- No severe chest trauma or pulmonary contusion
- No serious pulmonary infection
- No aspiration or severe sepsis
- Clear chest skiagram (exceptions may be there)
- No prolonged cardiac arrest (heart-lung only)
- Minimal pulmonary secretions
- Negative HIV status
- Negative Hepatitis B and C virus
- ABO identity*
- Similar total lung capacities
- Matched cytomegalovirus (CMV) serology*
- No previous thoracic surgery
- PaO₂ 300 mm Hg on FiO₂ 1.0, PEEP 5 cm H₂O (if patient on ventilator)
- Gram stain shows sputum sample free of bacteria, fungus, and significant number of WBC

*Not absolutely required.

lung transplant donors and recipients because of the short period that is available between an organ and the time of transplant (few hours only). Secondly, because of rare availability of the lungs this is not a feasible option. It is always better to use CMV negative donors for CMV negative recipients, otherwise the mismatching may lead on to CMV disease, in the later.[32] However, this is not always possible to select only matched donors due to widespread CMV exposure. Most transplant programs will not reject a CMV-positive donor for transplantation into a negative recipient. Ganciclovir is useful in this situation.

Since the available organ is quite precious, it is imperative to keep it in the optimal functional state. Fluid management in particular is important when both the kidneys and lungs are available for transplantation. It is perhaps the best to maintain a low central venous pressure (to avoid lung edema), and fluid replacement sufficient to maintain adequate blood pressure and adequate but not excessive urine output. After organ recovery, the lungs are usually flushed with donor blood or Eurocollins solution and then maintained in cold Eurocollins solution. This way, the organ can be preserved for 6 to 8 hours.[33] Pulmonary endothelium is the most susceptible compartment to preservation damage. Other solutions that are used for preservation are the Belzer (UWS) and a low-potassium solution (SPAL UP).[34]

SELECTION OF PATIENTS (RECIPIENTS)

Because of scarcity of donor organs, selection of the recipient is done very meticulously. Although every

transplant program has its own selection and rejection criteria, by and large the following are the selection criteria and contraindications for lung transplantation (Table 32.3 and 32.4).

The overall goal of selection of recipient is to identify individuals whose pulmonary function and prognosis justify transplantation and whose current health will not increase the risk of the operation unnecessarily or jeopardize its long-term success. Before a patient is taken up for lung transplantation, records are reviewed as an initial screening procedure. The screening data includes detailed medical history, nature and progression of lung disease, smoking history, prior surgery of the abdomen and thorax, medication history particularly that of steroids and exercise tolerance of the patient.

A thorough physical examination and laboratory tests of arterial blood gases, complete blood count, electrolytes, renal and hepatic function tests, electrocardiogram including echocardiography, chest X-ray, pulmonary

TABLE 32.3: Selection criteria of lung transplant recipients[2,3,15]

- Age < 60 years
- Life expectancy of < 12-24 months because of the disease (limited life expectancy)
- Untreatable end-stage pulmonary vascular or progressive lung disease
- Substantial limitation of daily activity
- Adequate right ventricular function and no coronary artery disease
- Patient not receiving corticosteroid therapy (patients receiving low dose corticosteroid therapy can be considered)
- Medically compliant patient with constant emotional support system
- Satisfactory psychological profile
- Ambulatory patient who is nutritionally stable with rehabilitation potential
- No contraindication for immunosuppressive therapy
- Adequate renal and hepatic function and no other systemic disease
- Sufficient financial support

TABLE 32.4: Contraindications of single lung transplantation

- Age > 60 years
- Active systemic or extra pulmonary infection, AIDS, or hepatitis
- Inadequate hepatic, or renal functions or other concomitant systemic disease
- Prolonged endotracheal intubation
- Severe malnutrition
- High dose corticosteroids used over a long time
- Cerebrovascular disease
- Obesity
- Peptic ulcer disease
- Ischemic heart disease or poor ventricular functions
- Emotional or social instability
- Smoking, alcoholism, or other drug abuse
- Severe chest wall deformity
- Malignancy
- Noncompliant patient

function tests and psychosocial assessment are carried out. Patients accepted for transplantation continue in an outpatient rehabilitation program till a suitable donor organ is available. A further detailed evaluation is done which includes pulmonary assessment (pulmonary function tests, $\dot{V}/\dot{Q}$ scans, CT scans if needed); cardiac assessment (MUGA, 2-D Echocardiogram, right heart catheterization, coronary angiograph in some cases); evaluation by social worker, physical therapist, and dietician. The patient should have the adequate psychological make up because he has to wait for few months to, as long as more than 1 year till a suitable donor organ is available. He has to wait for 24 hours a day. The cost involved is enormous. In a recent report, it is estimated that the median hospital charges for lung transplantation were $ 150,126 (Approx. 53 lakh Indian rupees); and this comes to about $ 710 (Rs 25,000) per day of life lived after lung transplantation.[35]

SURGICAL PROCEDURE

Very limited availability of organ donors, it is necessary to utilize the available organs more judiciously.[8,36] It seems logical to use lung-only transplants whenever possible. This allows the hearts to be used for those patients needing heart or heart-lung transplantations. Various possibilities those can be adopted are:
- Single lung transplantation (SLT)
- Sequential double lung transplantation (DLT)
- Heart-lung transplantation (HLT)
- Lobar lung transplantation (experimental at present)
- Retransplantation.

With the use of recent SLT in obstructive lung diseases and pulmonary vascular diseases, and the development of the bilateral sequential approach to double lung transplantation have widened the choice of procedure for end stage lung diseases. The general framework of selection of procedure is shown in Table 32.1.

Because of the complexity of the entire procedure, starting from selection of donors, recipients, operative and postoperative problems, certain transplant center characteristics are essential to enhance the success. The American Thoracic Society has outlined the ideal transplant center characteristics which are shown in Table 32.5.[2] Kumar et al have reviewed details of the surgical procedure and lung preservation methods recently.[37]

POSTOPERATIVE MANAGEMENT

Immediately after transplantation, there is high arterial-alveolar (A-a) gradient.[5] The transplanted lung is susceptible to fluid overload. This is because of total

TABLE 32.5: Ideal characteristics of transplant centers[2]

Standard features
- Well-qualified medical and surgical personnel
- Local and readily available support in all necessary areas (immunology, pulmonary medicine, infectious diseases, cardiology, rehabilitation, etc.)
- Adequate experience in transplantation medicine

Desirable features
- Qualified house staff available on a 24 hours basis
- Number of lung transplants performed is adequate to develop and maintain proficiency
- Active programes in basic and clinical research related to transplantation

disruption of lymphatic vessels and because of an increase in the extra vascular lung water.[38] It is therefore better to employ low-dose pressure support rather than volume infusion. Transcutaneous oximetry, arterial pressure, and pulmonary artery pressures are monitored continuously. Cardiac output and mixed venous saturation are also measured. Intraoperative and postoperative hemorrhage is a problem in some cases of double lung transplantation that may affect subsequent airway ischemia. Weaning from the ventilator should be done as early as possible to avoid prolonged intubation and colonization with microorganisms. Airway injury can be assessed with repeated bronchoscopies. Many patients may develop ileus following transplantation, which can be managed with intravenous fluid administration. Vigorous chest physiotherapy is essential to mobilize secretions in the tracheobronchial tree.

IMMUNOSUPPRESSIVE THERAPY FOR LUNG TRANSPLANTATION

Administration of immunosuppressive therapy in patients of lung transplantation is the most important step for successful end results. The immunosuppressive regimens for patients undergoing lung transplantation vary among centers and must be tailored to each patient. Cyclosporine, azathioprine, and prednisolone are the main drugs used for this purpose. A representative regimen is given in Table 32.6.[3,39]

COMPLICATIONS

According to the International Registry, the 1 year actuarial survival is approximately 70 percent, and most of the deaths occur within 30 days of transplantation.[40] The main cause of death during the first postoperative month is nonspecific graft failure secondary to ischemia/reperfusion injury.[40-44] Early graft failure after lung transplantation is given various names, such as

TABLE 32.6: Immunosuppressive therapy for lung transplantation[3]

Preoperative
1. Cyclosporine A, 4-8 mg/kg orally
2. Azathioprine, 4 mg/kg intravenously
3. Methyl prednisolone, 500 mg intravenously.

Postoperative
1. Horse antilymphocytic globulin, 10 mg/kg/day intravenously, 3-5 days
2. Cyclosporine A, 7.5 mg/kg/day in divided doses twice daily (day 1-7 postoperative). Subsequent dose adjustment is to be done (3-8 mg/kg/day) according to the serum cyclosporine level: 1st year—300-400 ng/ml; 2nd year—200-300 ng/ml; and 3rd year and afterwards—100-200 ng/ml.
3. Azathioprine, 0.5-1 mg/kg/day; check leukocyte count > 4500/mm^3
4. Methylprednisolone, 125 mg IV, 8 hourly day 1
5. Prednisolone, 20 mg/day, (begin day 7-14)

reimplantation edema, reperfusion edema, primary graft failure (PGF), or allograft dysfunction. Early and late dysfunction of the lung allograft remains the common and is responsible for a significant morbidity and mortality. At least 20 to 25 percent of lung transplant recipients are at risk of graft failure and death within 3 months of surgery, due to a variety of difficulties primarily related to early donor lung dysfunction, acute rejection, infection, and airway complications.[45,46] The clinical spectrum of early graft dysfunction is wide and ranges from mild hypoxemia with associated radiographic infiltrates to severe ARDS with hemodynamic instability. The condition manifests within 24 hours following transplant procedure. Nonspecific diffuse alveolar damage are the pathological changes. The primary graft dysfunction represents a syndrome consisting of elevated pulmonary vascular resistance, pulmonary edema, and hypoxemia. Some of the identifiable risk factors include prolonged graft ischemia time, increasing donor age, pulmonary hypertension in recipient, and use of cardiopulmonary bypass. Ischemia-reperfusion is the underlying pathophysiologic mechanism of primary graft failure. This phenomenon involves a complex cascade of interactions between pulmonary vascular endothelium, fragile type II pneumocytes, macrophages, and recipient neutrophils. This leads to increased pulmonary vascular permeability. The diagnosis remains on the occurrence of noncardiogenic pulmonary edema with impaired gas exchange. Four risk factors are identified: age, degree of gas exchange impairment, graft ischemia time, and severe early hemodynamic failure.[47] Post-transplant risk for mortality is three times greater in obese patients than in nonobese patients.[48,49]

The problem of lung transplantation is dehiscence and stenosis of the bronchial anastomosis. Dehiscence is now rare because of the advanced technology of interposing the omentum and avoidance of steroids before the patient is taken up for surgery. Bronchial stenosis may occur as a late complication, which can be managed by bronchial dilatation and by placement of stents.[50] Mechanical imbalance between the native diseased lung and the healthy transplanted lung, particularly in emphysema, can lead on to respiratory failure. However, this can now be managed very efficiently.[51] A radiological pattern of pulmonary edema without evidence of infection or rejection has been described as the pulmonary re-implantation response.[6,10,52] This complication is quite common and recovery is equally good. This is thought due to prolongation of graft ischemia.

With improved strategies for graft preservation, surgical techniques, and postoperative immunosuppression, early graft failures and airway complications have become uncommon and the major post-transplantation complications have been (i) *rejection* (ii) *infection* and (iii) *obliterative bronchiolitis*. The accurate diagnosis and effective treatment of early graft rejection and infection remain a significant step to improved patient survival.[53]

Rejection

While the acute rejection occurs during the first 4 to 6 days following transplantation, and the second episode of rejection commonly occurs after 2 to 3 weeks of surgery. It is very difficult to distinguish between the infection and rejection. Acute lung rejection is thought to represent a T-cell-mediated phenomenon in response to major histocompatibility complex antigen differences between donor and recipient.[54] *Rejection* is characterized by an abnormal chest radiograph with or without fever, gas exchange abnormalities, or worsening of pulmonary functions. The chest radiograph shows diffuse or patchy infiltrates, consolidation, nodular opacities, or pleural effusion. The radiograph may be normal in about 75 percent of the cases. Spirometry is often abnormal in the first several months after transplantation Spirometry is not of any use. Gas exchange abnormalities are nonspecific indicators of rejection. Perfusion scanning may show changes in blood flow to the transplanted lung.[55-57] Symptoms like cough, dyspnea or fever are nonspecific signs. Diagnosis of rejection is made on the basis of histologic evidence, which is not easy. For histological proof, transbronchial biopsy is very helpful. Although bronchoscopy in such sick patients is often very difficult, it can be done safely in these patients.[58,59] Broncoalveolar lavage fluid analysis may help in differentiating rejection and infection although it may not be accurate at times.[60] It is suggested that the donor-specific primed lymphocyte response of bronchoalveolar lavage cells is useful in the diagnosis of lung allograft rejection.[61] Presence of a perivascular monocytic infiltrate with or without submucosal inflammation, eosinophilic infiltration and interstitial involvement are features of rejection. The Lung Rejection Study Group of the International Society of Heart Transplantation has recommended a working formula for the standardization of nomenclature in the diagnosis of pulmonary rejection.[62] In this system, acute rejection has been graded from Grade 0 to Grade 4. Accordingly, the rejection can be classified as no significant abnormality, minimal acute rejection, mild acute rejection, moderate acute rejection, and severe acute rejection. According to this criteria, acute lung rejection occurs more frequently than clinically suspected early and late after transplantation and bronchoalveolar lavage lymphocytosis correlates with the presence and severity of histologically proven rejection.[63] Response to pulse methyl prednisolone (1 gm intravenously) with alleviation of symptoms and improvement of chest X-ray within 24 hours is another important evidence of acute rejection. Induction therapy with rabbit antithymocyte globulin significantly reduces the incidence of acute allograft rejection.[64]

Chronic rejection reaction of the transplanted lung is characterized by obliterative bronchiolitis with inflammation and obliteration of the distal bronchioles.[65-67] In the early era of heart-lung transplantation, the incidence of bronchiolitis obliterans was to the extent of 50 percent.[68] However, with the use of increased and better immunosuppressants, the incidence has decreased to around 20 percent with slowed disease progression.[69,70] The exact pathogenesis of bronchiolitis obliterans is not known. Available data suggest that the process is immunologically mediated against the epithelial cells of the airways and is an indicator of chronic graft rejection.[71,72] Those patients who developed more frequent, more histologically severe, and more persistent acute rejection are at increased risk for subsequent development of bronchiolitis obliterans.[65] The pathogenesis is similar to those observed in bone marrow and other solid organ transplantation. Other proposed pathogenic mechanisms include infectious agents such as cytomegalo virus infection, and postoperative ischemic airway injury. The Lung Rejection Study Group has further graded these changes into lymphocytic bronchitis, lymphocytic bronchiolitis, subtotal and total bronchiolitis obliterans (active and inactive), chronic

vascular rejection and vasculitis.[62] This complication can occur at any time following 2 months after transplantation, but the typical onset is 8 to 12 months following surgery.[73] Dry cough is an important symptom, which becomes increasingly productive and purulent. Other symptoms include recurrent bacterial infections of the airways and parenchyma, and increased breathlessness. The onset most often is heralded by an upper respiratory tract infection. The patient may also present asymptomatically. Radiological changes are nonspecific. The most characteristic feature is the development of an obstructive pulmonary dysfunction on spirometry, particularly FEV_1 and FEF^{24-74} percent.[66] Transbronchial lung biopsy can be used to confirm the diagnosis but the sensitivity of this test varies from 5 to 100 percent.[74] Because of these difficulties, a committee of the International Society for Heart and Lung transplantation defined and standardized a clinical staging of chronic graft dysfunction secondary to progressive airways disease for which there is no identifiable cause. This is referred to as bronchiolitis obliterans syndrome (BOS).[75]

Bronchiolitis obliterans has become *sine quo non* for chronic lung rejection in the lung transplant population. This presents clinically with an obstructive deterioration in pulmonary function and little change in chest radiograph. It develops more than 3 to 6 months following transplantation, usually at a mean of 16 to 20 months. Pathologically there is obliteration of the terminal bronchioles (constrictive bronchiolitis). Because it is difficult to make a reliable histologic diagnosis of bronchiolitis, the International Society for Heart Lung Transplantation has defined a bronchiolitis obliterans syndrome (BOS) staging system based on a deterioration of pulmonary function (FEV_1 reported as a percentage of post-transplant baseline values) with the performance of bronchoscopy to exclude alternative diagnoses such as acute rejection, infection, or anastomotic complications.[75] According to this system the syndrome is defined as follows:

Stage 0 (no obliterative bronchiolitis)	FEV_1 80 percent or more of baseline value
Stage 1 (mild obliterative bronchiolitis)	FEV_1 66-80 percent of baseline value
Stage 2 (moderate obliterative bronchiolitis)	FEV_1 51-66 percent of baseline value
Stage 3 (severe obliterative bronchiolitis)	FEV_1 less than 50 percent of baseline value

Each stage is further categorized as "a" or "b" according to whether pathologic changes are present or not. Since the sensitivity of transbronchial lung biopsy for the pathological diagnosis of BOS can be as low as 15 percent, in the majority of cases the diagnosis of BOS is made based on pulmonary function changes alone.[42] Home spirometry can detect pulmonary decline earlier than clinic spirometry and home spirometry can be a reliable and safe alternative to frequent pulmonary function testing in lung recipients.[76,77] Although numerous risk factors have been enumerated for the causation of BOS, the etiology remains unknown. The problem risk factors are: acute rejection, lymphocytic bronchiolitis, cytomegalo virus pneumonitis, CMV infection, organizing pneumonia, non-CMV infections, older donor age, prolonged ischaemia time, human leucocyte antigen mismatching, and donor antigen-specific reactivity.[78] Interestingly, the bilateral lung transplant group of patients has a significantly lower incidence of development of BOS (31.7%) than did the single lung transplant group.[79,80]

Once the changes of bronchiolitis obliterans occur, there is no effective treatment. However, some centers use the triple drug combinations (cyclosporine A, azathioprine, and prednisolone) to their maximally tolerated levels. Others add solumedrol or other lympholytic therapy with transient improvement.[65,66] Bronchodilators and aerosolized steroids may be of help as symptomatic therapy. However, the course is frequently progressive and re-transplantation is the only alternative. Re-transplantation may be tried in these cases with varying success.[8,81]

Infection

Infection is a very important and common complication of lung transplantation.[82,83] The primary determinant of early patient survival is infection. Bacterial pneumonias are the major infectious complications in the early, intermediate and late postoperative periods.[83,84] Most of the infections occur in the first 4 months after transplantation. The incidence of *bacterial pneumonia* is very high. The incidence may be as high as 35 percent during the first two weeks following surgery and the overall figure may be 67 percent in some series.[83] In this series, a pretransplant diagnosis of pulmonary hypertension or post-transplant occurrence of bronchial stenosis or dehiscence was associated with a higher rate of bacterial pneumonia. The underlying native lung may predispose to infection at that site.[85,86] *Staphylococcus aureus*, *Pseudomonas aeruginosa*, and other Gram-negative rods are the common pathogens. Other predisposing factors may include immunosuppression and alterations in the natural lung defense mechanisms induced by transplantation. In the late postoperative period the major predisposing factor is the presence of chronic rejection. Fever, cough, radiographic abnormalities, and breathlessness are the common features and every effort should be made to diagnose the condition. Examination of the tracheal secretions, culture of bronchial specimens, and the use of broad-spectrum antibiotics are helpful to decrease the incidence of infection. This approach is usually effective in most cases.

Cytomegalo virus (CMV) infection is the second most frequent cause of pneumonia. Seronegative organ recipients are more susceptible to the infection. The rate of infection will depend upon the serological status of the patient, the organ donor, and blood donors. CMV infection causes similar changes as in chronic rejection like obliterative bronchiolitis. This viral infection is because of immunosuppression and the susceptibility of the transplanted lung to CMV infection.[87,88] The infection is common from 30 to 120 days after transplantation. A rise in CMV titer or detection of viremia is suggestive of the infection and the definite diagnosis is made by isolation of the virus from the cells. Bronchoalveolar lavage can reliably detect CMV infection in the allograft, accurate diagnosis of CMV pneumonitis may require a lung biopsy. Transbronchial lung biopsy is a highly reliable technique to distinguish between CMV infection and disease.[89] It has been suggested that serum Neopterin/Creatinine ratio increases more than 3 weeks after transplantation, only in cases of infection and mostly CMV pneumonia.[90] Due to clinical impact of this infection, many lung transplant centers employ IV ganciclovir combined with CMV hyperimmuneglobulin as standard antiviral prophylaxis soon after surgery. Usually a prolonged course (3 months or more) of the drug is used. This approach is however, expensive and may lead to bone marrow suppression. Some others use a different regimen. A regimen of CMV prophylaxis employing 2 weeks of IV ganciclovir initiated 3 to 4 weeks after lung transplantation followed by virologic monitoring and pre-emptive therapy as needed provides good protection against CMV disease.[91] Other viruses like Herpes simplex, *Varicella zoster*, hepatitis virus, and Respiratory syncytial viruses can cause infection in these patients although less frequently than that of the CMV. *Fungal infections* are not common in lung transplant patients.[84,92] However, it is often difficult to differentiate colonization from true infection in immunocompromised patients. Candida and Aspergillus are the two most common fungal infections in these patients. Like any other immunocompromised patients, these subjects are susceptible to infections with *Pneumocystis carinii*. Prophylactic use of trimethoprim-sulfamethoxazole or aerosolized pentamidine is useful.[84]

CONCLUSION

Lung transplantation (LT) is offered to patients with progressive end-stage pulmonary disease to improve their quality of life. Patients who undergo transplantation, perioperative complications are quite common.[93,94] Such perioperative complications reported following lung transplantation range from 10 to 97 percent,[95-105] and include pulmonary edema/early graft failure,[95-98] respiratory infections,[94] airway complications,[99] cardiovascular events,[96,101] drug toxicity,[96] and phrenic nerve injury.[105] Commonly, many of the serious complications manifest as postoperative respiratory failure and are associated with a relatively high early mortality (5 to 29%).[42] Potential clinical predictors of poor perioperative outcome after lung transplantation have been identified as older age (> 60 years), underlying disease (other than COPD), and development of graft failure and infection.[93-98,101,103,104,106-108] Postoperative respiratory failure after the initial injury is often multifactorial and involves infections, muscle weakness, and cardiovascular complications. Respiratory failure after lung transplantation is common (55%) and is associated with high morbidity and mortality (45%). Respiratory failure often occurred in patients with operative technical complications, cardiovascular events, and postoperative ischemic reperfusion lung injury, which were observed most in patients requiring cardio-pulmonary bypass because of right ventricular dysfunction.[109]

Extensive research over the years has made lung transplantation possible in previously untreatable patients. The International Lung Transplant Registry which includes a total of more than 800 lung transplants procedures performed till 1991, reports a 1 year survival rate of 61 to 70 percent overall, and a 2 year survival rate single lung transplantation of 56 percent.[2] The current survival rates for 2002 for lung transplant recipients are 72 percent, 56 percent, and 43 percent respectively, at 1, 3, and 5 years as reported by the registry of the International Society of Heart Lung Transplantation (ISHLT). While for single lung transplantation patients the survival rates were 71 percent, 54 percent, and 40 percent at 1, 3, and 5 years respectively, the same were 72 percent, 58 percent, and 48 percent respectively for bilateral lung transplantation. There is varying degree of functional recovery.[110-116] The leading cause of mortality soon after is infection and early rejection and after the first year following transplantation is bronchiolitis obliterans, with an incidence of 30 to 50 percent. However, because of the high cost involved and the difficulty in obtaining donor organs, the procedure is still considered a luxury and is confined only in few centers of the world. Major efforts are needed to overcome the difficulties in the long-term management of these patients to improve the quality of life. Lung transplantation has been a reality now even in pediatric patients.[117] Introduction of legislations to identify brain death[118] may an early step towards the availability of more organs for transplantation is a right step towards such a treatment modality in many end stage lung diseases has become a reality in India not withstanding the various difficulties that may arise.

REFERENCES

1. Cooper JD. The St Louis International Lung Transplant Registry. April 1995 Update. St Louis, Missouri.
2. Report of the ATS workshop on lung transplantation. Lung transplantation. Am Rev Respir Dis 1993;147:772-76.
3. Tanoue LT. Lung transplantation. Lung 1992;170:187-200.
4. Toronto Lung Transplantation Group. Experience with single lung transplantation for pulmonary fibrosis. JAMA 1988;259:2258.
5. Kaiser LR, Cooper JD. Lung transplantation. In: Lenfant C, Dekker M (Eds). Lung biology in health and disease: Adult Respiratory Distress Syndrome. Inc, NewYork, Chapter 1991;22,491-538.
6. Reitz BA, Wallwork JL, Hunt SA, et al. Heart lung transplantation: Successful therapy for patients with pulmonary vascular disease. N Engl J Med 1982;306:557-64.
7. Cooper JD, Patterson GA, Grossman R, Maurer J. Double lung transplantation for advanced chronic obstructive lung disease. Am Rev Respir Dis 1989;139:303-07.
8. Estenne M, Knoop C. Lung re-transplantation. Eur Respir J 1993;6:1093-94.
9. Cooper JD. Current status of lung transplantation. Transplant Proc 1991;23:2107-14.
10. Sleiman Ch, Mal H, Fournier M, et al. Pulmonary reimplantation response in single-lung transplantation. Eur Respir J 1995;8:5-9.
11. Hardy JD, Webb WR, Dalton ML, Walker GR. Lung homotransplantation in man. JAMA 1963;186:1065-74.
12. Derom F, Barbier F, Ringoir S, et al. Ten month survival after lung homotransplantation in man. J Thorac Cardiovasc Surg 1971;61:835-46.
13. Cooper DKC, Keogh AM, Brink J, et al. Report of the xenotransplantation advisory committee of the International Society for Heart and Lung Transplantation: The present status of xenotransplantation and its potential role in the treatment of end-stage cardiac and pulmonary disease. J Heart Lung Transplant 2000; 19:1125-65.
14. Egan TM, Trulock EP, Boychuk J, et al. Analysis of referrals for lung transplantation. Chest 1991;99:867-70.
15. Egan TM, Kaiser LR, Cooper JD. Lung transplantation. Curr Prob Surg 1989;26:673-751.

16. Arcasoy SM, Kotloff RM. Medical progress: Lung transplantation. New Engl J Med 1999;340:1081-91.
17. Mal H, Andreassian B, Pamela F, et al. Unilateral lung transplantation in end-stage pulmonary emphysema. Am Rev Respir Dis 1989;140:797-802.
18. Trulock EP, Cooper JD, Kaiser LR, et al. The Washington-Barnes Hospital Experience with lung transplantation. JAMA 1991;266:1943-46.
19. Trulock EP, Egan TM, Kouchoukos NT, et al. Single lung transplantation for severe chronic obstructive pulmonary disease. Chest 1989;96:738-42.
20. Levine SM, Anzueto A, Gibbons WJ, et al. Graft position and pulmonary function after single lung transplantation for obstructive lung disease. Chest 1993;103:444-48.
21. D'Alonzo GE. Survival in patients with primary pulmonary hypertension. Results from a national prospective registry. Ann Intern Med 1991;115:343-49.
22. Egan TM. Lung transplantation in cystic fibrosis. Semin Respir Infect 1992;7:227-39.
23. Goldsmith MF. Which transplant technique will let cystic fibrosis patients breathe easier? JAMA 1990;264:9.
24. Ramirez JC, Patterson GA, Winton TA, et al. Bilateral lung transplantation for cystic fibrosis. J Thorac Cardiovasc Surg 1992;103:287-94.
25. Shennib H, Noirclerc M, Ernst P, et al. Double-lung transplantation for cystic fibrosis. Ann Thor Surg 1992;54:27-32.
26. The Registry of the International Society for Heart and Lung Transplantation. 10th official report-1993. J Heart Lung Transplant 1993;12:541-48.
27. Kerem E, Reisman J, Corey M, et al. Prediction of mortality in patients with cystic fibrosis. N Engl J Med 1992;326:1187-91.
28. Egan TM, Detterbeck FC, Mill MR, et al. Improved results of lung transplantation for cystic fibrosis. J Thorac Cardiovasc Surg 1995;109:224-35.
29. Ciriaco P, Egan TM, Cairns E, et al. Analysis of cystic fibrosis referrals for lung transplantation. Chest 1995;107:1323-27.
30. Goldsmith MF. Mother to child: First living donor lung transplant. JAMA 1990;264:2724.
31. Well D. Donor criteria in lung transplantation: An issue revisited. Chest 2002;121:2029-31.
32 Lawrence EC, Holland VA, Berger MG, et al. Lung transplantation: An emerging technology. Tex Med 1988;84:61-67.
33. Reitz BA. Heart and lung transplantation. In: Baumgartner WA, Reitz BA, Achuff SC (Eds): Heart and heart-lung transplantation. Philadelphia: WB Saunders 1990;319-46.
34. Spaggiari L, Regnard JF, Carbognani P, et al. Pulmonary endothelial cell viability by a new lung preservation solution. Chest 1995;108:170S.
35. Goodman WH, Hanrahan JP, Reilly JJ, et al. Quality of life and lung transplantation. Chest 1995; 108:170S.
36. Calhoon JH, Grover FL, Gibbons WJ, et al. Single lung transplantation. Alternative indications and techniques. J Thorac Cardiovasc Surg 1991;10:816-25.
37. Kumar A, Sharma SK, Chattopadhyay TK, Pande JN. Lung transplantation. Ind J Chest Dis All Sc 1995;37:127-66.
38. Cowan GS, Staub NC, Edmunds LH. Changes in the fluid compartments and dry weight of reimplanted dog lungs. J Appl Physiol 1976;40:962-70.
39. Ettinger NA, Trulock EP. Pulmonary considerations of organ transplantation. Part 3. Am Rev Respir Dis 1991;144:444-51.
40. Hosenpud JD, Bennett LE, Keck BM, et al. The registry of the International Society for Heart and Lung Transplantation: Sixteenth official report –1999. J Heart Lung transplant 1999;18:611-26.
41. Trulock EP. Lung transplantation. Am J Respir Crit Care Med 1997;155:789-818.
42. Khan SU, Sdalloum J, O'Donovan PB, et al. Acute pulmonary oedema following lung transplantation: The pulmonary reimplantation response. Chest 1999;116:187-94.
43. Christie JD, Bavaria JE, Palevsky HI, et al. Primary graft failure following lung transplanation. Chest 1998;114:51-60.
44. Duarte AG, Lick S. Predicting outcome in primary graft failure. Chest 2002;121:1736-38.
45. Kaye MP. The registry of the International Society for Heart and Lung Transplantation. Ninth Official Report. 1992. J Heart Lung Transplant 1992;11:599-606.
46. Madden B, Radley-Smith R, Hodson M, et al. Medium term results of heart and lung transplantation. J Heart Lung Transplant 1992;11:S241-S243.
47. Thabut G, Vinatier I, Stern JB, et al. Primary graft failure following lung transplantation. Predictive factors of mortality. Chest 2002;121:1876-82.
48. Kanasky WF Jr, Anton SD, Rodrigue JR, et al. Impact of body weight on long term survival after lung transplatation. Chest 2002;121:401-06.
49. Levine SM, Sako EY. Waiting to make the weight for lung transplantation. Chest 2002;121:317-8.
50. Neagos GR, Martinez FJ, Deeb GM, et al. Diagnosis of unilateral mainstem bronchial obstruction following single lung transplantation with routine spirometry. Chest 1993;103:1255-58.
51. Govazzeni V, Lapichino G, Mascheroni D, et al. Prolonged independent lung respiratory treatment after single lung transplantation in pulmonary emphysema. Chest 1993;103:96-100.
52. Kaplan JD, Trulock EP, Cooper JD, Schuster DP. Pulmonary vascular permeability after lung transplantation. Am Rev Respir Dis 1992;145:954-57.
53. Griffith BP, Hardesty RL, Trento A, et al. Heart-lung transplantation: Lessons learned and future hopes. Ann Thorac Surg 1987;43:6-16.

54. Krensky AM, Weiss A, Crabtree G, Davis MM, Parham P. T-lymphocyte-antigen interactions in transplant rejection. New Engl J Med 1990;322:510-17.

55. Williams TJ, Grossman RF, Maurer JR. Long-term functional follow up of lung transplant recipients. Clin Chest Med 1990;11:347-58.

56. Burke CM, Baldwin JC, Morris AJ, et al. Twenty-eight cases of human heart-lung transplantation. Lancet 1986;1:517-19.

57. Williams TJ, Patterson GA, Mcclean PA, Zamel N, Maurer JR. Maximal exercise testing in single and double lung transplant recipients. Am rev Respir Dis 1992;145:101-05.

58. Kurland G, Noyes BE, Jaffe R, et al. Broncoalveolar lavage and transbronchial biopsy in children following heart-lung and lung transplantation. Chest 1993; 104:1043-48.

59. Higgenbottam T, Stewart S, Penketh A, Wallwork J. Transbronchial lung biopsy for the diagnosis of rejection in heart-lung transplant recipients. Transplant 1988; 46:532-39.

60. Rabinowich H, Zeevi A, Yousem SA, et al. Alloreactivity of lung biopsy and bronchoalveolar lavage-derived lymphocytes from pulmonary transplant patients: Correlation with acute rejection and bronchiolitis obliterans. Clin Transplant 1990;4:376-84.

61. Rabinowich H, Zeevi A, Paradis IL, et al. Proliferative response of bronchoalveolar lavage lymphocytes from heart-lung transplant patients. Transplantation 1990; 49:115-21.

62. Yousem SA, Berry G, Brunt EM, et al. A working formulation for the standardization of nomenclature in the diagnosis of pulmonary rejection: Lung Rejection Study Group. J Heart Transplant 1990;6:593-600.

63. De Hoyos A, Chamberlain D, Schvartzman R, et al. Prospective assessment of a standardized pathologic grading system for acute rejection in lung transplantation. Chest 1993;103:1813-18.

64. Palmer SM, Miralles AP, Lawrence CM, et al. Rabbit antithymocyte globulin decreases acute rejection after lung transplantation. Results of a randomized, prospective study. Chest 1999;116:127-33.

65. Levine SM, Bryan CL. Bronchiolitis obliterans in lung transplant recipients. The "thorn in the side" of lung transplantation. Chest 1995;107:894-96.

66. Nathan SD, Ross DJ, Belman MJ, et al. Bronchiolitis obliterans in single lung transplant recipients. Chest 1995;107:967-72.

67. Keller CA, Cagle PT, Brown RW, Noon G, Frost AE. Bronchiolitis obliterans in single, double, and heart lung transplantation. Chest 1995;107:973-80.

68. Burke CM, Glanville AR, Theodore J, et al. Lung immunogenicity, rejection, and obliterative bronchiolitis. Chest 1987;92:547-49.

69. McCarthy PM, Starnes VA, Theodore J, et al. Improved survival after heart-lung transplantation. J Thorac Cardiovasc Surg 1990;99:54-60.

70. Glanville AR, Baldwin JC, Burke CM, et al. Obliterative bronchiolitis after heart-lung transplantation: Apparent arrest by augmented immunosuppression. Ann Intern Med 1987;107:300-04.

71. Griffith BP, Paradis Il, Zeevi A, et al. Immunologically mediated disease of the airways after lung transplantation. Ann Surg 1988;208:371-78.

72. Scott JP, Sharples L, Mullins P, et al. Further studies on the natural history of obliterative bronchiolitis following heart-lung transplantation. transplant proc 1991; 23:1201-02.

73. Anzueto A, Levine SM, Bryan CL, et al. Obliterative bronchiolitis in single lung transplant recipients. Am Rev Respir Dis 1992;145:A700.

74. Trulock EP. Management of lung transplant rejection. Chest 1993;103:1566-76.

75. Cooper JD, Billingham M, Egan T, et al. A working formulation for the standardization of nomenclature and for clinical staging of chronic dysfunction in lung allografts: International Society for Heart and Lung Transplantation. J Heart Lung Transplant 1993;12:713-16.

76. Finkelstein SM, Snyder M, Stibbe CE, et al. Staging of bronchiolitis obliterans syndrome using home spirometry. Chest 1999;116:120-26.

77. Levine SM. Can bronchiolitis obliterans syndrome be diagnosed by phone from the comfort of home? Chest 1999;116:5-6.

78. Estenne M, Maurer JR, Boehler A, et al. Bronchiolitis obliterans syndrome 2001: An update of the diagnostic criteria. J Heart Lung Transplant 2002;21:297-310.

79. Hadjiliadis D, Davis RD, Palmer SM. Is transplant operation important in determining posttransplant risk of bronchiolitis obliterans syndrome in lung transplant recipients? Chest 2002;122:1168-75.

80. Levine SM. Lung transplantation and bronchiolitis obliterans syndrome. Are two lungs better than one? Chest 2002;122:1112-14.

81. Novick RJ, Kaye MP, Patterson GA, et al. Redo lung transplantation: A North American-European experience. J Heart Lung Transplant 1993;12:5-16.

82. Herve P, Silbert D, Cerrina J, et al. Impairment of mucocilliary clearance in long-term survivors of heart/lung and double lung transplantation. Chest 1993; 103:59-63.

83. Horvath J, Dummer S, Loyd J, et al. Infection in the transplanted and native lung after single lung transplantation. Chest 1993;104:681-85.

84. Dauber JH, Paradis IL, Dummer JS. Infectious complications in pulmonary allograft recipients. Clin Chest Med 1990;11:291-308.

85. Frost AE, Keller CA, Noon GP, et al. Outcome of the native lung after single lung transplant. Chest 1995;107:981-84.

86. Deusch E, End A, Grimm M, et al. Early bacterial infections in lung transplant recipients. Chest 1993;104: 412-16.

87. Dummer JS, White LT, Ho M, et al. Morbidity of cytomegalovirus infection in recipients of heart or heart-lung transplants who received cyclosporine. J Infect Dis 1985;152:1182-91.

88. Duncan AJ, Dfummer JS, Paradis IL, et al. Cytomegalovirus infection and survival in lung transplant recipients. J Heart Lung Transplant 1991;10:638-46.

89. Paradis IL, Grgurich WF, Dummer JS, Dekker A, Dauber JH. Rapid detection of cytomegalovirus pneumonia from lung lavage cells. Am Rev Respir Dis 1988;138:697-702.

90. Humbert M, Delattre M, Cerrina J, et al. Serum neopterin after lung transplantation. Chest 1993; 103:449-54.

91. Brumble LM, Milstone AP, Loyd JE, et al. Prevention of cytomegalovirus infection and disease after lung transplantation. Results using a unique regimen employing delayed ganciclovir. Chest 2002;121:407-14.

92. End A, Helbich T, Wisser W, Dekan G, Klepetko W. The pulmonary nodule after lung transplantation. Cause and outcome. Chest 1995;107:1317-22.

93. Registry of the International Society for Heart and Lung Transplantation.17th annual report, April 2000. Available at: http://www.ishlt.org. Accessed December 2002.

94. Bando K, Paradis IL, Komatsu K, et al. Analysis of time-dependent risks for infection, rejection, and death after pulmonary transplantation. Thorac Cardiovasc Surg 1995;109,49-59.

95. King RC, Binns O, Rodriguez F, et al. Reperfusion injury significantly impacts clinical outcome after pulmonary transplantation. Ann Thorac Surg 2000;69,1681-85.

96. De Hoyos AL, Patterson GA, Maurer JR, et al. Pulmonary transplantation: Early and late results. Thorac Cardiovasc Surg 1992;103,295-306.

97. Christie JD, Bavaria JE, Palevsky HI, et al. Primary graft failure following lung transplantation. Chest 1998; 114,51-60.

98. Sleiman C, Mal H, Fournier M, et al. Pulmonary reimplantation response in single-lung transplantation. Eur Respir J 1995;8,5-9.

99. Cooper JD, Alexander-Patterson G, Trulock EP. Results of single and bilateral lung transplantation in 131 consecutive recipients. Thorac Cardiovasc Surg 1994;107,460-71.

100. Davis RD, Trulock EP, Manley J, et al. Differences in early results after single-lung transplantation. Ann Thorac Surg 1994;58,1327-35.

101. Khan SU, Salloum J, O'Donovan PB, et al. Acute pulmonary edema after lung transplantation: The pulmonary reimplantation response. Chest 1999;116, 187-94.

102. Anderson DC, Glazer HS, Semenkovich JW, et al. Lung transplantation edema: Chest radiography after lung transplantation: The first 10 days. Radiology 1995; 195,275-81.

103. Bando K, Keenan RJ, Paradis IL, et al. Impact of pulmonary hypertension on outcome after single-lung transplantation. Ann Thorac Surg 1994;58,1336-42.

104. Aeba R, Griffith BP, Kormos RL, et al. Effect of cardiopulmonary bypass on early graft dysfunction in clinical lung transplantation. Ann Thorac Surg 1994; 57:715-22.

105. Sheridan PH, Cheriyan A, Doud J, et al. Incidence of phrenic neuropathy after isolated lung transplantation. J Heart Lung Transplant 1995;14,684-91.

106. Date H, Triantafillou AN, Trulock EP, et al. Inhaled nitric oxide reduces human lung allograft dysfunction. Thorac Cardiovasc Surg 1996;111,913-19.

107. Glassman LR, Keenan RJ, Fabrizio MC, et al. Extracorporeal membrane oxygenation as an adjunct treatment for primary graft failure in adult lung transplant recipients. Thorac Cardiovasc Surg 1995; 110,723-7.

108. Boujoukos AJ, Martich GD, Vega JD, et al. Reperfusion injury in single-lung transplant recipients with pulmonary hypertension and emphysema. J Heart Lung Transplant 1997;16,439-48.

109. Chatila WM, Furukawa S, Gaughan JP, Criner GJ. Respiratory failure after lung transplantation. Chest 2003;123:165-73.

110. Dawkins KD, Jamieson SW, Hunt SA, et al. Long term complications after combined heart and lung transplantation. Circulation 1985;71:919.

111. William TJ, Grossman RF, Maurer JR. Long-term functional follow-up of lung transplant recipients. Clin Chest Med 1990;11:347.

112. Burke CM, Baldwin JC, Morris AJ, et al. Twenty-eight cases of human heart lung transplantations. Lancet 1986;1:517.

113. Dawkins KD, Jamieson SW. Pulmonary function of the transplanted human lung. Annu Rev Med 1988;37:263.

114. Williams TJ, Patterson GA, McClean PA, Zamel N, Maurer JR. Maximal exercise testing in single and double lung transplant recipients. Am Rev Respir Dis 1992;145:101.

115. Nixon PA, Fricker FJ, Noyes BE, et al. Exercise testing in pediatric heart, heart-lung, and lung transplant recipients. Chest 1995;107:1328-35.

116. Busschbach JJ, Horikx PE, Van den Bosch JMM, et al. Measuring quality of life before and after bilateral lung transplantation in patients with cystic fibrosis. Chest 1994;105:911-17.

117. Whitehead BF, de Leval MR. Paediatric lung transplantation. The agony and ectasy. Thorax 1994;49:437-39.

118. The Transplantation of Human Organs Bill, 1994; Act No. 42/1994; Govt of India.

Chapter 33

Pediatric Lung Diseases

Most of the pulmonary disorders discussed in earlier chapters are applicable to children and most of these disorders are also common in them. However, some diseases like chronic bronchitis and emphysema, lung cancer, interstitial lung diseases, occupational lung diseases including pneumoconioses, ARDS, collagen vascular diseases affecting the lungs, pulmonary vasculitides, etc. are distinctly uncommon, although may occur exceptionally in pediatric age group. Pathophysiology, and clinical presentation of most of the other diseases described earlier will be same in children. This section will describe only some peculiar problems confined to pediatric population and some other clinical problems relevant to children. Congenital disorders of the lung and respiratory system are described earlier. Pulmonary physiology in children, acute respiratory infections, tuberculosis, bronchial asthma, and hyaline membrane disease will be described in some detail.

VENTILATORY FUNCTION IN CHILDREN

In the section on development and growth of lungs, the transition of respiration from the intrauterine life to the newborn has been discussed. In brief, surfactant appears by about the 28th week of intrauterine life, which has the effect of lowering the surface tension at the air-tissue interface, and once this happens, the lungs are capable of normal expansion and supporting of life. Before birth, the lungs do not expand and have a relatively smaller blood supply, and respiratory function of gas exchange in the fetus takes place through the placenta. During birth, the situation alters because of expansion of the lungs and because of the occlusion of the placental circulation. The hemoglobin concentration of the fetus is higher than that in the adult life and the oxyhemoglobin dissociation curve is to the left compared to that in the adult. This physiological adaptation facilitates oxygen uptake by the fetus from the maternal blood. The process is assisted by the passage of acid substances across the placenta in the reverse direction.

After birth, there is a change in the blood flow mainly because of expansion of the lungs, which reduces the resistance of pulmonary blood flow, and occlusion of placental circulation increases the resistance in the systemic circulation. These changes result in the development of a pressure gradient between the left and right atria and leads to the closure of the foramen ovale. Ductus arteriosus is occluded by active constriction of the smooth muscle in its wall.

Many workers have studied lung function parameters in the newborn and some of them are cited in Table 33.1. At birth the functional residual capacity (FRC) becomes stabilized within the first few breaths. After that the minute ventilation, alveolar ventilation, and work of breathing are comparable to adults when adjusted to metabolic rate.[1-7] The FRC is less than expected and is associated with a relatively high frequency of breathing. The ventilation and oxygen consumption of oxygen are dependent on the weight of the baby. The consumption is less on the day of birth and subsequently increases. It diminishes when the baby is hypoxic and varies with the ambient and deep body temperatures.

The lungs of children are smaller and the muscles of respiration are relatively inefficient compared to adults. These differences affect the lung function parameters in them. However, the ratios like residual volume (RV)/total lung capacity (TLC) and the FEV_1/FVC are unaffected because of these differences.

TABLE 33.1: Approximate values of lung function in newborn (3 kg weight)

Parameter	Value
Respiratory rate (per min)	25-40
Expired gas volume (ml/min BTPS)	550
Tidal volume (ml)	17
Dead space (ml)	9
Oxygen consumption (ml/min)	23
Compliance (L/cm H_2O)	0.003-0.006
Resistance (cm H_2O/L/Sec)	20-40

The relationship of lung function and age is very poor in children and the best correlation is with the height. The difference is most marked at the age of 12 years because the acceleration of growth at puberty occurs earlier in some children than in others. However, such discrepancies can be avoided when the indices of lung function are related to body size. Up to the age of puberty, the values are similar for boys and girls, after which they differ significantly.

As discussed earlier, the parameters of various lung functions should be established for each laboratory and population group before applying them for clinical use. Although data is available for many western countries, such information is not available for many countries particularly India, but some parameters like peak expiratory flow rates are available for Indian children. Besides the ethnic differences, other factors that may affect lung function include climate, nutrition, physical fitness, and impact of the personality of the operator. Various parameters of ventilatory function are depicted in Table 33.2.[1-5] The data is mainly from the European children.

The total lung capacity and its subdivisions are smaller in children than in young adults. However, the RV/TLC is about 24 percent as in the latter. Airway resistance measured at functional residual capacity is greater in children than in adults because of the smaller airways diameter. Thus, the ventilatory capacity will be less compared with the maximum breathing capacity or the forced expiratory volume. The bellowing function of a child's lung is more efficient than in the adult. Thus,

TABLE 33.3: Respiratory rates per minute of normal children

Age	Sleeping Mean	Sleeping Range	Awake Mean	Awake Range
6-12 months	27	22-31	64	58-75
1-2 yrs	19	17-23	35	30-40
2-4 yrs	19	16-25	31	23-42
4-6 yrs	18	14-23	26	19-36
6-8 yrs	17	13-23	23	15-30

children can expire a larger proportion of their vital capacity in 1 second compared to adults. Similarly, the airways conductance expressed per unit of the thoracic gas volume is greater than it is in the adults because the airways remain relatively widely open in them. On the other hand, overall compliance of the lung is lower during childhood. However, specific compliance standardized for the size of the lung, is similar to that in the adults.

The different respiratory frequency in children and adults is mainly because of altered mechanical properties of the lungs. The rate is highest in the infants and decreases progressively during childhood. Normal values at different ages are shown in Table 33.3.

The tidal volume is small in small children. The relatively large dead space ventilation augments the minute ventilation and when standardized for the consumption of oxygen tends to be higher than in adults. However, alveolar ventilation when standardized for minute ventilation is relatively independent of age. The total surface area for the alveolar capillary membranes and their volume is less in children since they depend on the lung size. Accordingly, the transfer factor is less in children. However, when expressed per liter of lung volume as the diffusion constant, higher values are observed in children.

ACUTE RESPIRATORY INFECTIONS (ARI)

Acute respiratory infections (ARI) are major causes of morbidity and mortality in children worldwide, particularly in developing countries, second only to diarrheal diseases among the acute infectious diseases. While the mortality due to ARI is about 30 to 40 per 100,000 live births in developed countries, the same may be many more times in developing nations, the figures reaching as high as 1000 or more per 100,000 live births. In these countries, a child under the age of 5 years dies every 7 seconds because of an ARI. In both the developed and developing countries, in the average child, 20 to 30 episodes of ARI occur in the first 5 years of life. About four and a half million children die of this every year accounting for 30 percent of all deaths in childhood.

TABLE 33.2: Predicted values for lung function parameters. The regression relationship is drawn on the basis of height (h)

Parameter	Value	Standard deviation
Total lung capacity (L)	1.19 h	12.2%
Vital capacity (L)	0.907 h	12.6%
Functional residual capacity (L)	0.483 h	15.4%
Residual volume (L)	0.263 h	19.7%
FEV, (L)	$0.708 H^3 + 0.11$	9%
PEFR (L/min)	547 h - 460	13.4%
	-370.16 + 5.03 K*	Boys
	-252.08 + 3.93 H*	Girls
Airway resistance (cm $H_2O/l/sec$)	$antilog_{10}(1.599-0.0068 h)$	42%
Compliance (ml/cm H_2O)	41.0 h	32%
Transfer factor for the lung (ml/min/rnm Hg)	$antilog_{10} (0.656 h + 0.308)$ —	
Diffusing capacity of the alveolar capillary membrane (ml/min/mm Hg)	$antilog_{10}(0.855 h + 0.333)$	

* Value for Indian tribal children

Pneumonia unassociated with measles causes 70 percent of these deaths; post-measles pneumonia 15 percent; pertussis 10 percent; and bronchiolitis or croup 5 percent. The mortality rates are more in the developing than in the developed countries. This wide difference is mainly attributable to malnutrition, poverty, lack of health education, large family size, lateness in the birth order, crowding, low birth weight, vitamin A deficiency, lack of breastfeeding, pollution, young age, improper utilization of available health facilities and bacterial infections prevalent in these countries. About half of all illnesses in children below the age of 5 years are due to ARI and about a third in children in the age group of 5 to 12 years. Almost 25 percent of all pediatric admissions in developing countries are because of ARI. While most infections involve the upper respiratory tract, only about 5 percent involve the lower respiratory tract. However, death rates are higher in the latter group.[8-18]

ARI can be either classified on anatomical basis or on the basis of etiology. The classification is shown in Table 33.4.

Most of the ARI are restricted to the upper respiratory tract and Viruses cause more than 90 percent of these. Respiratory viral infections have a major impact on public health. Acute respiratory infections largely caused by viruses, are the most common illnesses experienced by otherwise healthy adults and children. Among the respiratory viruses, influenza viruses are known to cause outbreaks globally.

The etiology of pneumonias on the other hand is of bacterial origin particularly in developing countries. The most important bacterial agents are *Streptococcus pneumoniae*, *Haemophilus influenzae* and *Staphylococcus aureus*. The data on bacterial etiology of pneumonia during the first three months of life are limited, and almost no information on the role of chlamydia and pertussis in this age group is available. The distribution of viral pathogens in developing countries can be summarized as follows:

Respiratory syncytial virus	15-20 percent
Parainfluenza viruses	7-10 percent
Influenza A, B, and adenovirus	2-4 percent
Mixed viral and bacterial infections very frequent	

ARI in India

Acute viral respiratory infections causing significant morbidity are the most common illnesses experienced by otherwise healthy adults and children.[19] Mortality due to acute viral respiratory illness in economically-developed countries is less compared to the developing countries.[20] The mortality rate due to acute respiratory infection was estimated to be approximately 2707/

TABLE 33.4: Classification of ARI

I. Anatomical classification of ARI
Upper respiratory tract Infections
- Common colds
- Sinusitis
- Pharyngitis
- Tonsillitis
- Otitis media

Lower respiratory tract infections
- Laryngotracheobronchitis
- Epiglottitis
- Acute bronchitis
- Bronchiolitis
- Pneumonias

II. Etiological classification

A. *ARI of viral origin*	
Common cold (Coryza)	Rhinovirus, adenovirus, enterovirus, influenza, and parainfluenza viruses
Acute sinusitis and otitis media	Same as above
Sore throat	Adenovirus, influenza virus, enterovirus, parainfluenza virus, coxsackie virus
Infectious croup	Parainfluenza virus, adenovirus (mainly laryngotracheitis)
Bronchiolitis	Respiratory syncitial virus
Pneumonia	Parainfluenza virus, respiratory syncitial virus, influenza virus, rhinovirus
B. *ARI of bacterial origin*	
Acute sinusitis and otitis media	*Streptococcus pneumoniae*, *Haemophilus influenzae*, *Branhamella catarrhalis*
Sore throat	Beta hemolytic Group A Streptococcus
Infectious croup (Diphtheria, Epiglottitis, Bacterial tracheitis)	*Corynebacterium diphtheriae*, *Haemophilus influenzae*, *Staphylococcus aureus*
Pertussis	*Bordetella pertussis*
Pneumonia	*Streptococcus pneumoniae*, *Haemophilus influenzae*, *Staphylcoccus aureus*

1,00,000 children (under 1 yr) in rural India.[21] Monthly incidence of respiratory infections is 23 percent in urban area and 17.65 percent in rural area.[22] Outbreaks of respiratory tract infections are also common in tertiary care centers for the aged.[23]

Influenza viruses are known to cause frequent epidemics and periodic pandemics, and are unique with regard to their antigenic variability, seasonality and impact on general population. Though children are mainly affected during epidemics,[24] these are also responsible for substantial mortality in the aged and chronically ill persons.[25]

Studies on the etiology of acute respiratory infections have been carried out in many parts of India.[26,27] Seroepidemiological studies have been conducted during 1997 to 1999 in Pune.[28] Spectrum of influenza activity is not known in southern states of India except for a seroprevalence study conducted in Vellore. Influenza viral activity in Chennai, a coastal city with high humidity is not known.

While bacterial infection is less common than viral lower respiratory infections (LRI), the risk of death is far greater with the former. The estimated case fatality rate for bacterial pneumonia due to *Streptococcus pneumoniae,* and *Haemophilus influenzae* in developing countries is more than 50 times higher than that due to RSV or parainfluenza virus infection. Yet the estimated number of deaths due to bacterial pneumonia is only 2.7 times higher than the number due to the viral infections. Both the viral and bacterial infections are important contributors to the excessive ARI in developing countries. Nasopharyngeal secretions and throat-swab specimens from 809 children from a South Indian hospital below the age of 6 years with ARI-were examined by culture and indirect immunofluorescence for the presence of virus or viral antigens.[9] Blood and pleural fluid were examined to isolate bacteria in LRI. Viruses were detected in 495 of cases with LRI. RSV was the commonest agent isolated. Other viruses isolated were parainfluenza virus, adenovirus, and influenza virus. Outbreaks of infection due to RSV occurred during the period between August through October. Pneumonia was the commonest LRI and amongst children with pneumonia, viruses were detected in 37 percent of the cases and bacteria from 18 percent of the cases in the blood culture.

RSV and parainfluenza viruses are most frequently isolated infectious microorganisms in infants and children with LRIs. RSV is found in 40 to 80 percent of infants hospitalized with bronchiolitis and in 20 to 25 percent of infants hospitalized with pneumonia. Parainfluenza viruses are found in 10 to 15 percent of infants with bronchiolitis and pneumonia and in 40 percent of infants with croup. Parainfluenza virus type 1 is the most common cause of croup with the type 3 and parainfluenza type 2 are the second and third most frequent causes. Parainfluenza virus type 3 is also a common cause of pneumonia and bronchitis; type 1 and 2 are found less frequently. Bronchiolitis and pneumonia due to RSV occur commonly at the age of 2 to 3 months. Although the peak age of these diseases due to parainfluenza virus type 3 is 2 to 4 months, parainfluenza type 1 causing croup peaks at 9 to 24 months. As against RSV infection occurring in winter or early spring, outbreaks of parainfluenza virus type 1 infection occur every other year in the autumn. The seasonality of parainfluenza virus type 3 is more variable, and the virus can be endemic, with infections found throughout the year. This type 3 virus has tended to produce yearly outbreaks in the late winter and early spring.

Inoculation of the RSV and parainfluenza virus presumably occurs through the nasal mucosal surface. RSV can also be introduced through the conjunctiva. In the child who has not previously experienced infection with one of these viruses, inoculation is followed by an asymptomatic incubation period of 4 to 5 days for RSV and 2 to 4 days for parainfluenza virus. At the end of this period the child develops symptoms of upper respiratory tract infection (URI). This phase is characterized by rhinorrhea and progresses over several days to nasal obstruction, low-grade fever, and cough. The infection usually resolves slowly, the only common complication of such a URI being otitis because of obstruction of the eustachean tube. In more severely affected infants, the disease may spread to the lower respiratory tract. This spread of virus occurs presumably through aspiration of infected secretions. During peak of rhinorrhea in RSV infection, which usually precedes the onset of lower respiratory tract symptoms, secretions are profuse and large amounts of virus to the tune of 10^5 to 10^6 infectious units/ml of secretion. Thus, aspiration of even a small amount of secretion into the bronchi or bronchioles would increase the chance of lower respiratory tract infection. Bronchiolitis and pneumonia due to these viruses are diffuse and bilateral, therefore aspiration must also be diffuse and bilateral, and the virus spreads widely and quickly to involve all lobes and lobules soon after aspiration. Presumably, this spread occurs during the period of profuse rhinorrhea, although that can occur even before. During this period of viral activity, immune response of the body responds in the form of the appearance of a coating of IgA and IgM on virus-infected cells shed from the respiratory epithelium.

Detailed pathological changes are discussed subsequently.

Information on the activity of influenza virus in India is limited. A study was carried out to isolate and identify the influenza virus serotypes causing acute respiratory infection in children attending a tertiary care center at Chennai. During January to December 2002, convenient sampling included 240 children with acute respiratory infection attending the out patient clinic of Institute of Child Health. Throat swabs were collected from 4 to 5 cases every week. Isolation of influenza virus was attempted by inoculating the sample in Madin Darby Canine Kidney (MDCK) cell line. The isolates were typed by hemagglutination inhibition test and confirmed by immunofluorescence assay. Virus isolation was positive in 30 (12.5%) of the 240 samples. Influenza A/H3N2/Panama/2000/99 was the predominant serotype isolated accounting for 24 (80%) of the 30 isolates. Influenza B/Sichuan/379/99 was isolated in 4 (13.33%) and a combination of Influenza A/H3N2 and B/Sichuan in 2 (6.6%) of the isolates. The study concluded that isolation of influenza A and B viruses indicated a significant activity of these viruses in Chennai. Peak activity was observed during and after the first spell of rain. The predominance of A/H3N2/ Panama is an indication that the Indian scenario is similar to the global picture of influenza activity.[29]

A prospective study on 93 children admitted to Kasturba Medical College Hospital, Manipal and TMA Pai Rotary Hospital of Udupi and Karkala was carried out to find out the *Mycoplasma pneumoniae* infection in children. Blood samples from 93 children admitted to the ward with no respiratory illness were taken as age-matched controls for the inpatients; IgM antibody against Mycoplasma pneumoniae was detected using a commercial kit following the manufacturer's instructions. 23.96 percent of the inpatients with respiratory tract symptoms had IgM antibodies against *Mycoplasma pneumoniae*. The highest infection rate was found to be in the 2 to 5 and 5 to 10 year age group. The most common mode of presentation was an upper respiratory focus of infection with cervical lymphadenopathy. Bronchial breathing signifying pneumonic consolidation was significantly less in the Mycoplasma positive group (p = 0.006). There was no statistically significant difference in the radiological findings in the Mycoplasma positive and Mycoplasma negative groups.[30]

Various clinical entities due to different viruses are described in the chapter on pneumonias. A brief account of some of the other entities not covered in that chapter is presented here.

Acute Otitis Media

Although the infection may be self-limiting, most authors opine that prompt and appropriate antibiotic should be instituted. Viruses may cause mucosal damage. Amoxycillin or co-trimoxazole should be given for 10 to 14 days. Improvement is observed within 48 to 72 hours of institution of therapy. Persistence of severe otalgia, fever, and toxemia indicate immediate tympanocentesis and a change in antibiotics. Antihistamines and decongestants are not required and on the other hand, may produce unpleasant side effects.

Acute Sinusitis

Diagnosis of acute sinusitis in children is often difficult because of lack of specific symptoms and signs. This may constitute about 0.5 to 5 percent of all cases of ARI. Antibiotic therapy is needed for the condition to reduce complications like orbital and intracranial infections. Sinus aspiration will be needed if pain persists despite antibiotic therapy.

Sore Throat (Acute Pharyngitis/Tonsillitis)

Most common cause of sore throats is viral, although bacterial infections due to Beta-hemolytic streptococcus group A is isolated in 10 to 33 percent of cases. Lymph nodes are usually firmer and tenderness is less marked in viral sore throats compared to the sore throats due to bacteria. Petechiae and follicular pus points on the fauces favor bacterial etiology. Beta-hemolytic streptococcus infection has a more acute onset and involvement of the mucosa of the nose and eyes are more common in viral infections. However, at times the differentiation between the two is very difficult, although not impossible. In the tropics, infection with streptococcus can occur even in children younger than 4 years. Penicillin is the drug of choice and the duration of therapy is for 10 days. Shorter courses of therapy fail to eradicate the organism and increase the chances of recurrence.

Infectious Croup

The croup syndrome is characterized by inspiratory stridor, cough, and hoarseness and due to obstruction in the region of the larynx. Inflammatory edema and spasm are the causes of obstruction. The syndrome is potentially a life-threatening emergency. Acute laryngotracheitis, epiglottitis, diphtheria, and bacterial tracheitis are important causes of infectious croup. The latter three need antibiotic therapy. Maintenance of adequate airway is crucial to the management of such a patient.[31]

Laryngotracheitis is a viral infection due to parainfluenza type 1,3, RSV, and parainfluenza virus type 2 in that order. The disease is insidious in onset and brassy cough is the characteristic feature of the disorder. Downes score based on the presence of stridor, cough, retraction and nasal flaring, cyanosis, and inspiratory breath sounds can assess the severity.

Epiglottitis is a fulminant bacterial infection due to *Hemophilus influenzas* type B, which involves the epiglottis, arytenoids, aryepiglottic folds, and uvula. The child is very toxic and respiratory distress is very common.

Diphtheria is a bacterial infection and is usually seen in an unimmunized or incompletely immunized child. The disease rarely causes tracheitis without marked supraglottic involvement. The disease is characterized by a membrane formation in the pharynx and, sometimes, in and around the larynx. The child often looks ill and the toxicity is out of proportion to the fever. Sporadic croup is a sudden attack of croup during night times and allergy and virus infections are the causes of the disorder.

Bacterial tracheitis (pseudomembranous croup, membranous laryngotracheo-bronchitis) is mainly caused by *Staphylococcus aureus* and characterized by high fever, severe airways obstruction, toxicity, and subglottic narrowing. Pus will be seen coming out of the glottic opening.

LOWER RESPIRATORY TRACT INFECTIONS

Bronchiolitis and pneumonia are the two important components of lower respiratory tract infections. As discussed earlier, viruses are the most important causes of this disorder. Bacterial infections can cause pneumonias. In fact, bacteria are the most important cause of pneumonia in children from developing countries.

Bronchiolitis

Bronchiolitis is an acute lower respiratory tract infection of the small airways and occurs in children between the age group of 2 months to 2 years.[32] It consists of about 8.5 percent of total respiratory diseases seen in hospitalized children. Respiratory syncytial virus (RSV) is the main offending agent, although other viruses like adenovirus, enterovirus, parainfluenza virus (type 1 and 3), and rhinovirus can produce this syndrome. Amongst 116 children with bronchiolitis from a South Indian Hospital, 83 (72%) had viral infections and the commonest virus was RSV (81%).

The disease is characterized by necrosis of the epithelium in the bronchioles and peribronchiolar lymphocytic infiltrations. The submucosa may be edematous. Other pathological changes include epithelial damage associated with edema, epithelial sloughing, squamous metaplasia, goblet cell metaplasia, and fibrinous plugging of the small bronchioles. Bronchiolitis obliterans is an extreme consequence of a progressive formation of necrotic lesions that leads to permanent destruction of small airways. At autopsy only remnants of bronchioles or scar tissues adjacent to bronchial arteries can be identified. Other components including the alveoli are usually spared. Bronchioles of 75 to 300 µm in size are commonly affected, because of partial obstruction of bronchioles, air trapping occurs distal to the lesions resulting in over inflation of alveoli. Consequently, obstructive emphysema and patchy atelectasis occurs. Complete obstruction will lead to more atelectasis seen as multiple diffuse infiltrates, which may be patchy or lobar.

With recovery, bronchiolar epithelium regenerates within 3 to 4 days, but recovery of cilia takes much longer.

Since the overall airways resistance in children lies mostly in the peripheral airways compared to that in the adults; -bronchiolitis is more severe in the pediatric population. Secondly, because of smaller dimensions, same amount of cellular debris and edema will produce more obstruction as compared to older children. Inadequate development of collateral ventilation in infants contributes to the development of patchy atelectasis in some areas and overdistension in other areas. Moreover, the bronchiolar epithelium is more loosely attached in infants. Since the soft tissue is proportionately more, edema is much more. The dynamic compliance is decreased with increased airways resistance and thus, the work of breathing is increased considerably.

The usual clinical features include cough, dyspnea, chest retraction, rhonchi, crepitations, and tachycardia. Respiratory distress and cyanosis may be present in severe cases. Initial upper respiratory tract infection in the form of mild rhinorrhea, cough, low-grade fever, mild conjunctivitis, otitis media, and pharyngitis are usual. The causative RSV can be identified in the nasal washings by immunofluorescence technique within few hours. Culture of the virus takes about 3 to 4 days.

The first attack of bronchial asthma may be difficult to differentiate from bronchiolitis, which may be easier if there is history of more such attacks and there is a family history of bronchial asthma or atopy. Viral myocarditis may present with similar features, which can be differentiated by careful physical examination, chest X-ray, and electrocardiogram. Laryngeal obstruction and lobar emphysema may rarely be confused with this condition.

Generally, bronchiolitis is a mild, self-limiting illness requiring only supportive therapy and close observation. However, in about 5 percent of cases it may be severe enough to warrant hospitalization, few of which may require ventilatory support. The usual treatment for bronchiolitis includes oxygen therapy (in moderate and severe cases, 30 to 40% are usually adequate); and intravenous fluid administration in dehydrated cases at 1 to 1.5 times the maintenance requirements with care to avoid overhydration. Antimicrobials are usually not recommended except with rising fever, development of fever while on ventilator, or when there is sudden deterioration of the clinical condition with a suspicion of infection.

Aerosolized ribavirin gives good results and has been discussed earlier in greater details. Bronchodilators have no role in the management of bronchiolitis except when it is not possible to differentiate the condition from bronchial asthma. Some pediatricians use theophylline in severe cases. Corticosteroids have no beneficial effect. Ventilatory support is mandatory if the child is seriously ill. Continuous positive airways pressure (CPAP) ventilation can easily be given by nasal cannulation alone. Intermittent positive pressure breathing (IPPB) is indicated in the face of decreased responsiveness, and allergy, apneic spells, little spontaneous breathing, and hypercarbia of more than 60 mm Hg. Children tolerate carbon dioxide retention quite well. Since RSV is shed for many days after the onset of illness, the infants should be looked after in isolation and child-to-child contact should be avoided. Frequent hand washing prevents spread of the virus.

The response is usually very good even in hospitalized patients, although about 20 percent of cases may have a protracted course with persistent wheezing and hyperinflation of the chest, which may persist for many months. Obstructive collapse may not clear for several weeks. Occasionally pneumothorax and pneumomediastinum may develop, particularly in those who receive assisted ventilation. Sudden apnea may occur very rarely. The mortality varies from 1 to 8.3 percent and infants below the age of 6 months are more susceptible. Abnormal arterial blood gases and pulmonary function abnormalities may be present for as long as 12 months. These children are more prone to develop chronic obstructive lung disease in adult life. Although the relationship of bronchiolitis and subsequent development of bronchial asthma is not well defined, approximately one-third to one-half of these cases with bronchiolitis will develop bronchial asthma, particularly in those who are atopic and in those where there is family history of bronchial asthma.

Pneumonias

The etiology of pneumonia in childhood is discussed earlier. Viruses are the most common cause, although bacterial pneumonia also does occur.[33-42] The pathogenesis of pneumonia in children depends on both the etiologic agent and the immune defence mechanisms of the host. Host defence mechanisms have already been described in chapter 5. In brief, antigen-specific host protective factors include both humoral and cellular immunity. Nonspecific host defences include a normal flora, intact epithelium like the skin and mucosa, cilia, phagocytic cells, and soluble substances, particularly secretory IgA, lysozymes, and interferon. In respiratory infection, bacteria and viruses utilize proteases, adhesions, and surface structures to damage epithelial surface receptors. Adequate nutrition is required to maintain host defences. A deficient or impaired immune mechanism increases the susceptibility to fatal respiratory infections.[43,44]

It is proposed that malnutrition, especially vitamin A deficiency, is responsible for the high case fatality rate in the developing world. Vitamin A deficiency causes squamous metaplasia of the epithelial surfaces, particularly in the tracheobronchial tree. The deficiency impairs the integrity, differentiation, and regenerative capability of respiratory epithelium. Defective epithelium provides portal of entry for both viruses and bacteria. Deficiency of other micronutrients, particularly zinc (and vitamin A), impairs many immune functions. Infections in other systems like the urinary tract and the gastrointestinal tract are more in vitamin A deficient patients and the pathogenesis is same as in xerophthalmia. Some believe that vitamin A supplement will reduce the mortality from respiratory tract infection. Protein-calorie malnutrition produces lymphoid involution, particularly in the thymus. This lymphoid deficiency is associated with defective hypersensitivity, depression of CD4+ helper cells, loss of secretory IgA, decreased bactericidal activity of polymorphonuclear cells, and depressed complement system. This disorder has been termed as nutritionally acquired immunodeficiency syndrome (NAIDS) and is a worldwide problem. NAIDS currently claims more lives of children than does AIDS due to HIV.

Viral Infections

These begin with attachment of virions to the mucosal surface. In some cases, changes in the infected cell surface can aggregate cells into syncytial giant cells. Virus particles are then passed between contiguous cells. Once the virus is present inside the cell, it regulates the synthetic process in the cell and produces more virions. Cytolysis releases free virus particles, which infect additional cells. Systemic illness follows episodes of viremia. Viral pneumonia can manifest in three major forms:

   i. Bronchiolitis
  ii. Interstitial pneumonia
 iii. Pneumonia associated with viral inclusions.
   Bronchiolitis has been discussed in detail above.

Interstitial pneumonia: Lymphocytic infiltration occurs within the alveolar walls and around the smaller airways. There is also engorgement of the capillary bed, edema, and a cytopathic effect on the alveolar or bronchial cells. The presence of interstitial infiltrates with focal variations with the stage and severity of disease is the hallmark of viral pneumonia. Exudation and characteristic inclusion bodies may be seen. With progression of disease, thickened alveolar walls may be lined with pink proteinaceous material. These hyaline, refractory, eosinophilic membranes are characteristic but not specific of viral pneumonias.

Viral inclusions. Cytomegalo virus infection produces pathognomonic large infected cells, about 25 to 40 µm in diameter, which have characteristic owl's-eye appearance. The nuclei contain single, large, hematoxylin-positive inclusions surrounded by clear halos. Recently infected cells may have minute basophilic granules in the cytoplasm. Adenovirus produces amphophilic intranuclear inclusions with smudgy edges in bronchial and bronchiolar epithelial cells. RSV does not produce Syncytia in vivo. A minute basophilic inclusion in the cytoplasm has been described. Measles giant cells have eosinophilic nuclear inclusions with a halo. These cells may contain a few or a hundred nuclei per single syncytial giant cell. The measles virus may infect the lymphoid cells and, particularly cortical necrosis of the thymus, may contribute to the defective cellular immunity that provides an opportunity for a post measles bacterial or viral infections. Such post measles infections are fatal in malnourished children with marginal immune function. Giant cell pneumonia occurs exclusively in an immunodeficient host. Necrosis of the epithelial cells and the postmeasles immune deficit accounts for the high incidence of measles mortality in children. Vitamin A and zinc deficiency potentiates this problem.

Bacterial Pneumonias

The common bacteria causing pneumonia in children are *Streptococcus pneumoniae, Hemohilus influenzas,* and *Staphylococcus aureus,* particularly the community-acquired pneumonias. While the first two are the most common isolates, the latter is common in pneumonias that follow infections like influenza and measles.[32-41]

Five distinct histologic patterns of pneumonia occur:[45,46]

   i. Lobar pneumonia. This involves an entire lobe or lung segment and is most frequently associated with *Streptococcus pneumoniae*
  ii. Bronchopneumonia affects the airways and most common organism is *Staphylococcus aureus*
 iii. Necrotizing Gram-negative bacterial pneumonia frequently follows aspiration
 iv. Tuberculous pneumonia may resemble acute pyogenic pneumonia in the acute phase
  v. Bacterial superinfection following viral pneumonias, which includes interstitial and peribronchiolar lymphocytes with necrosis of epithelium and bronchopneumonia and/or aspiration pneumonia.

Precise contribution of bacteria in the etiology of pneumonia is difficult to determine because of many reasons. Isolation rates of the organisms in blood culture are low. Culture of a bacterial pathogen from the upper respiratory tract is no evidence that the organism is responsible for pneumonia because of the normal colonization of many organisms. Lung puncture is not routinely indicated in many cases. Rapid diagnostic tests like latex agglutination, and coagulatination and counterimmunoelectrophoresis (CIEP) may be helpful but are expensive and not easily available at all places.

Procaine penicillin is the drug of choice for the treatment of pneumonia at any level of primary health care service.[47-50] Adequate serum levels are achieved even after when given intramuscularly once a day and are effective against pneumonia due to *Streptococcus pneumoniae* and *H. influenzae.* Benzyl penicillin can be given intravenously in a dose of 50,000 units/kg/day in divided doses for a period of 5 to 7 days. Subsequently, this can be substituted by oral penicillin V in a dose of 250 mg six hourly. Recent reports indicate some concern regarding the penicillin resistance of pneumococcal pneumonia particularly in developing countries. Some prefers Amoxycillin and ampicillin in daily doses of 50 to 150 mg/kg as the first line of treatment in- community acquired pneumonia. When *Staphylococcal pneumonia* seems likely, cloxacillin in a dose of 50 mg/kg/day can be added. At present most of the Staphylococcal infections whether community acquired or hospital acquired are penicillin resistant. Therefore, initiation of therapy should be with the semisynthetic beta-lactamase resistant penicillins like methicillin, nafcillin, or oxacillin. Some advocate simultaneous administration of gentamycin for synergistic effect. In field conditions when injectables are not feasible, co-trimoxazole is a suitable alternative, since it is effective against pneumococcus, *H. influenzae,* and *S. aureus.* The drug is cheaper, and can be given twice daily and is well tolerated. However, it has not been used very frequently in neonates and young infants. Newer cephalosporins like cefaclor and cefuroxime axetil (100 mg/kg/day) can be used in severe infections. Erythromycin (50 mg/kg/day) and chloramphenicol (50 mg/kg/day) are other alternative drugs. The former is particularly useful in atypical pneumonias. The latter drug is an alternative to ampicillin for *H. influenzae* infection.

A detailed description of bacterial pneumonias is given in the chapter on pneumonias.

Mixed Pneumonia

Mixed viral and bacterial infection is more common than pneumonia due to virus alone. Viral infections promote epithelial cell desquamation and destruction of mucociliary defenses, which increase bacterial adherence and set the stage for secondary bacterial pneumonia. Type A and B influenza viruses specifically target ciliated epithelial cells. Regeneration of epithelial cells starts from the existing basal cell layer. Six days after the insult, transitional polyhedral epithelium appears. Columnar cells with cilia replace these cells. The restorative process may take several weeks and bacterial infection may cause death during these periods. Superinfection with *Streptococcus pneumoniae, Hemophilus influenzae,* and *Staphylococcus aureus* may follow influenza or measles. Giant cell pneumonia has been associated with subsequent adenovirus or herpes virus infection. Infection with RSV may be followed by *Streptococcus pneumoniae, or Hemophilus influenzae,* pneumonia. The histopathological features of both viral and bacterial pneumonia are observed in these mixed infections.

Supportive Therapy in ARI

Supportive therapy may be required in cases of ARI, although evidence as regards its effectiveness in all cases has not been tested by well-conducted controlled trials. Steam inhalation, cough suppressants/mucolytics, nasal decongestants, and antihistaminics have no proven

value. However, care should be taken to ensure that fluid intake is adequate and breastfeeding is continued. Forced feeding should be avoided. The child should be nursed in a neutral environment. Paracetamol in a dose of 10 to 15 mg/kg/ dose orally should be given every 6 hourly if the axillary temperature exceeds 38.5° C. Sponging with cold water is better avoided. Humidified oxygen (40%) by mask or intranasal catheter is indicated if: *(i)* the respiratory rate is more than 70; (ii) the child has wheeze; or *(iii)* cyanosis.

WHO Protocol for ARI Management

The overall objective of the program is to reduce the morbidity and mortality from ARI, the major emphasis being on the prevention of death from pneumonia.[51,52] The recommendations comprise of health education, standard case management, and immunization. Standard case management consists of discrimination of severity, use of antimicrobials at village level, and referral of severe cases. The recommendations are based on the studies of Leventhal and Shann. Tachypnea, chest indrawing and inability to drink are the three important signs that decide severity. In children with cough, a respiratory rate greater than 40 or 50 per minute or a qualitative impression of tachypnea is probably the best indicator of the need for starting antibiotic treatment by the village level health worker. The presence of fever is a poor guide to start antibiotic therapy. The presence of chest indrawing is, however, a reliable indicator in a child with cough for admission into a hospital. Cherian *et al* while studying about 700 children found that respiratory rates of over 50/min in infants and over 40 in children 12 to 35 months of age, as well as a history of rapid breathing and the presence of chest retraction in both age groups were found to be specific and sensitive indicators of lower respiratory tract infections (LRI). Increased respiratory rates and history of rapid breathing were also sensitive in diagnosing less severe LRI that did not necessitate admission to the wards, whereas chest retraction does not. All these clinical signs, however, had a low sensitivity in diagnosing LRI in children aged 36 months and over. An useful classification of ARI is shown in Tables 33.5 with appropriate suggested interventions.

Prevention of ARI

Some of the major bacterial and viral causes of morbidity and mortality due to ARI are amenable to control by vaccines.[53-55] Among the vaccine preventable serious ARI, diphtheria, pertussis, and measles immunization, in appropriately scheduled programs, can make an

TABLE 33.5: Classification of ARI and suggested management plan

Mild ARI
- Cough, hoarseness, wheeze or fever, respiratory rate < 50/min
- Stridor that goes away when the child is at rest, i.e. not crying or upset
- Red throat
- Blocked or runny nose
- Earache or discharge for more than 2 weeks
  Treatment: Supportive; no antimicrobials

Moderate ARI
- Cough and fast breathing with respiratory rate > 50/min, no chest indrawing
- Wheeze and fast breathing between 50-70/min
- Red ear drum, or ear discharge for less than 2 weeks (or ear ache if no otoscope available)
- Purulent pharyngitis with large, lender cervical lymph nodes
  Treatment: Antimicrobials at home plus supportive treatment

Severe ARI
- Cough and chest indrawing but no wheeze
- Wheeze and respiratory rate > 70/min
  Treatment: Needs admission and benzyl penicillin

Very severe ARI
- Cough or wheeze with cyanosis or unable to drink
  Treatment: Patient needs admission. Chloramphenicol to be added and oxygen therapy needed

immediate contribution to the reduction of severe ARI. Immunization against measles at the age of 9 to 11 months, with a 80 to 90 percent coverage, and with a 90 percent efficacy (seroconversion), 59 to 67 percent of measles cases and deaths can be achieved and overall reduction of 20 to 25 percent of ARI related deaths in children under the age of 5 years. Emerging technologies offer the promise of vaccines against bacterial and viral respiratory pathogens that are suitable for infants and children, particularly in the developing countries. These advances include the use of protein-polysaccharide conjugates of endemic serotypes for *Hemophilias influenzae* and *Streptococcus pneumoniae* vaccines. Other new approaches include the use of purified protein components or attenuated live virus with respiratory syncytial virus and paramyxovirus vaccines, which are expected to be available soon for evaluation.

Breastfeeding, correction of malnutrition, prevention of vitamin A deficiency, and a reduction of low birth weight babies are useful preventive measures to reduce ARI morbidity and mortality. It is also advisable that infants should not be taken to congregations and fairs as that increases the risk of exposure to infected persons. Similarly, harmful practices like instillation of oils into the nostrils and feeding of butter oil increases the chances of lipid pneumonia. Recent studies show that air pollution, both indoor and outdoor, increases the chances of respiratory tract infections. Indoor air pollution due to cooking with biomass fuel increases the chances of ARI. Passive smoking and overcrowding are other risk factors. All of these factors are avoidable, and thus, can contribute significantly in reducing the morbidity and deaths from ARI.

REFERENCES

1. Lung function at different stages in life, including normal values. In: Cotes JE (Ed): Lung Function: Assessment and Application in Medicine (2nd edn), Chapter 14, BlackwMl Scientific Publications, Oxford 1968;345.
2. Behera D, Behera A, Malik SK. Peak expiratory flow rate of school going tribal children (9-15 years) from Orissa. Ind Pediatr 1988;25:623-25.
3. Malik SK, Jindal SK, Sharda PK, Banga N. Peak expiratory flow rate of healthy school boys from Punjab. Ind Paediatr 1981;18:517-21.
4. Malik SK, Jindal SK, Sharda PK, Banga N. Peak expiratory flow rates of school age girls from Punjab (Second report) Ind Paediatr 1982;19:161-64.
5. Parmar VR. Kumar L, Malik SK. Normal values of peak expiratory flow rate in healthy north Indianschool children, 6-16 years of age. Ind Paediatr 1977;14:591-94.
6. Narang A, Singh S. Ventilatory therapy. Ind Paediatr 1988;25(Suppl):31-36.
7. Waring WW. The history and physical examination. In: Kendig and Chernlate (Eds): Disorders of the Respiratory Tract in Children. WB Saunders Co, Philadelphia 1983;pp63.
8. Berman S. Epidemiology of acute respiratory infections in children in developing countries. Rev Infect Dis 1991;13 (Suppl 6): S454-62.
9. John TJ, Cherian T, Steinhoff C, Simoes EAF, John M. Etiology of acute respiratory infections in tropical southern India. Rev Infect Dis 1991;13(suppl 6): S463-69.
10. Mclntosh K. Pathogenesis of severe acute respiratory infections in the developing world: Respiratory syncytial virus and parainfluenza viruses. Rev Infect Dis 1991;13(Suppl6):S492-500.
11. Ward JI, Cherry JD, Chang SJ, Partridge S, Lee H, Treanor J, Greenberg DP, Keitel W, Barenkamp S, Bernstein DI, Edelman R, Edwards K, APERT Study Group. Efficacy of an acellular pertussis vaccine among adolescents and adults. N Engl J Med 2005;353:1555-63.
12. Brooks WA, Santosham M, Naheed A, Goswami D, Wahed MA, Diener-West M, Faruque AS, Black RE. Effect of weekly zinc supplements on incidence of pneumonia and diarrhoea in children younger than 2 years in an urban, low-income population in Bangladesh: Randomised controlled trial. Lancet 2005; 366(9490):999-1004.

13. Bastien N, Robinson JL, Tse A, Lee BE, Hart L, Li Y. Human coronavirus NL-63 infections in children: A 1-year study. J Clin Microbiol 2005;43:4567-73.

14. Tewodros W, Kronvall G. M protein gene (emm type) analysis of group A beta-hemolytic streptococci from Ethiopia reveals unique patterns. J Clin Microbiol 2005;43:4369-76.

15. Calegari T, Queiroz DA, Yokosawa J, Silveira HL, Costa LF, Oliveira TF, Luiz LN, Oliveira RC, Diniz FC, Rossi LM, Carvalho CJ, Lima AC, Mantese OC. Clinical-epidemiological evaluation of respiratory syncytial virus infection in children attended in a public hospital in midwestern Brazil. Braz J Infect Dis 2005;9:156-61.

16. March Mde F, Sant'Anna CC. Signs and symptoms indicative of community-acquired pneumonia in infants under six months. Braz J Infect Dis 2005;9:150-55.

17. Viegas M, Mistchenko AS. Molecular epidemiology of human respiratory syncytial virus subgroup A over a six-year period (1999-2004) in Argentina. J Med Virol 2005;77:302-10.

18. Long SS. Emerging infections and children: Influenza and acute necrotizing encephalopathy. Adv Exp Med Biol 2005;568:1-9.

19. National Center for Health Studies. Benson V, Marano MA. Current estimates from the National Health Interview Survey, 1992. DHHS Publ. No. (PHS) 94-1517. Natl Center for Health Statistics, Hyattsville, MD, 1994.

20. Pio A, Leowski T, Ten Dam HG. The magnitude of the problems of acute respiratory infections. In: Douglas RM, Kerby EE (Eds). Acute respiratory infections in childhood. Proceedings of an International Workshop Sydney, Australia, August 1984. Adelaide: University of Adelaide 1984;3-17.

21. Office of the Registrar General of India. Survey on infant and child mortality, 1979, Ministry of Home Affairs, New Delhi 1981;54.

22. Deb SK. Acute respiratory disease survey in Tripura in case of children below five years of age. J Indian Med Assoc 1998;96:111-16.

23. Mark L, McGeer A, McArthur M, Peeling RW, Petric M, Simor AE. Surveillance for outbreaks of respiratory tract infections in nursing homes. Can Med Assoc J 2000;162:1133-37.

24. Rao BL. Epidemiology and control of Influenza. Natl Med J India 2003;16:143-49.

25. Townsend TF. History of influenza epidemics. Ann Med Hist 1933;5:533.

26. Mathur A, Singh UK, Tandon HO, Chaturvedi UC. Pattern of some viruses in acute respiratory illness during 1972-73 at Lucknow. Indian J Med Res 1979;69:546-52.

27. Kloene W, Bang FB, Chakraborty SM, Cooper MR, Kulemann H, Shah KV, et al. A two year respiratory virus survey in four villages in West Bengal. Am J Epidemiol 1970;92:307-20.

28. Yeolekar LR, Kulkarni PB, Chadha MS, Rao BL. Seroepidemiology of influenza in Pune, India. Indian J Med Res 2001;114:121-26.

29. Ramamurty N, Pillai LC, Gunasekaran P, Elango V, Priya P, Sheriff AK, Mohana. Influenza activity among the paediatric age group in Chennai. Indian J Med Res 2005;121:776-79.

30. Shenoy VD, Upadhyaya SA, Rao SP, Shobha KL. Mycoplasma pneumoniae infection in children with acute respiratory infection. J Trop Pediatr 2005;51:232-35.

31. Kumar L, Singh S. Croup syndrome. Ind Paediatr 1987;23(Suppl):69-80.

32. Kumar L, Singh S. Bronchiolitis. Ind Paed 1987;23(Suppl):61-68.

33. Shann F. Etiology of severe pneumonia in developing countries. Pediatr Infect Dis J 1985;5:247-52.

34. Denny FW, FA loda. Acute respiratory infections are the leading cause of death in developing countries. Am J Trop Med Hyg 1986;35:1-2.

35. Bulla W, Hitze KL. Acute respiratory infections. A review. Bull WHO 1978;56:481-98.

36. Pio A. Acute respiratory infections in children in developing countries: An international point of view. Paed Infect Dis 1986;5:179-83.

37. Kumar L. Acute respiratory infections. Ind Paed 1988;25:595-98.

38. Stansfield SM. Acute respiratory infections in the developing world: Strategies for prevention, treatment and control. Paed Infect Dis 1987;6:622.

39. Datta-Banik ND, Krishna R, Mane SIS, et al. A longitudinal study of morbidity and mortality pattern of children under the age of five years in an urban community. Ind J Med Res 1969;57:948-57.

40. Kamath KR, Feldman RA, Rao PS, Webb JK. Infection and disease in a group of South Indian families. II. General morbidity pattern in families and family members. Am J Epidemiol 1969;89:375-78.

41. Gupta KB, Walia BNS. A longitudinal study of morbidity in children in a rural area of Punjab. Ind J Paed 1980;47:297.

42. Narain JP. Epidemiology of acute respiratory infections. Ind J Paed 1987;54:153-60.

43. Busse WW. Pathogenesis and sequela of respiratory infections. Rev Infect Dis 1991;13(Suppl 6):S477-85.

44. Leigh MW, Carson JL, Denny FW Jr. Pathogenesis of respiratory infections due to influenza virus: Implications for developing countries. Rev Infect Dis 1991;13(Suppl 6):S501.

45. Aherene W, Bird T, Court SDM, Gardener PS, McQuillin J. Pathologic changes in virus infections of the lower respiratory tract in children. J Gin Pathol 1970;23:7-18.

46. Anderson VM, Turner T. Histopathology of childhood pneumonia in developing countries. Rev Infect Dis 1991;13(Suppl 6):S470-6.

47. Singh S, Kumar L. Inadequacies in management of acute respiratory infections. Ind J Pediatr 1987;54:183-87.

48. Kumar L, Walia BNS, Singh S. Acute respiratory infections. In: Wallace HM, Giri K (Ed). Health care of Women and Children in Developing Countries. Third Party Publishing Company, California 1990;349.

49. Leventhal JM. Clinical predictors of pneumonia as a guide to order chest roentgenograms. Clin Paed 1982;21:730-34.
50. Shann F, Hart K, Thomas D. Acute lower respiratory tract infection in children: Possible criteria for selection of patients for antibiotic therapy and hospital admission. Bull WHO 1984;62:749-53.
51. World Health Organization. Clinical management of acute respiratory infections in children—A WHO memorandum. Bull WHO 1981;59:707-16.
52. World Health Organization. Case management of acute respiratory infection in children in developing countries. Report of a working group, meeting, Geneva: WHO, Apr 3-6,1984.
53. World Health Organization. Programme for the control of acute respiratory infections. 1987 programme report. WHO/ARI/88.1.
54. Karzon DT. Control of acute lower respiratory illness in the developing world: An assessment of vaccine intervention. Rev Infect Dis 1991;13(Suppl 6):S571-77.
55. Mostow SR, Cate TR, Ruberi FL. Prevention of influenza and pneumonia. Am Rev Respir Dis 1990;142:487-88.

TUBERCULOSIS IN CHILDREN

EPIDEMIOLOGY

Tuberculosis has been dealt with extensively in previous chapters. In this section, some important differences as applicable to children will be discussed. They are the reservoir of the disease for later life. As children acquire infection with *Mycobacterium tuberculosis* from adults in their environment, the epidemiology of childhood tuberculosis (TB) follows that in adults. While global burden of childhood tuberculosis is unclear, in developing countries the annual risk of tuberculosis infection in children is 2 to 5 percent. Nearly 8 to 20 percent of the deaths caused by tuberculosis occur in children. It has been suggested that BCG vaccination is responsible for decrease in the occurrence of disseminated and severe disease. Localized forms of illness, e.g. intrathoracic lymphadenopathy, and localized CNS disease have been reported to occur with greater frequency in vaccinated children. Human immunodeficiency virus (HIV) infected children are at an increased risk of tuberculosis, particularly disseminated disease. Tuberculosis in children is an important public health marker for the community because they represent ongoing transmission of tuberculosis and, at least a partial failure of the tuberculosis control program in that country. The exact incidence and prevalence of tuberculosis in children is not known. Approximately

1200 new cases occur annually in children in the United States.[1] These increases are thought to be due to the prevalence of infection with the Human Immunodeficiency Virus (HIV). Although the exact burden of the disease in children in India is not known, in view of a large adult population with tuberculosis and with the rapid spread of HIV infection in this country, a sizable pediatric population will have tuberculosis. Infection rate is determined easily by tuberculin test, but it does not provide exact idea of the extent of disease, as infection is not invariably followed by disease. Death notifications are often incomplete, faulty, and incorrect. Another problem of estimation of the extent of the disease is the difficulty in surveys, which fail to provide requisite information, as children below the age of 5 years are invariably not included in radiographic surveys. Large majority of the children do not produce sputum. Therefore, estimates of pulmonary tuberculosis in children are not precise. Most of the figures available from this country are based on hospital figures rather than community surveys. Data on the burden of extrapulmonary tuberculosis is still obscure and surveys for estimating the problem in children is difficult and is not carried out.[2,3]

Average infection rates for the age group of 6 to 14 years was 14 percent in 1965 as computed by the Director General of Health Services. The figure was much higher in a survey of over 1.5 million children from west coast of India between 1950 and 1955. The infection rate was found to be 34.7 percent in children below the age of 6 years. The figure was 51 to 78 percent in children between 7 to 14 years of age. In Madras city the infection rates have been as follows:

- 0-2 years   5%
- 3-4 years   10%
- 5-9 years   22%
- 10-12 years   37%
- 0-12 years   20% (overall rate)

The rates on the whole, are little lower in the rural areas and in the females. In the poorly ventilated **chawls** of Bombay, about 34 percent of the children were tuberculin positive by the age of 6 years and the same was 80 percent by the age of 13 years. The infection rate does not depend *per se* on race, religion, or socioeconomic status, but mainly on the opportunity of getting the infection, as in congestion or overcrowding. In a survey from Delhi, it was found that in congested schools, 55 percent of the children in the age group of 5 to 15 years were infected, whereas the figure was 27 percent in schools situated in open surroundings and where children from higher income families are studying. In contrast, 75 percent of the children were infected when there was a sputum positive contact.

Tuberculosis infection and disease among children are much more prevalent in developing countries, where resources for control are scarce.[2] It is estimated that in developing countries the annual risk tuberculosis infection in children is 2 to 5 percent. The estimated lifetime risk of developing tuberculosis disease for a young child infected with *Mycobacterium tuberculosis* as indicated by positive tuberculin test is about 10 percent.[4] About 5 percent of those infected are likely to develop disease in the first year after infection and the remaining 5 percent during their lifetime. These rates increase about six-fold in HIV infected individuals. Nearly 8 to 20 percent of the deaths caused by TB occur in children.[5] The age of the child at acquisition TB infection has a great effect on the occurrence tuberculosis disease. Approximately 40 percent infected children less than 1 yr of age if left untreated develop radiologically significant lymphadenopathy or segmental lesions compared with 24 percent children between 1 to 10 yr and 16 percent of children 11 to 15 years of age.[6]

The incidence of infection (first infection amongst the previously noninfected) in children in India has been estimated to be between 2 to 3 percent per year. In contrast, in western countries the figure is less than 0.1 percent per year. The first National Sample Survey by the Indian Council of Medical Research reported the prevalence of the disease to be about 7 per 1000 in children between the age groups of 5 to 14 years of which 0.3 per thousand were infectious. Similar figures were reported from Delhi in a longitudinal survey of about 30,000 children. However, subsequent surveys from Delhi and Bangalore in the mid seventies had shown a significant and continuous decline in children during the last 10 years. Similarly, hospital admissions showed a downward trend, although they do not indicate precisely the total extent of the problem. The pattern of disease also varies from institution to institution in this country. About 30 percent of the freshly diagnosed tuberculosis in children have primary disease, 18 percent tuberculous lymphadenitis, 0.6 percent miliary tuberculosis, 4.8 percent pleurisy with effusion, 1.2 percent tuberculous meningitis, and 12 percent late postprimary tuberculosis (New Delhi Tuberculosis Centre, 1974). The figures are different in the Mehrauli Tuberculosis Hospital, Delhi, where 30 percent of the cases had primary disease, 60 percent had late post-primary tuberculosis, and in the remaining 10 percent there was miliary or meningeal tuberculosis. Data on mortality rates

from tuberculosis in children are still scarce and has been reported to be between 50 to 240 per 100,000 between the ages of 0 to 4 years. Some workers have reported a figure of 60 per 100,000 per year in children of 0 to 14 years of age.

In Indian children the disease is almost entirely caused by the human type of bacillus. Infection due to bovine bacillus has disappeared because of the practice of boiling and pasteurization of milk.

The number of cases of tuberculosis annually constitutes about 5 to 6 percent of the total number of cases in USA, majority of which occur in children below the age of 5 years. The interval between ages 5 and 14 years is known as "the favored age" for tuberculosis since children in this age group have a lower active case rate, although not the infection rate, than any other segment of the population. Data from that country shows that most cases occurred in children of Hispanic, black, Native American, and Asia/Pacific origin. Tuberculosis incidence rates for South-East Asian refugees were as much as 70 times higher than those for other persons living in USA.

The likelihood of a child developing tuberculous infection or disease is directly related to the likelihood of adults in the child's environment developing active disease. More than 80 percent of tuberculosis in children can be traced to an adult case in the household. Other environments such as prisons, nursing homes, shelters for the homeless, and day-care centers promote transmission. Malnutrition, and infection with measles are important contributory factors for the development of tuberculosis in children. A child with tuberculosis can rarely, if ever, infect other children. Therefore, for every child with tuberculous infection, there must be an adult in the environment with active and infective form of tuberculosis.

Tuberculosis infection and disease among children are much more prevalent in developing countries, where resources for control are scarce.[2] It is estimated that in developing countries the annual risk of tuberculosis infection in children is 2 to 5 percent. The estimated lifetime risk of developing tuberculosis disease for a young child infected with *Mycobacterium tuberculosis* as indicated by positive tuberculin test is about 10 percent.[3] About 5 percent of those infected are likely to develop disease in the first year after infection and the remaining 5 percent during their lifetime. These rates increase about six-fold in HIV infected individuals. Nearly 8 to 20 percent of the deaths caused by TB occur in children.[5] The age of the child at acquisition of TB infection has a great effect on the occurrence of tuberculosis disease.

Approximately 40 percent of infected children less than 1 yr of age if left untreated develop radiologically significant lymphadenopathy or segmental lesions compared with 24 percent of children between 1 to 10 years and 16 percent of children 11 to 15 years of ages.[7,8]

To estimate the annual risk of tuberculosis infection (ARTI) among children aged 1 to 9 years in the south zone of India, a survey was carried out recently in a representative sample of villages and census enumeration blocks of towns in four south Indian states, as a part of a nationwide tuberculin survey. Six districts were selected through systematic random sampling. Four hundred and twenty rural clusters and 180 urban clusters were selected from these districts on the basis of the rural-urban ratio in the entire zone. To obtain the required sample of 12,000 children without bacilli-Calmette-Guerin (BCG) vaccination, 51,000 had to be covered. Eighty-five children from each cluster were tuberculin tested and read for reaction sizes. The ARTI was computed from the estimated prevalence of TB infection among children without a BCG scar. Among 52,951 children registered for the study, 50,846 (96%) had a tuberculin test result. The BCG coverage for the study population was about 65 percent. Among 17,811 children without a BCG scar, the prevalence of infection was 5.9 percent (95% CI 4.0-7.7%); the corresponding ARTI was 1.0 percent (95%CI 0.7-1.4%) [Correction]. The estimated ARTI for the south zone is 1.0 percent, as compared to the national average of 1.7 percent used for program evaluation. This baseline information should be useful for the assessment of future trends.[9]

MORBIDITY AND MORTALITY

The actual global disease burden of childhood TB is not known, but it has been assumed that 10 percent of the actual total TB case load is found amongst children. Global estimates of 1.5 million new cases and 130,000 deaths due to TB per year amongst children is reported.[10,11] However these figures appear to be an underestimate of the size of the problem. Childhood TB prevalence indicates:

- Community prevalence of sputum smear-positive pulmonary tuberculosis (PTB)
- Age-related prevalence of sputum smear-positive PTB
- Prevalence of childhood risk factors for disease
- Stage of epidemic.

Proper identification and treatment of infectious cases will prevent childhood TB. However often childhood TB is accorded low priority by National TB Control programs. Probable reasons include:

- Diagnostic difficulties
- Rarely infectious
- Limited resources
- Misplaced faith in BCG
- Lack of data on treatment.

But this disregards the impact of tuberculosis on childhood morbidity and mortality. Children can present with TB at any age, but the majority of cases present between 1 and 4 years. Disease usually develops within one year of infection—the younger, the earlier and the more disseminated. PTB is usually smear-negative. PTB to extrapulmonary TB (EPTB) ratio is usually around 3:1. The PTB prevalence is normally low between the ages of 5 and 12 years, and then increases in adolescence when PTB manifests like adult PTB (post-primary tuberculosis).[12]

Clinical Features and Diagnosis

Diagnosis of childhood tuberculosis is difficult since cultures for mycobacteria are less frequently positive than they are in adults with active disease. Isolation of acid-fast bacilli is uncommon because cavities are rare and cough and sputum are not usually associated with tuberculosis in children. In the majority of cases, the diagnosis is established by a combination of history of exposure to an adult with active tuberculosis, a positive tuberculin skin test, a reasonable exclusion of other possible causes for the symptoms, chest radiograph and/or physical examination consistent with tuberculosis, and a response to antituberculosis drugs.

With tuberculous infection and development of primary complex, the tuberculin reaction becomes positive. Like in adults, a large majority of cases with primary complex are asymptomatic and the lesion is discovered accidentally on radiological examination in the form of "Ghon's focus". A small group of children will have systemic symptoms.

History of contact with a sputum positive tuberculosis case in a child with other features suggestive of the disease is an important pointer towards the diagnosis. Most often the symptoms and signs are not well correlated with the degree of radiological changes in many children with tuberculosis. About one-half of the children with moderate to severe radiological changes are asymptomatic at presentation. Young children, particularly infants less than one year of age, are more likely to be symptomatic. The initiation of the primary tuberculous infection is marked by low-grade fever and mild cough, which resolve spontaneously over several days. As hypersensitivity to tuberculous antigens increases and inflammation in the lungs progresses, nonspecific symptoms such as fever, cough, weight loss, and night sweats may occur. Failure to thrive is common in young infants. However, there is no specific presentation typical of tuberculosis.

Pulmonary signs are usually absent. Some children may have signs of distal air trapping with bronchial obstruction due to lymph nodes. In that event, wheezing, decreased air entry, tachypnea or rarely respiratory distress may be present. Signs of frank segmental or lobar collapse may be there with complete obstruction. Bacterial superinfection may play a role in pathogenesis. Other clinical features may include lymphadenitis, hepatosplenomegaly, phlyctenular conjunctivitis, erythema nodosum, and pleural effusion.

Acute miliary tuberculosis is a generalized hematogenous disease with formation of multiple tubercles. It usually occurs within the first 6 to 9 months of primary disease. It is more common in infants and young children. The onset is usually acute with high fever, hepatosplenomegaly, and choroidal tubercles. The child appears very ill and sometimes the picture resembles bronchiolitis.

Chronic pulmonary tuberculosis or adult-type or reinfection type of tuberculosis can occur in older children and adolescents. About one-third of the children with active tuberculosis have extrapulmonary manifestations. Whereas pulmonary disease is frequently silent clinically, extrapulmonary tuberculosis is usually evident. The most common extrapulmonary tuberculosis is tubercular lymphadenitis, meningitis, and disseminated disease besides pleural tuberculosis, although infections of other sites can occur as in adults. Cervical or supraclavicular lymphadenitis is the commonly affected nodes and the usual organism is M*ycobacterium tuberculosis*. The affected nodes are typically nontender, firm in consistency, and multiple. The overlying skin may develop erythema, or a purple hue. Sinus formation is unusual. Nontuberculous mycobacterial infection can also cause such lymphadenitis. Tuberculous meningitis is common in children who have not received BCG vaccination. The children are usually younger than 2 years. Initial symptoms and signs are nonspecific including fever, personality changes, listlessness, irritability, and delayed or loss of developmental milestones. Most or virtually all of these children will have some degree of hydrocephalus. Other common signs or symptoms include cranial nerve palsies, vomiting, lethargy, and convulsions. Rarely, a picture like encephalopathy may be there. Computed tomography usually reveals some degree of hydrocephalus and basal meningitis. The tuberculin skin test is usually negative in about 40 percent of the cases. The most important clue to the diagnosis is the history of exposure to an adult with active tuberculosis. Congenital tuberculosis is discussed in detail in the chapter in tuberculosis.

Widespread coverage with BCG vaccine has possibly led to modification in the pattern of clinical manifestations. It has been suggested that BCG vaccination is responsible for decrease in the occurrence of disseminated and severe disease. Localized forms of illness, e.g. intrathoracic lymphadenopathy, and localized CNS disease have been reported to occur with greater frequency[13] but these need confirmation from large epidemiological studies. A recent study from Spain[7] reported an increase number of children with single hilar adenopathy 32 percent for the period 1978 to 1987 to 43.4 percent for the period 1988 to 1997 in comparison with those with parenchymal involvement or a mixed pattern (62 vs 45%). The authors also reported a nonsignificant trend towards a lower rate of tubercular meningitis in the last decade.[14] Indian experience from a tertiary care referral center in north India suggests an increase in the proportion of cases of extrapulmonary TB over the last 3 decades. The increase was predominantly due to increase in lymph node TB. The severe form of tubercular meningitis decreased over the last three decades[15] form of tubercular meningitis decreased over the last three decades.[15]

HIV and Tuberculosis

It has been reported that HIV infection is probably one of the most important factors for the resurgence of TB in adults as well as in children. In 1990, 4.2 percent of tuberculosis cases worldwide occurred in HIV-infected individuals and estimates for the year 2000 were around 14 percent.[16] Adults with HIV infection are more likely to develop tuberculosis from latent infection, and those who encounter *M. tuberculosis* after HIV related immune suppression have a more rapid progression to disease.[17] The impact of the HIV epidemic on paediatric TB has been reported in several studies. A prospective cohort study of children with TB diagnosed in Addis Ababa from December 1995 to January 1997 in which HIV-positive children were compared with HIV negative children, reported that HIV-positive children were younger, more underweight and had a six-fold higher mortality than HIV-negative children.[11] The tuberculin skin test was less sensitive and chest radiography was less specific in HIV-infected patients. Adherence to treatment was high (96%), and the cure rate was 58 percent for HIV-positive and 89 percent for HIV-negative pediatric TB patients. The study concluded that HIV-positive children are at risk of diagnostic error as well as delayed diagnosis of TB. Clinical manifestations were more severe and progression to death was more rapid in HIV-positive children than in HIV-negative children. Weight for age may be used to identify children at high risk of a fatal outcome.[18] In a retrospective study of 118 culture proven tuberculosis patients in Durban, South Africa; 57 (48%) children were detected to be HIV-1 infected, 44 (37%) non-HIV-1-infected, and in 17 (14%) HIV-1 status was not determined.[12] In contrast to previous studies, this study has shown that TB-HIV coinfection in children is common (48% of all culture proven cases), the presentation of tuberculosis may be acute (43%), and supportive tests are individually useful in confirming the diagnosis in a-third of cases. All culture for *M. tuberculosis* were positive by 8 wk. Clubbing and age over 2 yr were the most reliable indicators of underlying HIV-1 disease in a child with tuberculosis, while clinical features, radiology and supportive tests were found to be similar between HIV-infected and non-infected TB cases. Hospital-related mortality was higher (17.5%) in HIV-1-infected children compared to that in noninfected group (11.4%). The changing pattern of presentation of childhood tuberculosis and the high prevalence of TB in HIV endemic areas have made it imperative to maintain a high index of suspicion, with culture evaluation being an important part of clinical practice.[19] There are not many studies from India on proportion of children co-infected with HIV and TB. In a small study from Mumbai,[20] 18 percent of children with disseminated tuberculosis (N = 50) were HIV sero-positive. Reported co-infection of HIV and TB in various Indian studies was 16 to 68 percent.[21-23] Since follow-up data of HIV infected children are not available, it is very difficult to estimate annual infection rate of tuberculosis in HIV positive patients.

The varying clinical manifestations of childhood tuberculosis have been described by several authors.[24-29]

Radiological changes of childhood tuberculosis can be of the following types: (i) Primary complex. This is the predominant radiological lesion of pulmonary tuberculosis in children, which consists of the Ghon's focus, lymphatics, and the draining lymph nodes in the mediastinum. Primary tuberculosis is the commonest form encountered in children. Chest radiography remains the initial imaging technique and the radiographic features are hilar or mediastinal lymphadenopathy, with or without opacities in the unilateral lung. Occasionally,

the chest radiograph may be normal and lymphadeno-pathy may be detected on computed tomography (CT), which is not evident radiographically. In addition, CT features such as low attenuation lymph nodes with peripheral enhancement, lymph node calcification, branching centrilobular nodules and miliary nodules are helpful in suggesting the diagnosis in cases where the radiograph is normal or equivocal. Other features such as segmental or lobar consolidation and atelectasis are nonspecific.[48] In a study by Kim *et al*,[30] CT [including high-resolution (HRCT) revealed lymphadenopathy, which was not demonstrated in 21 percent of radiographs, and parenchymal abnormalities, not seen on 35 percent of radiographs. HRCT is more sensitive than chest radiography for the detection of military TB. The HRCT findings are widespread multiple small (< 2 mm diameter) nodules.[50] The nodules may be so numerous that they coalesce to form larger nodules greater than 2 mm in diameter or even consolidation with air broncho-grams. Thickening of the interlobular septa may also be a feature. Mediastinal and hilar lymphadenopathy may also be present. Cavitation is reported to be rare on chest radiography in children with TB. However, children with both HIV and TB may have atypical radiographic features and cavitation has been reported.[51,52] CT may show areas of cavitation that are not apparent on chest radiography, which may raise the possibility of a previously unsuspected underlying immune disorder. Role of high-resolution and color Doppler ultrasono-graphy (US) in diagnosis of cervical lymphadenopathy has been reported.[53] Central irregular hyperechogenic areas, blurred margins and central necrosis were most frequent in bacterial, tuberculous and cat scratch disease. Though individual sonographic signs were not specific, the categorization and combination of findings might be highly suggestive of diagnosis of the underlying disease presenting with cervical lymphadenopathy.[31] TB of the spine is the most common site of osseous involvement and has a higher prevalence in developing nations with an increasing incidence in developed nations. There are few reports of TB spondylitis in pediatric population that include magnetic resonance imaging (MRI) findings.[31,32] In a retrospective review of patients' records and MRI scans, by three readers using a consensus method, of 53 patients below 13 yr of age, MRI showed contiguous involvement of two or more vertebral bodies in 85 percent.[54] An intraspinal or araspinal soft tissue mass or abscess was present in 98 percent. Subligamentous extension was noted in 64 percent patients. Ring enhancement of the soft tissue mass was shown in 65 percent patient after gadolinium.[31] Contrast enhanced

MRI is emerging as a very useful technique for diagnosing CNS tuberculosis, as it demonstrates the localized lesions, meningeal enhancement and the brain stem lesion.[33,34]

The parenchymal inflammation is usually not visualized in the chest radiograph but nonspecific infiltrates may be seen. Usually, one site of infection is present but in about a fourth of cases, multiple lung foci may be seen. The hallmark of initial tuberculous infection is the relatively large size and importance of hilar lymphadenitis compared to the insignificant size of the parenchymal focus. In most cases, the parenchymal infiltrates and hilar lymphadenitis resolve spontaneously with the child left with a positive tuberculin test, *(ii)* In some, particularly young infants, the lymph nodes continue to enlarge and bronchial obstruction develops. Common sequences of progressive lymph node enlargement are hyperaeration and atelectasis. The resulting radiological shadows have been called as "collapse consolidation", "segmental lesions" or "epituberculosis". These lesions are more common in infants than in older children and usually occur within months of the initial infection. Approximately 45 percent of the children below one year of age with tuberculous infection will develop such segmental lesions compared to only 16 percent of children at 11 to 15 years of age. With proper treatment, complete regression occurs. *(iii)* However, in a few, scarring and bronchiectasis develop. Other radiological changes in childhood tuberculosis include *(iv)* pleural effusion; *(v)* calcification; *(vi)* adult-type reactivation tuberculosis; *(vii)* bronchopneumonia; and *(viii)* miliary mottling. Calcification, when it occurs, results from caseation of the primary complex, especially the lymph nodes. The calcification develops about 6 months or more after inoculation. Extensive calcification is uncommon when treatment is instituted promptly.

The most important laboratory test for the diagnosis and management of tuberculosis is the demonstration of mycobacteria either in the smear or culture. However, the difficulty in the isolation of the organism in children is already highlighted. In children, therefore isolation of *M. tuberculosis* is not necessary in many cases of pulmonary tuberculosis if the epidemiologic, skin test, and radiographic information is compatible with the disease. If the adult source case culture and susceptibility results are known, culture from the child adds little to the management. However, all attempts should be made to demonstrate the bacilli. Younger children produce sputum rarely. Gastric aspirates yield the organism in 30 to 40 percent of cases. Some investigators even reported a yield of more than 80 percent of cases particularly in infants with extensive disease. Gastric aspirates are more likely to yield organisms than bronchial aspirates if they are obtained correctly. Aspiration should be done early in the morning as the child awakens, before the stomach empties itself of the overnight accumulation of secretions swallowed from the respiratory tract during night. A nasogastric tube needs to be inserted for aspiration and can be withdrawn immediately. Three consecutive morning stomach aspirates are to be collected and to be examined for acid-fast bacilli either using the Ziehl-Neelsen staining or fluorescent microscopy. The sample should be collected in saline-free fluid and the pH should be neutralized if the procedure of isolation is delayed for several hours. The traditional methods using LJ (Lowenstein-Jensen) and Middlebrook's media take 4 to 6 weeks for identification of the organism. However, with the availability of BACTEC radiometric system using ^{14}C can give the result within 7 to 10 days (details discussed previously). Little information is available about the BACTEC methodology for gastric aspirates.[35-41]

Analyses of infected body fluids—pleural, joint, and cerebrospinal—may be helpful which may show lymphocytic reaction, elevated proteins, and decreased glucose that may suggest tuberculosis. These fluids may be subjected to bacteriological examination. Routine laboratory tests such as complete blood counts, and white cell differentiation and erythrocyte sedimentation rates rarely aid in the diagnosis. Abnormalities of liver function tests may help suggest disseminated tuberculosis. White or red cell sedimentation of the urine may indicate renal tuberculosis. Aspiration cytology or surgical biopsy of superficial lymph nodes also will help in arriving at the diagnosis. Ultrasonographic or CT guided aspiration of lymph nodes either in the mediastinum or abdomen may be tried where such expertise are available.

The tuberculin skin test[42,43] is referred to earlier. A positive tuberculin skin test signifies either *(a)* immunity conferred by a prior effective BCG vaccination; *(b)* tuberculous infection; or *(c)* tuberculous disease. The duration of immunity following BCG vaccination tends to decrease after 3 years or so (it may last for as long as 8 years), after which a positive Mantoux test may actually denote a tuberculous infection. The drawbacks of tuberculin test are highlighted in the earlier chapter on tuberculosis. In the event of the Mantoux test being negative, and there is a strong clinical suspicion of tuberculosis, or the tuberculin material is unavailable, some physicians use BCG as a diagnostic test. They believe that it is more sensitive and specific than the Mantoux test and is safe even in patients with well-established tuberculosis. BCG is given intradermally in a dose of 0.1 ml in the left deltoid region as for vaccination. An induration of more than 5 mm during the next one-week period is considered as positive. A positive test denotes hypersensitivity and the implications are same as those for the Mantoux test.

The modern advent of immunochemistry and genetic engineering has recently been applied to the diagnosis of mycobacterial diseases.[44-50] Although these tests are not yet available for wide and general use, their development is imminent in the near future. Using a wide variety of complex antigens using PPD, BCG, mycobacterial antigens 5, and 6, and other polysaccharide and protein antigens have attempted serologic diagnosis. Of various serological methods, enzyme linked immunosorbent assay (ELISA) has been used most extensively in field trials of tubercular serology. The major problem, however, with all serological tests is their nonspecificity. There are too many false positive tests to recommend the techniques as definite diagnostic tools. Although, these tests may not be of much use in the diagnosis of adult pulmonary tuberculosis, their usefulness in childhood tuberculosis and extrapulmonary tuberculosis may be of tremendous help. Reports from Argentina in a smaller group of children with pulmonary tuberculosis indicated that ELISA yielded a sensitivity of 86 percent and a specificity of 100 percent using antigen 5. However, in tuberculous meningitis in children, ELISA is of not much help, although other systems had much higher success rates in the diagnosis of this condition. Other new advances in the diagnosis detect directly the components of products of the mycobacterium. The first such technique to be in widespread use involved DNA probes, which are complementary to specific ribosomal RNA or DNA sequences of the mycobacterium. A very promising advance in DNA technology is the polymerase chain reaction (PCR) to mycobacterial populations. The technology uses an enzyme to geometrically amplify DNA replication. Combined with a DNA probe, this technique will allow the detection of mycobacteria within 4 hours. This technique has been able to identify femtimole quantities of mycobacterial DNA. This technique is specifically useful for directly measuring the presence of mycobacterial DNA inpatient samples and is an exciting technology for diagnosing childhood tuberculosis. Other investigations have attempted to detect structural components of mycobacteria directly. The most common amongst these is the mycolic acid, particularly the tuberculostearic acid. Very minute quantities of mycolic acids can be detected by high-pressure liquid chromatography and gas chromatography. The technique has been used directly to sputum, serum, and cerebrospinal fluid with the sensitivity being greater than 95 percent. Another advantage of this technique is that each species of mycobacteria has its own 'fingerprint' mycolic acids allowing for very rapid speciation of the organism isolated from the patient sample.

Thus, the gold standard for diagnosis of tuberculosis is demonstration of mycobacteria from various body fluids. This is often not possible in children due to paucibacillary nature of illness. Significant improvement in understanding of molecular biology of *Mycobacterium tuberculosis* has led to development of newer diagnostic techniques of tuberculosis. Polymerase chain reaction (PCR) is an emerging diagnostic tool for diagnosis of TB in children. However, its role in day-to-day clinical practice needs to be defined. A negative PCR never eliminates possibility of tuberculosis, and a positive result is not always confirmatory. The PCR may be useful in evaluating children with significant pulmonary disease when diagnosis is not readily established by other means, and in evaluating immunocompromised children (HIV infection) with pulmonary disease. In the absence of good diagnostic methods for tuberculosis, a lot of interest has been generated in serodiagnosis. ELISA has been used to detect antibodies to various purified or complex antigens of *M. tuberculosis* in children. Despite a large number of studies published over the past several years, serology has found little place in the routine diagnosis of tuberculosis in children, even though it is rapid and does not require specimen from the site of disease. Sensitivity and specificity depend on the antigen used, gold standard for the diagnosis of tuberculosis and the type of tubercular infection. Though most of these tests have high specificity, their sensitivity is poor. In addition, these tests may be influenced by factors such as age, prior BCG vaccination and exposure to environmental mycobacteria. The serological tests, theoretically, may not be able to differentiate between infection and disease. At present, serodiagnosis does not appear to have any role in diagnosis of childhood pulmonary tuberculosis. A new test (Quantiferon-TB or QFT) that measures the release of interferon-gamma in whole blood in response to stimulation by purified protein derivative is comparable with the tuberculin skin testing to detect latent tubercular infection, and is less affected by BCG vaccination. It can also discriminate responses due to nontuberculous mycobacteria, and avoids variability and subjectivity associated with placing and reading the tuberculin skin test. Polymerase chain reaction based test for identification of katG and rpoB mutation which are associated with isoniazid and rifampicin resistance may help in early identification of drug resistance in mycobacterium.[51]

Treatment

The management of tuberculosis has undergone major changes since the early eighties.[57-76] Clinical trials in children have several difficulties: (i) establishment of the diagnosis in children is less precise since culture positivity is often less than 50 percent; (ii) definition of treatment failure and relapse are usually on clinical grounds because of low culture positivity; (iii) primary tuberculosis in children may improve even without treatment; (iv) well controlled trials may not always be possible because of the small number of patients at this age. However, during the past decade, there have been several major studies of six month multiple drug therapy for tuberculosis disease in children reported from a number of countries. These trials have used several different regimens with quite similar results. In contrast to the usually recommended 18 months duration of treatment for both adults and children with tuberculosis, these new regimens, "short course" chemotherapy, have been proved to be useful for the successful treatment of tuberculosis, in children, both pulmonary and extrapulmonary, as in adults. The duration of such therapy has been 6 to 9 months, the former being used more frequently. In all, experience is available in more than 1000 children with tuberculous disease treated with 6 month chemotherapy regimens. The success rates are high, with very few adverse reactions and number of relapses has been very few. The most popular regimen has been two months of daily isoniazid, rifampin and pyrazinamide followed by four months of daily or twice-a-week rifampin and isoniazid. This regimen gives cure rates of more than 98 percent. The rationale, duration, drugs, dosage, side effects, and effectiveness of such therapy has been dealt with in detail in the earlier chapter on tuberculosis.

There are many differences in the principle of treatment of tuberculosis in children. Traditionally, recommendations for treatment of children with tuberculosis have been extrapolated from studies of adults with pulmonary tuberculosis. However, the disease differs in children than that in the adults in many ways, that may greatly affect treatment. Tuberculous disease in children develops as an immediate complication of the primary infection, typically with closed caseous lesions with relatively small bacillary population in contrast to the large bacillary load in open cavitary lesions in adult form of the disease. As secondary resistance is proportional to the total bacillary load, children are less likely than adults to develop resistance during therapy even if the compliance is poor, although such resistance can definitely occur. Children also develop most extrapulmonary forms of tuberculosis, particularly the disseminated disease and meningitis. Therefore, while deciding about chemotherapy for children, drugs should be selected in such a way that they should have a good penetration to different tissues. Fortunately, isoniazid, rifampin, and pyrazinamide cross both the inflamed and uninflamed meninges adequately while streptomycin crosses only the inflamed meninges. The pharmacokinetics of antituberculous drugs also differs in children. Generally, children tolerate larger doses per kilogram of body weight and have fewer adverse reactions than adults. The higher serum concentrations so achieved, might be of some advantage, although this assertion is unclear.[77-79] The lower rates of toxicity in children help in better compliance. But, children with severe forms of the disease, particularly disseminated disease and meningitis, experience more hepatotoxicity reactions. Malnutrition also appears to be another risk factor. There are also difficulties in the form of medications to be given to the children. Since most of the antituberculous drugs are available in capsule or tablet forms, either they are to be divided or crushed. Fortunately, recently many liquid preparations are available neither, although many of them are either not standardized or well studied. Compliance is as big a problem as in adults. Information on the effectiveness of short course chemotherapy in extrapulmonary tuberculosis in children is scanty. Most nonserious forms of extrapulmonary tuberculosis respond well to six/nine months of chemotherapy. However, failure rates are high in joint and bone tuberculosis when short-course chemotherapy is used. Because of seriousness of the problem, short-course chemotherapy in tuberculous meningitis is not yet adequately studied, although many reports indicate effectiveness of regimens of 6 to 12 months duration. A study from Thailand compared three regimens in this disease in more than 300 children: 12 months of daily isoniazid, streptomycin, and ethambutol; 9 months of daily isoniazid, streptomycin, and rifampin; and 6 months of daily isoniazid, streptomycin, rifampin, and pyrazinamide. For mildly ill patients all the three were equipotent. However, in patients with initial severe impairment of consciousness, there were significantly fewer deaths with the 6-month regimen using pyrazinamide. Intensive initial therapy is important to minimize neurological sequelae.

Drug resistant tuberculosis in children should be treated on the same principle as in adults.[80]

Recent guidelines of Revised National Tuberculosis Control Programme (RNTCP) have advocated and recommended DOTS for children also (Annexures 1A and 1B).

Prevention

The methods of preventing tuberculosis consist of:

a. *Primary prevention*
   › Interruption of transmission
   › Case management, contact investigation
   › Environmental control—UV light, airflow vaccination

b. *Secondary prevention*
   › Chemotherapy[81-84]

The most important step in the prevention of tuberculosis in children is case finding. When a child is suspected or proved to have tubercular infection, a thorough search should be made to identify the contact. Similarly, when an adult is discovered to have tuberculosis, it is necessary to screen all the children in the immediate contact for evidence of infection. It is not enough to enquire about the parents alone. Other inmates, particularly old people, neighbors, schoolteacher, schoolbus driver, and helper looking after the baby are other important sources of contact. In some circumstances, it may not be possible to separate the baby from the infected mother. It is also debated whether breastfeeding should be continued during this period or not. However, it has been proved that provided home treatment of adult open case is carried out properly, risks to the contacts are not greater than if they are isolated. Therefore, the best course is for newborn infants of mothers with open tuberculosis to get BCG vaccination soon after birth and isoniazid prophylaxis along with vigorous treatment of the mother. With the use of rifampin containing regimens, the sputum convertibility is achieved fast.

Despite varying degrees of success of BCG vaccination, this is perhaps the most important and single most prophylactic measure used the world over. The United States and the Netherlands are the only two countries in the world who have not routinely used BCG vaccination as a method of tuberculosis control, where the emphasis has been on case management and contact investigation, coupled with isoniazid preventive therapy for infected individuals who have not yet developed active disease. Most countries still advocate the use of BCG vaccination of all children, although the schedule of vaccination varies. Studies from India and other countries have reported the effectiveness of the vaccination to be between 14 to 80 percent, except the recent Chingel put trial. Another encouraging finding in recent years in India and Africa is that if children are in apparently good health, direct BCG vaccination is absolutely safe, even if the child is Mantoux positive. All newborn children should be given BCG vaccination, although some pediatricians prefer to vaccinate the child at the age of 12 weeks. This can be, given at any time during this period. All preschool children should be given BCG wherever they can be got.

Use of isoniazid prophylactically in individuals with asymptomatic tuberculous infection in order to prevent development of potentially communicable disease is an established practice in the United States. In the fifties, investigations revealed that children with primary tuberculosis treated with isoniazid did not develop previously common complications of the infection. A study of 2,750 with asymptomatic primary tuberculosis showed that preventive therapy with isoniazid produced a 94 percent reduction in tuberculous complications during a year of treatment and a 70 percent reduction over the subsequent 9 years. Placebo controlled isoniazid prophylaxis involving more than 1,25,000 subjects have shown a median reduction in tuberculosis of 60 percent in the treated group during the period of observation. When the analysis was limited to subjects with good compliance, effectiveness reached 90 percent. In children, the effectiveness has been nearly 100 percent and the effect has lasted for at least 30 years. In India, although INH prophylaxis in adults has many limitations, however, in children it has a definite role and should be indicated in the following circumstances: (i) children who are Mantoux positive especially below the age of five years; *(ii)* children who show a strongly positive Mantoux reaction; *(iii)* children in contact with sputum positive parents; and *(iv)* children who have recently converted to a tuberculin positive state. The commonly used regimen of isoniazid prophylactic therapy is the use of 5 to 10 mg of the drug per kilogram of body weight not exceeding 300 mg per day in a single daily oral dose for 12 months. Treatment lasting for more than 12 months did not confer additional protection. The drug is well tolerated in children. Isoniazid-related hepatitis is extremely rare. Transient elevation of liver enzymes may occur which do not warrant cessation of therapy.

Some other investigators had made an attempt to develop a model of treatment for tuberculosis in children in lines with that suggested by World Health Organization for treatment of tuberculosis in adults. While preparing treatment protocol, recommendations of professional bodies and various reports of treatment of tuberculosis in children available in literature were also consulted. The authors have suggested the following categorization as shown in Table 33.6.[85]

The modifications in WHO guidelines included: inclusion of AFB negative patients in category 1. WHO guideline includes freshly diagnosed AFB positive and

TABLE 33.6: Clinical categories and clinical conditions in children

Categories	Suggested by WHO for adults	Suggested conditions in children	Suggested regimens
• Category I	• New sputum positive Pulmonary TB (PTB)	PPD, TBL Pleural effusion Abdominal TB	2HRZE 4 HR*
	• New smear-negative PTB with extensive parenchymal involvement • New cases of severe forms of extra-pulmonary TB	Osteoarticular TB Genitourinary TB CNS TB Pericardial TB	
• Category II	• Relapse • Treatment failure • Return after default (Interrupted treatment)	Relapse Treatment failure Interrupted treatment	2SHRZE 1HRZE 5HR
• Category III	• Sputum negative pulmonary with limited parenchymal involvement • Extrapulmonary TB (less severe forms)	Single lymph node Small effusion Skin TB PPC	2HRZ 4 HR
• Category IV	• Chronic cases	Resistant cases	**

PPC—Pulmonary Primary Complex, PPD—Progressive Primary Disease, TBL—Tubercular Lymphadenitis, CNS TB—Central Nervous System Tuberculosis, 2 HRZE 4 HR—2 months of isoniazid, rifampicin, pyrazinamide and ethambutol, followed by 4 months of isoniazid and rifampicin, 2 SHRZE 1 HRZE 5 HRE—first two months daily isoniazid, rifampicin, pyrazinamide, ethambutol and streptomycin followed by one month of isoniazid, rifampicin, pyrazinamide and ethambutol, followed by 5 months of isoniazid and ethambutol, 2 HRZ 4 HR—2 months of isoniazid, rifampicin and pyrazinamide, followed by 4 months of isoniazid and rifampicin.
*10 HR in cases of Osteoarticular and CNS tuberculosis.
**Treatment with at least 3 new drugs that patient has not received in the past and to continue the drugs for 24 months.

AFB negative but serious illness in category I. Since AFB positivity is less common in tuberculosis in children, the serious form of tuberculosis in children was defined as one that can be identified objectively based on X-ray film of chest in pulmonary tuberculosis and by other objective criteria depending on organs involved and subsequent outcome. Other important difference was treatment with daily regimens rather than intermittent regimen because the treatment in their study was not directly observed. Success of intermittent regimen has been demonstrated in various studies in children. With their observations of feasibility of categorization of tuberculosis in children into existing framework available for adults and efficacy of intermittent regimens, it should be feasible to include children as beneficiaries of the DOTS strategy. However, this will require appropriate formulations of antituberculosis drugs for children.

The other difference was prolonged duration of treatment up to 12 months when the illness was involving bone and joints and central nervous system. The recommended guidelines of professional bodies were followed. However, recent studies suggest that 6 months of treatment for CNS tuberculosis and 9 months of treatment in spinal tuberculosis may be sufficient. Ethambutol was used for all age groups in categories I and II. It was based on the reports and recommendations that it can be used

in doses of 15 to 20 mg/kg in young children without significant increase in the ocular toxicity.

In that study, the diagnosis was often based on indirect evidence of infection due to *Mycobacterium tuberculosis* as AFB could be demonstrated only in 11 percent of the patients. Poor yield of AFB in tuberculosis in children may be due to paucibacillary nature of illness and inability of young children to give appropriate sputum samples. Children in that study were investigated and treated on ambulatory basis and no extra effort was made for isolation of AFB. The yield of AFB in children with pulmonary tuberculosis can be improved by induction and collection of sputum.

Revised National TB Control Program and Treatment of Pediatric Tuberculosis[86,87]

India has had a National Tuberculosis Programme (NTP) in operation since 1962. In 1992, a joint Government of India/World Health Organization review found that despite the existence of the NTP, TB patients were not being accurately diagnosed and that the majority of diagnosed patients did not complete treatment. Based on the recommendations of the review, the Revised National Tuberculosis Control Programme (RNTCP), incorporating the internationally recommended DOTS strategy, was developed. In 1993, RNTCP was started in pilot areas covering a population of 18 million. Large-scale implementation of the RNTCP began in 1998, with a World Bank credit of Rs 604 crore.

Since 1998, the RNTCP has been rapidly expanding and to date covers over 740 million of the population. RNTCP is the fastest expanding TB control program in the history of DOTS, and nationwide coverage is planned by 2005. In 2002, over 6.2 lakh patients were initiated on treatment under RNTCP. Of these, almost 2.5 lakh were infectious new sputum smear positive pulmonary TB. Over 70,000 patients are now being placed on treatment each month. By March 2006, the entire country is covered under RNTCP-DOTS program.

Good data on the burden of all forms of TB amongst children in India are not available. Most surveys conducted have focused on pulmonary TB and no significant population based studies on extrapulmonary TB are available. Pulmonary TB is primarily an adult disease and it has been estimated that the 0 to 19 year old population contains only 7 percent of the total prevalent cases.

In 2002, of the 2,45,051 new smear positive PTB cases initiated on treatment under RNTCP, 4,159 (1.7%) were aged 0 to 14 years. From a survey of RNTCP implementing districts, Pediatric cases were seen to make up 3 percent of the total load of new cases registered under RNTCP. Lymph node (LN) TB cases predominated (>75%) amongst the pediatric EPTB cases registered under RNTCP. Many EPTB cases (> 40% of LN cases) were diagnosed on clinical grounds with no confirmatory examinations performed. An almost equivalent number of Pediatric TB cases were being diagnosed in the same health facilities, but were not being registered under RNTCP. Of those Pediatric cases treated under RNTCP, cure and completion rates were both above 90 percent. Comparative figures for those cases not treated under RNTCP were 80 percent and 70 percent, with default rates between 27 to 33 percent. (Central TB Division. Unpublished data).

Hence for RNTCP, there are the issues of under diagnosis and under registration of Pediatric TB cases in the program. To seek consensus on improved case detection and improved treatment outcomes for all diagnosed pediatric TB cases, a workshop on the "Formulation of guidelines for diagnosis and treatment of Pediatric TB cases under RNTCP" was held in New Delhi on 6th and 7th August 2003. In attendance were National and International Pediatricians, TB experts and TB Control Program Managers.

1. Diagnosis

Suspect cases of PTB will include children presenting with: fever and/or cough for more than 3 weeks, with or without weight loss or no weight gain; and history of contact with a suspected or diagnosed case of active TB disease within the last 2 years. Diagnosis to be based on a combination of clinical presentation, sputum examination wherever possible, Chest X-ray (PA view), Mantoux test (1 TU PPD RT23 with Tween 80, positive if induration >10 mm after 48-72 hours) and history of contact. Diagnosis of TB in children should be made by a Medical Officer. Where diagnostic difficulties are faced, referral of the child should be made to a Pediatrician for further management. The existing RNTCP case definitions will be used for all cases diagnosed. The use of currently available scoring systems is not recommended for diagnosis of pediatric TB patients.

2. Treatment of Pediatric TB

DOTS is the recommended strategy for treatment of TB and all Pediatric TB patients should be registered under RNTCP. Intermittent short course chemotherapy given

Category of treatment	Type of patients	TB treatment regimens Intensive phase	Continuation phase
Category I	• New sputum smear-positive PTB • Seriously ill* sputum smear-negative PTB • Seriously ill extra-pulmonary TB	$2H_3R_3Z_3E_3$***	$4H_3R_3$
Category II	• Sputum smear-positive relapse • Sputum smear-positive treatment failure	$2S_3H_3R_3Z_3E_3/$ $1H_3R_3Z_3E_3$	$5H_3R_3E_3$
Category III	• Sputum smear-negative and Extra-pulmonary TB, not seriously ill**	$2H_3R_3Z_3$	$4H_3R_3$

TABLE 33.7: RNTCP treatment regimens

*Seriously ill sputum smear-negative PTB includes all forms of PTB other than primary complex; seriously ill EPTB includes TB meningitis (TBM), disseminated/miliary TB, TB pericarditis, TB peritonitis and intestinal TB, bilateral or extensive pleurisy, spinal TB with or without neurological complications, genitourinary tract TB, bone and joint TB. **Not-seriously ill EPTB includes lymph node TB and unilateral pleural effusion. ***Prefix indicates month and subscript indicates thrice weekly.

under direct observation, as advocated in the RNTCP, should be used in children (Table 33.7).

In patients with TBM on Category I treatment, the four drugs used during the intensive phase should be HRZS or HRZE. Continuation phase of treatment in TBM and spinal TB with neurological complications should be given for 6 to 7 months, extending the total duration of treatment to 8 to 9 months.

Steroids should be used initially in hospitalized cases of TBM and TB pericarditis and reduced gradually over 6 to 8 weeks.

In all instances before starting a child on Category II treatment, the patient should be examined by a Pediatrician or TB expert, wherever available. As recommended by WHO and in view of the growing evidence that the use of ethambutol in young children is safe, ethambutol is to be used as per RNTCP regimen for all age groups.[3,7]

To assist in calculating required dosages and administration of anti-TB drugs for children, the medication should be made available in the form of combipacks in patient wise-boxes, linked to the child's weight.

3. Chemoprophylaxis

Asymptomatic children under 6 years of age, exposed to an adult with infectious (smear-positive) tuberculosis, from the same household, will be given 6 months of isoniazid (5 mg per kg daily) chemoprophylaxis.

4. Monitoring and Evaluation

Pediatric-focused monitoring may preferably be an integral part of the program. Wherever possible, follow-up sputum examination is to be performed with the same frequency as in adults. Clinical or symptomatic improvement is to be assessed at the end of the intensive phase of treatment and at the end of treatment. Improvement should be judged by absence of fever or cough, a decrease in the size of lymph node(s), weight gain. Radiological improvement is to be assessed by chest X-ray examination in all smear-negative pulmonary TB cases at the end of treatment.

A review of the RNTCP existing treatment card will be undertaken as the collecting of additional information in relation to Pediatric TB patients, such as the basis for starting treatment along with categorization, documentation of clinical and radiological monitoring is required. Until this review is completed, the remarks section in the current card should be used to document diagnostic and clinical data as needed. Also there will be an evaluation of the need for modification in other RNTCP formats and registers to facilitate drug ordering of pediatric formulations and potential analyses of data by age groups.

5. General Issues

A revision of the RNTCP training modules will be undertaken to include Pediatric TB issues. District TB Control Societies should include representatives from the local bodies of Pediatricians. In coordination with the Indian Academy of Pediatrics (IAP), RNTCP should organize sensitization of Pediatricians regarding the program.

6. Operational Research Issues

Identified operational research should be prioritized and conducted. Topics include: development of, and implementation of a multicentric field evaluation of a Pediatric TB diagnostic scoring system; feasibility of using mothers as DOT providers for children with TB; examination of the Pediatric TB case yield if the children who have a history of contact with smear negative patients are additionally screened.

A committee, including representatives of the Indian Academy of Pediatrics, will be set up to monitor the implementation of these recommendations.

Subsequent to that development work on pediatric patient-wise boxes (PWBs) has been completed and recommendation have been made. The treatment is based on the child's body weight and by weight bands. There are two generic Pediatric PWBs-6 to 10 kgs and 11 to 17 kgs weight bands. This is a unique global achievement for RNTCP, as no other DOTS program in the world has such PWBs for the treatment of children with tuberculosis.

The initial RNTCP training material has been revised to include details of new pediatric guidelines and revised records and reports. Staff already trained under RNTCP, are being given updates on the revised diagnostic and treatment guidelines, and the recording and reporting formats.

The Salient features of the Pediatric TB program are as follows:

* Children < 6 years of age, who are contacts of sputum smear positive PTB cases, will continue to receive 6 moth chemoprophylaxis with isoniazid.
* For diagnosis of pulmonary and extra pulmonary TB in children, the existing facilities, in terms of laboratory, X-ray and staff, in the respective district would be utilized.

- Tuberculin will be supplied to the districts by RNTCP for diagnosis.
- Tuberculin will be procured from the open market by RNTCP and supplied to the respective districts.
- The cold chain system already available with the districts will be utilized for storage.
- The BCG laboratory at Guindy would provide Quality Control Services to RNTCP in relation to procurement of said tuberculin from the open market.

REFERENCES

1. Starke JR. Current concepts of epidemiology, diagnosis and treatment of childhood tuberculosis in the United States. Ind Pediatr 1991;28:335-55.
2. Udani PM, Pamra SP. Size and extent of problem and sources of infection. Tuberculosis in children. In: Textbook of Tuberculosis. The Tuberculosis Association of India 1981;359.
3. Job CK, Webb JKC. Pathology. Tuberculosis in children. In: Textbook of tuberculosis. The Tuberculosis Association of India 1981;363.
4. Comstock GW, Livesay VT, Woolpert SF. The prognosis of a positive tuberculin reaction in childhood and adolescence. Am J Epidemiol 1974;99:131-38.
5. Munoz FM, Starke JR. Tuberculosis in children. In: Tuberculosis : A comprehensive international approach, (2nd edn) NewYork: Marcell Dekker Inc.; 2000;553-95.
6. Miller FM, Seale RME. Tuberculosis in children, Bostan, Little Brown & Co 1963.
7. Kabra SK, Lodha R, Seth V. Some current concepts on childhood tuberculosis. Indian J Med Res 2004;120:387-437.
8. Donald PR. Childhood tuberculosis: Out of control? Curr Opin Pulm Med 2002;8:178-82.
9. Kolappan C, Gopi PG, Subramani R, Chadha VK, Kumar P, Prasad VV, Appegowda BN, Rao RS, Sashidharan R, Ganesan N, Santha T, Narayanan PR. Estimation of annual risk of tuberculosis infection (ARTI) among children aged 1-9 years in the south zone of India. Int J Tuberc Lung Dis 2004;8: 418-23.
10. Kochi A. The global tuberculosis situation and the new control strategy of the World Health Organisation. Tubercle 1991;72:1-6.
11. World Health Organisation (WHO). WHO report on the Tuberculosis epidemic. Geneva: WHO 1996.
12. WHO. Treatment of tuberculosis. Guidelines for National Programs. Geneva: WHO; 2003 (WHO/CDS/TB 2003.313).
13. Udani PM. BCG vaccination in India and tuberculosis in children: Newer facets. Indian J Pediatr 1994;61:451-62.
14. Sanchez-Albisua I, Baquero-Artigao F, Del Castillo F, Borque C, Garcia-Miguel MJ, Vidal ML. Twenty years of pulmonary tuberculosis in children: What has changed. Pediatr Infect Dis J 2002;21:49-53.
15. Kabra SK, Lodha R, Seth V. Tuberculosis in children, what has changed in last 20 years. Indian J Pediatr 2002; 69 (Suppl):S5-10.
16. Raviglione MC, Snider DE Jr, Kochi A. Global epidemiology of tuberculosis. Morbidity and mortality of a worldwide epidemic. JAMA 1995;273:220-26.
17. Antouucci G, Girardi E, Raviglione MC, Ippolito G, for the Gruppo Italiano di Studio Tubercoloise AIDS (GISTA). Risk factors for tuberculosis in HIV-infected persons: A prospective cohort study. JAMA 1995; 274:143-48.
18. Palme IB, Gudetta B, Bruchfeld J, Muhe L, Giesecke J. Impact of human immunodeficiency virus-1 infection on clinical presentation, treatment outcome and survival in a cohort of Ethiopian children with tuberculosis. Pediatr Infect Dis J 2002;21:1053-61.
19. Jeena PM, Pillay P, Pillay T, Coovadia HM. Impact of HIV-1 co-infection on presentation and hospital-related mortality in children with culture proven pulmonary tuberculosis in Durban, South Africa. Int J Tuberc Lung Dis 2002;6:672-78.
20. Merchant RH, Shroff RC. HIV seroprevalence in disseminated tuberculosis and chronic diarrhoea. Indian Pediatr 1998;35:883-87.
21. Merchant RH, Oswal JS, Bhagwat RV, Karkare J. Clinical profile of HIV infection. Indian Pediatr 2001;38:239-46.
22. Lodha R, Singhal T, Jain Y, Kabra SK, Seth P, Seth V. Pediatric HIV infection in a tertiary care center in north India: Early impressions. Indian Pediatr 2000;37:982-86.
23. Dhurat R, Manglani M, Sharma M, Shah NK. Clinical spectrum of HIV infection. Indian Pediatr 2000;37:831-36.
24. Manchanda SS, Lai H, Gupta S. Clinical manifestations. Tuberculosis in children. In: Textbook of Tuberculosis. The Tuberculosis Association of India 1981;368.
25. Snider DE Jr, Rieder HC, Combs D, Bloch AB, Hayden CH, Smith MH. Tuberculosis in children. Paediatr Infect Dis 1988;7:271-78.
26. Schuitj KE, Powel DA. Mycobacterial lymphadenitis in childhood. Am J Dis Child 1978;132:675-77.
27. Jones EM, Rafferty TN, Willis HS. Primary tuberculosis. Am Rev Tuberc 1942;46:392.
28. Morrison JB. Natural history of segmental lesions in primary pulmonary tuberculosis. Arch Dis Child 1973;48:90.
29. Daly JF, Brown DS, Lincoln EM, Wilking VN. Endobronchial tuberculosis in children. Dis Chest 1952;22:380.
30. Kim WS, Moon WK, Kim IO, Lee HJ, Jm JG, Yeon KM, et al. Pulmonary tuberculosis in children: Evaluation with CT. Am J Roentgenol 1997;168:1005-09.
31. Papakonstantinou O, Bakantaki A, Passpalaki P, Charoulakis N, Gourtsoyiannis N. High-resolution and

color Doppler ultrasonography of cervical lymph-adenopathy in children. Acta Radiol 2001;42:470-76.

32. Andronikou S, Jadwat S, Douis H. Patterns of disease on MRI in 53 children with tuberculous spondylitis and the role of gadolinium. Pediatr Radiol 2002;32:798-805.

33. Uysal G, Kose G, Guven A, Diren B. Magnetic resonance imaging in diagnosis of childhood central nervous system tuberculosis. Infection 2001;29:148-53.

34. Panchatcharam M, John E, Raj CM, Santhanakrishnan BR. Radiological criteria for the diagnosis of pulmonary forms of tuberculous infection. Ind J Paediatr 1985;52:357-63.

35. Heifets LB. Rapid automated methods (BACTEC system) in clinical mycobacteriology. Semin Respir Infect1986;242-49.

36. Neff TA. Bronchoscopy and BACTEC for the diagnosis of tuberculosis. State of the art, or a brief desertation on the efficient search for the tubercle bacillus? Am Rev Respir Dis 1986;133:962.

37. Somu N, Subramanyan L. Childhood Tuberculosis—A Practical Approach. Siva and Co, Madras 1991;130.

38. Daniel TM, Debanne SM. The serodiagnosis of tuberculosis and other mycobacterial diseases by enzyme-linked immunosorbent assay. Am Rev Respir Dis 1987;135:1137-51.

39. Danniel TM, Debanne SM, Van der Kuyp F. Enzyme-linked immunosorbent assay using Mycobacterium tuberculosis antigen 5 and PPD for the serodiagnosis of tuberculosis. Chest 1985;88:388-92.

40. Mohan C, Kumar A, Agarwal SC. Serodiagnosis of pulmonary and extrapulmonary tuberculosis by ELISA or IgG antibodies using BCG "pressate" antigen. Ind J Med Res 1987;85:367-73.

41. Aide SL, Pinasco HM, Pelosi FR, Budani HF, Palma-Beltrah OH, Gonzalez-Montaner LJ. Evaluation of an enzyme linked immunosorbent assay using an IgG antibody to Mycobacterium tuberculosis antigen 5 in the diagnosis of active tuberculosis in children. Am Rev Respir Dis 1989;139:748-51.

42. Snider DE Jr. The tuberculin skin test. Am Rev Respir Dis 1982;175:108-18.

43. Kent DC, Schwartz R. Active pulmonary tuberculosis with negative tuberculin skin reactions. Am Rev Respir Dis 1967;95:411-18.

44. Roberts MC, McMillan C, Coyle MB. Whole chromosomal probes for rapid identification of Mycobacterium tuberculosis and Mycobacterium avium complex. Clin Microbiol 1987;25:1239-43.

45. Tenover FC. Diagnostic deoxyribonucleic acid probes for infectious diseases. Clin Microbiol Rev 1988;1:82-101.

46. Brisson-Noel A, Gicquel B, Lecossier D, et al. Rapid diagnosis of tuberculosis by amplification of myco-bacterial DNA in clinical samples. Lancet 1989;1:1069-71.

47. Eisenach KD, Cave MD, Bates JH, Crawford JT. Polymerase chain reaction amplification of a repetitive DNA sequence specific for Mycobacterium tuberculosis. J Infect Dis 1990;161:977-81.

48. Patel RJ, Fries JW, Piessens WF, Wirth DF. Sequence analysis and amplification by polymerase chain reaction of a cloned DNA fragment for identification of Mycobacterium tuberculosis. J Clin Microbiol 1990;28:513-18.

49. Hermanns PWM, Schuietma ARJ, Van Soolingen D Verstynen CP, Bik EM, Thole JE, Kolk AH, Van Embden JD. Specific detection of Mycobacterium tuberculosis complex strains by polymerase chain reaction. J Clin Microbwl 1990;28:1204-13.

50. French GL, Chan CY, Cheung SW, Oo KT. Diagnosis of pulmonary tuberculosis by detection of tuberculo-stearic acid in sputum by using gas chromatography-mass spectrometry with selected ion monitoring. Infect Dis 1987;156:356-62.

51. Lodha R, Kabra SK. Newer diagnostic modalities for tuberculosis. Indian J Pediatr 2004;71:221-27.

52. Mitchison DA. Basic mechanisms of chemotherapy. Chest 1979;76(Suppl):771-81.

53. Fox W. Whither short course chemotherapy? Br J Di Chest 1981;75:331.

54. Treatment of childhood tuberculosis: Consensus Statement Recommendations of Indian Academy of Pediatrics. Indian Pediatr 1997;34:1093-96.

55. Anonymous. Short-course therapy for tuberculosis in infants and children. Infectious Diseases and Immunization Committee, Canadian Paediatric Society. CMAJ 1994;150:1233-39.

56. Scientific Committee of IUATLD: Tuberculosis in children: Guideline for diagnosis, prevention and treatment. Bull Int Union Tuberc Lung Dis 1991;66:61-67.

57. American Thoracic Society: Medical Section of The American Lung Association: Diagnostic standard and Classification of Tuberculosis. Am Rev Respir Dis 1990;142:725-35.

58. Treatment of Tuberculosis: Guideline for National Programmes. World Health Organization: Geneva 1993.

59. Verma K, Kapila K. Aspiration cytology for the diagnosis of tuberculosis perspective in India. Indian J Pediatr 2002;69 (supplement): S39-S43.

60. Seth V, Kabra SK, Lodha R. Management of tuberculosis. In: Seth V, Kabra SK (Eds): Essentials of Tuberculosis in Children (2nd edn). Delhi; Jaypee Brothers 2001;349-54.

61. Al-Dossary FS, Ong LT, Correa AG, Starke JR. Treatment of childhood tuberculosis with a six month directly observed regimen of only two weeks of daily therapy. Pediatr Infect Dis J 2002;21:91-97.

62. Gocmen A, Ozcelic U, Kiper N, Toppare M, Kaya S, Cengizlier R, Cetinkaya F. Short course intermittent chemotherapy in childhood tuberculosis. Infection 1993;21:324-27.

63. Kumar L, Dhand R, Singhi PD, Rao KL, Katariya S. A randomized trial of fully intermittent vs. daily followed by intermittent short course chemotherapy for childhood tuberculosis. Pediatr Infect Dis J 1990;9:802-06.

64. Biddulph J. Short course chemotherapy for childhood tuberculosis. Pediatr Infect Dis J 1990;9:794-801.

65. Jawahar MS, Sivasubramanian S, Vijayan VK, Ramakrishnan CV, Paramasivan CN, Selva-kumar V, et al. Short course chemotherapy for tuberculous lymphadenitis in children. BMJ 1990;301:359-62.

66. van Loenhout-Rooyackers JH, Keyser A, Laheij RJ, Verbeek AL, van der Meer JW. Tuberculous meningitis: Is a 6-month treatment regimen sufficient? Int J Tuberc Lung Dis 2001;5:1028-35.

67. Donald PR, Schoeman JF, Van Zyl LE, De Villiers JN, Pretorius M, Springer P. Intensive short course chemotherapy in the management of tuberculous meningitis. Int J Tuberc Lung Dis 1998;2:704-11.

68. Rajeswari R, Balasubramanian R, Venkatesan P, Sivasubramanian S, Soundarapandian S, Shanmuga-sundaram TK, et al. Short-course chemotherapy in the treatment of Pott's paraplegia: Report on five year follow-up. Int J Tuberc Lung Dis 1997;1:152-58.

69. Jacobs RF, Sunakorn P, Chotpitayasunonah T, Pope S, Kelleher K. Intensive short course chemotherapy for tuberculous meningitis. Pediatr Infect Dis J 1992;11: 194-98.

70. Abernathy RS, Dutt AK, Stead WW, Moers DJ. Short-course chemotherapy for tuberculosis in children. Paediatrics 1983;72:801-06.

71. Varudkar BL. Short-course chemotherapy for tuberculosis in children. Ind J Paediatr 1985;52:593-97.

72. Starke JR, Taylor-Watts KT. Six month chemotherapy of intrathoracic tuberculosis in children. Am Rev Respir Dis 1989;139:A314.

73. Medical Research Council Tuberculosis and Chest Diseases Unit. Management and outcome of chemotherapy for childhood tuberculosis. Arch Dis Child 1989;64:1004.

74. Khubchandani RP, Kumta NB, Bharucha NB, Ramakantan R. Short-course chemotherapy in childhood pulmonary tuberculosis. Am Rev Respir Dis 1990; 141:A338.

75. Biddulph J. Short-course chemotherapy for childhood tuberculosis. Paediatr Infect Dis 1990;9:794-801.

76. Iseman MD, Sbarbaro JA, Manalo F, Tan P. Community based short-course treatment of pulmonary tuberculosis in a developing nation. Am Rev Respir Dis 1990;141:A432.

77. Holdiness MR. Clinical pharmacokinetics of antituberculous drugs. Clin Pharmacol 1984;9:511.

78. Stein MT, Liang D. Clinical hepatotoxicity of isoniazid in children. Paediatrics 1979;64:499.

79. O'Brien RJ, Long MW, Cross FS, Lyle MA, Snider DE Jr. Hepatotoxicity from isoniazid and rifampin among children treated for tuberculosis. Paediatrics 1983; 72:491-99.

80. Steiner P, Rao M, Mitchell M. Primary drug-resistant tuberculosis in children. Correlation of drug-susceptibility pattern of matched patient and source-case strains of Mycobacterium tuberculosis. Am J Dis Child 1985;139:780-82.

81. Ferbec SH. Controlled chemoprophylaxis trials in tuberculosis. A general review. Adv Tuberc Res 1970;17:28.

82. Hsu KH. Thirty years after isoniazid. Its impact on tuberculosis in children and adolescents. JAMA 1984;251:1283-85.

83. IUAT Committee on prophylaxis. Efficacy of various durations of isoniazid preventive therapy for tuberculosis: Five years of follow-up in the IUAT trial. Bull WHO 1982;60:555-64.

84. Snider DE Jr, Caras GJ, Kaplan JP. Preventive therapy with isoniazid. Cost effectiveness of different durations of therapy. JAMA 1986;255:1579-83.

85. Kabra SK, Lodha R, Seth V. Category based treatment of tuberculosis in children. Indian Pediatrics 2004; 41:927-37.

86. Chauhan LS, Arora VK. Management of Pediatric Tuberculosis under the Revised National Tuberculosis Control Program (RNTCP)". Based on a Workshop for Formulation of guidelines for diagnosis and treatment of Pediatric TB cases under RNTCP" held at LRS Institute of TB and Respiratory Diseases, New Delhi, 6-7 August 2003. Indian Pediatrics 2004;41:901-05.

87. Chauhan LS, Arora VK. Management of Pediatric Tuberculosis Under the Revised National Tuberculosis Control Programme. Indian J Pediatr [serial online] 2004 [cited 2005 Oct 27];71:341-3.

ANNEXURE 1A

Schedule of Requirement

Product Code	Product Description	Strength	Unit
Product Code 13	Treatment box for pediatric category (6-10 kg). Each treatment box containing 24 combi-packs of Schedule-5 in one pouch and 18 multi-blister calendar combi-pack of Schedule-6 in another pouch	Each combi-pack of **Schedule-5 containing** 1 R Tab. of 75 mg 1 H Tab. of 75 mg 1 E Tab. of 200 mg 1 Z Tab. of 250 mg Each multi-blister calender combi-pack of **Schedule-6 containing** 3 R Tabs. of 75 mg each 3 H Tabs. of 75 mg each 4 Pyridoxine Tabs of 5 mg each	Treatment boxes
Product Code-14	Treatment box for pediatric category (11-17 Kg). Each treatment box containing 24 combi-packs of Schedule-7 in one pouch and 18 multi-blister calendar combi-pack of Schedule-8 in another pouch	Each combi-pack of **Schedule-7 Containing** 1 R Tab. of 150 mg 1 H Tab. of 150 mg 1 E Tab. of 400 mg 1 Z Tab. of 500 mg Each multi-blister calender combi-pack of **Schedule-8 containing** 3 R Tabs. of 150 mg each 3 H Tabs. of 150 mg each 4 Pyridoxine Tabs of 5 mg each	Treatment Boxes
Product Code-15 Treatment box for prolongation of intensive phase of pediatric cases (18-25 kg)	Treatment box for prolongation of intensive phase of pediatric cases (18-25 kg). Each box containing 5 pouches and each pouch containing 12 blister combipack of Schedule-5	Each combi-pack of **Schedule-5 Containing** 1 R Tab. of 75 mg 1 H Tab. of 75 mg 1 E Tab of 200 mg 1 Z Tab. of 250 mg	Treatment Boxes
Product Code-16 Treatment box for prolongation of intensive phase of pediatric cases (18-25 kg and 26-30 kg)	Treatment box for prolongation of intensive phase of pediatric cases (18-25 kg and 26-30 kg). Each box containing 5 pouches and each pouch containing 12 blister combi-pack of Schedule-7	Each combi-pack of **Schedule-7 Containing** 1 R Tab. of 150 mg 1 H Tab. of 150 mg 1 E Tab of 400 mg 1 Z Tab. of 500 mg	Treatment Boxes

ANNEXURE 1B

Guidelines for use of Pediatric Patient Wise Boxes Under the Revised National Tuberculosis Control Programme

The Revised National Tuberculosis Control Programme (RNTCP), which was initiated in 1997, included the treatment of pediatric cases according to body weight. Until now, the same strategy has been continued. The regimen recommended for treating the pediatric cases had been $2R_3H_3Z_3/4R_3H_3$ for children less than 6 years of age. For all children above 6 years, the same regimen was recommended as for adults. In early 2004, in consultation with Indian Academy of Pediatrics, the recommendations were revised whereby Ethambutol was included for treatment of pediatric cases even under 6 years of age.

The Programme had been getting feedback in regard to the difficulty in administering the drugs to smaller children as the available formulations needed to be broken up to meet the patients' individual weights. To overcome these problems, RNTCP in consultation with IAP, has taken steps to make the pediatric drugs available in patient-wise boxes (PWBs) similar to those supplied for adult patients under RNTCP. With the availability of pediatric PWBs, all new pediatric patients diagnosed and registered for treatment under RNTCP, would be initiated on pediatric patient wise boxes. This will enable optimum dosage for the patients, without resorting to further breaking of the tablets, as per the respective weight bands. Further, Rifampicin would be available in tablet form, which will enable easier swallowing of the drug by the pediatric patients.

The new formulations to be used in RNTCP are:
- Rifampicin—75/150 mg
- Isoniazid—75/150 mg
- Ethambutol—200/400 mg
- Pyrazinamide—250/500 mg

For the purpose of treatment, the pediatric population is divided into four weight bands:
- 6 to 10 kg
- 11 to 17 kg
- 18 to 25 kg
- 26 to 30 kg

The anti-TB drugs for pediatric patients will be available in the form of 2 generic patient wise boxes, i.e. Product Code 13 and Product Code 14. Product Code 15 and 16 would be available for the prolongation of the intensive phase, if required and also to facilitate conversion of the boxes into Category II and for reconstitution, if required.

The composition of product codes 13 to 16 is given below:

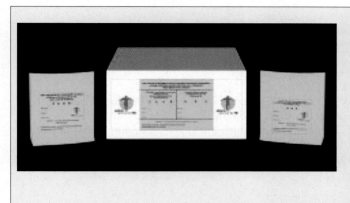

Product Code 13: Treatment box for pediatric weight band category (6-10 kg). Each treatment box containing 24 Combi-packs of Schedule-5 in one pouch and 18 multi-blister calendar Combi-pack of Schedule-6 in another pouch.

The intensive phase consists of Isoniazid, Rifampicin, Pyrazinamide and Ethambutol to be given under direct observation thrice a week on alternate days for 2 months (24 doses).

The continuation phase consists of 4 months (18 weeks; 54 doses) of Isoniazid and Rifampicin given thrice a week on alternate days—the first dose of every weekly blister being directly observed.

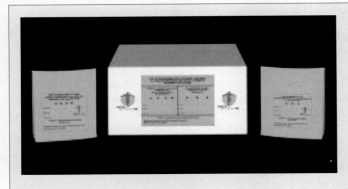

Product Code 14: Treatment box for pediatric weight band category (11-17 kg). Each treatment box containing 24 Combi-packs of Schedule 7 in one pouch and 18 multi-blister calendar Combi-pack of Schedule-8 in another pouch.

The intensive phase consists of Isoniazid, Rifampicin, Pyrazinamide and Ethambutol to be given under direct observation thrice a week on alternate days for 2 months (24 doses).

The continuation phase consists of 4 months (18 weeks; 54 doses) of Isoniazid and Rifampicin given thrice a week on alternate days—the first dose of every weekly blister being directly observed.

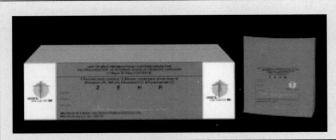

Product Code 15: Treatment box for prolongation of intensive phase of pediatric cases (6-10 kg and 18-25 kg). Each box containing 5 pouches and each pouch containing 12 blister Combi-pack of Schedule-5.

The pouch consists of Isoniazid, Rifampicin, Pyrazinamide and Ethambutol to be given under direct observation thrice a week on alternate days for 1 month (12 doses).

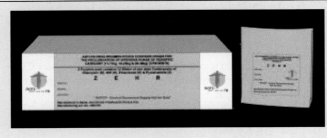

Product Code 16: Treatment box for prolongation of intensive phase of pediatric cases (11-17 kg, 18-25 kg and 26-30 kg). Each box containing 5 pouches and each pouch containing 12 blister Combi-packs of Schedule-7.

Prolongation Pouch consists of Isoniazid, Rifampicin, Pyrazinamide and Ethambutol to be given under direct observation thrice a week on alternate days for 1 month (12 doses).

The composition of all Product Codes is enclosed at Annexure—1A

The generic patient wise boxes, i.e. product code 13 and 14, according to weight band would be used for the pediatric patients in the following manner.
— A patient weighing 6 to 10 kg would require 1 box of Product Code 13.
— A patient weighing 11 to 17 kg would require 1 box of Product Code 14.
— A patient weighing 18 to 25 kg would require 1 box of Product Code 13 and 1 box of Product Code 14.
— A patient weighing 26 to 30 kg would require 2 boxes of Product Code 14.

The boxes have been designed to suit the requirements of Category I cases which are expected to dominate the patients belonging to pediatric age group. In case, any patients are to be placed on Category II or III, the following steps will have to be taken to convert the generic boxes into a Category II or III box:

Category II—Re-treatment Cases

For children to be placed on Category II, PPs would be added for prolongation of IP. For the extra 1 month of CP, a PP would be added after removing the Pyrazinamide tablets from the PP. For the other 4 months of CP blisters, Ethambutol tablets will need to be added which can be used from the supplies of loose drugs under the Program.

SM Inj (750 mg) supplied under the program shall be used for such patients and the dosage would be as per body weight.

Category III Cases

For children who are to be put on Category III, the Ethambutol tablets will be removed from the IP blisters.

Categorization and Duration of Therapy

Categorization of pediatric cases will be as per RNTCP policy. The treatment regimens recommended under RNTCP are the same for adult and pediatric cases. The duration of therapy will be as per the treatment regimen. If required, the duration of therapy may be extended within the current RNTCP guidelines.

Use of Prolongation Pouches

Sputum positivity in the pediatric patients of lower weight categories is usually not found and it is also difficult to get a sputum sample in such children. However, for the older patients, sputum samples can be obtained and prolongation of intensive phase may be required. For such patients, prolongation pouches will be required. In addition, PP would also be required for the purpose of reconstitution of the PWBs of patients who have died, defaulted, transferred out and indoor patients who also would be treated under RNTCP using PPs.

Chemoprophylaxis

Asymptomatic children under 6 years of age, exposed to an adult with infectious (smear positive) tuberculosis from within the same household, are to be given 6 months of Isoniazid (5 mg per kg daily) as chemoprophylaxis. Loose tablets of INH 100 mg would continue to be supplied for this purpose as was previously done.

Use of Pediatric Patient Wise Boxes for Under Weight Adult Patients (< 30 kg)

One adult patient < 30 kg would require two generic boxes of the PC 14. These boxes would be used according to the category of the patient, if required, after making alterations in the boxes as given above.

BRONCHIAL ASTHMA

PREVALENCE

International Scene

A worldwide rise in the prevalence of asthma is being reported with increase in wheeze at an alarming rate of 5 percent per year. From 1983 onwards an increase in asthma mortality and morbidity has been noticed worldwide.[1] Data on prevalence of bronchial asthma on children are few from most countries but many from countries like Australia and UK.[2] Table 33.8 shows the prevalence of current asthma, diagnosed asthma, wheeze ever, airway hyperresponsiveness, and atopy in children.

There are large differences in the prevalence among the rich, partly rich, and poor populations, with the highest prevalence found in Australia. It is possible that the differences may be as a consequence of responses to different allergens, to different allergen loads, or to other factors in the environment in the affluent and not-so-affluent populations. There are some suggestions that patients with high levels of parasitic infections are less atopic, although there is no convincing experimental confirmation. This protection of parasitic infections against asthma may be a cause of less prevalence of the later in many developing countries (Hygiene hypothesis). Diet may also be a factor. Exposure to allergens may be important although the most common allergen, the house dust mite has been found everywhere it has been looked for. However, these mites are mainly found in bedding and it is possible that steeping on a bed rather than on a floor, which many poor children do, increases exposure to them.

There was considerable concern that the prevalence of asthma and allergic diseases is increasing in Western and developing countries. However, the etiology of these conditions remains poorly understood, despite a large volume of clinical and epidemiological research within populations that has been directed at explaining why some individuals and not others develop asthma and allergies. Little is known about such worldwide variations in the prevalence of asthma and allergic diseases. More authentic data was available from the International Study of Asthma and Allergies in Childhood (ISAAC) designed in late 90s.[3] The study allowed comparisons between populations in different countries. ISAAC Phase One used standardized simple surveys conducted among representative samples of school children from centers in most regions of the world. Two age groups (13-14 yrs and 6-7 yrs) with approximately 3,000 children in each group were studied in each center. The 13 to 14 year olds (n = 463,801) were studied in 155 centres (56 countries) and the 6 to 7 year olds (n = 257,800) were studied in 91 centres (38 countries). There were marked variations in the prevalence of asthma symptoms with up to 15-fold differences between countries. The prevalence of wheeze in the last 12 months ranged from 2.1 to 32.2 percent in the older age group and 4.1 to 32.1 percent in the younger age group and was particularly

Country	Number	Age	Current asthma	Diagnosed asthma	Wheeze ever	Airway Hyper-responsiveness	Atopy (SPT)
TABLE 33.8: Prevalence of asthma in children in different countries							
Australia	1,487	8-10	5.4	11.10	21.7	10.1(H)	29.3
	I,217	8-11	6.7	17.3	26.5	10.0(1-1)	31.9
	1,575	8-11	9.9	30.8	40.7	16.0(H)	37.9
New Zealand	813	9	11.1	27.0		22.0(M)	45.8
	1,084	6-11	9.1	14.2	27.2	20.0(H)	
	873	12	8.1	16.8	26.6	12.0(E)	
England	1,613		8.0		14.8*	?(H)	
Wales	965		5.3	1.2	22.3	8.0(E)	
Germany	5,768	9-11	4.2	7.9			?
Denmark	527	7-16	5.3			16.0(H)	31
Spain	2,216	9-14	?		?	6.9(E)	
Indonesia	406	7-15	1.2	2.3	14.5	2.2(H)	
China	3,067	11-17	1.9	2.4	6.3	4.1(H)	?30
Papua New Guinea	257	6-20	0	0	1.7	1.0(H)	17
Kenya	402	9-12	3-3	11.4		10.7(E)	
Australia Indigenous Aborigines	215	7-12	0.1	0	1.4	1.8(H)	20.5

Current asthma: Airway hyperresponsiveness (AHR) + wheeze in the last 12 months; Diagnosed asthma: asthma ever diagnosed; H: histamine; M: methacholine; E: exercise; All figures are a percentage of the population tested.

high in English speaking countries and Latin America. A video questionnaire completed in the older age group in 99 centers (42 countries) showed a similar pattern.

The major differences between populations found in the International Study of Asthma and Allergies in Childhood Phase One are likely to be due to environmental factors. The results provide a framework for studies between populations in contrasting environments that are likely to yield new clues about the etiology of asthma.[3] Self completed wheezing questionnaire data in 13 to 14 years and 6 to 7 years old age group from different regions of the world are shown in Tables 33.9 and 33.10.

The ISAAC study has demonstrated, by means of simple standardized questionnaires, that there are large variations in the prevalence of asthma symptoms throughout the world (Fig. 33.1). The self-reported 12 months prevalence of wheezing among 13 to 14 year olds between countries ranged from 2.1 percent in Indonesia to 32.2 percent in the UK. Parental reported 12 months prevalence of wheezing in 6 to 7 year olds ranged from 4.1 percent in Indonesia to 32.1 percent in Costa Rica. The highest values for 12 month prevalence of wheeze were found in developed English-speaking countries (e.g.

Peru and Costa Rica). There were considerable variations within regions, e.g. the 12 months prevalence in the 13 to 14 year old age group varied within Europe from < 5 percent in Centers in Albania, Georgia, Greece, Italy, Romania and Russia; to > 30 percent in the UK; and within Latin America from <10 percent in centers in Argentina, Chile and Mexico to > 25 percent in center in Brazil and Peru.

The analysis shows that there is consistently more variation between countries than within countries. Three countries with a very large number of centers were represented across the range of prevalence, India with 14 centers representing the low prevalence group, Italy with 14 centers representing the middle prevalence group and the UK with 15 centers representing the high prevalence group. However, it must be remembered that the countries, and centers within countries were self-selected, and it is possible that countries with larger within country variation did not participate.

The only other comparable international survey of asthma is the European Community Respiratory Health Survey (ECHRS),[4,5] which studied males and females aged 20 to 44 years, mainly from European centers. Among the 13 centers 10 countries that were reported in

TABLE 33.9: Twelve months prevalence of bronchial asthma (%) in school going children 13-14 years old age group

Region	Wheeze	≥4 Attacks	Severe wheeze	Exercise wheeze	Night cough	Ever had asthma	Number studied
Africa	11.7	3.4	5.4	23.3	23.3	10.2	20475
Asia Pacific	8	2.2	1.8	16	17.8	9.4	83826
Eastern Mediterranean	10.7	2.9	3.8	16.9	20.2	10.7	28468
Latin America	16.9	3.4	4.5	19.1	28.6	13.4	52549
North America	24.2	7.6	9.2	30.9	33.7	16.5	12460
Northern and Eastern Europe	9.2	1.9	1.8	12.3	12.2	4.4	60819
Oceania	29.9	9.9	8.1	39.0	29.3	25.9	31301
South East Asia	6.0	1.6	3.0	9.5	14.1	4.5	37171
Western Europe	16.7	4.6	4.2	20.0	27.1	13.0	1,35,559
Grand Total (All World)	**13.8**	**3.7**	**3.8**	**18.8**	**22.3**	**11.3**	**4,63,801**

TABLE 33.10: Twelve months prevalence of bronchial asthma (%) in school going children 6-7 years old age group

Region	Wheeze	≥4 Attacks	Severe wheeze	Exercise wheeze	Night cough	Ever had asthma	Number studied
Asia Pacific	9.6	2.2	1.5	5.0	17.6	10.7	39476
Eastern Mediterranean	6.8	1.7	1.7	4.0	13.6	6.5	12853
Latin America	19.6	4.0	4.5	9.1	30.6	12.4	36264
North America	17.6	5.5	3.0	9.6	25.1	14.7	5755
Northern and Eastern Europe	8.8	2.0	1.5	3.6	11.4	3.2	23827
Oceania	24.6	8.9	4.6	15.9	29.4	26.8	29468
South East Asia	5.6	1.5	1.9	3.6	12.3	3.7	31697
Western Europe	8.1	1.9	1.5	3.7	16.1	7.2	68460
Grand Total (All World)	**11.8**	**3.1**	**2.4**	**6.2**	**19.1**	**10.2**	**2,57800**

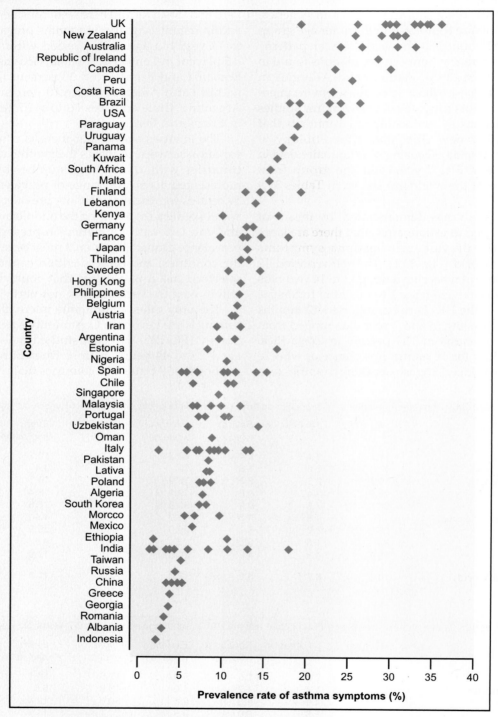

FIGURE 33.1: Worldwide variation in prevalence of asthma symptoms

International Study of Asthma and Allergies in Children (ISAAC)
Source: Lancet 1998;351:1225. In India there is wide variation in different regions.

both studies, the ranking of prevalence of wheeze in the last 12 months was similar, with the English-speaking countries (Australia, New Zealand, Republic of Ireland and the UK) having the highest and Italy and Greece the lowest rates. Subsequent other studies from different parts of the world also show similar trends.[6-14]

Indian Scene

The ISAAC data from 12 different parts of the country shows wide variability in the history of wheeze over a 12 months period in children between 13 to 14 year old age group (Table 33.11). In Akola the prevalence was 1.6 percent whereas the highest figures was reported from Kottayam (17.8%) in the South. The children from this town also had history of "Ever had asthma" of 12.4 percent. The prevalence was also the highest 24.6 percent from Kottayam in the 6 to 7 year old age group

(Table 33.12). There is a difference in the prevalence of asthma in children from Northern and Southern part of the country. From the Northern part of the country the figure varied between 5.4 to 6.9 percent in the 6 to 7 yr old age group. The figures from the Western part were less compared to those from the Northern and Southern regions.[5] Another hospital based study from South India, Bangalore on 20,000 children under the age of 18 years from 1979, 1984, 1989, 1994 and 1999 in the city of Bangalore showed a prevalence of 9 percent, 10.5 percent, 18.5 percent, 24.5 percent and 29.5 percent respectively. The increased prevalence correlated well with demographic changes of the city. Further to the hospital study, a school survey in 12 schools on 6550 children in the age group of 6 to 15 years was undertaken for prevalence of asthma and children were categorized into three group depending upon the geographical

TABLE 33.11: Twelve months prevalence of bronchial asthma (%) in school going children 13-14 years old age group in different parts of India

Region	Wheeze	≥ 4 Attacks	Severe wheeze	Exercise wheeze	Night cough	Ever had asthma	Number studied
Akola	1.6	0.5	1.0	2.7	3.8	2.6	2138
Bombay (area 1)	1.9	1.2	1.0	2.6	6.5	3.6	4225
Bombay (area 2)	10.6	1.8	3.2	11.1	22.4	6.5	2226
Bombay (area 3)	3.6	1.0	1.4	7.4	14.9	5.2	3178
Borivali	3.4	0.6	1.6	5.3	10.2	5.9	3878
Chandigarh	4.2	1.5	2.7	8.0	8.0	3.3	3139
Jodhpur	10.7	3.5	4.8	15.9	18.4	6.4	1094
Kottayam	17.8	1.7	13.5	17.9	32.2	12.4	2047
Madras (area 1)	8.4	1.9	2.9	7.7	14.6	2.8	1903
Madras (area 2)	6.0	3.3	3.6	7.4	11.5	1.8	3086
New Delhi	13.0	3.0	4.8	18.4	25.8	5.3	3026
Neyveli	6.0	1.9	2.5	23.2	16.9	2.4	3281
Orissa	3.8	0.8	2.1	6.8	13.5	2.8	1248
Pune	1.8	0.8	1.3	4.0	9.4	4.9	2702

TABLE 33.12: Twelve months prevalence of bronchial asthma (%) in school going children 6-7 years old age group in different parts of India

Region	Wheeze	≥ 4 Attacks	Severe wheeze	Exercise wheeze	Night cough	Ever had asthma	Number studied
Akola	5.6	1.5	1.9	3.6	12.3	3.7	31697
Bombay (area 1)	0.8	0.6	0,6	1.0	3.3	1.3	2030
Bombay (area 2)	3.8	1.3	1.6	3.0	12.6	3.8	3967
Bombay (area 3)	1.8	0.7	0.7	1.8	8.3	2.3	3568
Borivali	5.2	2.0	1.7	3.1	12.3	3.4	1672
Chandigarh	5.4	1.9	2.8	3.8	10.7	2.8	2891
Jodhpur	3.5	1.3	1.4	2.9	13.6	4.1	1104
Kottayam	24.6	4.7	7.5	13.3	27.0	14.4	2156
Madras (area 1)	7.2	2.1	1.4	2.5	16.4	1.4	1406
Madras (area 2)	8.5	2.4	2.5	3.8	15.4	2.2	2491
New Delhi	6.9	1.4	1.6	4.1	14.6	3.7	2938
Neyveli	1.5	0.1	0.3	1.4	8.1	1.0	1498
Orissa	4.1	1.4	2.2	3.8	8.7	3.8	1520
Pune	2.3	1.0	1.3	2.5	9.5	4.2	3248

situation of the school in relation to vehicular traffic and the socioeconomic group of children. Group I –Children from schools of heavy traffic area showed prevalence of 19.34 percent, Group II–Children from heavy traffic region and low socioeconomic population had 31.14 percent and Group III–Children from low traffic area school had 11.15 percent respectively. A continuation of study in rural areas showed 5.7 percent in children of 6 to 15 areas. The persistent asthma also showed an increase from 20 to 27.5 percent and persistent severe asthma 4 to 6.5 percent between 1994-99.[15] Another study from Delhi in 1999 revealed the prevalence of current asthma was 11.9 percent while past asthma was reported by 3.4 percent of children. Exclusive exercise-induced asthma was reported by 2.1 percent while that associated with colds by 2.4 percent of children. Boys had significantly higher prevalence of current asthma as compared with girls (12.8% and 10.7%, respectively). Multiple logistic regression analysis showed that male sex, a positive family history of atopic disorders, and the presence of smokers in the family were significant factors influencing the development of asthma while economic class, air pollution (total suspended particulates), and type of domestic kitchen fuel were not. The prevalence of current asthma in children in Delhi is 11.9 percent. Significant risk factors for its development are male sex, a positive family history of atopic disorders, and the presence of smokers in the family.[16] A more recent study from Chandigarh, North India examined the prevalence of asthma and its association with environmental tobacco smoke exposure among adolescent school children. Using a previously standardized questionnaire, data from 9090 students in the 9 to 20 year age range were analyzed. There were 4367 (48%) boys, in whom the observed prevalence of asthma was 2.6 percent. Among 4723 (52%) girls, asthma was present in 90 (1.9%) students. 31 percent students reported presence of one or more respiratory symptoms. More students with asthma had either parents or other family members smoking at home as compared to non-asthmatics (41% vs. 28%, p < 0.0001). The odds ratio for being asthmatic for patients exposed to ETS compared to those not exposed to ETS was 1.78 (95% confidence interval 1.33-2.31). ETS was also positively associated with prevalence of all the respiratory symptoms, with odds ratios varying between 1.6 and 2.25.[17]

Risk Factors

A number of risk factors have been identified for the causation of bronchial asthma in children. They include male sex a positive family history of atopic disorders, and the presence of smokers in the family,[16] urbanization, air pollution, environmental tobacco smoke,[15,17] and other socio environmental factors.[18]

Intrauterine Exposure

Some studies have suggested a link to maternal, not paternal, allergy in the development of allergy and asthma. While it has been suggested that preferential acquisition of the mother's genes (genomic imprinting) may account for this phenomenon, such an occurrence is excessively uncommon and the intrauterine environment is a more likely cause.

A positive relationship has been found between greater head circumference at birth and the later development of allergy and high serum IgE levels. At first, such an association may sound strange, but placental and nutritional factors that increase brain growth in the last trimester of pregnancy may well influence the maturation of the thymus gland, the origin of the immune system. It has been suggested that after 26 week's gestation, the fetus adopts a T'hl-like immune-phenotype, to prevent maternal rejection and that, in the last trimester, with increased IFN-γ production, this phenotype converts to a more T'hl picture. IL-4 is produced by the human amnion epithelium throughout pregnancy, and IL-10, a cytokine that inhibitors have been found in human placenta. If, on account of factors, the Th2 mode is maintained rather than converting to a Thl mode, an allergic diathesis might be expected to occur. Such a mechanism might also be invoked as a factor in sudden infant death syndrome in which mast cell tryptase and eosinophils are encountered in the lung and circulation.

It is also possible that allergens crossing the placenta may be involved in subsequent development of allergy and asthma since mothers exposed to high concentrations of allergens, such as birch pollen, during the last trimester of pregnancy are more likely to have children who develop allergy and asthma. It is not known, however, how minute amounts of allergen taken in by the mother can cross the placenta to sensitive offspring. However, it has been shown, that children who subsequently develop allergy or asthma, have impaired cord blood T-lymphocyte production of IFN-γ at birth in response to exposure to specific allergens. This impaired response suggests an impaired inhibitory mechanism for shutting down a Th2 response rather than one that primarily enhances it. Other environmental factors that may direct the placental-fetal relationship towards a Th2 response include young maternal age and smoking during pregnancy.

Several studies have reported an increased prevalence of respiratory symptoms like cough, wheeze and reduction in lung function in children or adolescents who were born as premature infants or who had a low birth weight.[19,20]

Viral Infection

It has long been recognized that viral infections, especially the common cold viruses, can lead to deterioration of asthma lasting several weeks. In infants, respiratory syncytial virus (RSV) is responsible for most wheezing illnesses. These observations have suggested that viral infections may be intimately involved in the development of asthma and allergy. It has been shown that over 80 percent of acute asthma exacerbations in school children and about 60 percent in adults result from viral infections (mostly common cold viruses). One explanation of the susceptibility of the asthmatic airway to viral inflammation is that persistent allergic mast cell and eosinophil-driven inflammation stimulates the release of cytokines such as tumor necrosis factor-alpha, which cause an increase in the expression of receptors for human respiratory viruses on the airway lining epithelium. In the case of most rhinoviruses, the receptor is an adhesion molecule, intracellular adhesion molecule-1. Once the virus enters the epithelial cells, it replicates and is able to generate wide variety of proinflammatory cytokines, which further enhance eosinophil and mast cell inflammation.

Protective Infections

Curiously, an important additional socioeconomic factor may be a reduction in early childhood infections (viral, bacterial, or parasitic) associated with improved living conditions. While viral infections can undoubtedly cause deterioration of established asthma, there is evidence that viral or bacterial Infection during the first 3 years of life may serve a protective function against the development of allergic diseases (Hygiene hypothesis).

One of the most consistent risk factors for allergy relates to family size. The prevalence of mucosal allergy and positive skin tests in children declines markedly in the last-born child with increasing numbers of siblings. A working hypothesis is that over the past 30 years, opportunities for acquiring infections from siblings or playmates in early childhood have declined with reduction in average family size, vaccination programs, and higher standards of personal hygiene. Most viruses and some bacteria are able to evoke a Thl like protective response with the generation of IFN-α and IL-12. Thus, if multiple infections occur during the first few years of life, high concentrations of these Th1, cytokines could inhibit the release of Th2 cytokines, thereby biasing the mucosal immune response away 'for this hypothesis is seen in an African study of, from allergen sensitization. Support adolescents infected with measles during the first year of life compared to those vaccinated later. Those infected early had a 63 percent lesser chance of developing positive skin tests to common aeroallergens. Repeated Bacille Calmette-Guerin (BCG) vaccination in young Japanese children also exerts a protective effect against the development of allergy. Both measles and BCG are potent stimulators of the Th1 cytokine response.

It has also been suggested that the increase in asthma and allergy with movements to urban centers may be related to the decrease in early exposure to parasitic infections common in some rural areas. One study tested the effect of anti-helminthic treatment on the allergic reactivity of children in a slum area of Caracas, Venezuela. One group was treated for 22 months while a second group who declined treatment was used as a control. Active treatment eliminated worms in children (from 68-5%) and resulted in a decrease in total serum IgE levels (from 2,543 to 1,124 IU/ml) but was accompanied by an increase in skin test reactivity to house dust mite (from 17-68%). In contrast, in the untreated group, parasite colonization continued to increase (43-70%), IgE levels increased (1,649-3,697 IU/ml), but dust mite sensitization fell (26-16%). Further testing showed that polyclonal stimulation of IgE synthesis by the parasites resulted in mast cell receptor saturation and suppression of specific IgE antibody synthesis. From a public health stand point; high levels of nonspecific IgE may protect rural dwellers exposed to parasites from allergy and asthma. It follows that eradication of parasites or reduced opportunities for infection could, in part, explain the rural to urban differences in the prevalence of allergic diseases.

Some investigators believe that early childhood respiratory symptoms are a risk factor for asthma.[21] This inference however, is weakened by the possibility of recall bias. Perhaps, respiratory symptoms reported by parents very early in life are not significantly associated with future asthma, but those symptoms that begin at or persist through age 3 to 4 years are likely to be associated with asthma.[22]

Diet

As societies become affluent, the dietary habits change and such changes are linked with increased prevalence of asthma observed in recent years.[23-25] Prospective studies have shown that breastfeeding has a transient beneficial effect on the incidence of eczema, food allergy, atopic sensitization, and wheezing illness in the first three years of life.[26,27] However, there is little evidence for a persistent protective effect of breastfeeding on the incidence of childhood asthma.[28-30] In the UK, the amount of salt eaten with food seems to be correlated with bronchial hyperreactivity and asthma mortality.[31] The severity of asthma—not its inception—has been linked to increased salt intake, but only in males.[32] Recent studies have shown lower prevalence of asthma and bronchial hyperresponsiveness in children with a high intake of fresh oily fish,[33] a source of polyunsaturated oils. Other studies also have shown an association of a, high fish consumption and improved baseline FEV_1.[34] Children who eat fish regularly consume more omega-3 fatty acids, which may protect them from bronchial hyperresponsiveness.

Air Pollution

Air pollution has been cited as – a causal factor in the development of asthma. The US Environmental Protection Agency concludes that[35] passive exposure to tobacco smoke is causally related to:

i. An increased risk of lower respiratory tract infections, such as bronchitis and pneumonia in infants and young children
ii. A small but significant dose-dependent reduction in pulmonary function
iii. Additional episodes and increased severity of asthma symptoms in asthmatic children.

Exposure to tobacco smoke is also considered to be a risk factor for the development of new cases of asthma in children.[36] Trucson Children's Respiratory Study has shown that maternal smoking is related to both transient early wheezing and persistent wheezing.[37] The role of sulphur dioxide and particulate matters in the causation of asthma is not well established.[38-41] Traffic pollutions[42] and effects of ozone may also be of consequence for childhood asthma.[43]

Evolution of Asthma

Asthma may develop during the first few months of life, but it is often difficult to make a definite diagnosis until the child is older. In infants, the most common cause of wheezing is respiratory viral infections. However, there is a correlation of early wheeze with reduced lung function before the onset of symptoms, which suggests that small lungs may be responsible for some infant wheeze that resolves with the child's growth. Those children with asthma continue to wheeze in later childhood. Recurring exacerbations of asthma may be associated with exposure to allergens. In the susceptible

infant, atopy may predispose the airways to sensitization by environmental allergens or irritants and the child experiences recurrent episodes of wheezing. In particular, early exposure to Alternaria, house-dust mite, and animal allergens in high quantities appears to be important as discussed above.

During early childhood, wheezing and cough may occur at infrequent intervals. In some infants wheezing becomes more frequent and asthma is well established at an early age. It is reported that the majority of 7 year old children with airway hyperresponsiveness suffered from atopy during their infancy.[44] Asthma also affects development of the lung. Asthma in infancy can result in a decrease in lung function by approximately 20 percent in adulthood,[45] although subsequent studies did not confirm the same.[46]

The predominant feature associated with asthma in children is allergy, and house dust mite represent major allergens worldwide in, both affluent and partly affluent countries.[47] The role of viral infection in the causation of asthma in older children is less clear, although in atopic children viral infection is clearly important triggers of asthma exacerbations. By the age of 8 years, a proportion of children develop airway hyperresponsiveness and the associated symptoms of moderate to severe persistent asthma, while others continue to have mild intermittent asthma.[48] Lung growth is unaffected in most children with asthma, but it can be reduced throughout childhood and adolescence in those with severe and persistent symptoms. A longitudinal study in New Zealand concluded that improved spirometric function was impaired in children with airway hyper-responsiveness and/or allergy to house dust mite or cat allergen.[49]

Although childhood asthma has long been considered as a single, easily recognizable disease characterized by reversible airflow limitations,[50] recent findings have challenged this concept. Martinez et al studied the natural history of children (0-6 years) and found that approximately half of them experienced wheezing at some time during the study period. They recognized three patterns of wheezing:

1. *Transient early wheezing.* Wheezing occurred in life but resolves by the age of three years
2. *Late onset wheezing.* Some experience wheezing between the ages of three and six years
3. *Persistent wheezing.* Wheezing illness throughout the entire study period.

The outcomes of these patterns are associated with different risk factors. Children with transient early wheezing had reduced pulmonary function as measured by functional residual capacity shortly after birth and before any lower respiratory tract illness had occurred. The risk also increases in children of mothers who smoked during pregnancy, had lower lung function values compared to those whose mothers did not smoke. Thus, the authors concluded that congenitally smaller airways might predispose children to wheeze illness later in life. Persistent and late onset wheezing is more likely associated with atopy with their mothers being asthmatics. Lung function in persistent wheezers is also less.

The long-term prognosis of childhood asthma is a matter of controversy and of major concern. It has often been believed that the child grows out of its asthma when he or she reaches adulthood (asthma disappears). However, epidemiological studies are less convincing.[46,51,52] Although there are methodological difficulties it is estimated that asthma disappears in 30 to 50 percent of children at puberty, but often reappears in adult life. Up to two-third of children with asthma continue to suffer from the disorder through puberty and adulthood. Even when asthma symptoms disappear, the lung function frequently remains altered or airway hyperresponsiveness or cough persists. The prognosis of asthma becomes worse when the child has eczema or there is a family history of eczema. Wheezing in the first year of life is not a prognostic indicator for asthma or for more severe asthma or for more severe asthma later in childhood. About 5 to 10 percent of children with asthma that is considered trivial will have severe-asthma in later life. Therefore, childhood asthma should never be neglected with the hope that the child will grow out of it. Children with mild asthma are likely to have a good prognosis, but those with a moderate to severe asthma probably continue to have some degree of airway hyperresponsiveness and will be at risk of the long-term effects of asthma throughout life.[53] Some, clinical studies have reported that up to 80 percent of asthmatics become asymptomatic during puberty.[54,55] In a cohort study of Australian school children[56] tested initially at the age of 8 to 10 years and then again at 12 to 14 years of age, the persistence if bronchial hyperresponsiveness at 12 to 14 years of age was found to be related to the severity of disease at 8 to 10 years of age, the atopic status of the child, and the presence of asthma in the parents. Most of the children who had a slight or mild degree of bronchial hyperresponsiveness at 8 to 10 years of age lost their increased response by the age of 12 to 14 years. However, only 15.4 percent of children with severe or moderate bronchial hyperresponsiveness at initial assessment had normal levels of bronchial responsiveness at the later assessment. There are several factors why asthma often goes unrecognized and tends to be under treated in teenagers because usually this is a period of turmoil, awkwardness, rebelliousness, and intolerability.[53-59]

Notwithstanding the factors described above as the factors responsible for the induction of asthma in childhood, occurrence of asthma within families is the strongest risk factor for the development of asthma in children.[60-63]

DIAGNOSIS

Various symptoms and signs of bronchial asthma are not different than those in adults as discussed earlier. However, in children there is more chance of under diagnosis in this age group. This is a frequent problem and occurs most often when young children who wheeze only when they have respiratory infections and are dismissed as having wheezy bronchitis, asthmatic bronchitis, bronchitis, bronchiolitis, or pneumonia, despite evidence that the signs and symptoms are most compatible with a diagnosis of bronchial asthma.

Although, recurrent episodes of cough and wheezing are almost always due to asthma in both children and adults, it is to be remembered that all that wheezes is not asthma always. There are other causes of airways obstruction leading to wheezing. The differential diagnosis will be as follows.

Infants and Children

Obstruction in the Large Airways

1. Foreign body in trachea, bronchus
2. Vascular rings
3. Laryngotracheomalacia
4. Enlarged lymph nodes or tumors
5. Laryngeal webs
6. Tracheal stenosis
7. Bronchial stenosis.

Obstruction Involving Both Large and Small Airways

1. Bronchial asthma
2. Viral bronchiolitis
3. Cystic fibrosis
4. *Chlamydia trachomatis* infection
5. Obliterative bronchiolitis
6. Bronchopulmonary dysplasia
7. Aspiration
8. Vascular engorgements
9. Pulmonary edema.

Miscellaneous

1. Primary ciliary dyskinesia syndrome
2. Primary immune deficiency
3. Congenital heart disease
4. Congenital malformations causing narrowing of intrathoracic airways.

Asthma in childhood can present a particularly difficult problem largely because episodic wheezing and cough are among the most common symptoms encountered in childhood illnesses, particularly in the under 3 year old. Although health care professionals are increasingly encouraged to make a positive diagnosis of asthma whenever recurrent wheezing, breathlessness, and cough occur (particularly if associated with nocturnal and early morning symptoms), the underlying nature of the disorder's process may differ in infants from that in older children and adults. The use of the label "asthma" to describe such children has important clinical consequences. It implies a syndrome in which there is airway inflammation and for which there is a specific protocol of management. The younger the child, particularly below ages 5, the greater the possibility of an alternative diagnosis for recurrent wheeze as described above. Chest radiography is important as a diagnostic test to exclude alternative causes. Features such as a neonatal onset of symptoms, associated failure to thrive, vomiting-associated symptoms, and localized lung or cardiovascular signs all suggest an alternative diagnosis and indicate the need for investigations, such as a sweat test to exclude cystic fibrosis, measurements of immune function, and reflux studies.

Among those with no alternative diagnosis, there is the possibility that the problem does not have a uniform underlying pathogenesis. Nonetheless, there are two general patterns of wheezing in infancy. Some infants who have recurrent episodes of wheeze associated with acute viral respiratory infections, often with a first episode in association with respiratory syncytial virus (RSV) bronchiolitis, come from nonatopic families and have no evidence of atopy themselves. These infants usually outgrow their symptoms in the preschool years and have no evidence of subsequent asthma, though they may have minor defects of lung function and airway hyperresponsiveness. This syndrome may have more to do with airway geometry than airway inflammation, and thus may differ mechanistically from the more established chronic inflammatory condition that underlies asthma in older children and adults.

Other infants with asthma have an atopic background often associated with eczema and develop symptoms later in infancy that persists through childhood and into adult life. In these children, characteristic features of airway inflammation can be found even in infancy. However, there are no practical clinical tests that can be done to establish the presence of airway inflammation. Only associated atopic problems can be used as a guide to prognosis. Early age (less than 2 years) of onset of wheeze is a poor predictor of continuing problem in later childhood.

It is likely that the issue of asthma associated with recurrent virus-related episodes and the later development of persistent asthma requires further study. Apart from the confusion over etiological mechanisms of asthma in childhood, there is also considerable reluctance in establishing a diagnosis and, as a consequence, initiating appropriate therapy. Because lower respiratory tract symptoms similar to symptoms of asthma are so common in childhood (and frequently occur in association with upper respiratory tract symptoms), either a correct diagnosis is not made or an inappropriate diagnosis is given, thereby, depriving the child of anti-asthma medication.

Although in these young children there is the possibility of over treatment, the episodes of wheezing may be foreshortened and reduced in intensity by the effective use of anti-inflammatory drugs and bronchodilators rather than antibiotics, and it is for this reason that health care professionals are encouraged to use the word "asthma" rather than other terminology to describe this syndrome.

Asthma in all age groups may present only as repeated coughing especially at night, with exercise, and with viral illness, but these are particularly common forms of presentation of asthma in childhood. The presence of recurrent nocturnal cough in an otherwise healthy child should raise awareness of asthma as a probable diagnosis. Although repeated infections of the sinuses, tonsils, and adenoids may explain nocturnal coughing, the occurrence of this symptom awaking the child in the early hours of the morning is almost always diagnostic of asthma.

Under the age of 5 years, the diagnosis of asthma has to rely largely on clinical judgment based on a combination of symptoms and physical findings. Because the measurement of airflow limitation and airway hyperresponsiveness infants and small children requires complex equipment and is difficult, it can therefore only be recommended as a research tool. A trial of treatment is probably the most confident way in which a diagnosis of asthma can be secured in children (and in many adults as well). Prognostic features include a family history of asthma or eczema and presence of eczema in a young child with respiratory symptoms. Children aged 4 to 5 can be taught to use a peak expiratory flow (PEF) meter and obtain reliable readings. However, unless there is careful parental supervision over when and how the measurements are made, PEF recording in childhood can be unreliable.

Some children with asthma only present with exercise-induced symptoms. In this group, or when there is doubt over the existence of low-grade asthma in childhood, exercise testing is helpful. A 6 minute running protocol is easily performed in clinical practice, and when used in-conjunction with measurements of airflow limitation (FEV or PEF), it can be most helpful in establishing a firm diagnosis, especially if the cough produced by the exercise is similar to that occurring spontaneously at night.

MANAGEMENT OF ASTHMA IN CHILDREN

Several guidelines have been published since 1990 with the aim of improving management of asthma both in children and adults. However a systematic analysis of guidelines till 1995 had brought out several controversial-issues as well as gaps in knowledge. In May 1997, an expert committee of the National Heart Lung and Blood Institutes of USA published guidelines about management of asthma where they have tried to overcome many of the previous lapses. These guidelines along with the recent British thoracic society guideline have been discussed in previous chapters.

The need for similar guidelines has always been felt amongst the physicians managing children in India, but no uniform guidelines are available for the disease as seen in India. It was felt that the guidelines originating in India would have much more relevance to the ground situation and the status of health services. To set up the process of achieving consensus, towards suitable guidelines, a Consensus Conference was held on April 17 and 18, 1998 at the Advanced Paediatric Centre of the Post Graduate Institute of Medical Education and Research, Chandigarh in which, 15 experts who manage asthma patients and have published papers in this field, participated. Recent evidence was accessed using searches on Medline, Embase, Index Medicus and Excerpta Medica. Some of the contentious issues were resolved with the help of the Cochrane Library.[64] Since the consumer of health care in India is not sufficiently literate, physicians have been assigned a lot of responsibility in decision making for the patients. The guidelines are required to be updated periodically and provide flexibility to individualize patients. Since in a large area

in our country, all the recommended modalities may not be available then suitable improvisations must be made. The objectives of the conference were:
i.   To reach at a uniform treatment approach towards children with asthma keeping in mind the limitations of resources in the Indian context and to develop guidelines based on available evidence for the pediatricians.
ii. To prepare a consensus document for management of children with asthma which would provide guidelines to a general pediatricians managing asthma in India.

Various components discussed included pathogenesis, definition, classification of severity, measure of assessment and monitoring, referral, control of factors contributing to asthma in seventy, pharmacological therapy and education of patient, family and health professionals regarding asthma care.

The Expert Group I recommended that for the diagnosis of asthma in children a detailed medical history, careful physical examination and peak-expiratory flow rate (PEFR) measurement to demonstrate obstruction with reversibility of variable airflow obstruction are needed. To establish the diagnosis of asthma the clinician must determine that:
i.   Episodic symptoms of airflow obstruction, more than 3 episodes are present
ii. Airflow-obstruction is at least partially reversible
iii. Alternative diagnoses are excluded.

Physicians who care for children with asthma should be well versed in (PEFR) monitoring. They should perform spirometery wherever possible.

Measures of Assessment and Monitoring

A child with asthma is to be monitored for clinical signs and symptoms of asthma with the help of asthma diary given to the patients/parents and record of PEFR with a standardized peak flow meter. PEFR must be monitored at the physician's office, asthma clinics (where spirometry should be available) and in the emergency room, and patients must be encouraged and trained to monitor their PEFR at home once a day routinely and twice a day if the morning reading is abnormal to determine their PEFR variability. Patient's personal best should be assessed and used subsequently. Spirometry has been kept optional, and emphasis must be given to patient's quality of life. Emphasis must be on self-management but physician's supervision must still be the prima mode. Patients must be given a written crisis management plan where literate. Otherwise verbal communication at each contact must continue.

Classification of Asthma Severity

Asthma severity classification was accepted as changed to be mild intermittent, mild persistent, moderate persistent and severe persistent asthma (Table 33.13). Since spirometry is not routinely available to pediatricians in this country it was felt that more emphasis be placed on PEFR measurement, especially at the physician's office. Patient's personal best be used as the standard but in its absence expected PEFR according to norms published on children in India must be used.[65] It was also mentioned that a severe form of asthma requiring daily oral steroids or stronger treatments like immunosuppressants is extremely uncommon in Indian children, and most of the children get controlled with inhaled medications.

The presence of one of the features is sufficient to place a patient in that category. A child should be assigned to the most severe category in which any feature occurs. An individual classification may change over a period of time.

Goals of Asthma Therapy

The goals of asthma therapy are:
- Prevent chronic and troublesome symptoms
- Maintain near normal (PEFR)
- Maintain normal activity levels (including exercise and physical activity)
- Prevent recurrent exacerbations of asthma and minimize the need for emergency room visits and hospitalization
- Provide optimal pharmacotherapy with minimal side effects
- Meet patient's and family's expectations of satisfaction with asthma care.

Pharmacological Therapy

Pharmacological therapy is the cornerstone of management. It must be instituted with proper environmental control measures. Medications are classified into two broad categories: (i) long-term control medications or the preventatives, and (ii) medications or rescue medications. Long-term control medications, are, inflammatory compounds. Early intervention with inhaled steroids can improve control and normalize lung function, and preliminary studies show that it might prevent irreversible airway injury. These are to be administered with the help of a metered dose inhaler (MDI) and a spacer (in patients who cannot afford the spacers a homemade spacer can be used). Another cheaper alternative is a dry powder inhaler (transparent rotahaler). A step care approach management of asthma starting at a higher level and then stepping down as control is established (Table 33:14). Table 33.15 gives details of assessment of severity of asthma in children and Table 33.16 and 33.17 outline management of asthma exacerbation.

Referral

Patients must be refereed to a special clinic of asthma if any of the following problems arise:
- Failure to meet the goals of therapy
- Atypical signs or symptoms or uncertain diagnosis
- Presence of complications
- Need for additional diagnostic testing like skin tests, pulmonary function tests endoscopy, incremental growth assessment, etc.
- Severe symptoms such as step 4 care
- Nonadherence to therapy

	TABLE 33.13: Classification of asthma severity		
Guide	Symptoms	Night-time symptoms	Lung function
Severe persistent Step 4	Continual symptoms Limited physical activity Frequent exacerbations	Frequent	PEFR < 60% Predicted
Moderate persistent Step 3	Daily symptoms Daily use of beta-agonist Exacerbation affecting activity, ≥ 2/weeks, lasting days	> 1 time/week	PEF > 60 to < 80% Predicted
Mild persistent Step 2	Symptoms > 2/week but < 1/day Exacerbation may affect activity	> 2 time/month	PEF ≥ 80% predicted
Mild intermittent Step 1	Symptoms ≤ 2/week Exacerbation brief, Asymptomatic between exacerbations	≤ 2 time/month	PEF ≥ 80%

TABLE 33.14: Stepwise approach in long-term management of children with asthma

Grade	Long-term	Quick relief	Education
Severe pesistent Step 4	Daily therapy. High dose inhaled, steroid (BDP 1200 µg or BUD > 600 or FP* 200-400 µg + Long acting beta sympathomimetic or SR Theophylline or oral steroids. For infants $\leq$ 2 years inhaled medication with spacer and/or mask	Short-acting bronchodilator. Infants as in step 1	Step 1 + self-monitoring Group education
Moderate pesistent step 3	Daily therapy. Medium dose inhaled steroid (BDP 600-1200 µg or BUD 400-600 or FP 100-200 µg) or Low-medium dose inhaled steroid + SR Theophylline or long acting beta sympathomimetic. For infants inhaled medication with spacer and mask	Short-acting bronchodilator Infants as in step 1	Step 1 + self monitoring Group education/ counselling
Mild persistent Step 2	Daily medication NSAIDs like Cromolyn (1-5 mg/dose Or) or low-dose inhaled steroid (BDP 200-600 or BUD 100-400 or FP50-100 µg) and Theophylline 5-15 mg/kg spacer and Mask for infants $\leq$ 2 years	Short-acting bronchodilator. Infants as in step 1	step 1 + self-monitoring Group education
Mild intermittent. Step 1	No daily medications needed	Short-acting bronchodilator, inhaled β_2-agonists SOS use of β_2-agonist > 2 times/week indicates need for for preventative drugs. For infants (< 2 years) bronchodilator as needed for symptoms. Use facemask with holding chamber or nebuliser or oral β_2-agonist.	Basic facts about asthma, inhaler technique,discuss role of medication, self-management and action plans, environmental control

Abbreviation

BDP—beclomethasone dipropionate, BUD—budesonide, FP—fluticasone propionate, SR—sustained release
FP is recommended for children older than 4 years.

- Need for good asthma education
- Significant psychosocial or psychiatric problems

Environmental Control and Prevention of Asthma

Allergen Avoidance

Indoor allergens: Cockroach, house dust mite, fungal spores, animals (pets) are the main sources. Skin testing can be used, for the diagnosis. Following control measures are suggested.

Cockroaches: Leave no food uncovered. Traps are better than the anti-cockroach chemicals.

House dust mite: Sun the bedding weekly. No carpets or stuffed belongings, in the house. Proper mapping of the country needs to be done to see where dust mite is an important allergen-expected in warm, humid climate.

Pets: Pets like dogs, cats or birds should not be kept. Reports on pets are very few in this country. If pets are already in the house contact with the patients should be minimized or they should be kept out of the premises.

Moulds or indoor fungal spores: Prevent seepage of water through rooms or walls during the rainy season. Keep rooms well ventilated and allow sunlight in.

Seasonal exposure to pollens and fungi can be reduced by keeping the doors and windows closed from every morning till evening. Wherever affordable, air-conditioning can be used. In case an allergen is found to contribute significantly to patient problem, he or she should be referred to a specialist for skin testing and if required, for immunotherapy. In children less than 5 to 6 years of age immunotherapy is avoided.

Irritants or Chemicals

Avoid tobacco smoke, strong odors, fumes from various kinds of stoves/chullah, using kerosene, wood, cowdung.

In high risk families (atopy on both sides or even one side), exclusive breastfeed to continue for 4 to 6 months and mother to avoid well-known allergenic food in diet while baby is exclusively breastfed.

TABLE 33.15: Classifying severity of asthma exacerbations

	Mild	Moderate	Severe	Respiratory arrest imminent
Symptoms				
Breathlessness	While walking	While talking (infant-softer, shorter cry; difficult feeding)	While at rest (infant-stops feeding)	
	Can lie down	Prefers sitting	Sits upright	
Talks in	Sentences	Phrases	Words	
Alertness	May be agitated	Usually agitated	Usually agitated	Drowsy/confused
Signs				
Respiratory rate	Increased	Increased	often > 30/min	

(Guide to breathing rates in awake children):

Age	Normal rate
< 2months	< 60/niin
< 2-12 months	< 50/n-dn
1-5 years	< 40/n-dn
6-8 years	< 30/min

	Mild	Moderate	Severe	Respiratory arrest imminent
Use of accessory muscles: Suprasternal retractions	Usually not	Commonly	Usually	Paradoxical thoraco-abdominal movement
Wheeze	Moderate often only end expiratory	Loud; throughout exhalation	Usually loud; throughout inhalation and exhalation	Absence of wheeze
Pulse/min	< 100	100-120	> 120	Bradycardia

(Guide to heart rate in normal children):

Age	Normal rate
2-12 months	< 160 min
1-2 years	< 120 min
2-8 years	< 110 min.

Psychosocial Aspects of Asthma Management in Children

Children with chronic illnesses are at an increased risk for developing psychological disturbances.

Children with severe asthma have been found to be three times more likely to develop emotional/behavioral problems as compared to healthy children. It was decided at the meeting that the primary physician to the patient be able to deliver the necessary preventive services like explaining the basic facts about the disease and try to improve the quality of life by optimum care. Mental health workers can provide important services to asthmatic children, who have obvious psychological or behavioral problems, experience school difficulties and are noncompliant with treatments.

Family therapy aimed at modifying family interaction problems and parent-child relationships can help in improved management of asthma and also improve the overall quality of life. Hence, family therapy is considered an adjunct to the conventional treatment in asthma in children with severe disease. It is important that psychologists be part of the multidisciplinary treating team in order to provide comprehensive services to children with asthma.

Health Education

The experts stressed the need for health education not only in asthma clinic or hospital but also on TV, radio and other communication media. The attitudes and practices concerning this disease demonstrate a high degree of ignorance and misinformation. Written material containing information regarding basic facts of asthma should be made available to the patient and the parent at the time of transmission of information regarding the diagnosis. Special measures were recommended to be taken to educate the people about the harms of passive smoking.

TABLE 33.16: Management protocol for acute exacerbation of childhood asthma emergency room

Ask and record
1. Duration of present episode
2. Medications already being used
3. Time of last aminophylline dose (if taking)
4. Precipitating factors—infections, exercise, drugs, stress, seasonal, etc.
5. Severity of previous episodes of treatment required

Examine for
1. Sensorium
2. Respiratory rate, heart rate, color, use of accessory muscles, breath sounds intensity, wheeze
3. Saturation-SaO$_2$ if pulse oxymeter is available
4. Peak expiratory flow rate

Treatment Phase-I - Ist one hour
1. Oxygen by mask to achieve saturation > 90 percent (minimum 5 L/min through simple facemask)
2. Start β$_2$ sympathomimetic nebulization 0.15 mg/kg/dose (minimum dose 2.5 mg) every 20 min for 3 doses. For delivery dilute aerosols to mnimum of 4 ml of saline at flow of 6-8 L/minutes or β$_2$ sympathomimetic through MDI and spacer with/without facemask 4 to 8 puffs every 20 minutes (10-20 puffs in one hour).
   In case of nonavailability of nebuliser or MDI and spacer or where the patient cannot move the needle of the peak flowmeter - parenteral beta-agonists (adrenaline/ terbutaline) should be given in the dose of 0.01 mg/kg up to 0.3 to 0.5 mg every 20 minutes for 3 doses in the first hour subcutaneously.
3. All children presenting with acute exacerbation should receive systemic steroids. Prednisolone 2 mg/kg/dose or methylprednisolone 1-2 mg/kg/dose or hydrocortisone 10 mg/kg/dose. At the end of hour repeat assessment with more emphasis on symptoms and signs, PEFR done if possible. In interpreting PEFR value is compared with predicted value of Indian children or personal best of the child if available. From the assessment 2 groups are identified:

A. *Good response*
   Physical examination normal (decrease in heart rate from the previous value, respiratory rate, pulses paradoxus < 10 mm Hg, no usage of accessory muscles, alert sensorium) O$_2$ saturation >90 percent, PEFR > 70 percent.
B. *Incomplete response/poor response*
   Mild to moderately severe symptoms and signs (see Table above) for mild, moderate and severe classification of symptoms/ signs, PEFR < 50 to < 70 percent.

Phase II-Management

A Good response group
- Discharge home, continue treatment with β$_2$-agonist and course of oral systemic corticosteroid 1-2 mg/kg/ day maximum 60 mg/ day in a single or 2 divided doses for 3-10 days.
- Patient education, review medicine use, initiate action plan, recommend close medical follow-up
B Incomplete/poor responders
- Continue O$_2$, β$_2$ sympathomimetic inhalation every 20 mts. Continuous nebulization can also be used under strict monitoring for heart rate and blood potassium levels.
- Continue systemic steroids
- Add ipratropium bromide nebulization 250 micrograms every 20 mts for three doses, May mix in same nebulizer with β$_2$ sympathomimetic.
- If no response, aminophylline infusion, (0.25 mg/ kg/hr) can be tried
- IV Magnesium sulphate 50 percent 50 mg/kg/dose IV infusion in 30 ml normal saline/30 mts can be given before transfer to ICU

Continue to assess every one-hour, continue same treatment for 4 hours
Improvement—at end of 6 hours since initiation of treatment decrease the frequency of β$_2$ sympathomimetic inhalations every 1 to 4 hrs as needed, stop parenteral aminophylline, continue systemic steroids 1-2 mg/kg/day in 2 divided doses for 3-10 days
If no deterioration continue same treatment
If deterioration, follow intensive care of the child with asthma in pediatric ICU for possible intubation and mechanical ventilation in presence of
i. Exhaustion, shallow respiration, confusion or drowsiness
ii. Coma/respiratory arrest
iii. Worsening or persisting hypoxia

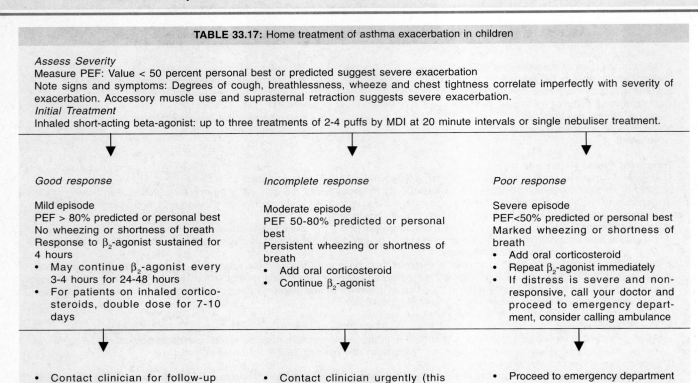

TABLE 33.17: Home treatment of asthma exacerbation in children

Assess Severity
Measure PEF: Value < 50 percent personal best or predicted suggest severe exacerbation
Note signs and symptoms: Degrees of cough, breathlessness, wheeze and chest tightness correlate imperfectly with severity of exacerbation. Accessory muscle use and suprasternal retraction suggests severe exacerbation.
Initial Treatment
Inhaled short-acting beta-agonist: up to three treatments of 2-4 puffs by MDI at 20 minute intervals or single nebuliser treatment.

Good response	*Incomplete response*	*Poor response*
Mild episode	Moderate episode	Severe episode
PEF > 80% predicted or personal best	PEF 50-80% predicted or personal best	PEF<50% predicted or personal best
No wheezing or shortness of breath	Persistent wheezing or shortness of breath	Marked wheezing or shortness of breath
Response to β_2-agonist sustained for 4 hours	• Add oral corticosteroid	• Add oral corticosteroid
• May continue β_2-agonist every 3-4 hours for 24-48 hours	• Continue β_2-agonist	• Repeat β_2-agonist immediately
• For patients on inhaled cortico-steroids, double dose for 7-10 days		• If distress is severe and non-responsive, call your doctor and proceed to emergency depart-ment, consider calling ambulance
• Contact clinician for follow-up instructions	• Contact clinician urgently (this day) for instructions	• Proceed to emergency department

Future Directions for Research

The data presented indicates gross inadequacy of information regarding basic facts of asthma to patients and their parents. Intervention in the form of written material significantly improves the knowledge of these individuals. More studies need to be done to assess the knowledge, attitudes and practices of these patients and specific materials developed to improve the baseline information and change attitudes towards inhalational therapy. All the participants felt that there was a local social stigma attached to the disease, and parents of the patients were specially concerned about the inhalational therapy having potential for producing drug dependence. Why incidence of asthma is relatively less in India and the disease is less severe as compared to some of the western countries, information regarding it is not available. More data need to be generated towards epidemiology of asthma in this country. Research into usefulness of yogic breathing exercises and role of Ayurveda needs to be evaluated, although at present they have no proven scientific value.

The new GINA Guidelines are shown in Annexure 2.

REFERENCES

1. Global Strategy for Asthma Management and Prevention. NHLBI/WHO Workshop report. Global Initiative for asthma. NIH Publication No. 95-3659; January 1995, reprinted 1996; Epidemiology; Chapter 2;11-24.
2. Gergen PJ, Mullay DY, Evans RM. National Survey of prevalence of asthma among children in the United States, 1976 to 1980. Pediatrics 1988;81:1-7.
3. The International study of asthma and allergies in childhood (ISAAC) Steering Committee. Worldwide variations in the prevalence of asthma symptoms: The International study of Asthma: The International study of asthma and allergies in childhood (ISAAC). Eur Respir J 1998;12:315-35.
4. Burney PGJ, Luczynska C, Chinn S, Jarvis D. The European Community Respiratory Health Survey. Eur Respir J 1994;7:954-60.
5. European Community Respiratory Health Survey (EC-RHS). Variations in the prevalence of respiratory symptoms, self-reported asthma attacks, and use of asthma medication in the European Community Respiratory Health Survey (ECRHS). Eur Respir J 1996;9:687-95.
6. Habbick BF, Pzzichini MM, Taylor B, Rennie D, Senthilselvan A, Sears MR. Prevalence of asthma, rhinitis and eczema among children in 2 Canadian cities: In: International Study of Asthma and Allergies in Childhood. CMAJ 1999;160:1824-28.
7. Shamssain MH, Shamsian N. Prevalence and severity of asthma, rhinitis, and atopic eczema in 13 to 14 year

old schoolchildren from the northeast of England. Ann Allergy Asthma Immunol 2001;86:428-32.

8. El-Sharif NS, Nemery B, Barghuthy F, Mortaja S, Qasrawi R, Abdeen Z. Geographical variations of asthma and asthma symptoms among schoolchildren aged 5 to 8 years and 12 to 15 years in Palestine: The International Study of Asthma and Allergies in Childhood (ISAAC). Ann Allergy Asthma Immunol 2003;90:63-71.

9. Al-Dawood K. Epidemiology of bronchial asthma among schoolboys in Al-Khobar city, Saudi Arabia: Cross-sectional study. Croat Med J 2000;41:437-41.

10. Al-Riyami BM, Al-Rawas OA, Al-Riyami AA, Jasim LG, Mohammed AJ. A relatively high prevalence and severity of asthma, allergic rhinitis and atopic eczema in schoolchildren in the Sultanate of Oman. Respirology 2003;8:69-76.

11. Trakultivakorn M. Prevalence of asthma, rhinitis, and eczema in Northern Thai children from Chiang Mai (International Study of a Asthma and Allergies in Childhood, ISAAC). Asian Pac J Allergy Immunol 1999;17:243-48.

12. Shohat T, Golan G, Tamir R, Green MS, Livne I, Davidson Y, Harari G, Garty BZ. Prevalence of asthma in 13-14 yr-old schoolchildren across Israel. Eur Respir J 2000;15:725-29.

13. Crane J, Mallol J, Beasley R, Stewart A, Asher MI. International study of Asthma and Allergies in Childhood Phase I study group. Agreement between written and video questions for comparing asthma symptoms in ISAAC. Eur Respir J 2003;21:455-61.

14. Beasley R, Ellwood P, Asher I, International patterns of the prevalence of pediatric asthma in ISAAC program. Pediatr Clin North Am 2003;50:539-53.

15. Paramesh H. Epidemiology of asthma in India. Indian J Pediatr 2002;69:309-12.

16. Chhabra SK, Gupta CK, Chhabra P, Rajpal S. Risk factors for development of bronchial asthma in children in Delhi. Ann Allergy Asthma Immunol 1999;83:385-90.

17. Gupta D, Aggarwal AN, Kumar R, Jindal SK. Prevalence of Bronchial Asthma and Association with Environmental Tobacco Smoke Exposure in Adolescent School Children in Chandigarh, North India. Journal of Asthma 2001;38:501-07.

18. Palmer LJ, Valinsky IJ, Pikora T, Zubrick SR, Landau LI. Environmental factors and asthma and allergy in schoolchildren from Western Australia. Eur Respir J 1999;14:1351-57.

19. Chan KN, Elliman A, Bryan E, et al. Respiratory symptoms in children of low birth weight. Arch Dis Child 1989,64:1294-304.

20. Chan KN, Noble-jamieson Cm, Elliman A, et al. Lung function of children of low birth weight. Arch Dis Child 1989;1284-393.

21. Burrows B, Taussig ML. "As the twig is bent, the tree inclines" (perhaps). Am Rev Respir Dis 19K-122.813-16.

22. Dodge R, Martinez FD, Cline MG, et al. Early childhood respiratory symptoms and the subsequent diagnosis of asthma. J Allergy Clin Immunol 1996,98.48-54.

23. Roberson CF, Heycock E, Bishop J, et al. Prevalence of asthma in Melbourne school-children—changes over 26 years. BMI 1991;302:1116-18.

24. Ninan T, Ryssekk G. Respiratory symptoms and atopy in Aberdeen school children – Evidence from two surveys 25 years apart-BMI 1992;304,873-75.

25. Peat JK, van den Berg RH, Green WF, et al. Changing prevalence of Asthma in Australian children. BMJ 1994308:1591-96.

26. Chandra RK. Prospective studies of the effect of breast feeding on incidence of infection and allergy. Acta Paediatr Scand 1979;68:691-94.

27. Fergusson DK, Horwood JL, Shannon FT, et al. Breast-feeding gastrointestinal and lower respiratory illness in the first two years. Aust Paediatr J 1981;17-191-95.

28. Burr ML, Limb ES, Maguire MJ, et al. Infant feeding wheezing, and allergy—A prospective.study. Arch Dis Child 19930:724-28.

29. Poysa L, Korppi M, Remes K, et al. Atopy in childhood and diet in infancy—A nine-year follow-up study-I - clinical manifestations. Allergy Proc 1991;12:107-11.

30. Rust GS, Thompson CJ, Minor P, Davis-Mitchell W, Holloway K, Murray V. Does breastfeeding protect children from asthma? Analysis of NHANES III survey data. J Natl Med Assoc 2001;93:139-49.

31. Burney P. A diet rich in sodium may potentiate asthma-epidemiology evidence for a new hypothesis. Chest l987;91(Suppl):143S-48S.

32. Carey OJ, Locke C, Cooksoh JB. Effect of alterations of dietary sodium on the severity of asthma in men. Thorax 1993;48:714-18.

33. Peat JK, Hodge-T, Salome CM, et al. Dietary fish intake and asthma in children. Am J Respir Crit Care Med 1995;151(Suppl):A469.

34. Schwartz J, Weiss ST. The relationship of dietary fish intake to level of pulmonary function in the first National Health and Nutrition Survey (NHANES). Eur Respir J 1994;7.1821-24.

35. National Research Council, Environmental tobacco smoke—Exposures and assessing effects. Washington: National Academy Press 1986.

36. Cunningham J, O'Connor GT, Dockery DW, et al. Environmental tobacco smoke, wheezing and asthma children in 24 communities. Am I Respir Crit Care Med 1996;153:218-24.

37. Martinez FD, Wright AL, Taussig LM, et al. Asthma and wheezing in the first six years of life. N 1995;332:133-38.

38. Von Mutius E, Sherrill DL, Fritzsch C, et al. Air pollution and upper respiratory-symptoms in children from East Germany. Eur Respir J 1995;8:23-28.

39. Braback L, Breborowicz A, Knutpson A, et al. Atopic sensitisation and respiratory symptoms, and Swedish school children. Clin Exp Allergy 1994;24:826-35.

40. Behera D, Sood P, Singhi S. Passive smoking, domestic fuels, and lung function in North India Children. Ind J Chest Dis All Sci 1998;40:89-98.

41. Behera D, Sood P, Singhi S. Respiratory, symptoms in Indian children exposed to different cooking fuels. J Assoc Phys India 1998;46:182-18.

42. Wjst M, Reitmeir P, Dold S, et al. Road traffic and adverse effects on respiratory health in children. BMJ 1993;307-596-600.

43. Weinmann GG, Bowes SK, Gerbase MW, et al. Response to acute ozone exposure in healthy men. Results of a screening procedure. Am J Respir Crit Care Med 1995;151:33-40.

44. Clough JB, WAHom JD, Holgate ST. Effect of atopy on the natural history of flow, and bronchial, hyper-responsiveness in 7- and 8-year-old children with asthma. Respir Dis 1991;143:755-60.

45. Martin AJ, Landau LI, Phelan PD. Lung functions in young adults who had asthma in childhood. Am Respir Dis 1980;122:609-16.

46. Gerritsen J. Prognosis of asthma from childhood to adulthood. Am Rev Respir Dis 1989;140:1325-30.

47. Peat JK, Wookock AJ. Sensitivity to common allergens; Relation to respiratory symptoms and bronchial hyperesponsiveness in children from different climatic areas of Australia. Clin Expt Allergy 1991-21:573-81.

48. van Asperen PP, Kemp AS, Mukhi A. Atopy in infancy predicts the severity of bronchial hyperresponsiveness in later childhood. J Allergy Cline Immune 1990; 85:790-95.

49. Sherril D. The effect of airway hyperresponsiveness, wheezing and atopy on longitudinal pulmonary function in children—A six ear follow-up study. Pediatr Pulmonol 1992;13:78-85.

50. Murphy S. Asthma: An inflammatory disease: In: Hillman BC (Ed): Paediatric Respiratory Disease: Diagnosis and Management. Philadelphia: WB Saunders 1993;621-26.

51. von Mutius E. Progression of allergy and asthma through childhood to adolescence. Thorax 1996; 51(suppl 1):S3-S6.

52. Kelly WJ. Childhood asthma and adult lung function. Am Rev Respir Dis 1988;138:26-30.

53. Martin AJ, Landau LI, Phelan PD. Asthma from childhood at age 21-the patient and his (or her) disease. Br Med J 1982;284:380-82.

54. Williams H, McNicol KN. Prevalence, natural history, and relationship of wheez bronchitis and asthma in children. An epiden-dologic study. Br Med J 1969;4;321-25.

55. Park ES, Golding J, Carswell F, et al. Pre-school wheezing and prognosis at 10. Arch Dis Child 1986;61:642-46.

56. Balfour-Lynn. Childhood asthma and puberty. Arch Dis Child 1985;60:231-35.

57. Peat JK, Salome CM, Segwick CS, et al. A prospective study of bronchial hyperresponsiveness and respiratory symptoms in a population of Australian school children. Clin Expt Allergy 1989;19:299-306.

58. Roorda RJ. Prognostic factors for the outcome of childhood asthma in adolescence. Thorax 1996;51(suppl 1):S7-Sl2.

59. Price JF. Issues in adolescent asthma: What are the needs? Thorax 1996;51(suppl 1):Sl3-Sl7.

60. Ownby DR. Environmental factors versus genetic determinants of childhood inhalant allergies. J Allergy Clin Immunol 1990;86:279-87.

61. Frischer T, Kuehr J, Meinert R, et al. Risk factors for childhood asthma and recurrent wheezy bronchitis. Eur J Pediatr 1993;152:771-75.

62. Sherman CB, Tosteson TD, Tager IB, et al. Early childhood predictors of asthma. Am I Epidemiol 1990;132:83-95.

63. Sibbald B, Horn MEC, Gregg I. A family study of the genetic basis of asthma and wheezy bronchitis. Arch Dis Child 1980;55:354-57.

64. The Cochrane Library: Update Soft Ware, Oxford, UK.

65. Parmar V, Kumar L, Malik SK. Normal values of peak expiratory flow rate in healthy north Indian school children 6-16 years of age. Ind Pediatr 1977;14,591-94.

ANNEXURE 2

WHAT IS KNOWN ABOUT ASTHMA?

Unfortunately...asthma is one of the most common chronic diseases worldwide. The prevalence of asthma symptoms in children varies from 1 to more than 30 percent in different populations and is increasing in most countries, especially among young children.

Fortunately... asthma can be effectively treated and most patients can achieve good control of their disease. When asthma is under **control** children can:
- Avoid troublesome symptoms night and day
- Use little or no reliever medication
- Have productive, physically active lives
- Have (near) normal lung function
- Avoid serious attacks

- Asthma causes recurring episodes of **wheezing, breathlessness, chest tightness,** and **coughing,** particularly at night or in the early morning.
- Asthma is a **chronic inflammatory disorder** of the airways. Chronically inflamed airways are **hyperresponsive;** they become obstructed and airflow is limited (by bronchoconstriction, mucus plugs, and increased inflammation) when airways are exposed to various risk factors.
- Common **risk factors** for asthma symptoms include exposure to allergens (such as those from house dust mites, animals with fur, cockroaches, pollens, and molds), occupational irritants, tobacco smoke, respiratory (viral) infections, exercise, strong emotional expressions, chemical irritants, and drugs (such as aspirin and beta blockers).
- A **stepwise approach** to pharmacologic treatment to achieve and maintain control of asthma should take into account the safety of treatment, potential for adverse effects, and the cost of treatment required to achieve control.
- Asthma **attacks** (or exacerbations) are episodic, but airway inflammation is chronically present.
- For many patients, **controller** medication must be taken daily to prevent symptoms, improve lung function, and prevent attacks. **Reliever** medications may occasionally be required to treat acute symptoms such as wheezing, chest tightness, and cough.
- To reach and maintain asthma control requires the development of a **partnership** between the person with asthma and his or her health care team.
- Asthma is not a cause for shame. Olympic athletes, famous leaders, other celebrities, and ordinary people live **successful lives** with asthma.

DIAGNOSING ASTHMA

Asthma can often be diagnosed on the basis of a patient's **symptoms** and **medical history** (Table A2.1).

TABLE A2.1: Is it asthma?

Consider asthma if any of the following signs or symptoms are present:
• Frequent episodes of wheezing—more than once a month
• Activity-induced cough or wheeze
• Cough particularly at night during periods without viral infections
• Absence of seasonal variation in wheeze
• Symptoms that persist after age 3
• Symptoms occur or worsen in the presence of:
  − Animals with fur
  − Aerosol chemicals
  − Changes in temperature
  − Domestic dust mites
  − Drugs (aspirin, beta blockers)
  − Exercise
  − Pollen
  − Respiratory (viral) infections
  − Smoke
  − Strong emotional expression
• The child's colds repeatedly "go to the chest" or take more than 10 days to clear up
• Symptoms improve when asthma medication is given

Measurements of **lung function** provide an assessment of the severity, reversibility, and variability of airflow limitation, and help confirm the diagnosis of asthma in patients older than 5 years.

Spirometry is the preferred method of measuring airflow limitation and its reversibility to establish a diagnosis of asthma.

- An increase in FEV_1 of ≥12% (or ≥ 200 ml) after administration of a bronchodilator indicates reversible airflow limitation consistent with asthma (However, most asthma patients will not exhibit reversibility at each assessment, and repeated testing is advised).

Peak expiratory flow (PEF) measurements can be an important aid in both diagnosis and monitoring of asthma.

- PEF measurements are ideally compared to the patient's own previous best measurements using his/her own peak flow meter.
- An improvement of 60 L/min (or ≥ 20% of the prebronchodilator PEF) after inhalation of a bronchodilator, or diurnal variation in PEF of more than 20% (with twice-daily readings, more than 10%), suggests a diagnosis of asthma.

Do all children who wheeze have asthma?

No. Most children who develop wheezing after age 5 have asthma. However, diagnosis of asthma in children 5 years and younger presents a particularly difficult problem. Episodic wheezing and cough are also common in children who do not have asthma, particularly in children younger than age 3. The younger the child, the greater the likelihood that an alternative diagnosis may explain recurrent wheeze.

Although there is the possibility of overtreatment, episodes of wheezing may be shortened and reduced in intensity by effective use of anti-inflammatory medications and bronchodilators rather than antibiotics.

Alternative but very rare causes of recurrent wheezing, particularly in early infancy, include chronic rhino-sinusitis, cystic fibrosis, gastroesophageal reflux, recurrent viral lower respiratory tract infections, bronchopulmonary dysplasia, tuberculosis, congenital malformation causing narrowing of the intrathoracic airways, foreign body aspiration, primary ciliary dyskinesia syndrome, immune deficiency, and congenital heart disease.

In children 5 years and younger, the diagnosis of asthma has to be based largely on clinical judgment and an assessment of symptoms and physical findings. A useful method for confirming the diagnosis in this age group is a trial of treatment with short-acting bronchodilators and inhaled glucocorticosteroids. Marked clinical improvement during the treatment and deterioration when treatment is stopped supports a diagnosis of asthma.

Children 4 to 5 years old can be taught to use a PEF meter, but to ensure accurate results parental supervision is required. Other diagnostic considerations in children include:

- Diary cards to record symptoms and PEF (in children older than 5 years) readings are important tools in childhood asthma management.
- Allergy skin tests, or the measurement of specific IgE in serum, can help in the identification of risk factors so that appropriate environmental control measures can be recommended.

CLASSIFICATION OF ASTHMA BY LEVEL OF CONTROL

Traditionally, the degree of symptoms, airflow limitation, and lung function variability have allowed asthma to be classified by **severity** (e.g. as intermittent, mild persistent, moderate persistent, or severe persistent).

However, it is important to recognize that asthma severity involves both the severity of the underlying disease and its responsiveness to treatment. In addition, severity is not an unvarying feature of an individual patient's asthma, but may change over months or years.

Therefore, for ongoing management of asthma, **classification of asthma by level of control** is more relevant and useful (Table A2.2).

Examples of validated measures for assessing clinical control of asthma include:

- Asthma Control Test (ACT): http://www.asthmacontrol.com
- Asthma Control Questionnaire (ACQ): http://www.qoltech.co.uk/Asthma1.htm
- Asthma Therapy Assessment Questionnaire (ATAQ): http://www.ataqinstrument.com
- Asthma control scoring system

FOUR COMPONENTS OF ASTHMA CARE

The **goal of asthma care is to achieve and maintain control** of the clinical manifestations of the disease for prolonged periods. When asthma is controlled, patients can prevent most attacks, avoid troublesome symptoms day and night, and keep physically active.

			TABLE A2.2: Levels of asthma control

Characteristic	Controlled (All of the following)	Partly controlled (Any measure present in any week)	Uncontrolled
Daytime symptoms	None (twice or less/week)	More than twice/week	**Three or more features of partly controlled asthma present in any week**
Limitations of activities	None	Any	
Nocturnal symptoms/ awakening	None	Any	
Need for reliever/rescue treatment	None (twice or less/week)	More than twice/week	
Lung function (PEF or FEV1)‡	Normal	< 80% predicted or personal best (if known)	
Exacerbations	None	One or more/year*	One in any week†

* Any exacerbation should prompt review of maintenance treatment to ensure that it is adequate.
† By definition, an exacerbation in any week makes that an uncontrolled asthma week.
‡ Lung function testing is not reliable for children 5 years and younger.

To reach this goal, four interrelated components of therapy are required:

Component 1. Develop patient/family/doctor partnership

Component 2. Identify and reduce exposure to risk factors

Component 3. Assess, treat, and monitor asthma

Component 4. Manage asthma exacerbations

Component 1: Develop patient/family/doctor partnership

With the help of everyone on the health care team, children and their families can be actively involved in managing asthma to prevent problems and enable children to live productive, physically active lives. They can learn to:

• Avoid risk factors
• Take medications correctly
• Understand the difference between "controller" and "reliever" medications
• Monitor asthma control status using symptoms and, if available, PEF in children older than 5 years of age
• Recognize signs that asthma is worsening and take action
• Seek medical help as appropriate.

Education should be an integral part of all interactions between health care professionals and patients. Using a variety of methods—such as discussions (with a physician, nurse, outreach worker, counselor, or educator), demonstrations, written materials, group classes, video or audio tapes, dramas, and patient support groups—helps reinforce educational messages.

Working together, you and the child and their family/caregiver should prepare a **written personal asthma action plan** that is medically appropriate and practical. A sample asthma plan is shown in Table A2.3.

Additional self-management plans can be found on several Websites, including:

http://www.asthma.org.uk

http://www.nhlbisupport.com/asthma/index.html

http://www.asthmanz.co.nz

TABLE A2.3: Example of contents of an action plan to maintain asthma control

Your Regular Treatment:

1. Each day take _____

2. Before exercise, take _____

WHEN TO INCREASE TREATMENT
Assess your level of Asthma Control

In the past week have you had:

Daytime asthma symptoms more than 2 times ?	No	Yes
Activity or exercise limited by asthma?	No	Yes
Waking at night because of asthma?	No	Yes
The need to use your [rescue medication] more than 2 times?	No	Yes
If you are monitoring peak flow, peak flow less than_____?	No	Yes

If you answered *Yes* to three or more of these questions, your asthma is uncontrolled and you may need to step up your treatment.

HOW TO INCREASE TREATMENT

STEP UP your treatment as follows and assess improvement every day:
_____[Write in next treatment step here]

Maintain this treatment for _____days [specify number]

WHEN TO CALL THE DOCTOR/CLINIC

Call your doctor/clinic _____[provide phone numbers]

If you don't respond in _____days [specify number]

_____[optional lines for additional instruction]

EMERGENCY/SEVERE LOSS OF CONTROL

• If you have severe shortness of breath, and can only speak in short sentences
• If you are having a severe attack of asthma and are frightened
• If you need your **reliever medication** more than every 4 hours and are not improving.

1. Take 2 to 4 puffs _____ [reliever medication]

2. Take_____mg of_____ [oral glucocorticosteroid]

3. Seek medical help: Go to_____; Address_____Phone: _____

4. Continue to use your _____ [**reliever medication**] until you are able to get medical help.

Component 2: Identify and Reduce Exposure to Risk Factors

To improve control of asthma and reduce medication needs, patients should take steps to avoid the risk factors that cause their asthma symptoms (Table A2.4). However, many asthma patients react to multiple factors that are ubiquitous in the environment, and avoiding some of these factors completely is nearly impossible. Thus, medications to maintain asthma control have an important role because patients are often less sensitive to these risk factors when their asthma is under control.

Physical activity is a common cause of asthma symptoms but patients **should not avoid exercise.** Symptoms can be prevented by taking a rapid-acting inhaled β_2-agonist before strenuous exercise (a leukotriene modifier or cromone are alternatives).

Children over the age of 3 with severe asthma should be advised to receive an **influenza vaccination** every year, or at least when vaccination of the general population is advised. However, routine influenza vaccination of children with asthma does not appear to protect them from asthma exacerbations or improve asthma control.

TABLE A2.4: Strategies for avoiding common allergens and pollutants

Avoidance measures that improve control of asthma and reduce medication needs:

- **Tobacco smoke:** Stay away from tobacco smoke. Patients and parents should not smoke.

- **Drugs, foods, and additives:** Avoid if they are known to cause symptoms.

  Reasonable avoidance measures that can be recommended but have not been shown to have clinical benefit:

- **House dust mites:** Wash bed linens and blankets weekly in hot water and dry in a hot dryer or the sun. Encase pillows and mattresses in airtight covers.

  Replace carpets with hard flooring, especially in sleeping rooms. (If possible, use vacuum cleaner with filters. Use acaricides or tannic acid to kill mites—but make sure the patient is not at home when the treatment occurs).

- **Animals with fur:** Use air filters. (Remove animals from the home, or at least from the sleeping area. Wash the pet).

- **Cockroaches:** Clean the home thoroughly and often. Use pesticide spray—but make sure the patient is not at home when spraying occurs.

- **Outdoor pollens and mold:** Close windows and doors and remain indoors when pollen and mold counts are highest.

- **Indoor mold:** Reduce dampness in the home; clean any damp areas frequently.

Component 3: Assess, Treat, and Monitor Asthma

The goal of asthma treatment—to achieve and maintain clinical control—can be reached in most patients through a continuous cycle that involves
- Assessing asthma control
- Treating to achieve control
- Monitoring to maintain control

Assessing Asthma Control

Each patient should be assessed to establish his or her current treatment regimen, adherence to the current regimen, and level of asthma control. A simplified scheme for recognizing controlled, partly controlled, and uncontrolled asthma is provided in Table A2.2.

Treating to Achieve Control

For children over age 5, each patient is assigned to one of the treatment "steps" (Fig. A2.1).

At each treatment step, **reliever medication** should be provided for quick relief of symptoms as needed. (However, be aware of how much reliever medication the patient is using—regular or increased use indicates that asthma is not well controlled).

At Steps 2 through 5, patients also require one or more regular **controller medications,** which keep symptoms and attacks from starting. Inhaled glucocorticosteroids (Fig. A2.6) are the most effective controller medications currently available.

For most patients newly diagnosed with asthma or not yet on medication, treatment should be started at Step 2 (or if the patient is very symptomatic, at Step 3). If asthma is not controlled on the current treatment regimen, treatment should be stepped up until control is achieved.

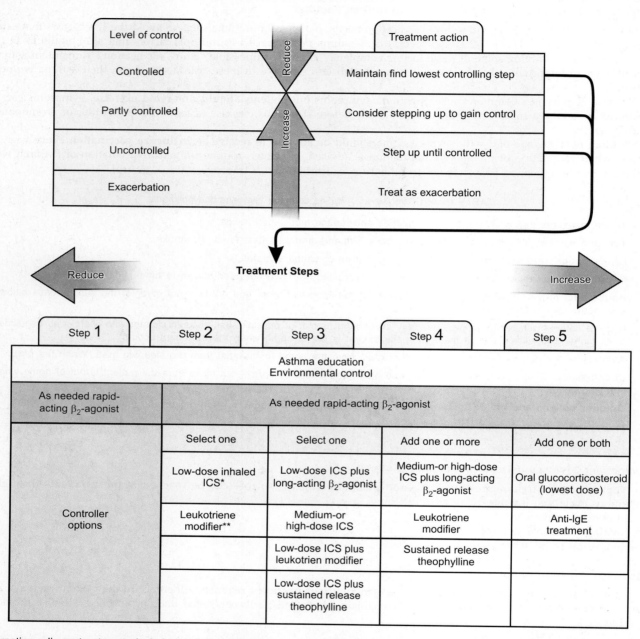

Alternative reliever treatments include inhaled anticholinergics, short-acting oral β₂-agonists, some long-acting β₂-agonists, and short-acting theophylline. Regular dosing with short and long-acting β₂-agonist is not advised unless accompanied by regular use of an inhaled glucocorticosteroid.

FIGURE A2.1: Management approach based on control for children older than 5 years, adolescents and adults

For **children age 5 and younger,** a low-dose inhaled glucocorticosteroid is the recommended initial controller treatment (Box A2.1). If this treatment does not control symptoms, an increase in the glucocorticosteroid dose is the best option.

BOX A2.1: Management approach based on control (children 5 years and younger)

The available literature on treatment of asthma in children 5 years and younger precludes detailed treatment recommendations. The best documented treatment to control asthma in these age groups is inhaled glucocorticosteroids and at step 2, a low-dose inhaled glucocorticosteroid is recommended as the initial controller treatment. Equivalent doses of inhaled glucocorticosteroids, some of which may be given as a single daily dose, are provided in Table A2.5.

TABLE A2.5: Estimated equipotent doses[†] of inhaled glucocorticosteroids for children

Drug	Low daily dose (µg)	Medium daily dose (µg)	High daily dose (µg)[‡]
Beclomethasone dipropionate	100-200	> 200-400	> 400
Budesonide*	100-200	> 200-400	> 400
Budesonide-Neb inhalation suspension	250-500	> 500-1000	> 1000
Ciclesonide*	80-160	> 160-320	> 320
Flunisolide	500-750	> 750-1250	> 1250
Fluticasone	100-200	> 200-500	> 500
Mometasone furoate*	100-200	> 200-400	> 400
Triamcinolone acetonide	400-800	> 800-1200	> 1200

[†] Comparisons based on efficacy data.
[‡] Patients considered for high daily doses except for short periods should be referred to a specialist for assessment to consider alternative combinations of controllers. Maximum recommended doses are arbitrary but with prolonged use are associated with increased risk of systemic side effects.
* Approved for once-daily dosing in mild patients.

Additional Notes
- The most important determinant of appropriate dosing is the clinician's judgment of the patient's response to therapy. The clinician must monitor the patient's response in terms of clinical control and adjust the dose accordingly. Once control of asthma is achieved, the dose of medication should be carefully titrated to the minimum dose required to maintain control, thus reducing the potential for adverse effects.
- Designation of low, medium, and high doses is provided from manufacturers' recommendations where possible. Clear demonstration of dose-response relationships is seldom provided or available. The principle is therefore to establish the minimum effective controlling dose in each patient, as higher doses may not be more effective and are likely to be associated with greater potential for adverse effects.
- **As CFC preparations are taken from the market, medication inserts for HFA preparations should be carefully reviewed by the clinician for the correct equivalent dosage.**

A variety of controller (**Appendix 1**) and reliever (**Appendix 2**) medications for asthma are available. The recommended treatments are guidelines only. Local resources and individual patient circumstances should determine the specific therapy prescribed for each patient.

Inhaled medications are preferred because they deliver drugs directly to the airways where they are needed, resulting in potent therapeutic effects with fewer systemic side effects.
- Devices available to deliver inhaled medication include pressurized metered-dose inhalers (pMDIs), breath-actuated MDIs, dry powder inhalers (DPIs), and nebulizers. Spacer (or valved holding-chamber) devices make inhalers easier to use and reduce systemic absorption and side effects of inhaled glucocorticosteroids.
- Teach children and their parents how to use inhaler devices. Different devices need different inhalation techniques.
  - Give demonstrations and illustrated instructions.
  - Ask patients to show their technique at every visit.
  - Information about use of various inhaler devices is found on the GINA Website.

- For each child, select the most appropriate device. In general:
  - Children younger than 4 years of age should use a pMDI plus a spacer with face mask, or a nebulizer with face mask.
  - Children aged 4 to 6 years should use a pMDI plus a spacer with mouthpiece, a DPI, or, if necessary, a nebulizer with face mask.
  - For children using spacers, the spacer must fit the inhaler.
  - Children of any age over 6 years who have difficulty using pMDIs should use a pMDI with a spacer, a breath-actuated inhaler, a DPI, or a nebulizer. DPIs require an inspiratory effort that may be difficult to achieve during severe attacks.
  - Children who are having severe attacks should use a pMDI with a spacer or a nebulizer.
  - Particularly among children under age 5, inhaler techniques may be poor and should be monitored closely.

Monitoring to Maintain Control

Ongoing monitoring is essential to maintain control and establish the lowest step and dose of treatment to minimize cost and maximize safety.

Typically, patients should be seen one to three months after the initial visit, and every three months thereafter. After an exacerbation, follow-up should be offered within two weeks to one month.

At each visit, ask the questions listed in Table A2.6.

TABLE A2.6: Questions for monitoring asthma care

IS THE ASTHMA MANAGEMENT PLAN MEETING EXPECTED GOALS?

Ask the patient:	**Action to consider:**
Has your asthma awakened you at night? Have you needed more reliever medications than usual? Have you needed any urgent medical care? Has your peak flow been below your personal best? Are you participating in your usual physical activities?	Adjust medications and management plan as needed (step up or step down). But first, compliance should be assessed.

IS THE PATIENT USING INHALERS, SPACER, OR PEAK FLOW METERS CORRECTLY?

Ask the patient:	**Action to consider:**
Please show me how you take your medicine.	Demonstrate correct technique. Have patient demonstrate back.

IS THE PATIENT TAKING THE MEDICATIONS AND AVOIDING RISK FACTORS ACCORDING TO THE ASTHMA MANAGEMENT PLAN?

Ask the patient, for example:	**Action to consid er:**
So that we may plan therapy, please tell me how often you actually take the medicine. What problems have you had following the management plan or taking your medication? During the last month, have you ever stopped taking your medicine because you were feeling better?	Adjust plan to be more practical. Problem solve with the patient to overcome barriers to following the plan.

DOES THE PATIENT HAVE ANY CONCERNS?

Ask the patient:	**Action to consider:**
What concerns might you have about your asthma, medicines, or management plan?	Provide additional education to relieve concerns and discussion to overcome barriers.

Adjusting Medication

- If asthma is **not controlled** on the current treatment regimen, **step up** treatment. Generally, improvement should be seen within 1 month. But first review the patient's medication technique, compliance, and avoidance of risk factors.

- If asthma is **partly controlled, consider stepping up** treatment, depending on whether more effective options are available, safety and cost of possible treatment options, and the patient's satisfaction with the level of control achieved.
- If **control is maintained** for at least 3 months, **step down** with a gradual, stepwise reduction in treatment. The goal is to decrease treatment to the least medication necessary to maintain control.

Monitoring is still necessary even after control is achieved, as asthma is a variable disease; treatment has to be adjusted periodically in response to loss of control as indicated by worsening symptoms or the development of an exacerbation.

Consult with an asthma specialist when other conditions complicate asthma, if the child does not respond to therapy, or if asthma remains uncontrolled with treatment at step 3.

Component 4: Manage Exacerbations

Exacerbations of asthma (asthma attacks) are episodes of a progressive increase in shortness of breath, cough, wheezing, or chest tightness, or a combination of these symptoms.
- **Do not underestimate the severity of an attack;** severe asthma attacks may be life threatening.
- Children/adolescents at high risk for asthma-related death require closer attention and should be encouraged to seek urgent care early in the course of their exacerbations. These patients include those:
  - With a history of near-fatal asthma
  - Who have had a hospitalization or emergency visit for asthma within the past year, or prior intubation for asthma
  - Who are currently using or have recently stopped using oral glucocorticosteroids
  - Who are overdependent on rapid-acting inhaled β_2-agonists
  - With a history of psychosocial problems or denial of asthma or its severity
  - With a history of noncompliance with asthma medication plan.

Patients should immediately seek medical care if...
- The attack is severe (Table A2.7):
  - The patient is breathless at rest, is hunched forward, talks in words rather than sentences (infant stops feeding), agitated, drowsy or confused, has bradycardia, or a respiratory rate greater than 30 per minute
  - Wheeze is loud or absent
  - Pulse is greater than:
        160/min for infants
        120/min for children 1-2 years
        110/min for children 2-8 years
  - PEF is less than 60 percent of predicted or personal best even after initial treatment
  - The child is exhausted
- **The response to the initial bronchodilator treatment is not prompt** and sustained for at least 3 hours
- **There is no improvement within 2 to 6 hours** after oral glucocorticosteroid treatment is started
- **There is further deterioration.**

Mild attacks, defined by a reduction in peak flow of less than 20%, nocturnal awakening, and increased use of rapid-acting β_2-agonists, can usually be treated at home if the patient is prepared and has a personal asthma management plan that includes action steps.

Moderate attacks may require, and severe attacks usually require, care in a clinic or hospital.
Asthma attacks require prompt treatment:
- Oxygen is given at health centers or hospitals if the patient is hypoxemic (achieve O_2 saturation of 95%).
- Inhaled rapid-acting β_2-agonists in adequate doses are essential (Begin with 2 to 4 puffs every 20 minutes for the first hour; then mild exacerbations will require 2 to 4 puffs every 3 to 4 hours, and moderate exacerbations 6 to 10 puffs every 1 to 2 hours
- Oral glucocorticosteroids (0.5 to 1 mg of prednisolone/kg or equivalent during a 24 hour period) introduced early in the course of a moderate or severe attack help to reverse the inflammation and speed recovery.
- Methylxanthines are not recommended if used in addition to high doses of inhaled β_2-agonists. However, theophylline can be used if inhaled β_2-agonists are not available. If the patient is already taking theophylline on a daily basis, serum concentration should be measured before adding short-acting theophylline.

TABLE A2.7: Severity of asthma exacerbations*

Parameter	Mild	Moderate	Severe	Respiratory arrest imminent
Breathless	Walking	Talking Infant—softer, shorter cry: difficulty feeding	At rest infant stops feeding	
	Can lie down	Prefer sitting	Hunched forward	
Talks in	Sentences	Phrases	Words	
Alertness	May be agitated	Usually agitated	Usually agitated	Drowsy or confused
Respiratory rate	Increased	Increased	Often > 30/min	

Normal rates of breathing in awake children:

Age	Normal rate
< 2 months	< 60/min
2-12 months	< 50/min
1-5 years	< 40/min
6-8 years	< 30/min

Parameter	Mild	Moderate	Severe	Respiratory arrest imminent
Accessory muscles and suprasternal retractions	Usually not	Usually	Usually	Paradoxical thoraco-abdominal movements
Wheeze	Moderate, often only and expiratory	Loud	Usually loud	Absence of wheeze
Pulse/min	< 100	100-120	> 120	Bradycardia

Guide to limits of normal pulse rate in children:

Infants	2-12 months	— Normal rate < 160/min
Preschool	1-2 years	— Normal rate < 120/min
School age	2-8 years	— Normal rate < 110/min

Parameter	Mild	Moderate	Severe	Respiratory arrest imminent
Pulsus paradoxus	Absent < 10 mm Hg	May be present 10-25 mg Hg	Often present > 25 mm Hg (adult) 20-40 mm Hg (child)	Absence suggests respiratory muscle fatigue
PEF after initial bronchodilator % predicted or % personal best	Over 80%	Approx 60-80%	< 60% predicted or personal best (< 100 L/min adolescents) or response lasts < 2 hrs	
PoO$_2$ (on air)[†]	Normal Test not usually necessary	> 60 mm Hg	< 60 mm Hg Possible cyanosis	
and/or paCO$_2$[†]	< 45 mm Hg	< 45 mm Hg	> 45 mm Hg; Possible respiratory failure (see text)	
SaO$_2$% (on air)[1]	> 95%	91-95%	< 90%	

Hypercapnia (hypoventilation) develops more readily in young children than in adolescents.

*Note: The presence of several parameters, but not necessarily all, indicates the general classification of the exacerbation.
†Note: Kilopascals are also used internationally, conversion would be appropriate in this regard.

Therapies not recommended for treating attacks include:
- Sedatives (strictly avoid).
- Mucolytic drugs (may worsen cough).
- Chest physical therapy/physiotherapy (may increase patient discomfort).
- Hydration with large volumes of fluid for adults and older children (may be necessary for younger children and infants).
- Antibiotics (do not treat attacks but are indicated for patients who also have pneumonia or bacterial infection such as sinusitis).
- Epinephrine (adrenaline) may be indicated for acute treatment of anaphylaxis and angioedema but is not indicated during asthma attacks.
- Intravenous magnesium sulphate has not been studied in young children.

Monitor Response to Treatment

Evaluate symptoms and, as much as possible, peak flow. In the hospital, also assess oxygen saturation; consider arterial blood gas measurement in patients with suspected hypoventilation, exhaustion, severe distress, or peak flow 30-50 percent predicted.

Follow-up

After the exacerbation is resolved, the factors that precipitated the exacerbation should be identified and strategies for their future avoidance implemented, and the patient's medication plan reviewed.

SPECIAL CONSIDERATIONS IN MANAGING ASTHMA

Special considerations are required in managing asthma in relation to:

Surgery. Airway hyperresponsiveness, airflow limitation, and mucus hypersecretion predispose patients with asthma to intraoperative and postoperative respiratory complications, particularly with thoracic and upper abdominal surgeries. Lung function should be evaluated several days prior to surgery, and a brief course of glucocorticosteroids prescribed if FEV_1 is less than 80% of the patient's personal best.

Rhinitis, Sinusitis, and Nasal Polyps. Rhinitis and asthma often coexist in the same patient, and treatment of rhinitis may improve asthma symptoms. Both acute and chronic sinusitis can worsen asthma, and should be treated. Nasal polyps are associated with asthma and rhinitis, often with aspirin sensitivity and most frequently in adult patients. They are normally quite responsive to topical glucocorticosteroids.

Respiratory infections. Respiratory infections provoke wheezing and increased asthma symptoms in many patients. Treatment of an infectious exacerbation follows the same principles as treatment of other exacerbations.

Gastroesophageal reflux. Gastroesophageal reflux is nearly three times as prevalent in patients with asthma compared to the general population. Medical management should be given for the relief of reflux symptoms, although this does not consistently improve asthma control.

Anaphylaxis. Anaphylaxis is a potentially life-threatening condition that can both mimic and complicate severe asthma. Prompt treatment is crucial and includes oxygen, intramuscular epinephrine, injectable antihistamine, intravenous hydrocortisone, and intravenous fluid.

APPENDIX 1

APPENDIX 1

Glossary of asthma medications – Controllers

Name and also known as	Usual doses	Side effects	Comments
Glucocorticosteroids: Adrenocorticoids Corticosteroids Glucocorticoids **Inhaled (ICS):** Beclomethasone Budesonide Ciclesonide Flunisolide Fluticasone Mometasone Triamcinolone	**Inhaled:** Beginning dose dependent on asthma control then titrated down over 2-3 months to lowest effective dose once control is achieved.	**Inhaled:** High daily doses may be associated with skin thinning and bruises, and rarely adrenal suppression. Local side effects are hoarseness and oropharyngeal candidiasis. Low to medium doses have produced minor growth delay or suppression (av. 1 cm) in children. Attainment of predicted adult height does not appear to be affected.	**Inhaled:** Potential but small risk of side effects is well balanced by efficacy. Valved holdingchambers with MDIs and mouth washing with DPIs after inhalation decrease oral Candidiasis. Preparations not equivalent on per puff or µg basis.
Tablets or syrups: Hydrocortisone Methylprednisolone Prednisolone Prednisone	**Tablets or syrups:** For daily control use lowest effective dose 5-40 mg of prednisone equivalent in a.m. or qod. For acute attacks 40-60 mg daily in 1 or 2 divided doses for adolescents or 1-2 mg/kg daily in children.	**Tablets or syrups:** Used long-term, may lead to osteoporosis, hypertension, diabetes, cataracts, adrenal suppression, growth suppression, obesity, skin thinning or muscle weakness. Consider coexisting conditions that could be worsened by oral glucocorticosteroids, e.g. herpes virus infections, Varicella, tuberculosis, hypertension, diabetes and osteoporosis.	**Tablet or syrup:** Long-term use: alternate day a.m. dosing produces less toxicity. Short-term: 3-10 day "bursts" are effective for gaining prompt control.
Sodium cromoglycate cromolyn cromones	MDI 2 mg or 5 mg 2-4 inhalations 3-4 times daily. Nebulizer 20 mg 3-4 times daily.	Minimal side effects. Cough may occur upon inhalation.	May take 4-6 weeks to determine maximum effects. Frequent daily dosing required.
Nedocromil cromones	MDI 2 mg/puff 2-4 inhalations 2-4 times daily	Cough may occur upon inhalation.	Some patients unable to tolerate the taste.
Long-acting β2-agonists beta-adrenergis sympathomimetics LABAs **Inhaled:** Formoterol (F) Salmeterol (Sm)	**Inhaled:** DPI-F: 1 inhalation (12 µg) bid. MDI-F: 2 puffs bid. DPI-Sm: 1 inhalation (50 µg) bid. MDI-Sm: 2 puffs bid.	**Inhaled:** Fewer, and less significant, side effects than tablets. Have been associated with an increased risk of severe exacerbations and asthma deaths when added to usual therapy.	**Inhaled:** Salmeterol not to be used to treat acute attacks. Should not use as monotherapy for controller therapy. Always use as adjunct to ICS therapy. Formoterol has onset similar to salbutamol and has been used as needed for acute symptoms.
Sustained-release Tablets: Salbutamol (S) Terbutaline (T)	**Tablets:** S: 4 mg q12h. T: 10 mg q12h.	**Tablets:** May cause tachycardia, anxiety, skeletal muscle tremor, headache, hypokalemia.	**Tablets:** As effective as sustained-release theophylline. No data for use as adjunctive therapy with inhaled glucocorticosteroids.

Contd...

Contd...

Name and also known as	Usual doses	Side effects	Comments
Combination ICS/LABA Fluticasone/ salmeterol (F/S) Budesonide/ formoterol (B/F)	DPI-F/S 100, 250, or 500 µg/50 µg 1 inhalation bid MDI-F/S 50, 125, or 250 µg/25 µg 2 puffs bid DPI-B/F 100 or 200 µg/6 µg 1 inhalation bid MDI-B/F 80 or 160 µg/4.5 µg 2 puffs bid	Similar to those described above for individual components of the combination	In moderate to severe persistent asthma, combination more effective than doubling the ICS dose. Budesonide/formoterol has been approved for adjustable as needed dosing in addition to regular dosing in some countries. Dosing is dependent on level of control. Limited data in children 4-11 yrs. No data in children < 4 yrs.
Sustained-release Theophylline Aminophylline Methylxanthine Xanthine	Starting dose 10 mg/kg/day with usual 800 mg maximum in 1-2 divided doses.	Nausea and vomiting are most common. Serious effects occurring at higher serum concentrations include seizures, tachycardia, and arrhythmias	Theophylline level monitoring is often required. Absorption and metabolism may be affected by many factors, including febrile illness.
Antileukotrienes Leukotriene modifiers Montelukast (M) Pranlukast (P) Zafirlukast (Z) Zileuton (Zi)	Adolescents: M 10 mg qhs P 450 mg bid Z 20 mg bid Zi 600 mg qid Children: M 5 mg qhs (6-14 y) M 4 mg qhs (2-5 y) Z 10mg bid (7-11 y).	No specific adverse effects to date at recommended doses. Elevation of liver enzymes with Zafirlukast and Zileuton and limited case reports of reversible hepatitis and hyperbilirubinemia with Zileuton and hepatic failure with Zafirlukast	Antileukotrienes are most effective for patients with mild persistent asthma. They provide additive benefit when added to ICSs though not as effective as inhaled long-acting β_2-agonists
Immunomodulators Omalizumab Anti-IgE	Adolescents: Dose administered subcutaneously every 2 or 4 weeks dependent on weight and IgE concentration	Pain and bruising at injection site (5-20%) and very rarely anaphylaxis (0.1%).	Need to be stored under refrigeration 2-8°C and maximum of 150 mg administered per injection site

Glossary of asthma medications – Relivers

Name and also known as	Usual doses	Side effects	Comments
Short-acting β₂-agonists Adrenergics β₂-stimulants Sympathomimetics Albuterol/salbutamol Fenoterol Levalbuterol Metaproterenol Pirbuterol Terbutaline	Differences in potency exist but all products are essentially comparable on a per puff basis. For prn symptomatic use and pretreatment before exercise 2 puffs MDI or 1 inhalation DPI. For asthma attacks 4-8 puffs q2-4h, may administer q20min x 3 with medical supervision or the equivalent of 5 mg salbutamol by nebulizer.	**Inhaled:** Tachycardia, skeletal muscle tremor, headache, and irritability. At very high dose hyperglycemia, hypokalemia. Systemic administration as **Tablets or Syrup** increases the risk of these side effects.	Drug of choice for acute bronchospasm. Inhaled route has faster onset and is more effective than tablet or syrup. Increasing use, lack of expected effect, or use of > 1 canister a month indicate poor asthma control; adjust long-term therapy accordingly. Use of ≥ 2 canisters per month is associated with an increased risk of a severe, life-threatening asthma attack.
Anticholinergics Ipratropium bromide (IB) Oxitropium	IB-MDI 4-6 puffs q6h or q20 min in the emergency department. Nebulizer 500 µg q20 min x 3 then q2-4 hrs for adolescents and 250-500 µg for children.	Minimal mouth dryness or bad taste in the mouth.	May provide additive effects to β₂-agonist but has slower onset of action. Is an alternative for patients with intolerance for β₂-agonists.
Short-acting theophylline Aminophylline	7 mg/kg loading dose over 20 min followed by 0.4 mg/kg/hr continuous infusion.	Nausea, vomiting, headache. At higher serum concentrations: seizures, tachycardia, and arrhythmias.	Theophylline level monitoring is required. Obtain serum levels 12 and 24 hours into infusion. Maintain between 10-15 µg/mL.
Epinephrine/ adrenaline injection	1:1000 solution (1 mg/mL) .01 mg/kg up to 0.3-0.5 mg, can give q20 min x 3.	Similar, but more significant effects than selective β₂-agonist. In addition: hypertension, fever, vomiting in children and hallucinations.	In general, not recommended for treating asthma attacks if selective β₂-agonists are available.

HYALINE MEMBRANE DISEASE

Hyaline membrane disease (HMD) or idiopathic respiratory distress syndrome (IRDS) is a disease of the newborn infants and mainly occurs in children who are born prematurely. It is a leading cause of death in low birth weight infants worldwide and even in the western countries. Although precise incidence of the disease is difficult to determine, it has been estimated that HMD occurs in 14 to 60 percent of premature deliveries at gestational ages between 28 to 35 weeks. HMD and associated complications of prematurity may account for up to 75 percent of neonatal deaths. About 15 years ago, the death rates attributable to HMD was estimated to be 23 per 1000 live births in USA. Although chances of survival have improved over the years because of advances in the management techniques, it remains a major cause of death.[1-3] The disease occurs in about 0.5 to 1 percent of all deliveries and in about 10 percent of all preterm infants. The male: female ratio is about 1.7:1. It is seen exclusively in preterm infants born before 37 weeks of gestation and the more preterm the infant, the greater is the likelihood of developing HMD. Other risk factors include infants of diabetic mothers, the second of twins, and cesarian section. The degree of maturity of the infant and the indication of cesarian section are more important than the cesarian section itself. Conditions associated with birth asphyxia, such as antepartum hemorrhage associated with prematurity are also important factors.

The disease is more common in India than is generally believed. It has been reported that the incidence of IRDS is higher in India than in the western countries possibly because of the higher incidence of prematurity. Modern management has resulted in prolonged survival for several sick infants, some of whom may have a delayed death. As more infants with the disease survive, permanent serious sequelae of the disorder itself or its associated complications continue to increase.[4] In a report from Northern India, the incidence, etiology and the outcome of respiratory distress in 243 consecutive liveborn very low birth weight neonates (VLBW) were analyzed. One hundred and forty six (60%) VLBW neonates developed respiratory distress. Hyaline membrane disease, congenital pneumonia and transient tachypnea of the newborn were the major underlying causes (35.6%, 28.1%, and 27.4% respectively). The mortality rate was significantly higher in neonates with respiratory distress (72 of 146, 49.3%) than in those without distress (28 of 97, 28.8%) (p < 0.05). This difference was more sharply reflected in the 1000 to 1249 birth weight group and in the 29 to 32 weeks gestation group. Respiratory distress is a significant determinant of VLBW mortality.[5] The incidence of neonatal respiratory distress (RD) ranges from 2.2 to 7.6 percent in developed countries and from 0.7 to 8.3 percent in India. A study conducted in Pondicherry, India, found the incidence of neonatal RD to be 6.7 percent. The leading cause of neonatal RD is transient tachypnea (50-60% of RD cases) followed by infections (pneumonia, sepsis, or meningitis), meconium aspiration, and hyaline membrane disease (HMD). Significant predictors of neonatal RD include prematurity, malpresentation, abnormal delivery, premature rupture of membranes, fetal distress, multiple pregnancy, male sex, and low apgar score at birth. The case fatality rate for RD in India is 30 to 40 percent. In the Pondicherry study, it was 19 percent. Case fatality is highest for newborns with HMD (20-40% in developed countries and 50-75% in India). It ranges from 14.3 to 30.37 percent for meconium aspiration-related RD deaths. RD incidence and subsequent infant mortality can be reduced by improved prenatal care, early detection and referral of high risk pregnancies, closer links between referral hospitals and health centers, close monitoring of labor to detect fetal distress, and early intervention when indicated. In cases of RD, adequate and immediate resuscitation, oxygen supplementation, maintenance of optimal temperature, and time referral if RD lasts beyond two hours will reduce mortality. In cases of HMD and meconium aspiration, adequate ventilatory support and surfactant therapy will reduce mortality.[6]

Etiology

The most important underlying cause for development of HMD is a relative deficiency of surfactant, either quantitatively or qualitatively. The surfactant must not only be present at birth but must also be capable of being regenerated at a rate equal to its metabolism. This means that Type II pneumocytes, which secrete these substances, must be viable and active. Tissue storage of surfactant is detectable at about 24 weeks of gestation and certainly by the 26th week. Thus, surfactant can be detected well before the period of viability and has been detected in fetuses weighing as little as 200 to 500 gms. The surfactant is delivered to the alveoli at about the 30th week. However, adequate amounts are produced at about 35 to 36 weeks, although the timing is variable and production may occur as early as 30 weeks or as late as 38 weeks. For an equivalent period of gestation, females have higher indexes of pulmonary maturity than did male infants, which may account for a higher incidence of HMD in the latter.[7] The disease can rarely occur in full term babies.[8] The risk of hyaline membrane disease in neonates at < 32 weeks of gestation is increased in patients with preeclampsia. This supports the contention that fetal lung maturity is not accelerated in pre-eclampsia.[9]

The discovery of surfactant deficiency in lungs of infants who died of hyaline membrane disease (hence their description of these lungs at autopsy as "liver-like") and subsequent observation of the absence of foam in the airways after death has established the cause and effect relationship since the 50's.[10,11] The material with specific activity is a phospholipid, which has the unique property that the film formed by it on the surface of a watery liquid, changes its surface activity with increasing or decreasing surface area. On expiration, when the surface area of the lungs is decreased, the surfactant becomes more highly active and thus, reduces the surface tension to very low levels; on inspiration it rapidly reverts to low activity and higher tension. Since the pressure required expanding a lung or maintaining its aeration is largely a function of surface tension, this changing surface activity results in higher pressure required inflating lungs than to maintain the air content on deflation. This is responsible for the hysteresis of the pressure-volume curve. The normal stability of aeration, maintaining a considerable amount of residual air within lungs through expiration into the next inspiratory phase, is because of this peculiarity of pulmonary surfactant. If its activity is abnormally low, or if it is expelled from the lungs during expiration, the lung collapses at expiration. At each inspiration then, the infant must take a first and deep breath, which explains the excessive inspiratory effort. Thus, in HMD, alveoli lacking surfactant collapse on expiration because of high internal wall pressure and absence of a mechanism for reducing surface tension. Adjacent alveoli overinflate during inspiration. Inadequate surfactant leads to progressive expiratory collapse, the lung compliance falls and the work of breathing increases. The resultant hypoxemia and alveolar hypoventilation result in acidosis. The resultant reduced pulmonary blood flow and inhibition of the enzyme system further impair surfactant synthesis and a vicious circle continues.

The sequence of structural and functional events in the lungs in infants with HMD has been well studied. The earliest change was shown to be an interstitial edema with localized necrosis and desquamation of alveolar cells and absence of osmiophilic granules in the Type II pneumocytes. It is recognized that hyaline membranes can develop in some cases despite normal lung surfactant and also, lack of surfactant can rarely occur in term infants. Studies on the control of fetal lung development have thrown new light on the possible etiopathogenesis of HMD. Recent work on rabbit indicates that normal mammalian lung growth requires the integration of neuromuscular and secretory activities. Secretion of lung liquid provides a moulding force for the developing lobule enhanced by swings in intrathoracic pressure associated with fetal respiratory movements. Corticosteroids could modulate some of these activities. Other agents can also help in the maturation of the lungs. Diversion of substrates to surfactant production can reduce the quantity available for cell proliferation. There is a biological advantage in the lung remaining functionally immature, which is thought to protect against development of HMD, although there are some evidences to the contrary. To allow efficient transition to an air-breathing state it is postulated that one or more early warning systems exist to trigger biochemical lung maturation. HMD possibly arises as a result of failure to activate these systems or the inability of the target tissue to respond. Endogenous glucocorticoid is capable of inducing enzymes necessary for surfactant synthesis and specific cortisol receptors have been identified in the fetal lung. There is also evidence to suggest that thyroxin and autonomic nervous system can promote lung maturation. Alterations in any one of these systems/control mechanisms can lead to HMD.

Recently the role of various proinflammatory cytokines has been examined in the pathogenesis of hyaline membrane disease.[12-18] Deficient expression of the counterregulatory cytokine IL-10 by lung inflammatory cells may facilitate chronic inflammation and the pathogenesis of hyaline membrane disease (HMD), in premature infants. Deficient expression of the counter-regulatory cytokine IL-10 by lung inflammatory cells may facilitate chronic inflammation and the pathogenesis of hyaline membrane disease (HMD), in premature infants. In cell culture IL-1α expression was inhibited by rIL-10 in a dose-dependent fashion while IL-8 expression was inhibited by higher concentrations of rIL-10. IL-10 protein was undetectable from BAL fluid of the premature infants sampled over 28 days. The results demonstrate that lung inflammatory cells, which do not express IL-10 *in vivo*, are capable of responding to rIL-10 in cell culture with reduction of IL-1α and IL-8 expression. These data support the rationale for the development of rIL-10 as a potential antiinflammatory agent in the treatment of HMD.

Pathology

Four stages of the disease can be identified. These stages are:[19]

- Acute stage (0-3 days)
- Healing stage (4-10 days)
- Transition stage (10-20 days)
- Bronchopulmonary dysplasia (1 month).

Pathological changes are quite characteristic of each stage. In the *acute stage*, the lungs are uniformly red-purple and moderately firm in consistency, although in some cases they may be pale brown. The weight is not significantly increased. The histological changes include atelectasis with dilatation of the terminal bronchiolar air passages, necrosis of their epithelium, hyaline membrane lining exclusively or predominantly the terminal air passages, pulmonary edema, capillary and venous congestion, dilatation of the pulmonary lymphatics, and paucity or absence of osmiophilic granules in the alveolar epithelial cells (Fig. 33.6). *Healing stage* is seen between 4 to 10 days after onset of HMD. The lungs are grossly yellow-brown to red-brown in color and firmer than normal. Microscopically the walls of the terminal air passage are still denuded of epithelium and some may show signs of regeneration. Hyaline membranes are present focally. There is a mixed pattern of alveolar expansion. Some may be atelectatic, some are emphysematous, and some may be normally expanded. The alveolar lumina may contain histiocytes and cuboidal metaplasia will be present in the alveolar epithelium. *Transition stage* is usually seen between 10 to 20 days after the onset and pathological changes are intermediate between the healing stage and those seen in bronchopulmonary dysplasia. *Bronchopulmonary dysplasia* is seen in infants who continue to have respiratory problem and require hospitalization beyond 1 month with oxygen therapy. The alveoli show a mixed picture of atelectasis, hyperinflation or emphysematous changes. The most striking change is the hypertrophy and proliferation of fibroblasts, and smooth muscles with deposition of collagen. The lining cells of the alveoli are cuboidal and large and bizarre nuclei. Squamous metaplasia of the bronchiolar and bronchial epithelium is common. There will be proliferation of bronchial, smooth muscles and medial hypertrophy of pulmonary arteries. Interstitial fibrosis can also be present. The type II cells proliferate.

Clinical Features

Some infants may appear normal at birth, but may have evidence of intrapartum asphyxia with depressed Apgar scores. However, signs of respiratory distress become apparent soon. The clinical characteristics of respiratory distress syndrome due to HMD include:[20-22]

- Increased respiratory rate (> 60/min) Progressive intercostal, suprasternal, supracostal, and substernal retractions Cyanosis
- Decreased breath sounds nasal flaring
- Expiratory grunting present one hour after birth and lasting beyond 4 hours
- Chest X-ray taken within 6 hours of birth showing reticulogranular appearance with air bronchogram.

The radiological features are fairly characteristic of HMD. There is a diffuse, fine reticulo-granular pattern, which involves both the lung fields. Air bronchograms may be seen extending up to the periphery. With severe HMD, there may be uniform granularity or even a total "white out" with the air bronchogram being the only visible lung markings.

The above four stages represent a systematized version of the probable sequence of events and are not distinctive clinicopathological entities. Some overlap between the consecutive stages is expected. Clinical symptoms reach a peak within 2 to 3 days after birth following which gradual recovery is seen in those infants who survive. In the absence of assisted ventilation, progressive deterioration occurs during the first 24 to 48 hours and highest mortality occurs within the first 72 hours. Approximately 50 percent of all deaths occur during the first 24 hours; 70 percent within 48 hours; and 90 percent within 72 hours.[23,24]

Management

Over the last few years' dramatic improvement has occurred in the field of management of these cases. Lecithin/sphingomyelin (L/S) ratio is a useful test for a precise diagnosis of the condition. Measuring pharyngeal L/S ratios could make an accurate diagnosis of HMD. The correlation of L/S ratio with gestational age and weight for the risk of development of HMD is presented in the Table 33.18.

More refined biochemical tests are available now in the prediction of HMD by looking at the presence of

TABLE 33.18: Correlation of L/S ratio with gestational age and birth weight for development of HMD

L/S ratio	Gestational age (weeks) 32 or less	> 32	Birth weight (gms) 1500 or less	>1500
1.7 or less	97%	74%	100%	72%
1.8	50%	14%	33%	26%
1.9 or more	4%	5%	7%	4%

phosphatidyl glycerol in the amniotic fluid, which is a more reliable indicator of the state of lung maturity.

The aim of management of HMD is to *(i)* control and if possible normalization of blood gases; *(ii)* the control and, if possible normalization of biochemical and physiological abnormalities generally seen in these cases in an ICU namely, hypotension, hypothermia, electrolyte imbalance, oliguria, paralytic ileus etc.; and *(iii)* the prevention if possible, but otherwise the control of side-effects both of the treatment and the disease — like patent ductus arteriosus, and bronchopulmonary dysplasia. Oxygenation can be maintained by increasing the inspired oxygen concentration enough to keep the arterial PaO_2 between 60 to 90 mm Hg. It is possible by means of a mechanical ventilator with monitoring of the arterial blood gas, which can be done on blood drawn from an umbilical arterial catheter. If the above said blood gas level is maintained, there is no risk of development of retrolental fibroplasia.

Assisted ventilation: The indications for need for assisted ventilation are as follows:[25-33]

- PaO_2 of 50 mm Hg or less while breathing 100%
- Oxygen
- $PaCO_2$ of 70 mm Hg or more
- pH < 7.20.

Two simple bedside tests are also available to predict infants with HMD who will require ventilatory assistance. One is the *Foam stability test* (FST); and the other is the *Hyperoxia test*. The foam stability test is based on the capacity of pulmonary surfactant to form highly stable surface films or bubbles. Either the amniotic fluid obtained by amniocentesis or gastric aspirate collected from the infant after birth is mixed with an equal volume of 95% ethanol, and the mixture is shaken in air. Bubbles indicate the presence of surfactant. The test is rapid, simple, and inexpensive. In the hyperoxia test, the infant breathes 100% oxygen for 10 to 15 minutes and the test is carried out between the first and the sixth hours of life. It can define high-risk infants when it yields a PaO_2 of 200 mm Hg or less.

A constant positive airway pressure (CPAP) as low as 6 cm of H_2O is useful to maintain oxygenation in spontaneously breathing infants with HMD. The same can be also achieved by constant negative pressure (CNP). Both CPAP and CNP increase transpulmonary pressure and the functional residual capacity of the lungs. The tendency of atelectasis at end expiration is counterbalanced and oxygen exchange is enhanced between the alveoli and pulmonary capillaries. About a third of neonates with HMD and respiratory failure can be treated with constant distending pressure during

spontaneous respiration as the only form of ventilatory assistance with excellent survival.

Over the years there are refinements in the ventilatory care of infants with HMD. Mechanical ventilators are mainly of three types: Positive pressure, negative pressure, and high frequency oscillator devices. However, for neonates positive pressure ventilators are more commonly used. The ventilators may be either pressure cycled or volume cycled. The ventilator should ideally be set at a rate of 30 to 40 minute, with peak inspiratory pressure (PIP) of 15 to 20 cm of H_2O and peak end expiratory pressure (PEEP) being 3 to 5 cm of H_2O. It is preferable to have an inspiratory: expiratory ratio of 1:1 and an oxygen concentration of 0.4 to 1.0, which is just sufficient to keep the baby pink. Majority of the babies can be ventilated satisfactorily without the use of any muscle paralytic agents. However, a small minority may fight the ventilator and a muscle relaxant, like pancuronium has been shown to be useful. Other advantages of the drug include the reduction of complications of ventilator like pneumothorax,[34,35] and intraventricular hemorrhage. However, the drug may induce hypotension.

Ventilation of the neonates is a formidable task requiring technical skills, proper facilities, and willing workers. With the availability of ventilators, a number of other problems have come. Some of the more frequent complications associated with severe HMD requiring assisted ventilation include:

- Intraventricular or intrapulmonary hemorrhage
- Pneumothorax and pneumomediastinum
- Kernicterus
- Problems associated with endotracheal intubation
- Retrolental fibroplasia
- Bronchopulmonary dysplasia.

While mechanical ventilation plays an important role, they are net the major determinants of outcome. In addition to pulmonary ventilation management, other supportive care involves management of circulation, fluid and electrolyte balance, caloric intake, prevention and treatment of infections, and maintenance of optimal thermal conditions, which will mainly decide the outcome. The skill of the attending physician, nurses, and supportive staff is also of paramount importance.

Surfactant Therapy

Some obstetricians in England, France and Germany in the second half of the 18th century published the first observations on neonatal respiratory distress syndrome (RDS). The concept that RDS might involve the absence of something stems from the observations of a Swiss physiologist, Kurt von Neergaard, who published an article in 1929 about a fundamental principle of respiratory mechanics: the surface tension in the alveoli. Further early descriptions of the existence, composition, and synthesis of the surfactant complex and its physiologic role in maintaining alveolar stability were dependent on the pioneering contributions of Radford, Macklin, Pattle, and Clements (among others). But, the final link, describing surfactant deficiency as a cause of RDS, came from Avery and Mead in 1959, when they showed lung extracts from babies with hyaline membrane disease deficient in surfactant. Understanding surfactant composition, function and therapeutic usefulness has increased exponentially over the last 50 years and subsequent observations reorganize the steps of the research in this field until nowadays. Most of the concerns are the fundamental role of lung surfactant in RDS of premature infants, and the success of exogenous surfactant replacement in the clinical therapy of this disease.[36]

Since pulmonary surfactant deficiency is associated with HMD, attempts have been made during the past decade to treat these cases with surfactant replacement therapy.[37-43] There are at least 15 good clinical trials available in the subject. Some of these trials have used surfactant as a "prophylactic treatment" and others have used surfactant as "rescue treatment". In the prophylactic treatment surfactant is given at birth and in the rescue treatment surfactant is given to babies with HMD requiring ventilators. Many preparations of surfactants have also been available, although their availability is limited to certain countries only. Surfactant TA (extracted from homogenized cow's lungs), Calf lung surfactant; Porcine surfactant (from minced pig lungs); artificial lung expanding compound (from dipalmitoyl-phosphatidyl-choline and unsaturated phosphaticlyl glycerol in a ratio of 7:3, weight by weight); human surfactant (extracted from amniotic fluid); and Exosurf (dipalmitoylphosphatidylcholine 108 mg, tyloxapol 8 mg, hexadecanol 12 mg in 10 ml saline without protein) are some of the naturally occurring and synthetic surfactants used in clinical trials. Their usefulness have been stressed in the form of improvement in oxygenation, reduced mortality, bronchopulmonary dysplasia, and periventricular hemorrhage. The surfactant treatment has been shown to benefit babies less than 30 weeks' gestation. However, the only problem with rescue treatment was an increase in the patent ductus arteriosus. Prophylactic treatment is also beneficial and is apparently harmless. Observations in autopsied infants with HMD suggested a possible acceleration of epithelial cell regeneration in those receiving surfactant.[39] Exogenous surfactant treatment of hyaline membrane disease is known to modify the pattern of radiological changes on the chest radiograph. Asymmetrical clearing of chest radiographs, sometimes patchy, after surfactant treatment requires exclusion of pneumothorax or infection but has no influence on clinical outcome.[40]

One of the major concerns is the development of sensitization to proteins in the surfactant, although evidence for production of antibodies to such proteins is lacking. It is suggested that artificial surfactant may not be as effective as natural surfactant because, it lacks the apoproteins; results of trials have shown that it reduces the incidence of complications and improves the outcome in babies of less than 30 weeks of gestation. Surfactants most likely to have longer-term benefits are human surfactant, calf lung surfactant, and artificial lung expanding compound used prophylactically and porcine surfactant used in rescue treatment. However, the decision will depend upon its possible side effects, ease of preparation available, and the cost. Exogenous lung surfactant has transformed HMD therapy in developed countries, but an equivalent benefit has not been accomplished in developing countries due to a variety of factors. Porcine surfactant is an inexpensive alternative to other surfactants and had similar clinical effects than bovine surfactant in the oxygenation and ventilation variables, with no significant differences. The incidences of hyaline membrane disease, pulmonary interstitial emphysema, hemorrhagic necrosis and parenchymal degeneration of the liver and kidney are all higher in nonresponders, whereas the incidences of bronchopulmonary dysplasia and pneumonia are higher in responders. Prior to treatment, acidosis and hypothermia are significantly more severe in nonresponders, and perinatal complications, such as fetal distress and intrauterine infection, are observed more often in nonresponders. Substantial degradation of vital organs has already occurred during the early postnatal or intrauterine life of the nonresponders, which would be expected to interfere with the clinical response to instilled surfactant. It is anticipated that in the future improved monitoring of immature fetuses will be indispensable to improve intrauterine fetal management and to achieve better control over the timing and mode of delivery. A recent metaanalysis of surfactant replacement therapy[43] was carried out to determine (i) the efficacy of surfactant therapy in the reduction of short-term morbidity and long-term outcome in terms of bronchopulmonary dysplasia (BPD) and mortality; (ii) whether there are differences in efficacy between modified natural surfactant and synthetic surfactant; (iii) the effectiveness of prophylactic surfactant therapy; and (iv) whether there are differences in efficacy between the prophylactic approach and the rescue strategy. The analysis included studies in which infants with birth weights between 500 and 1500 gm were eligible. Studies were grouped into the following categories: (i) rescue therapy with modified natural surfactant; (ii) rescue therapy with synthetic surfactant; (iii) prophylaxis with modified natural surfactant; (iv) prophylaxis with synthetic surfactant; (v) prophylaxis versus rescue studies; (vi) modified natural surfactant versus Exosurf studies. The relative risk ratios, corrected for study size, were calculated for the outcome variables (pneumothorax, incidence of BPD, survival, survival without BPD, prevention of hyaline membrane disease [HMD], and intraventricular hemorrhage [IVH]). Surfactant therapy was found to be efficacious in reducing the risk for pneumothorax and increasing the chance for survival without BPD. Synthetic surfactant was not efficacious in the prevention of HMD. Modified natural surfactant was more effective in reducing the risk of pneumothorax and increasing the chance for survival without BPD than is synthetic surfactant. These data did not support the use of either synthetic or modified natural surfactant for routine prophylaxis.

Glucocorticoids have been shown to be effective in increasing surfactant synthesis and in reducing oxygen toxicity and lung inflammation. Therefore, trials were made to prevent the development of HMD.[44-50] Results are conflicting. A double blind, collaborative study was initiated in 1976 to evaluate the effect of dexamethasone to mothers as a method of preventing neonatal respiratory distress syndrome. Five centers in USA enrolled 696 women at risk for premature delivery. Up to 20 mg of dexamethasone phosphate (5 mg every 12 hours) or placebo was administered intramuscularly. The overall incidence of respiratory distress syndrome was different in the control group (18.0%) and steroid treated mothers (12.6%) (p = 0.05). The effect was, however, mainly attributable to discernible differences among singleton female infants (p < 0.001), whereas no treatment effect was observed in male infants (p = 0.96). Non-Caucasians were improved whereas Caucasians showed little benefit. Fetal and neonatal mortality and maternal postpartum infection rates were not different. Neurological examination at 40 weeks' gestation demonstrated no significant difference in the rate of abnormal outcomes in the neonatal steroid group. Thus, a marginal benefit was observed in female infants. Another study evaluated the effect of early postnatal dexamethasone therapy in premature infants with severe respiratory distress syndrome in double blind, controlled manner in 57 infants of less than 2000 gm of weight. It

was concluded that early postnatal dexamethasone therapy improves pulmonary status, facilitates removal of the endotracheal tube, and minimizes lung injury in premature infants with severe respiratory distress syndrome. Thus, corticosteroids have some beneficial effect in preventing the development of respiratory distress syndrome in premature infants. Another study examined (a) perinatal factors affecting condition at birth in very preterm infants (23-32 weeks) and (b) the relationship between poor condition at birth and neonatal respiratory morbidity and mortality. Convenience sample (n = 479) was drawn from a geographic population inception cohort. It was observed that antenatal steroid use reduced the risk of pH < or = 7.20 [Adjusted Odds Ratio 0.29 (95% CI 0.17, 0.50)], one minute Apgar < 4 [0.54 (0.33, 0.88)], and 5 min Apgar < 7 [0.44 (0.23, 0.84)]. Gestational age was significantly related to Apgar score but not cord arterial acid-base status. No other perinatal factor was significant. Poor condition at birth was associated with an increase in the incidence and severity of hyaline membrane disease and death. These effects were lessened in those exposed to steroids. The authors concluded that antenatal steroid use is associated with improved condition at birth and reduces the deleterious effects of poor condition at birth on early respiratory morbidity and mortality. Maternal administration of corticosteroids before preterm delivery results in a decrease in the incidence and severity of respiratory distress syndrome and a decrease in neonatal mortality rate among premature neonates born to treated versus untreated mothers at 26 to 34 weeks' gestation as was reported in Tunisian women. Antenatal steroids given to the mother in imminence of premature birth are for real benefit in reducing neonatal mortality, increasing the number of survivors among small prematures and improving their quality of life. Even, life threatening distress from other causes seem to be less severe, and even an incomplete course therapy conduces to decrease of distress severity. The single or the multiple courses of antenatal steroids did not apparently increase neonatal sepsis in patients with preterm delivery.[48]

Inhaled nitric oxide (NO) clearly decreased pulmonary vascular resistance in pediatric patients with pulmonary hypertension, regardless of the underlying origin of the pulmonary hypertension. In persistent pulmonary hypertension of the neonate (PPHN) and CHD, the use of inhaled NO appears to improve the outcome of these patients. In acute respiratory distress syndrome (ARDS) and surfactant deficiency the role of inhaled NO therapy remains unclear. The use of inhaled NO is safe in a carefully monitored setting with a delivery system designed to minimize the generation of NO_2.[51,52] Other experimental drugs are also being tried recently.[53]

REFERENCES

1. Farrell PM, Avery ME. Hyaline membrane disease. Am Rev Respir Dis 1975;111:657-88.
2. Farrell PM, Wood RM. Epidemiology of hyaline membrane disease in the United States. Analysis of national mortality statistics. Paediatrics 1976;58:167.
3. Inselman LS. Respiratory distress syndrome. Paediatr Ann 1978;7:34.
4. Webb JKG, John TJ, Jadhav M, Graham MD, Walter A. The incidence of hyaline membrane syndrome in south India Ind Paediatr Soc 1962;193.
5. Bhakoo ON, Narang A, Karthikeyan G, Kumar P. Spectrum of respiratory distress in very low birthweight neonates. Indian J Pediatr 2000;67:803-04.
6. Kumar A, Bhat BV. Respiratory distress in newborn. Indian J Matern Child Health. 1996;7:8-10.
7. Wigglesworth JS. Aetiology of hyaline membrane disease. Arch Dis Childhood 1979;54:835-37.
8. Goraya JS, Nada R, Ray M. Hyaline membrane disease in a term neonate. Indian J Pediatr. 2001;68:771-73.
9. Chang EY, Menard MK, Vermillion ST, Hulsey T, Ebeling M. The association between hyaline membrane disease and preeclampsia. Am J Obstet Gynecol 2004;191:1414-17.
10. Avery ME, Mead J. Surface properties in relation to atelectasis and hyaline membrane disease. Am J Dis Child 1959;97:517-23.
11. Avery ME. Surfactant deficiency in hyaline membrane dsease: The story of discovery. Am J Respir Crit Care Med 2000;161:1074-75.
12. de Waal Malefyt, Abrams J, Bennett B, Figdor CG, deVries JE. Interleukin-10 (IL-10) inhibits cytokine synthesis by human monocytes. J Exp Med1 991; 174:1209-20.
13. Kwong KYC, Jones CA, Cayabyab R, Lecart C, Khuu N, Rhandhawa I, Hanley JM, Ramnathan R, deLemos RA, Minoo P. The effects of IL-10 on proinflammatory cytokine expression (IL-1α and IL-8) in hyaline membrane disease (HMD). Clin Immunolo Immunopath 1998;88:105-13.
14. Ogden BE, Murphy S, Saunders GC, Johnson JD. Lung lavage of newborns with respiratory distress syndrome: Prolonged neutrophil influx is associated with bronchopulmonary dysplasia. Chest 1983;83:31–33.
15. Rozycki HJ. Bronchoalveolar lavage interleukin-1β in infants on day 1 of life. South Med J 1994;84:991-96.
16. Groneck P, Gotae-Speer B, Oppermann M, Eiffert H, Speer CP. Association of pulmonary inflammation and increased microvascular permeability during the development of bronchopulmonary dysplasia: A sequential analysis of inflammatory mediators in respiratory fluids of high risk preterm neonates. Pediatrics 1994;93:712-18.
17. Bagchi A, Viscardi RM, Taciak V, Ensor JE, McCrea KA, Hasday JD. Increased activity of interleukin-6 but not tumor necrosis factor-α in lung lavage of premature infants is associated with the development of bronchopulmonary dysplasia. Pediatr Res 1994;36:244-52.
18. Jones CA, Cayabyab RG, Kwong KYC, Stotts C, Wong B, Hamdan H, Minoo P, deLemos RA. Undetectable interleukin (IL)-10 and persistent IL-8 expression early in hyaline membrane disease: A possible developmental basis for predisposition to chronic lung inflammation in preterm newborns. Pediatr Res 1996;39:966–75.
19. Joshi VV. Pathology of idiopathic respiratory distress syndrome of newborn infants. Bull Post Grad Med Inst 1975;9:178.
20. Robertson NRC. Management of hyaline membrane disease. Arch Dis Childhood 1979;54:838.
21. Gluke L, Kulovich MV, Borer RC, et al. Diagnosis of the respiratory distress syndrome by amniocentesis. Am J Obstet Gynecol 1971;109:440.
22. Pieper CH, Smith J, Brand EJ. The value of ultrasound examination of the lungs in predicting bronchopulmonary dysplasia. Pediatr Radiol 2004;34:227-31.
23. Kamper J. Long-term prognosis of infants with severe idiopathic respiratory distress syndrome. Neurological and mental outcome. Acta Paediatr Scand 1978;67:61-69.
24. Reynolds EO, Taghizadeh A. Improved prognosis of infants mechanically ventilated for hyaline membrane disease. Arch Dis Childhood 1974;49:505-15.
25. Hakanson DO, Stern L. Respiratory distress syndrome of the newborn. Current status of ventilatory assis tance. Post Grad Med 1975;58:200-06.
26. Tarnow-Mordi W, Wilkinson A. Mechanical ventilation of the newborn. Br Med J 1986;292:575-76.
27. Millar D, Kirpalani H. Benefits of Non Invasive Ventilation. Indian Pediatr 2004 7;41:1008-17.
28. Kamlin CO, Davis PG. Long versus short inspiratory times in neonates receiving mechanical ventilation. Cochrane Database Syst Rev 2004;18;(4):CD004503.
29. Mathur NB. Effect of stepwise reduction in minute ventilation on PaCO$_2$ in ventilated newborns. Indian Pediatr 2004;41:779-85.
30. Riyas PK, Vijayakumar KM, Kulkarni ML. Neonatal mechanical ventilation. Indian J Pediatr 2003;70:537-40.
31. Muller W, Pichler G. Results of mechanical ventilation in premature infants with respiratory distress syndrome. Wien Med Wochenschr 2002;152:5-8.
32. Karthikeyan G, Hossain MM. Conventional ventilation in neonates: experience from Saudi Arabia. Indian J Pediatr 2002;69:15-18.
33. Thompson PJ, Greenough A, Gamsu HR, Nicolaids KH. Ventilatory requirements for respiratory distress syndrome in small-for-gestational-age infants. Eur J Paediatr 1992;151:528-31.
34. Madanasky DL, Lawson EE, Chernick V, Teusch HW Jr. Pneumothorax and other forms of air leak in newborns. Am Rev Respir Dis 1979;120:729-37.

35. Monin P, Vert P. Pneumothorax. Clin Perinatal 1978;5:335.
36. Parmigiani S, Solari E. The era of pulmonary surfactant from Laplace to nowadays. Acta Biomed Ateneo Parmense. 2003;74:69-75.
37. Victorin LH, Deverajan LV, Curstedt T, Robertson B. Surfactant replacement in spontaneously breathing babies with hyaline membrane disease — A pilot study. Biol Neonate 1990;58:121-26.
38. Morley CJ. Surfactant treatment for premature babies— A review of clinical trials. Arch Dis Childhood 1991;66: 445-50.
39. Gonda TA, Hutchins GM. Surfactant treatment may accelerate epithelial cell regeneration in hyaline membrane disease of the newborn. Am J Perinatol 1998;15:539-44.
40. Slama M, Andre C, Huon C, Antoun H, Adamsbaum C. Radiological analysis of hyaline membrane disease after exogenous surfactant treatment. Pediatr Radiol 1999; 29:56-60.
41. Nicolson M, Fleming J, Spencer I. Hyaline membrane and neonatal radiology—Ian Donald's first venture into imaging research. Scott Med J 2005;50:35-37.
42. Shima Y, Takemura T, Akamatsu H, Kawakami T, Yoda H. Clinicopathological analysis of premature infants treated with artificial surfactant. J Nippon Med Sch 2000;67:330-34.
43. Kresch MJ, Clive JM. Meta-analyses of surfactant replacement therapy of infants with birth weights less than 2000 grams. J Perinatol 1998;18:276-83.
44. Collaborative group on antenatal steroid therapy, effect of antenatal dexamethasone administration on the prevention of respiratory distress syndrome. Am J Obstet Gynecol 1981;141:276-87.
45. Yeh TF, Torre JA, Rastogi A, Aneybuno MA, Pildes RS. Early postnatal dexamethasone therapy in premature infants with severe respiratory distress syndrome: A double blind, controlled study. J Paediatr 1990;17:273-83.
46. Danders RJ, Cox C, Phelps DL, Sinkin RA. Two doses of early intravenous dexamethasone for the prevention of bronchopulmonary dysplasia in babies with respiratory distress syndrome. Pediatr Res. 1994;36:122-28.
47. Ee L, Hagan R, Evans S, French N. Antenatal steroids, condition at birth and respiratory morbidity and mortality in very preterm infants. J Paediatr Child Health 1998; 34:377-83.
48. Driul L, Furlan R, Macagno F, Pezzani I, Plaino L, Ianni A, Casarsa S, Zavarise D, Marchesoni D. Induction of fetal lung maturation in the prevention of hyaline membrane disease: The connection with neonatal sepsis. Mi nerva Ginecol 2003;55:37-42.
49. Fekih M, Chaieb A, Sboui H, Denguezli W, Hidar S, Khairi H. Value of prenatal corticotherapy in the prevention of hyaline membrane disease in premature infants. Randomized prospective study. Tunis Med 2002 ;80: 260-65.
50. Paduraru L, Paduraru D, Stamatin M. Antenatal corticosteroid therapy and the effects on complications of prematurity. Rev Med Chir Soc Med Nat Iasi 2001;105: 521-26.
51. Nelin LD, Hoffman GM. The use of inhaled nitric oxide in a wide variety of clinical problems. Pediatr Clin North Am 1998;45:531-48.
52. Storme L, Zerimech F, Riou Y, Martin-Ponthieu A, Devisme L, Slomianny C, Klosowski S, Dewailly E, Cneude F, Zandecki M, Dupuis B, Lequien P. Inhaled nitric oxide neither alters oxidative stress parameters nor induces lung inflammation in premature lambs with moderate hyaline membrane disease. Biol Neonate 1998;73:172-81.
53. Danan C, Franco ML, Jarreau PH, Dassieu G, Chailley-Heu B, Bourbon J, Delacourt C. High concentrations of keratinocyte growth factor in airways of premature infants predicted absence of bronchopulmonary dysplasia. Am J Respir Crit Care Med. 2002;165: 1384-87.

Critical Care in Pulmonary Medicine

Intensive care (ICU) or critical care is a branch of medicine, which has grown rapidly in recent years. This specialized service is required for critically ill patients, who otherwise cannot be managed in the general wards. This is growing rapidly from a privileged service in few developed countries to a more widely available super-speciality. Intensive care has been defined by the King's fund panel (UK) as "a service for patients with potentially recoverable disease who can benefit from more detailed observation and treatment than is available generally in the standard wards and departments".[1] Although there is a tug-of-war who should manage the ICU—the anesthetist or the pulmonary physician—it is best managed by "intensivists". It is teamwork, where both the pulmonary physician and the anesthetist besides other specialists including cardiologists, internists, nephrologists, etc. play useful roles. Moreover, it is the convenience of the hospital which decides who should actually manage an ICU or critical care. There are institutions, which offer critical care fellowships and degrees so that the person should be able to manage the critically ill patient. While intensive care in many developed countries has made rapid advances with planned formal training programs, it is still considered a luxury in poor and developing countries where provision of basic health needs is more important. It is perhaps a formidable challenge for these socially and economically strained countries to develop an intensive care service, which is appropriate, affordable, and sustainable. Nonetheless, many such countries have developed their own ICUs, although to a very limited extent.[2]

Critical care represents the challenge of high technology medicine. They make heavy demands in terms of staff, equipment, and other resource, yet they have the potential to save lives and increase the chances of survival where alternative therapies have failed or have nothing more to offer. While they undoubtedly bring benefit to the patient, ICUs also result in loss of the patient's dignity, privacy and autonomy. Cost-benefit ratios are difficult to calculate and have different meaning in different circumstances and different socioeconomic milieu.

It must be very clear that ICU is a place, and not a form of therapy or treatment, which provides special skills and experience of medical, and nursing staff for the care of the critically ill patient and particularly in those in whom there is expectation of failure of one or more organ systems. It also provides a center for physiological measurements, nursing procedures, and therapeutic maneuvers which are not practicable in the general wards. Procedures undertaken in the ICU are done with an assumption that the concentration of special facilities and expertise gives better results and reduces cost. The type of care provided in an ICU varies according to the activities of the hospital and the predominant mix of patients admitted for intensive attention.

The task force on guidelines of the society of Critical Care Medicine has put forth the guidelines for categorization of services for the critically-ill patients and has defined what an "intensivist" is.[3,4] According to the group, critical care units appropriately concentrate critically ill patients in a specified area in the hospital, which is well equipped not only with machineries and supplies, but also has the personnel with special training and expertise in the care of critically ill. A multidisciplinary team led by an intensivist must design the unit.

In addition to delivery of excellent patient care, the provider has the important administrative and quality assurance duties.

Two levels of critical care have been advocated. Level I units represent delivery of care to the desperately ill patients with complicated needs requiring continuous availability of sophisticated equipments, specialized nurses, and physicians trained in the critically ill. Level 1C units represent this high level of clinical care. Level IA units in addition, are committed to education and research in the field of critical care medicine. Level II units are usually run by hospitals with limited resources. The requirements of a critical care unit include some basic components. These include medical staff organization; unit organization; bioethical committee; round-the-clock coverage by the physician; nursing availability; respiratory therapy; fully equipped service to cover all the physiological needs; and the supportive laboratory service 24 hours a day.

Criteria of Admission into an ICU

The practice of critical care medicine is hospital based, dedicated to and defined by the needs of critically ill patients. Such patients are those who are physiologically unstable, requiring continuous, coordinated, physician, nursing, and respiratory care, necessitating particular attention to detail, and those who are at increased risk for physiologic decompensation and thus, require constant monitoring. ICU should be given primarily to those where there is an expectation of benefit when these are achieved within a cost-benefit manner. It should not be given to those in whom possible harms outweigh the remote possibilities of benefit. Within a group of patients, the outcome of such a care is of major concern. The King's Fund Panel recommends a simple 5 point scale.

- Expected to survive
- Potentially recoverable (a good chance)
- Prognosis uncertain
- Death probable shortly whatever may be done
- Death apparently imminent.

The panel recommends that ICU should be provided for the first two categories, although it is a highly debatable question whether others can be denied the opportunity to get this facility. Potential organ donors may be admitted to the ICU who fulfil the criteria of brain stem death or are expected to do so because mechanical ventilation will keep the organs in good condition. The ideal thing is that the hospital or the ICU should set up its own guidelines for admission.

Most of the intensive care involves temporary maintenance of the function of one or more organs. It may be ventilation for respiratory failure or dialysis for renal failure. Best results are achieved with single organ failure. It is also used to monitor, to detect and to respond rapidly to any serious complications in patients judged to be at risk of becoming critically ill.

The intensive care areas demand specific skills and abilities from the respiratory care provider (RCP) in providing therapy, support, and management of patients who are seriously ill and at highest risk for complications. To optimize the quality of respiratory care provided, specific staffing standards and RCP expectations have been established.[5-11]

The RCPs are expected to maintain adequate skills to function in any of the ICUs, which include: Surgical/ Trauma, Burn, and CCU/ Medicine. Additional pediatric training and competency check off is necessary for therapists assigned to any pediatric patient in the ICU. However, every hospital/institution has its own policy of providing care to different categories of patients. As workload demands, any RCP may also be assigned to the medical floors at the discretion of the team leader. In emergency situations the RCP exhibits a high degree of skill compromising events. He should be able to organize workday and set priorities to insure essential tasks are performed, exhibits good time management skills so the RCP time at the bedside is maximized. He also should be able to communicate well with others during shift report, able to effectively interact with attending consultants, house staff, nursing, and peers. The RCP by virtue of interest, desire, commitment to excellence in care, and advanced level skills and abilities is scheduled to primarily work in a specific ICU area. All RCPs are expected to work in collaboration with the RCP Technical Director and ICU Coordinator to formulate and implement patient care plans as well as assist in policy development, to a greater degree the Clinical Specialist will be relied upon as an expert in the unit they are primarily assigned. RCPs are eligible for Clinical Specialist assignments if they meet the established criteria like a desire to primarily work in a specific ICU area and meet the minimum job requirements as outlined in the job description.

The Respiratory Care provider working in ICU is not only expected to be fully ICU qualified in the standard skills of their profession but must also demonstrate acceptable knowledge and skills that are required to perform efficiently in ICU. The care provider must be able to transport, critically ill patients; must have training for resuscitation and intubation procedures; should be proficient in ventilator management; must be aware of patient care plan assessments and interventions; and must have knowledge in other areas like hemodynamic monitoring, ABG drawing and interpretation, indications and use of BiPAP able to do bronchoscopy or assistance, airway assessment, monitoring, and proper suctioning technique, setup and administration of oxygen, heliox, nitric oxide, and metabolic systems. He or she should possess a working knowledge of pulmonary and cardiac anatomy and pathophysiology as well as oxygen transport and delivery. Further, they will be responsible for knowing the indications, contraindictions, and hazards of all respiratory medications, equipments, and procedures.

The staffing pattern in the ICU is different than that is in the general wards or areas as patients are critical and need help in every aspect including handling and taking care of various instruments. Most ICUs will have a nursing ratio of 1:1 with that of the patient round the clock.

In the ICU, nursing staff and respiratory care provider will work as a team in coordinating patient care. Joint responsibility includes verification of appropriate respiratory therapy administered; airway maintenance and suctioning; infection control; patient assessments during acute changes; sputum collection; communication with patient, other physicians, and family; patient rounds/report; patient positioning; patient transport; ventilator and respiratory treatment order; coordinating respiratory care plan; drawing ABGs ; and able to carry out electrocardiograms.

CRITICAL CARE IN PULMONARY DISEASES

Any patient having pulmonary disease might need critical care. Respiratory failure is the most common pulmonary problem which needs ICU care. Bronchial asthma during acute severe attacks needs critical care. Similarly, fulminant pneumonia, acute respiratory distress syndrome, massive hemoptysis, septicemia, drug toxicities, and acute exacerbations of COPD, all of which will need careful monitoring and management even if it does not mean the use of a ventilator. Most of the medical disorders requiring ICU care are because of respiratory disorders. Besides basic equipments like ventilators, nebulizers and other inhalation devices, other facilities those should be available in a respiratory ICU will include the following:[4-11]

- Continuous monitoring of ECG
- Continuous arterial monitoring
- Central venous pressure monitoring
- Equipment to maintain the airway including laryngoscope, Endotracheal tubes
- Equipment to ventilate including ventilators
- Noninvasive ventilators
- IPPB (intermittent positive pressure breathing) facilities
- Metered dose inhaler to be delivered through the ventilators
- Ambubag
- Oxygen, and compressed air

- Emergency resuscitation set
- Equipments to monitor hemodynamics, including infusion pumps, blood warmers, pressure bags, blood filters
- Ultrasonic nebulization
- Transport monitor
- Adjustable beds
- Suction facilities
- Hhypo-, hyperthermia blankets scale
- Temporary pacemaker
- Temperature monitoring device
- Pulmonary pressure monitoring device
- Cardiac output monitoring
- Continuous oxygen monitoring facilities in the ventilators
- Central catheters
- All emergency drugs
- Dialysis
- Capnography
- Transcutaneous oxygen monitoring or pulse oxymetry for all patients receiving oxygen therapy
- Access to CT scanner
- Cardiac catheter laboratory
- Nuclear imaging
- Bronchoscopy both fiber-optic and rigid
- Radiology with fluoroscopy
- Intracranial pressure monitoring
- Extracorporeal membrane oxygen
- Left heart assist devices
- Hyperbaric chamber
- Computerized data management system
- Respiratory physiotherapist
- Twenty-hours availability of laboratory services for standard analysis of blood, urine and body fluids, blood typing and cross matching, coagulation studies, blood banking service, blood gas determination, electrolyte determination, microbiology help and toxicology screening.

The purpose of a critical care service is to provide continuous titrated medical care, and to avoid fragmentation among various consultants and health care providers.

Many ICUs in the leading centers have their own set guidelines/protocols of management of patients like who should do what and defined criteria for applying a particular form of therapy/procedure.[12] Many of the ICUs in various hospitals have their own policies and guidelines for everyone working in the area. Some of the broad guidelines of some important procedures are described below:

I. OXYGEN ADMINISTRATION

- Each ICU bed should be equipped with an oxygen flowmeter and nipple adapter.
- The ICU staff usually sets up and discontinues oxygen therapy as per physician's order or per protocol.
- Respiratory Care Provider may administer oxygen, at their discretion, to any patient demonstrating signs of life threatening hypoxemia.
- ICU nursing staff may initiate oxygen delivery utilizing a nasal cannula if respiratory care is not readily available. However, nursing staff must inform the physician incharge of a new start so that an assessment, appropriate monitoring and documentation of use is performed.

II. AIRWAY MANAGEMENT

All airway maintenance is a joint responsibility of the nursing staff and RCP, requiring interaction between them to coordinate airway care. Although the following tasks are actually the responsibility of both of them, they have been specified as follows to assist in insuring they are performed:

The RCP has primary responsibility for:
- Assisting/doing the intubation
- Airway suctioning during ventilator check period if needed
- Airway suctioning following a treatment
- Placement of oral airway to protect ETT (endotracheal tube)
- Documentation of ETT cm mark
- ET tube manipulation as per MD
- Changing catheter system every 72 hours
- Measuring and documenting cuff pressure every shift and when required
- Extubation
- Patient assessment to determine, if alternative secretion clearance plan vs. airway management is indicated.

Usually the nursing staff has primary responsibility for:
- Trach care, stoma site, and trach ties
- ET care, oral hygiene, and tape change
- Airway suctioning when indicated
- Checking cuff pressure and volume when clinically indicated
- Communicating complications to the physician
- Coordinating tube feeding with airway manipulations.

It is recognized that patients with artificial airways require a specialized level of care. Of primary importance is the maintenance of a patient's airway, adequate hydration, and to minimize complications associated with artificial airways. The staff should check all non-ventilated patients with artificial airways no less than every 8 hours. The following things need to be noted:[13,14]
- Resuscitation bag/mask at bedside with patient label
- Neurological status
- Respiratory rate
- Heart rate
- Breath sounds
- Airway site
- Airway indications
- Airway size
- Airway length
- Airway refer point
- Cuff pressure
- Suction
- Sputum production
- Sputum consistency
- Sputum color
- Change in breath sounds
- Adverse reaction
- Activity outcome.

For intubation; low pressure/high volume cuffs should be utilized and MOV (minimal occluding volume) technique be utilized to set cuff pressure. Equipment attached to the Endotracheal tube is to be properly supported to minimize airway torque, pressure exerted on the soft tissues, and to reduce the potential for inadvertent extubation. This may include the use of: Swivel adapters and 4" flex tubes between the ET/trach tube and ventilator "Y", Support arms on all ventilator systems to hold the weight of the tubing; velcro type tube holders secured to the patients gown or other anchor that moves with the patient; Smaller pediatric patients may not use the swivel adapters/4" flex tubes to prevent excessive CO_2 rebreathing. Any problems with airway occlusion, placement, function, will be reported to the responsible nurse and physician. Although there may be some variance in airway management policy to meet the specific needs of patients in a particular area, the general approach is the same for all.

III. AIRWAY SUCTIONING

I. Suctioning of the airway should be performed when clinically indicated with the objective to remove secretions from the airway. Indications include:[15-17]
- Coarse rhonchi
- Visible secretions in the airway

- Coughing
- Increase in PIP (positive inspiratory pressure)
- Concern regarding airway patency
- Desaturation
- TCPV ventilator mode with decrease in tidal volume
- Suspected aspiration of gastric or upper airway secretions.

Some patients may not demonstrate the above indications until the airway is actually suctioned. It should be evaluated if the patient requires suctioning at a specific frequency in addition to when it is indicated.

II. A period of at least 15 minutes should elapse between suctioning and the drawing of an arterial blood gases to minimize the reflection of alterations in blood gas values that may be the direct result of suctioning.

III. In those patients in which a disconnect for suctioning may place the patient at greater risk for acute compromise, a closed system should be utilized that enables the patient to remain connected to the ventilator while being suctioned. This group of patients include any of the following clinical situations:
- Bradycardia/arrhythmia upon disconnect
- Desaturation while bagging with 100 percent oxygen
- PEEP > 10
- FiO_2 > 60
- PIP > 50.

IV. Vacuum regulator pressure should be set at 80 to 100 mm Hg for children and 100 to 120 mm Hg for adults. The system should have the ability to achieve these pressure levels with the tubing and suction catheter attached and the thumb/vacuum valve occluded.

V. Sterile technique should always be utilized. This includes sterile gloves and a fresh catheter for each series of suction passes. The upper airway should be cleared last. Sterile suction supplies are single use only, and then discarded.

VI. All patients should be preoxygenated at 100 percent for a period of at least 30 seconds prior to suctioning maintained on 100 percent for the duration of the procedure, and for a period of 30 seconds after the procedure. This may be accomplished by adjusting the FiO_2 setting on the mechanical ventilator.

VII. Each pass of the suction catheter should not exceed 15 seconds in duration. Failure of the patient to return to presuction levels of SaO_2 should be viewed seriously and may require some modification in the pre/post oxygenation durations.

VIII. Hand resuscitators should be available at the bedside and capable of delivering 100 percent oxygen if needed. Bagging is not routinely required in adults, but may be useful to minimize ventilator asynchrony as a result of coughing and, in certain patients, help facilitate secretion removal. If the evaluation of the patient indicates increased airway resistance (peak plateau > 5 cm H_2O) in which secretions are suspected and less than 5 ml is returned via suction, the clinician should evaluate if bagging will result in improved secretion return. Bagging may also be considered in the event the patient becomes desaturated and/or asynchronous with the ventilator during suctioning that is minimized by bagging. Bagging is best performed with two individuals, one bagging while the other suctions.

In pediatric patients with non-cuff tubes bagging is required to provide additional volume that may be offset by a pressure leak around the tube and to provide immediate modifications in ventilation in response to changes in patient condition during suctioning.

IX. Instillation of solutions into the airway is not routinely performed when suctioning. When secretions are thick and difficult to remove at vacuum pressures of 120 mm Hg, instillation of 5 to 10 ml of normal saline may be of benefit. Adequate hydration and humidity should rarely require supplemental instillation to decrease sputum viscosity. If the evaluation of the patient indicates increased airway resistance (peak-plateau > 5 cm H_2O) in which secretions are suspected and less than 5 ml is returned via suction, the clinician should evaluate if instillation will result in improved secretion return. Perhaps its greatest role is to facilitate a cough to move secretions into the larger airways within the reach of the suction catheter. Instillation in the amounts of 5 to 10 ml of normal saline just prior to insertion of the suction catheter may be performed.

X. In pediatric patients vacuum pressure should be 80 to 100 mm Hg and instillation is not performed unless requested by the physician in which the quantity should be specified. Pediatric suctioning is a two-person procedure, which targets reducing the time the patient is not oxygenated and control of the airway.

XI. Procedure:
- Explain the procedure to the patient.

- Preoxygenate at 100 percent.
- Prepare suction equipment, to include goggles, mask, and other appropriate equipment for Standard Precautions, sterile gloves over washed hands, attaching suction catheter to vacuum, and sterile water for catheter irrigation between passes.
- As indicated, disconnect ET adaptor or utilize closed system to introduce the catheter into the airway. Without applying suction, advance the catheter gently beyond the distal tip of the ET/trach tube (except for PTEs) until resistance is felt, then pull back slightly and apply suction. Apply intermittent suction. Apply intermittent suction and rotate the catheter during withdrawal.
- Remove the catheter from the airway and insure the patient is being ventilated and oxygenated adequately. Total time for a single pass in and out of the airway should not exceed 15 seconds. If multiple passes are necessary, provide recovery period between each pass.

  Evaluate for complications associated with suctioning, which include:
- Hypoxemia
- Tissue trauma
- Tachycardia/bradycardia
- Hypotension/hypertension
- Bronchoconstriction/bronchospasm
- Bleeding
- Increased ICP
- Tissue trauma to the tracheal and/or bronchial mucosa.
XII. Document that suctioning was performed, the results of the procedure, and any adverse response observed. Patients with bleeding complications may require a softer rubber catheter for suctioning.

IV. INTUBATION-ENDOTRACHEAL[18-20]

Before intubation, one should identify patient and determine the need for intubation.

Infection control precautions are to be observed.

Hands must be washed prior to and after any respiratory modality or anytime contamination is suspected.

One should observe universal precautions at all times

Other precautions are:
- Obtain equipment and supplies
- Resuscitation bag or mask to mouth system
- Oxygen source
- Wall

- Cylinder
- Suction set-up
- Suction kit
- Yankauer
- Laryngoscope with appropriate sized blade (curved and straight)
- Endotracheal tube (ETT)
- Stylet
- Syringe 10 ml
- Oral airway
- McGil forceps
- Lubrication gel (K-Y jelly)
- 2 percent Xylocaine jelly
- CO_2 detector
- Adhesive tape: Twill, cloth, or anesthesia
- Tincture of benzoin
- Stethoscope
- Glove, appropriate mask, and protective eyewear.

Prior to beginning the intubation procedure have the following equipment ready:
Endotracheal tube
Determine ETT size – High volume-low pressure cuff for an adult. Tube size that are available: 6.0, 6.5, 7.0, 7.5, 8.0, 8.5 and, 9.0. Tube size of the adult patient depends on tracheal anatomy. 6.0 is very small, 9.0 very large, 7.5 to 8.0 are most commonly used.

Check tube for cuff leaks. Keep tube inside sterile wrapper. Add air to cuff, squeeze the cuff without contaminating it.

Insert stylet if desired. Make sure the stylet does not extend beyond the tip of tube.

Bend extra length of stylet over the top of adapter to prevent sliding during intubation.

Attach 10 ml syringe to pilot balloon, or have immediately available.

LARYNGOSCOPE

Determine proper blade size. Curved blade (Macintosh) or Straight blade (Miller).

Check that it snaps as it locks into position, fit should be snug.

Check light source at end of blade, (if light does not illuminate, tighten bulb or change batteries in handle if necessary).

Oxygen source: Assure that patient is being hand ventilated with oxygen flowmeter at flush, 100 percent oxygen. Visualize oxygen supply tubing for proper connection.

Suction set-up: Set-up suction with Yankauer suction tip with pressure set to full to suction oral secretions.

Endotracheal tube tape or twill.

Pulse oximeter and ECG monitor if available.

Lower head of bed, adjust height of bed if necessary, and remove headboard from bed if indicated.

Ventilate patient with 100 percent oxygen by bag-mask ventilation to ensure proper oxygenation. Use oral airway if unable to maintain open airway. Remove dentures or bridges from mouth. Clear secretions from mouth and glottic area with Yankauer, if necessary.

Resume bag-mask ventilations for approximately one minute, if oral suction is necessary.

Attempt to intubate patient not exceeding 30 seconds. If monitoring with saturation monitor, resume bag-mask ventilations with 100 percent oxygen, when oxygen saturation is less than 90 percent. In the event the patient has a chronic disease, i.e. cystic fibrosis or emphysema, intubation attempts should cease if the saturation falls to < 85 percent. Resume ventilations with 100 percent oxygen before reattempting intubation. If RCP is unsuccessful after two attempts, the RCP shall ask a healthcare worker to call the ER Physician stat.

Hold laryngoscope in the left hand and the blade is inserted into the mouth in a right to left sweeping motion as to optimize visualization of the vocal cords. The blade when inserted properly should end up in the center of the mouth.

Note: If the curved blade is used, the tip is placed in the vallecula above the epiglottis. If a straight blade is used, its tip is passed below the epiglottis to rest above the glottic opening.

Exert blade traction upward in the direction of the long axis of the handle to displace the base of the tongue and the epiglottis anteriorly, exposing the glottis.

Hold the prepared ET tube in the right hand and pass it along side the laryngoscope under direct visualization. Place the tube from the right side of the mouth, (the channel of the blade should be used for visualization during tube placement), into the tracheal orifice and through the vocal cords.

Note: The patient should never be intubated blindly. Always visualize the proper landmarks before attempting an intubation. Advance cuff just distal to the vocal cords.

Inflate cuff to a minimal or no leak conditions, while holding the tube in place. Remove stylet, (if used), resuscitate with 100 percent oxygen. Check immediately for bilateral air exchange movement with chest auscultation and direct visualization. (Listen for the absence of breath sounds). Listen with stethoscope over the stomach to rule out esophageal intubation.

End Tidal CO_2 are available and must be used as an additional means to document tube placement. CO_2 detectors are placed between ETT and resuscitation bag while ventilating patient. Purple to yellow change occurs in presence of exhaled CO_2, verifying proper placement.

Tape the tube securely in place, noting the cm mark at teeth or gums.

Verify tube placement as soon as possible with chest X-ray and reposition tube as necessary to achieve proper position.

V. ARTERIAL PUNCTURE FOR BLOOD GAS ANALYSIS[21-24]

Purpose

- To obtain arterial blood sample to measure pH, PO_2, and PCO_2 to provide a means of assessing the adequacy of oxygenation and ventilation and the acid base status of a patient
- To quantitate the response to therapeutic intervention (e.g. supplemental oxygen administration, mechanical ventilation) and/or diagnostic evaluation (e.g. exercise desaturation)[1-3]
- The need to monitor severity and progression of documented disease processes.

Procedure

Gather equipment needed:
- Prepackaged ABG kit containing
- 3 ml heparinized syringe
- 22 gauge needle
- Rubber cube for corking needle
- Rubber stopper for syringe.

Additionally:
- Betadine swab
- Alcohol swab
- 2 × 2 gauze pad
- Transport bag with ice and water (slush)
- Patient label
- Lab slip.

Place all items on a firm surface close to you. It is helpful to open the betadine, alcohol and gauze pad before you begin.
- Wash hands
- Introduce yourself and explain the procedure
- Apply clean gloves.

Evaluate pulses for optimal site. Examine site for skin rash, scarring, trauma or abnormalities. If present choose alternate site.

For radial sticks, perform an Allen's test by obliterating radial and ulnar pulse simultaneously at the wrist then have patient clench and unclench fist until blanching occurs. Release pressure on the ulnar then watch for return of the skin color. If negative, choose alternate site.

For radial sticks, raise patient's bed to a level that is comfortable.

For radial sticks, position patient's arm extended flat with the palm up and a rolled towel underneath the wrist to assist in flexing.

Cleanse the skin at the puncture site with betadine, let dry, then cleanse again with alcohol.

With your nondominate hand, palpate the artery with your index finger and locate the point of maximal pulsation.

While palpating the pulse, take the barrel of the sampling syringe in your dominate hand, holding the syringe like a pencil with the bevel up, slowly penetrate the skin aiming the end of the needle toward the pulsing artery.

Advance the needle in a straight line until you see a flash of blood in the hub of the syringe.

If you miss the artery, withdraw the needle to just below the level of the skin. Reevaluate the artery's position and redirect the needle and try again.

Never change the angle of the needle while the needle is deep under the skin as laceration of tissue, veins, muscle, nerves, and even periosteum could occur.

When a flash of blood appears in the hub of the syringe, stop advancing the needle and hold the position until 1.5 to 2 cc has filled the syringe.

Remove the needle from the wrist, foot or groin area and quickly place a gauze pad over the puncture site applying firm pressure for approximately 5 minutes or until bleeding ceases.

Expel any air bubbles then cork the needle in the rubber cube, gently rotate the syringe to mix blood with heparin, and then place in slush.

Place a label with the patient ID onto the barrel of the syringe.

Observe puncture site again to assure bleeding has stopped.

Within 10 minutes deliver the sample to the lab or inform nurse to arrange for delivery.

Information needed on ABG lab slip:
- Patient's name and location
- Physician ordering sample
- Time of sampling
- Patient temperature
- FiO_2 and device
- Vent settings (if applicable)
- Sampling site
- Document procedure in CliniVision.

VI. VENTILATOR SUPPORT

A. To initiate ventilator support the following points are to be taken into account:
- Modes of ventilation
  - Assist control
  - SIMV
  - Spontaneous ventilation
  - Pressure control (PCV)
  - Bi level ventilation
- Setting of rate
- Tidal volume or inspiratory pressures
- FiO_2
- PEEP or CPAP
- Pressure support

B. In addition to the above settings, the other parameters to be taken care are:
- Inspiratory time
- Flow (volume ventilation)
- Flow acceleration percentage
- Flow trigger (for synchronization with patient's spontaneous efforts)
- Flow waveform pattern ("ramp" unless otherwise specified)
- Expiratory sensitivity (to declare end of inspiration during a pressure Support breath)
- Apnea parameters (match to previous ventilator settings)
- Alarms (following P and P guidelines for mechanical ventilation)

C. Initiation of ventilation may be done utilizing the following guidelines and the desired parameters may be adjusted subsequently:
- Indication
- A/C Mode
- Volume ventilation
- Flow trigger
- Rate 10 to 12 breaths per minute
- Tidal volume 10 ml/kg lean body weight
- Flow rate = 50 LPM or adjusted to achieve an I:E ratio of 1:3
- "Ramp" flow waveform
- Flow sensitivity = 3.0 lpm
- FiO_2 = 1.0
- PEEP = 0 cm H_2O
- P circ max (Maximun Circuit Pressure) = 40 cm H_2O
  - All ventilated patients shall have a resuscitation bag/mask attached to an O_2 flowmeter with a patient label and filter. Filters will be changed every 24 hours if in use (noted by soiling or if filter packaging is torn). Any

patient on > 5 of PEEP should have a PEEP valve attached to the resuscitator bag with a manometer to monitor PEEP level.

- In the event the ventilator is discontinued, the flex tube/ ETT adapter should be covered with a rubber glove and the entire ventilator should be covered with a large sized clear plastic bag which are kept in the utility areas of each ICUs. The ventilator will be covered before transporting the ventilator from the ICU.
- If apnea should occur on low rate SIMV: Initiate volume or pressure ventilation using the same FiO_2 and tidal volume with a rate of 8 to 12 breaths per minute.
- Impending cardiac arrest or during a code: Manually ventilate with self inflating manual resuscitation bag with oxygen flow at 15 L/min at a pressure that matches ventilator delivery.
- Patient clinically not tolerating advancement: Revert to previous settings or place patient on 100 percent O_2 if necessary.

Auto-PEEP measurements are performed using the "Exp Hold" expiratory hold key. During the pause, the most recently selected graphics are displayed and frozen, so the operator can follow and assess when expiratory pressure stabilizes.

Inspiratory Pause ("Insp Pause") During this maneuver the ventilator seals the patient's breathing circuit after the end of the gas delivery phase of a designated, volume- or pressure-based mandatory inspiration. The ventilator performs two types of pause maneuver: automatic, which is initiated by a momentary pressing of the Insp Pause key, and manual, which the practitioner controls by holding the key down. The automatic pause lasts 0.5 to 2.0 seconds. The manual pause lasts no longer than 7 seconds. The maneuver provides a way to measure the patient's static lung thoracic compliance (C), static resistance (R) (only of square wave, volume control breath), and plateau pressure (Ppl) or to maintain the inflated state of the lung.

I. Circuit Disconnect is declared when the patient circuit is disconnected at the ventilator or the patient side of the "y". Adjusting the "D sens" can set the sensitivity of the Circuit Disconnect alarm. The "D sens" sets the allowable loss (in%) of delivered volume, which, if exceeded, causes the ventilator to detect a Circuit Disconnect alarm. The greater the setting, the more returned volume must be lost before a Circuit Disconnect is detected. The default for "New Patient Value" is 75 percent. There is no ventilation during a Circuit Disconnect alarm.

Expiratory Sensitivity ("E sens"). The E sens setting defines the percentage of the projected peak inspiratory flow at which the ventilator cycles from inspiration to exhalation. When inspiratory flow falls to the level defined by E sens, exhalation begins. E sens is active during every spontaneous breath. The respiratory practitioner can adjust the E sens setting. The higher the E sens setting, the shorter is the inspiratory time. The default value for E sens is 30 percent.

A. A new ventilator flowsheet should be started at the initiation of mechanical ventilation. Up to three days of flow sheet information should remain at the bedside for reference after which the form should be placed in the patient permanent medical record.

II. Flowsheet header.

III. Clinical Assessment:

A. Neuro status: Awake, sleeping, comatose, paralyzed are general descriptive terms that are acceptable for entry.

B. HR:Heart rate from the ECG.

IV. Physical Examination:

A. The RCP should enter data related to chest physical examination, any adverse response, and assessment of physiologic data no less than once per shift. In addition this section is to note specific rational for ventilator changes. Each entry should start with a time which may correlate with the ventilator check.

V. Volume:

A. Mode(s): Indicate the mode selected on the ventilator, include all modes currently active. (Ex. SIMV/PSV or CMV/TCPV or PCV+, etc.).

B. Tidal volume-set: Record the set inspired tidal volume.

C. Exhaled-Digital: The digital exhaled tidal volume from a mandatory breath.

D. Exhaled-Spontaneous: Record the exhaled spontaneous tidal volume reading average volume over 10 to 20 seconds.

E. Minute-Total: Record the total minutes ventilation displayed. Includes both mandatory and spontaneous components.

F. Minute-Spontaneous: Record the spontaneous minutes ventilation displayed.

VI. Rate:

A. Set: Record the breathing frequency in breaths per minute for set breaths (control of SIMV rate).

B. Total: The total breaths per minute. Count the total number of breaths per minute by timed observation. The digital reading on any ventilator is a running average of prior breath to breath intervals. The displayed rate may therefore not be a true representation of the patient rate especially if a mechanical breath has just been delivered in the SIMV mode.

VII. FiO_2:
 A. Set from 21 to 100 percent.

VIII. Pressure:
 A. PIP: Record the peak inspiratory pressure as displayed on the 7200 or if using the Bear or Sechrist as observed on the pressure manometer.
 B. PEEP/CPAP: Record the observed amount of pressure for PEEP/CPAP, the manometer is the most accurate indicator of PEEP/CPAP on any ventilator.
 C. MAP: Record the Mean airway pressure as indicated on the digital readout.
 D. Pressure Support: Record the value programmed into the ventilator for the level of pressure support. Remember that the pressure support entered is that pressure that is above PEEP setting. The peak pressure observed on the manometer should be PEEP plus the pressure support level.

IX. TCPV:
 A. The respiratory therapist in the ICU will be involved in the assessment, evaluation, and communication of appropriate respiratory therapy care plans.

VII. OTHER SUPPORTIVE MEASURES IN ICU

In intensive care medicine, there is a shortage of "gold standard" randomized controlled trial evidence to support (or not support) therapeutic decisions. In addition, even when well-conducted randomized trials have been performed, there are still with unanswered questions.[25] In the last few years, several clinical trials have yielded positive results with a number of interventions being shown to improve outcomes. Actually, the intensive care medicine literature has included more negative trials than positive trials. A number of therapeutic strategies have not been shown to be helpful in patients with severe sepsis and septic shock, including high doses of corticosteroids, ibuprofen, antitumor necrosis factor (TNF) antibodies, TNF receptors, interleukin-1 receptor antagonist, and various platelet-activating factor antagonists. Likewise, many studies have been negative in the field of the management of acute lung injury (ALI) or ARDS, including the administration of nitric oxide by inhalation, the administration of surfactant, or the use of different modes of mechanical ventilation. Some interventions have even resulted in worse outcomes, including the use of a TNF receptor in patients with severe sepsis, excessive doses of dobuta-

mine in acutely ill patients, the administration of hemoglobin solutions in trauma patients, and the administration of growth factors. IV fluids, including albumin and RBC transfusions, have been areas of hot debate over the last few years, and even monitoring systems, especially the pulmonary artery catheter, have created controversy. Even some routine practices like mechanical ventilation and sedation may result in worse outcomes.

In the last 5 years, however (finally), some more positive strides have been made in clinical trial results, with a number of interventions having been shown to result in better outcomes.

Noninvasive Mechanical Ventilation

Endotracheal intubation is associated with a number of complications and may unduly prolong the need for mechanical ventilation. A number of studies have emphasized that the use of noninvasive mechanical ventilation could result in lower morbidity rates and even lower mortality rates in patients with COPD.[26,27] The use of noninvasive mechanical ventilation can also significantly reduce the incidence of ventilator-associated pneumonia.[28-30] This technique has found a significant place in modern ICUs, although the benefits in hypoxemic respiratory failure are less well-established.

Induced Hypothermia After Cardiac Arrest

Hypothermia can substantially decrease cellular oxygen demand, including that of the neurons, and these observations have led to a number of attempts to induce hypothermia following severe neurologic insults. Although the place of induced moderate hypothermia in patients with severe brain injury has not been clearly established, two studies.[31,32] have indicated that hypothermia, when induced as soon as possible after cardiac arrest, may improve neurologic outcomes. Hypothermia in these conditions should be instituted as early as possible and for at least 12 h.

Intensive Insulin Therapy in Critically Ill Patients

In a landmark study, Van den Berghe et al[33] randomized > 1,500 ICU patients to conventional management of hyperglycemia vs intensive management aimed at keeping blood sugar levels within tight limits of 80 to 110 mg/dL. This intensive strategy decreased mortality rates from 8.0 to 4.6 percent (p < 0.04). Moreover, the intensive treatment was associated with significantly fewer patients staying for > 14 days in the ICU, a lower requirement for renal replacement therapy, a lower incidence of hyperbilirubinemia, fewer bloodstream infections, fewer ICU neuropathies, and a reduced need for transfusion.

Blood Transfusions

A key multicenter Canadian study published by Hebert et al[34] changed the blood transfusion practice. In this prospective randomized control trial involving 25 Canadian centers, patients with a hemoglobin concentration below 9 g/dL were randomized to either a liberal blood transfusion strategy (i.e. maintaining hemoglobin levels at > 10 g/dL) or a restricted blood transfusion strategy (i.e. maintaining hemoglobin levels at > 7 g/dL).[34] The former group received a mean amount of 5.6 U RBCs to raise the hemoglobin concentration from 8.2 to 10.7 g/dL, whereas the latter group received a mean amount of 2.6 U RBCs to raise the mean hemoglobin concentration from 8.2 to 8.5 g/dL. These were critically ill patients with an APACHE II score of about 21. The hospital mortality rate was 28 percent in the liberal transfusion group but only 22 percent in the restricted transfusion group, leading to a statistically significant difference (p = 0.05). Clearly, the differences in short-term outcome could not be related to different incidences of transfusion-related infections, but they could be due to more subtle alterations in immune function, perhaps resulting in a greater risk of subsequent infections. These results were later confirmed in a large European study including > 3,500 patients, the Anemia and Blood Transfusion in the Critically Ill study.[35] In this study, which was performed in November 1999, transfusions were associated with a worse outcome in a multivariable analysis. Blood transfusions came before hemoglobin concentration in this multivariable analysis, indicating that it is the blood transfusion, rather than the anemia, that is associated with a worse outcome. Moreover, the use of a propensity score to match patients who did or did not receive a blood transfusion indicated significant differences in mortality rates (22.7 vs 17.1%). However, a more recent European study, the Sepsis Occurrence in Acutely Ill Patients study[36] also including > 3,000 patients and conducted in May 2002, failed to identify a worse outcome in transfused patients. These differences could be due to changes in the risks of blood transfusions and, in particular, to the now widely implemented leukodepletion programs. Indeed, the Canadian experience with universal leukoreduction programs indicated a reduction in mortality rates in patients after cardiac surgery or repair of hip fracture, or in those who required intensive care following a surgical intervention or multiple trauma.[37] as well as a reduction in neonatal morbidity.[38]

Development of Drotrecogin Alfa (Activated) in Severe Sepsis/Septic Shock

Several studies have emphasized the complex interplay between coagulation and inflammation in the development of organ failure following sepsis. In one study[39] the administration of drotrecogin alfa (activated) resulted in significant decreases in mortality rates in patients with severe sepsis and septic shock. The results of this study showed that the safety profile was certainly acceptable. Moreover, the results of a large study of > 2,300 patients, the ENHANCE trial[40] which were presented at the 2003 American College of Chest Physicians meeting; support the beneficial effects of drotrecogin alfa (activated) on outcome. The mode of action of drotrecogin alfa (activated) has not been entirely elucidated, but it is clearly more than just an anticoagulant effect, especially in view of the negative results from studies with two other natural anticoagulants, antithrombin[41] and tissue factor pathway inhibitor.[42] The results of ongoing studies[43,44] have suggested that its mechanism of action includes antiinflammatory and antiapoptotic protective effects on endothelial cells.

Other Interventions in Severe Sepsis

Another intervention that led to controversial results is bactericidal permeability-increasing protein. This natural substance that is released by leukocytes can combine with endotoxin to eliminate it. It was, therefore, natural to look for a homogeneous disease state characterized by a massive endotoxin release (e.g. meningococcemia) to test this agent. In the largest study involving acutely ill children[45] 393 patients were randomized to receive either recombinant bactericidal permeability-increasing protein or placebo. This study missed the end point of a significant reduction in mortality rates, but the mortality rate was only 9.9 percent in the placebo group vs 7.4 percent in the treated group (p = 0.48). In this study, the number of patients with full functional recovery was only 66.3 percent in the placebo group but was 77.3 percent in the treated group (p = 0.02).

Steroids in Septic Shock

The initial studies[46] investigating the effects of massive doses of methylprednisolone (30 mg/kg) in patients with septic shock did not show any benefit. More recent studies have indicated that patients with septic shock may have relative adrenal sufficiency and, therefore, may benefit from moderate doses of hydrocortisone (around 200 mg/d). A French RCT by Annane and coworkers[47] indicated that such a strategy may decrease mortality rates in patients with septic shock.

Vasopressin Administration in Septic Shock

The important concept of relative vasopressin deficiency was introduced by Landry et al[48] in 1997 when they observed that vasopressin levels were remarkably elevated in patients who were in cardiogenic shock but not in those in septic shock. A number of subsequent observations[49,50] have indicated that vasopressin administration could raise BP in septic shock patients and help to decrease the need for norepinephrine therapy. Some studies in animals[51] and in patients[49] also have suggested an improvement in urine output with this therapeutic strategy. Actually, a number of critical care physicians have already adopted this strategy and have used vasopressin in patients with severe septic shock.

Early Goal-directed Therapy in Severe Sepsis and Septic Shock

How to optimize the treatment of severe sepsis and septic shock has been an important question, especially after the disappointing results of strategies aimed at raising oxygen delivery to supranormal levels.[52] In a single-center RCT, Rivers et al[53] randomized patients with sepsis, arterial hypotension, and/or hyperlactemia to a standard resuscitation regimen or to so-called *early goal-directed therapy* (EGDT) guided by continuous measurements of oxygen saturation in the superior vena cava ($ScvO_2$) using a modified central venous catheter that was equipped with fiberoptic fibers. In addition to the standard oxygenation, fluid infusion, and vasoactive drug strategies, the authors maintained $ScvO_2$ at least at 70 percent in the EGDT group using additional fluids, blood transfusions, or dobutamine administration. In the first 6 h following resuscitation, there was no difference in the number of patients receiving vasopressors or mechanical ventilation, but the quantity of IV fluid was significantly greater in the EGDT group. Patients in the intervention group also received blood transfusions and dobutamine more commonly. Interestingly, the total amount of fluid administered during the first 72 h was similar in the two groups of patients, and the number of patients requiring vasopressor therapy, mechanical ventilation, or monitoring with a pulmonary artery catheter was lower in the EGDT group than in the control group.

Selective Decontamination of the Digestive Tract

The routine administration of an antibiotic mixture in the form of an oral paste to reduce the risk of nosocomial infections in ICU patients started initially in Groningen,

the Netherlands,[54] but it has led to great controversy. Moreover, the topical antibiotic administration must optimally be accompanied by the systemic administration of a broad-spectrum antibiotic like a third-generation cephalosporin. Several meta-analyses have indicated that selective decontamination of the digestive tract (SDD) may be associated with reduced morbidity rates, and even reduced mortality rates, and yet this strategy has not been implemented largely because of the risk of the emergence of resistant organisms. Recently, de Jonge et al[55] published the results of an impressive prospective RCT including 934 patients. In this study, the ICU mortality rate was 23 percent in the control group but was only 15 percent in the SDD group (p = 0.002). Most interestingly, the incidence of resistant Gram-negative organisms was 26 percent in the control group but only 16 percent in the treated group (p = 0.001).

ARDS Management

As outlined above, there is little proof that anything can reduce mortality among ARDS patients. Maybe the application of open-lung strategies, as proposed by Amato et al[56] may improve outcomes, but the optimal setting of positive end-expiratory pressure is still controversial. An important study by the ARDS Network[57] including 361 patients, showed that ventilating patients with ALI/ARDS with a tidal volume of 6 mL/kg resulted in better outcomes than when a tidal volume of 12 mL/kg was used (mortality rate, 31.0 vs 39.8%, respectively).

Rounds at the Bedside: The Role of the Intensivist

Studies have consistently indicated that the presence of a properly trained critical care physician can have a significant impact on outcome.[58-60] Pronovost et al[61] also have indicated that rounds at the bedside may result in better outcomes. For effective bedside rounds, a battery of questions should be raised systematically in front of each patient (Table 34.1).

TABLE 34.1: Questions that should be systematically raised at the bedside[25]
If the patient is mechanically ventilated, can he/she be weaned from mechanical ventilation?
Is pain controlled, is sedation well titrated, and does the patient need restraints?
Is nutrition adequate?
Is the head of the bed elevated?
Is deep venous thrombosis prophylaxis implemented?
Is ulcer prophylaxis implemented?

Criteria for Discharge from ICU

The patient can be discharged from the ICU if he is recovered and stable. If the immediate threat has been taken care of but the patient remains at risk unless under close observation, he can be discharged or retained depending upon the needs of other patients and the availability of facilities in other areas of the hospital. Patient whose immediate threat has been taken care of but he is expected to die shortly can be discharged although in some cases the family may show resentment. When death is imminent even if intensive care is continued withdrawal of life support is always difficult. However, this question has both ethical and medicolegal aspects, which are to be weighed before such a decision is taken.

Problems of Critical Care

Even if critical care has come up as a new branch in medicine and has made tremendous progress over the past few years and had a good impressive impact on saving hundreds of thousands of lives with good quality care, a number of other issues have also cropped up. The prohibitory cost because of obvious reasons are beyond the reach of many and could not be afforded to by all. Further, the type of investment required leads to the demand of more and more hospital beds. Another important problem is the ICU-acquired infection and antibiotic resistance.

ANTIBIOTIC RESISTANCE IN ICU

The risk of emergence antibiotic resistance depends on three factors genetic selection, antibiotic pressure, risk of cross infection. Genetic mechanisms responsible for AB resistance include mutations; plasmids, transposons and integrons mediated resistance. Transposons are mobile unit of DNA that can jump from plasmid or chromosome of a bacterium to another without site specificity transferring resistance genes. Integrons are mobile genetic elements, which capture and spread genes by site-specific recombination can cause interspecies spread of resistance genes at alarming rates.[62,63]

Beta Lactamases

They are major defense of Gram-negative bacilli (GNB) against β lactam antibiotics and have coevolved with introduction of newer drugs. They spread from Staphylococci initially to *H. Influenzae* and *N. gonorrhea*, but with overuse of third generation cephalosporins (3GCS) in last 2 decades have led to emergence of "new" extended spectrum beta lactamases (ESBL), and carbapenemases, which are capable of neutralizing newer AB to produce

multidrug resistant bacteria (MDR). There are more than 100 different ESBL named variously as TEM, SHV, CTX, OXA type enzymes.

Diagnosing ESBL production in the microbiology laboratory is difficult as most do not routinely screen for ESBL production and there is no universal marker for ESBL. Some authors have suggested that ceftazidime resistance be used as a "surrogate" marker. Bacteria having ceftazidime MIC > 2 µg /ml are likely ESBL producers and should be tested further by double disk approximation, three dimensional agar test, ESBL card or strip test (last two are investigational). Authors have recommended screening for ESBL K pneumoniae and E coli with reduced susceptibility to 3GCS. In addition due to "inoculum effect", a drug sensitive *in vitro* may fail *in vivo* due to increase in MIC with increased bacterial load of the ESBL producing organism *in vivo*.

To give an example of the alarming situation Linezolid, a glycopeptide antibiotic was approved for use in Vancomycin resistant enterococci (VRE) and Methicillin resistant *Staphylococcus aureus* (MRSA) in 2001. Emergence of linezolid resistant VRE and MRSA were documented within a year of its use. It is imperative that the drug must be used with caution in poor penetration sites (infected foreign body) and must not be used in lengthy or repeated courses (cystic fibrosis and CRF on hemodialysis), if further resistance is to be curbed.

COMBATING ANTIBIOTIC RESISTANCE

Combating antibiotic resistance involves two strategies applied concurrently throughout the hospital and in the surrounding medical facilities:
    i. Improve infection control practices
    ii. Reduce selective antibiotic pressure.

INFECTION CONTROL PRACTICES

Hand Hygiene

Enterococci contaminate hands of caregivers and are carried on uniforms and stethoscopes. The single most important measure to reduce nosocomial transmission of infection is regular hand washing in between patients. However, compliance rates are low in best of centers (30-60%). Alcohol based hand rubs are useful alternative as they are bactericidal and reduce. When colonization pressure is high (> 50%) these measures cannot prevent transmission and universal use of gowns and gloves for contact with infected patients followed by disinfections with alcohol rubs are recommended.

Active Surveillance (AS)

This provides data on local bacterial flora and resistance patterns in the ICU. Routine cultures must be obtained from suspected sites before empirical antibiotics are started. Routine surveillance cultures from respiratory and perianal region help in detection of colonized patients and institution of cohort nursing. Molecular epidemiology methods help in deciding the mechanism of resistance development due to lax hygiene policy or to antibiotic pressure or exogenous introduction of bacteria or both and appropriate corrective measures can be instituted.

REDUCING ANTIBIOTIC PRESSURE

These strategies can be readily be incorporated into day-to-day practice and can be implemented by the following principles.

1. Restricting the use of Antibiotics (AB)

To minimize the unnecessary AB exposure, AB should be used in proper dosage, intervals and for optimal duration, using AB based on local guidelines drawn by hospital infection control committee consisting clinicians and microbiologists which are audited regularly. Colonization with nosocomial pathogens is very common in critically ill patients and should never be treated as it promotes drug resistance.

2. Using Narrow Spectrum AB

For nonlife threatening infections such as community-acquired pneumonias, urinary tract infections narrow spectrum older drugs (penicillin, gentamicin, trimethoprim) should be used instead of broad spectrum agents. This reduced incidence of *Clostridium difficile* infections and minimized resistance of bacteria to cephalosporins, quinolones, and aminoglycosides in some studies.

3. Rationalize AB Prescription Practices

Restriction of use of antibiotic by using order forms or concurrent feedback to senior physicians prior to initiating AB. Hospital formulary based restriction of drugs in situations such as emergence of ESBL producers (3GCS) and VRE (Vancomycin) to control their further propagation. Computer based antibiotic prescription have reduced hospital expenditure, and resistance rates without adverse effects on clinical outcomes.

4. AB Rotation or Cycling Policy

Cycling or rotation means AB class are withdrawn for a defined period and reintroduced later, has potential for reducing resistance as bacterial isolates regain sensitivity to those classes of AB. The optimal duration of cycles not yet established. Authors have rotated class of drugs (3GCS, Fluoroquinolone, carbapenems, Piperacillin-tazobactam) for empiric therapy for periods of 3 to 4 months and found reduction in prevalence of resistant organisms (MRSA, VRE and ESBL producing bacteria)

5. Selective Decontamination of Digestive Tract (SDD)

SDD aims to selectively eliminate aerobic GNB and yeast from the oral cavity and GIT in order to reduce the occurrence of nosocomial infections. It employs four components, topical antibiotics and antifungals (aminoglycoside, Amphotericin B), systemic antibiotics (3GCS), infection control policies and surveillance cultures. Two meta-analysis involving 8500 patients have shown SDD to be effective in reducing lower airway infection or 0.35 (0.29-0.41) and mortality or 0.80 (0.69-0.93) and 6 percent overall mortality reduction from 30 to 24 percent without any increase in infection due to resistant bacteria. However, controversial issues are whether benefits of SDD are due to enteral or parenteral drugs and are medical patients likely to benefit as most series with surgical and trauma patients and some studies have shown emergence of resistant strains of MRSA, VRE. Due to fear of antibiotic resistant strains, SDD has not gained popularity in most centers.

Based on the available evidence and experience with SDD and the likelihood of emergence of resistant bacteria, the routine clinical use of SDD cannot be recommended at the present time.

HOSPITAL ACQUIRED PNEUMONIA (HAP)

Early onset HAP: Pneumonia occurring within 4 days after hospitalization is usually caused by sensitive community acquired pathogens.

Late onset HAP: After 5 days of hospitalization caused by MDR pathogens, and carries high morbidity and mortality.

Early onset HAP associated with following risk factors is likely to be due to MDR pathogens and needs to be treated aggressively.

Risk factors for HAP
- Antimicrobial therapy in preceding 90 days
- Current hospitalization of 5 days or more
- High frequency of antibiotic resistance in the community/hospital
- Immunosuppressive disease and/or therapy.

Risk factors for Health care associated pneumonia (HCAP)
- Hospitalization for 2 days or more in the preceding 90 days
- Residence in a nursing home or extended care facility
- Home infusion therapy (including antibiotics)
- Chronic dialysis within 30 days.

Diagnosis of VAP is difficult in critically ill patients and mimicks include atelectasis, pulmonary hemorrhage, drug reaction, pulmonary edema, ARDS and pulmonary embolism. Nosocomial tracheobronchitis (NTB) is associated with purulent tracheal secretions with normal radiograph and is not associated with increased mortality. A new biomarker, soluble triggering receptors expressed on myeloid cells (sTREM-1) in BAL (rapid immuno-blot) may make the bedside diagnosis easy in future and facilitate early initiation of AB therapy.

VAP is associated with attributable mortality of 33 to 50 percent, which increases further in infections due to Acinetobacter, Pseudomonas SP, presence of bacteremia, inappropriate empirical antibiotics, and delayed antibiotic therapy. The subject has been discussed in detail in earlier chapter.

Empiric Antibiotic Therapy

Prompt appropriate antibiotic therapy is associated with greatest mortality benefit therefore empiric AB have to be chosen and started early. Most accurate criteria for starting Empiric AB are new or progressive radiological infiltrates, with 2 of 3 clinical features, fever >38 C, leucocytosis or leucopenia, purulent tracheal secretions. Microbiological cultures of lower respiratory tract secretions should be used to confirm the diagnosis and guide further therapy after 48 to 72 hours.

Empiric AB therapy should take into consideration the time of onset of HAP, presence of risk factors for drug resistant pathogens, local microbiological flora and resistance patterns. Tracheal aspirate gram stain have been used to guide initial therapy and use of broad spectrum AB combination reduce chances of inappropriate AB therapy to < 10 percent.

Avoid changing AB before 48 to 72 hours, which is the time, required for clinical response unless rapid deterioration occurs. Prompt de-escalation of AB therapy once results of microbiological cultures are available

should be attempted. This strategy, reduces unnecessary expenditure, side effects and development of resistance

Antibiotic therapy recommended for HAP
- Early onset HAP—ceftriaxone/cefotaxime or levofloxacin/moxifloxacin or Amoxycillin-clavulanic acid
- Late onset—HAP or with risk factors for HCAP
- Cefepime, ceftazidime or
- Imipenem or Meropenem or
- Piperacillin–tazobactam (for antipseudomonal cover) plus
- Ciprofloxacin or levofloxacin or Amikacin, gentamicin, or tobramycin plus
- Linezolid or vancomycin (if MRSA is suspected).

Duration of AB therapy of 7 to 8 days is recommended for uncomplicated HAP with good clinical response to treatment except for nonlactose fermenting GNB (Pseudomonas and Acinetobacter) where longer duration (10-14 days) is advised to prevent relapses and complications.

Combination therapy is recommended as initial empiric therapy for late onset HAP/with risk factors for MDR pathogens as inadequate therapy associated with mortality. Pseudomonas HAP in neutropenic host, combination therapy has synergistic effect and prevents emergence of antibiotic resistance. Monotherapy with Quinolones/carbapenems/piperacillin-tazobactam is recommended for cases of early HAP with no risk factors for MDR pathogens, documented gram-positive HAP (MRSA), mild HAP (clinical pulmonary infection score CPIS < 6).

CONCLUSIONS

Combating antibiotic resistance involves simultaneous application infection control practices and reduction of selective antibiotic pressure. Hand hygiene is the simplest most cost effective measure to reduce nosocomial infections. Avoiding antibiotics unless strong clinical or microbiological evidence of infection exists is possibly the best method of reducing antibiotic pressure.

Early and appropriate therapy based on local data of bacterial infections and resistance patterns is associated with reduced mortality from nosocomial pneumonias. Prompt de-escalation of therapy once results of microbiological cultures are available should be done in all cases.

Some of the typial X-ray pictures and photographs of different diseases as seen typically in an ICU (Figs 34.1 to 34.9).

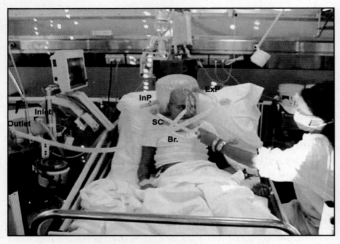

FIGURE 34.1: Helmet mask. Typical view of a patient in the ICU with tubes and other equipments

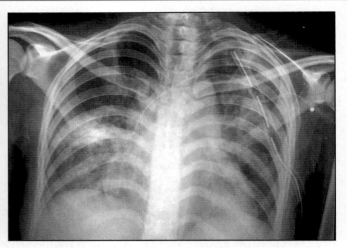

FIGURE 34.4: Case of ARDS with pneumothorax in the ICU

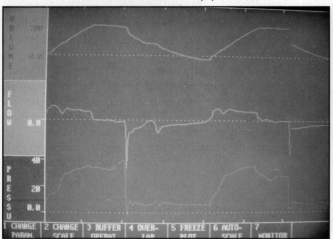

FIGURE 34.2: Monitoring of different parameters in a patient on ventilator

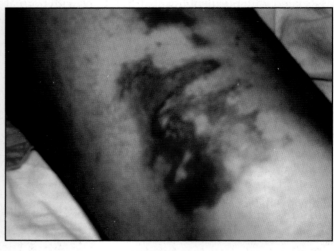

FIGURE 34.5

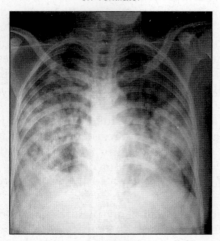

FIGURE 34.3: Peripartum pneumonia developing ARDS

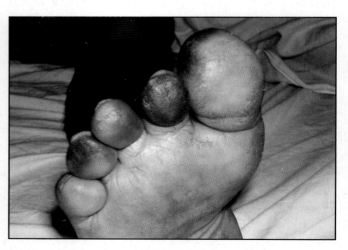

FIGURE 34.6

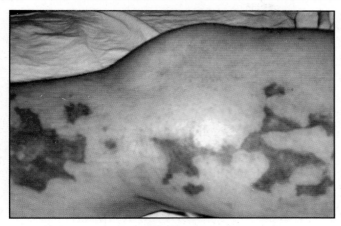

FIGURE 34.7

FIGURES 34.5 to 7: Purpura fulminans in a case of septicemia

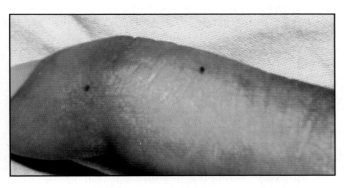

FIGURE 34.8: A case of snakebite with fang marks developing respiratory muscle paralysis and DIC. The patient required ventilatory support

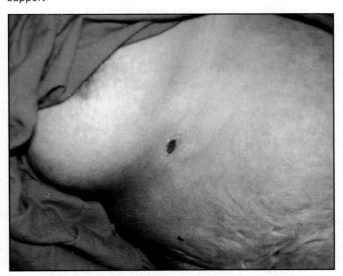

FIGURE 34.9: Rickettsial eschar. The patient developed ARDS

REFERENCES

1. Intensive care in the United Kingdom: Report from the King's Fund Panel. Anaesthesia 1989;44:428-31.
2. Batra YK, Praveen BV, Singh H. Intensive care in India: Experience of a major teaching hospital. Int Care World 1991;8:186-90.
3. Task Force on Guidelines, Society of Critical Care Medicine: Guidelines for categorization of services for the critically ill patient. Crit Care Med 1991;19:279-85.
4. Guidelines Committee. Society of Critical Care Medicine. Guidelines for the definition of an intensivist and the practice of critical care medicine. Crit Care Med 1992;20:540-42.
5. AARC Clinical Practice Guideline: In: Hospital transport of the mechanically ventilated patient—2002 revision and update. Respiratory Care 2002;47:721-23.
6. American Association of Respiratory Care, AARC Clinical Practice Guideline-Patient-Ventilator System Checks, http://www.rcjournal.com/online resources/cpgs/mvsccpg.html (Accessed on Oct. 2005).
7. American Association of Respiratory Care, AARC Clinical Practice Guideline-Removal of the Endotracheal Tube, http://www.rcjournal.com/online resources/cpgs/mvsccpg.html (Accessed on Oct. 2005).
8. American Association of Respiratory Care, AARC Clinical Practice Guideline-Metabolic Measurement using Indirect Calorimetry during Mechanical Ventilation. http://www.rcjournal.com/online resources/cpgs/mvsccpg.html.
9. American Association of Respiratory Care, AARC Clinical Practice Guideline-Endotracheal Suctioning of Mechanically Ventilated patients with Artificial Airways, http://www.rcjournal.com/online resources/cpgs/mvsccpg.html.
10. American Association of Respiratory Care, AARC Clinical Practice Guideline-Fiberoptic Bronchoscopy Assisting. http://www.rcjournal.com/online resources/cpgs/mvsccpg.html.
11. Yu, 1998, Contributions of Respiratory Care Practitioners to Intensive Care: A Review.http://www.ncbi.nlm.nih.gov/entrez/query.fcgi?cmd = Retrieve & db = PubMed.
12. The Department of Respiratory Care. University of California, San Diego. Accessed at http://www-respcare.ucsd.edu/index.php (Accessed on Oct. 2005).
13. Airway management is a crucial area of critical care practice, 2004, Crit Care Med, http://www.ncbi.nlm.nih.gov/entrez/query.fcgi? cmd = Retrieve & db = PubMed &dop=Citation&list_uids= 15343051.
14. American Association of Respiratory Care, 2003 AARC Clinical Practice Guideline-Bland Aerosol Administration.
15. Bostick J, Wendelgass ST. Normal saline instillation as part of the suctioning procedure: Effects on PaO2 and amount of secretions. Heart Lung 1987;16:532-37.

16. American Association of Respiratory Care, AARC Clinical Practice Guideline-Endotracheal Suctioning of Mechanically Ventilated patients with Artificial Airways Demers RR. Complications of endotracheal suctioning procedures. Respir Care 1982;27:453-57.

17. Centers for Disease Control. Update: Universal Precautions for prevention of transmission of human Immunodeficiency virus, hepatitis B virus, and other blood borne pathogens in health care settings. MMWR 1988;37:377-99.

18. American Association of Respiratory Care, AARC Clinical Practice Guideline-Endotracheal Suctioning of Mechanically Ventilated patients with Artificial Airways http://www.rcjournal.com/online_resources/cpgs/cpg_index.asp.

19. American Association of Respiratory Care, AARC Clinical Practice Guideline- Removal of the Endotracheal Tube, http://www.rcjournal.com/online_resources/cpgs/cpg_index.asp.

20. Egan's Fundamentals of Respiratory Care. Scanlon, Spearman and Sheldon (7th edn), Mosby Publishing 2003;612-14.

21. Shapiro BA, Peruzzi WT, Kozelowski-Templin R. Clinical application of blood gases (5th edn). St Louis: Mosby-Year Book Inc 1994.

22. Raffin TA. Indications for arterial blood gas analysis. Ann Intern Med 1986;105:390-98.

23. Browning JA, Kaiser DL, Durbin CG Jr. The effect of guidelines on the appropriate use of arterial blood gas analysis in the intensive care unit. Respir Care 1989;34:269-76.

24. National Committee for Clinical Laboratory Standards (NCCLS). Procedures for the collection of arterial blood specimens, 1999. Available from NCCLS: phone 610-688-0100; Fax 610-688-0700; e-mail exoffice@nccls.org.

25. Vincent JL. Evidence-Based Medicine in the ICU*. Important Advances and Limitations. Chest 2004;126:592-600.

26. Brochard L, Mancebo J, Wysocki M, et al. Noninvasive ventilation for acute exacerbations of chronic obstructive pulmonary disease. N Engl J Med 1995;333,817-22.

27. Plant PK, Owen JL, Elliott MW. Early use of non-invasive ventilation for acute exacerbations of chronic obstructive pulmonary disease on general respiratory wards: A multicentre randomised controlled trial. Lancet 2000;355,1931-35.

28. Antonelli M, Conti G, Rocco M, et al. A comparison of noninvasive positive-pressure ventilation and conventional mechanical ventilation in patients with acute respiratory failure. N Engl J Med 1998;339, 429-35.

29. Nourdine K, Combes P, Carton MJ, et al. Does noninvasive ventilation reduce the ICU nosocomial infection risk?: A prospective clinical survey. Intensive Care Med 1999;25,567-73.

30. Girou E, Schortgen F, Delclaux C, et al. Association of noninvasive ventilation with nosocomial infections and survival in critically ill patients. JAMA 2000;284,2361-67.

31. Bernard SA, Gray TW, Buist MD, et al. Treatment of comatose survivors of out-of-hospital cardiac arrest with induced hypothermia. N Engl J Med 2002;346, 557-63.

32. Hypothermia after Cardiac Arrest Study Group. Mild therapeutic hypothermia to improve the neurologic outcome after cardiac arrest. N Engl J Med 2002; 346,549-56.

33. Van den Berghe G, Wouters P, Weekers F, et al. Intensive insulin therapy in the critically ill patient. N Engl J Med 2001;345,1359-67.

34. Hebert PC, Wells G, Blajchman MA, et al. A multicenter, randomized, controlled clinical trial of transfusion requirements in critical care. N Engl J Med 1999;340,409-17.

35. Vincent JL, Baron JF, Reinhart K, et al. Anemia and blood transfusion in critically ill patients. JAMA 2002;288,1499-1507.

36. Vincent JL, Sakr YL, Carlet J, et al. Sepsis occurrence in acutely ill patients (SOAP): Results of a large European multicenter study. Am J Respir Crit Care Med 2003;167:A837.

37. Hebert PC, Fergusson D, Blajchman MA, et al. Clinical outcomes following institution of the Canadian universal leukoreduction program for red blood cell transfusions. JAMA 2003;289,1941-49.

38. Fergusson D, Hebert PC, Lee SK, et al. Clinical outcomes following institution of universal leuko-reduction of blood transfusions for premature infants. JAMA 2003;289,1950-56.

39. Bernard GR, Vincent JL, Laterre PF, et al. Efficacy and safety of recombinant human activated protein C for severe sepsis. N Engl J Med 2001;344,699-709.

40. Wheeler AP, Doig C, Wright T, et al. Baseline characteristics and survival of adult severe sepsis patients treated with drotrecogin alfa (activated) in a global, single-arm, open-label trial (ENHANCE). Chest 2003;124(suppl),91S.

41. Warren BL, Eid A, Singer P, et al. Caring for the critically ill patient: High-dose antithrombin III in severe sepsis; A randomized controlled trial. JAMA 2001;286,1869-78.

42. Abraham E, Reinhart K, Opal S, et al. Efficacy and safety of tifacogin (recombinant tissue factor pathway inhibitor) in severe sepsis: A randomized controlled trial. JAMA 2003;290,238-47.

43. Joyce DE, Grinnell BW. Recombinant human activated protein C attenuates the inflammatory response in endothelium and monocytes by modulating nuclear factor-kappaB. Crit Care Med 2002;30,S288-S293.

44. Esmon CT. The protein C pathway. Chest 2003;124 (suppl),26S-32S.

45. Levin M, Quint BA, Goldstein B, et al. Recombinant bactericidal/permeability-increasing protein (rBPIZ1) as

adjunctive treatment for children with severe meningo-coccal sepsis: A randomised trial. Lancet 2000;356, 961-67.

46. Bone RC, Fisher CJ, Clemmer TP, et al. The methyl-prednisolone severe sepsis study group: A controlled clinical trial of high-dose methylprednisolone in the treatment of severe sepsis and septic shock. N Engl J Med 1987;317,353.

47. Annane D, Sebille V, Charpentier C, et al. Effect of treat-ment with low doses of hydrocortisone and fludro-cortisone on mortality in patients with septic shock. JAMA 2002;288,862-71.

48. Landry DW, Levin HR, Gallant EM, et al. Vasopressin deficiency contributes to the vasodilation of septic shock. Circulation 1997;95,1122-25.

49. Patel BM, Chittock DR, Russell JA, et al. Beneficial effects of short-term vasopressin infusion during severe septic shock. Anesthesiology 2002;96,576-82.

50. Malay MB, Ashton RC Jr, Landry DW, et al. Low-dose vasopressin in the treatment of vasodilatory septic shock. J Trauma 1999;47,699-703.

51. Sun Q, Dimopoulos G, Nguyen DN, et al. Low-dose vasopressin in the treatment of septic shock in sheep. Am J Respir Crit Care Med 2003;168,481-86.

52. Hayes MA, Timmins AC, Yau EH, et al. Elevation of systemic oxygen delivery in the treatment of critically ill patients. N Engl J Med 1994;330,1717-22.

53. Rivers E, Nguyen B, Havstad S, et al. Early goal-directed therapy in the treatment of severe sepsis and septic shock. N Engl J Med 2001;345,1368-77.

54. Stoutenbeek CP, van Saene HK, Miranda DR, et al. The effect of selective decontamination of the digestive tract on colonisation and infection rate in multiple trauma patients. Intensive Care Med 1984;10,185-92.

55. de Jonge E, Schultz MJ, Spanjaard L, et al. Effects of selective decontamination of the digestive tract on mortality and the acquisition of resistant bacteria in intensive care patients. Lancet 2003;362,1011-16.

56. Amato MB, Barbas CS, Medeiro DM, et al. Effect of a protective-ventilation strategy on mortality in the acute respiratory distress syndrome. N Engl J Med 1998; 338,347-54.

57. The ARDS Network. Ventilation with lower tidal volumes as compared with traditional tidal volumes for acute lung injury and the acute respiratory distress syndrome. N Engl J Med 2000;342,1301-08.

58. Pronovost PJ, Angus DC, Dorman T, et al. Physician staffing patterns and clinical outcomes in critically ill patients: A systematic review. JAMA 2002;288,2151-62.

59. Higgins TL, McGee WT, Steingrub JS, et al. Early indicators of prolonged intensive care unit stay: Impact of illness severity, physician staffing, and pre-intensive care unit length of stay. Crit Care Med 2003;31,45-51.

60. Blunt MC, Burchett KR. Out of hours consultant cover and case-mix-adjusted mortality in intensive care. Lancet 2000;356,735-36.

61. Pronovost PJ, Jenckes MW, Dorman T, et al. Orga-nizational characteristics of intensive care units related to outcomes of abdominal aortic surgery. JAMA 1999;281,1310-17.

62. Guidelines for the management of adults with hospital-acquired, ventilator-associated, and healthcare-associated pneumonia. The Official statement of ATS & IDSA. Am J Respir Crit Care Med 2005;171:388-416.

63. Weinstein RA. Antibiotic resistance in hospitals and intensive care units: The problem and potential solutions. Semi Resp Crit Care Med 2003;24:113,120.

Index